D0217832

99⁰⁰
7/7

Rehabilitation of the hand

REHABILITATION OF THE HAND

EDITORS

JAMES M. HUNTER, M.D.

Professor of Orthopaedic Surgery,
Jefferson Medical College of Thomas Jefferson University,
and Chief, Hand Surgery Service,
Department of Orthopaedics,
Thomas Jefferson University Hospital,
Philadelphia, Pennsylvania

LAWRENCE H. SCHNEIDER, M.D.

Clinical Associate Professor of Orthopaedic Surgery,
Department of Orthopaedics,
Jefferson Medical College of Thomas Jefferson University,
Philadelphia, Pennsylvania

EVELYN J. MACKIN, L.P.T.

Director of Hand Therapy,
Hand Rehabilitation Center,
Philadelphia, Pennsylvania

ANNE D. CALLAHAN, M.S., O.T.R.

Assistant Director of Hand Therapy,
Hand Rehabilitation Center,
Philadelphia, Pennsylvania

SECOND EDITION

With 1397 illustrations, including 26 in color

The C. V. Mosby Company

ST. LOUIS • TORONTO • PRINCETON   1984

A TRADITION OF PUBLISHING EXCELLENCE

Editor: Eugenia Klein
Developmental editor: Kathryn Falk
Manuscript editors: Stephen C. Hetager, Carl Masthay
Design: Gail Morey Hudson
Production: Linda R. Stalnaker, Barbara Merritt, Margaret B. Bridenbaugh

SECOND EDITION

Copyright © 1984 by The C.V. Mosby Company

All rights reserved. No part of this publication may be
reproduced, stored in a retrieval system, or transmitted, in
any form or by any means, electronic, mechanical, photocopying,
recording, or otherwise, without prior written permission from
the publisher.

Previous edition copyrighted 1978

Printed in the United States of America

The C.V. Mosby Company
11830 Westline Industrial Drive, St. Louis, Missouri 63146

Library of Congress Cataloging in Publication Data

Main entry under title:

Rehabilitation of the hand.

  Includes bibliographies and index.
  1. Hand—Wounds and injuries. 2. Hand—Surgery.
3. Physically handicapped—Rehabilitation. I. Hunter,
James M. [DNLM: 1. Hand injuries—Rehabilitation.
2. Rehabilitation. 3. Hand. WE 830 R345]
RD559.R43 1984   617′.575   83-19523
ISBN 0-8016-2355-3

GW/MV/MV 9 8 7 6 5 4 3   01/D/036

Contributors

URSULA ALBION, P.T., O.T.
Victoria Hospital and the University of Western Ontario, London, Ontario, Canada

PETER C. AMADIO, M.D.
Consultant in Orthopedics, Mayo Clinic; Assistant Professor of Orthopedics, Mayo Medical School, Rochester, Minnesota

PAT L. AULICINO, M.D.
Assistant Professor of Orthopaedic Surgery, Eastern Virginia Medical School, Norfolk, Virginia

MELANIE S. BALLARD, O.T.R.
Occupational Therapist, Hand Rehabilitation Center, Inc., Philadelphia, Pennsylvania

LOIS M. BARBER, O.T.R., F.A.O.T.A.
President, LMB Hand Rehab Products, Inc., San Luis Obispo, California; Clinical Instructor, School of Occupational Therapy, University of Southern California, Los Angeles, California

J.V. BASMAJIAN, M.D., F.A.C.A., F.R.C.P.(C.)
Professor of Medicine and Director of Rehabilitation Medicine, Department of Medicine (Division of Rehabilitation Medicine), McMaster University, Hamilton, Ontario, Canada

PATRICIA L. BAXTER, O.T.R.
Director of Return to Work Program, Hand Rehabilitation Center; Clinical Assistant Professor, Department of Occupational Therapy, Temple University, Philadelphia, Pennsylvania

JANE BEAR-LEHMAN, M.S., O.T.R.
Consultant in Hand Therapy, Henry Bernstein, M.D., Ltd., Elmwood Park, Illinois

ROBERT W. BEASLEY, M.D.
Professor of Surgery (Plastic Surgery) and Director of Hand Surgery Service, New York University School of Medicine, New York, New York

JUDITH A. BELL, O.T.R., F.A.O.T.A.
Clinical Research Therapist and Chief of Hand Therapy, Rehabilitation Research Department, U.S. Public Health Service Hospital, Carville, Louisiana

HARRY T. BERGTHOLDT, M.S., R.P.T.
Chief, Physical Therapy Department, U.S. Public Health Service Hospital, Indian Health Service, Shiprock, New Mexico; formerly Assistant Chief, Physical Therapy, National Hansen's Disease Center, Carville, Louisiana

SIDNEY J. BLAIR, M.D.
Chief, Section of Hand Surgery, Department of Orthopaedics and Rehabilitation, Loyola University Medical Center, Maywood, Illinois

ANNE B. BLAKENEY, M.S.O.T., O.T.R.
Assistant Professor, Department of Medical Allied Health Professions, The Medical School, University of North Carolina at Chapel Hill, Chapel Hill, North Carolina; formerly Staff Occupational Therapist, National Hansen's Disease Center, Carville, Louisiana

JOHN A. BOSWICK, Jr., M.D.
Professor of Surgery and Chief, Hand Surgery Service, Department of Surgery, University of Colorado Health Sciences Center, Denver, Colorado

PAUL W. BRAND, M.D.
Chief, Rehabilitation Branch, National Hansen's Disease Center, Carville, Louisiana; Clinical Professor of Orthopaedics and Surgery, Louisiana State University Medical School, New Orleans, Louisiana

PAULA BREME, R.P.T.
Hand Rehabilitation Center, Philadelphia, Pennsylvania

D. MICHAEL BROWN, O.T.R.
Director, Hand Rehabilitation Center of Atlanta, Inc., Atlanta, Georgia

STERLING BUNNELL, M.D.†

WILLIAM E. BURKHALTER, M.D.
Professor of Orthopaedics, Department of Orthopaedics and Rehabilitation, University of Miami School of Medicine; Chief, Division of Hand Surgery, Jackson Memorial Hospital, Miami, Florida

---

†Deceased.

ANNE D. CALLAHAN, M.S., O.T.R.
Assistant Director of Hand Therapy, Hand Rehabilitation Center, Philadelphia, Pennsylvania

CATHERINE A. CAMBRIDGE, M.S., R.P.T.
Hand Therapy of Wilmington, Wilmington, Delaware

MARGARET S. CARTER, O.T.R.
Director, Hand Rehabilitation Unit, Hand Surgery Associates, Phoenix, Arizona

GAYLORD L. CLARK, M.D.
Assistant Professor of Orthopaedic Surgery, Department of Orthopaedic Surgery, Johns Hopkins University School of Medicine; Attending Hand Surgeon, Raymond M. Curtis Hand Center, The Union Memorial Hospital, Baltimore, Maryland

JUDY C. COLDITZ, O.T.R.
Director, Raleigh Hand Rehabilitation Center, Raleigh, North Carolina; formerly Director, Occupational Therapy Department, Wake County Medical Center, and Hand Therapist, Raleigh Orthopaedic Clinic, Raleigh, North Carolina

CARL R. COLEMAN, M.D.
Clinical Professor and Co-director, Hand Service, Department of Surgery, Division of Orthopedic Surgery, Ohio State University College of Medicine; Director of Orthopedic Education, Riverside Methodist Hospital, Columbus, Ohio

RAYMOND M. CURTIS, M.D.
Associate Professor of Orthopaedic Surgery and Associate Professor of Plastic Surgery, Johns Hopkins University School of Medicine, Baltimore, Maryland

GLORIA L. DeVORE, O.T.R.
Director, Hand Therapy Associates; Associate, Department of Surgery, University of Arizona College of Medicine, Tucson, Arizona

ADOLPH DIODA
Instructor in Sculpture, Pennsylvania Academy of Fine Arts, Philadelphia, Pennsylvania

THEODORE E. DuPUY, M.D.
Associate Professor of Orthopaedic Surgery, Eastern Virginia Medical School, Norfolk, Virginia

ROBERT J. DURAN, M.D.
Clinical Professor and Co-director, Hand Service, Department of Surgery, Division of Plastic Surgery, Ohio State University College of Medicine, Columbus, Ohio

WILLIAM J. ERDMAN II, M.D.
Professor and Chairman, Department of Physical Medicine and Rehabilitation, University of Pennsylvania, School of Medicine, Philadelphia, Pennsylvania

ELAINE EWING FESS, M.S., O.T.R., F.A.O.T.A.
Founder and formerly Director, Hand Rehabilitation Center of Indiana, Zionsville, Indiana

VINCENT G. FIETTI, Jr., M.D.
Assistant Clinical Professor, Department of Orthopaedic Surgery, Columbia University College of Physicians and Surgeons; Assistant Attending Orthopaedic Surgeon, St. Luke's–Roosevelt Hospital, New York, New York

SHARON L. FRIED, C.O.T.A.
Hand Rehabilitation Center, Philadelphia, Pennsylvania

CHERYL MUELLER FRIEDMAN, R.N., C.N.O.R.
Nursing Care Coordinator of the Operating Room, Thomas Jefferson University Hospital, Philadelphia, Pennsylvania

GARY K. FRYKMAN, M.D.
Associate Professor, Department of Orthopaedic Surgery, School of Medicine, Loma Linda University; Medical Director, Hand Rehabilitation Center, Loma Linda, California

CARL GÖRAN-HAGERT, M.D.
Department of Orthopaedic Surgery, University of Göteborg, Göteborg, Sweden

ROSEMARIE SAVINELLI HECKER, O.T.R.
Department of Occupational Therapy, Sacred Heart General Hospital, Eugene, Oregon

BRENDA C. HILFRANK, R.P.T.
Hand Therapist and Clinical Assistant Professor, Department of Orthopedics and Rehabilitation, University of Vermont College of Medicine, Burlington, Vermont

ROBERT G. HOUSER, M.D.
Clinical Assistant Professor of Surgery, Division of Plastic Surgery, Ohio State University College of Medicine, Columbus, Ohio

JAMES M. HUNTER, M.D.
Professor of Orthopaedic Surgery, Jefferson Medical College of Thomas Jefferson University, and Chief, Hand Surgery Service, Department of Orthopaedics, Thomas Jefferson University Hospital, Philadelphia, Pennsylvania

RICHARD S. IDLER, M.D.
Attending Hand Surgeon, St. Vincent Hospital and Health Center and Methodist Hospital, Indianapolis, Indiana

SCOTT H. JAEGER, M.D.
Clinical Associate Professor, Orthopaedic Surgery, Jefferson Medical College of Thomas Jefferson University, Philadelphia, Pennsylvania

MARY C. KASCH, O.T.R.
Supervisor, Hand Therapy, Hand Surgery Associates, Sacramento, California

LOIS SUSAN KEMPIN, B.A.
Hand Rehabilitation Center, Philadelphia, Pennsylvania

S.L. KOLUMBAN, M.A., R.P.T.
Formerly Chief Physical Therapist, Schieffelin Leprosy
Research and Training Center, Tamil Nadu, India

L. LEE LANKFORD, M.D.
Clinical Professor, Department of Orthopaedic Surgery, The
University of Texas Health Science Center at Dallas, Dallas,
Texas

GEORGIANN F. LASETER, O.T.R.
Director, Hand Rehabilitation Services, Dallas, Texas

VALERIE HOLDEMAN LEE, R.P.T.
Director, Hand Rehabilitation Associates, Phoenix, Arizona

ROBERT D. LEFFERT, M.D.
Associate Professor of Orthopaedic Surgery, Harvard Medical
School, Boston, Massachusetts

JUDY LEONARD, O.T.R.
Occupational Therapist, Regional Hand Rehabilitation Service,
Grand Rapids, Michigan

EVA McCORMICK, O.T.R.
Director, Occupational Therapy Department, Loyola University
Medical Center, Maywood, Illinois

PAMELA M. McENTEE, O.T.R.
Occupational Therapist, Hand Rehabilitation Center,
Philadelphia, Pennsylvania

ROBERT M. McFARLANE, M.D.
Professor and Chief, Division of Plastic Surgery, Department of
Surgery, University of Western Ontario; Chief, Department of
Surgery, Victoria Hospital, London, Ontario, Canada

CAROL McGOUGH, M.S., O.T.R.
Director of Occupational Therapy, Sharp Rehabilitation Center,
San Diego, California

EVELYN J. MACKIN, L.P.T.
Director of Hand Therapy, Hand Rehabilitation Center,
Philadelphia, Pennsylvania

JOHN W. MADDEN, M.D.
Clinical Professor of Orthopaedics, University of New Mexico
School of Medicine, Albuquerque, New Mexico

LORETTA M. MAIORANO, O.T.R.
Prosthetics Coordinator, Hand Rehabilitation Center,
Philadelphia, Pennsylvania

WANDRA K. MILES, O.T.R.
Occupational Therapist, Hand Rehabilitation Center,
Philadelphia, Pennsylvania

ERIK MOBERG, M.D.
Emeritus Professor, Department of Orthopaedic and Hand
Surgery, University of Göteborg, Göteborg, Sweden

CHRISTINE A. MORAN, M.S., R.P.T.
Clinical Instructor, Department of Physical Therapy, Old
Dominion University, Norfolk, Virginia; Assistant Clinical
Professor, Graduate Studies in Physical Therapy, Medical
College of Virginia, Richmond, Virginia; Director, The
Richmond Upper Extremity Center, Richmond, Virginia

ALBIE MORRIS, R.N.
Unit Specialist in Hand Surgery, Thomas Jefferson University
Hospital, Philadelphia, Pennsylvania

MARIA MUSUR-GRIEVE, Ph.D., P.T.
Formerly Hand Research and Rehabilitation Unit, Rehabilitation
Department, Institute of Rheumatology, Warsaw, Poland

EDWARD A. NALEBUFF, M.D.
Clinical Professor of Orthopedic Surgery, Tufts University
School of Medicine; Chief of Hand Surgery, New England
Baptist Hospital, Boston, Massachusetts

ARTHUR J. NELSON, Ph.D.
Professor, Department of Physical Therapy, School of
Education, Health, Nursing and Arts Professions, New York
University, New York, New York

ELVERT F. NELSON, M.D.
Hand Fellow, Department of Orthopaedic Surgery, Loma Linda
University School of Medicine, Loma Linda, California

VERNON L. NICKEL, M.D.
Medical Director of Rehabilitation, Sharp Rehabilitation Center;
Professor of Surgery, Department of Orthopaedics and
Rehabilitation, University of California, San Diego, California

BONNIE L. OLIVETT, O.T.R.
Director, Upper Extremity Rehabilitation, and Clinical
Instructor, University of Colorado Health Sciences and Research
Center, Denver, Colorado

GEORGE E. OMER, Jr., M.D., M.S. (Orthopaedic Surgery)
Professor of Orthopaedics and Chairman, Department of
Orthopaedics and Rehabilitation; Professor of Surgery and
Chief, Division of Hand Surgery; Medical Director, Physical
Therapy Program; Professor of Anatomy; The University of
New Mexico School of Medicine, Albuquerque, New Mexico

SHIRLEY OLLOS PEARSON, M.S., O.T.R.
President, Hand Rehabilitation Center, Inc., Miami, Florida

RICHARD L. PETZOLDT, M.D.
Hand Surgery Consultant, Santa Clara Valley Medical Center;
Department of Orthopaedic Surgery, Stanford University
Medical Center, Palo Alto, California

CYNTHIA A. PHILIPS, M.A., O.T.R.
Hand Therapist, Hand Surgical Associates, Brookline,
Massachusetts, and New England Baptist Hospital, Boston,
Massachusetts

JEAN PILLET, M.D.
Director, Centre de Prosthèse Plastique, Paris, France

KAREN HULL PRENDERGAST, M.A., R.P.T.
Clinical Director, Hand Management Center; Instructor,
Department of Surgery, Medical College of Virginia, Virginia
Commonwealth University, Richmond, Virginia

R. GUY PULVERTAFT, C.B.E., M.D., M.Chir., F.R.C.S.
Orthopaedic Surgeon Emeritus, Derbyshire Royal Infirmary,
Derby, England

HELEN WOOD RAMSAMMY, L.O.T.R., F.A.O.T.A.
Formerly Chief, Occupational Therapy, National Hansen's
Disease Center, Carville, Louisiana

RICHARD READ, R.P.T.
Physical Therapist, Hand Rehabilitation Center, Philadelphia,
Pennsylvania

SANDY REEVES, O.T.R.
Occupational Therapist, Burn Program, Shands Teaching
Hospital, Gainesville, Florida

C. CHRISTOPHER REYNOLDS, R.P.T.
Physical Therapist, Hand Surgery Associates, Phoenix, Arizona

ERIK A. ROSENTHAL, M.D.
Associate Clinical Professor of Orthopedic Surgery, Tufts
University School of Medicine, Boston, Massachusetts;
Director, Hand Surgery Service, Baystate Medical Center,
Springfield, Massachusetts

ROGER E. SALISBURY, M.D.
Professor of Surgery and Chief of Plastic and Reconstructive
Surgery, New York Medical College; Director, Burn Center,
Westchester County Medical Center, Valhalla, New York

RODNEY W. SCHLEGEL, P.T.
Director of Hand Rehabilitation and Chief Physical Therapist,
The Union Memorial Hospital, Baltimore, Maryland

LAWRENCE H. SCHNEIDER, M.D.
Clinical Associate Professor, Department of Orthopaedic
Surgery, Jefferson Medical College of Thomas Jefferson
University, Philadelphia, Pennsylvania

STANTON N. SMULLENS, M.D.
Associate Professor of Surgery and Chief of Vascular
Laboratory, Thomas Jefferson University Hospital, Philadelphia,
Pennsylvania

RUTH ANNE SNYDER, O.T.R.
Patient Care Coordinator for Hand Occupational Therapy,
Raymond M. Curtis Hand Center of The Union Memorial
Hospital, Baltimore, Maryland

MORTON SPINNER, M.D.
Clinical Professor of Orthopaedic Surgery, Albert Einstein
College of Medicine, Yeshiva University, New York, New York

JAMES B. STEICHEN, M.D.
Clinical Professor of Orthopaedic Surgery, Department of
Orthopaedic Surgery, Indiana University School of Medicine;
Attending Hand Surgeon, St. Vincent Hospital and Health Care
Center, Indianapolis, Indiana

MARY G. STOVER, M.S., O.T.R.
Columbus, Ohio

JAMES W. STRICKLAND, M.D.
Chief, Section of Hand Surgery, Department of Orthopaedics,
St. Vincent Hospital and Health Care Center; Clinical Professor,
Department of Orthopaedic Surgery, Indiana University School
of Medicine, Indianapolis, Indiana

ALFRED B. SWANSON, M.D.
Professor of Surgery, Michigan State University, Lansing,
Michigan; Chief of Orthopaedic and Hand Surgery Training
Program, Blodgett and Butterworth Hospitals, Grand Rapids,
Michigan; Chief, Orthopaedic Research, Blodgett Memorial
Hospital, Grand Rapids, Michigan

GENEVIEVE de GROOT SWANSON, M.D.
Assistant Clinical Professor of Surgery, Michigan State
University, Lansing, Michigan

JAMES E. SWEIGART, C.P.O.
Director, Orthotic/Prosthetic Department, The Pennsylvania
State University, Elizabethtown Hospital and Rehabilitation
Center, Elizabethtown, Pennsylvania

MARIE TRUSKOWSKY, R.N.
Account Representative/Rehabilitation Supervisor, International
Rehabilitation Associates, Inc., Wayne, Pennsylvania

ROBERT L. WATERS, M.D.
Chief, Surgical Services, Rancho Los Amigos Hospital,
Downey, California; Clinical Professor of Orthopedics,
University of Southern California School of Medicine, Los
Angeles, California

JANET WAYLETT, O.T.R.
Supervising Therapist, Hand Rehabilitation Center, Loma Linda University Medical Center; Clinical Instructor, Department of Occupational Therapy, Loma Linda University, Loma Linda, California

GEORGE T. WELCH
President, International Institute of Rehabilitation; Consultant in Health Care and Rehabilitation, Paoli, Pennsylvania

JILL G. WHITE, M.A., O.T.R.
Chief Hand Therapist, Hand Surgery Associates, New York, New York

DOROTHY J. WILSON, O.T.R., F.A.O.T.A.
Clinical Assistant, University of Southern California School of Medicine, Los Angeles, California, and Rancho Los Amigos Hospital, Downey, California

ROBERT LEE WILSON, M.D.
Chief, Hand Surgery Service, Maricopa County Medical Center, Phoenix, Arizona; Associate in Surgery, University of Arizona College of Medicine, Tucson, Arizona

PHYLLIS WRIGHT, L.P.T.
Physical Therapy Department, North Carolina Memorial Hospital, Chapel Hill, North Carolina

DEDICATION TO THE SECOND EDITION

To Raymond M. Curtis, M.D.

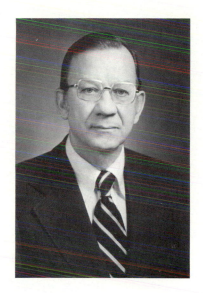

The second edition of *Rehabilitation of the Hand* will reach an ever-expanding worldwide team of hand surgeons and therapists. The book has a definite personality that blends teamwork, scholarship, imagination, and compassion. It is with great pleasure that we dedicate this volume to a man we hold in high esteem, Dr. Raymond M. Curtis, because to enumerate those qualities is to describe Dr. Curtis—the surgeon and the man. We are grateful for his countless contributions to hand surgery and rehabilitation. This dedication is our way of thanking him for the contribution he has made to the professional lives of hand surgeons and hand therapists.

DEDICATION TO THE FIRST EDITION

To Paul W. Brand, M.D.

It is with great pride that we dedicate our book to Dr. Paul W. Brand. This devout man has unselfishly used his extraordinary skills and high standards of medicine in his service and devotion to God.

Therapists and surgeons who seek to know the origin and philosophy of hand rehabilitation centers should know that the idea began in the mind and heart of this humble, gentle man.

Born in India, the son of missionaries, Paul Brand was aware at an early age of the frustration that beset those stricken with Hansen's disease. With no hope of help, these persons merely existed as outcasts in the dark corners of their little world. Dr. Brand's efforts through reconstructive surgery restored useless hands and gave persons with Hansen's disease the opportunity to be educated and to work and live with dignity.

When Dr. Brand began his work in India, there were no hand centers or hand therapists. He trained young Indian men in specific phases of treatment, such as sensory evaluation or muscle training. After years of performing their specialties, they developed amazing expertise, and when physical therapy schools were established these young men were the first to be admitted and graduated as physical therapists.

The first hand center was an old shack, but it was the birthplace of the hand rehabilitation team—surgeons, therapists, and patients working together. The center provided an environment where patients could have surgery, treatment, and training in a workshop. Having been a carpenter during his early years of life, Dr. Brand recognized the value of woodworking and other purposeful activities in treatment of the hand. Thus he employed concepts of occupational therapy to help restore crippled fingers to useful function.

We shall be forever indebted to the fates that led this quiet man to his great work in India with patients with Hansen's disease and later at the U.S. Public Health Service Hospital in Carville, Louisiana. Their good fortune has become ours because he has given us a precious charge. Surgeons and therapists together in hand centers throughout the world can build upon the work he started. As we try to emulate the high standards he has set for us, we offer this book in honor of Dr. Paul Brand.

JAMES M. HUNTER

Foreword TO THE SECOND EDITION

Over the past few decades, advances in the treatment of lesions of the hand and upper extremity have been tremendous. This is the result of many factors, including the development of hand surgery as a specialty; the growth of knowledge of the functional anatomy of the hand, wound healing, and nerve physiology; new concepts in the treatment of tendon, nerve, bone, and joint problems; and the development of microsurgery.

However, the growth of the concept of centers combining hand surgeons and hand therapists in the same unit is perhaps the most significant advance of all. In these centers all the ingredients contributing to functional recovery after a hand lesion are synthesized.

The hand serves as both a receiver of information and an executor of the response. These two functions are closely intertwined and influence each other. The mobility of the fingers is indispensable for tactile identification of objects. The way the hand grips an object is directly influenced by the sensory input of the individual, and especially by the sensibility of the hand.

Thus the treatment of hand lesions cannot be accomplished without the combination of repair of the involved tissues and sensory and motor reeducation. A perfect anatomical repair without a functional recovery is useless.

I believe that this new philosophy of a "global approach" to the treatment of hand problems has not been better presented than in *Rehabilitation of the Hand*. The four editors have formed a hand rehabilitation center, consisting of both surgeons and therapists, that has served as a model around the world. Their experience, devotion, and contagious enthusiasm are evident in all their symposia and writings. In this work they have gathered together the most prestigious authors in all areas involving problems of the hand.

The first edition of this book immediately enjoyed a huge success. This new edition has been considerably revised and expanded. There are 25 more chapters than in the first edition, and the book covers all aspects of rehabilitation, from the evaluation of function and impairment to the management of replanted parts and the use of the newer limb prostheses and orthoses. This book will be invaluable for those who read the previous edition, physicians and therapists alike, and for anyone, from student to specialist, who is interested in hand rehabilitation.

RAOUL TUBIANA

Foreword TO THE FIRST EDITION

The successful management of the crippled hand depends on accurate preoperative assessment, skilled surgery, and devoted aftercare. This trinity is the rock on which modern hand surgery is built. As surgeons, we look to physical therapists to assist us in the assessment and preparation of the patient as well as in the aftercare. It matters not whether we are engaged in the reconstruction of the mutilated hand or concerned with the palsy of leprosy, the stiff hand, or the tetraplegic patient. All require the coordinated effort of the team.

It was this concept that led to the Symposium on Rehabilitation of the Hand held in Philadelphia, in March, 1976. This, the first combined meeting of its kind, set a pattern for the future and a standard that will be difficult to surpass. From this union has arisen a new body, the American Society of Hand Therapists, which had its first meeting in February, 1978.

During the closing session of the symposium, the thought came of presenting the work to a wider audience. All will be grateful to the editors, on whom the burden of publication has fallen. The table of contents speaks for itself. In these pages is gathered the wisdom of a galaxy of talents, for all who contributed are leaders in their respective fields. The subjects range from basic principles and techniques, which need to be stated again and again, to the latest thoughts on some difficult problems. Pervading the entire volume is the personal experience of hand therapists in the widest sense of the word who have given years of practice to their subject. It is fitting that the words of Sterling Bunnell should be included, for no one has done more to raise surgery of the hand from the unknown to the position it holds today, and his words are still relevant. We welcome, also, the tribute to Paul Brand, who has shown that the same principles apply when the material is unpromising and the odds are long, provided there is the determination and the compassion to win through.

There is no need to wish success to this work, for it is assured a special place in the libraries of all who aspire to care for the wounded hand.

R. GUY PULVERTAFT

Preface

During the five years following the publication of the first edition of *Rehabilitation of the Hand,* the specialty of hand surgery and hand rehabilitation has continued to grow both nationally and internationally. Special recognition is given in this second edition to the American Society of Hand Therapists, founded in 1978; to the hand centers throughout the world where surgeon and therapist collaborate as a team; to the First and Second Congresses of the International Federation of Societies for Surgery of the Hand; and to the surgeons and therapists who have contributed so much through education and literature—a testimony to their profession's achievements and scientific knowledge.

In 1978, with the encouragement and support of the American Society for Surgery of the Hand, a group of enthusiastic physical and occupational therapists founded the American Society of Hand Therapists. The Society has grown from 58 founding members in 1978 to a membership of 232 in 1983. The high standards the therapists set for themselves both professionally and personally are the keystone upon which the Society has continued to build and grow during the past five years.

The wide vision of Sterling Bunnell lifted hand surgery to a special field. His influence as founder of the American Society for Surgery of the Hand gave direction to all the hand surgeons who followed him. His system for the management of hand injuries in regional hospital centers during World War II is the principle behind today's hand center, which gathers together under one roof a hand rehabilitation team—hand surgeon, hand therapist, and patient. In 1978 there were 75 hand centers in the United States. During the past five years the number has increased to 145, nearly doubling.

One of the important events in the expansion of this specialty was the meeting of the First Congress of the International Federation of Societies for Surgery of the Hand, in Rotterdam, The Netherlands, in June 1980. The Federation was founded in 1966 to coordinate the activities of member hand societies and to promote the full and free exchange of knowledge between them to improve the quality of care for conditions affecting the hand and upper extremity. It was during this Congress that the American Society of Hand Therapists held its first international meeting. Enthusiastic surgeons and therapists from many countries crowded into a meeting room at the Erasmus University medical facility in Rotterdam to hear papers presented by the hand therapists. At the termination of the meeting, it was clear that surgeons and therapists had begun an alliance to advance the concept of the hand rehabilitation team on a global scale.

As was noted in the first edition of *Rehabilitation of the Hand,* the impetus for our book grew out of a unique experience—the "first" meeting on hand surgery correlated with hand rehabilitation, sponsored by the Hand Rehabilitation Foundation of Philadelphia, in 1976. Over 4000 surgeons and therapists from the United States and 18 foreign countries (Australia, Brazil, Canada, Chile, China, France, Great Britain, Israel, Japan, Mexico, The Netherlands, New Zealand, Panama, Saudi Arabia, Scotland, Sweden, Switzerland, and Venezuela) have attended the annual symposium, Rehabilitation of the Hand, in Philadelphia since the 1976 meeting. This response and the participants' enthusiasm have reinforced the continuation of our efforts through our annual symposium and the publication of the second edition of *Rehabilitation of the Hand.*

The papers presented in the first edition were contributed by the faculty of the 1976 meeting. In the second edition we have eliminated repetition, revised chapters, and added new authors and topics. Only a few chapters from the first edition have been carried over with little or no revision. Most chapters have been revised extensively. The number of chapters has increased from 70 to 95. Thirty-six chapters are devoted to new topics; most have been contributed by new authors.

We wish to thank all of the authors who, by generously contributing their time, effort, and knowledge, have made the second edition of *Rehabilitation of the Hand* possible.

We wish to express our gratitude to Judith A. Bell, OTR, FAOTA, who coedited the first edition of *Rehabilitation of the Hand.* Her editorial assistance in the first edition and her contributions to the second edition reflect her many skills and professionalism.

We are privileged to include Sterling Bunnell's "The Management of the Nonfunctional Hand—Reconstruction vs. Prosthesis," published posthumously in *Artificial Limbs* in 1957. This article is deserving of a careful review by all interested in rehabilitation of the hand.

We appreciate the permission to reprint certain articles or chapters of special interest—"Psychological Aspects of Hand Injury," by R. Guy Pulvertaft; "Wound Healing: The Biological Basis of Hand Surgery," by John W. Madden; and the major parts of two chapters on pathogenesis and pathomechanics of arthritis from the book by Alfred B. Swanson, *Flexible Implant Resection Arthroplasty in the Hand and Extremities.*

The editors appreciate the special consideration of CIBA Pharmaceutical Company in permitting us to publish five hand anatomy plates of Frank H. Netter in the section on anatomy.

Certain groups and persons have helped to make the second edition of *Rehabilitation of the Hand* an even more significant contribution to the field of hand surgery and hand rehabilitation than the first edition has been, and they are gratefully acknowledged: We thank Mr. Earl Spangenberg, Department of Visual Aids of Thomas Jefferson University, for his photographic assistance and for his excellent audio-visual assistance in our annual symposia. For its continued support, we thank the Department of Orthopaedic Surgery, Jefferson Medical College of Thomas Jefferson University. Special thanks go to Miss Dorothy Malin, the Hand Therapy Department secretary, and to Mrs. Kathryn Maynes, Hand Rehabilitation Foundation secretary, for their many hours of yeoman labor in typing and organizing manuscripts as well as their efficient assistance at the annual symposia. These acknowledgments would not be complete without our expression of warm and sincere thanks to Mrs. Dorothy B. Kaufmann for her support and belief in the dreams of the Hand Rehabilitation Foundation. Finally, we wish to thank the many friends and patients of the Hand Rehabilitation Center of Philadelphia, whose motivation and spirit have provided the strengths upon which the concept of a hand rehabilitation center began and continued to grow. They have provided the impetus for the past eight annual symposia, future planned symposia, and, most of all, the second edition of *Rehabilitation of the Hand*.

JAMES M. HUNTER
LAWRENCE H. SCHNEIDER
EVELYN J. MACKIN
ANNE D. CALLAHAN

Contents

I

BASIC CONSIDERATIONS
management by objectives, physiologic aspects, and anatomy

1

Hand rehabilitation—management by objectives

PAUL W. BRAND

Hand surgery has been around a long time. The American Society for Surgery of the Hand has worked for 30 years "to improve and develop surgery of the hand" in response to the energy and foresight of Sterling Bunnell and with the purpose of promoting better understanding and better professional standards in surgery of the hand. This society, along with other similar societies around the world, has been influential in that more and more surgeons are devoting themselves wholly or mainly to this one specialization—surgery of the hand. Specialization really gets results. By the time one surgeon has operated on a thousand cases of flexor tendon injury in the finger and has listened and discussed the techniques and problems with a dozen others who have done the same, he or she really must be able to do a far better job than the finest general surgeon who does one hand case a month and one flexor tendon case per year.

However, specialization also has its dangers. It tends to narrow our vision and to magnify the significance of small factors that are of statistical significance in those overall results we publish from time to time, which tend to become an index of our professional success. We may see a patient simply as our six-hundredth flexor tendon case with our eighty-fifth use of primary repair in the proximal segment and our fifth use of the newest suture material or prophylactic antibiotic.

If asked about our objective for the case, we might say that we want to assess the effect of wide excision of the tendon sheath at the suture site. The patient probably also has an objective, and this may affect the outcome even more than our objective. He may want to get back to work as fast as he can, or he may want to penalize his employer and maximize his financial compensation. I recently had a patient with the late results of a high nerve injury, and my objective was to use a new pattern of tendon transfers. This would require careful postoperative reeducation. The patient was an inmate of the state penitentiary, and he had his own overriding objective, which was to use his period of postoperative hospitalization to escape from prison. His success depended in part on his ability to remove his splints and use his operated hand to manipulate and remove his shackles and then to keep one jump ahead of the police. The strong motivation he had to use his hand and the fact that I had used synergistic tendon transfers and strong tendon suture techniques allowed our apparently diverse objectives to reinforce each other, so that when we met many months later he had an almost perfect result.

Hand rehabilitation is bigger than hand surgery. It takes into account all factors that are important to the patient as well as those local factors that are amenable to the surgeon's knife and the therapist's skill. It recognizes that the surgeon in his proper preoccupation with his art may miss or underrate the most significant elements of the case and that good teamwork must include not only the skilled and experienced allied health personnel but also the owner of the hand himself—that previously uninformed, fearful, and apprehensive person on whose faith, courage, and determination the success of the whole operation depends.

Since we are discussing management by objectives, we should start at the beginning and determine priorities. What are the first objectives for a hand surgeon developing a hand surgery unit into a hand rehabilitation program? I will mention two that concern patterns of staff and space and two that refer to patient care.

STAFF AND SPACE
The team

Therapists as team members. From my personal experience and from what I have seen elsewhere, the first objective is to have a team, and the first step in attaining that objective is to have one therapist work with the surgeon. This objective is not attained by having therapists available in some other department or organization, unless some very special understanding and commitment are reached. Physical therapy at one time had a bad image among the older hand surgeons. The reason was that standardized methods of therapy, suitable perhaps for backs and hips, have sometimes been disastrous for fingers. Many a hand, moving slowly toward mobility, has been turned back to stiffness by an enthusiastic therapist who was unfamiliar with the case and probably unfamiliar with the stern disciplines that are second nature to a therapist who works mainly with hands.

In large medical centers, where all physical and occupational therapists are in a separate department under a physiatrist, and in private practice, where a number of therapists work out of their own joint office, it may be difficult for a surgeon to know who is to be assigned to any given case. It may even be that different therapists handle the same case on different days. Such an arrangement does not fulfill the objective of a team and may sometimes be worse than not using a therapist at all. The right thing for the surgeon to do in these circumstances is to take the time to achieve full understanding and cooperation with the physiatrist or chief therapist so that a certain therapist or two may be set aside for the hand cases and may be given the time and freedom to consult fully with the surgeon at every preoperative and postoperative stage. If a physiatrist has the time and interest to sit in on these discussions and to accept responsibility as a member of the team, then this is still better, but continuity of the physiatrist is still not as significant as continuity of the therapist. It is the *touch* of the therapist's hands that helps a patient to relax and to make progress. At every fresh pair of hands he tightens up again until further experience allows him to relax, develop confidence, and start to progress again. For the same reason, I like the concept of the "hand therapist" rather than simply physical therapists and occupational therapists. A hand therapist may start his or her professional life as either a physical therapist or an occupational therapist and then learn by experience the aspects of the skills of the other discipline that are applicable to hands. There is no need for a therapist to confine himself or herself to hands; it is just a matter of special interest and special skills. In a unit that is large enough to employ several therapists, there may be room for the retention of some special distinctions. For example, one occupational therapist may make and adapt most of the splints. Even so, I think a patient does better with continuity of responsibility with one individual therapist.

Team interaction. After the identification of a therapist as a member of the team, the next step is to develop a working relationship in which there is true team interaction. It is sometimes difficult for a surgeon, or any physician, to get over the feeling that he or she alone is the source of all wisdom. Some knowledge comes from books, more comes from experience; in the case of the hand most comes by touch—by skin-to-skin, eye-to-eye dynamic interaction, whereby a good therapist comes to know just how a patient feels and reacts. Many times I have planned an operation and then, as the therapist works on the preoperative hand, have been told firmly that in this particular case the planned procedure would be a waste of time or that it would be better if it were postponed or modified. More often than not the therapist has been right. I am indebted to a succession of therapists whose insights have contributed at least as much to my education as I have been able to contribute to theirs. It is good for hand therapists to come into the operating room and observe the actual placement of transferred tendons and to see the kinds of problems that may contribute to scar formation. This need not be a routine, but it is helpful in the training stages and for difficult cases.

There are probably therapists who work in a situation in which they have little or no access to the surgeon and in which teamwork does not exist. My advice to them is to keep good records, especially graphs of range of motion, swelling, and the temperature of joints. When such graphs show a plateau that suggests a change of treatment is needed, the therapist should go to the prescribing surgeon armed with the graphs and ask for advice. The chances are the surgeon will be impressed with the fact that the therapist can contribute clear, pertinent, factual information about the patient, and he or she will probably begin asking for this kind of help with other patients. Teamwork can develop in many ways.

Time and space

The next objective concerns time and space. I believe that many hands become stiff from a dangerous mixture:

$$\left.\begin{array}{l}\text{Overtreatment—30 minutes}\\\text{Disuse—23½ hours}\end{array}\right\}\text{daily}$$

This situation stems from hospital and clinic routines, in which therapists have a timetable and in which charges are made per session. A therapist knows that he or she has just 20 minutes or so to *do* something to improve range of motion or get a tendon gliding. He or she is likely to work too fast or push too hard. The patient also feels that those minutes are critical, and when they are over, he will relax his hand into immobile disuse. Human tissue cells, however, have no consciousness of timetables. They respond to sudden intense stress by inflammation and an outpouring of fibrinogen. Then they occupy the idle hours of disuse by sitting there knitting the strands of fibrin into a fabric that will resist further joint movement.

The present new generation of hand rehabilitation centers is being organized in a different way. They do not need more staff, but they use more space. The idea is that patients pay by the day or week rather than by the minute or hour. Then they are free to come to the center in the morning and stay all day if they like. This may fit in with family programs, since a family member can drop the patient off on the way to work or school and pick him up on the way home. The therapists do not attempt to work with the patient all the time; rather they set him up with an exercise program or some therapeutic job or form of recreation. The therapists move around checking on progress and keeping activity going. New patients may be paired with older ones, and rheumatoid arthritics can exchange ideas on how to handle the activities of daily living without causing painful stress on their joints. This sort of program requires more room than the older type of program. There should be space for straight exercise programs and electronic, diagnostic, and stimulation apparatus. There must be room for a splint workshop or bench. A variety of benches and tables is needed for different types of manual tasks and a few games. There should be a rest area and, if I had my choice, a garden. In almost any condition of sickness and disability it is therapeutic to mind and body to be part of a living system where seeds are sprouting and worms and bees are about their business. Life and growth are infectious.

PATIENT OBJECTIVES

If staff and space are available, what about objectives for the individual patient? This book will suggest many objectives related to surgery, therapy, and splinting. Two should be mentioned in relation to the patient as a whole—the man or woman to whom the hand is attached and who will have to live with it when we have finished.

Responsibility and competence

The first objective is to establish responsibility and competence. We all know that the most successful results occur when the patient is determined to do well and believes that he can do well. He accepts advice, but he does things himself. Yet we all have a tendency to build up the importance and significance of what we as professionals can do for the patient, thereby downplaying his own contribution. We would like the patient to leave his hand with us in the morning and pick it up in the evening. We take credit for the improvements and blame the patient for poor results.

For real rehabilitation, from the very start we need to make the patient feel that he is doing it all himself. Only the surgery is done while he is asleep. Even that is something he has understood, asked for, and agreed to. Now as he starts to move his postoperative hand, he must understand what makes his hand swell, what makes it heal, and how tendons move. Above all we must teach him the significance of pain. It is not an enemy. It is his own living cells keeping him informed about the limits within which he must stay. Each patient must see his own graph of changing range of motion at each joint, and he must be encouraged to feel responsible for improvement or to wonder why it got worse. He must see his hand volume measurements and perhaps measure the volume himself. This process is like biofeedback because he quickly recognizes that when he hangs his hand down, his volume graph goes up; when the volume level comes down, his range of motion improves. He should see how the temperature of his joints is assessed by a touch of the thermistor probe—how it goes up and down with good activity but goes up and stays up if he pushes his exercises too hard. He may check the tension of the rubber bands of his splint and make sure they do not slip. He must see the dial of his dynamometer as he tests his improving strength. When the time comes for the therapist to use some passive motion, there must be such close rapport that the patient knows that he is not going to be subjected to a force against his will. As I hold and stroke a hand with my eyes on the face of the patient, I can soon get to feel that his nerve endings cross the interface between his hand and mine and that I feel his pain as soon as he does. As we talk together and I respond to his fear and build up his confidence, we soon get the feeling that he is in control of his own hand, and I am acting only in place of his damaged or paralyzed muscle tendon units. Each time we sit together and hold hands the symbiotic synergistic feeling increases until there is ideally an absolute mutual confidence and respect that is quite an exhilarating experience. I have become a new strength for the patient, but it is his strength now, not mine, and he can pick up from there and do things himself.

This is the great value of a rehabilitation center as compared with a hospital ward. When I had my gallbladder removed several years ago, I was exposed for the first time to the full impact of the system of hospital medical care in this country. My overwhelming impression was that of being reduced to a cog in a remorseless machine—an incompetent cog at that. My sterile prison cell was visited by an assembly line of technicians who entered and left, each with his own competence and superiority: "Roll up your sleeve," "Pull down your pants," "I'm doing this again because your first blood clotted"—with a frown that implied it was poor-quality blood. The cumulative effect of a long succession of total strangers gathering data that were never shared with me produced the feeling that I was the only totally incompetent person on the ward. My bowels were one person's responsibility and my blood another's responsibility, while a third person took care of my mind by keeping up the proper level of pain medication. If I as a doctor could be given that feeling, what is the hope for a nonmedical person? So let's minimize hospitalization and maximize the patient's sense of personal competence. "It's my hand—I can do it!"

Patient's overall goals

We should always be ready to reevaluate and modify our minor and technical objectives in a flexible response to our understanding of the patient's overall goals for life. It is good to set ourselves measurable objectives. The tip of the finger should reach the distal crease of the palm after tendon grafting. Pinch strength in this hand should reach 2 kg. Metacarpophalangeal range of motion should be 80 degrees after Silastic joint replacement. These measurements are good because they set targets for the patient, and we can plot the progress on a graph for all to see. However, the danger of narrow objectives is that we forget the overall view. I recently had to stop and reevaluate the situation as I found myself prescribing more therapy to perfect the opposition of the thumb in a 68-year-old retired patient who could already use his hand for all ordinary activities. My objective of perfection was a matter of my professional pride. How long was this patient's expectation of life? What percentage of his remaining months should be spent on his thumb? What did he ask of his thumb?

CONCLUSION

The real trouble with management by objectives is that the most important goals in life and health are not amenable to measurement at all. We tend to fasten on things that we can measure and feed into a computer. We glorify technical progress and let the spirit languish. In agriculture, we maximize the harvest but lose the soil that is the basis of future harvests. In medicine we kill germs and mend bones, but we need to learn to combat fear and build confidence. A good surgeon will mend a lacerated hand, choosing what can be saved and what cannot. A good rehabilitation team will mobilize it as far as it can be mobilized, and then will convince the patient that life is still good and achievement still possible in spite of what has been lost.

It is here that teamwork has its greatest value. Not all of us inspire the kind of confidence that encourages a patient to speak his fears and shyly expose the inner ambitions or resentments that make up the very essence of who he is and where he is aimed. It may be the therapist or the social worker who gets the best insights, but he or she can help the other group members to adjust their sights and match their tempo to a new rhythm.

Like Thoreau, we all march better if we sense the beat of our own drum. However, we have to learn to subdue our own rhythm and listen for the drummer who is real to the patient.

2

Psychological aspects of hand injuries

R. GUY PULVERTAFT

Our President has asked me to undertake a task for which I feel inadequately equipped. Psychology is defined in the Oxford Dictionary as "The science of the nature, function and phenomenon of the human mind and conduct." It would not be fitting for me to attempt a description of the physiological and pathological patterns of behaviour. To those of you who wish to study the subject from a psychiatric viewpoint, I commend an Article written by Cone and Hueston [2] which appeared in the Medical Journal of Australia last January. What I have to say to you comes not from a knowledge of psychology but from a lifetime of surgical practice with its failures and its successes. I can do no more than draw your attention to some of the conditions which may be initiated or influenced by the patient's and the doctor's mental attitude. Human relationship is a matter of fundamental importance in the care of the patient, whether he be a child or an adult. You have all been through a long and arduous training designed to fit you for the many decisions and actions you are called upon to make. Few, if any, of you will have had formal instruction in the art of rapport. This has been left to your own personality and the attitudes you have observed in your teachers. I know that I feel deep gratitude to the men and women I served as student, house surgeon and registrar and to the many others whom I have been privileged to know throughout my life. Albert Schweitzer said, "One other thing strikes me when I look back on my youthful days. The fact that so many people gave me something, or were something to me, without knowing it. Much that I would otherwise not have felt so clearly or done so effectively was felt or done as it was, because I stood under the sway of these people. If we had before us those who have thus been a blessing to us and could tell them how it came about, they would be amazed to learn what had passed over from their life to ours."

It is often said that rehabilitation commences at the moment of injury. It is also true that the words spoken by the emergency surgeon can engender a feeling of confidence and trust, particularly for the patient who has suffered a mutilating injury of the hand; who sees his skills destroyed, his career ruined and his family's future placed in jeopardy. The same feeling of despair must enter the minds of parents when their child is born with a severe malformation. I do not mean to infer that it is right to be unduly optimistic and give promises which cannot be honoured. There are ways in which we can combine sympathy with truth.

The best service that we can give is to get on with the job as effectively as we can and see the patient through the ensuing weeks and months personally, with the assistance of the Social Worker and the Department of Physical Medicine. In Orthopaedic and Plastic Surgery there is a tradition of continuing personal care and the same is seen in those who practise Hand Surgery. The Resettlement Service for the Disabled is doing a most valuable work. I quote the words of George Cochrane, Director of Physical Medicine in Derby, with whom I have worked for many years. "Rehabilitation begins with the appraisal of clinical problems at the outset and the defining for all, and this includes the patient and his relatives, the problem and the expected outcome and what we should aim to achieve in various stages on the way to this. Well before the end of treatment, the District Resettlement Officer is advised of his abilities, limitations, interests and past skills and charged to seek out work for him."

I need hardly remind you that in the animal world a weak or wounded animal may be deserted or attacked by other members of the herd. The same may be seen in a more subtle form in the human race. It is our duty to see that the infirm are supported spiritually as well as physically. A man may react to a physical disaster by a determination to overcome or he may fold up and withdraw into himself. The response, no doubt, depends primarily upon the patient but it can be influenced by the personality of the doctor. As Cone put it "an unresponsive surgeon will find that he has an unresponsive patient." We may take encouragement from the knowledge that few give up whilst we can remember many who have been victorious.

This lad of 16 years (Fig. 2-1), whom Douglas Reid will remember, never lost heart and despite his disability qualified as a surveyor and now holds a responsible post. I recall the day when he demonstrated to us how he could lift the ash from a cigarette with his double hook without breaking it; a trick which none of us could do with our normal hands. This man (Fig. 2-2) suffered gross damage from the same cause—fireworks—at the age of 13. He, also, lost the other hand. In the surviving hand two stumps provided his sole grip. He has steady employment as a clerk.

One of the most remarkable stories of physical handicap

Reprinted with permission from *The Hand; 1975 Journal of the British Society for Surgery of the Hand*, Longman Group, Ltd., **7**:93-103.

overcome is that of Howard Blackburn,[5] who while fishing from a dory on the Newfoundland Banks was caught in a blizzard and was unable to rejoin his schooner. He rowed for two days through the intense cold and reached Newfoundland but frostbite destroyed all fingers and part of his thumbs. Some years later, Blackburn made a solo voyage from Goucester, Massachusetts, to Gloucester, England, in a 30 foot open boat under sail. Two years later, he made another Atlantic crossing to Lisbon in a smaller boat.

While working in a Leprosy Hospital last year I was much struck by a patient who had lost one foot and numerous fingers. I came across him on my night rounds, when I found him surrounded by the other men in the ward playing rummy with great merriment. He was an inspiration to his friends and, though little did he know it, to the Staff as well. It was only later that I learned he read to the ward from the Bible every day.

The spirit in man can rise above the evils that can harm the body.

Although our prime objective is to restore function, the

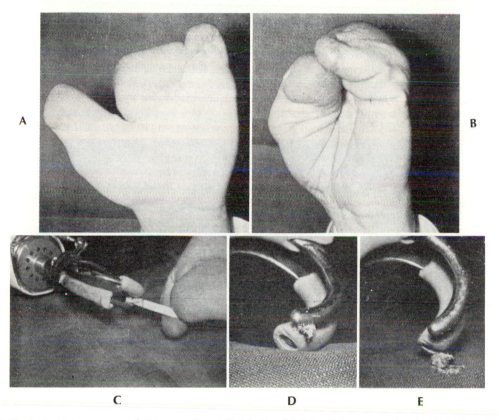

FIG. 2-1. Explosive injury at age of 16 years. **A** and **B,** Mutilated left hand (reconstruction by D.A.C. Reid). **C, D,** and **E,** Precision control of prosthesis, right hand.

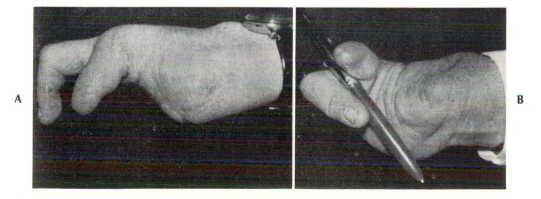

FIG. 2-2. Explosive injury at age of 13 years. **A** and **B,** Mutilated right hand. Left hand amputated. Reproduced from British Journal of Bone and Joint Surgery by permission of the Editor.

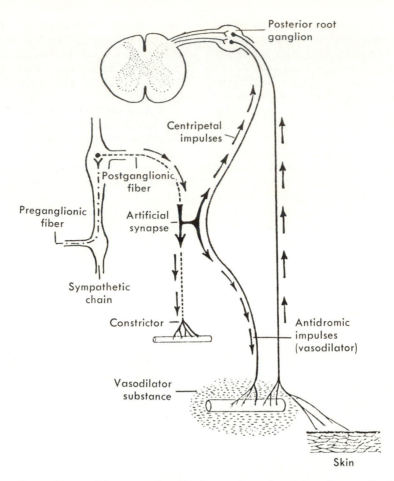

FIG. 2-6. The pain pathways in causalgia as postulated by Doupe. Reproduced from Barnes, R., in Peripheral Nerve Injuries, M.R.C. Special Report Series No. 282, by permission of the Author and the Controller of H.M. Stationery Office.

salgia'' as Seddon[12] put it, such as are seen after amputations, digital nerve divisions and some plexus injuries. These syndromes may arise from a variety of causes, whereas causalgia is most commonly a result of high velocity missile wounds. The nerve interruption is often complete in irritative lesions, but in causalgia it is usually incomplete. Irritative lesions may occur in any nerve, whilst causalgia as a rule arises from injuries to the median and tibial nerves and the brachial plexus.

This is not the occasion to discuss the management of these conditions, except to stress that the temptation to lose patience with those who suffer from them must be resisted. The subject is fully reviewed by Seddon, and Cullen's work on causalgia[3] should also be studied.

Hysteria

Hysteria is a functional disturbance in which symptoms are assumed for a personal advantage without the patient being fully conscious of this motive. In making this diagnosis, it is essential to exclude organic disease and this may be difficult when hysteria is superimposed upon an organic disorder. In a limb the presenting features are usually an anaesthetic area and alternatively paralysis which do not

accord with anatomy, unless the patient has a knowledge of anatomy. In a case of long standing there may be secondary trophic changes such as oedema, shiny skin and joint stiffening. The diagnosis is made after a thorough neurological examination including electrodiagnosis. A reasoned explanation to the patient may be sufficient to direct thought in the right direction and avoid prolonged incapacity. Aubrey Lewis[8] has said that common sense on the part of the physician is as important as psychological understanding and that too much treatment is as harmful as too little treatment. In a resistant case, there should be no hesitation in seeking psychiatric advice.

Malingering

There are those who deliberately set out to deceive, and the border line between true hysteria and malingering is sometimes difficult to determine. I have avoided the term when composing a medical report and have used a phrase such as ''I am unable to find a satisfactory explanation for this man's complaints.'' When a remark of this kind follows an examination which clearly has been thoroughly performed, the reader of the report or the Judge may safely be left to draw his own conclusions. In my experience, no useful purpose is served by arguing with the patient about symptoms and signs which are manifestly not genuine. Repeat the examination quietly and without undue comment until you are convinced of the sincerity or otherwise of the patient and the unreality of the physical signs. Many years ago I came across the expression "Profitable Humbug." Francis Walshe,[15] in discussing these situations pointed out that we do not see this phenomenon arising after injuries sustained at sport. The sportsman, when injured, is expected to resume the game with the least possible delay and is not well regarded if he does not do so. No such code applies to the victim of an accident upon the roads or in industry, nor does he lose face if he behaves in the most extravagant fashion after the most trifling or injuries and claims disability for months or years. Sir Francis recalls that he was once asked by the Judge in a High Court action:—"Doctor, when these people kid themselves that they are ill, do they know that they are kidding themselves?" I give his reply verbatim:—"This is a difficult question to answer without qualification, but my view is that at some time in his 'illness,' if perhaps not all the time, the subject is aware that he is exploiting the situation for a known end. Possibly, as the months go by, the still small voice of conscience becomes less frequent and more still and finally falls silent. By this time the story of the accident has been rehearsed so many times in the circle of relatives and friends and to solicitor and doctors that the patient does not clearly know what is fact and what is legend. That the entire illness is determined and maintained by factors in the unconscious of the patient, I am not able to believe; willing as I am to credit these patients with a high capacity for self-deception."

The self-inflicted injury

You will meet these puzzling and worrying problems in many forms. For those of you who are not familiar with the life of Baron Munchausen I suggest you read "Singular Travels and Adventures of Baron Munchausen" published by the Cresset Press. To illustrate his remarkable initiative, I will relate one of his unpublished experiences. While riding alone through a Polish forest, Munchausen was thrown from his horse and was obliged to spend the night in that wolf infested place. Aware that wolves attack in single file, he stationed himself with his back to a tree and awaited the onslaught. It was not long before Munchausen observed their eyes gleaming in a long line and he braced himself for the attack. As the leading wolf sprang he, with great presence of mind, thrust his right arm through the jaws of the beast and seized its anus; then leaning back he withdrew his arm, thus turning the animal inside out. Naturally, the wolf made off in the opposite direction closely followed by the rest of the pack.

Sometimes, it seems that the symptoms to which we are obliged to listen rival these tales in their imaginative content. I think of a young lass of eight who presented with a weeping finger. The slightly frothy fluid appeared to ooze from a fault in the nail. We were mystified until it occurred to us that the simplest explanation should not be overlooked— placing the finger in the mouth. Mother found it difficult to believe that her daughter could behave in this manner, even when the finger remained dry it if was protected by a cov-

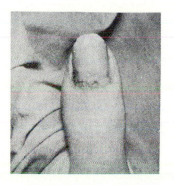
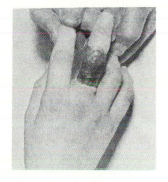

Fig. 2-7. Self-inflicted paronychia.   Fig. 2-8. Self-inflicted burn.

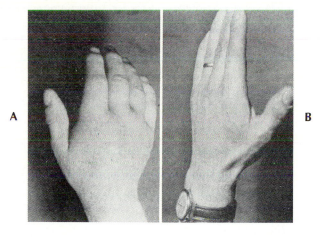

A   B

Fig. 2-9. Secretan's syndrome. A, Right hand. B, Normal left hand.

ering. Another child came with a persistently swollen hand for no reason that her parents nor her doctor could detect. We could find no evidence that a constriction band had been used. However, admission to hospital and elevation of the limb allowed the oedema to disperse and a plaster cast prevented its recurrence. The parents accepted the evidence and it remained to cure the habit without causing the child to lose face. This was done to everyone's satisfaction and the trouble did not return. I believe that we should endeavour to resolve these situations in an understanding way. This may try our patience in a busy Clinic, but an early redirection of a young person may avoid worse trouble later.

Here is a case of chronic paronychia (Fig. 2-7) caused by deliberate insertion of thorns. Nineteen were removed. This unusual burn (Fig. 2-8) was caused by an encircling bandage soaked in some corrosive fluid. The physical defect was cured but, undefeated, this woman continued to haunt the out-patient department for years with a variety of self-inflicted injuries. Psychiatric treatment has failed to relieve her of these strange tendencies.

Peritendinous fibrosis of the dorsum of the hand (Fig. 2-9) which Secretan described in 1911[11] is a curious condition in which the extensor tendons become surrounded by a mass of organising fibrous tissue containing macrophages and haemosiderin. It probably results from repeated minor contusions of the hand and the suspicions of self-infliction should enter your mind. It is interesting to note that Secretan states that he had not seen a patient suffering from this condition who did not have some possible claim for occupational injury.

Attempted suicides demand the immediate help of the Psychiatrist and, indeed, this is a standing requirement in the National Health Service.

Sudeck's atrophy

Sudeck in 1900 described a syndrome of osteoporosis of the bones of the hand accompanied by oedema in the early stages, stiffness, pain, muscle atrophy and skin changes.[13] The cause remains unknown, but it appears to be an acute autonomic dystrophy occurring after injury, usually of a minor nature, surgery or inflammation. It is said to be more commonly seen in women than in men although a recent report by Kleinert[7] indicates otherwise. It tends to occur more often in persons who are introspective and apprehensive. Symptoms usually develop within a few weeks of the exciting cause, but the onset may be delayed for several months.

I have nothing to add to what is already known except to emphasize two lessons which experience has taught me; the importance of early recognition and the imperative need for immediate and determined treatment before the condition progresses to a state from which the hand may never fully recover. The early danger signs are oedema and pain, and when either of these present in the absence of a simple explanation action should be taken. The temptation is to compromise by advising physical treatment in the hope of seeing an improvement at the next visit. The patient should be admitted to hospital for elevation of the limb and for a full programme of physical treatment which can only be given effectively as an inpatient. It may be difficult to convince the patient that this action be necessary for to him the early signs do not appear to warrant this inconvenience. He must be told that a week's delay at this stage may mean a month's delay in final recovery. I have never had cause to regret insisting upon this course, but have regretted it when I have been complacent. I need hardly add that the psychological management of these situations is not unimportant. Strict observance of these rules may avoid the need for sympathetic block or sympathectomy later.

• • •

We commenced the day with "Evolution of the Hand." We have moved on through anatomy and treatment to the forefront of progress in the accomplishments of micro-surgery. We have been warned of the complications of surgery and I have spoken of psychological complications. I will conclude with some sound advice which you will find in the Book of Proverbs. "Wisdom is the principle thing; therefore get wisdom; and with all thy getting get understanding."[10]

ACKNOWLEDGEMENTS

My thanks are due to Barry Wilks and his staff of the Department of Medical Illustration at the Derbyshire Royal Infirmary for their assistance.

REFERENCES

1. Barnes, R. (1954) Causalgia. A Review of 48 Cases. Peripheral Nerve Injuries. Medical Research Council Special Report Series 282. London, H.M. Stationery Office, p. 156.
2. Cone, J., and Hueston, J.T. (1974) Psychological Aspects of Hand Injury. Medical Journal of Australia, 1:104-108.
3. Cullen, C.H. (1948) Causalgia. Diagnosis and Treatment. Journal of Bone and Joint Surgery, 30-B:467-477.
4. Doupe, J., Cullen, C.H. and Chance, G.Q. (1944) Post-Traumatic Pain and The Causalgic Syndrome. Journal of Neurology, Neurosurgery and Psychiatry, 7:33-48.
5. Garland, J.E. (1963) Lone Voyager. Boston, Little, Brown and Company.
6. Jones, R., and Lovett, R.W. (1923) Orthopaedic Surgery. London, Oxford University Press, p. 525.
7. Kleinert, H.E., Cole, N.M., Wayne, L., Harvey, R., and Kutz, J.E. (1972) Post-Traumatic Sympathetic Dystrophy. Journal of Bone and Joint Surgery, 54-A:899.
8. Lewis, A. (1956) Price's Textbook of the Practice of Medicine. Ed. Hunter, D. London, Oxford University Press, p. 1975.
9. Mitchell, S.W. (1894) Traumatic Neuralgia. Section of Median Nerve, American Journal of the Medical Sciences, 135:2-29.
10. Proverbs, chapter 4, verse 7.
11. Secretan, H. (1901) Oedeme dur et Hyperplasie Traumatique du Metacarpe Dorsal. Revue Médicale de la Suisse Romande, 21:409-416.
12. Seddon, H.J. (1972) Surgical Disorders of the Peripheral Nerves. Edinburgh and London, Churchill Livingstone, pp. 139-152.
13. Sudeck, P. (1900) Uber die acute entzündliche Knochenatrophie. Archiv. Fur Klinische Chirurgie, 62:147-156.
14. Sunderland, S. (1968) Nerves And Nerve Injuries. Edinburgh and London, E & S. Livingstone Ltd., p. 425.
15. Walshe, F.M.R. (1958) The Role of Injury, of the Law and of the Doctor in the Aetiology of the so-called Traumatic Neurosis. The Medical Press, 239:493-496.

3

Practical functional anatomy

J. V. BASMAJIAN

Proper rehabilitation of injuries and deformities of the hand requires an extraordinary knowledge of the fine function and anatomy of its bones, joints, muscles, nerves, and vessels. Even the skin and subcutaneous tissues take on a special importance in the hand that they do not have in any other parts of the body. In this brief chapter one cannot hope to cover all the complex functional anatomy adequately; rather, an attempt will be made to present the anatomic highlights of particular importance in rehabilitation of the hand, with an emphasis on the dynamic aspects. The latter are described on the basis of electromyographic findings from extensive studies by the author and his colleagues and by others.[1] The extensor tendons are more fully discussed in Chapter 28. For a thorough description of structure as seen in exquisite detail by an anatomist who has spent his professional life on the study of the hand, the reader must consult the *Atlas of Anatomy of the Hand* by Landsmeer.[9]

MUSCLES AND MOVEMENTS
Movements of the five digits

A line drawn through the middle finger, middle metacarpal, and capitate is the axial line of the hand. Movement of a finger away from this axial line is abduction; movement toward it is adduction. These take place at the metacarpophalangeal joints. The thumb, set at right angles to the other digits, can be abducted and adducted, but the movements take place not at its metacarpophalangeal joint but at its multiaxial carpometacarpal joint; the movement forward (anteriorly) is abduction, and backward (posteriorly), adduction. The thumb owes its remarkable functions to the unique movements of medial and lateral rotation at its carpometacarpal joint.

Hand muscles

Three thenar muscles. The most superficial of the three thenar muscles (Fig. 3-1), the abductor pollicis brevis, draws the thumb forward (that is, abducts it); the movement takes place at the saddle-shaped carpometacarpal joint. Its removal uncovers a fleshy sheet that pronates or medially rotates the whole thumb and flexes its metacarpophalangeal joint. The portion inserted into the metacarpal is named the opponens pollicis; the portion inserted into the phalanx (largely via the radial sesamoid embedded in the palmar ligament) is the flexor pollicis brevis.

Three hypothenar muscles. The hypothenar muscles (Fig. 3-2) act on a metacarpophalangeal joint, but, of course, opposition of the little finger is impossible.

Adductor pollicis. A transverse head arises from the palmar border of the middle metacarpal, and an oblique head arises from the corresponding carpal bone (the capitate). It is inserted into the base of the first phalanx of the thumb along with the ulnar insertion of the flexor brevis. Obviously, the adductor draws the thumb to the palm.

Opposition. Bringing the pad of the thumb to the pad of a finger and holding it there, as in pinching, writing, holding a cup by its handle, fastening a button, and almost all other delicate actions performed by the hand, involve opposition. The movements executed almost simultaneously are circumduction, rotation, and flexion. Rotation takes place principally at the metacarpophangeal joint but also at the carpometacarpal joint, while the trapezium moves on the scaphoid and the scalphoid angulates forward. The three joints of the opposing finger (or fingers) are flexed by the profundus, the superficialis, a lumbrical and two interossei.

Without two muscles supplied by the median nerve (opponens and flexor pollicis brevis), there would be no rotation. Without two muscles supplied by the ulnar nerve (adductor pollicis and an interosseus), the grip would be weak. An interosseus muscle is required to steady (that is, to prevent ulnar deviation of) the finger against which the adductor pollicis is exerting pressure. In the case of the index finger, it is the first dorsal interosseus. Hence ulnar paralysis results in weak opposition.

Palmar aponeurosis. The palmaris longus tendon (Fig. 3-1) adheres to the front of the flexor retinaculum, enters the palm, and divides into four broad, diverging bands. These descend to the roots of the four fingers, there to blend with subcutaneous tissues. In the distal half of the palm the aponeurosis sends fibrous septa dorsally to the palmar ligaments (plates), which are thickenings of the joint capsules, and to the deep fascia.

Long flexors of the digits. The tendons of a superficialis muscle and a profundus muscle (Fig. 3-2) descend deep to the palmar aponeurosis. In front of the head of a metacarpal bone each pair enters a fibrous digital sheath. Each sheath extends from the palmar ligament of a metacarpophalangeal joint to the insertion of a profundus tendon into the base of a distal phalanx. Each sheath, therefore, crosses three joints.

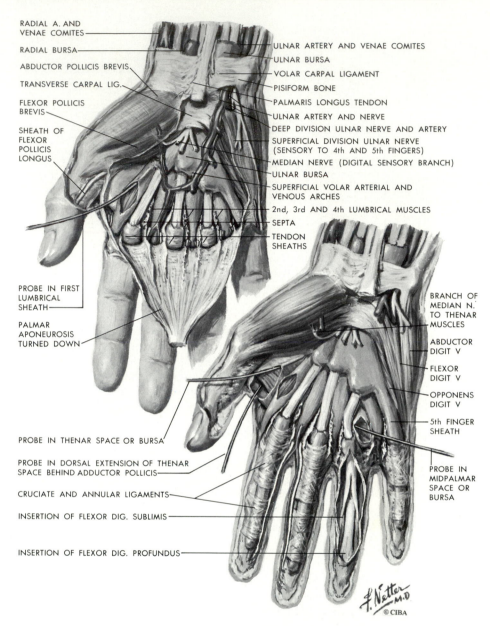

RADIAL A. AND VENAE COMITES
RADIAL BURSA
ABDUCTOR POLLICIS BREVIS
TRANSVERSE CARPAL LIG.
FLEXOR POLLICIS BREVIS
SHEATH OF FLEXOR POLLICIS LONGUS

ULNAR ARTERY AND VENAE COMITES
ULNAR BURSA
VOLAR CARPAL LIGAMENT
PISIFORM BONE
PALMARIS LONGUS TENDON
ULNAR ARTERY AND NERVE
DEEP DIVISION ULNAR NERVE AND ARTERY
SUPERFICIAL DIVISION ULNAR NERVE (SENSORY TO 4th AND 5th FINGERS)
MEDIAN NERVE (DIGITAL SENSORY BRANCH)
ULNAR BURSA
SUPERFICIAL VOLAR ARTERIAL AND VENOUS ARCHES
2nd, 3rd AND 4th LUMBRICAL MUSCLES
SEPTA
TENDON SHEATHS

PROBE IN FIRST LUMBRICAL SHEATH
PALMAR APONEUROSIS TURNED DOWN

BRANCH OF MEDIAN N. TO THENAR MUSCLES
ABDUCTOR DIGIT V
FLEXOR DIGIT V
OPPONENS DIGIT V
5th FINGER SHEATH
PROBE IN MIDPALMAR SPACE OR BURSA

PROBE IN THENAR SPACE OR BURSA
PROBE IN DORSAL EXTENSION OF THENAR SPACE BEHIND ADDUCTOR POLLICIS
CRUCIATE AND ANNULAR LIGAMENTS
INSERTION OF FLEXOR DIG. SUBLIMIS
INSERTION OF FLEXOR DIG. PROFUNDUS

Figs. 3-1 and **3-2.** Anatomy of the palm. (© Copyright 1969 CIBA Pharmaceutical Company, Division of CIBA-GEIGY Corporation. Reproduced with permission from *Clinical Symposia;* illustrated by Frank H. Netter, M.D. All rights reserved.)

In front of the joints the sheath, for mechanical reasons, must be pliable and thin.

Each profundus tendon is inserted into the anterior aspect of the base of a distal phalanx. Each superficialis tendon splits in front of a proximal phalanx into medial and lateral halves that ultimately insert on the margins of a middle phalanx. Each profundus tendon passes through a perforation in a superficialis muscle. The intricate perforation remains so widely open that you can easily thread a cut profundus tendon through it again.

The *seven interossei* (four dorsal and three palmar) arise from the metacarpal bodies and pass behind the deep transverse ligaments to insert on the proximal phalanges as well as the extensor expansions. The four lumbricals arise in the palm from the profundus tendons. They lie behind the digital vessels and nerves, and they accompany them in front of the deep transverse ligaments of the palm to the radial side of the fingers, where they join the extensor expansions distal to the attachments of the interossei.

Synovial sheaths. A synovial sheath (Fig. 3-3) may extend 2 or 3 cm proximal to and distal to the site of friction. But this depends on the excursion the tendon makes, as does the probability of disappearance of the mesotendon. Every tendon lying within a synovial sheath has a mesotendon—a double layer of synovial membrane that attaches a tendon to the wall of its sheath and conveys vessels to it. The very

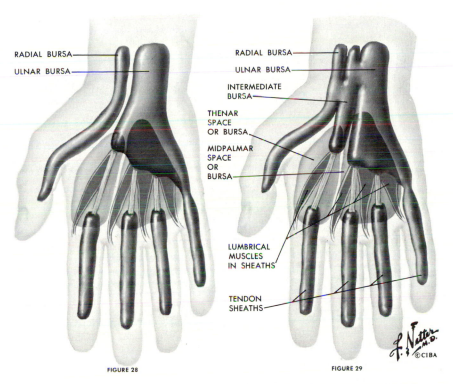

RADIAL BURSA
ULNAR BURSA

RADIAL BURSA
ULNAR BURSA
INTERMEDIATE BURSA
THENAR SPACE OR BURSA
MIDPALMAR SPACE OR BURSA
LUMBRICAL MUSCLES IN SHEATHS
TENDON SHEATHS

FIGURE 28   FIGURE 29

Fig. 3-3. Synovial sheaths of the palm and wrist. (© Copyright 1969 CIBA Pharmaceutical Company, Division of CIBA-GEIGY Corporation. Reproduced with permission from *Clinical Symposia;* illustrated by Frank H. Netter, M.D. All rights reserved.)

end portions of the original mesotendons of the long flexors remain as triangular folds, the vincula brevia; several thread-like portions persist in front of the proximal phalanges as vincula longa. Each vinculum conveys blood vessels to the tendons and, therefore, must be so offset as to avoid constant pressure between the tendon and its surroundings.

The long flexor tendons require synovial sheaths where they pass first through the carpal tunnel and then through the digital tunnels—that is, carpal synovial sheaths and digital synovial sheaths. The thumb obviously has the freest range of movement; this and the shortness of the metacarpals of the thumb and of the fifth digit result in their carpal and digital sheaths being continuous (Fig. 3-3). Those of the thumb probably always unite; those of the little finger fail to unite in about 10% of persons.

The carpal sheaths of the four superficialis and four profundus tendons usually become one, the common synovial sheath of the digital flexors. The carpal sheath of the flexor pollicis longus commonly joins, too. Thus an infection starting in the sheath of the little finger may spread by this route to the thumb.

Palmar spaces. In the palm there are four closed fascial spaces, which are important because of potential closed infections. The thenar muscles occupy (create) one, the thenar space (Fig. 3-4); the hypothenar muscles occupy another, the hypothenar space. Between these two there is a large, triangular central space that contains the tendons of the fingers. Its anterior wall is the palmar aponeurosis. Its posterior wall is formed by the three medial metacarpals, the palmar and deep transverse ligaments, and the fascia covering the medial interossei and the adductor pollicis. Its

side walls are the backward-turned edges of the palmar aponeurosis, which fuse with the thenar and hypothenar fasciae. The fourth space is located between the adductor pollicis in front and the two lateral intermetacarpal spaces behind.

In the distal half of the palm, the central space has eight subdivisions or tunnels (Fig. 3-5). The septa separating the tunnels are derived from the palmar aponeurosis. The tendons of the lumbrical muscles prolong the spaces downward onto the dorsum of the digits. It is by this lumbrical route that infection in the central palmar space may spread to the dorsum of the hand.

Extensors of the wrist

The extensor tendons occupy the lateral side as well as the back of the wrist and, lying in bony grooves, are held in place by a transverse band of fibrous tissue called the extensor retinaculum. From the deep surface of the extensor retinaculum a series of fibrous partitions passes to the margins of the bony grooves, thus producing six compartments in which lie the 12 extensor tendons (Figs. 3-6 and 3-7).

Since the contributions that extensor digitorum itself makes to the extensor expansions can be traced no farther than the bases of the middle phalanges, the muscle can have no power to extend the terminal phalanges. Indeed, its principal action is to extend the metacarpophalangeal joints, and for them it is the sole extensor. The extensors carpi ulnaris, carpi radialis brevis, and carpi radialis longus extend the wrist and, acting with their companion flexors, produce side-to-side motion at the wrist (adduction and abduction).

The three deep outcropping extensor muscles of the thumb

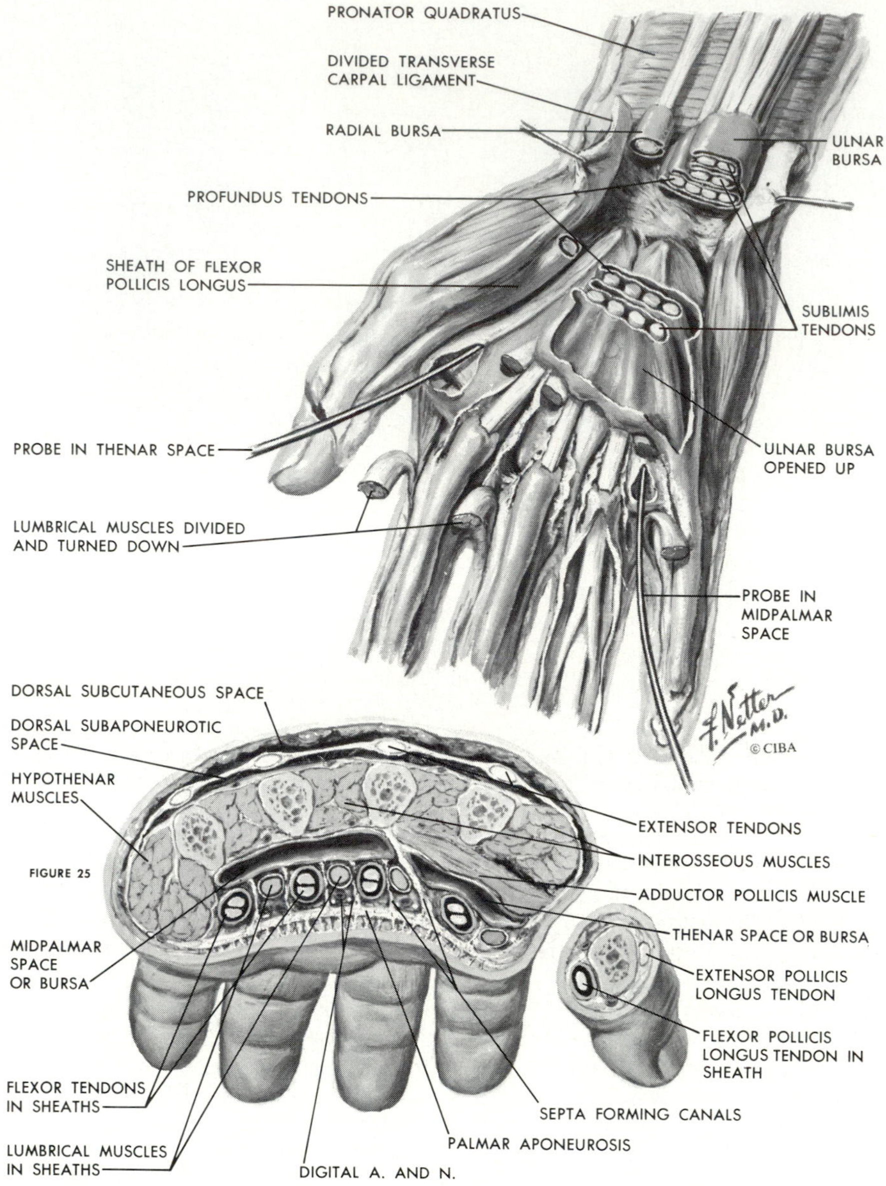

PRONATOR QUADRATUS

DIVIDED TRANSVERSE
CARPAL LIGAMENT

RADIAL BURSA

PROFUNDUS TENDONS

SHEATH OF FLEXOR
POLLICIS LONGUS

PROBE IN THENAR SPACE

LUMBRICAL MUSCLES DIVIDED
AND TURNED DOWN

ULNAR
BURSA

SUBLIMIS
TENDONS

ULNAR BURSA
OPENED UP

PROBE IN
MIDPALMAR
SPACE

DORSAL SUBCUTANEOUS SPACE

DORSAL SUBAPONEUROTIC
SPACE

HYPOTHENAR
MUSCLES

FIGURE 25

MIDPALMAR
SPACE
OR BURSA

FLEXOR TENDONS
IN SHEATHS

LUMBRICAL MUSCLES
IN SHEATHS

DIGITAL A. AND N.

PALMAR APONEUROSIS

SEPTA FORMING CANALS

EXTENSOR TENDONS

INTEROSSEOUS MUSCLES

ADDUCTOR POLLICIS MUSCLE

THENAR SPACE OR BURSA

EXTENSOR POLLICIS
LONGUS TENDON

FLEXOR POLLICIS
LONGUS TENDON IN
SHEATH

FIGS. 3-4 and 3-5. Palmar spaces. (© Copyright 1969 CIBA Pharmaceutical Company, Division of CIBA-GEIGY Corporation. Reproduced with permission from *Clinical Symposia*, illustrated by Frank H. Netter, M.D. All rights reserved.)

are almost exclusively devoted to what may properly be called "supination of the thumb." This movement is contrary to the movement performed when the thumb is "pronated" in order to oppose it to the other digits in such an everyday action as picking up a pencil. (A fourth and lowest extensor muscle is present and joins the tendon of the extensor digitorum of the index finger; it can, of course, produce only extension of the index finger.)

In sequence from above downward, the outcropping muscles to the thumb are the abductor pollicis longus, extensor pollicis brevis, and extensor pollicis longus (Fig. 3-6). Their actions depend on the sites of insertion of their tendons and the direction of pull. Hold your wrist constantly straight

with the palm facing the floor and draw the thumb laterally and backward to point at the ceiling. The tendon of extensor pollicis longus will be seen running to its insertion on the dorsum of the base of the distal phalanx of the thumb, and it can be traced in back of the lower end of the radius, which it uses as a pulley to set the direction of its pull.

Next, stretch the thumb into the position of its widest span. This usually reveals the tendon of extensor pollicis brevis crossing the lateral aspect of the wrist (where it is held in a compartment of the extensor retinaculum) to its insertion on the base of the proximal phalanx. If the thumb is carried on through an arc until its tip stretches toward the floor, the tendon of abductor pollicis longus can be felt and

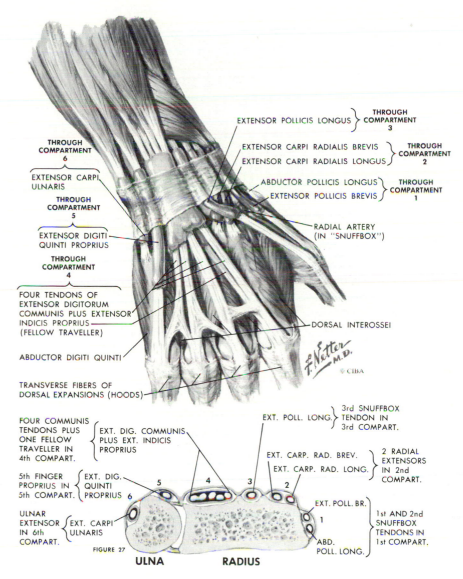

THROUGH COMPARTMENT 3 — EXTENSOR POLLICIS LONGUS

THROUGH COMPARTMENT 2 — EXTENSOR CARPI RADIALIS BREVIS / EXTENSOR CARPI RADIALIS LONGUS

THROUGH COMPARTMENT 1 — ABDUCTOR POLLICIS LONGUS / EXTENSOR POLLICIS BREVIS

RADIAL ARTERY (IN "SNUFFBOX")

THROUGH COMPARTMENT 6

EXTENSOR CARPI ULNARIS

THROUGH COMPARTMENT 5

EXTENSOR DIGITI QUINTI PROPRIUS

THROUGH COMPARTMENT 4

FOUR TENDONS OF EXTENSOR DIGITORUM COMMUNIS PLUS EXTENSOR INDICIS PROPRIUS (FELLOW TRAVELLER)

DORSAL INTEROSSEI

ABDUCTOR DIGITI QUINTI

TRANSVERSE FIBERS OF DORSAL EXPANSIONS (HOODS)

FOUR COMMUNIS TENDONS PLUS ONE FELLOW TRAVELLER IN 4th COMPART. { EXT. DIG. COMMUNIS PLUS EXT. INDICIS PROPRIUS }

5th FINGER PROPRIUS IN 5th COMPART. { EXT. DIG. QUINTI PROPRIUS }

ULNAR EXTENSOR IN 6th COMPART. { EXT. CARPI ULNARIS }

3rd SNUFFBOX TENDON IN 3rd COMPART. — EXT. POLL. LONG.

EXT. CARP. RAD. BREV. / EXT. CARP. RAD. LONG. — 2 RADIAL EXTENSORS IN 2nd COMPART.

EXT. POLL. BR. / ABD. POLL. LONG. — 1st AND 2nd SNUFFBOX TENDONS IN 1st COMPART.

FIGURE 27

ULNA   RADIUS

FIGS. 3-6 and **3-7.** Extensor tendon anatomy and relation of the extensor tendons at the wrist. (© Copyright 1969 CIBA Pharmaceutical Company, Division of CIBA-GEIGY Corporation. Reproduced with permission from *Clinical Symposia;* illustrated by Frank H. Netter, M.D. All rights reserved.)

seen as the most lateral tendon on the anterior aspect of the wrist. Its insertion is on the base of the first metacarpal. At the wrist, its tendon is in a compartment of the extensor retinaculum, which is far enough forward for the muscle to abduct the thumb, to flex the wrist, and to assist the extensors of the wrist and thumb in their stabilizing functions, one of the most significant being that of preventing the hand from being forced ulnarward (as in holding a heavy jug by its handle).

Of the two radial extensors of the wrist, the extensor carpi radialis brevis is much more active during pure extension than the extensor carpi radialis longus, whether the movement is slow or fast. Actually, except with fast extension, the extensor carpi radialis longus is essentially inactive. However, the roles of the two muscles are completely reversed during prehension or fist making; now the extensor

carpi radialis longus is very active as a synergist. The two muscles are both quite active during abduction of the wrist, as one would guess from their positions.

During simple extension of the wrist, there is a reciprocal innervation between extensors and flexors. The three extensors of the wrist as well as the extensor digitorum work synchronously; none seems to be the prime mover. During forced extreme flexion of the wrist, there is a reactive co-contraction of the extensor carpi ulnaris, apparently to stabilize the wrist joint; this does not occur with the extensor digitorum and radial extensors.

Flexors of the wrist

The three flexors of the superficial layer, flexors carpi radialis and ulnaris and palmaris longus, act only on the wrist and carpal joints (Figs. 3-8 and 3-9). As one would

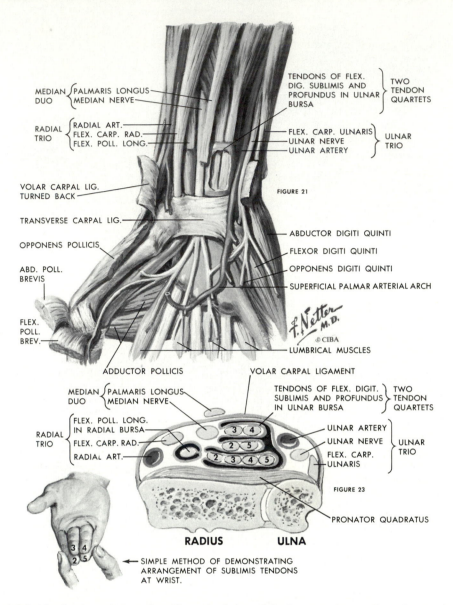

FIGS. 3-8 and **3-9.** The flexor tendons at the wrist and relation of the flexor tendons at the wrist. (© Copyright 1969 CIBA Pharmaceutical Company, Division of CIBA-GEIGY Corporation. Reproduced with permission from *Clinical Symposia;* illustrated by Frank H. Netter, M.D. All rights reserved.)

expect, they are inserted not on the mobile carpal bones but on the relatively fixed bases of the metacarpals. The one flexor of the middle layer, that is, flexor digitorum superficialis, reaches the middle phalanges and acts on all intermediate joints in passing. The two flexors of the deep layer, that is, flexor digitorum profundus and flexor pollicis longus, reach the terminal phalanges and similarly act on the intermediate joints.

The flexor carpi radialis, palmaris longus, and flexor carpi ulnaris all flex the wrist, although the flexor palmaris longus is not very powerful. The flexor carpi radialis is not an important abductor of the wrist; for that matter, the wrist can be abducted very little from "neutral." However, the flexor carpi ulnaris is an important adductor, acting in con-

cert with the extensor carpi ulnaris. All the muscles of the wrist are quite important for their synergistic use in stabilizing the wrist so that the fingers and fist work to the best advantage.

During flexion of the wrist, the flexors carpi radialis, ulnaris, and superficialis act synchronously; none is the sole prime mover. The flexor digitorum profundus plays no role. Two possible muscles in the antagonist position (the radial extensors of the wrist and the extensors of the fingers) are passive, even in extreme flexion of the wrist, but the extensor carpi ulnaris shows marked activity as an antagonist.

In abduction and adduction the appropriate flexors and extensors act reciprocally as one might expect, the antagonist muscles relaxing. The extensor digitorum contracts during abduction (radial abduction), but this contraction is not limited to the radial part of the muscle; the flexor digitorum superficialis may be active too. Apparently this type of activity has a synergistic function. Similarly, there is antagonist activity in the flexors when the wrist is extended and the metacarpophalangeal joints hyperextended.

Postures of the thumb and the little finger

During extension produced by the extensors, only the opponens pollicis and abductor pollicis brevis muscles show reciprocal activity. During abduction, the same two muscles show marked activity on the average, whereas the activity of the flexor pollicis is slight. During flexion, the mean activity of the flexor pollicis brevis is moderate to marked; the opponens pollicis is only slightly active, and the abductor pollicis brevis is essentially inactive.

The occurrence of equal levels of activity in both the abductor pollicis brevis and the opponens pollicis during extension and abduction of the thumb cannot be rationalized on the basis of their insertions. Their insertions are such that these muscles would be expected to move the thumb in opposite directions, especially during extension and to a lesser extent during abduction. Stabilization of the part in order to produce a smooth, even movement results from the significant activities of these muscles.

Not all thenar muscles are active during extension and flexion of the thumb. During flexion the abductor pollicis brevis exhibits negligible activity; the opponens pollicis, slight activity on the average; and the flexor pollicis brevis, moderate-to-marked activity. Indeed, in the position of flexion, most persons have little activity in both the opponens and abductor, while the flexor is significantly active.

In one other position there is coincident activity and inactivity in the thenar muscles. During firm pinch between the thumb and the side of the flexed index finger, only negligible activity is recorded from the abductor pollicis brevis. Yet the opponens pollicis and, in particular, the flexor pollicis brevis are significantly active.

During extension of the little finger, all three hypothenar muscles are rather inactive on the average. During abduction, although the abductor digiti minimi fulfills the function indicated by its name and is the dominant muscle, with strong activity, the other hypothenar muscles are also significantly active. During flexion, considerable activity occurs in all three hypothenar muscles.

The abductor digiti minimi is very active during flexion of the little finger at the metacarpophalangeal joint. (The participation of this muscle in this position of the finger is obvious by palpation.) Part of the explanation for this activity depends on the insertion of the muscle into the ulnar side of the base of the proximal phalanx. The abductor digiti minimi is also significantly active when the thumb is held opposed to either the ring or little finger. Some of this activity is possibly associated with the small degree of flexion at the fifth metacarpophalangeal joint that is required when the thumb and little finger are opposed. Yet such flexion is obviously not required during opposition of the thumb and ring finger. Some of the activity of the abductor digiti minimi may be to provide stability, and simple ab-

duction of the little finger may be the least important function of the abductor of this finger.[3]

Positions of opposition

During soft opposition of the thumb to the side or tip of each finger, the opponens is the most active of the thenar muscles and the flexor is the least active. The hypothenar muscles are recruited when the opposition is to the ring and little fingers. Then the opponens digiti minimi is the most active hypothenar muscle, but the thenar muscles are generally more active than the hypothenar muscles.

When opposition is firm, the flexor pollicis brevis replaces the opponens pollicis as the dominant muscle, particularly in forceful opposition to the index and middle fingers. In forceful opposition to the ring and little fingers, the activity of the opponens pollicis approaches and then equals that of the flexor pollicis brevis. During opposition to any finger the abductor pollicis brevis is the least active of the thenar muscles. With forceful opposition, higher levels of activity occur with firm opposition of the thumb to the side of any finger as compared with the activity during tip-to-tip opposition with the same finger.

Firm pinch between the thumb and the index and middle fingers is a grip position of day-to-day importance. The great power of the thumb, which enables this digit to balance the combined power of the fingers, has been attributed to the flexor pollicis brevis and to the mechanically advantageous position of the adductor pollicis.[3]

As medial rotation of the first metacarpal is increased, the tendency of the head of the fifth metacarpal to be drawn in an anterolateral (volar-radial) direction is similarly increased. The opponens digiti minimi is mainly responsible for this movement of the fifth metacarpal, and its action is almost reflexive in nature. The more active the opponens pollicis is in medially rotating the first metacarpal, the more active the opponens digiti minimi becomes. The opponens pollicis is always the more active muscle. It is possible that beyond a certain degree of medial rotation of the first metacarpal, the two opponens muscles begin to act in unison to form the transverse metacarpal arch. Indeed, this might be expected when one views the two opponens muscles, with the flexors retinacula between, linking up the first and fifth metacarpal bones.

Positions of grip

The important role of the flexor pollicis brevis in firm grasp is illustrated in the positions of firmly clasping a dowel (or rounded handle) and of holding a cup of water. Although the flexor pollicis brevis is the most active muscle while a dowel is being grasped firmly, this is not the case when a glass of water is being held firmly; both the opponens pollicis and the abductor pollicis brevis are then more active. Therefore the more the thumb is abducted (as in holding a glass), the less the flexor brevis contributes to a firm grip. The activity of this muscle, which provides firmness of grip when only a small degree of abduction exists (as in holding the cup), is replaced by that of the opponens when a large amount of abduction is present. In the absence of significant flexor activity, this activity of the opponens coupled with that of the abductor provides the power of a firm grip.

In summary, not all thenar muscles are active in all thumb postures, but all hypothenar muscles are active in the three basic postures of the little finger. Two somewhat different patterns of activity occur when the thumb is first softly and then firmly opposed to each of the fingers in a sequence that begins at the index and ends at the little finger. The flexor pollicis brevis is dominant in firm grip, particularly in grip between the thumb and two radial fingers, but a large degree of abduction of the thumb might possibly be a limiting factor in the activity of this muscle. The two opponens muscles seem to act as a unit in opposition of the thumb to both the ring and little fingers. Certain activity in some of the six muscles, which is inexplicable on a morphologic basis, probably serves to provide stability.

Flexor pollicis brevis versus adductor pollicis

Patterns of activity occur for each part of the flexor brevis and adductor muscles. There are marked differences between the role of the transverse head of the adductor and the superficial head of the flexor during most functions. Most of the time, but not always, the two heads of each muscle act in concert. My colleagues, Forrest and Khan,[4] found that the oblique adductor often acted differently from the adjacent part of the flexor brevis; this justifies the view that they are clearly different muscles belonging to adduction and flexion, respectively. Forrest and Khan showed that in very fine functions each part of the two muscles is a functional entity with precise influence on the stabilization of the thumb. Khan[8] also found that in their direction of fibers and observed activity, the deep flexor is more flexor than adductor; similarly, the oblique adductor is more adductor than flexor.

Adductors are more active than flexors during combined adduction–lateral axial rotation of the thumb. Conversely, flexors are more active than adductors during combined abduction–flexion–medial axial rotation of the thumb.[8]

The introduction of moderate resistance to a series of positions of simple pinch between the thumb and first two fingers resulted in no appreciable increase of activity in all muscles except the superficial flexor muscles. This may be evidence, although inconclusive in this study, that the prime function of some of the intrinsic muscles of the thumb is to move and position it, not to provide it with strength.[8]

Flexors are quite active during opposition of the thumb to the little finger and medial side of the hand, but significant adductor activity in this situation does not occur unless pressure is exerted by the thumb.

A small decrease in the activity of each of the four muscles apparently occurs as the thumb exerts moderately firm pressure against a series of objects requiring gradually increasing abduction of the thumb. Future studies should deal with the role of the thumb and its muscles during grips of the hand.

Intrinsics versus extrinsics

In a complex study of the intrinsic and extrinsic muscles, my associates Johnson and Forrest[7] first compared the abductor pollicis brevis and the abductor pollicis longus. The abductor pollicis brevis is usually more active than the abductor pollicis longus; this was true in simple abduction of the thumb and in movements of the thumb having abduction

as one component, with or without a load applied. This includes postures of the thumb described as opposition and lateral pinch. In thumb extension, however, the abductor pollicis longus is more active than the abductor pollicis brevis when no load is applied; with a load, activities are equal.

In comparing the flexor pollicis brevis (superficial head) and longus, the flexor pollicis brevis is usually more active than the flexor pollicis longus in various postures of the hand requiring flexion–medial rotation of the thumb. In full flexion of the thumb (in which medial rotation is minimal) the flexor pollicis longus is more active than the flexor pollicis brevis. The two flexors flex the metacarpophalangeal joint of the thumb either independently or together, depending on the position of the interphalangeal joint or the load applied.

The position of the distal phalanx in movements of the thumb apparently determines to some extent the interrelationships of these two muscles with respect to their action on the metacarpophalangeal joint of the thumb.[6] As the interphalangeal joint is increasingly flexed, the flexor pollicis longus becomes the prime mover of the metacarpophalangeal joint. This is particularly evident when the thumb is flexed and when its tip is positioned near the bases of the two radial fingers. When the thumb is positioned near the distal ends of fingers, the short flexor appears to act as the prime mover of the proximal phalanx at the metacarpophalangeal joint.

Most daily activities involving the thumb require that it be positioned near the tips of the fingers. The relatively high levels of activity seen in the short flexor as the thumb assumes these positions (no load applied) indicate that its primary role may be to position the thumb with the assistance of other thenar muscles and the adductor pollicis. Throughout these movements, Johnson[6] found that the long flexor remains relatively quiet and is probably only minimally involved in these positioning activities.

The long flexor appears to provide much of the force necessary in overcoming moderate loads applied to the thumb while its tip is positioned near the tips of fingers. This is true regardless of the position of the distal phalanx. With a load applied to the thumb during movements such as opposition to the tips of fingers, activity in the long flexor increases sharply—more so than in the short flexor. This conclusion is further reinforced by a morphologic characteristic of this muscle. Some of its tendinous fibers insert onto the midportion (palmar surface) of the distal phalanx. As the distal phalanx is flexed, this factor apparently brings about an increase in the muscle's line of application of force to the center of rotation of the joint.[1,6]

Interplay of extrinsics of the thumb

During adductory movements of the thumb, the intrinsic muscles seem to require the assistance of the flexor pollicis longus and the extensor pollicis longus when a load is applied. In the process of balancing the other muscle's tendency to flex or extend the thumb, the resultant action, apparently, of the two muscles is to adduct the thumb.[6] The abductor longus is not only a primary mover in abduction of the carpometacarpal joint of the thumb, it also appears to bring about some flexion of the joint.

The extensor pollicis longus and brevis muscles are the prime movers in extension of the thumb. Perhaps their most valuable contribution to the function of the thumb lies in their ability to assist the abductor muscles in repositioning the thumb from positions of opposition or, by continued action, to spread the thumb out widely in order that the hand may grasp large objects. These muscles evidently act also to stabilize the interphalangeal and metacarpophalangeal joints of the thumb during some movements of opposition, perhaps enabling the thumb to perform fine, smooth, and precise movements.

NERVES AND ARTERIES
Ulnar nerve

The ulnar nerve (Fig. 3-1) enters the hand by passing vertically between the pisiform bone and the hook of the hamate in front of the flexor retinaculum and the pisohamate ligament. It is covered first by a slip of deep fascia and then by the palmaris brevis, which is a superficial sheet of muscle that passes from the retinaculum to the skin at the ulnar border of the hand. Between the pisiform and hamate bones the nerve divides into a deep branch and a superficial branch.

The superficial branch supplies the cutaneous branches to the medial one and one-half fingers and the motor branch to the palmaris brevis, and it usually communicates with the median nerve. The deep branch supplies the three muscles of the hypothenar eminence and then curves around the lower edge of the hook of the hamate into the depths of the palm, where it supplies all the short muscles of the hand, except the five usually supplied by the median nerve.

Median nerve

Crossing the midpoint of the skin crease of the wrist, the median nerve (Fig. 3-8) enters the palm through the carpal tunnel adhering to the deep surface of the flexor retinaculum. It appears in the palm deep to the prolongation of the palmaris longus called the palmar aponeurosis, so it is fairly superficially placed. At once it begins to break up into "recurrent" and digital branches. These are distributed to five muscles and to the skin of the lateral three and one-half digits, to the joints of these digits, and to the local vessels.

The five muscles supplied by the median nerve are the three thenar muscles (by the recurrent branch) and the two lateral lumbrical muscles (by the palmar digital branches).

The standard, or textbook, pattern of motor innervation to the hand just described is commonly departed from either by the ulnar nerve encroaching on median nerve territory or vice versa. Thus in 226 hands the ulnar nerve supplied the flexor pollicis brevis partially in 15% and completely in 32% of the hands; it supplied the abductor pollicis brevis in 3% and all three thenar muscles in 2% of the hands. Conversely, the median nerve supplied the adductor pollicis in 3% and the adductor pollicis plus first dorsal interosseus in 1% of the hands. Neither the musculocutaneous nerve nor the radial nerve has been proved to supply a thenar muscle.[10] Forest[2] confirmed the variability of thenar nerve supply, but electrical stimulation and electromyography re-

vealed that 85% of the flexor pollicis brevis muscles in 25 hands are supplied by both median and ulnar nerves. Morphologic studies by Harness and Sekeles[5] provide overwhelming confirmation.

The three common palmar digital nerves descend to the three interdigital clefts, protected by the tough palmar aponeurosis and crossed by the superficial palmar arch. The two digital branches to the thumb accompany the flexor pollicis longus tendon. The ulnar nerve commonly extends its influence to median nerve territory and vice versa through communicating branches to the palm. The palmar digital branches of the median and ulnar nerves lie on the sides of the fibrous digital sheaths.

Arteries

The blood supply from the ulnar and radial arteries is good, and the anastomoses are excellent through four transversely placed arterial arches. The superficial palmar arch lies deep to the palmar aponeurosis. The deep palmar, dorsal carpal, and palmar carpal arches lie on the skeletal plane.

Superficial palmar arch. The superficial palmar arch is the largest and most distal. It is the continuation of the ulnar artery completed by one or other of the palmar or digital branches of the radial artery. (The deep branch of the ulnar artery accompanies the deep branch of the ulnar nerve and completes the deep arch.) The superficial palmar arch supplies the medial three and one-half digits, leaving the lateral one and one-half digits to the care of the deep palmar arch. Palmar digital arteries and nerves run on the sides of the flexor tendons in their fibrous sheaths, the nerve being anteromedial to the artery.

Radial artery. After giving off the palmar radial carpal and superficial palmar arteries, the radial artery turns around the lateral border of the wrist and descends vertically through the anatomic snuffbox to reach the proximal end of the first intermetacarpal space, where it passes between the two heads of the first dorsal interosseus muscle and enters the palm to become the deep palmar arch (Fig. 3-6).

The radial artery crosses the radial collateral ligament of the wrist, the scaphoid, and the trapezium; in turn, it is crossed by the three tendons that bound the snuffbox, branches of the radial nerve to the thumb, and the dorsal venous arch. While in the snuffbox, the radial artery gives off the dorsal radial carpal artery and sends small branches, dorsal digital arteries, to the sides of the lateral one and one-half digits.

Deep palmar arch. The radial artery, continued into the palm, is completed by the deep branch of the ulnar artery. Palmar digital branches run to the lateral one and one-half digits. There are also three palmar metacarpal arteries, three perforating arteries, and several recurrent branches.

Palmar carpal arch. The palmar carpal arch is more accurately a rete or network formed by the union of the palmar carpal branch of the ulnar artery and the palmar branch of the radial artery. It receives twigs of the anterior interosseous artery and recurrent branches of the deep palmar arch.

The *dorsal carpal arch* is applied to the dorsal surface of the carpal bones, and its branches have many anastomoses.

ACKNOWLEDGMENT

Illustrations for this chapter were drawn by the well-known medical artist Frank Netter, M.D., and were supplied through the courtesy of the CIBA Pharmaceutical Co. The numbers used in the figures are as they appeared in the *CIBA Symposium on Surgical Anatomy of the Hand,* published originally in December 1951.

REFERENCES

1. Basmajian, J.V.: Muscles alive: their functions revealed by electromyography, ed., 4, Baltimore, 1979, The Williams & Wilkins Co.
2. Forrest, W.J.: Motor innervation of human thenar and hypothenar muscles in 25 hands: a study combining electromyography and percutaneous nerve stimulation, Can. J. Surg. 10:196-199, 1967.
3. Forrest, W.J., and Basmajian, J.V.: Function of human thenar and hypothenar muscles: an electromyographic study of 25 hands, J. Bone Joint Surg. 47A:1585-1594, 1965.
4. Forrest, W.J., and Khan, M.A.: Electromyography of the flexor pollicis brevis and adductor pollicis in twenty hands: a preliminary report, Electromyogr. Clin. Neurophysiol. 8(Suppl. 1):49-53, 1968.
5. Harness, D., and Sekeles, E.: The double anastomotic innervation of thenar muscles, J. Anat. 109:461-466, 1971.
6. Johnson, D.R.: An electromyographic study of extrinsic and intrinsic muscles of the thumb, M.Sc. Thesis, Queen's University, Canada, 1970.
7. Johnson, D.R., and Forrest, W.J.: An electromyographic study of the abductors and flexors of the thumb in man (abstract), Anat. Rec. 166:325, 1970.
8. Khan, M.A.: Morphology and electromyography of the flexor pollicis brevis and adductor pollicis muscles, M.Sc. Thesis, Queens' University, Canada, 1969.
9. Landsmeer, J.M.F.: Atlas of anatomy of the hand, Edinburgh, 1976, Churchill Livingstone.
10. Rowntree, T.: Anomalous innervation of the hand muscles, J. Bone Joint Surg. 31B:505-510, 1949.

II

EVALUATION

4

Clinical examination of the hand

PAT L. AULICINO and THEODORE E. DuPUY

Clinical examination of the hand is a basic skill that should be mastered by both the surgeon and the therapist. To master this skill, it is necessary to have an understanding of the functional anatomy of the hand. A thorough history, a systematic examination, and knowledge of disease processes that affect the hand will leave the examiner with few diagnostic dilemmas. Radiographs, electrodiagnostics, and specialized laboratory tests are ancillary tools that only confirm a diagnosis that has been made on a clinical basis.

An organized approach and clear, concise records are of paramount importance. Either line drawings of the deformities or clinical photographs should be prepared for each new patient evaluated. Range of motion of the affected parts should be recorded and dated in a table format. If there is a discrepancy between active and passive motion, this should also be noted. A good hand examination is useless if the results are not recorded accurately.

This chapter will outline one approach to examination of the hand. The most important points have already been made: perform a systematic, organized clinical examination, and record the results accurately and clearly.

HISTORY

Prior to examination of a patient's hand, an accurate history must be taken. The patient's age, hand dominance, occupation, and avocations are elicited. If the patient has had an injury, the exact mechanism as well as the time and date of the injury and prior treatment are recorded. Prior surgical procedures, infections, medications, and prior therapy are also noted. Once this background data is obtained, the patient is questioned specifically regarding his involved extremity. Does he have pain? What is the character of the pain? When does it occur? Is it work related, or constant? Does it occur at night or during the day? What relieves the pain, and what exacerbates it? What is the patient not able to do now that he could do prior to his injury? What does the patient desire from you? This last question is extremely important. The patient's reply will assist you in determining whether the patient has a realistic understanding of the true nature of his injury. Unrealistic expectations can never be fulfilled. They result in both an unhappy patient and an unhappy surgeon. During this interview it is also important to assess the impact that the injury or disease process has upon the patient's family, economic, and social life. Patients who have litigation pending or significant secondary gain are usually poorly motivated and are not optimum candidates for elective hand surgery. Successful hand surgery requires precise surgical techniques followed by expert hand therapy in conjunction with a well-motivated, compliant patient.

The patient's pertinent past medical history is now obtained. Does he have rheumatoid arthritis or some other progressive collagen-vascular disease? Is the patient taking systemic steroids or some other medication? Does the patient have any other chronic systemic illness that would make him a poor surgical risk? The history is completed only after the surgeon or therapist has a complete understanding of the patient's problem and how this affects the patient physically, psychologically, and economically.

PHYSICAL EXAMINATION
General inspection

When examining a patient's upper extremity, one must be able to observe the shoulder, arm, forearm, and hand. Therefore, the patient should be disrobed. The gross appearance of the entire extremity is noted. Are the shoulder muscles atrophied? Does the patient have a normal-appearing upper extremity or is there a traumatic or congenital anomaly? Are there any scars? How does the patient carry this limb? Can he move his shoulder and arm without pain? Is the patient able to place his hand? If the hand cannot be placed in a functional position, a brilliantly reconstructed hand is useless.

After the general appearance of the limb has been noted, the attention is directed to the integument. The color, tone, and moisture of the skin are noted. Are the normal skin creases present (Fig. 4-1)? Is there any edema of the hand? Are the nails ridged, pitted, or deformed? Is there correct rotational alignment of the nail plates (Fig. 4-2)? Are there any obvious deformities of the hand? Do the thenar or hypothenar muscles appear atrophied? Are there any contractures? When the patient's injured extremity is being inspected, the uninjured extremity should also be inspected for comparison. The attitude of the hand is then noted. Normally with the hand resting and the wrist in neutral, the fingers are progressively more flexed from the radial to the ulnar side of the hand. A loss of the normal attitude of the hand can indicate a tendon laceration, a contracture, or possibly a peripheral nerve injury (see Fig. 4-3).

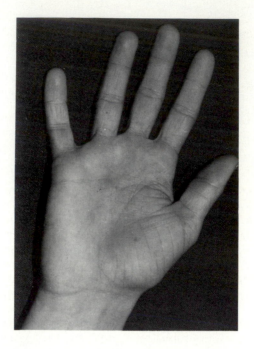

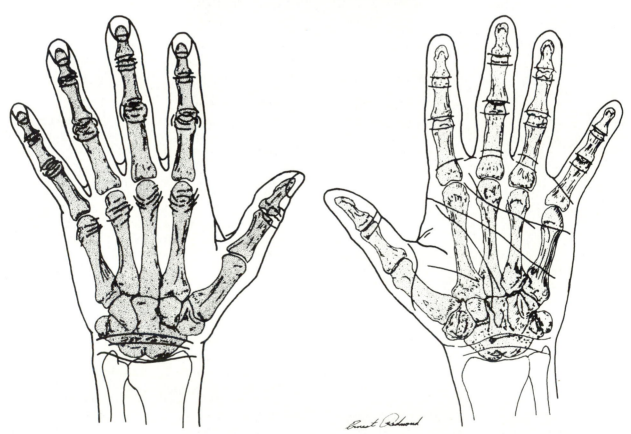

FIG. 4-1. Clinical photograph and diagramatic illustrations of the relationship of the volar and dorsal skin creases to the underlying joints. The absence of a volar skin crease may indicate the presence of an underlying joint anomaly and thus the inability of the patient to flex that digit, as is seen in congenital symphalangism. The absence of both volar and dorsal skin creases is seen in conditions that cause edema, or as a result of the atrophic phase of a reflex sympathetic dystrophy. (Redrawn from Chase, R.A.: Atlas of hand surgery, Philadelphia, 1973, W.B. Saunders Co.)

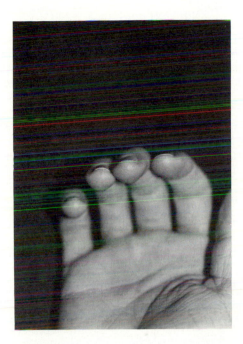

FIG. 4-2. Normal rotational alignment of nail plates.

Part of the general inspection is noting how the patient treats his injured limb. Does he cradle his injured hand and stare at it as if it did not belong to him, or does he appear relatively unhampered by his injury? All observations are, of course, assiduously recorded.

Range of motion

The motion of the entire extremity should be measured and compared to the opposite side. As previously stated, discrepancies between active and passive motion should be noted. Fixed deformities are also noted.

The shoulder should be tested for forward flexion, extension, abduction, and internal and external rotation. Elbow extension and flexion and forearm supination and pronation are also checked and recorded. Wrist dorsiflexion, volar flexion, and ulnar and radial deviation are recorded. Thumb extension, flexion, opposition, adduction, carpometacarpal extension, and carpometacarpal abduction are measured and recorded. A finger goniometer should be used to make each of these measurements.[35] If motion is lacking, the distance from the tip of the finger to the distal palmar crease is measured. If the finger touches the palm but does not reach the crease, as in a profundus tendon disruption, this should be noted and the distance from the tip of the finger to the distal palmar crease should be recorded; how-

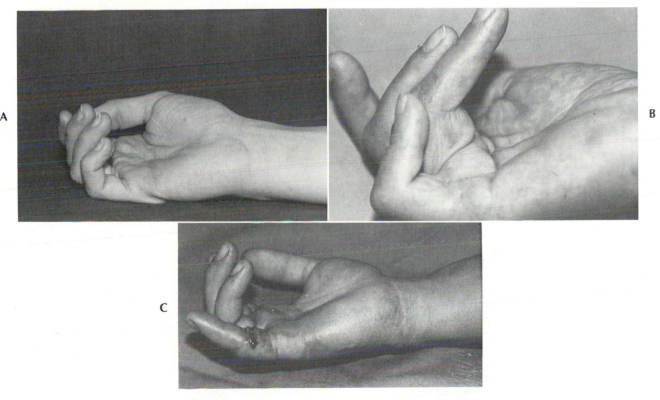

FIG. 4-3. A, Normal attitude of the hand in a resting position. Notice that the fingers are progressively more flexed from the radial aspect to the ulnar aspect of the hand. In **B** this normal attitude is lost because of flexion contractures of the digits as a result of Dupuytren's disease. **C,** Loss of the normal attitude as a result of a laceration of the flexor tendons to the fifth digit.

ever, it should be stated that the finger did touch the palm, but did not reach the distal palmar crease (see Fig. 4-4).

Once all active and passive motions have been examined, the wrist is flexed and extended to see if the normal tenodesis effect is present. In an uninjured hand, when the wrist is flexed the fingers and the thumb will extend, and as the wrist is extended the fingers will assume an attitude of flexion and the thumb will oppose the fifth digit (see Fig. 4-5). The alignment of the digits is then inspected. As stated before, the nail plates should all be parallel to one another and their alignment should be similar to that of the other hand. Each finger should point individually to the tuberosity of the scaphoid, and the longitudinal axis of all fingers when flexed should point in the direction of the scaphoid (see Fig. 4-6).

Muscle testing

The hand is powered by intrinsic and extrinsic muscles. The extrinsic muscles have their origin in the forearm and the tendinous insertions in the hand. The extrinsic flexors are located on the volar side of the forearm and flex the digits and the wrist. The extrinsic extensors originate on the dorsal aspect of the forearm and extend the fingers, thumb, and wrist. The intrinsic muscles originate and insert in the hand. These include the thenar and hypothenar muscles as well as the lumbricals and the interossei. The thenar and hypothenar muscles help to position the thumb and the fifth finger and also aid in opposition of the thumb and in pinch. The interossei assist in abduction and adduction of the digits. The lumbricals flex the metacarpophalangeal joints and extend the interphalangeal joints. The interossei also have the

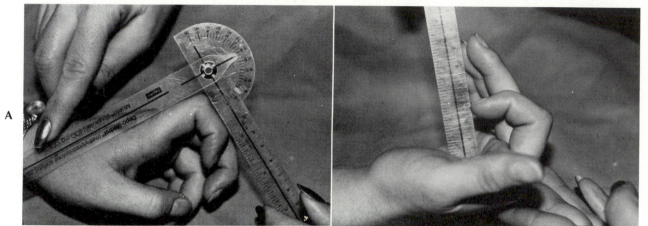

FIG. 4-4. A, A finger goniometer is utilized to measure the range of motion of the proximal interphalangeal joint of the index finger. **B,** A ruler is then used to measure the distance of the pulp of the finger from the distal palmar crease. Active as well as passive motions should be noted and recorded.

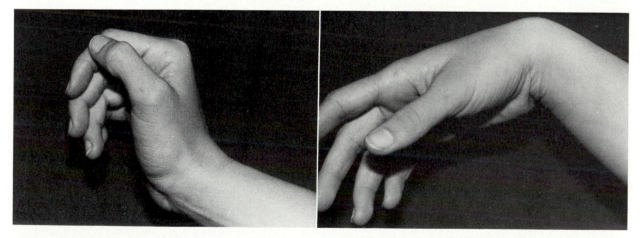

FIG. 4-5. Tenodesis of the hand. In an uninjured hand, on wrist dorsiflexion the fingers and thumb will flex and on flexion of the wrist the thumb and fingers will extend. In the presence of a tendon laceration, contractures of the joints, or adhesions of the flexor or extensor systems, the normal tenodesis effect will be lost. This test can be performed actively by the patient or passively by the examiner.

function of flexing the metacarpophalangeal joints and, by and large, are much stronger than the lumbricals. The function and testing of the intrinsic muscles will be discussed later in this chapter.

Extrinsic muscle testing—the extrinsic flexors. As each specific extrinsic muscle-tendon unit is tested, its strength should be graded and recorded. Strength should be graded from 0 to 5, with 5 being normal. In grade 0, there is no evidence of contractility. In grade 1 (trace), there is slight evidence of contractility and no joint motion. In grade 2 (poor), there is complete range of motion with gravity eliminated. In grade 3 (fair), there is complete range of motion against gravity. In grade 4 (good), there is complete range of motion against gravity with some resistance. In grade 5 (normal), there is complete range of motion against gravity with full resistance.

The flexor pollicis longus (long flexor of the thumb) flexes the interphalangeal joint of the thumb. This muscle is tested by asking the patient to actively flex the last joint of his thumb (Fig. 4-7).

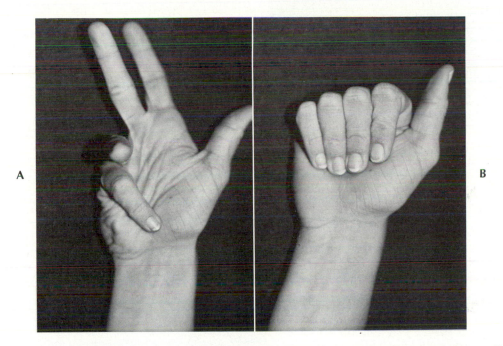

FIG. 4-6. A, On flexion the tip of the fifth finger will point directly to the tuberosity of the scaphoid, as will all the fingers when individually flexed. **B,** When all the digits are flexed simultaneously, the longitudinal axes of all fingers converge at an area proximal to the tuberosity of the scaphoid, because of crowding of the adjacent digits. If there is a malunited fracture, the rotational alignment will be off and often there will be crossover of the digits.

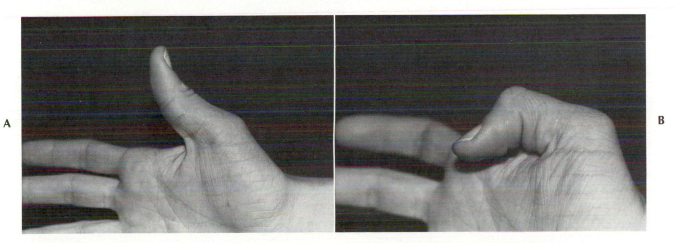

FIG. 4-7. Testing the flexor pollicis longus. With the thumb in a position of full extension at the interphalangeal joint **(A),** the patient is asked to actively flex this joint **(B).** The range of motion and grade of strength are recorded. It is also important to note whether the motion is obtained with or without blocking of the preceding joint by the examiner. This applies not only to testing the flexor pollicis longus, but to testing all other flexor systems, since more power and motion can be obtained when blocking is utilized.

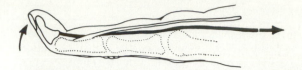

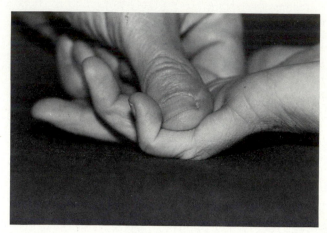

FIG. 4-8. Profundus test. The flexor digitorum profundus tendon flexes the distal interphalangeal joint. With the metacarpophalangeal joint and the proximal interphalangeal joint held in extension by the examiner, the patient is asked to flex the distal interphalangeal joint. (Redrawn from Hoppenfeld, S.: Physical examination of the spine and extremities, New York, 1976, Appleton-Century-Crofts.)

FIG. 4-9. Superficialis test. The flexor digitorum superficialis tendon flexes the proximal interphalangeal joint. The examiner must hold the adjacent fingers in full extension while asking the patient to flex the finger being tested. If the flexor system is functioning normally, the proximal interphalangeal joint will flex, while the distal interphalangeal joint remains in extension. (Redrawn by permission from Hoppenfeld, S.: Physical examination of the spine and extremities, New York, 1976, Appleton-Century-Crofts.)

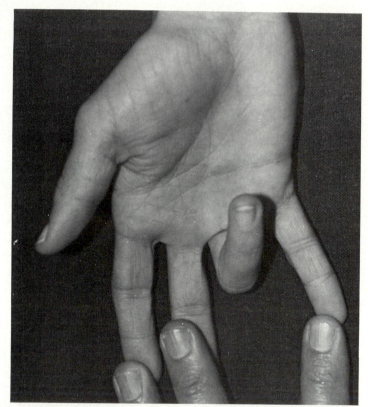

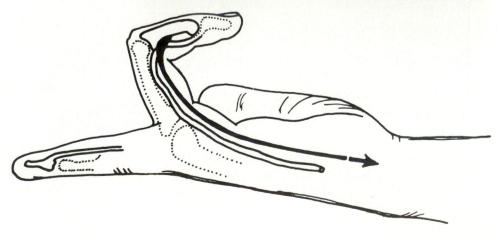

The flexor digitorum profundus of each finger is then tested, in sequence, by having the patient flex the distal interphalangeal joint of the finger being tested while the examiner holds the digit in full extension and blocks motion at the proximal interphalangeal joint and the metacarpophalangeal joint. During the testing of each profundus tendon, the other fingers are maintained in a slightly flexed position (see Fig. 4-8).

The flexor digitorum superficialis of each finger is then tested. The examiner must hold the adjacent fingers in full extension. The proximal interphalangeal joint of the finger being tested is not blocked (see Fig. 4-9). If the flexor system is functioning properly, the proximal interphalangeal joint will flex, and the distal interphalangeal joint will remain in extension. The fifth finger often has a deficient superficialis.[3] That is, it is not strong enough to flex the interphalangeal joint: on testing, the metacarpophalangeal joint will flex and the distal interphalangeal joint and the proximal interphalangeal joint will remain in extension.

The flexors of the wrist can be tested by having the patient flex the wrist against resistance in a radial and then in an ulnar direction, while the examiner palpates each tendon. The flexor carpi radialis is palpated on the radial side of the wrist, and the flexor carpi ulnaris is palpated on the ulnar side of the wrist. The palmaris longus tendon can be palpated just ulnar to the flexor carpi radialis tendon.

Extrinsic muscle testing—the extensors. As was previously stated, the extensors of the digits and the wrist originate on the dorsal aspect of the forearm and pass through six discrete retinacular compartments at the dorsum of the wrist prior to their insertions in the hand.

In the first dorsal compartment the abductor pollicis longus and the extensor pollicis brevis tendons pass. The abductor pollicis longus usually has multiple tendon slips and inserts on the base of the first metacarpal and often has insertions on the trapezium. The extensor pollicis brevis and abductor pollicis longus function in unison and are responsible for abduction of the first metacarpal and extension into the plane of the metacarpals. These muscle-tendon units are tested by asking the patient to bring the thumb ''out to the side and the back.'' Pain in the area of the first dorsal compartment and radial styloid is common and often a result of stenosing tenovaginitis of these tendons. This was first described by de Quervain in 1895 and now is a well-established clinical entity, which bears his name. Finkelstein, in 1930, stated that acute flexion of the thumb and deviation of the wrist in an ulnar direction would produce excruciating pain at the first dorsal compartment, near the radial styloid, in patients who had stenosing tenovaginitis. This examination is now universally known as Finkelstein's test (Fig. 4-10).[13]

The extensor carpi radialis longus and brevis run in the second dorsal compartment. The longus inserts on the base of the second metacarpal and the brevis on the third. These are tested by asking the patient to make a tight fist and to strongly dorsiflex the wrist. The two tendons are then palpated by the examiner (Fig. 4-11).

The extensor pollicis longus runs in the third compartment. This tendon extends the interphalangeal joint of the thumb as well as adducts the first ray. The tendon passes sharply around Lister's tubercle, and may rupture spontaneously after a Colles fracture or in rheumatoid arthritis.[37] Its function is tested by placing the patient's hand flat on the examining table and having him lift only the thumb off the table. The extensor pollicis longus can be visualized and palpated (Fig. 4-12).

The area of the wrist just distal to the radial styloid and bounded by the extensor pollicis longus ulnarly and the abductor pollicis longus and extensor pollicis brevis radially is known as the anatomic snuffbox. In this area runs the deep branch of the radial artery. The carpal scaphoid can be palpated in the base of the snuffbox. Tenderness in this area is suggestive of an acute scaphoid fracture or a painful scaphoid nonunion.

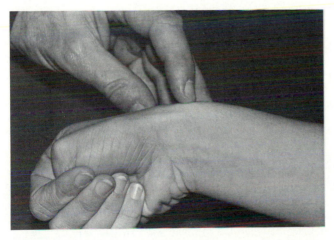

FIG. 4-10. Finkelstein's test for de Quervain's stenosing tenovaginitis of the first dorsal compartment. Acute flexion of the thumb and deviation of the wrist in an ulnar direction will produce excruciating pain at the first dorsal compartment, near the radial styloid, in patients who have this pathologic entity.

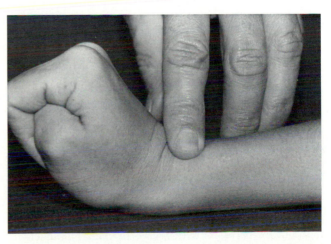

FIG. 4-11. On dorsiflexion of the wrist, the examiner can palpate the extensor carpi radialis longus, inserting on the base of the second metacarpal, and the extensor carpi radialis brevis, inserting on the base of the third metacarpal.

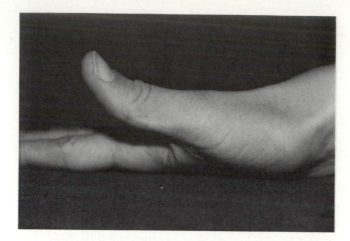

FIG. 4-12. The extensor pollicis longus tendon is tested by placing the patient's hand flat on the examining table and asking him to lift the thumb off the table. The extensor pollicis longus can then be visualized and palpated.

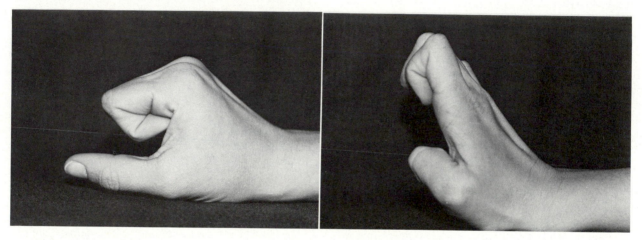

FIG. 4-13. The extensor digitorum communis tendons are tested by having the patient extend the metacarpophalangeal joints, with the proximal interphalangeal joints flexed.

The fourth dorsal compartment contains the extensor indicis proprius and the extensor digitorum communis. These tendons are responsible for extension of the metacarpophalangeal joints of the fingers. The extensor indicis proprius allows independent extension of the index metacarpophalangeal joint. The extensor indicis proprius is tested by having the patient extend the index finger while the other fingers are flexed into a fist. The mass action of the extensor digitorum communis tendons is tested by having the patient extend the metacarpophalangeal joints (Fig. 4-13). This test is performed with the interphalangeal joints flexed, since the proximal interphalangeal joints are extended by the intrinsic muscles and not the long extensors of the hand. This may be a source of confusion to an uninitiated examiner, especially in a patient who has a high radial nerve palsy yet is still able to extend his interphalangeal joints.

The fifth dorsal compartment contains the extensor digiti quinti, which is responsible for independent extension of the metacarpophalangeal joint of the little finger. It is tested by having the patient extend the fifth finger while the others

are flexed. Since the extensor digiti quinti and the extensor indicis proprius work independently of the communis tendons, most examiners test them simultaneously by having the patient extend the index and fifth fingers while the middle and ring fingers are flexed (Fig. 4-14).

The sixth dorsal compartment contains the extensor carpi ulnaris, which inserts into the base of the fifth metacarpal and helps dorsiflex the wrist in an ulnar direction. This is tested by having the patient pull the hand dorsally and in an ulnar direction while the examiner palpates the tendon (Fig. 4-15).

Intrinsic muscle testing. The intrinsic musculature of the hand consists of the thenar and hypothenar muscles, as well as the lumbricals and the interossei. All of these muscles originate and insert within the hand. There is a delicate balance between the intrinsic and extrinsic muscles, which is necessary for normal functioning of the hand.

The thenar muscles consist of the abductor pollicis brevis, the flexor pollicis brevis, the opponens pollicis, and the adductor pollicis. These muscles position the thumb and help perform the complex motions of opposition and ad-

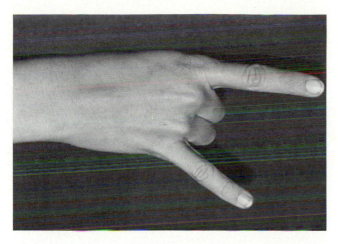

FIG. 4-14. The extensor digiti quinti and the extensor indicis proprius work independently of the communis tendons; they are tested by asking the patient to extend the index and fifth fingers while the middle and ring fingers are flexed.

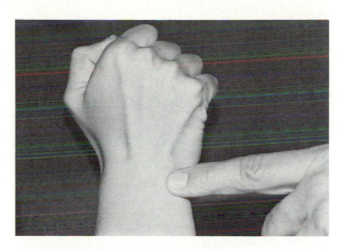

FIG. 4-15. The extensor carpi ulnaris can be visualized and palpated as it inserts on the base of the fifth metacarpal, while the patient dorsiflexes the wrist in an ulnar direction.

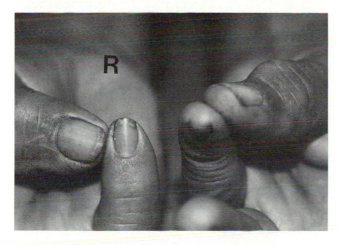

FIG. 4-16. Hands of a patient with a low median nerve palsy on the right, resulting from a long-standing carpal tunnel syndrome. Notice that in attempted opposition, the nail plate is perpendicular to the plane of the metacarpals on the affected side, while the nail plate is parallel to the plane of the metacarpals on the normal side. Tip-to-tip pinch is impossible on the side with the loss of opposition.

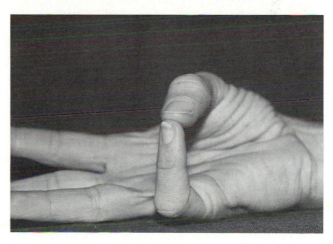

FIG. 4-17. Opposition of tip of thumb to tip of fifth digit. Notice tip-to-tip pinch and the relationship of the nail plate of the thumb to the plane of the metacarpals.

duction of the thumb.[27] Opposition, according to Bunnell, takes place in the intercarpal, carpometacarpal, and metacarpophalangeal joints.[7] All three of these joints contribute to the angulatory and rotatory motions that produce true opposition. If one observes the thumb during opposition, it first abducts from the hand, and then it follows a semicircular path. The thumb pronates and the proximal phalanx angulates radially on the first metacarpal. If the nail plate is observed, one can see that prior to beginning opposition, the thumbnail is perpendicular to the plane of the metacarpals. At the end of opposition, the thumbnail is parallel to the plane of the metacarpals. During adduction, the thumb sweeps across the palm without following the semicircular path. The nail plate remains at all times perpendicular to the plane of the metacarpals. Since opposition is median nerve innervated and adduction is usually ulnar nerve innervated, one can easily see the difference between these two motions by comparing the hands of a patient with a long-standing low median nerve palsy on one side (Fig. 4-16).

Opposition is tested by having the patient touch the tip of the thumb to the tip of the little finger (Fig. 4-17). At the end of opposition, the thumbnail should be parallel to the nail of the little finger as well as parallel to the plane of the metacarpals.

The abductor pollicis brevis, which is the most radial and

superficial of the thenar muscles, is usually the first to atrophy with a low median nerve palsy, such as that resulting from a long-standing carpal tunnel syndrome. This muscle can be tested by having the patient abduct the thumb while the examiner palpates the muscle.

Thumb adduction is performed by the adductor pollicis, which is an ulnar nerve–innervated muscle. This muscle, in combination with the first dorsal interosseus, is necessary for strong pinch. The adductor stabilizes the thumb during pinch and also helps extend the interphalangeal joint of the thumb through its attachment into the dorsal apparatus. Thumb adduction can be tested by having the patient forcibly hold a piece of paper between his thumb and the radial side of the proximal phalanx of the index finger. When adduction is weak or nonfunctional, the interphalangeal joint of the thumb flexes during this maneuver; this is known as Froment's sign (1915).[25] Froment's sign is an indication of weak or absent adductor function. Jeanne's sign (1915) is hyperextension of the metacarpophalangeal joint of the thumb during pinching grip.[25] (See Fig. 4-18.)

The hypothenar muscles consist of the abductor digiti minimi, the flexor digiti minimi, and the opponens digiti minimi. The abductor and flexor aid in abduction of the fifth digit and in metacarpophalangeal joint flexion of that digit. The deeper opponens digiti minimi aids in adduction and in rotating the fifth metacarpal during opposition of the thumb to the fifth finger. This helps cup the hand during grip and opposition. The hypothenar muscles are tested as one unit by having the patient abduct the little finger while the examiner palpates the muscle mass (Fig. 4-19).

The anatomy of the interossei is very complex, with much variation in their origins and insertions. There are seven interossei, four dorsal and three palmar. These muscles arise from the metacarpal shafts, but have variable insertions. The palmar interossei almost always insert into the dorsal apparatus of the finger. The first dorsal interosseus almost always inserts into bone. The remaining dorsal interossei have varying insertions. (Refer to the work of Eyler and Markee for a more detailed description of the anatomy.[12])

The interossei are usually ulnar nerve–innervated, with a few exceptions.

There are four lumbricals, which originate on the radial side of the profundus tendons and usually insert on the dorsal apparatus. Occasionally a few fibers insert into the base of the proximal phalanges. Since these muscles are a link between the extrinsic flexor and extrinsic extensor mechanisms, they act as a modulator between flexion and extension of the interphalangeal joints.[28]

The interossei are much stronger than the lumbricals; however, both muscle groups work in conjunction. All of these muscle groups are of fundamental importance in extension of the interphalangeal joints and flexion of the metacarpophalangeal joints. The interossei also abduct and adduct the fingers. It is believed that the dorsal interossei are the primary abductors and the volar interossei the primary adductors of the fingers.

The preceding statements are an oversimplification of the anatomy and functional significance of the interossei and the lumbricals. The clinical examination of these two groups of muscles is, however, rather easy.

To test interossei function, one can ask the patient to spread his fingers apart. This is best done with the hand flat on the examining table to eliminate the action of the long extensors, which can simulate the function of the dorsal interossei (see Fig. 4-20). To supplement this test, one can have the patient radially and ulnarly deviate the middle finger while it is flexed. This cannot be performed if the interossei are paralyzed; this test is known as Egawa's sign (1959).[25]

The first dorsal interosseus is a very strong radial abductor of the index finger and plays an important role in stabilizing that digit during pinch. It can be tested separately by having

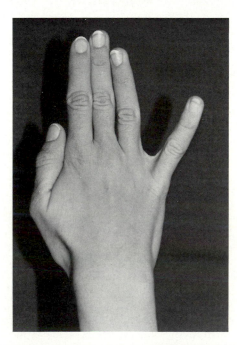

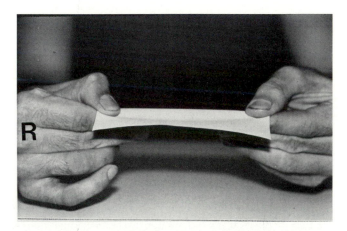

FIG. 4-18. Patient with low ulnar nerve palsy on the right. Weakness of pinch is demonstrated by Froment's and Jeanne's signs on the affected side.

FIG. 4-19. Testing function of the hypothenar muscles by having patient abduct fifth digit.

the patient strongly abduct the index finger in a radial direction while the examiner palpates the muscle belly (Fig. 4-21). The interphalangeal extension function of the lumbricals and interossei is tested by having the patient extend the proximal interphalangeal joints of the digits while the metacarpophalangeal joints are held in flexion by the examiner (Fig. 4-22).

If all the interossei and lumbricals are functioning properly, the patient will be able to put his hand into the "in-trinsic-plus position"; that is, the metacarpophalangeal joints are flexed and the proximal interphalangeal joints are in full extension. J.I.P. James has recommended this as the position of immobilization for the injured hand.[17]

Injuries to the median or ulnar nerves, or both, or a crushing injury to the hand can result in paralysis or contractures of the intrinsic muscles. A hand without intrinsic function is known as the "intrinsic-minus hand."[8,14] This hand will have lost the normal cupping of the hand. The

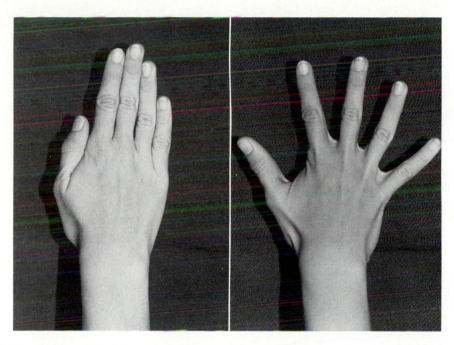

FIG. 4-20. Testing function of the interossei. With the hand flat on a table, the patient is asked to spread his fingers apart. Abduction and adduction are assessed from the relationship of the digits to the axis of the third metacarpal.

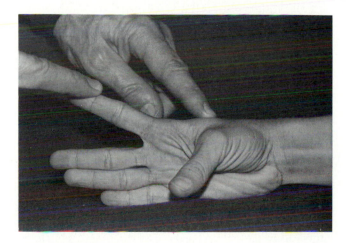

FIG. 4-21. On abduction of the patient's index finger, the examiner can palpate the first dorsal interosseus. This is the last muscle to receive innervation from the ulnar nerve.

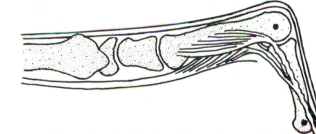

FIG. 4-22. The intrinsic muscles, by means of their attachment into the lateral bands and proximal phalanges, produce flexion of the metacarpophalangeal joints and extension of the proximal interphalangeal joints. The function of the lumbricals and interossei is tested by having the patient extend the proximal interphalangeal joints of the digits while the metacarpophalangeal joints are held in flexion by the examiner. (Redrawn from Tubiana, R.: The hand, Philadelphia, 1973, W.B. Saunders Co.)

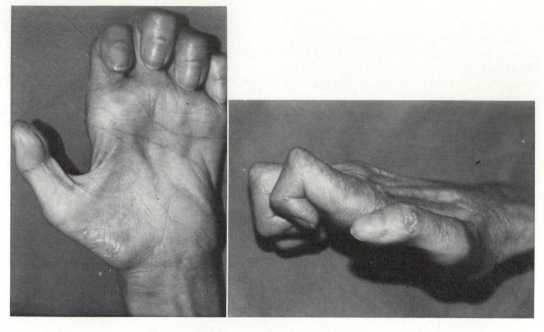

FIG. 4-23. Intrinsic-minus hand resulting from a long-standing low median and ulnar palsy. Notice loss of normal arches of the hand and wasting of all intrinsic musculature.

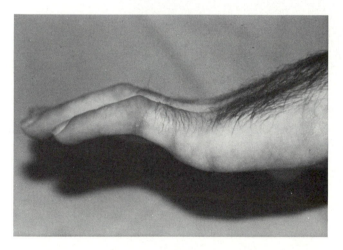

FIG. 4-24. Ulnar claw hand resulting from ulnar nerve laceration at the wrist. Notice hyperextension of the metacarpophalangeal joints and flexion of the proximal and distal interphalangeal joints because of an imbalance of the extrinsic flexor and extensor systems as a result of paralysis of the ulnar innervated intrinsic muscles.

arches of the hand will disappear, and there will be wasting of all intrinsic musculature (Fig. 4-23). There will be clawing of the fingers, as described by Duchenne in 1867.[25] The claw deformity is defined as hyperextension of the metacarpophalangeal joints and flexion of the proximal and distal interphalangeal joints (Fig. 4-24). This is the result of an

imbalance between the intrinsic and extrinsic muscles of the hand.[47] The extrinsic extensors hyperextend the metacarpophalangeal joints, and the extrinsic flexors flex the proximal and distal interphalangeal joints. The flexion vector, induced by the intrinsics, across the metacarpophalangeal joint is lost.[29] In time, the volar capsular-ligamentous structures will stretch out and the claw deformity will increase in severity.[32]

Injury to the intrinsics, which can be due to ischemia, crushing injuries, or other pathologic states (such as rheumatoid arthritis), can result in tightness of the intrinsic muscles. A test for intrinsic tightness was first described by Finochetto in 1920.[53] Later, Bunnell and then Littler redescribed this test.[9] The intrinsic tightness test is performed by having the examiner hold the patient's metacarpophalangeal joint in extension (stretching the intrinsics) and then passively flexing the proximal interphalangeal joint. Then the metacarpophalangeal joint is held in flexion (relaxing the intrinsics), and the examiner passively flexes the proximal interphalangeal joint again. If the proximal interphalangeal joint can be passively flexed more when the metacarpophalangeal joint is in flexion than when it is in extension, there is tightness of the intrinsic muscles.[9,44,53] (See Fig. 4-25.) In patients with rheumatoid arthritis, intrinsic tightness is common and may result in a swan-neck deformity.[34] The swan neck is a result of the strong pull of the contracted intrinsics on the lateral bands, which subsequently sublux dorsal to the axis of rotation of the proximal interphalangeal joint. The resultant deformity is one of hyperextension at the proximal interphalangeal joint and flexion at the distal

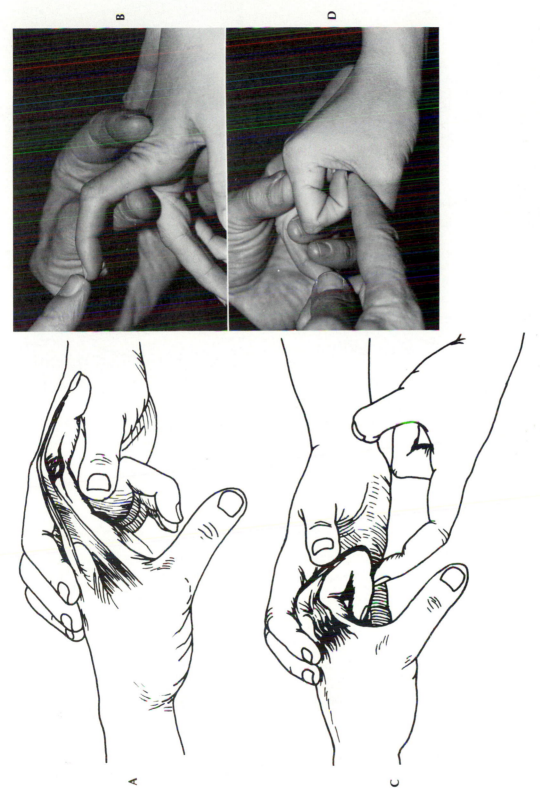

Fig. 4-25. Intrinsic tightness test. In A and B, the intrinsics are put on stretch by the examiner, who then passively flexes the proximal interphalangeal joint. The intrinsics are then relaxed by flexing the metacarpophalangeal joint (C and D). If the proximal interphalangeal joint can be passively flexed more with the metacarpophalangeal joint in flexion than when it is in extension, there is tightness of the intrinsic muscles. (Redrawn from Hoppenfeld, S.: Physical examination of the spine and extremities, New York, 1976, Appleton-Century-Crofts.)

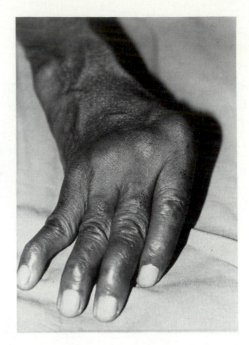

FIG. 4-26. Swan-neck deformity in a patient with rheumatoid arthritis. The swan-neck deformity is due to intrinsic tightness, which causes the lateral bands to sublux dorsal to the axis of rotation of the proximal interphalangeal joint.

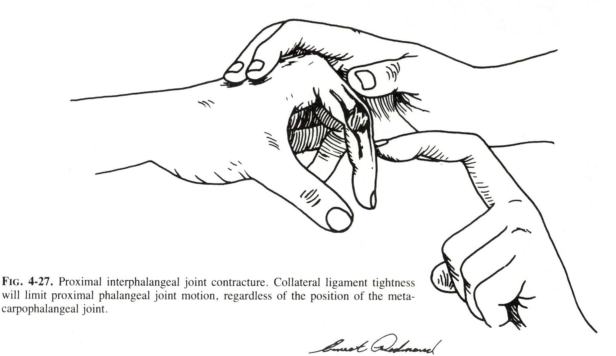

FIG. 4-27. Proximal interphalangeal joint contracture. Collateral ligament tightness will limit proximal phalangeal joint motion, regardless of the position of the metacarpophalangeal joint.

interphalangeal joint (Fig. 4-26). The boutonnière deformity may also occur in patients with rheumatoid arthritis.[33,52]

Occasionally there is confusion as to the cause of limited proximal interphalangeal joint motion. Is the condition due to intrinsic tightness, to extrinsic tightness (for example, scarring of the long extensors proximal to the proximal interphalangeal joint), or to the joint itself (that is, collateral ligament tightness)? Three simple tests will clarify the situation. The intrinsic tightness tests will help one either rule out or identify intrinsic muscle problems. The extrinsic

tightness test is just the opposite of the intrinsic test. Again the examiner holds the metacarpophalangeal joint in extension and passively flexes the proximal interphalangeal joint and notes the amount of flexion. He or she then flexes the metacarpal phalangeal joint and passively flexes the proximal interphalangeal joint again. If there is extrinsic tightness (because, for example, the long extensors are scarred), there will be more passive flexion of the proximal interphalangeal joint when the metacarpophalangeal joint is held in extension than when it is held in flexion. Holding the metacarpophalangeal joint in extension functionally lengthens the extrinsic extensor, while holding it in flexion relatively shortens it. If the motion of the proximal interphalangeal joint is unchanged regardless of the position of the metacarpophalangeal joint, then there is a joint contracture (Fig. 4-27).

OBLIQUE RETINACULAR LIGAMENT TEST

Occasionally a patient will exhibit a lack of flexion at the distal interphalangeal joint. This loss of flexion may be due to a joint contracture or to a contracture of the oblique retinacular ligament.[21] The oblique retinacular ligament arises from the volar lateral ridge of the proximal phalanx and has a common origin with the distal A2 and C1 pulleys. It

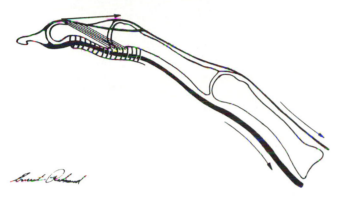

FIG. 4-28. Oblique retinacular ligament. (Redrawn from Tubiana, R.: The hand, Philadelphia, 1981, W.B. Saunders Co.)

then traverses distally and dorsally to attach to the dorsal apparatus near the distal interphalangeal joint (see Fig. 4-28). As pointed out by Schrewsbury and Johnson, the tendon varies in its development and occurrence.[43] It is, however, consistently made taut by flexion of the distal interphalangeal joint. If this ligament is contracted, passive distal interphalangeal motion will be limited. The oblique retinacular ligament tightness test is performed by passively flexing the distal interphalangeal joint with the proximal interphalangeal joint in extension, and then repeating this with the proximal interphalangeal joint in flexion. If there is greater motion when the proximal interphalangeal joint is flexed than when it is extended, there is a contracture of the ligament (see Fig. 4-29). Equal loss of flexion indicates a joint contracture.

GRIP AND PINCH STRENGTH

The next step after evaluation of intrinsic and extrinsic musculature of the hand is determination of gross grip and pinch strength of the injured hand versus the noninjured hand. There are several commercially available devices for objective measurement of grip strength. The grip dynamometer (Fig. 4-30) with adjustable handle spacings provides an accurate evaluation of the force of grip.[4] This dynamometer has five adjustable spacings—at 1, 1½, 2, 2½, and 3 inches. The patient is shown how to grasp the dynamometer and is requested to grasp it with his maximum force. The grip is measured at each of the five handle spacings. The right and left hands are tested alternately, and the force of each is recorded. The test is paced at such a rate as to eliminate fatigue. According to Bechtol, there is usually a 5% to 10% difference between the dominant hand and the nondominant hand.[4] Patients who use a less than maximal effort can be identified in two ways. First, if the test is repeated, a patient who applies less than maximal effort is usually not able to duplicate his previous perfor-

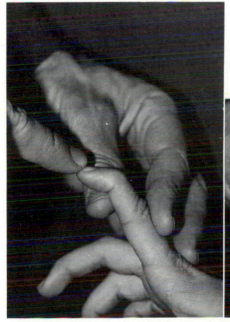
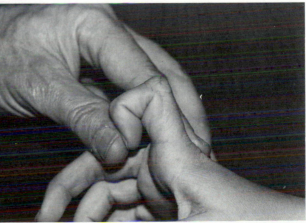

FIG. 4-29. The oblique retinacular ligament tightness test. The distal interphalangeal joint is passively flexed with the proximal interphalangeal joint held in extension. The distal interphalangeal joint is then passively flexed with the proximal interphalangeal joint flexed. If there is greater motion when the proximal interphalangeal joint is flexed than when it is extended, there is a contracture of the ligament. Equal loss of distal interphalangeal joint motion regardless of proximal interphalangeal joint position indicates a joint contracture.

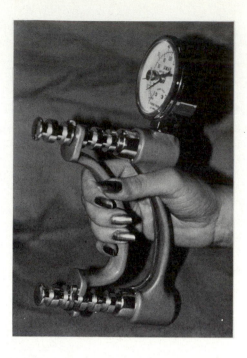

FIG. 4-30. Jamar grip dynamometer with five adjustable spacings (Asmow Engineering Co., Los Angeles, Calif.).

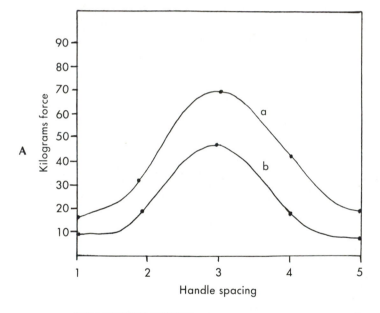

A

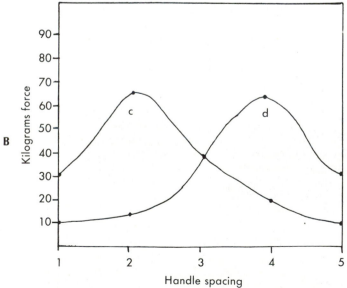

B

FIG. 4-31. A, The grip strengths of a patient's uninjured hand *(a)* and injured hand *(b)* are plotted. Despite the patient's decrease in grip strength because of injury, curve *b* maintains a bell-shaped pattern and parallels that of the normal hand. These curves are reproducible in repeated examinations, with minimal change in values. A great fluctuation in the size of the curve or the absence of a bell-shaped pattern casts doubt on the patient's compliance with the examination and may indicate malingering. **B,** If the patient has an exceptionally large hand, the curve will shift to the right *(d);* with a very small hand, the curve will shift to the left *(c).* Notice, however, that the bell-shaped pattern is maintained despite the curve's shift in direction.

mance. The discrepancy will be greater than 20% and sometimes as great as 100%.[4] Second, there is a normal bell curve of grip strength; the strength is greatest at the middle spacings and weakest at each end (for example, level I, 20 pounds; level II, 25 pounds; level III, 35 pounds; level IV, 25 pounds; and level V, 20 pounds). A patient who applies less than maximal effort will usually have a flat curve, with all values being approximately the same. If a patient has pain in the hand or forearm, of course the strength will be decreased. However, the bell curve pattern is usually still present. (See Fig. 4-31.)

There are three basic types of pinch: chuck, or three-fingered pinch; lateral, or key pinch; and tip pinch (see Fig. 4-32). These can be tested with a pinch meter (Fig. 4-33). Many disease processes can affect pinch power: basilar arthritis of the thumb, ulnar nerve palsy, and anterior interosseus nerve palsy, to mention a few.

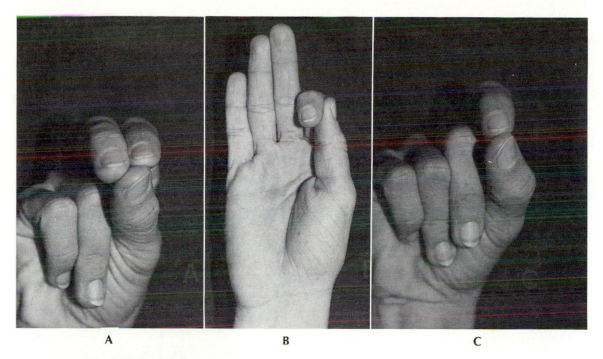

FIG. 4-32. A, Chuck, or three-fingered, pinch. **B,** Lateral, or key, pinch. **C,** Tip pinch.

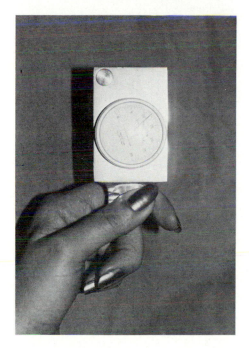

FIG. 4-33. Preston pinch gauge (J.A. Preston Corp., New York, N.Y.).

NERVE SUPPLY OF THE HAND—MOTOR AND SENSORY MOTOR

Three nerves provide motor and sensory function to the hand: the median, radial, and ulnar nerves (Fig. 4-34). The motor and sensory innervation of the hand is also subject to much variation, as pointed out by Rowntree.[40] However, we will discuss the usual, textbook innervation and ignore the variations.

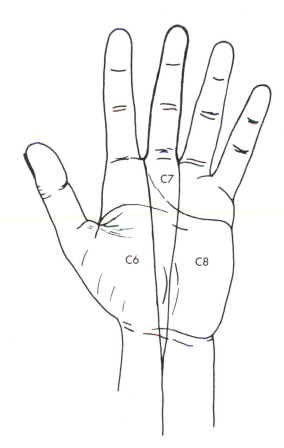

FIG. 4-34. Sensory dermatomes of the hand, by neurologic levels. (Redrawn from Hoppenfeld, S.: Physical examination of the spine and extremities, New York, 1976, Appleton-Century-Crofts.

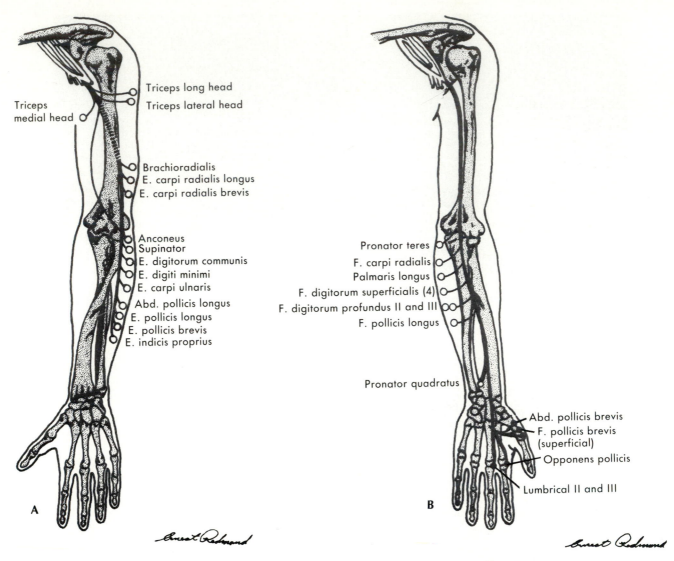

FIG. 4-35. Terminal branches of the radial **(A)**, median **(B),** and ulnar **(C)** nerves. (Redrawn from American Society for Surgery of the Hand: The hand, examination and diagnosis, Aurora, Colo., 1978, The Society.)

The median, radial, and ulnar nerves are peripheral branches of the brachial plexus. The radial nerve is formed from the C6 and C7 nerve roots. The median nerve is formed by branches of the C7, C8, and T1 nerve roots. The ulnar nerve is formed from branches of the C8 and T1 nerve roots. The terminal branches of the median, radial, and ulnar nerves are shown in Fig. 4-35. It is necessary to have a fundamental knowledge of the branches and their sequence of innervation, in order to appropriately place the level of an injury or to follow the path of a regenerating nerve.

These three nerves enter the forearm through various muscle and fascial planes and have multiple potential sources of entrapment. Entrapment of these nerves results in classic clinical presentations, with loss of motor function and paresthesias in the distribution of each nerve.

The median nerve may be entrapped as it enters the forearm at the level of the pronator teres muscle, the lacertus fibrosus, or the superficialis arch.[15,18,46] As it enters the hand,

it may be entrapped at the level of the carpal tunnel.[38] This common neuropathy has been termed "carpal tunnel syndrome." Patients with carpal tunnel syndrome often complain of numbness in the thumb and the radial two and one-half fingers, as well as night pain, weakness of grip, and dropping of objects. With a long-standing compression, there will be marked thenar atrophy and loss of thumb opposition.[36,38,49]

Compression of the median nerve at the wrist was first described by Paget in 1854.[36] Numerous authors since then have reported this entity and have recommended division of the transverse carpal ligament. Phalen has most clearly defined this entity as a syndrome; in 1966 he reported his experience with 654 cases of carpal tunnel syndrome.[36] Phalen found that in a very high percentage of cases, the wrist flexion test, now commonly known as Phalen's test, had a positive result and that Tinel's sign was present.

When performing Phalen's test, the patient holds his fore-

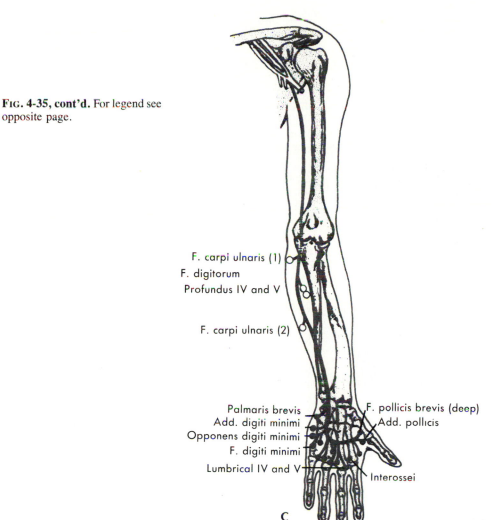

FIG. 4-35, cont'd. For legend see opposite page.

F. carpi ulnaris (1)
F. digitorum
Profundus IV and V

F. carpi ulnaris (2)

Palmaris brevis
Add. digiti minimi
Opponens digiti minimi
F. digiti minimi
Lumbrical IV and V

F. pollicis brevis (deep)
Add. pollicis

Interossei

C

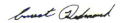

arms vertically and allows both hands to drop into complete flexion at the wrist for approximately 1 minute. In this position, the median nerve is compressed between the transverse carpal ligament and the adjacent flexor tendons. This maneuver causes almost immediate aggravation of numbness and paresthesias in the fingers.

Percussion of the median nerve at the wrist will produce paresthesias in the distribution of the nerve; this result is known as Tinel's sign (Fig. 4-36). Tinel's sign will be present not only in compressive neuropathies of nerves but also in partial and complete lacerations of nerves, and in areas where neuromas have formed.[19,31,50]

The presence of thenar atrophy, paresthesias in the median nerve distribution, a positive Phalen's test, and Tinel's sign, in association with a history of night pain, is pathognomonic for a compressive neuropathy of the median nerve in the carpal tunnel.

The ulnar and radial nerves are also subject to compression as they enter the arm and hand. The ulnar nerve can be compressed near the medial intermuscular septum, the cubital tunnel, or at the wrist (in Guyon's canal).[16,20,42,51] The radial nerve is subject to compression at the radial tunnel and as it passes between the two heads of the supinator muscle in an area known as the arcade of Frohse, or

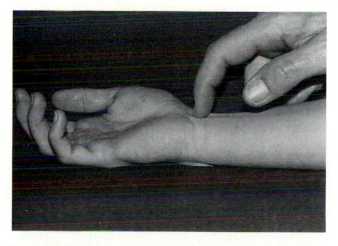

FIG. 4-36. Percussion of the median nerve at the wrist will elicit Tinel's sign in the presence of carpal tunnel syndrome.

it can be compressed superficially at the wrist.* As with compression of the median nerve, patients will complain of paresthesias in the sensory distribution of the irritated nerve and may have Tinel's sign. In long-standing or severe acute compressive neuropathies, there will be severe atrophy or even paralysis of the muscles innervated distal to the area

*See references 6, 23, 24, 39, 41, and 45.

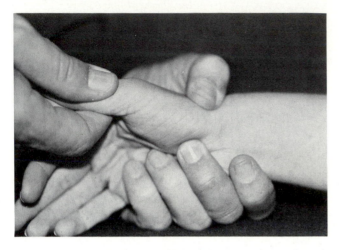

FIG. 4-37. The "grind test." Mild axial compression and gentle rotation of the thumb will elicit pain in the trapezial metacarpal joint if osteoarthritis is present.

of compression. If one is aware of the sequence of innervation or each nerve and performs a good manual motor examination, it is usually not hard to make a diagnosis of a nerve entrapment.

Patients with carpal tunnel syndrome, especially postmenopausal women, may have pain at the base of the thumb, which may be thought to be due to a compressive neuropathy. In this particular patient population, osteoarthritis of the metacarpal trapezial joint is frequent. The diagnosis can be made by performing the "grind test" and of course by radiographic examination. The grind test (Fig. 4-37) is performed by manipulating the patient's thumb with mild axial compression and gentle rotation. This maneuver will induce pain in the metacarpal trapezial joint if degenerative joint disease is present. Often carpal tunnel syndrome and metacarpal trapezial arthritis will coexist, and it is sometimes difficult to separate the pain-causing lesion. The test performed for carpal tunnel syndrome and the grind test will help clarify the situation.[48]

CUTANEOUS SENSIBILITY

Normal sensibility is a prerequisite to normal hand function. A patient with a median nerve injury has essentially a "blind hand" and is greatly disabled, even if all motor function is present. The assessment of sensibility is therefore an integral and important part of the examination of the hand.

The distribution of sensory nerves is subject to as much variation as the distribution of the motor branches.[40] The

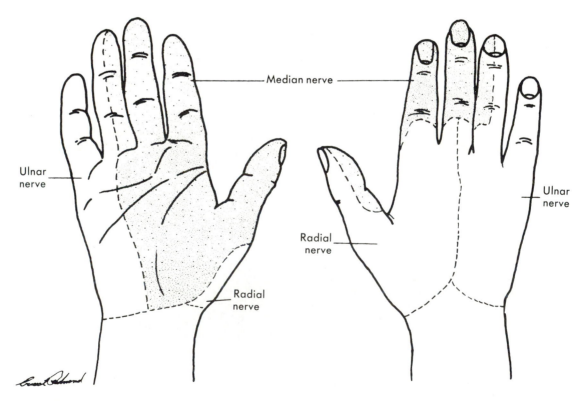

FIG. 4-38. Sensory distribution of the median, radial, and ulnar nerves in the hand. (Redrawn from Weeks, P.M., and Wray, R.C.: Management of acute hand injuries: a biological approach, St. Louis, 1973, The C.V. Mosby Co.)

classic distribution of the median, ulnar, and radial nerves is shown in Fig. 4-38.

There are many ways to assess sensibility: von Frey filaments, Moberg's "picking up test," Seddon's coin test, the moving two-point discrimination test described by Dellon, and Weber's two-point discrimination test, just to mention a few.[5,11,22,30] Each test has its supporters and detractors. Other chapters in this book will deal with sensibility testing and sensory reeducation in detail.

From a practical standpoint, an adequate sensibility examination can be performed by utilizing the two-point discrimination test and by careful examination of the patient's skin. Skin that has been deinnervated has lost its autonomic input and sudomotor function (that is, it does not sweat). The finger pulp becomes atrophic, smooth, and dry, with

relative loss of dermal ridges. Deinnervated skin will not wrinkle when placed in warm water (the "wrinkle test").[30] Tinel's sign will be present at the site of a nerve injury. (See Fig. 4-39.)

The two-point discrimination test is performed with a paper clip that has been bent into a caliper. With the patient's eyes closed and his hand cradled in the examiner's, the examiner gently places the caliper on the skin in a longitudinal direction—that is, on either the ulnar or the radial side of the digit. The ends of the paper clip must touch the skin lightly, just to the point of blanching. The ends should be smooth and not barbed. The patient is then asked whether he feels one point or two. Gradually the points are brought closer together and reapplied until the patient feels only one point. Normal two-point discrimination at a fingertip is 6

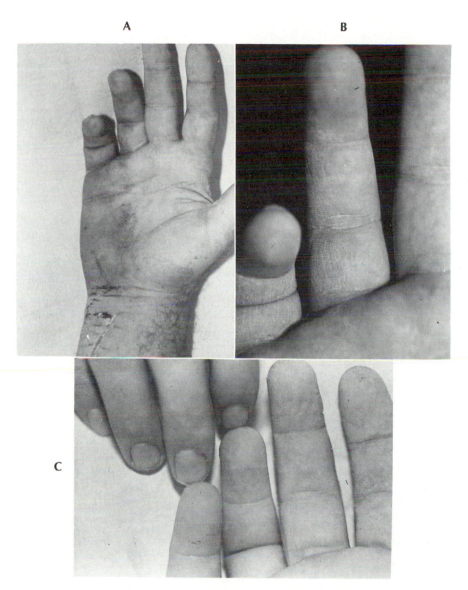

FIG. 4-39. Photographs illustrating loss of autonomic function after a peripheral nerve injury. **A,** The injury level to the ulnar nerve at the wrist is seen. The accumulated dry skin after the first postoperative dressing change can be seen in the classic ulnar nerve distribution. **B,** Closer view of the dry skin, which indicates a loss of sudomotor function. Notice how the fourth ray is split. **C,** Positive result of "wrinkle test" in same patient.

mm or less. (See Fig. 4-40.) Although this is not the most sensitive of tests and the result does not correlate with function of the hand, it is an adequate screening test and is much less time consuming than the more involved tests described above.

VASCULARITY OF THE HAND

The vascular supply of the hand is usually extensive; however, it should be carefully evaluated prior to any surgery of the hand. The primary blood supply to the hand is through the radial and ulnar arteries. In some individuals, the dominant blood supply to the hand can be from one artery. The ulnar artery gives rise to the superficial palmar arch, and the radial artery gives rise to the deep arch. These arches usually have extensive anastomoses.[10,26] The superficial palmar arch gives rise to four common digital arteries, which then branch to form the proper digital arteries. The superficial arch may supply blood to the thumb, or the thumb may be completely vascularized by a branch of the radial artery known as the princeps pollicis artery. To assess blood supply to the hand, one should check the color of the hand (pale, red, or cyanotic), digital capillary reflux, and the radial and ulnar pulses at the wrist, and perform Allen's test. Allen, in 1929, described a simple clinical test to determine the patency of the radial and ulnar arteries in thromboangiitis obliterans.[1] This test is performed by having the patient make a tight fist to exsanguinate the hand. The examiner occludes the radial and ulnar arteries at the wrist with digital pressure. The patient then opens his hand, which will be white and blanched. The examiner then releases either the ulnar or the radial artery and watches for revascularization of the hand. If the hand does not flush, the artery is occluded. This test is then repeated with the opposite artery. (See Fig. 4-41.)

A modification of Allen's test can be performed on a single digit.[2] The steps are the same as just outlined, except that the examiner occludes and releases the radial and ulnar digital arteries.

CONCLUSION

In this brief chapter, we have attempted to present an organized approach to clinical examination of the hand. The books and articles listed at the end of this chapter will provide more detailed descriptions of the tests and clinical entities that have been superficially presented here. Clinical examination is an art that will improve with practice and experience.

ACKNOWLEDGMENTS

We would like to thank Cynthia DuPuy for her assistance in preparation of the illustrations and Mavis Stinus for her secretarial assistance in the preparation of this chapter.

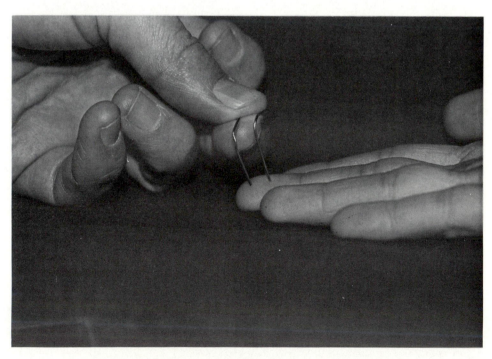

FIG. 4-40. Two-point discrimination test utilizing a bent paper clip.

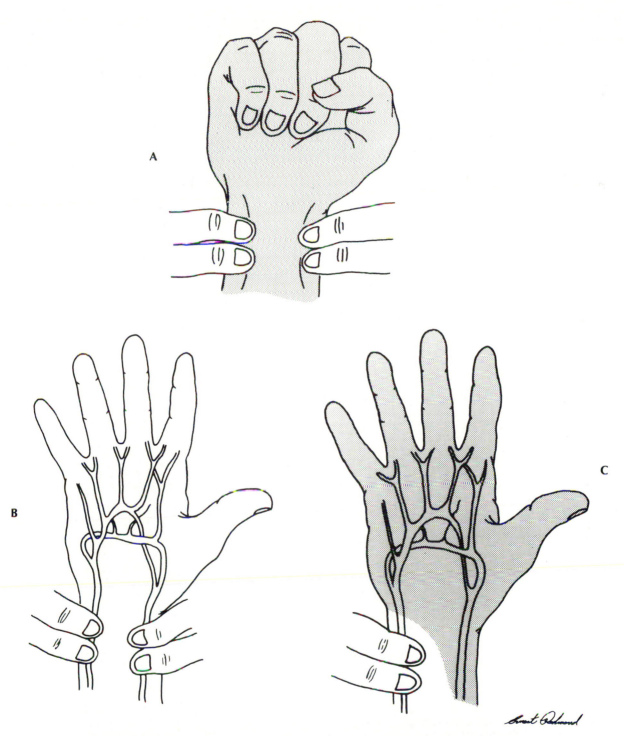

FIG. 4-41. Allen's test for arterial patency. **A,** The examiner places his fingers over the ulnar and radial arteries at the wrist. The patient then forcibly opens and closes his hand to exsanguinate it while the examiner occludes the radial and ulnar arteries **(B).** The patient then opens his hand, and the examiner releases one artery and observes the flushing of the hand **(C).** The steps are then repeated, and the other artery is tested for patency. (Redrawn from American Society for Surgery of the Hand: The hand, examination and diagnosis, Aurora, Colo., 1978, The Society.)

REFERENCES

1. Allen, E.: Thromboangitis obliterans: methods of diagnosis of chronic occlusive arterial lesions distal to the wrist with illustrative cases, Am. J. Med. Sci. **178:**237-244, 1929.
2. Ashbell, T., Kutz, J., and Kleinert, H.: The digital Allen test, Plast. Reconstr. Surg. **39:**311-312, 1967.
3. Baker, D., Gaul, J., Williams, V., and Graves, M.: The little finger superficialis—clinical investigation of its anatomical and functional shortcomings. J. Hand Surg. **6:**374-378, 1981.
4. Bechtol, C.: Grip test: the use of a dynamometer with adjustable handle spacings, J. Bone Joint Surg. **36A:**820-824 and 832, 1954.
5. Bowden, R., and Napier, J.: The assessment of hand function after peripheral nerve injuries, J. Bone Joint Surg. **43B:**481-492, 1961.
6. Braidwood, A.: Superficial radial neuropathy, J. Bone Joint Surg. **57B:**380-383, 1975.
7. Bunnell, S.: Opposition of the thumb, J. Bone Joint Surg. **20:**269-284, 1938.
8. Bunnell, S.: Surgery of the intrinsic muscles of the hand other than those producing opposition of the thumb, J. Bone Joint Surg. **24:**1-31, 1942.
9. Bunnell, S.: Ischaemic contracture, loca!, in the hand. J. Bone Joint Surg. **35A:**88-101, 1953.
10. Coleman, S., and Anson, B.: Arterial patterns in the hand based upon a study of 650 specimens, Surg. Gynecol. Obstet. **113:**408-424, 1961.
11. Dellon, A.: The moving two-point discrimination test: clinical evaluation of the quickly adapting fiber-receptor system, J. Hand Surg. **3:**474-481, 1978.
12. Eyler, D., and Markee, J.: The anatomy and function of the intrinsic musculature of the fingers, J. Bone Joint Surg. **36A:**1-9 and 18-20, 1954.
13. Finkelstein, H.: Stenosing tenovaginitis at the radial styloid process, J. Bone Joint Surg. **12:**509-514, 1930.
14. Harris, C., and Riordan, D.: Intrinsic contracture in the hand and its surgical treatment, J. Bone Joint Surg. **36A:**10-20, 1954.
15. Hartz, C., Linscheid, R., Gramse, R., and Daube, J.: The pronator teres syndrome: compressive neuropathy of the median nerve, J. Bone Joint Surg. **63A:**885-890, 1981.
16. Hunt, J.R.: Occupation neuritis of the deep palmar branch of the ulnar nerve: a well-defined clinical type of professional palsy of the hand, J. Nerv. and Ment. Dis. **35:**673-689, 1908.
17. James, J.I.P.: The assessment and management of the injured hand, Hand **2:**97-105, 1970.
18. Johnson, R.K., Spinner, M., and Shrewsbury, M.M.: Median nerve entrapment syndrome in the proximal forearm, J. Hand Surg. **4:**48-51, 1979.
19. Kaplan, E.: Translation of J. Tinel's "Four millement" paper. In Spinner, M.: Injuries to the major branches of peripheral nerves of the forearm, ed. 2, Philadelphia, 1978, W.B. Saunders Co., pp. 8-13.
20. Kleinert, H., and Hayes, J.: The ulnar tunnel syndrome, Plast. Reconstr. Surg. **47:**21-24, 1971.
21. Landsmeer, J.M.F.: The anatomy of the dorsal aponeurosis of the human finger and its functional significance, Anat. Rec. **104:**31-43, 1949.
22. Levin, S., Pearsall, G., and Ruderman, R.: Von Frey's method of measuring pressure sensibility in the hand: an engineering analysis of the Weinstein-Semmes pressure aesthesiometer, J. Hand Surg. **3:**211-216, 1978.
23. Linscheid, R.: Injuries to radial nerve at the wrist, Arch. Surg. **91:**942-946, 1965.
24. Lister, G.D., Belsole, R.B., and Kleinert, H.E.: The radial tunnel syndrome, J. Hand Surg. **4:**52-59, 1979.
25. Mannerfelt, L.: Studies on the hand in ulnar nerve paralysis: a clinical-experimental investigation in normal and anomalous innervation, Acta Orthop. Scand. [Suppl.] **87:**1-176, 1966.
26. Markee, J., and Wray, J.: Circulation of the hand: injection-corrosion studies, J. Bone Joint Surg. **41A:**673-680, 1959.
27. McFarlane, R.: Observations on the functional anatomy of the intrinsic muscles of the thumb, J. Bone Joint Surg. **44A:**1073-1088, 1962.
28. Mehta, H., and Gardner, W.: A study of lumbrical muscles in the human hand, Am. J. Anat. **109:**227-238, 1961.
29. Micks, J., Reswick, J., and Hager, D.L.: The mechanism of the intrinsic-minus finger: a biomechanical study, J. Hand Surg. **3:**333-341, 1978.
30. Moberg, E.: Objective methods for determining the functional value of sensibility in the hand, J. Bone Joint Surg. **40B:**454-476, 1958.
31. Moldaver, J.: Tinel's sign: its characteristics and significance, J. Bone Joint Surg. **60A:**412-414, 1978.
32. Mulder, J., and Landsmeer, J.: The mechanism of the claw finger, J. Bone Joint Surg. **50B:**664-668, 1968.
33. Nalebuff, E., and Millender, L.: Surgical treatment of the boutonniere deformity in rheumatoid arthritis, Orthop. Clin. North Am. **6:**753-763, 1975.
34. Nalebuff, E., and Millender, L.: Surgical treatment of the swan-neck deformity in rheumatoid arthritis, Orthop. Clin. North Am. **6:**733-752, 1975.
35. Noer, H., and Pratt, D.: A goniometer designed for the hand, J. Bone Joint Surg. **40A:**1154-1156, 1958.
36. Phalen, G.: The carpal tunnel syndrome: seventeen years' experience in diagnosis and treatment of 654 hands, J. Bone Joint Surg. **48A:**211-228, 1966.
37. Riddell, D.: Spontaneous rupture of the extensor pollicis longus: the results of tendon transfer, J. Bone Joint Surg. **45B:**506-510, 1963.
38. Robbins, H.: Anatomical study of the median nerve in the carpal tunnel and etiologies of the carpal tunnel syndrome, J. Bone Joint Surg. **45A:**953-966, 1963.
39. Roles, N., and Maudsley, R.: Radial tunnel syndrome: resistant tennis elbow as a nerve entrapment, J. Bone Joint Surg. **54B:**499-508, 1972.
40. Rowntree, T.: Anomalous innervation of the hand muscles, J. Bone Joint Surg. **31B:**505-510, 1949.
41. Shaw, J., and Sakellarides, H.: Radial nerve paralysis associated with fractures of the humerus: a review of forty-five cases, J. Bone Joint Surg. **49A:**899-902, 1967.
42. Shea, J., and McClain, E.: Ulnar nerve compression syndromes at and below the wrist, J. Bone Joint Surg. **51A:**1095-1103, 1969.
43. Shrewsbury, M., and Johnson, R.: A systematic study of the oblique retinacular ligament of the human finger: its structure and function, J. Hand Surg. **2:**194-199, 1977.
44. Smith, R.: Non-ischemic contractures of the intrinsic muscles of the hand, J. Bone Joint Surg. **53A:**1313-1331, 1971.
45. Spinner, M.: The arcade of Frohse and its relationship to posterior interosseous nerve paralysis, J. Bone Joint Surg. **50B:**809-812, 1968.
46. Spinner, M.: The anterior interosseous nerve syndrome with special attention to its variations, J. Bone Joint Surg. **52A:**84-94, 1970.
47. Srinivasan, H.: Clinical features of paralytic claw fingers, J. Bone Joint Surg. **61A:**1060, 1063, 1979.
48. Swanson, A.: Disabling arthritis at the base of the thumb: treatment by resection of the trapezium and flexible (silicon) implant arthroplasty, J. Bone Joint Surg. **54A:**456-471, 1972.
49. Tanzer, R.: The carpal tunnel syndrome: a clinical and anatomical study, J. Bone Joint Surg. **41A:**626-634, 1959.
50. Tinel, J.: Le signe du "fourmillement" dans les lesions des nerfs peripheriques, Press. Med. **47:**388-389, October 1915.
51. Uriburu, I., Morchio, F., and Marin, J.: Compression syndrome of the deep motor branch of the ulnar nerve (Piso-Hamate hiatus syndrome), J. Bone Joint Surg. **58A:**145-147, 1976.
52. Vaughn-Jackson, O.: Rheumatoid hand deformities considered in the light of tendon imbalance, J. Bone Joint Surg. **44B:**764-775, 1962.
53. Zancolli, E.: Structural and dynamic basis of hand surgery, Philadelphia, 1968, J.B. Lippincott Co., pp. 136-154.

5

Documentation: essential elements of an upper extremity assessment battery

ELAINE EWING FESS

"I often say that when you can measure what you are speaking about and express it in numbers, you know something about it; but, when you cannot measure it in numbers your knowledge is of a meagre and unsatisfactory kind; it may be the beginning of knowledge but have scarcely in your thought advanced to the stage of science whatever the matter may be."

LORD KELVIN

Objective measurements provide a foundation for hand rehabilitation efforts by delineating baseline pathology from which patient progress and treatment methods may be evaluated. A thorough and unbiased assessment procedure furnishes information that assists in predicting the rehabilitation potential of the diseased or injured hand, provides data to which subsequent measurements may be compared, and allows the medical specialist to plan and evaluate treatment programs and techniques. Conclusions gained from evaluation procedures aid in ordering treatment priorities, provide both patient and staff incentive, and define functional capacity when rehabilitative efforts reach an end point. Assessment, through analysis and integration of data, also serves as the vehicle for professional communication, eventually influencing the comprehensive body of knowledge of the profession.

Because the quality of information depends on the level of sophistication, predictability, and accuracy of the instruments used in gathering data, it is of utmost importance to choose assessment tools with care and forethought. Dependable, precise tools allow the clinician to reach conclusions that are minimally skewed by extraneous factors or biases, thus diminishing the chances of subjective error and facilitating an objective and more accurate level of understanding. An instrument that measures diffusely produces undelineated and nonspecific data, while an instrument that has been proved to measure with precision yields more accurate and selective information (Fig. 5-1).

In addition to knowledge of the specific characteristics of assessment tools, it is important to identify how the manner in which they are used may affect resultant data. First and foremost, in order to maintain validity it is critical that assessment instruments never be used as practice tools for patients in therapy. Information obtained from a tool

that has been used as part of the training process is radically skewed, rendering it invalid and meaningless. Other factors that may alter test results include patient fatigue, the patient's potential for physiologic adaptation, the degree of difficulty, and the length of time required to complete the test. To avoid possible tainting of test data through physiologic adaptation, sensory testing should be completed prior to the evaluation of gross grasp or pinch; and if appropriate rest periods are not provided, fatigue may diminish test scores. In addition, frustration thresholds can be inadvertently exceeded if difficult portions of the testing battery are scheduled early in the assessment session. The testing procedure must, therefore, reflect understanding of testing protocol as well as instrumentation requirements.

Although many variables influence the selection and use of assessment instruments, the underlying rationale for conducting evaluation procedures is communication. The acquisition and transmission of knowledge, which are fundamental to patient treatment and professional growth, can be enhanced through the development and use of a common professional language based on strict criteria for assessment instrument selection. In an age of consumer awareness and accountability it is no longer sufficient to rely on "homebrewed," nonvalidated evaluation tools, which almost universally produce meaningless splinter data (Fig. 5-2). Thus the purposes of this chapter are (1) to define testing terminology and criteria, (2) to identify key factors that influence the development of an upper extremity assessment battery, (3) to review currently utilized hand assessment instruments, and (4) to provide samples of assessment forms. It is not within the scope of this chapter to recommend the use of one test or instrument over another; instead readers are encouraged to choose those instruments or protocols that will best meet the specific needs of their own practices.

49

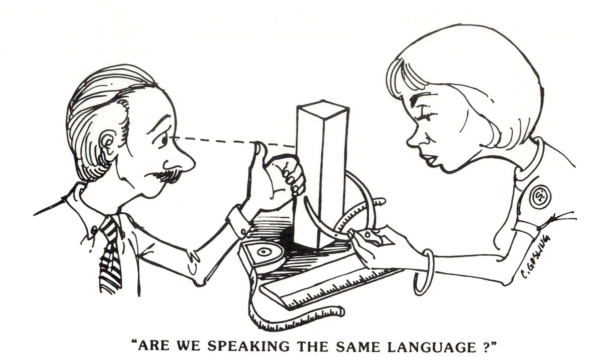

"ARE WE SPEAKING THE SAME LANGUAGE ?"

FIG. 5-1. Assessment with calibrated instruments provides accurate information and leads to a more thorough understanding of what is measured.

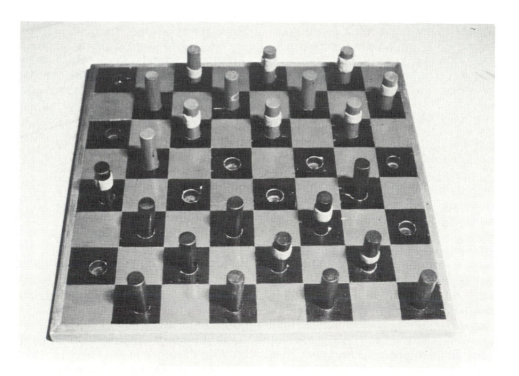

FIG. 5-2. Tests should be statistically proved to be reliable and valid before they are used for clinical assessment. "Home-brewed" tests should not be relied on to document patient progress.

ASSESSMENT TERMINOLOGY AND CRITERIA

Standardized tests, which represent the most sophisticated level of assessment tools, have been statistically proved to be both valid and reliable. This means that they measure what they purport to measure and that they measure consistently between examiners and from trial to trial. The few standardized tests currently available in the field of hand rehabilitation are limited to instruments that evaluate hand coordination, dexterity, and work tolerance; and unfortunately only a small number of these meet all the requirements of standardization. The remaining hand assessment instruments fall at varying levels along the validity and reliability continuums according to how closely their inherent properties coincide with those of standardized tools.

To qualify as a standardized test, an instrument must have all of the following elements: (1) a statement that defines the purpose or intent of the test, (2) correlation statistics or another appropriate measure of instrument validity, (3) correlation statistics or another appropriate measure of instrument reliability, (4) detailed descriptions of the equipment utilized in the test, (5) normative data, drawn from a large population sample, which is divided into categories according to appropriate variables, such as hand dominance, age, sex, or occupation, and (6) specific instructions for administering, scoring and interpreting the test. A bibliography of related literature may also be included. It is important to note that although they claim to be standardized, many tests lack true validity and reliability coefficients, relying instead on mean or ''average'' values. Such tests are not standardized and actually have no foundation for justifying their consistency of measurement and their ability to assess that for which they were designed. Since relatively few hand evaluation tools fully meet standardization criteria, instrument selection should be predicated on satisfying as many of the standardization requisites as possible, thus ensuring an identifiable level of quality control.

Through interpretation, standardized tests provide information that may be used to deduce or predict how a patient will perform in normal daily tasks. For example, if ''patient no. 3'' achieves ''X'' functional rating on a standardized test, it may be predicted that he should be able to perform at an equivalent of the ''75th percentile'' of ''normal assembly line workers.'' Standardized hand function tests also allow the clinician to make statements about changes in patient status: ''Yes, this patient's hand dexterity is improved as the result of this tendon transfer.''

Other types of tests also provide significant information when they are used properly. Most important are the observational tests, producing responses on a yes-no performance continuum. An activities-of-daily-living (ADL) evaluation is an example of an observational test; it consists of various tasks, and the patient is graded on whether he can accomplish the tasks under specific conditions (for example, independent, independent with equipment, needs assistance). The ADL test tells the examiner ''Yes, the patient can pick up a 12-ounce aluminum beer can with his right hand.'' This knowledge, however, cannot be used to predict the patient's performance in picking up potatoes or opening a ketchup bottle. An observational test is used to assess progress through comparisons of subsequent testing trials, and it is limited to longitudinal, item-to-item contrast: ''The patient is now able to accomplish 'task Z,' which he was unable to do three weeks ago.'' Further assumptions or predictions are invalid and meaningless. Observational tests have a definite role in an upper extremity assessment battery, as long as they are used appropriately.

DEVELOPMENT OF AN ASSESSMENT BATTERY
General considerations

Development of an upper extremity assessment battery cannot be undertaken without a thorough understanding of the conditions that will influence its use. The types of patients to be evaluated, expectations about the acquired data, the way the data will be used, and administrative factors such as personnel, budget, and physical setting must be carefully considered to ensure that an assessment battery meets the unique needs of a particular hand practice. Age, diagnosis, intelligence, socioeconomic background, language, and other patient population variables are important in the selection of assessment instruments. For example, tests requiring high degrees of patient cooperation may not be appropriate for a practice that deals primarily with young children, mentally retarded individuals, or persons whose language skills are limited. The intent or reason for gathering information also plays a significant role in the creation of an assessment battery. Because the need for exacting precision and sophistication in the collection of research data is paramount, requirements are often more stringent for research evaluation instruments than for instruments used in daily clinical testing. An assessment battery should reflect the scope and demands of the practice, including staff qualifications, physical plan, and fiscal parameters. In addition, through licensure regulations, state or federal legislation is frequently influential in determining the selection of test instruments.

Specific considerations

To be complete, an assessment battery should address the total spectrum of upper extremity performance and condition, including physical status, motion, sensation, and function. A history is also an important part of the patient's permanent record. This information not only is essential to identifying and understanding a pathologic condition, but provides the medical specialist with pertinent occupational and vocational facts that allow subsequent intervention to be tailored to meet the specific needs of the patient. In addition, an assessment battery may contain relevant administrative information (Fig. 5-3) and specialized tests such as an upper extremity prosthetic checkout for a splint evaluation (Fig. 5-4).

Since there is no universal hand assessment instrument, the clinician must rely on a variety of tools to measure the various parameters of hand condition and performance. The four main divisions—physical status, motion, sensation, and function—should be represented through the selection of a minimum of one instrument per area. Although this minimum-requirement assessment battery is sufficient for a cursory evaluation, it is preferable, in those practices specializing in hand dysfunction, to include several instruments

Text continued on p. 57.

SPLINTING AND HAND THERAPY REFERRAL

Name: _____

Address: _____

Phone number: _____

Diagnosis:

Referral for extremity: ☐ Right ☐ Left

 ☐ Evaluation and report
 ☐ Evaluation and treatment
  ☐ Range of motion
  ☐ Strengthening
  ☐ Dexterity
  ☐ Sensory reeducation
  ☐ Desensitization
  ☐ Activities of daily living
  ☐ Work/home evaluation
  ☐ Joint protection (arthritic program)
  ☐ Upper extremity prosthetic training
  ☐ Upper extremity Jobst garment measurement and fitting
  ☐ Transcutaneous stimulation
  ☐ Upper extremity Jobst pump
  ☐ Other (specify): _____
 ☐ Splint fabrication:

A

FIG. 5-3. Administrative forms are essential to the organization of a hand rehabilitation center. Forms such as these may also be helpful in retrieval of data for research purposes. **A,** Referral form. **B,** Daily patient log. (**A** from Fess, E., Gettle, K., and Strickland, J.: Hand splinting: principles and methods, St. Louis, 1981, The C.V. Mosby Co.)

SPLINTING AND HAND THERAPY REFERRAL—cont'd

Check joints desired to be incorporated in splint*:

Immobilize (specify position of joint in degrees)						Mobilize				
					Elbow					
					Ext					
					Flex					
					Wrist					
					Ext					
					Flex					
					UD					
					RD					
				TH		**TH**				
					CMC					
					Ext					
					Flex					
					Abd					
Ind	**Long**	**Ring**	**Sm**	**Th**		**Th**	**Ind**	**Long**	**Ring**	**Sm**
					MP					
					Ext					
					Flex					
				▮	RD	▮				
				▮	UD	▮				
					PIP (IP)					
					Ext					
					Flex					
					DIP					
				▮	Ext	▮				
				▮	Flex	▮				

*Ext, Extension; Flex, flexion; RD, radial deviation; UD, ulnar deviation; MP, metacarpophalangeal; PIP, proximal interphalangeal; DIP, distal interphalangeal; ABD, abduction; Th, thumb; Ind, index; Sm, small.

A

Continued.

FIG. 5-3, cont'd. For legend see opposite page.

SPLINTING AND HAND THERAPY REFERRAL — cont'd

Describe the function you would like the splint or splints to provide:

A

The correct fabrication of the splint is important. Therefore, please call for any specific instructions (phone number _____).

FIG. 5-3, cont'd. For legend see p. 52.

DATE: _____ am
                        pm

UPPER EXTREMITY ASSESSMENT BATTERY
DAILY PATIENT LOG

		NAME									

E	VOLUME
V	TEMPERATURE
A	RANGE OF MOTION
L	MUSCLE TEST
U	SENSIBILITY
A	COORDINATION
T	ADL/HOMEMAKING
I	EMPLOYMENT
O	PROSTHETIC
N	SPLINT
	JOBST MEASUREMENT
	EMG
	NCV
	OTHER
	INITIAL
	PROGRESS
	FINAL

T	
R	PASSIVE EXERCISE
E	ACTIVE EXERCISE
A	RESISTIVE EXERCISE
T	FUNCTIONAL ACTIVITY
M	EARLY MOBILIZATION
E	JOINT MOBILIZATION
N	DESENSITIZATION
T	SENSORY REEDUCATION
	DEBRIDEMENT
	JOINT PROTECTION
	HOME PROGRAM
	OTHER

M	
O	BIOFEEDBACK
D	ELEC STIMULATION
A	TNS
L	WHIRLPOOL
I	HOT PACKS
T	PARAFFIN
I	FLUIDOTHERAPY
E	INTERMIT PRESSURE
S	OTHER

S	
P	IMMOBILIZATION
L	MOBILIZATION
I	SIMPLE
N	COMPOUND
T	COMPLEX
S	
	EQUIPMENT
	OTHER

THERAPIST: _____

FIG. 5-3, cont'd. For legend see p. 52.

UPPER EXTREMITY FUNCTIONAL ASSESSMENT BATTERY

Upper extremity amputee prosthesis checkout

Amputee type: R _____ L _____ BE _____ AE _____ SD _____ WD _____ ED _____ Other _____

	Test	Performance	Standard
I	Conformance to prescription		Conform to written prescription
II	Workmanship and appearance		
III	Control system efficiency	Hook Hand	
	1. Force applied at terminal device	_____ lb _____ lb	B/E should be 70% or greater.
	2. Force applied at harness	_____ lb _____ lb	A/E should be 50% or greater.
	3. Efficiency = $\dfrac{\text{Force at T.D.}}{\text{Force at harness}}$	_____ % _____ %	
IV	Compression fit and comfort		Socket compression should cause no pain or discomfort.
V	Tension stability	_____ in displacement	50 lb (or ⅓ body weight) axial pull should not displace socket more than 1 in. Harness should not fail.
VI	Terminal device—opening and closing	Hook Hand	Full opening and closing should be obtained with forearm at 90°.
	1. Mechanical range	_____ in _____ in	
	2. Active range (forearm at 90°)	_____ in _____ in	B/E 70% (A/E 50%) opening at mouth and waist.
	3. Active range (waist)	_____ in _____ in	
	4. Active range (mouth)	_____ in _____ in	

Date: _____   Patient: _____

A

Upper extremity amputee prosthesis checkout

Additional below-elbow specifications

VII	Amount of forearm	Prosthesis off _____ Prosthesis on _____	Should be within 10° of range with prosthesis off, except for very short stumps
VIII	Amount of forearm rotation	Prosthesis off _____ Prosthesis on _____	Total rotation with prosthesis should be half that with prosthesis off (Practical only for long B/E and W/D)
IX	Placement of artificial elbow		Should be not more than below normal elbow on adult
X	Range of glenohumeral motion with prosthesis on	Abduction Flexion Extension Rotation	90° 90° 30° } Prosthesis on Variable
XI	Glenohumeral flexion required to flex forearm fully	_____ °	Should not exceed 45°
	Prosthetic elbow—mechanical range	_____ °	To 135°
	Prosthetic elbow—active range	_____ °	To 135°
XII	Force required to initiate forearm flexion from a position of 90° flexed	_____ lb	Should not exceed the force necessary to open terminal device or 10 lb
XIII	Socket rotation stability		Resist force of 3 lb 12 in from elbow center Applied laterally and medially

Prosthesis passed _____   Prosthesis rejected _____

Returned for following reasons: _____

_____

_____

Patient _____

FIG. 5-4. An assessment battery may contain specialized forms such as, **A,** upper extremity prosthetic checkout, designed by Prosthetic-Orthotic Department at Northwestern University, Chicago, or, **B,** splint check-out. (**B** from Fess, E., Gettle, K., and Strickland, J.: Hand splinting: principles and methods, St. Louis, 1981, The C.V. Mosby Co.) *Continued.*

SPLINT CHECKOUT FORM

	Yes	No	Comments
DESIGN			
Does the splint meet general design concepts, including adaptation for:			
1. Individual patient factors			
2. Total utilization time			
3. Simplicity			
4. Optimum function			
5. Optimum sensation			
6. Efficient construction and fit			
7. Ease of application and removal			
8. Exercise regimen			
Does the splint meet specific design concepts, including adaptation for:			
9. Influencing key joints			
10. Attaining purpose			
a. Augment passive motion			
b. Substitute for active motion			
11. Types of forces used			
12. Surface of application			
13. Anatomic variables			
14. Material properties			
MECHANICS			
Does the splint meet specific mechanical concepts, including adaptation for:			
1. Reduction of pressure			
2. Increased mechanical advantage (Ratio of FA to RA)			
3. Optimum rotational force (90°)			
4. Torque			
5. Variance of passive mobility of successive joints			
6. Optimum utilization of parallel forces			
7. Material strength			
8. Elimination of friction			

B

FIG. 5-4, B, cont'd. For legend see p. 55.

SPLINT CHECKOUT FORM—cont'd

	Yes	No	Comments
CONSTRUCTION			
Has the splint been fabricated appropriately to provide:			
1. Good cosmesis			
2. Rounded corners			
3. Smooth edges and surfaces			
4. Stable joints			
5. Finished rivets			
6. Ventilation			
7. Secure padding			
8. Secure straps			
FIT			
Has the splint been fitted appropriately to adapt to:			
1. Bony prominences			
2. Dual obliquity			
3. Ligamentous stress			
4. Arches			
5. Joint axis alignment			
6. Skin creases			
7. Kinematic changes			
8. Kinetic concepts			

B

FIG. 5-4, B, cont'd. For legend see p. 55.

within each category, producing gradation and verification of information.

The American Society for Surgery of the Hand (ASSH)[2] and the American Society of Hand Therapists (ASHT)[14] have established guidelines for clinical assessment of the hand; these guidelines include recommendations for measurement of range of motion, strength, sensation (ASSH), volume (ASHT), dexterity and coordination (ASHT), and vascular status (ASSH). Representing the first major steps taken by recognized professional hand societies toward creating a common assessment language, these recommendations are milestones in the history of hand rehabilitation. To enhance the quality of professional communication and understanding of hand dysfunction, it is important that individuals responsible for developing evaluation protocols seriously consider these guidelines and generate assessment batteries that reflect the recommendations of these two societies.

TIMING AND USE OF ASSESSMENT TESTS

Not all patients who are evaluated need to be given all of the tests within an assessment battery. Most hand specialists use a few quick tests to check hand function initially and add the more sophisticated testing procedures as dictated by the patient's condition. For example, if on interrogation the patient reports no loss of sensation, and this is verified by a normal two-point discrimination test, in most instances it is not necesary to administer the remainder of the sensory tests. To conserve time and decrease frustration levels, tests within each area should be ordered according to type of information provided and degree of difficulty of administration, beginning with an easy, dependable test that will supply basic data and working toward the more esoteric instruments.

Initial and final evaluations are usually comprehensive in scope, while the intervening evaluations are less formal and concentrate on assessing progress in specific areas of dysfunction according to the problems exhibited by each patient. The frequency of reevaluation sessions depends entirely upon the patient, the progress that he demonstrates, and the nature of the test itself. It is not unusual to measure range of motion in an early postoperative tenolysis patient three or four times a day. However, measurement of grip strength in the same patient may not be appropriate, because of wound healing and tensile strength limitations,[21] until 7 or 8 weeks postoperatively, and then strength, because of the time required to effect change, would not be measured as frequently as would motion.

The actual recording of assessment data also varies with the situation. For the tenolysis patient described above, unless significant problems were encountered and frequent documentation was necessary to demonstrate lack of cooperation or other mitigating variables, only one set of range-of-motion measurements would usually be recorded per day even though multiple readings were taken. As change occurs less rapidly, motion values may be recorded two or three times a week, eventually decreasing to once every 2 weeks, once a month, and so on. The important concept is that change in status be documented with objective measurements at appropriate intervals.

HISTORY AND PHYSICAL STATUS
History

In addition to noting the patient's current condition, the initial history should contain information regarding how and when the injury occurred, including specifics as to time and place. Questions about how the patient's vocational, avocational, and ADL skills have been changed by his disability are important, as is close observation of the patient's spontaneous use of the extremity during the evaluation session. The patient's subjective assessment of his pain may also provide insight into his attitude and his ability to cope with his situation, and it is helpful to attempt to determine the cause of pain and its perceived intensity.

Obtaining a history is not only the amassing of facts; it is the time in which the first steps are taken toward building a firm foundation of trust and communication between the patient and the examiner. Each must feel that the other is being honest and open. Genuine concern and an unhurried manner on the part of the examiner will facilitate discussion, eventually netting returns in cooperation and understanding as the patient participates in his rehabilitation process.

Examination

The detail in which this portion of the assessment battery is pursued, and by whom, depends upon the clinical setting in which patients are evaluated, and to a large extent upon the division of duties between the surgeons and the therapists. Regardless of who is responsible for conducting the intake evaluation, each patient is assessed for general configuration of the extremity; condition of skin and soft tissue; skeletal stability; articular motion and integrity; tendon continuity and glide; neurovascular status, including isolated muscle function, sensation, and vessel patency; and finally for general function, coordination, and dexterity.(Refer to Chapter 4 for further details.)

It is the combination of careful clinical examination and precise measurement (Fig. 5-5) that allows the examiner to identify and make judgments about the patient's rehabilitative potential and the need for therapeutic intervention. Assessment instruments outline the problem in terms of data expressed as specific numerical values, quantifying and adding dimension to knowledge and understanding. Without measurement, perceptions are diffuse and unclear.

CURRENT HAND ASSESSMENT INSTRUMENTS

Hand evaluation instruments may be divided into four basic groups according to the entity measured: extremity condition, motion, sensibility, and function. Condition involves the neurovascular system as it pertains to tissue viability, nutrition, patency of vessels, and arterial, venous, and lymphatic flow. Through noninvasive monitoring of hand volume, skin temperature, and arterial pulses, important clues are provided about the status of the skin and subcutaneous tissues and about neurovascular function. The measurement of motion is dependent upon muscle-tendon continuity, contractile and gliding capacity, neuromuscular communication, and volitional control. Techniques for evaluating hand motion include goniometric measurements and the determination of isolated muscle strength. Relying upon neural continuity, impulse transmission, receptor acuity, and cortical perception, assessment of sensibility may be divided into sudomotor or sympathetic response and the abilities to detect, discriminate, quantify, and recognize stimuli.[19] Hand function reflects the integration of all systems and is measured in terms of grip and pinch, coordination and dexterity, and ability to participate in ADL and vocational and avocational tasks.

Condition assessment instruments

The volumeter, as designed by Brand and Wood,[7] is based on Archimedes' principle of water displacement; it measures composite hand mass (Fig. 5-6). Commercially available in several dimensions,[9] volumeters may be used to assess changes in hand size, including atrophy, local swelling, and generalized edema, provided that immersion of the extremity in water is not contraindicated. Waylett and Seibly[37] found a commercial hand volumeter to be accurate to within 10 ml when used according to the manufacturer's specifications. Variables that were implicated in reducing accuracy included use of an aerated hose or faucet to fill the tank, wrist or forearm motion once the hand is immersed in the tank, inconsistency of pressure applied to the horizontal stop rod, and inconsistent placement of the volumeter during successive measurements. Normal comparison values may be obtained by measuring the contralateral extremity. Measurements from both extremities should be recorded in the chart initially, and successive measurements of the symptomatic extremity should be noted at appropriate intervals (Fig. 5-7).

Circumferential measurements, by means of a flexible tape measure, are also employed to evaluate upper extremity size. Although the accuracy of this technique depends upon consistency of placement[32] and tension of the tape, circumferential measurement provides a quick means of assessment; it is especially applicable in situations in which the

TENDON
   FUNCTION
      Connect motor to support system
      Glide = Active motion

| | | EVALUATION | |
ETIOLOGY OF DYSFUNCTION	SYMPTOM	MEASUREMENT	OBSERVATION
Loss of continuity	Loss of AROM	A & P ROM	Posture/use
Early inflammation	Swelling/edema	Volume/circum	Dec. wrinkling
	Decreased motion	A & P ROM	Posture/use
Loss of motor	Loss of AROM	A & P ROM	Posture/use
	Weakness	EMG	"
		Manual Muscle	
		Dynamometer	
		Pinchometer	
Denervation	Atrophy (late)	Volume/circum	Trophic changes
Adhesion	Decreased AROM	A & P ROM	Posture/use
	Tenodesis effect	"	
Change of position,	Bowstringing	"	
angle of pull	Subluxation	"	
	Dislocation	"	
	Decreased motion	"	Posture/use
Inflammation	Swelling/edema	Volume/circum	Dec. wrinkling
	Decreased motion	A & P ROM	Posture/use
	Crepitation		Palpation
	Triggering		"
	Tenodesis effect		"
	Pain		"
Infection	Swelling/edema	Volume/circum	Dec. wrinkling
	Decreased motion	A & P ROM	Posture/use
	Pain		Palpation

Note: The above tendon problems influence composite hand function and
        may require dexterity/coordination, ADL or vocational assessment.

FIG. 5-5. Clinical examination and objective measurements are combined to provide better understanding of underlying pathologic condition.

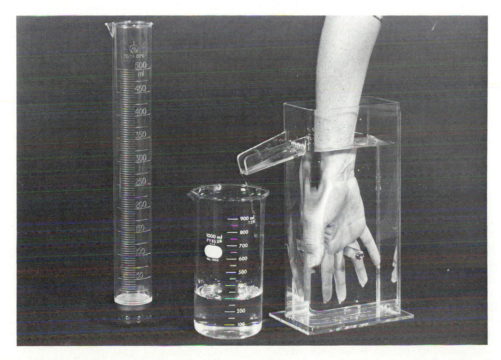

FIG. 5-6. Volumeter accuracy has been shown to be within 10 ml when used according to instructions.

UPPER EXTREMITY ASSESSMENT BATTERY

VOLUME

VOLUMETER MEASUREMENTS:

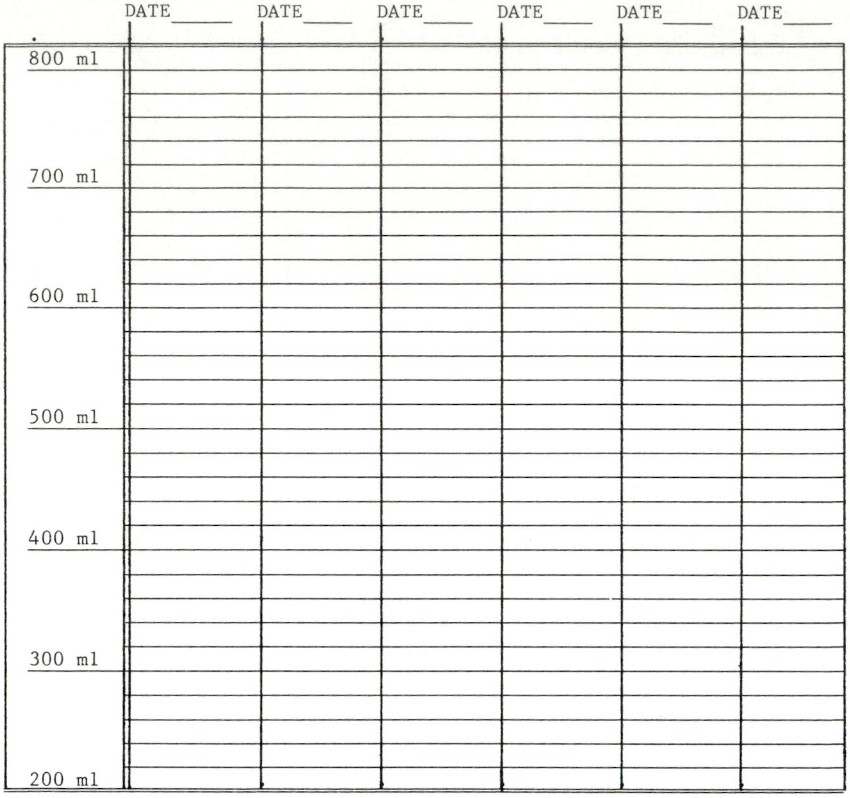

	DATE____	DATE____	DATE____	DATE____	DATE____	DATE____
800 ml						
700 ml						
600 ml						
500 ml						
400 ml						
300 ml						
200 ml						

NORMAL VOLUME (opposite hand):_____ml.

CIRCUMFERENCE / DIAMETER [c]:
    Biceps*   _____ _____ _____ _____ _____ _____
    Forearm*   _____ _____ _____ _____ _____ _____
    DPC   _____ _____ _____ _____ _____ _____
    Digit(_____)_____ _____ _____ _____ _____ _____

    NORMAL MEASUREMENT (opposite hand):
        Biceps _____   Forearm _____   DPC _____   Digit _____

[c] Circle method used.

* 10cm. above/below the medial
  epicondyle of the humerus

Name:_____
Number:_____
Hand:_____

FIG. 5-7. Recording of volumetric data on a graph facilitates explanations of progress for patients and students.

use of a volumeter would be awkward or inappropriate. Serial measurements should be taken and recorded (Fig. 5-7) at appropriate intervals, as dictated by patient requirements and progress.

An external caliper, calibrated in millimeters, offers an additional method of assessing localized swelling—measuring the diameter of a segment. As with circumferential measurement, the accuracy of diameter readings is subject to error through inconsistent placement and tension. This technique provides greater measurement reliability on smaller-diameter segments; it is usually employed to evaluate changes in digital size. (Refer to Chapter 11 for further details.)

Because skin temperature is directly related to digital

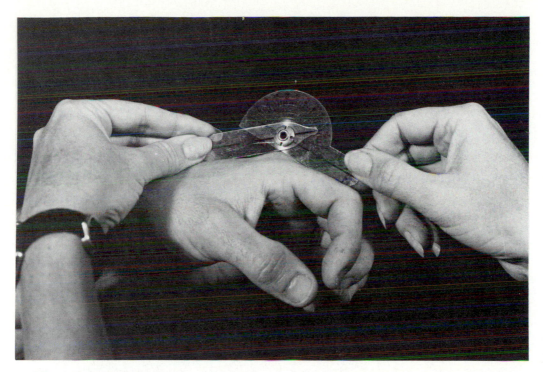

FIG. 5-8. A shortened goniometer facilitates range-of-motion measurements on the small joints of the hand.

vessel patency, it is a valuable indicator of tissue viability; temperature is used to monitor the status of revascularized hands or digits during the early postoperative period. Cutaneous temperature gauges are placed on the dressing, on a revascularized digit, and on a normal adjacent or corresponding digit, to monitor room temperature, the temperature of the area in question, and the temperature of a matching, normal area. It is important to note any decrease in temperature in the revascularized segment, with critical temperature considered to be 30° C; lower readings indicate possible vascular compromise. Normal digital temperature ranges between 30° and 35° C.[8]

A Doppler scanner is used to map arterial flow through audible ultrasonic response to arterial pulsing. Although inconsistencies continue to plague attempts to quantify Doppler readings, to date the scanner is accepted as an important noninvasive tool in the evaluation of arterial patency.

Motion assessment instruments

Goniometric evaluation of the upper extremity is essential to monitoring articular motion and musculotendinous function (Fig. 5-8). Passive range-of-motion measurements reflect the ability of a joint to be moved through its normal arc of motion; limitations in passive motion are generally indicative of problems within the joint itself or involvement of capsular structures surrounding the joint. Active range-of-motion measurements reflect the muscle's ability to effect motion via its tendinous link to the osseous kinetic chain. Limitations in active motion may be caused by lack of tendon continuity; adhesions between the tendon and surrounding structures; constriction of the tendon sheath; in-

flammation of the tendon; subluxation, dislocation, or bowstringing of the tendon; or tendon attenuation. In the presence of diminished articular motion (passive), active range of motion may seem to be impaired even though tendon amplitude and muscular contraction are normal. Conversely, normal joint motion may seem to be limited when tendon gliding is reduced. Because active motion cannot exceed the passive capacity of joint motion, it is essential that both active and passive range of motion be assessed and recorded (Fig. 5-9) in a patient with upper extremity dysfunction. It is also important that the etiology of the limitation be analyzed and thoroughly understood, thus providing proper direction for therapeutic intervention. Although goniometric measurement is not technically a standardized assessment tool, it does provide reliable and accurate information for which norms have been established.[1]

As an adjunct to the recording of individual joint motion, composite digital motion values may be computed as "total active motion" (TAM) and "total passive motion" (TPM).[2] TAM equals the sum of active flexion measurements of the metacarpophalangeal, proximal interphalangeal, and distal interphalangeal joints of a digit, minus the active extension deficits of the same three joints (Fig. 5-10). TPM is computed in a similar manner, except that passive flexion and extension measurements are used. In addition TAM and TPM are expressed as a single numerical value, "total motion," which reflects both the extension and the flexion capacities of a single digit and thus provides a comprehensive assessment of function. (Refer to Chapter 6 for further details.)

The determination of isolated muscle strength through manual muscle testing[17] (Fig. 5-11) may be used to evaluate

UPPER EXTREMITY ASSESSMENT BATTERY

RANGE OF MOTION

HAND

DATE: _____	THUMB	CHANGE +/−	INDEX	CHANGE +/−	LONG	CHANGE +/−	RING	CHANGE +/−	SMALL	CHANGE +/−
MP	( ) ( )	IP	( ) ( )	( ) ( )	( ) ( )	( ) ( )	( ) ( )
PIP	( ) ( )	CMC	( ) ( )	( ) ( )	( ) ( )	( ) ( )	( ) ( )
DIP	( ) ( )		( ) ( )	( ) ( )	( ) ( )	( ) ( )	( ) ( )
TAM (TPM)	( ) ( )		( ) ( )	( ) ( )	( ) ( )	( ) ( )	( ) ( )

DATE: _____	THUMB	CHANGE +/−	INDEX	CHANGE +/−	LONG	CHANGE +/−	RING	CHANGE +/−	SMALL	CHANGE +/−
MP	( ) ( )	IP	( ) ( )	( ) ( )	( ) ( )	( ) ( )	( ) ( )
PIP	( ) ( )	CMC	( ) ( )	( ) ( )	( ) ( )	( ) ( )	( ) ( )
DIP	( ) ( )		( ) ( )	( ) ( )	( ) ( )	( ) ( )	( ) ( )
TAM (TPM)	( ) ( )		( ) ( )	( ) ( )	( ) ( )	( ) ( )	( ) ( )

DATE: _____	THUMB	CHANGE +/−	INDEX	CHANGE +/−	LONG	CHANGE +/−	RING	CHANGE +/−	SMALL	CHANGE +/−
MP	( ) ( )	IP	( ) ( )	( ) ( )	( ) ( )	( ) ( )	( ) ( )
PIP	( ) ( )	CMC	( ) ( )	( ) ( )	( ) ( )	( ) ( )	( ) ( )
DIP	( ) ( )		( ) ( )	( ) ( )	( ) ( )	( ) ( )	( ) ( )
TAM (TPM)	( ) ( )		( ) ( )	( ) ( )	( ) ( )	( ) ( )	( ) ( )

KEY:

Active: extension/flexion

Passive: (extension/flexion)

Thumb CMC: adduction/abduction

Change: record in red

Name:_____

Number:_____

Hand:_____

FIG. 5-9. Active and passive range-of-motion and total-motion values should be recorded at appropriate intervals. Improvements or losses in motion may be expressed as plus or minus the amount of change, such as +15 or −5.

UPPER EXTREMITY ASSESSMENT BATTERY

RANGE OF MOTION

WRIST, FOREARM, ELBOW, SHOULDER

		DATE: ______	CHANGE +/-	DATE: ______	CHANGE +/-	DATE: ______	CHANGE +/-
WRIST	EXTENSION	( )	( )	( )	( )	( )	( )
	FLEXION	( )	( )	( )	( )	( )	( )
	RADIAL DEVIATION	( )	( )	( )	( )	( )	( )
	ULNAR DEVIATION	( )	( )	( )	( )	( )	( )
FOREARM	SUPINATION	( )	( )	( )	( )	( )	( )
	PRONATION	( )	( )	( )	( )	( )	( )
ELBOW	EXTENSION	( )	( )	( )	( )	( )	( )
	FLEXION	( )	( )	( )	( )	( )	( )
SHOULDER	EXTENSION	( )	( )	( )	( )	( )	( )
	FLEXION	( )	( )	( )	( )	( )	( )
	ABDUCTION	( )	( )	( )	( )	( )	( )
	INTERNAL ROTATION	( )	( )	( )	( )	( )	( )
	EXTERNAL ROTATION	( )	( )	( )	( )	( )	( )

KEY:
Active: #°
Passive: (#°)
Change: Record in red

Name: ______
Number: ______
Extremity: ______

FIG. 5-9, cont'd. For legend see opposite page.

DATE: 6-1-82	THUMB	CHANGE +/-	INDEX	CHANGE +/-	LONG	CHANGE +/-	RING	CHANGE +/-	SMALL	CHANGE +/-
MP	( )	( )	10/30 ( )	( )	( )	( )	( )	( )	( )	( )
PIP	IP ( )	( )	30/45 ( )	( )	( )	( )	( )	( )	( )	( )
DIP	CMC ( )	( )	0/75 ( )	( )	( )	( )	( )	( )	( )	( )
TAM (TPM)	( )	( )	110 ( )	( )	( )	( )	( )	( )	( )	( )

FIG. 5-10. Total motion provides a single numerical value for composite digital motion: summation of digit flexion (30 + 45 + 75 = 150); summation of digit-extension deficits (10 + 30 + 0 = 40); flexion sum minus extension deficit sum (150 − 40 = 110); total active motion of digit = 110 degrees.

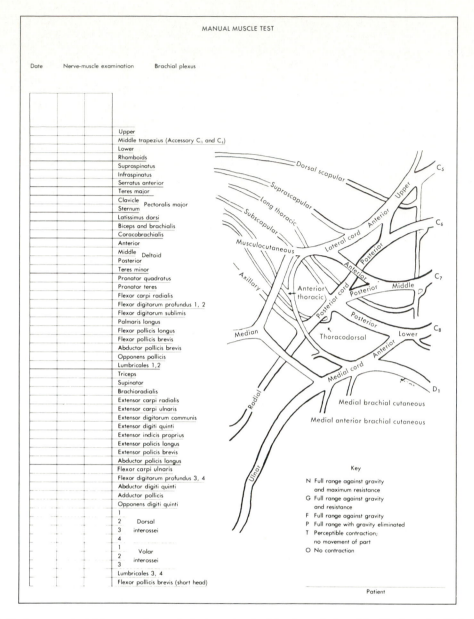

MANUAL MUSCLE TEST

Date   Nerve-muscle examination   Brachial plexus

Upper
Middle trapezius (Accessory C₃ and C₄)
Lower
Rhomboids
Supraspinatus
Infraspinatus
Serratus anterior
Teres major
Clavicle   Pectoralis major
Sternum
Latissimus dorsi
Biceps and brachialis
Coracobrachialis
Anterior
Middle   Deltoid
Posterior
Teres minor
Pronator quadratus
Pronator teres
Flexor carpi radialis
Flexor digitorum profundus 1, 2
Flexor digitorum sublimis
Palmaris longus
Flexor pollicis longus
Flexor pollicis brevis
Abductor pollicis brevis
Opponens pollicis
Lumbricales 1,2
Triceps
Supinator
Brachioradialis
Extensor carpi radialis
Extensor carpi ulnaris
Extensor digitorum communis
Extensor digiti quinti
Extensor indicis proprius
Extensor policis longus
Extensor policis brevis
Abductor policis longus
Flexor carpi ulnaris
Flexor digitorum profundus 3, 4
Abductor digiti quinti
Adductor pollicis
Opponens digiti quinti
1
2   Dorsal
3   interossei
4
1
2   Volar
3   interossei
Lumbricales 3, 4
Flexor pollicis brevis (short head)

Key
N Full range against gravity
   and maximum resistance
G Full range against gravity
   and resistance
F Full range against gravity
P Full range with gravity eliminated
T Perceptible contraction;
   no movement of part
O No contraction

Patient

FIG. 5-11. Basic concept of this manual muscle test was inspired by form designed by Dr. Lorraine F. Lake, Ph.D., Assistant Professor of Physical Therapy and Anatomy and Associate Director of Irene Walter Johnson Institute of Rehabilitation Medicine, Washington University School of Medicine, St. Louis, Mo.

peripheral nerve lesions and the regeneration of nerves after injuries, and for preoperative evaluation for potential tendon transfers. Although criteria for grading muscle strength have been improved, eliminating much of the chance for subjective error, portions of the test continue to be subject to interpretation by the examiner. To increase interrater reliability, concentrated efforts should be made to establish a common method of conducting and interpreting manual muscle examinations. Various grading systems exist, but the two most frequently used are a numerical system (from 0 to 5) established by Seddon[32] and the ratings of "zero," "trace," "poor," "fair," "good," and "normal," recommended by the Committee on After-Effects, National Foundation for Infantile Paralysis.[17] The latter is further refined by a plus-minus system, involving the determination of half-ranges. It is important to note that because of fluctuation of muscle tone and altered reflex activity, testing of isolated muscle strength is of little value in upper motor neuron lesions such as cerebral palsy or cerebrovascular accidents.

Sensibility assessment instruments

Volitional participation is required for motor, sensibility, and dexterity testing, but the problem is compounded in the assessment of sensibility because the stimulus, when received, is also interpreted by the patient, resulting in test information that is vulnerable to bias. Although the majority of patients are cooperative occasions arise when one is dealing with children, patients who have language problems or who exhibit mental confusion, or patients whose motives may be suspect, in which the use of a test that relies on sudomotor or sympathetic response may be helpful.[23,32,35]

The ninhydrin test identifies areas of disturbance of sweat secretion after peripheral nerve disruption. Because of the involvement of sympathetic fibers in a peripheral nerve injury, denervated skin does not produce a sweat reaction, resulting in dry skin in the distribution area of the involved nerve. Ninhydrin spray is a clear colorimetric agent that turns purple when it reacts with a small concentration of sweat. Unfortunately, sympathetic return after a peripheral nerve injury is variable, and on long-term follow-up sudomotor response does not correlate with sensibility return.[25]

The wrinkle test[26] is based on a similar concept of sympathetic fiber involvement in peripheral nerve injuries, in that denervated palmar skin, as opposed to normal skin, does not wrinkle when soaked in warm water. As with sweating, palmar wrinkling has diminishing correlation to sensory function as the postinjury period increases, and has no correlation to sensory capacity in nerve compression injuries.[27] Inclusion of a sympathetic response test in an assessment battery (Fig. 5-12) for use with specific patients is helpful, but it should not be relied upon as a primary sensibility assessment instrument.

The ability to detect a punctate stimulus is the initial and most simple level of function in the hierarchy of sensibility capacity of the hand. *Detection* requires that the patient be able to distinguish a single-point stimulus from normally occurring atmospheric background stimuli. The normal touch force threshold (using Semmes-Weinstein monofilaments[33]) (Figs. 5-13 and 5-14) is considered to be approximately 4.86 gm/sq mm (note: this is pressure, not force); to be completely valid, a touch force assessment instrument should be able to produce stimuli that measure less than the normal threshold level. As testing instruments the monofilaments are unique in their abilities to actually control the amount of force applied, and as such are important to the hand specialist's assessment armamentarium[4] (Fig. 5-15). Although the monofilaments produce the most sensitive and reliable data of all the clinical sensibility assessment instruments currently available, they are not without problems, including variance in tip geometry,[5] force changes with atmospheric conditions,[20,22] and discrepancies between filament sets.[20]

The Dellon-Curtis evaluation[11] consists of four categories, which assess moving touch, constant touch, flutter (30 cps vibration), and vibration (256 cps vibration). Controversy exists concerning this examination, with some neurophysiologists and neurologists questioning the use of vibration, because of a lack of stimulus specificity, to evaluate nerve status in a relatively small and confined space such as the hand.[12,19] Physicists also report that the use of a tuning fork in attitudes other than perpendicular to the surface of application changes the fine harmonic vibratory stimulus to a compression stimulus,[22] which may elicit a pain response.

Discrimination is the second level in the sensibility assessment continuum. The ability to perceive that stimulus A differs from stimulus B involves the capacity to detect each stimulus as a separate entity and to distinguish between

them. Discrimination requires finer reception acuity and more judgment on the part of the patient than does detection, which is the first level in the continuum.

The two-point discrimination test[2,34] is the most commonly used method of assessing sensibility of the hand. In the performance of the test, there is some disagreement as to whether it is preferable to begin the test with a great distance or a small distance between the two points, and the number of correct responses required varies slightly among examiners. Moving two-point discrimination, described by Dellon,[10] adds the variable of motion to the test.

The two-point discrimination tests have some problems in regard to instrumentation criteria. Bell and Buford[6] found that even among experienced hand surgeons and therapists, the differences between the amount of force applied to the one point and that applied to two points easily exceeded the resolution or sensitivity threshold for normal sensation (Fig. 5-16). They also discovered that because of the varying pressures applied, interrater reliability was poor, perhaps explaining the lack of agreement in reporting, and the multiplicity of current clinical sensibility assessment tools.

The Ridge device[28,30] introduces the important concept of control of the amount of tissue displacement instead of control of applied force. Sensibility instruments should control either the force variable or the displacement variable; and while most aesthesiometers are oriented toward regulation of force, the ridge device is unique among currently available assessment tools because of its displacement design. Consisting of a rectangular piece of plastic, from the center of which a narrow ridge gradually rises to a height of 1.5 mm, the ridge device is felt to be useful in identifying patients whose two-point discrimination is between 8 mm and 12 mm. Instrumentation problems with the ridge device include validity and reliability issues. Renfrew[30] reported that intelligence directly skewed test results, with more intelligent patients achieving better scores. Additionally, a lack of specificity relating to measurement of the amount of tissue deformation is a detracting factor, in that the ridge rises from 0 to 1.5 mm without interruption, significantly decreasing the potential for accuracy and precision of readings and thus limiting interrater reliability.

Quantification is the third level of the sensory capacity; it involves the organizing of tactile stimuli according to degree. For example, a patient may be asked which of several alternatives is roughest, most irregular, or smoothest. Recognition, the final and most complicated sensibility level, is the ability to identify objects. Currently there are no sensibility instruments specific to these two areas, although some of the sensory reeducation methods that are used as treatment techniques incorporate the basic concepts of quantification and recognition.

The Moberg picking-up test[23] requires the patient to pick up a series of 10 to 12 small objects of various sizes from a table surface and place them in a small container, using first the normal hand and then the symptomatic hand. The picking-up test, which may be adapted to include recognition variables, is an excellent example of a timed observational test in which the patient is his own normal.

The major problem in assessing sensibility is cortical

Text continued on p. 74.

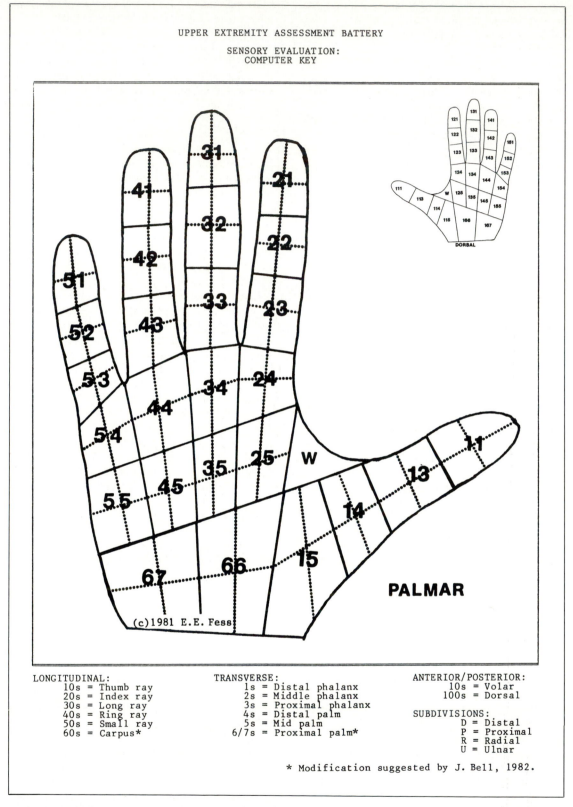

UPPER EXTREMITY ASSESSMENT BATTERY

SENSORY EVALUATION:
COMPUTER KEY

PALMAR

(c)1981 E.E. Fess

DORSAL

LONGITUDINAL:	TRANSVERSE:	ANTERIOR/POSTERIOR:
10s = Thumb ray	1s = Distal phalanx	10s = Volar
20s = Index ray	2s = Middle phalanx	100s = Dorsal
30s = Long ray	3s = Proximal phalanx	
40s = Ring ray	4s = Distal palm	SUBDIVISIONS:
50s = Small ray	5s = Mid palm	D = Distal
60s = Carpus*	6/7s = Proximal palm*	P = Proximal
		R = Radial
		U = Ulnar

* Modification suggested by J. Bell, 1982.

FIG. 5-12. A range of sensibility tests provides a more thorough understanding of the level of dysfunction.

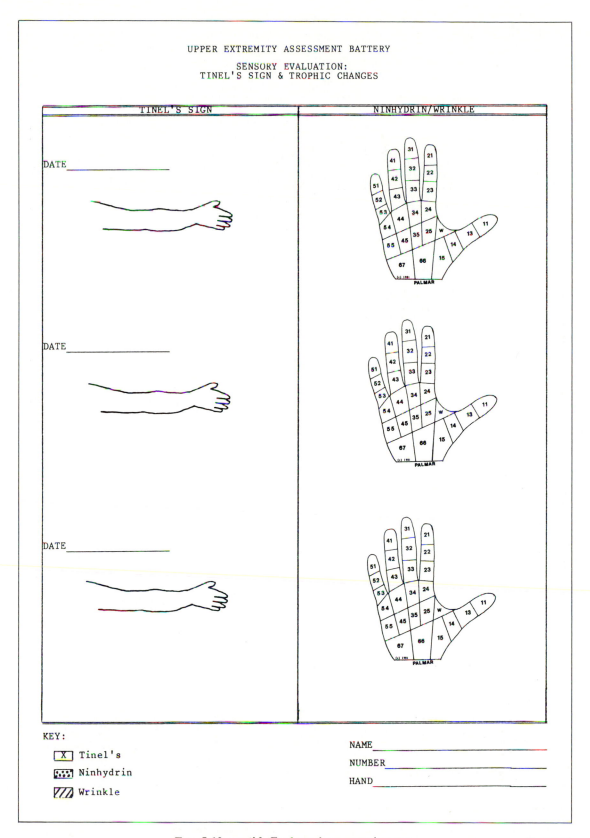

FIG. 5-12, cont'd. For legend see opposite page.   *Continued.*

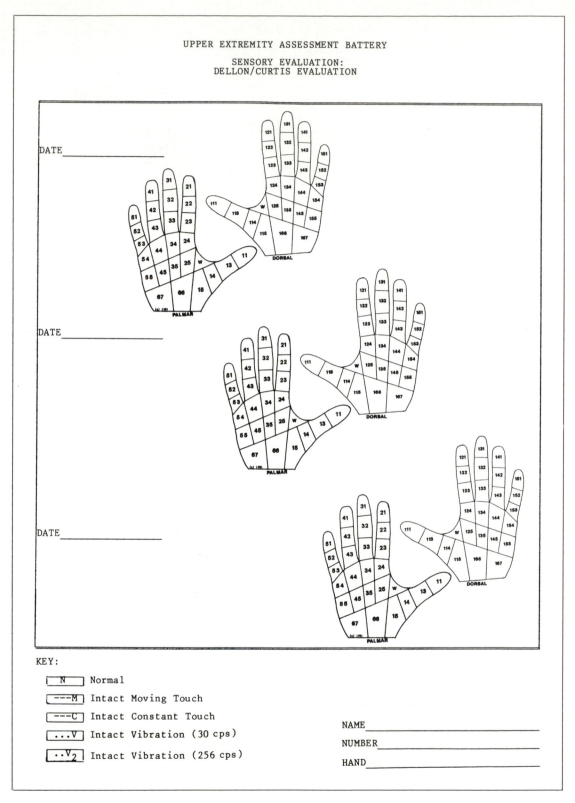

UPPER EXTREMITY ASSESSMENT BATTERY

SENSORY EVALUATION:
DELLON/CURTIS EVALUATION

DATE_____

DATE_____

DATE_____

KEY:

N	Normal
---M	Intact Moving Touch
---C	Intact Constant Touch
...V	Intact Vibration (30 cps)
..V₂	Intact Vibration (256 cps)

NAME_____

NUMBER_____

HAND_____

FIG. 5-12, cont'd. For legend see p. 66.

UPPER EXTREMITY ASSESSMENT BATTERY

SENSORY EVALUATION:
SEMMES-WEINSTEIN CALIBRATED MONOFILAMENTS

PALMAR/DORSAL (circle):

DATE:	THUMB 1		INDEX 2		LONG 3		RING 4		SMALL 5	
	U	R	U	R	U	R	U	R	U	R
1										
2										
3										
4										
5										
6/7	///		6				6			

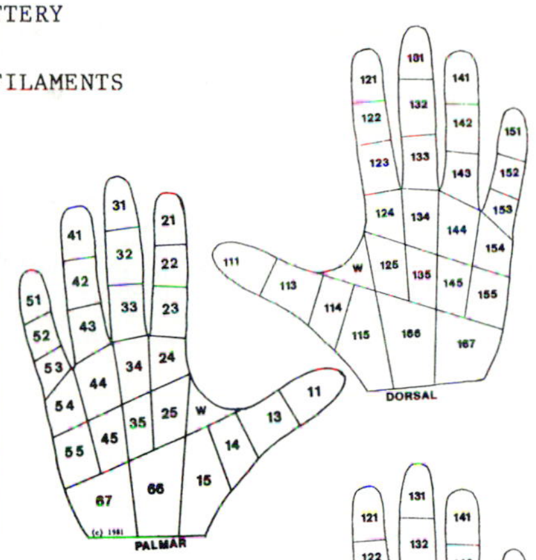

PALMAR/DORSAL (circle):

DATE:	THUMB 1		INDEX 2		LONG 3		RING 4		SMALL 5	
	U	R	U	R	U	R	U	R	U	R
1										
2										
3										
4										
5										
6/7	///		6				6			

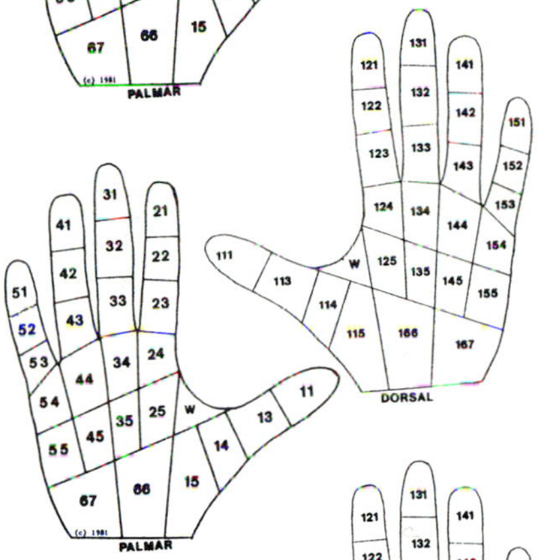

PALMAR/DORSAL (circle):

DATE:	THUMB 1		INDEX 2		LONG 3		RING 4		SMALL 5	
	U	R	U	R	U	R	U	R	U	R
1										
2										
3										
4										
5										
6/7	///		6				6			

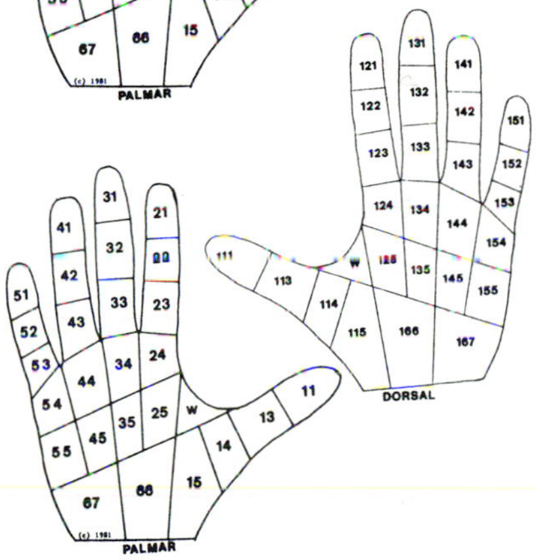

KEY:*

		Filament	Pressure (gm/mm^2)
	Normal	1.65-2.83	1.45- 4.86
Blue	Diminished light touch	3.22-3.61	11.1 - 17.7
Purple	Diminished protective sensation	3.84-4.31	19.3 - 33.1
Red	Loss of protective sensation	4.56-6.65	47.3 -439.0
Red-lined	Untestable	6.65	439.0

*Levine, S., Pearsall, G., & Ruderman, R.: J Hand Surg, 3:211, 1978.

NAME _____

NUMBER _____

HAND _____

Continued.

FIG. 5-12, cont'd. For legend see p. 66.

UPPER EXTREMITY ASSESSMENT BATTERY

SENSORY EVALUATION:
2 POINT DISCRIMINATION

PALMAR/DORSAL (circle):

DATE:	THUMB 1		INDEX 2		LONG 3		RING 4		SMALL 5	
	U	R	U	R	U	R	U	R	U	R
1										
2										
3										
4										
5										
6/7	/////		6				6			

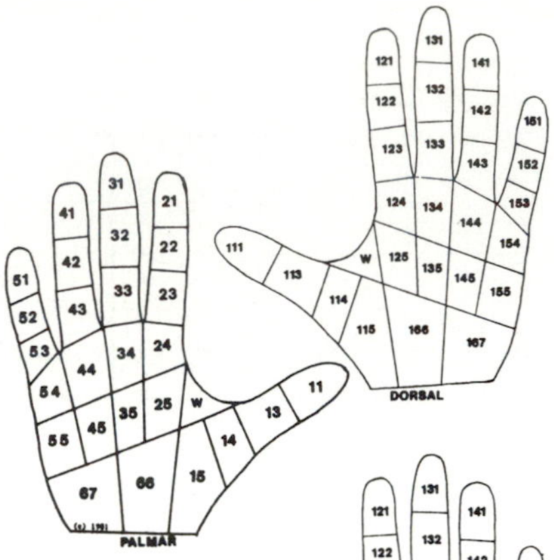

PALMAR/DORSAL (circle):

DATE:	THUMB 1		INDEX 2		LONG 3		RING 4		SMALL 5	
	U	R	U	R	U	R	U	R	U	R
1										
2										
3										
4										
5										
6/7	/////		6				6			

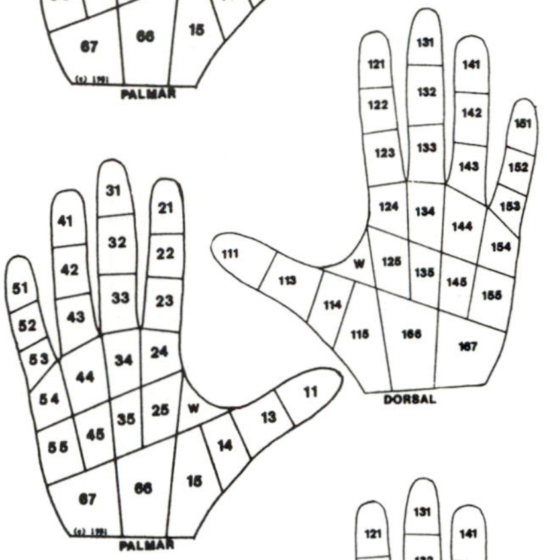

PALMAR/DORSAL (circle):

DATE:	THUMB 1		INDEX 2		LONG 3		RING 4		SMALL 5	
	U	R	U	R	U	R	U	R	U	R
1										
2										
3										
4										
5										
6/7	/////		6				6			

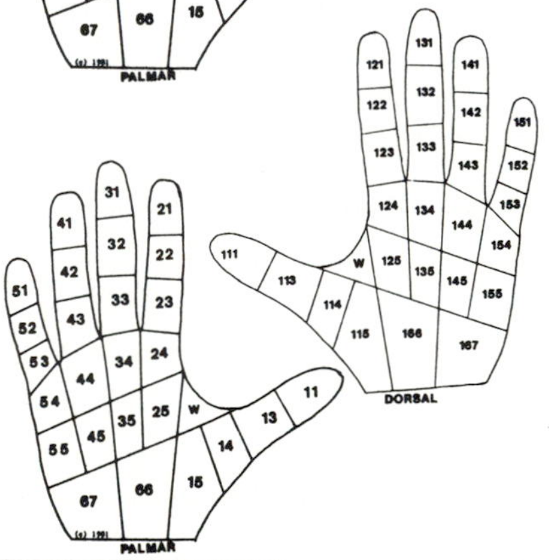

KEY:*

	Normal	Less than 6mm
Blue	Fair	6-10 mm
Purple	Poor	11-15 mm
Orange	Protective	One point perceived
Orange-lined	Anesthetic	No point perceived

*ASSH: The hand — examination and diagnosis, Aurora, Colorado, 1978.

NAME_____

NUMBER_____

HAND_____

FIG.5-12, cont'd. For legend see p. 66.

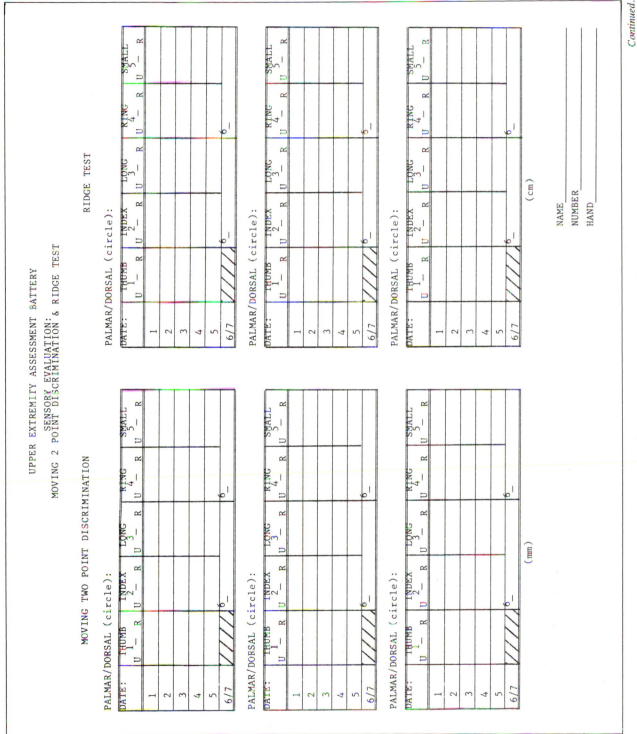

FIG. 5-12, cont'd. For legend see p. 66.

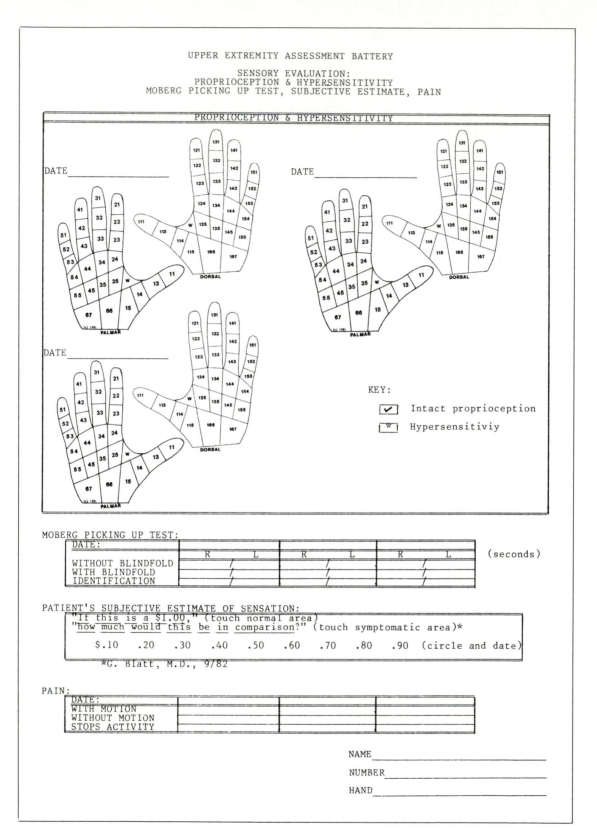

UPPER EXTREMITY ASSESSMENT BATTERY

SENSORY EVALUATION:
PROPRIOCEPTION & HYPERSENSITIVITY
MOBERG PICKING UP TEST, SUBJECTIVE ESTIMATE, PAIN

PROPRIOCEPTION & HYPERSENSITIVITY

DATE_____

DATE_____

DATE_____

KEY:

| ✓ | Intact proprioception |
| * | Hypersensitiviy |

MOBERG PICKING UP TEST:

DATE:							
	R	L	R	L	R	L	(seconds)
WITHOUT BLINDFOLD							
WITH BLINDFOLD							
IDENTIFICATION							

PATIENT'S SUBJECTIVE ESTIMATE OF SENSATION:
"If this is a $1.00," (touch normal area)
"how much would this be in comparison?" (touch symptomatic area)*

$.10   .20   .30   .40   .50   .60   .70   .80   .90   (circle and date)

*G. Blatt, M.D., 9/82

PAIN:

DATE:			
WITH MOTION			
WITHOUT MOTION			
STOPS ACTIVITY			

NAME_____

NUMBER_____

HAND_____

FIG. 5-12, cont'd. For legend see p. 66.

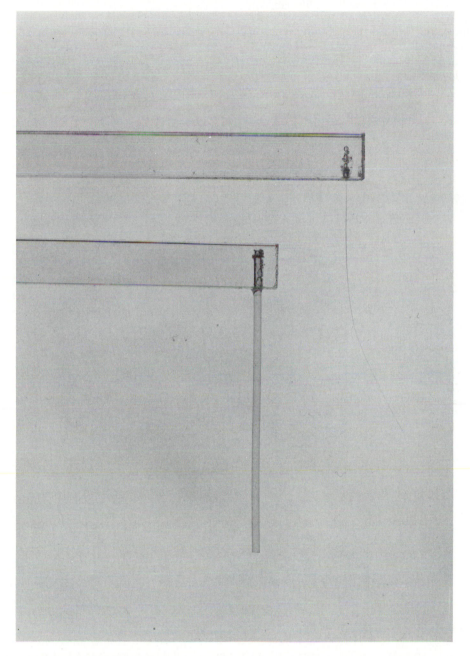

FIG. 5-13. The 20 Semmes-Weinstein calibrated monofilaments are graded in diameter, producing a large range of touch pressure (smallest and largest filaments).

modification of thresholds. With the exception of the sudomotor tests, all of the clinical sensibility evaluation instruments currently available have the potential for producing subjective, biased information. Another variable is callous formation (Fig. 5-17) or the hardness of the cutaneous surface. Influencing the amount of force transferred to sensory receptors, keratin layers decrease the applied force of a stimulus by increasing the area of force application. Therefore, the patient's occupation becomes a factor in the assessment of hand sensibility. Age and intelligence should also be considered. In addition, recent studies indicate that specific receptors cannot be isolated with the unrefined assessment instruments of today's technology.[6,12]

Sensibility assessment instrumentation is in an early developmental phase. Representing a final frontier that should be given a high priority, the generation of instruments that better evaluate sensibility of the hand will significantly influence the scope and direction of the profession in the next several decades. The inherent properties of instruments, current and future, must be analyzed and evaluated in terms of statistical reliability and validity. In order to progress, we must first be able to measure. In order to measure, we must look carefully at our tools. (Refer to Chapters 34, 35, and 36 for specific test protocols.)

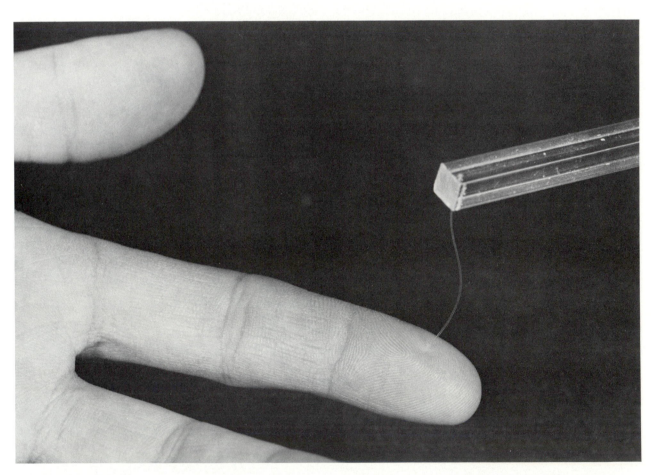

FIG. 5-14. The monofilament collapses when a given force, dependent on filament diameter, is reached, controlling the magnitude of applied touch pressure.

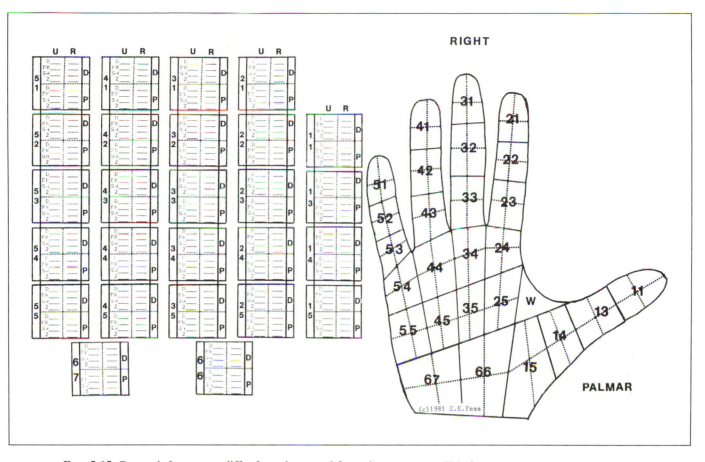

FIG. 5-15. Research forms may differ from those used for patient treatment. This form, used for a sensibility instrumentation study, requires explicit data on four instruments. Data from follow-up evaluations for research are often recorded on separate forms, while clinical follow-up data are included in an adjacent area on the form used for the initial evaluation.

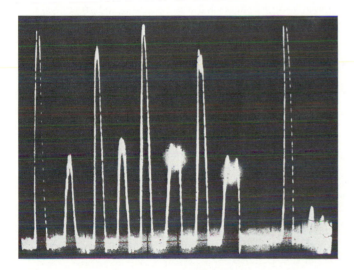

FIG. 5-16. Monitoring the applied force between one and two points, a transducer and oscilloscope graphically show the discrepancies in amount of force applied between one and two points in a two-point discrimination test by an experienced hand specialist using skin deformation and lack of blanching as clinical criteria. (Courtesy Judith A. Bell and W. Buford, Carville, La.)

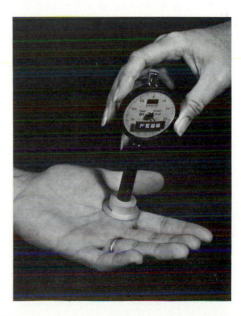

FIG. 5-17. A search for an instrument that will measure skin hardness involves instrumentation studies for reliability and validity.

Function assessment instruments

Grip strength may be measured with a commercially available hydraulic dynamometer (Fig. 5-18). Developed by Bechtol[3] and recommended in a study of grip assessment instruments by the California Medical Association,[18] the Jamar dynamometer has been shown to be a reliable test instrument.[3,18,31] Schmidt and Toews[31] reported proportional correlations between grip strength and height, weight, and age, and noted that the grip strength of the minor hand was equal to or stronger than that of the dominant hand in 28% of the normal population. Pryce[29] studied the effects of wrist position on grip strength and found that the strongest grips occurred with the wrist in 0° to 15° extension. In 1978 the Clinical Assessment Committee of the American Society for Surgery of the Hand recommended that the second handle position be used in determining grip strength and that the average of three trials be recorded[2] (Fig. 5-19). Fatigue has been shown not to be an influencing factor in protocols using the three-trial system with multiple handle readings, if a 5-minute rest is provided after completion of each three-trial series.[13] Of significant importance is the concept that grip strength changes according to the size of the object being grasped. Normal adult grip values for the five consecutive handle positions consistently create a bell-shaped curve, with the first position being the least advantageous for strong grip, followed by the fifth and fourth positions; the strongest grip values occur at the third and second handle positions.[3,13,24] If inconsistent handle positions are used to assess patient progress, normal alterations in grip readings may be erroneously interpreted as advances or declines in progress. Knowledge of this normal grip curve may also be of assistance in identifying patients whose motivation is questionable. Stokes and Murray[24] describe a clinical cor-respondence between ''flat'' handle position curves and patients who were found to have ''significant personality problems.''

The Jaymar's capacity as an evaluation instrument, the effects of protocol, and the ramifications of the instrument's use have been analyzed by many investigators over the years. Although not a standardized assessment tool, it does provide consistent and accurate information, when calibration is maintained. A major drawback is the lack of large population norms for the commercially available model. Unfortunately, the Schmidt-Toews study of 1200 subjects was based on Jaymar dynamometers that were altered with an application of a sand-paint mixture to the handles. This invalidates the use of the resultant norms, except when compared with values from a similarly altered dynamometer.

Pinch strength may be measured with a commercially available pinchometer. Three types of pinch are usually assessed: (1) prehension of the thumb pulp to the lateral aspect of the index middle phalanx (key, lateral, or pulp-to-side); (2) pulp of the thumb to pulps of the index and long fingers (three-jaw chuck, three-point chuck); and (3) thumb tip to the tip of index finger (tip-to-tip). Lateral is the strongest of the three types of pinch, followed by three-jaw chuck. Tip-to-tip is a positioning pinch used in activities requiring fine coordination rather than power. As with grip measurements, the mean value of three trials is recorded, and comparisons are made with the opposite hand.

Standardized tests for assessing manual dexterity and coordination are available in several levels of difficulty, allowing the examiner to screen and choose instruments that best suit the needs and abilities of individual patients. When a standardized instrument is being used, it is imperative not to deviate from the method, equipment, and sequencing delineated in the test instructions. The calibration, reliability, and validity of the test are determined using defined items and techniques, and any change in the stipulated pattern renders the resultant information invalid and meaningless. Utilizing a standardized test as a teaching or training device in therapy also excludes its use as an assessment instrument, because of skewing of data.

Of the tests available, the Jebson[16] hand function test requires the least amount of extremity coordination, and it is inexpensive to assemble and easy to administer and score. The test consists of seven subtests: (1) writing, (2) card turning, (3) picking up small objects, (4) simulated feeding, (5) stacking, (6) picking up large light-weight objects, and (7) picking up large heavy objects. The Jebson norms are categorized according to maximum time, hand dominance, age, and sex. The capacity to measure gross coordination makes this test an excellent instrument to assess individuals whose severity of involvement precludes the use of many of the other coordination tests, which often require very fine prehension patterns.

Based on placing blocks into spaces on a board, the Minnesota Rate of Manipulation Tests (MRMT) include five activities: (1) placing, (2) turning, (3) displacing, (4) one-hand turning and placing, and (5) two-hand turning and placing. The MRMT, originally designed for assessment of personnel for jobs requiring arm-hand dexterity, is another

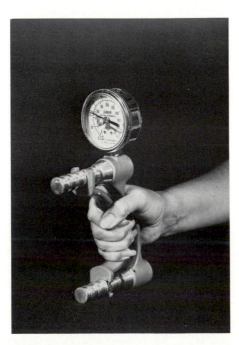

FIG. 5-18. The Jaymar dynamometer provides reliable and accurate measurement of grip strength.

excellent example of a test that measures gross coordination and dexterity, making it applicable to many of the needs encountered in hand rehabilitation. The norms of this instrument are based on more than 11,000 subjects.

Requiring prehension of small pins, washers, and collars, the Purdue Pegboard[36] evaluates finer coordination than the previously discussed instruments. This test's assessment categories are (1) right hand, (2) left hand, (3) both hands, (4) right, left, and both, and (5) assembly. The normative data are presented in categories based on sex and type of job: male and female applicants for assembly jobs, male and female applicants for general factory work, female applicants for electronics production work, male utility service workers, and so on.

In terms of a psychomotor taxonomy, all of the previously described tests assess activities that are classified as skilled movements. Evaluating compound adaptive skills, the Crawford Small Parts Dexterity Test adds another dimension to hand function assessment by introducing tools into the test protocol. Increasing the level of difficulty, this test requires subjects to control implements in addition to their hands. The test involves the use of tweezers and screwdriver to assemble pins, collars, and small screws on the test board. This test is related to activities requiring very fine coordination, such as engraving and the assembly or adjustment of clocks, watches, office machines, and other intricate devices.

Other hand coordination and dexterity testing instruments are available. These should be carefully evaluated in terms of the criteria for standardization previously outlined in this chapter, to ensure that they have been proved to measure appropriately and accurately. Although many tests claim to be standardized, close scrutiny often indicates that they are not. (Refer to Chapter 7.)

The extent to which activities of daily living are assessed depends on the type of clientele treated by the particular rehabilitation center. In a situation oriented toward treatment of trauma injuries, the need for extensive ADL evaluation and training would not be as great as it would in a center whose case load consisted primarily of arthritic patients. To date, ADL tests have not been standardized, and they are limited to observational types of tests, the results of which may be quantified by timing specific tasks. A general ADL test may easily be refined to include only those activities that require the use of the upper extremities. If this is done, however, it is important to make provisions for assessment and treatment of lower extremity problems noted during the course of the test.

Assessment of a patient's potential to return to work is generally based on a combination of standardized and observational tests, knowledge of the specific work situation, insight into the patient's motivational and psychological references, and understanding of the complexities of normal and disabled hands in general. Although its importance has been acknowledged in the past, vocational assessment of the upper extremity injury patient is being given a higher priority in many of the major hand centers in the country. Treatment no longer ends with the achievement of skeletal stability, wound healing, and a plateau of motion and sensibility. This shift in emphasis has been due, in large part, to the contributions of the Hand Rehabilitation Center in Philadelphia, and to the hand therapist who is in charge of its physical capacity area, Patricia Baxter, O.T.R. Chapters 7 and 84 in this book describes the specific programs that she has been instrumental in developing.

CONCLUSION

Evaluation with instruments that measure accurately allows physicians and therapists to correctly identify hand pathology and dysfunction, assess the effects of treatment, and realistically apprise patients of their progress. Accurate assessment data also permit analysis of treatment modalities for effectiveness, provide a foundation for professional communication through research, and eventually influence the scope and direction of the profession as a whole. Because of their relationship to the kind of information obtained, assessment tools cannot be chosen irresponsibly, for the choice of tools will directly influence the quality of individual treatment and the quality of understanding between hand specialists. Criteria exist for identifying instruments that can be depended upon to measure accurately when used by different evaluators, and from session to session. Unless the results of a "home-brewed" test are statistically analyzed, the test is tried on large numbers of normal subjects, and the results are analyzed again, it is naive to assume that such a test provides meaningful information. Current tools may be better understood by checking their reliability and validity levels with bioengineering technology, and statisticians may be of assistance in devising protocols that will lead to more refined and accurate information. We as hand specialists have a responsibility to our patients and to our colleagues to continue to critique the instruments we use in terms of their capacities as measurement tools. Without assessment, we cannot treat, we cannot communicate, and we cannot progress.

REFERENCES

1. American Academy of Orthopedic Surgeons: Joint motion—method of measuring and recording, Chicago, 1965, The Academy.
2. American Society for Surgery of the Hand: The hand—examination and diagnosis, Aurora, Colorado, 1978, The Society.
3. Bechtol, C.D.: Grip test: use of a dynamometer with adjustable handle spacing, J. Bone Joint Surg. **36A:**820, 1954.
4. Bell, J.: Sensibility evaluation. In Hunter, J., Schneider, L., Mackin, E., and Bell, J., editors: Rehabilitation of the hand, St. Louis, 1978, The C.V. Mosby Co.
5. Bell, J.: Symposium: assessment of levels of cutaneous sensibility, United States Public Health Service Hospital, Carville, Louisiana, 1980.
6. Bell, J., and Buford, W.: The force/time relationship of clinically used sensory testing instruments. Presented at the thirty-seventh annual meeting of the American Society for Surgery of the Hand, New Orleans, 1982.
7. Brand, P., and Wood, H.: Hand volumeter instruction sheet, U.S. Public Health Service Hospital, Carville, Louisiana.
8. Bright, D., and Wright, S.: Postoperative management in replantation. In American Academy of Orthopedic Surgeons: Symposium on microsurgery: practical use in orthopaedics, St. Louis, 1979, The C.V. Mosby Co.
9. Creelnan, G.: Report on hand volumeter—accuracy and sensitivity of measurements, Idyllwild, Calif., 1979, Engraving Experts, Medical Supply Division.
10. Dellon, A.: The moving two-point discrimination test: clinical evaluation of the quickly-adapting fiber receptor system, J. Hand Surg. **3:**474, 1978.

11. Dellon, A., Curtis, R., and Edgerton, M.: Reeducation of sensation in the hand after nerve injury and repair, Plast. Reconstr. Surg. **53:**297, 1974.

12. Dyck, P.J., O'Brien, P.C., Bushek, W., and others: Clinical vs quantitative evaluation of cutaneous sensation, Arch. Neurol. **33:**651, 1976.

13. Fess, E.: The effects of Jaymar dynamometer handle position and test protocol on normal grip strength, Proceedings of the American Society of Hand Therapists, J. Hand Surg. **7:**308, 1982.

14. Fess, E., and Moran, C.: Clinical assessment recommendations, Indianapolis, 1981, American Society of Hand Therapists.

15. Hines, M., and O'Connor, J.: A measure of finger dexterity, Personnel J. **4:**379, 1926.

16. Jebson, R., Taylor, N., Triegchmann, R., and others: An objective and standardized test of hand function, Arch. Phys. Med. Rehabit. **50:**311, 1969.

17. Kendall, H., Kendall, F., and Wadsworth, G.: Muscle testing and function, Baltimore, 1971, The Williams & Wilkins Co.

18. Kirkpatrick, J.: Evaluation of grip loss: a factor of permanent partial disability in California, Industr. Med. Surg. **26:**285, 1957.

19. LaMotte, R.: Symposium: assessment of levels of cutaneous sensibility, United States Public Health Service Hospital, Carville, Louisiana, 1980.

20. Levin, S., Pearsall, C., and Ruderman, R.: Von Frey's method of measuring pressure sensibility in the hand: an engineering analysis of the Weinstein-Semmes pressure aesthesiometer, J. Hand Surg. **3:**211, 1978.

21. Madden, J., and Arem, A.: Wound healing: biologic and clinical features. In Sabiston, J.: Davis-Christopher textbook of surgery, ed. 12, Philadelphia, 1981, W.B. Saunders Co.

22. Mitchell, E.: Symposium: assessment of levels of cutaneous sensibility, United States Public Health Service Hospital, Carville, Louisiana, 1980.

23. Moberg, E.: Objective methods of determining the functional value of sensibility in the hand, J. Bone Joint Surg. **40B:**454, 1958.

24. Murray, J.: The patient with the injured hand. Presidential address, American Society for Surgery of the Hand, J. Hand Surg. **7:**543, 1982.

25. Onne, L.: Recovery of sensibility and sudomotor activity in the hand after severe injury, Acta Chir. Scand. [Suppl.]:300, 1962.

26. O'Rain, S.: New and simple test for nerve function in the hand, Br. Med. J. **3:**615, 1973.

27. Phelps, P., and Walker, E.: Comparison of the finger wrinkling test results to establish sensory tests in peripheral nerve injury, Am. J. Occup. Ther. **31:**565, 1977.

28. Poppen, N., and others: Recovery of sensibility after suture of digital nerves, J. Hand Surg. **4:**212, 1979.

29. Pryce, J.: The wrist position between neutral and ulnar deviation that facilitates maximum power grip strength, J. Biomech. **13:**505, 1980.

30. Renfrew, S.: Fingertip sensation: a routine neurological test, Lancet **1:**396, 1969.

31. Schmidt, R., and Toews, J.: Grip strength as measured by the jaymar dynamometer, Arch. Phys. Med. Rehabil., June 1970, p. 321.

32. Seddon, H.: Surgical disorders of the peripheral nerves, ed. 2, New York, 1975, Churchill Livingstone.

33. Semmes, J., Weinstein, S., Ghent, L., and Teaber, H.L.: Somatosensory changes after penetrating brain wounds in man, Cambridge, 1960, Harvard University Press.

34. Smith, R.: Clinical examination. In Lamb, D., and Kuezynski, K., editors: The practice of hand surgery, Boston, 1981, Blackwell Scientific Publications, Inc.

35. Sunderland, S.: Nerves and nerve injuries, ed. 2, New York, 1978, Churchill Livingstone.

36. Tiffin, J., and Asher, E.: The Purdue Pegboard: norms and studies of reliability and validity, J. Appl. Psychol. **32:**234, 1948.

37. Waylett, J., and Seibly, D.: A study to determine the average deviation accuracy of a commercially available volumeter. J. Hand Surg. **6:**300, 1981.

38. Weber, E.: Data cited by Sherrington, C.S., in Shafer's textbook of physiology, Edinburgh, 1900, Young, J., Pentland.

6

Range-of-motion measurements of the hand

CATHERINE A. CAMBRIDGE

Rarely, if ever, is assessment of hand function discussed without some reference to the range of motion (ROM) of the involved extremity. In *Rehabilitation of the hand,* both chapters on evaluation included range of motion as essential components.[4,19] Swanson and others relied significantly on limitation of motion in assessing impairment of the hand.[2] Fess and others gave range of motion prominence in their chapter, ''Evaluation of the Hand by Objective Measurement.''[4] In *The Hand—Examination and Diagnosis,* by the American Society for Surgery of the Hand, and in *Clinical Assessment Recommendations,* published by the American Society of Hand Therapists, joint motion measurements are given considerable consideration.[5,7] Why? Because range of motion is considered by many clinicians to be a measurable, definable entity. Norms for motion of the various joints have been established in *Joint Motion: Method of Measuring and Recording,* allowing the examiner to compare readily the involved joint with the patient's own uninvolved contralateral joint or established values.[12]

But is the range of motion really reliable as an assessment tool? Does it really meet the criteria of being objective, measurable, and unbiased? Is the use of a goniometer necessary or are estimated motion measurements as reliable?[12] If a goniometer is used, does dorsal or lateral positioning change the measurement? Many such questions arise when health professionals involved in evaluation and treatment of patients with hand injuries discuss the role of range-of-motion measurements. One needs to answer these questions to determine the role of range of motion in the battery of assessment tools available to help evaluate the injured hand. My goal in this chapter is to address some of the questions about range of motion and to describe some of the more common methods used to determine range of motion in the hand and wrist.

REVIEW OF THE LITERATURE
Range of motion—examiner estimation versus use of a goniometer

Opinions about the importance of the use of a goniometer in measuring joint range of motion vary.[13,14] In the literature little information was found comparing the accuracy of joint motion measured with and without a goniometer. In *Joint Motion: Method of Measuring and Recording,* the use of a goniometer is left up to the surgeon's discretion.[12] In *The Reliability of Joint Measurement,* 50 examiners estimated

and then measured a fully flexed elbow and a completely extended wrist. The mean error in estimated elbow flexion was 9.3 degrees, compared to a 5-degree mean error in measured flexion. The mean estimated error for wrist extension was 12.8 degrees, with the measured mean error being 7.8 degrees.[13] No statistical analysis was completed to determine the level of significance of the variances. More research needs to be done before any firm conclusions can be reached, but the indication from this starting point is that reliability is improved by use of a goniometer, at least at the wrist and elbow.

The reliability of range-of-motion measurements made with a goniometer has been assessed by more researchers than the previous topic. One of the earlier works was ''Reliability of Goniometry,'' which found that a skilled observer varied 3 degrees or less in 70% of his or her measurements and 7 degrees or less in 95% of measurements when 780 paired observations were compared. The eight representative physical therapists used were found to be within 7 degrees or less of their first measurements in duplicate trials in 62% to 72% of their observations. Statistical comparisons showed the average therapist to be reliable in duplicating measurements made by a highly skilled observer.[8] Hamilton and Lachenbruch also found a statistically significant level of reliability among investigators measuring the joint motion of the metacarpophalangeal (MP), proximal interphalangeal (PIP), and distal interphalangeal (DIP) joints of the hand.[6] ''Reliability of Goniometric Measurements,'' by Boone and co-workers, compared four testers' measurements taken at the shoulder, elbow, and wrist and the hip, knee, and foot. They found reliability was greater for the three upper extremity movements than for the lower extremity movements. Their upper-extremity-motions intratester reliability compared favorably with the earlier work by Hellebrandt and others, ''*Reliability of Goniometry.*''[1,8]

Lateral goniometer placement compared to dorsal goniometer placement

Only one study that compared lateral and dorsal goniometric measurements of the hand was found. Hamilton and Lackenbruch investigated three types of goniometers: a 180-degree finger goniometer for dorsal placement, a 360-degree universal goniometer for lateral placement, and a pendulum type of goniometer that is also placed dorsally on the digit. Statistical analysis indicated equal reliability among all three goniometers. The authors then discussed factors such as edema and deformity that would influence the choice of instrument and may make one type more reliable than another given such complications. Choice of lateral or dorsal placement should be based on the experience of the tester and considerations of the injury, such as edema, dressing, and deformity.[6]

Intratester error compared to intertester error

The four studies previously mentioned were in agreement that the margin of error was greater when more than one tester was used to measure range of motion on the same patient.[1,6,8,13]

The intertester error averaged for measurement of the shoulder, elbow, and wrist by Boone and co-workers was comparable to the Hellebrandt findings.[1,8] Both intratester and intertester errors in the Boone and co-workers and the Hellebrandt studies were less than in the Low work.[1,8,13] The difference is not surprising because both Boone's and Hellebrandt's testers had definite protocols to follow, while Low allowed each tester to use whatever technique the tester wished.

The conclusion drawn by the authors of the papers cited is that intratester reliability is greater than intertester reliability and that, whenever possible, serial measurements of a joint should be done by the same examiner. The greater degree of intertester error in Low's study appears to indicate that the more specific the protocol used by the various testers for measuring joint motion, the lesser the degree of intertester error.[1,6,8,13]

Total active motion, total passive motion, and fingertip to distal palmar crease measurements

Total-motion values allow one number to represent the total motion capacity of a finger. The total extension deficits of a finger, including hyperextension, are added. This sum is subtracted from the total flexion capacity. The joint-flexion measurements are taken with the fingers in the "fisted" position of maximum MP, PIP, and DIP flexion. The extension-motion measurements are taken with all three joints in extension.[5]

The difference between total active motion and total passive motion is in the force causing the movement. The term "active motion" indicates the motion achieved by the patient's own muscle power, while "passive motion" refers to the freedom of movement at a joint when an external force is applied.[10] Because the fisted position is used to measure both total active and total passive range of motion, the total passive range-of-motion readings may not correlate with the sum of passive motion measurements taken where each joint was evaluated individually. An example would be a patient with a shortened extrinsic flexor tendon to the index finger. The passive range of motion in degrees could be MP, 0/90; PIP, 0/95; and DIP, 0/70, indicating that each joint has the capacity for full extension. The total passive extension deficit as measured in degrees in the completely extended position of the finger could be MP, 20; PIP, 30; and DIP, 20, equal to a total of 70 degrees. Then the sum of 70 degrees is subtracted from the sum of MP, 90; PIP,

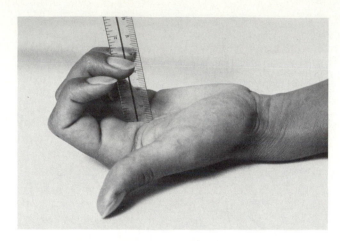

FIG. 6-1. Measuring from pulp of distal phalanx to distal palmar crease gives an easily understood value indicating the limitation of total finger flexion.

95; and DIP, 70 (total passive flexion in degrees), giving a total passive motion of 185 degrees. Each type of measurement gives a specific type of information. The passive range-of-motion figures tell us that the joints are not inherently stiff, while the total passive motion figures indicate that as a functioning unit the finger lacks full motion. Total active and passive motion sums also facilitate statistical analysis of range-of-motion progression or regression for an entire finger because only one numerical value per finger is involved. However, as the Clinical Assessment Committee of the American Society for Surgery of the Hand points out, total active motion values are not valid as part of a comparison of movement in determining a percentage of the norm.[4]

Another measurement technique that illustrates the lack of overall finger flexion is measuring the distance from the finger pulp to the distal palmar crease with the hand fisted.[5] This measurement gives an approximation of the total digital motion and is more comprehensible to many patients than motion measured in degrees.[4] Centimeters or inches can be used to record the distance, with zero indicating full flexion to the distal palmar crease (Fig. 6-1).

TECHNIQUES FOR MEASURING RANGE OF MOTION OF WRIST AND HAND USING A GONIOMETER
General considerations for all joints

The patient should be as comfortable as possible without sacrificing joint positioning or musculotendinous dynamics. A clear understanding of the motion he is to perform during active range of motion is necessary if the patient is to cooperate. He should also know that the movement is to take place only in the assigned joints so as to avoid substitution motions.[10,15] During passive range of motion he should be as relaxed as possible, avoiding the problem of tensing muscles around the joint being measured.

The force exerted on a joint during passive motion should be minimal and consistent from one test to another. Swanson

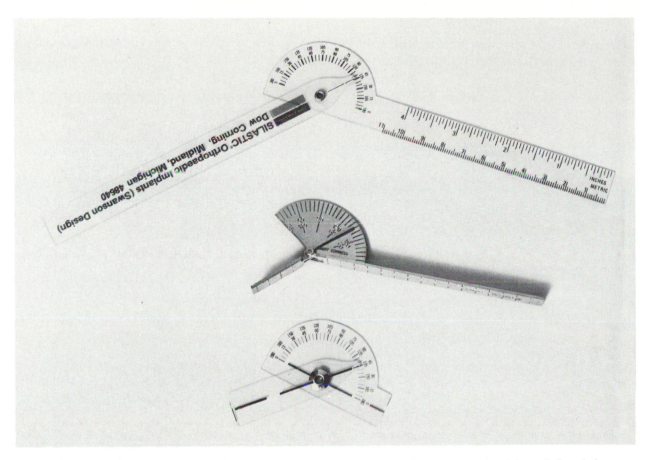

FIG. 6-2. Goniometer size and design should be appropriate for size of joint being measured and the technique being used.

suggests that a pressure of 1 pound applied to the middle of the adjacent distal phalanx is adequate for evaluation of passive motion in the fingers.[18] Brand has suggested that a therapist should check the amount of pressure that he or she is applying to the moving segment by using a pressure-gauging device. Such a check helps ensure consistent, gentle pressure.[2]

Range of motion—appropriateness of active and passive motion measurements. According to Hurt, "There are two primary purposes in measuring joint motion: to determine the degree of motion which can be accomplished in a joint by the active contraction of the governing muscle, and to determine the freedom existing at a joint by measuring the range through which it can be moved when all the muscles are relaxed."[10] Unless there are medical contraindications to active motion, the patient is first instructed in active motion to determine the available range of the joint when powered by its own musculature.[10] When the patient has full active excursion of a joint, passive motion values need not be taken. A joint that has full active range will have full passive range as well. However, if the patient cannot actively move through the full range, the passive motion measurements become necessary to gain an accurate picture of a joint's movement.[10,15]

Goniometer size and placement. Goniometers are man-

ufactured in a variety of forms and sizes. The size of the goniometer should be appropriate for the joint being measured. The wrist and forearm motions are adequately measured with a standard 14.5 cm length arm.[3,4] The finger joints are more easily measured by use of a commercially available finger goniometer made for dorsal alignment, or by shortening of the arms on a small goniometer. Such an adapted goniometer is suitable for lateral or dorsal measurements of the finger joints (Fig. 6-2).

When a lateral measurement is being made, the goniometer needs to be placed so that the arms are parallel to the long axis of the adjacent bones forming the joint. The fulcrum should be as close to the axis of motion of the joint as possible[3,10] (Fig. 6-3). When a goniometer is being placed dorsally on a digit, the fulcrum should be centered over the joint, with the arm lying dorsally along the long axis of the adjacent bones.[10]

In the case of a multiarticular joint complex such as the wrist, an anatomic landmark often is used for an approximate axis of motion. In the wrist, the styloid process of the radius laterally and the capitate dorsally and volarly are such landmarks.

Limiting the effects of positioning on range-of-motion values. Hurt states further that "the resting length of a 2-

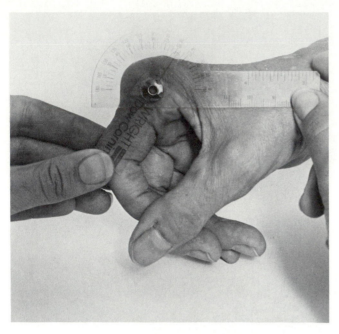

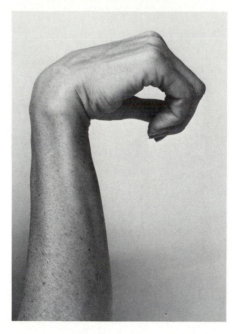

FIG. 6-3. Lateral placement of goniometer to measure active meta-carpophalangeal flexion of a patient with rheumatoid arthritis.

FIG. 6-4. Because of elongation of the extrinsic finger extensors over the fully flexed wrist, the remaining available excursion is inadequate to allow for full finger flexion.

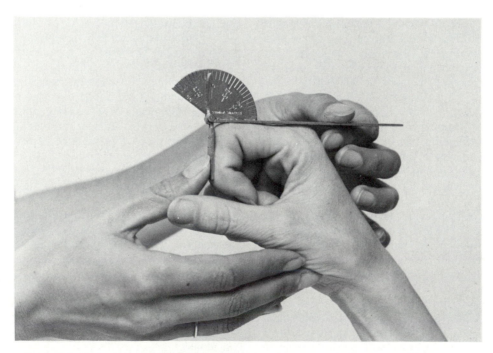

FIG. 6-5. Taking digital motion measurements with wrist in neutral and forearm in pronation eliminates possible effects of normal tendon-excursion limitation on range-of-motion measurements.

joint muscle is insufficient to allow full motion in the direction away from itself simultaneously in both joints over which it passes''[9] (Fig. 6-4). However, full motion is available at either joint with relaxation of the other.[9] The extrinsic finger flexors and extensors cross one or more finger joints and the wrist as well. In the case of the flexor digitorum superficialis, extensor digitorum communis, and the flexor pollicis longus the elbow is crossed as well just distal to their origins. To avoid having a resting-length insufficiency interfere with range-of-motion readings, *Clinical Assessment Recommendations* suggests that the wrist should be neutral when digital motion measurements are being taken. They also suggest that to limit the influence of forearm positioning on wrist measurements the forearm should be pronated[4] (Fig. 6-5).

Recording range-of-motion measurements. Lack of uniformity exists regarding how range-of-motion measurements should be recorded so that other professionals can accurately interpret the results. Several authors cited in this chapter comment on the importance of clearly defining a motion as being within the realm of normal flexion and extension or as an abnormal movement, such as hyperextension,[3,7,12,17-19] but exact guidelines for unequivocal interpretation are not given. The American Academy of Orthopaedic Surgeons[12] and the American Society for Surgery of the Hand[7] recommend a system of notation in which all motions are measured from a 0-degree (neutral) starting position. Flexion measurements are recorded as positive numbers; extension and hyperextension beyond the 0-degree starting position are recorded as negative numbers. Thus, 15/110 passive motion of the PIP joint indicates a 15-degree flexion contracture and full passive flexion. Similarly, −15/110 indicates 15-degree hyperextension and full passive flexion. Written statements can be used to indicate rotation and alignment deformities.[18-20]

Because of the lack of uniformity in recording motion measurements, it is important that a statement accompany range-of-motion records explaining the notation system being used. Otherwise, accurate data could be interpreted in an inaccurate manner.

Methods for measuring joint motion

Pronation and supination of the forearm. Measuring rotational movements at the radioulnar joints is difficult because of the long axis of movement, and the lack of stable anatomic lever arms with which to align the goniometer. The method used by Downer of the Ohio State University incorporates the salient points of other techniques and does not require special equipment other than a standard goniometer.[3,10,15]

The patient may be sitting or standing, but the elbow must be flexed to 90 degrees with the arm close to the side of the body. The arm position is important to avoid substitution movements of the shoulder.[3,11] The forearm should be in midposition with the palm vertical in relation to the floor. This position is defined as zero degrees.[12]

For measurement of supination, the patient rotates the hand and forearm to its maximum palm-up position without extending the elbow or abducting the upper arm. The stationary arm of the goniometer is aligned with the humerus

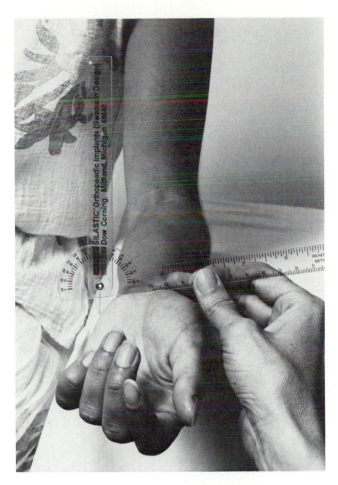

FIG. 6-6. Abduction of shoulder or extension of elbow will allow substitution of shoulder movement for true supination or pronation.

or held perpendicular to the floor.[3] The movable arm is placed on edge across the volar aspect of the wrist at the level of the ulnar styloid. The axis of the goniometer is just medial to the ulnar styloid (Fig. 6-6). Normal range of motion in supination is 0 to 80 or 90 degrees.[12]

The starting position for pronation is the same as for supination. The patient rotates the hand and forearm into the maximum palm-down position. The stationary arm again is aligned with the humerus or perpendicular to the floor. The only change is the position of the movable arm, which is now on the dorsum of the wrist at the level of the styloid processes.[15] Normal motion is from 0 to 80 or 90 degrees.[12]

Motion at the wrist. The wrist motions usually measured are flexion, extension, and radial and ulnar deviation. Wrist circumduction cannot be accurately measured.[12]

Flexion. Wrist flexion can be measured with the goniometer placed dorsally on the wrist,[5,18] or laterally along the radial border of the forearm and second metacarpal.[11,15] Placement of the goniometer along the ulnar border of the wrist and the fifth metacarpal also has been suggested.[3,15] However, the mobility of the carpometacarpal joints of the fourth and fifth metacarpals could skew the measurements of wrist flexion when an ulnar placement is used.[5]

For measurement of wrist flexion (volar flexion) on the

radial aspect of the forearm, the elbow is flexed and the forearm and wrist are placed in neutral for the starting position. The wrist is flexed, and the stationary arm of the goniometer is aligned with the radius while the movable arm is aligned with the second metacarpal.[11] The axis of motion of the goniometer is approximately at the level of the radial styloid (Fig. 6-7).

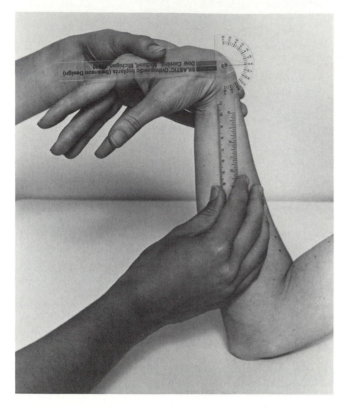

FIG. 6-7. Lateral measurement on radial aspect of wrist is preferred because of stability of second carpometacarpal joint.

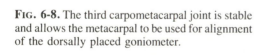

FIG. 6-8. The third carpometacarpal joint is stable and allows the metacarpal to be used for alignment of the dorsally placed goniometer.

Wrist flexion (volar flexion), with the goniometer placed dorsally, requires the elbow to be flexed and the forearm in pronation with the wrist in neutral as the starting position. The wrist is flexed with the fingers relaxed. The stationary arm of the goniometer is aligned with the long axis of the forearm while the movable arm is aligned with the third metacarpal.[5] The fulcrum of the goniometer is approximately at the level of the capitate (Fig. 6-8). According to *Joint Motion: Method of Measuring and Recording*, the normal arc of motion for wrist flexion is 0 to 80 degrees.[12]

Extension. For measuring wrist extension (dorsiflexion) using the lateral placement, the wrist is extended with the fingers allowed to flex passively.[11] The normal arc of motion is 0 to 70 degrees.[12]

For measurement of wrist extension with the goniometer volarly placed, the starting position of the arm is the same as for wrist flexion. However, goniometer placement is different. Once the wrist is extended, the stationary arm is aligned with the long axis of the forearm on the volar surface and the movable arm is aligned with the volar surface of the third metacarpal.[5] The fingers should be relaxed (Fig. 6-9).

Radial and ulnar deviation. The starting positions for taking measurements of radial and ulnar deviation are the same. The forearm is in pronation and the goniometer is placed dorsally.[5] The zero position is with the wrist in neutral.[12] The stationary arm is aligned in midposition along the forearm. The capitate and lateral epicondyle of the elbow can be used as reference points for the stationary arm, and the movable arm is placed along the third metacarpal[15] (Fig. 6-10). In both radial and ulnar deviation, wrist flexion and extension need to be avoided. The wrist is angled toward the thumb for radial deviation (Fig. 6-11) or angled toward the fifth finger for ulnar deviation.[3,11,15] The normal range of radial deviation is 0 to 20 degrees and for ulnar deviation 0 to 30 degrees.[12]

Motion of the fingers. The wrist should be in neutral to

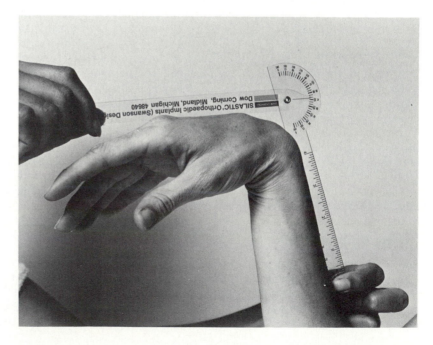

allow full tendon excursion of the long finger flexors and extensors when one is measuring the motion of the metacarpophalangeal, proximal interphalangeal, and distal interphalangeal joints.[5] This is true for both active and passive motion studies. At the Hand Rehabilitation Center in Philadelphia, active range-of-motion values for flexion are taken with all three joints of each finger actively flexed to their maximum. For the measurement of extension, all three joints actively extended to their maximum. Simultaneous flexion or extension of the finger joints during measurement gives the examiner a better picture of the musculotendinous limitations affecting active motion of the joints.

Passive motion is measured on a joint-by-joint basis with the adjacent joint or joints in neutral so that the musculotendinous effects are minimized and only the excursion of the joint is being measured.[10]

Metacarpophalangeal joint. Metacarpophalangeal joint motion can be measured laterally or dorsally. The landmarks used for lateral measurement of joint flexion and extension are the same. For lateral placement of the goniometer on the index or middle fingers, the stationary arm is aligned with the lateral longitudinal axis of the second metacarpal. The moving arm is aligned with the lateral longitudinal axis of the first phalanx (Fig. 6-12). In the case of the middle finger, this requires the examiner to have the index metacarpophalangeal joint slightly extended so that the middle finger can be clearly sighted (Fig. 6-13). The ring and little fingers are measured from the ulnar border of the hand with the same techniques.

Dorsal placement of the goniometer to measure metacarpophalangeal joint flexion and extension is the same for both. The stationary arm is placed over the dorsum of the metacarpal, the fulcrum is superior to the joint axis, and the movable arm is placed over the dorsum of the adjacent

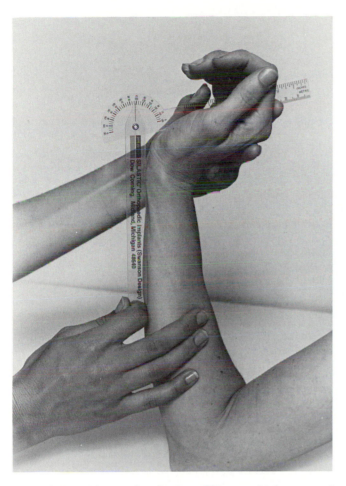

FIG. 6-9. Movable arm of goniometer will be over third metacarpal bridging palmar arc.

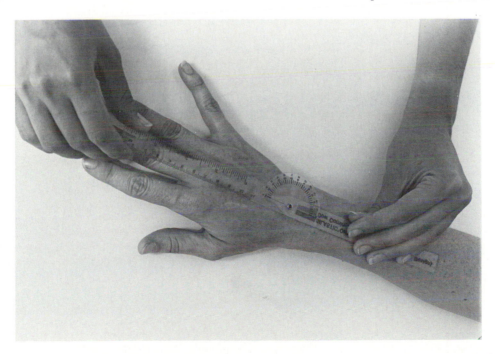

FIG. 6-10. Starting position for measurement of radial and ulnar deviation requires wrist to be in neutral in both planes of motion—flexion-extension and radial and ulnar deviation.

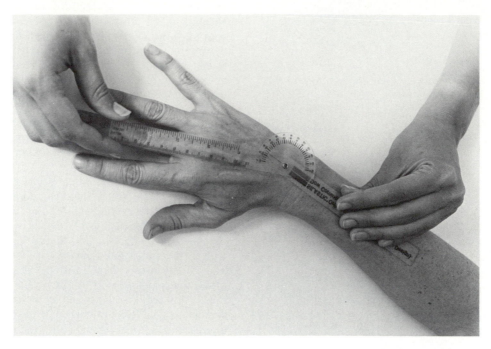

FIG. 6-11. It is important that movable arm be aligned with third metacarpal and not third finger.

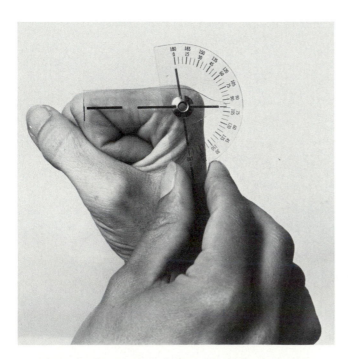

FIG. 6-12. Thumb should be held in abduction or adduction and slight extension when one is laterally measuring metacarpophalangeal motion of index finger, so as not to block full metacarpophalangeal flexion of index finger.

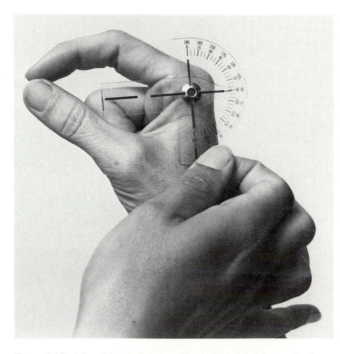

FIG. 6-13. Movable phalanx needs to be sighted as clearly as possible for an accurate measurement.

phalanx.[11] The arc of motion usually evaluated when one is measuring metacarpophalangeal joint motion is 0 to 90 degrees, but hyperextension of up to 45 degrees is also normal.[12]

Flexion and extension of the proximal and distal interphalangeal joints. The techniques used for measurement of joint motion at the proximal interphalangeal and distal interphalangeal joints are very similar; therefore they will be described together. The use of a commercially available finger goniometer for dorsal placement or a small goniometer in which the arms have been shortened for dorsal or lateral placement helps with the measurement of the finger joints[4] (Fig. 6-2).

For lateral measurements, the stationary arm is placed along the long axis of the proximal phalanx and the moving arm is placed along the long axis of the adjacent distal phalanx. The fulcrum approximates the axis of motion of the joint[16] (Fig. 6-14). The metacarpophalangeal joints may have to be extended slightly when one is measuring the distal interphalangeal flexion to allow the goniometer to clear the palm during full active flexion.

When one is measuring extension of the proximal inter-

phalangeal and distal interphalangeal joints, the same goniometer placement along the lateral long axis of the adjacent phalanges is used after the joints have been extended.

Dorsal measurements of proximal interphalangeal and distal interphalangeal flexion are made by placing the stationary arm on the dorsal long axis of the proximal phalanx and the movable arm on the dorsum of the adjacent distal phalanx.[3,11] The examiner should keep the goniometer in as complete contact with the dorsal finger surface as possible to avoid errors in measurement[16] (Fig. 6-5). As with lateral placement, slight metacarpophalangeal extension may be necessary for measurement of the distal interphalangeal flexion if total active flexion is complete or nearly so (Fig. 6-15).

The placement of the arms of the goniometer remains the same when one measures the extension of the proximal and distal interphalangeal joints, except that the joints are in maximum extension dorsally.[11] The range of motion of the proximal interphalangeal joints is 0 to 110 degrees and that of the distal interphalangeal joints 0 to 60 or 70 degrees.[12]

Abduction and adduction of the metacarpophalangeal joints. Joint Motion: Method of Measuring and Recording does not give norms for finger abduction and adduction. It suggests measuring the distance from fingertip to fingertip in inches or centimeters. These measurements can be used

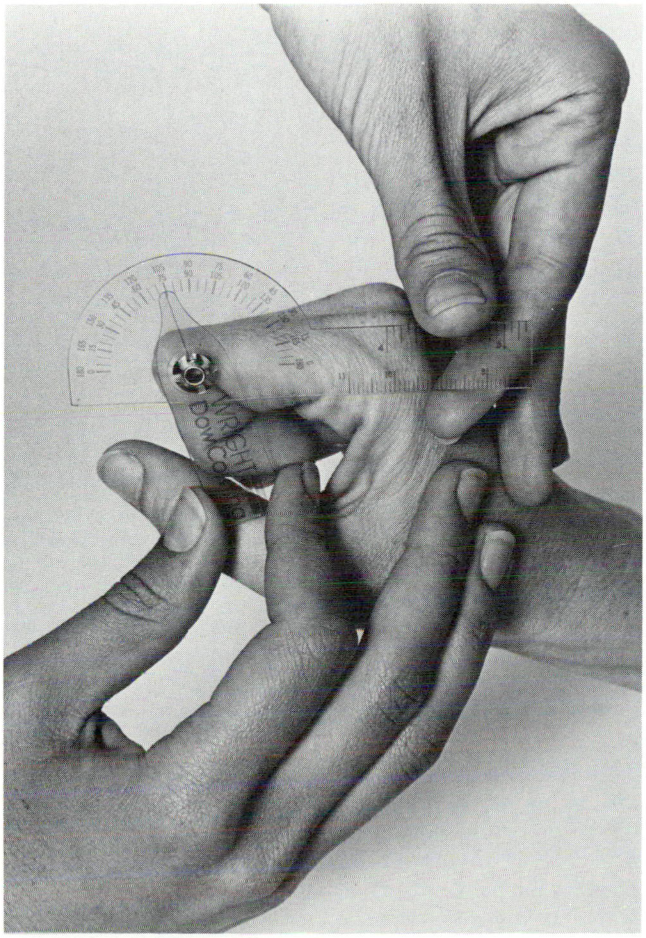

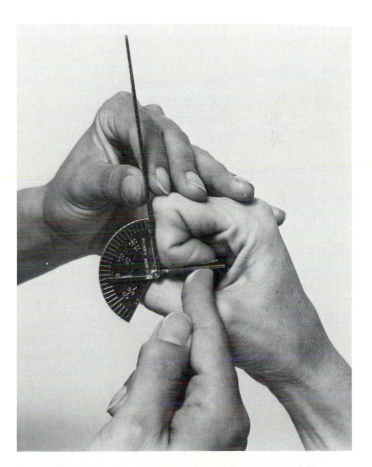

FIG. 6-14. Lateral placement of goniometer with shortened arms is suitable for finger joint measurements.

FIG. 6-15. Slight metacarpophalangeal extension allows full excursion of goniometer without interference by touching palm.

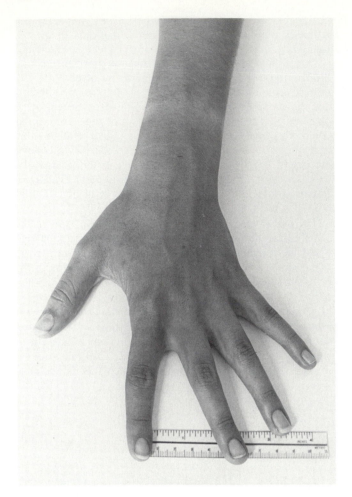

FIG. 6-16. Measuring distance between midpulps of adjacent maximally abducted fingers will allow for comparisons of abduction to help in evaluation of treatment effectiveness.

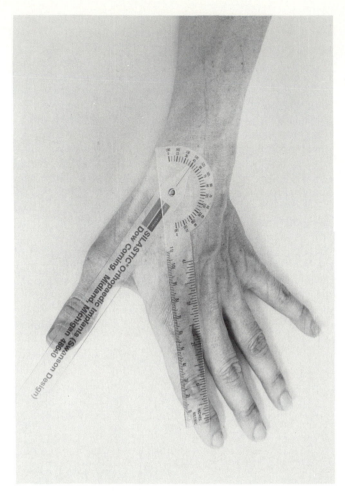

FIG. 6-17. Measurement of thumb extension is done with thumb in plane of palm. (From American Academy of Orthopaedic Surgeons: Joint motion: method of measuring and recording, Chicago, 1965, The Academy.)

for pretreatment and posttreatment comparisons only[12] (Fig. 6-16).

Thumb motions. The thumb's movement pattern is the most complex of all the digits because of its highly mobile carpometacarpal (CMC) joint. Flexion describes the movement across the palm that terminates with the tip of the thumb at the base of the fifth finger. It involves flexion of the carpometacarpal, metacarpal and interphalangeal joints for full excursion. Extension of the thumb involves the same joints in a movement away from the second metacarpal, again in the plane of the palm.[12]

Thumb flexion and extension can be measured with a goniometer placed laterally or dorsally along the appropriate adjacent bones. Carpometacarpal flexion requires the stationary arm to be aligned with the lateral or dorsal long axis of the radius with the movable arm aligned with the first metacarpal. The approximate axis of motion is level with the anatomic snuffbox. Flexion of the carpometacarpal joint is 15 degrees.[12] Carpometacarpal extension can be measured with the stationary arm aligned with the second metacarpal and the movable arm aligned over the first metacarpal (Fig. 6-17). Metacarpophalangeal and interphalangeal flexion and

extension can be measured with the same lateral or dorsal technique appropriate for the index-finger metacarpophalangeal and proximal interphalangeal joints. Thumb metacarpophalangeal motion is 0 to 50 degrees and interphalangeal excursion is 0 to 80 degrees.[12] The interphalangeal joint of the thumb has varying degrees of hypertension and should be compared with the contralateral thumb if a pathologic condition is suspected.

Thumb abduction and adduction occur in a plane perpendicular to the palm and involve only movement of the carpometacarpal joint normally. Norms for abduction have not been established by the American Academy of Orthopaedic Surgeons, but the measurement can be compared with that of the contralateral hand. Adduction is defined as the thumb in line with the radius lying immediately beside the second metacarpal, while abduction is the angle that occurs as the thumb moves perpendicularly away from the plane of the palm.[12] This angle can be measured in degrees with a goniometer. The stationary arm is aligned with the lateral aspect of the second metacarpal, and the moving arm is placed dorsally along the long axis of the first metacarpal.[11] An alternative method is to measure in inches or

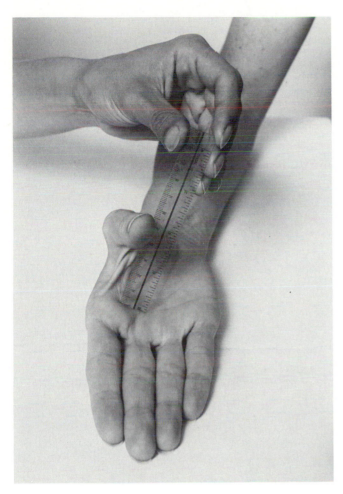

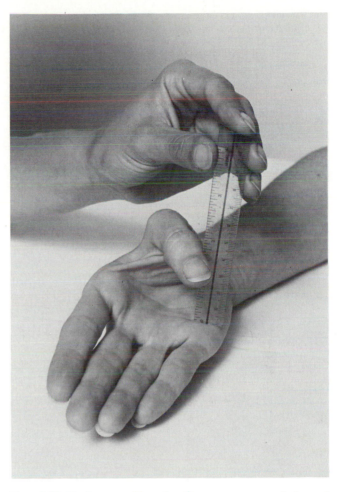

FIG. 6-18. Thumb abduction is measured in a plane perpendicular to palm. (From American Academy of Orthopaedic Surgeons: Joint motion: method of measuring and recording, Chicago, 1965, The Academy.)

FIG. 6-19. During opposition, thumb must move out of plane of palm while approaching fifth finger.

centimeters the distance from the distal palmar crease of the index finger to the pulp or interphalangeal crease of the thumb[12] (Fig. 6-18). Other methods of measurement, using special measuring devices such as dental calipers, have been suggested in the hand literature and may be helpful in specific circumstances.[17]

Thumb opposition is a composite motion comprising abduction, rotation, and flexion. Measurement of opposition is usually done in inches or centimeters between the thumb-tip and the tip or base of the fifth finger[12] (Fig. 6-19). For true opposition and not just thumb flexion, the thumb must move out and away from the plane of the palm with the thumbnail approximately parallel to the plane of the palm.

CONCLUSION

The limited research done on assessment of the reliability of measuring joint motion by use of a goniometer indicates that it can be an accurate, reproducible method for evaluation of motion. The use of the same tester for serial motion studies increases the reliability. When the same tester is not available, the use of the same goniometric technique may

help improve reliability. The single study that evaluated lateral versus dorsal goniometer placement in the fingers did not find one method more accurate than the other.

The methods for measuring joint motion presented in this chapter are for the evaluation of hands without major deformities that cause excessive joint deviations, subluxations, and dislocations, such as advanced rheumatoid arthritis. Refer to the chapters on arthritis and specifically to those written by Swanson for the evaluation of the arthritic hand.

REFERENCES

1. Boone, D.C., Azen, S.P., Lin, C.M., and others: Reliability of goniometric measurements, Phys. Ther. **58**:1355, 1978.
2. Brand, P., and Costa, P.: Principles of dynamic splinting, Symposium and Workshop on Hand Rehabilitation Correlated with Hand Surgery, March 1981.
3. Downer, A.: Goniometry: measurement of joint range of motion, Columbus, 1982, Ohio State University Press (unpublished).
4. Fess, E.E., and others: Evaluation of the hand by objective measurement. In Hunter, J.M., Schneider, L.H., Mackin, E.J., and Bell, J.A., editors: Rehabilitation of the hand, St. Louis, 1978, The C.V. Mosby Co.
5. Fess, E.E., and Moran, C.A.: Clinical assessment recommendations, Aurora, Colo., 1981, American Society of Hand Therapists.

6. Hamilton, G.F., and Lachenbruch, P.A.: The reliability of goniometry in assessing finger joint angle, Phys. Ther. **49:**465, 1969.

7. The hand—examination and diagnosis, Aurora, Colo., 1978, American Society for Surgery of the Hand.

8. Hellebrandt, F.A., Duvall, E.N., and Moore, M.L.: The measurement of joint motion. Part III. Reliability of goniometry, Phys. Ther. Rev. **29:**302, 1949.

9. Hurt, S.P.: Considerations in muscle function and their application to disability evaluation and treatment, Am. J. Occup. Ther. **1:**69, 1947.

10. Hurt, S.P.: Considerations in muscle function and their application to disability evaluation and treatment: joint measurement. Part I, Am. J. Occup. Ther. **1:**209, 1947.

11. Hurt, S.P.: Considerations in muscle function and their application to disability evaluation and treatment: joint measurement. Part II, Am. J. Occup. Ther. **1:**281, 1947.

12. Joint Motion: method of measuring and recording, Chicago, 1965, American Academy of Orthopaedic Surgeons.

13. Low, J.L.: The reliability of joint measurement, Physiotherapy **62:**227, 1976.

14. Moore, M.L.: The measurement of joint motion. Part I. Introductory review of the literature, Phys. Ther. Rev. **29:**195, 1949.

15. Moore, M.L.: The measurement of joint motion. Part II. The technic of goniometry, Phys. Ther. Rev. **29:**256, 1949.

16. Perry, J.F., and Bevin, A.G.: Evaluation procedures for patient with hand injuries, Phys. Ther. **54:**593, 1974.

17. Swanson, A.B., Göran-Hagert, C., and Swanson, G.: Evaluation of impairment of hand function. In Hunter, J.M., Schneider, L.H., Mackin, E.J., and Bell, J.A., editors: Rehabilitation of the hand, St. Louis, 1978, The C.V. Mosby Co.

18. Swanson, A.B.: Flexible implant resection arthroplasty in the hand and extremities, St. Louis, 1973, The C.V. Mosby Co.

19. Swanson, A.B., Swanson, G., and Leonard, J.: Postoperative rehabilitation program in flexible implant arthroplasty of the digits. In Hunter, J.M., Schneider, L.H., Mackin, E.J., and Bell, J.A., editors: Rehabilitation of the hand, St. Louis, 1978, The C.V. Mosby Co.

7

Evaluation of the hand by functional tests

PATRICIA L. BAXTER and MELANIE S. BALLARD

Functional assessment of the patient with a hand disability is carried out most effectively through the use of a variety of testing instruments. The therapist should rely on standardized test instruments that have been proved to measure precisely and accurately and produce consistent, dependable information.[1] The tests that are discussed include the Jebson Hand Function Test, the Minnesota Rate of Manipulation Test, the Purdue Pegboard Test, and various Valpar Work Samples. The work samples to be discussed include the Valpar Whole Body Range of Motion, the Upper Extremity Range of Motion, the Small Tools (Mechanical), the Eye-Hand-Foot Coordination, the Simulated Assembly, and the Clerical Comprehension and Aptitude.

JEBSON HAND FUNCTION TEST

The Jebson Hand Function Test measures unilateral functional hand skills. It also is an assessment of a person's ability to write, manage eating utensils, manipulate small objects, and manipulate both lightweight and heavy large objects (Fig. 7-1). The test evaluates dominant functional skills versus nondominant functional skills. The test utilizes materials that are common objects that must be assembled by the therapist. A stopwatch is needed to record the time a person takes to perform each of the seven subtests. R.H. Jebson describes step-by-step test administration in "An Objective and Standardized Test of Hand Function."[3] This article describes the dimensions of a testing board that the clinician would need to construct in order to administer the test.

The first subtest measures a person's ability to write sentences composed of 20 letters (Fig. 7-2). A pen and various cards with sentences printed on them are needed. The second subtest measures one's functional ability in simulated page turning using five 3 × 5–inch cards. The third subtest requires that the person pick up six small objects—two pennies, two paper clips, and two bottle caps—and place them in a container. The fourth subtest requires the person to stack four standard-sized checkers. The fifth subtest requires the person to perform five simulated eating tasks by manipulating a kidney bean onto a spoon and placing it into an empty 3-pound can. The sixth and seventh subtests require the person to grasp five cans and place them onto the testing board.

Standardized forms have been developed. These forms offer norms for males and females in two differing age groups. Each subtest is timed for both the dominant and the nondominant hand. The test should be administered in a relatively quiet area, free from distraction. The person tested should be seated at a table in a sturdy, comfortable chair directly across from the test administrator. All seven subsections of the test are administered, with the nondominant hand being timed first. Testing protocol is followed and standardized instructions are read to the patient. The test administrator should carefully adhere to the standardized instructions regarding the placement of the testing board and testing objects. Depending on the severity and type of disability of the individual being tested, the time for administration of the test ranges between 15 and 30 minutes.

An advantage of the Jebson Hand Function Test is that it emphasizes functional activities and documents changes of ability within each category of hand function. This test can be administered in a short time. Testing materials can be assembled quickly and inexpensively.

One disadvantage of the Jebson Hand Function Test is that it does not test bilateral hand function. A second disadvantage of the test is that the score of the individual is based on the speed of performance and does not consider altered prehension patterns. Independently of the evaluation, the therapist must note deficits of prehension that might be an important consideration for surgical intervention in such cases as rheumatoid arthritis or peripheral nerve palsy.

MINNESOTA RATE OF MANIPULATION TEST

The Minnesota Rate of Manipulation Test (MRMT) was designed to measure manual dexterity to provide employers with an instrument that would improve the efficiency of personnel selections for jobs requiring hand-and-arm dexterity.[2] Originally the test was standardized on older adults, unemployed during the Depression. To administer the test, the therapist would need a standard stopwatch and the Minnesota Rate of Manipulation testing board, disks, and instrument manual. Instructions are read to the patient, who is seated in a sturdy chair at a table located in a quiet, well-lighted room. The test involves moving 58 disks from one place to another, either placing or turning and placing the disks (Fig. 7-3). A broad range of shoulder motion is required (Fig. 7-4). The patient is given one practice trial for each of five subtests. The five subtests are the unilateral placing test, turning test, displacing test, and turning and placing test and the bilateral turning and placing test.

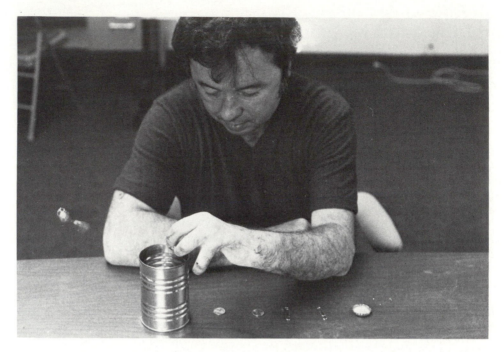

FIG. 7-1. Patient manipulating objects in Jebson Hand Function Test.

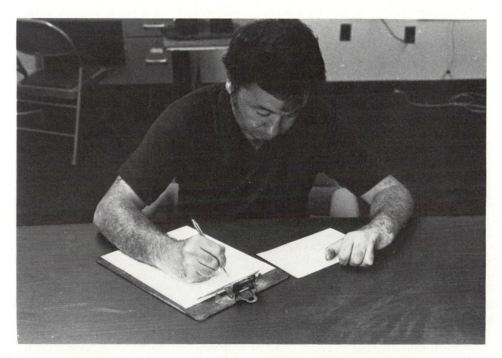

FIG. 7-2. Jebson test component for handwriting administered to patient.

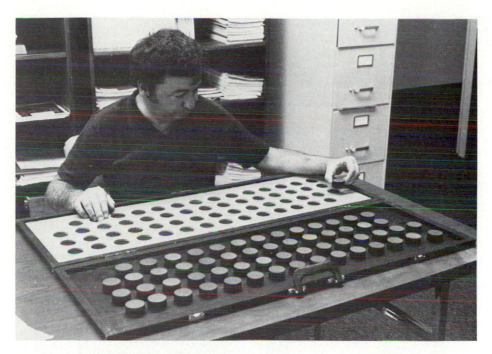

FIG. 7-3. Unilateral placing test is one subtest of the MRMT.

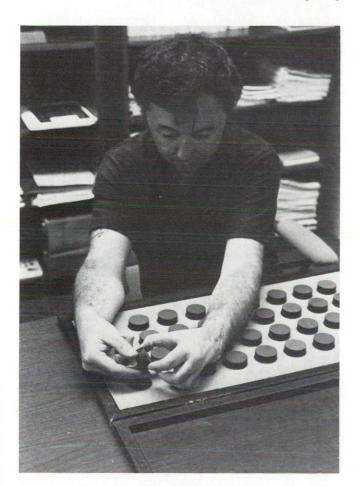

FIG. 7-4. Active motion of the upper extremity, including shoulder motion is required in the MRMT. Bilateral turning and placing test is another subtest of the MRMT.

The test board consists of two 30 × 9–inch boards connected by hinges. Each board contains 58 holes, approximately 1½ inches in diameter. Administering each test requires approximately 10 minutes. Three tests, the bilateral turning and placing test and the unilateral test for the right and left upper extremities, are used in most instances. Usually one practice trial and four test trials are given.

Positive features of the Minnesota Rate of Manipulation Test are the following: (1) individuals or groups can be tested; (2) the test can be given in a short period of time; (3) the patient's endurance can be observed when several tests are given; and (4) substitution patterns and incoordination from sensory loss, muscle weakness, poor tendon gliding, or amputation of digits can be observed.

Disadvantages of the Minnesota Rate of Manipulation Test are the following: (1) this test is not a comprehensive overview of functional hand skills; (2) alone, the Minnesota Rate of Manipulation Test cannot predict job success; and (3) upper extremity and trunk mobility are required in conjunction with the ability to manipulate small objects throughout the testing procedure.

PURDUE PEGBOARD TEST

The Purdue Pegboard Test was designed to test dexterity unilaterally and bilaterally. It measures dexterity for two types of activities, one involving gross movements of the hands, fingers, and arms and the other involving what might be called "fingertip" dexterity.[4] The Purdue Pegboard Test has been standardized on male and female adults and on school children. The test board and a standard stopwatch are required to administer this test. The testing board has two rows of holes and four recessed bowls so that all assembly components can be stored under a sliding removable

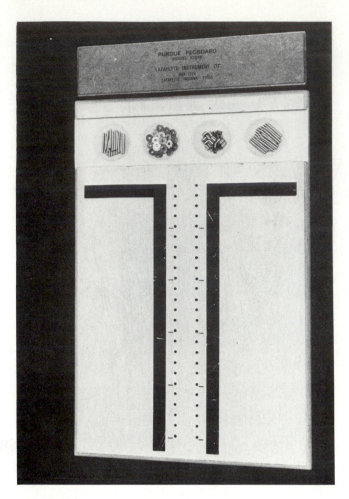

FIG. 7-5. Purdue Pegboard.

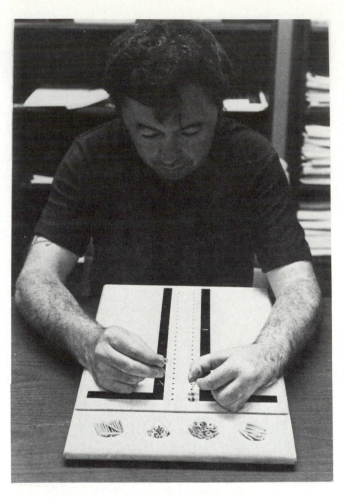

FIG. 7-6. Patient places small pins into the rows of holes on the Purdue Pegboard.

top (Fig. 7-5). Bowls 1 and 4 store the pins, and bowls 2 and 3 store either the washers or the collars. The board has two vertical columns of holes into which the assembly components are inserted. After every five holes there is a mark on the board enabling the therapist to tabulate the scores more easily. Complete instructions for the administration of the test are included in the manual. There are four subtests: (1) right-hand prehension test, (2) left-hand prehension test, (3) prehension test with both hands, and (4) assembly test.

The patient sits at a chair with the Purdue Pegboard directly in front of him. The right-hand and left-hand tests involve placing pins, one at a time, into the column of holes on the board. The test should be administered to the dominant hand first. The prehension test is timed for 30 seconds. The assembly test involves using both hands to form assemblies of a pin, a collar, and two washers (Fig. 7-6). The assembly test is timed for 1 minute. The patient's score can be calculated by either one or three repetitions of each subtest. Total test administration time may be 10 to 15 minutes. The therapist should be familiar with the administration manual so that the test can be adequately demonstrated to the patient.

The Purdue Pegboard Test offers the therapist an oppor-

tunity to look at fine prehension ability and to observe sensibility problems in the fingertips or the thumb. The test primarily assesses digital nerve function or median nerve innervated functional sensibility and/or motor function. The test can be given to groups or individuals, and separate scores for dominant versus nondominant hands are available. A disadvantage of the Purdue Pegboard Test is that the adult patient scores cannot be compared to a random sample, but rather to a specific population such as factory workers.

VALPAR WORK SAMPLE SERIES

The Valpar Work Sample Series* provides the therapist with a standardized means of assessing a person's ability to perform various work-related tasks or to perform the motions required for specific job tasks. Five of the Valpar Work Sample Series are discussed.

Valpar Whole Body Range of Motion Work Sample

The Valpar Whole Body Range of Motion Work Sample measures the agility of a person's gross body movements

---

*Valpar Corp., 3801 East 34th Street, Suite 105, Tucson, Ariz.

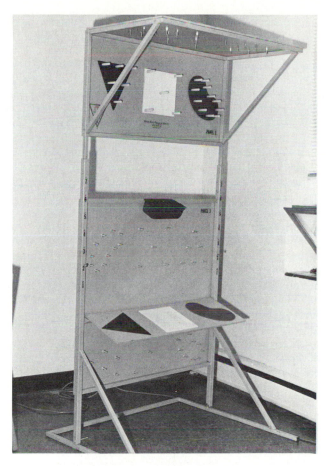

FIG. 7-7. Valpar whole body range of motion.

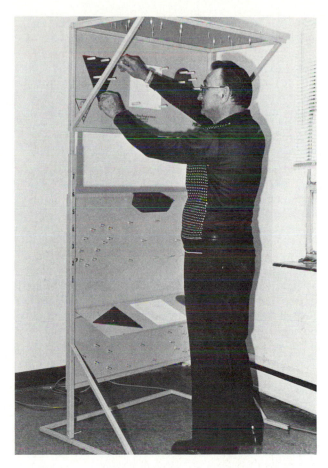

FIG. 7-8. Patient transfers Plexiglass forms onto five panels at varied heights.

of the trunk, arms, hands, legs, and fingers as they relate to the functional ability to perform job tasks. This work sample assesses the patient's ability to bilaterally manipulate small objects as he is required to reach overhead, stoop, and crouch. At times the patient must perform tasks with his vision occluded. The work sample is designed to give the therapist a means of assessing the relationship of gross body movement and fine manual dexterity required in many different work situations.

This work sample consists of a large free-standing, two-part, height-adjustable, metal frame consisting of five panels (Fig. 7-7). The height of the frame is adjustable at 3-inch intervals from 5 feet, 9 inches to 7 feet 3 inches. The frame measures 35 inches in width and is made of square steel tubing. Three panels are attached to the frame. A fourth diagonal panel is attached to the bottom work panel and separates that panel into two work areas. On the diagonal panel are three permanently mounted Plexiglas (acrylic plastic) forms. This panel is positioned such that the patient's vision is occluded from the fifth panel. Freely movable Plexiglas forms consisting of a black triangle, a white square, and a red kidney form are secured to a panel with a total of 22 booted nuts. A nut tray is attached to the steel

frame at the top center of the panel. A stopwatch is necessary for administration of the evaluation.

The patient stands in front of the work sample with the frame adjusted so that the top panel is approximately 6 inches above his or her head (Fig. 7-8). The patient is timed while taking three colored shapes, one at a time, and transferring them from shoulder level to a panel overhead. The patient then transfers the shapes to a panel at waist level. The Plexiglas forms are transferred a third time at knee level, thereby requiring the patient to crouch or kneel. The final timed transfer is performed when the patient transfers the forms from knee level back to shoulder height. During each transfer the patient must maneuver a total of 22 nuts, replacing them onto each of the three colored shapes, using both hands to perform the task. The shapes are positioned such that trunk rotation is required as the colored shapes are transferred. A total of four transfers are made, requiring the patient to remove and replace 176 nuts.

The administration time for the Valpar Whole Body Range of Motion Work Sample varies from 15 to 30 minutes. The patient is timed for each of the four transfers, and the time is recorded in seconds on the score sheet.

Advantages of the Valpar Whole Body Range of Motion

Work Sample are that (1) norms are available for the employed worker; (2) the evaluation is easy to administer and score; (3) the patient is observed performing dexterity tasks while working in a variety of postures and while working with vision occluded; and (4) after each transfer the patient is questioned regarding his subjective assessment of the type and location of discomfort or fatigue he experiences.

Valpar Upper Extremity Range of Motion Work Sample

This work sample is designed to measure the patient's range of motion and work tolerance as related to the upper extremities. This includes the patient's use of shoulders, upper arms, forearms, elbows, wrists, and hands. The Valpar Upper Extremity Range of Motion Work Sample is particularly useful to the therapist to assist in providing insight into the patient's level of fatigue, finger dexterity, and sense of touch.

This work sample consists of two major parts: Part 1 is a five-sided square box measuring 12 × 12 inches. In the front of the box is a 5-inch circular opening. The back of the box is open to allow the therapist an unobstructed view of the patient's work. The five sides of the box are lined with machine bolts whose heads are on the outside of the box with the threads exposed inside the box (Fig. 7-9). The inside of the box is divided into two equal sections, one red and one blue. Part 2 of the work sample is a covered tray measuring 8 × 11 × 2½ inches. The nut tray contains the hex nuts used in the completion of the sample. There are 42 ¾-inch no. 10 nuts and 42 ¼-inch no. 20 hex nuts. Both nuts and bolts are zinc plated and rustproof. The box and tray are fabricated of ½-inch particle board covered with plastic laminate.

The work sample weighs approximately 37 pounds. Included with this work sample are a manual, score pads, and upper extremity body chart pads. A stopwatch is needed for the administration of the test.

This work sample is administered in two separately timed sections: assembly and disassembly. During the assembly section, the patient is required to pick up one nut at a time, reach through the opening in the front of the box, place the nut on the bolt and screw the nut down snugly against the box. The assembly section of the test is divided into eight sections; bottom panel, top panel, side panel, and front panel for each hand. With each hand the patient is required to reach across the midline of the body to perform the sections of the test. The patient completes the test components for the dominant hand in one colored section of the box before beginning the test for the nondominant hand in the other colored section. After performing the assembly section, the patient is asked for a subjective assessment of his physical reaction to the test. The disassembly section is then performed by the patient in one timed session. He is required to remove all the nuts and bolts before the timed session is completed. Through the open back of the box, the therapist can observe the patient's spatial and perceptual skills, coordination, and endurance.

The total time to administer this test ranges from approximately 30 to 45 minutes, depending on the patient's performance. Each section of the assembly test is timed separately and identically. Timing begins when the patient has been told to begin work. Timing stops when all nuts have been placed on every bolt in the section being timed. The disassembly section of the work sample has one timed score only. Timing begins in this section when the patient is instructed to begin work and ends when all nuts have been removed from the bolts and the last nut has been placed in the nut tray.

Assembly and disassembly test components are scored separately. Only time scores are available for this work sample. There are no error scores. Therapists are referred to the accompanying manual for instructions in obtaining a time-percentile and performance-percentile score for the assembly section. For the disassembly section only a time-percentile score is obtained.

Advantages of the Valpar Upper Extremity Range of Motion Work Sample are that (1) norms are available for the employed worker; (2) the test is easy to administer and score; (3) the test requires the patient to perform dexterity activities with his wrist in several positions; and (4) the test offers a means of assessing the patient's endurance to perform manipulative tasks.

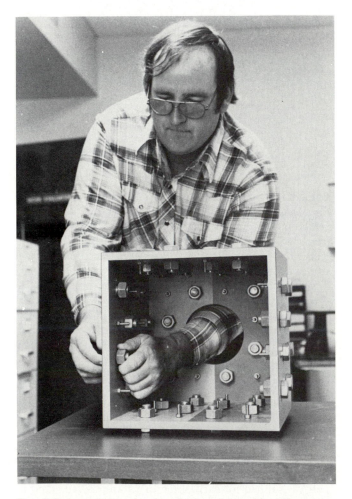

FIG. 7-9. As patient works, therapist can observe his performance.

Valpar Small Tools (Mechanical) Work Sample

The Valpar Small Tools Mechanical Work Sample provides a measure of a person's ability to understand and work with small tools, such as screwdrivers, pliers, and wrenches. Dexterity, though it varies in importance from one occupation to another, is fundamental to one's ability to function in many occupations. The use of small tools is particularly important to positions in such occupations as small-appliance repair, bicycle and auto repair, jewelry making, and assembly tasks in a wide variety of manufacturing settings. This work sample meaures a person's ability to perform repetitive tasks for prolonged periods of time using one's hands in a small space. A nonmedical measure of the patient's perseverance and frustration tolerance may also be assessed because the sample may require 1½ hours to complete. The work sample consists of two boxes, both construction of ½-inch Formica-covered particle board. Box 1 is a 12 × 12–inch five-sided hinged cube. Box 2 is a tool-and-parts box measuring 3½ × 10 × 17 inches (Fig. 7-10). This box contains all the hand tools and hardware required for participation in this work sample. The tools include three types of screwdrivers, eight different wrenches, a nutdriver, and a pair of pliers. In addition, the work sample manual and a pad of scoring sheets are included. A stopwatch is needed for administration of this test. The box can be opened up for easy viewing of parts for the disassembly portion of the evaluation. For assembly portions of the evaluation, the patient works through a square hole in the front of the box with visual observance of the task being performed prohibited. One side of the box is open to enable the therapist to view the patient's approach to the task and his usage of tools.

Instructions for administration of this test are included in the manual. The test should be administered in an environment that is well lit, clean, and relatively free of noise and visual distraction. The patient may sit or stand as he performs this work sample. The work box is placed on a table with the edge of the box approximately 3 inches from the edge of the table. The small square opening is facing the patient. The patient works through a square hole in the front of the work sample. This intentionally blocks the patient's view of some of the work he is doing and simulates many common working situations where work cannot be seen (Fig. 7-11). The patient works on each of the five panels. Each panel requires a different set of tools to insert fasteners such as screws, bolts, and hitch-pin clips. The evaluation is administered in two sections—assembly and disassembly. Five separately timed sections of the assembly component correspond to each panel of the box. Panel 1 requires the use of a Phillips screwdriver and a ¾-inch blade screwdriver. Phillips-head screws and round-head screws are provided in the toolbox. Panel 2 requires the use of pliers and hitch-pin clips. An Allen wrench and a ⁷/₁₆-inch nutdriver are used for the completion of panel 3. Three different-sized wrenches are used in panel 4 to assemble washers and nuts on various-sized bolts. The fifth and final panel requires the use of a blade screwdriver, a ¼-inch wrench, nuts, washers, and bolts. The disassembly section is performed with the box opened up and all parts easily viewed for manipulation.

Each section of the assembly component is timed separately, and times are recorded in total seconds. Timing begins immediately after the patient is told to begin a work panel. Timing ends when the patient has placed all the hardware on a panel. Five to 10 minutes are required for

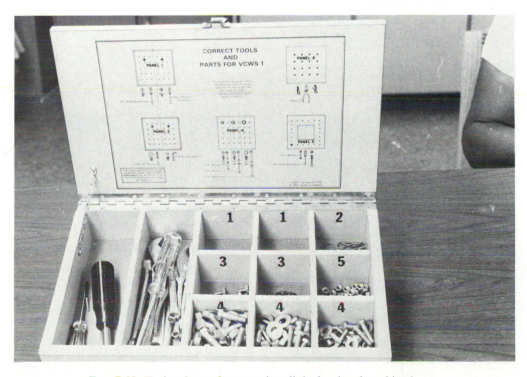

FIG. 7-10. Tool and parts box contains all the hand tools and hardware.

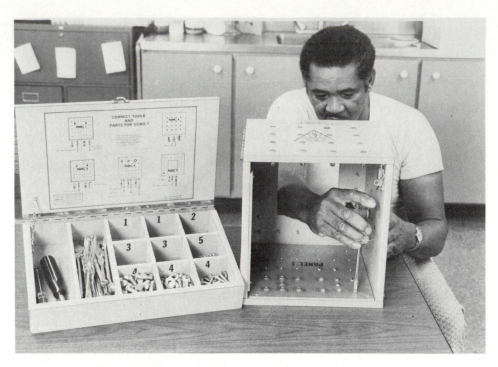

FIG. 7-11. Patient works in confined area with mechanical tools.

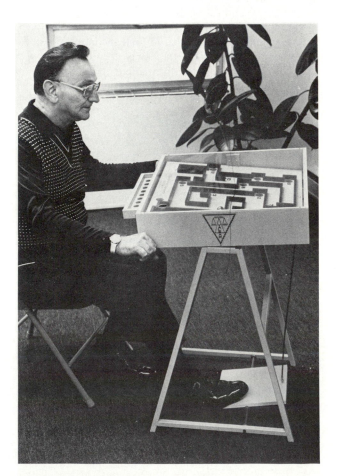

FIG. 7-12. Eye-hand-foot coordination is required to manipulate steel balls through a 13-point maze.

the completion of each panel. Panels may be given independently. If the entire test is administered, the time of administration varies from 45 minutes to 1½ hours. Forms available with the test are used to record time and a subjective assessment of worker characteristics.

Time scores and error scores are recorded. Motion time measurements are used to evaluate the patient's time scores. These scores relate to the patient's speed of performance as compared to the employed normal population. Error scores are used to determine the patient's accuracy of performance.

Advantages of the Valpar Small Tools Mechanical Work Sample are the following: (1) scoring is easily understandable; (2) the test gives indications of endurance when several panels are given; (3) the patient's performance may indicate his potential to do bench-work activities. Disadvantages of the Valpar Small Tools Mechanical Work Sample are the following: (1) small tools are included in the work sample; therefore occupations that require handling of larger hand tools cannot be tested; (2) the hardware of the test (that is, washers and nuts) are easily misplaced.

Valpar Eye-Hand-Foot Coordination Work Sample

The Valpar Eye-Hand-Foot Coordination Work Sample (Fig. 7-12) measures a person's ability to use simultaneously his eyes, hands, and feet to perform a skilled task in a coordinated manner. It gives the therapist an opportunity to observe the patient's concentration, reaction time, and planning and learning capacity as these relate to the task.

This work sample consists of a 21 × 21 × 4⁵⁄₁₆–inch box made with ½-inch Formica-covered particle board. The work box is covered with clear Plexiglas and mounted on a ¾-inch tubular metal frame. Beneath the cover is a maze containing 13 holes. There is a ball tray mounted on the front panel of the box and a ball drawer behind and underneath the front panel. Wooden handles are attached to the sides of the box. The ball tray and drawer allow for storage of nine chrome-steel balls. There is a foot pedal attached to the bottom of the frame with a ¼-inch metal rod attached to the pedal and to the maze. An instruction manual and a scoring pad are included with this work sample. A stopwatch is necessary for the administration of the evaluation.

The patient is required to sit in front of the test instrument on a sturdy chair. The patient must maneuver nine steel balls, one at a time, through a 13-point maze through which the steel balls may drop. Instruction in the method to operate the instrument and move the balls is given. Trials are given. To move the ball, the patient tilts the maze left and right with his hands and forward and back with his feet and tracks the movement of the ball with his eyes. The patient takes one ball at a time, places it through the hole in the glass top, where it drops to the starting point. Timing begins at this point. The patient's objective is to manuever the ball through the maze, avoiding 12 holes so that the ball will fall into the thirteenth hole and a higher score will be obtained. Because each hole is numbered, if the ball falls in a lower-numbered hole, the score will be less than if the ball falls through a higher-numbered hole. The patient repeats this task until all nine balls are moved through the maze to complete the first timed section. There are three timed sessions in this work sample, which are added together for a cumulative time score. Both a time score and an accuracy score are calculated for this test.

Advantages of the Valpar Eye-Hand-Foot Coordination Work Sample are the following: (1) patients usually respond to this test as a nonthreatening experience, and (2) the test is easily scored.

Disadvantages of this Work Sample are the following: (1) patients may focus on accuracy (attaining a higher score) and sacrifice speed of performance, and (2) occupations such as truck driving are not accurately simulated because minimal physical exertion is required to participate in this test.

Valpar Clerical Comprehension Work Sample

The Valpar Clerical Comprehension Work Sample measures a person's ability to perform various clerical tasks and ability to learn these clerical tasks. Tasks included in this work sample are telephone answering, alphabetical filing, bookkeeping, and typing. The patient must classify, file, sort correspondence, report verbal and written information, transcribe with a typewriter, and prepare numerical records (Fig. 7-13).

This Work Sample consists of a cassette tape recorder with a recorded tape and an adding machine. A modified typewriter with a keyboard of 10 Greek letters is provided, enabling an individual with no previous typing experience to participate in the test. A regular typewriter can be used, but it is not included in the work sample equipment. A hinged box made of ½-inch Formica-covered particle board measuring 17 × 13 × 10¼ inches is also supplied. The top of the box has 12 compartments. The bottom of the box has a lid and contains 258 items used in the test, such as message pads and cards used for filing.

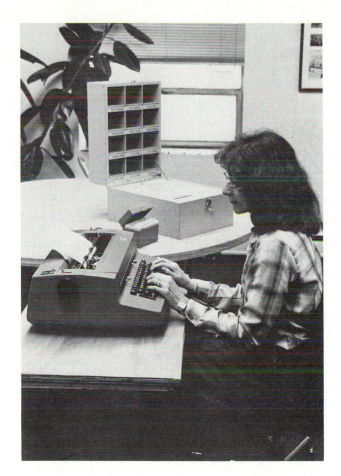

FIG. 7-13. Basic clerical tasks are evaluated.

There are three sections to this work sample. The first section encompasses general clerical skills. The second section provides an assessment of bookkeeping skills, and the third section tests typing ability. The test begins with a person sorting mail while simultaneously answering the telephone as a precorded tape plays a series of phone conversations at selected intervals, requiring the person to stop sorting mail and record messages.

The second part of the general clerical section requires that the person perform an alphabetical filing task again while simultaneously answering the telephone. In the bookkeeping section of the work sample the patient uses an adding machine to perform three selected tasks. This section emphasizes basic math skills. The patient is required to complete a disbursement ledger sheet, a daily log, and a payroll ledger.

The third section of the task evaluates a person's ability to type or his aptitude to learn typing. In the first typing task, the patient must type the home keys with each hand for a 30-second test. The second section of this typing component requires the patient to again perform three timed typing tasks of 30 seconds each. Only this time all 10 keys are used for the typing requirements. On the third section, the patient must alternate the use of his fingers of each hand to complete the test. Three timed sessions are recorded. No corrections of errors are permitted in the typing component, and a subjective assessment of the patient's characteristics are recorded by the therapist.

Scores for this work sample include time, error, and performance percentile scores for mail sorting, general clerical, and bookkeeping. The typing section includes an accuracy score and a speed of performance percentile score. Scoring is in both Method Time Motion Standards and employed worker norms.

The advantages of the Valpar Clerical Comprehension Work Sample are the following: (1) experienced and inexperienced people can be evaluated for clerical aptitude, and (2) this work sample offers patients the opportunity to evaluate their personal interests and reactions to the job demands of clerical occupations. The disadvantages are the following: (1) the manual typewriter is difficult for the hand-injured patient to operate, (2) scoring procedures are confusing, and (3) testing apparatus (adding machine, typewriter, and tape recorder) may be subject to frequent use and need regular upkeep and possible repair.

CONCLUSION

The standardized tests described in this chapter, when used with other evaluative proedures, provide the therapist with a means of providing a functional assessment of a patient with a hand disability. By relying on standardized tests and procedures, the therapist can be confident that the information obtained from these tests has been proved to measure precisely and accurately that which each test purports to measure.

REFERENCES

1. Fess, E.E., and Moran, C.A.: Clinical assessment recommendations, Aurora, Colo., 1981, American Society of Hand Therapists.
2. Instructions for the 32023 (4207) Minnesota Manual Dexterity Test: Lafayette Instrument Co., Sagamore and North Ninth Street, Lafayette, Ind.
3. Jebson, R.H., Taylor, N., Trieschman, R.B., and others: An objective and standardized test of hand function, Arch. Phys. Med. Rehabil. **50:**311-319, 1969.
4. Tiffin, J.: Purdue Pegboard examiner manual, Chicago, 1968, Science Research Associates, Inc.

BIBLIOGRAPHY

Bolton, B., editor: Measurements and evaluation in rehabilitation, Baltimore, 1976, University Park Press.

Cromwell, F.: A procedure for pre-vocational evaluation, Am. J. Occup. Ther. **13**(1):1-4, 1959.

Fess, E.E., Harmon, K.S., Strickland, J.W., and Steichen, J.B.: Evaluation of the hand by objective measurement. In Hunter, J.M., Schneider, L., Mackin, E., and Bell, J., editors: Rehabilitation of the hand, St. Louis, 1978, The C.V. Mosby Co.

Rosenberg, B., and Wellerson, T.: A structured pre-vocational program, Am. J. Occup. Ther. **14:**57-60, 1960.

Swanson, A.B., Göran-Hagert, C., and Swanson, G.: Evaluation of impairment of hand function. In Hunter, J., Schneider, L., Mackin, E., and Bell, J., editors: Rehabilitation of the Hand, ed. 2, St. Louis, 1983, The C.V. Mosby Co.

Tiffin, J., and Asher, E.J.: The Purdue Pegboard: norms and studies of reliability and validity, J. Appl. Psychol. **32:**234-47, 1948.

8

Evaluation of impairment of hand function

ALFRED B. SWANSON, CARL GÖRAN-HAGERT, and
GENEVIEVE DE GROOT SWANSON

There are millions of persons in the world who are suffering the residual effects of injury or destructive diseases to the hand and upper extremity. Physicians interested in treating disabilities of the hand should accept the responsibility for accurate evaluation of the patient's physical condition, both local and general, and be able to compute the permanent anatomic and functional impairment resulting from these deficiencies. This evaluation is usually limited to the analysis of the anatomic, functional, and cosmetic effect loss after optimal surgical and physical rehabilitation have been achieved. The physician is responsible for a medical evaluation of impairment, not a rating of disability. The latter is an administrative function that relates to the patient's ability to engage in gainful activity as this affects his social and economic standard of living.

Determination of treatment programs and proper evaluation of the results depend on accurate and complete patient records. Records of examinations, operations, and treatment on these patients are increasingly under review. Insurance companies, law courts, and other judicial bodies are frequently required to evaluate the results of trauma and disease to the hand. Techniques for recording the history and for measuring anatomic, functional, and cosmetic deficits should be standard and routine and are facilitated by an orderly and convenient method of examination. Evaluations should be made after consistent and thorough histories are taken and careful observations, examinations, and tests are performed.

The proper evaluation of impairment of the injured limb presumes a knowledge of the normal functional anatomy of the part. It requires an appraisal of the resultant loss of function as it relates to activities of daily living and work and the more specialized hand activities. It is usually a determination of loss of structure, limitation, motion, strength, pain, and/or loss of sensibility as compared to the opposite normal limb; if both are impaired, comparison with an average limb is made.

EVALUATION METHODS

Methods of evaluation of the condition of the upper extremity can be arbitrarily divided into anatomic, cosmetic, and functional categories. We believe that a combination of these methods is necessary to show an accurate profile of the patient's condition. Their effect on the patient's psychologic, sociologic, environmental, and economic status must also be considered. The *physical evaluation* is necessary to determine the anatomic impairment for preoperative and postoperative surgical considerations. It is based on the history and a detailed examination of the upper extremity and patient. The *cosmetic evaluation* concerns the patient's and society's reaction to his impairment or the result of the surgical treatment. The *functional evaluation* is much more involved and of the greatest importance; it relates to the quality of function and the ability to perform activities of daily living. Functional evaluation studies are becoming increasingly sophisticated and may add greatly to the evaluation process.

A complete and detailed examination of the upper extremity is facilitated by the use of a printed chart that lists the various tests and measurements in an orderly fashion. A sketch of the hand with dorsal and palmar views simplifies the description of loss of parts and the location of scars or other defects. The printed charts used for hand evaluation for both the traumatized and rheumatoid hand are shown in Fig. 8-1. The evaluation record includes a checklist for the common information necessary in recording the history, type of disease, onset, duration, distribution of disease process, laboratory tests, and treatment. Organized columns are provided for recording the range of motion and strength of each joint, prehensile patterns, ability to perform activities of daily living, and ambulatory status. Specific clinical abnormalities such as ulnar drift or lateral deviation, rotation, subluxation, and deformities secondary to tendon loss or imbalance are recorded through the use of a coded number system. Arbitrary classifications—mild, moderate, and severe—were devised to help determine the degree of involvement or index of severity of each particular deformity (see boxed material on p. 104). For example, a moderate degree of ulnar drift is recorded as 7-b. A special section is provided in this record to describe the previous and current medical and surgical treatment.

PRINCIPLES AND METHODS OF HISTORY TAKING

History taking should record the necessary information: identification, vital statistics, diagnosis, and history of the disease. Additionally, in the case of trauma, it should narrate the accident, how and where it happened, the mechanics of

A

RHEUMATOID ARTHRITIS EVALUATION RECORD
PREOPERATIVE SILASTIC[R] IMPLANTS

Name _____ Sex: ☐ Male ☐ Female Date _____ Birth date _____

Address _____

Occupation _____ Dominant hand: ☐ R ☐ L ☐ Hospital _____ Examiner _____

Diagnosis: ☐ Juvenile rheumatoid ☐ Adult rheumatoid ☐ Erosive arthritis ☐ Osteoarthritis ☐ Psoriatic arthritis
  ☐ Ankylosing spondylitis ☐ Sjögren's syndrome ☐ Systemic lupus erythematosus ☐ Trauma

Onset date _____ Sedimentation rate: ☐ Wintrobe ☐ Westergren ☐ Rourke _____ Rheumatoid test ☐ (+) ☐ (−)

Onset distribution ☐ Peripheral ☐ Central ☐ Both: Remission ☐ Yes ☐ No: Anemia ☐ Yes ☐ No: Family Hx ☐ (+) ☐ (−)

Check if the following has been completed: ☐ X-rays ☐ Photographs ☐ Movies ☐ Cineradiography

Range of motion (ROM) use neutral = zero method of American Academy of Orthopedic Surgeons 1965.

Codes 1-25 represent observed and measured abnormalities. Use as indicated in appropriate sections.

Severity indices mild, moderate, and severe are represented by a, b, & c and further categorize codes 1-25.

The code 1-25 is below on this sheet. Severity indices are on separate detachable sheet.

This evaluation record has been designed for computer analysis. Responses must be complete.

Thumb	Codes to use for thumb 1, 2, 3, 9-14, 19, & 22		Abd (Angle between 1 & 2 metacarp) Add (tip misses 5th MCP joint) Opp (tip from 3rd MCP joint)			
	Code		Joints	ROM		
	R	L		R	L	
			MC Abd			
			See Add			
			above Opp			
			MP			
			IP			

Finger codes 3-15, 19, 22-25				ROM		
Index			MP			
			PIP			
			DIP			
Flex DIP crease to palmar crease (cm)						
Middle			MP			
			PIP			
			DIP			
Flex DIP crease to palmar crease (cm)						
Ring			MP			
			PIP			
			DIP			
Flex DIP crease to palmar crease (cm)						
Little			MP			
			PIP			
			DIP			
Flex DIP crease to palmar crease (cm)						

Wrist	Codes 3, 7-14, 19, 20, 22, 23				
			Flex		
			Ext		
			U. Dev		
			R. Dev		

Prehensile patterns: Check if able to perform

Grasp:			R	L
Cylinders	2.5 cm			
	5 cm			
	7.5 cm			
	10 cm			
Spheres	5 cm			
	7.5 cm			
	10 cm			
	12.5 cm			

Strength: ☐ Lb ☐ Kg ☐ mm Hg		R	L
Pulp pinch	Index		
	Middle		
	Ring		
	Little		
Lateral or key pinch			
Grip			

ADL: I = Independent A = Assisted U = Unable

Dressing	I	A	U	Hygiene	I	A	U
Upper ext				Teeth			
Trunk				Hair			
Lower ext				Shave			
Bath				Pickup coin			
Shower				Turn key			
Eating				Doorknob			
Toilet				Car door			
Telephone				Screw top jar			
Typewrite				Aerosol can			
Write				Fasteners			

Ambulatory status:
☐ Independent ☐ Wheelchair with partial walking
☐ Assisted walk ☐ Bedfast

Code for clinical abnormality

1—Thumb swan neck
2—Thumb boutonniere
3—Subluxation—dislocation
4—Swan neck, finger
5—Boutonniere, finger
6—Intrinsic tightness
7—Ulnar drift
8—Radial drift
9—Ankylosis
10—Instability
11—Tendon rupture
12—Constrictive tenosynovitis
13—Synovial hypertrophy
14—Crepitation with motion
15—Extensor tendon subluxation
16—Varus angle

17—Valgus angle
18—Rotational deformity
19—Erosions
20—Joint narrowing
21—Subchondral sclerosis
22—Painful joint with motion
23—Nerve compression—M, U, R
24—Vasculitis
25—Nodules

Severity index
a—Mild
b—Moderate
c—Severe

Ambulatory status:

☐ Independent ☐ Wheelchair with partial walking
☐ Assisted walk ☐ Bedfast

Palm R   Palm L

Sketch implant into appropriate site

FIG. 8-1. Preoperative evaluation record. **A,** This form is designed for evaluation of rheumatoid and arthritic hands. **B,** This form is designed for posttraumatic conditions and other disorders of the hand. (From Swanson, A.B.: Flexible implant resection arthroplasty in the hand and extremities, St. Louis, 1973, The C.V. Mosby Co.)

HAND EVALUATION RECORD

Name _____ Age _____ Date _____ Major hand _____
Occupation _____ X-rays _____ Photographs _____
History:

Shoulder:	L	R	Wrist:				Circ:		
For	___	___		DF	___ ___		Biceps	___	___
Back	___	___		PF	___ ___		Forearm	___	___
Abd	___	___		RD	___ ___		Grip: L	___	___
Add	___	___		UD	___ ___		R	___	___
Rotation Int	___	___	Elbow:	Ext	___ ___		Forearm: Pro	___	___
Ext	___	___		Flex	___ ___		Sup	___	___

		MP	IP			% Impairment
Thumb	Ext			Abd (angle 1st-2nd metacarp.)		
	Flex			Add (tip misses 5th MCP joint)		
	Ankylosis			Opp (tip from 3rd MCP joint)		

		MP	PIP	DIP	Flex pulp to midpalmar crease	
Index	Ext					
	Flex					
	Ankylosis					
Middle	Ext					
	Flex					
	Ankylosis					
Ring	Ext					
	Flex					
	Ankylosis					
Little	Ext					
	Flex					
	Ankylosis					

Chart:
1. Amputations
2. Scars
3. Skin—subcutaneous loss
4. Nail bed injury
5. Major nerve loss: R, M, U
6. Digital bundle loss
7. Neuroma
8. Pain and tenderness
9. Bone damage
10. Joint damage
11. Flexor tendon loss
12. Extensor tendon loss
13. Ligament injury
14. Sensibility—pickup
        two-point
        Ninhydrin
15. Prehension:
    Grasp—small
            large
    Pinch—pulp
            tip
            lateral
    Hook—distal
            proximal
    Scoop
16. Maximum improvement
17. Rehabilitation needed
18. Further treatment
19. Classification
NOTE: Degrees of motion
    recorded as left/right

Total % _____

Dorsum R hand
or
Palmar L hand

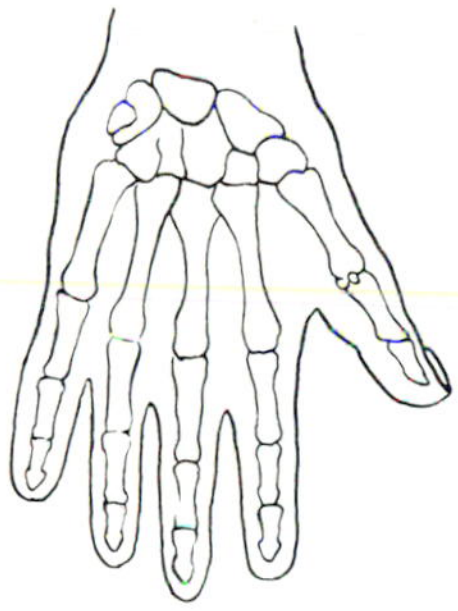

Dorsum L hand
or
Palmar R hand

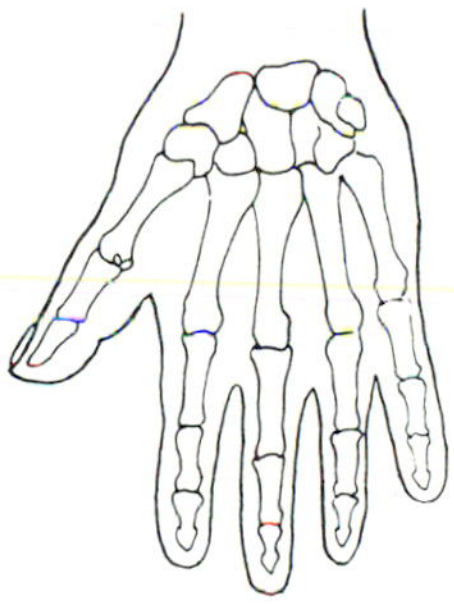

B

FIG. 8-1, cont'd. For legend see opposite page.

**Severity index arbitrarily classifies common deformities and degree of involvement
as mild, moderate, or severe**

1. Thumb swan neck—flexion limit of MCP joint
   a. Mild = MCP ROM +10° to 50°
   b. Moderate = MCP ROM +20° to 30°
   c. Severe = MCP ROM +30° to 10°
2. Thumb boutonnière—extension limit MCP joint
   a. Mild = MCP −5° to −20°
   b. Moderate = MCP −20° to −40°
   c. Severe = MCP more than −40°
3. Subluxation to dislocation
   a. Mild = capable of reduction manually
   b. Moderate = incomplete reduction manually
   c. Severe = irreducible dislocation
4. Swan-neck fingers—flexion limit of PIP joint
   a. Mild = PIP ROM +10° to 50°
   b. Moderate = PIP ROM +20° to 30°
   c. Severe = PIP ROM +30° to 10°
5. Boutonnière, finger—extension limit PIP joint
   a. Mild = PIP ext limit −5° to 10°
   b. Moderate = PIP ext limit −10° to −30°
   c. Severe = PIP ext limit more than −30°
6. Intrinsic tightness—with MCP joint extended
   a. Mild = PIP flexion more than 60°
   b. Moderate = PIP flexion 20° to 60°
   c. Severe = PIP flexion less than 20°
7. Ulnar drift—joint measured in maximum active extension
   measure metacarpophalangeal angle
   a. Mild = 0° to 10°
   b. Moderate = 10° to 30°
   c. Severe = more than 30°
8. Radial drift—joint measured in maximum active extension
   measure metacarpophalangeal angle
   a. Mild = 0° to 10°
   b. Moderate = 10° to 30°
   c. Severe = more than 30°
9. Ankylosis—record angle of ankylosis under ROM
   c. Severe, when present
10. Instability—measure excess of passive mediolateral motion compared to that of a normal joint
    a. Mild = 0° to 10°
    b. Moderate = 10° to 20°
    c. Severe = more than 20°
11. Tendon rupture
    c. Severe, complete
12. Constrictive tenosynovitis
    a. Mild = inconstant triggering during active ROM
    b. Moderate = constant triggering during active ROM
    c. Severe = prevents active ROM
13. Synovial hypertrophy
    a. Mild = visual increase in joint size
    b. Moderate = palpable increase in joint size
    c. Severe = more than 10% increase in joint size by measure

14. Crepitation with motion
    a. Mild = inconstant during active ROM
    b. Moderate = constant during active ROM
    c. Severe = constant during passive ROM
15. Extensor tendon subluxation
    a. Mild = subluxation in MCP flexion
    b. Moderate = tendon dislocated into intermetacarpal grove during MCP flexion but can be reduced
    c. Severe = tendon remains in intermetacarpal groove
16. Varus angle—clinical or x-ray measure
    a. Mild = 0° to 10°
    b. Moderate = 10° to 20°
    c. Severe = more than 20°
17. Valgus angle—clinical or x-ray measure
    a. Mild = 10° to 20°
    b. Moderate = 20° to 30°
    c. Severe = more than 30°
18. Rotational deformity
    Fingers
    a. Mild = 5° to 15°
    b. Moderate = 15° to 30°
    c. Severe = more than 30°
19. Erosions—x-ray exam
    a. Mild = one erosion
    b. Moderate = two erosions
    c. Severe = three or more erosions
20. Joint narrowing—x-ray exam
    a. Mild = $1/3$ narrowing
    b. Moderate = $2/3$ narrowing
    c. Severe = obliteration of joint space
21. Subchondral sclerosis
    a. Mild, when present
22. Painful joint with motion
    a. Mild = pain with active motion
    b. Moderate = pain with active motion which interferes with activity
    c. Severe = pain at rest and prevents activity
23. Nerve compression—median, ulnar or radial
    a. Mild = sensory disturbances
    b. Moderate = sensory disturbances and motor weakness
    c. Severe = sensory and motor paralysis
24. Vasculitis
    a. Mild = paronychial hemorrhages and/or
    b. Moderate = peripheral neuropathy
    c. Severe = cutaneous gangrene of an extremity
25. Nodules
    a. Mild = one nodule, mobile, and nontender
    b. Moderate = two nodules, fixed and tender
    c. Severe = more than three nodules, fixed, tender and with skin breakdowns

the injury, the degree of the injury, and the time sequence of treatment as to emergency care, definitive care, and postoperative therapy. The present complaint of how the residual difficulty affects the patient's activities should be recorded in his own words. Any history of previous difficulty in the same extremity should also be noted. Any general condition that would influence the patient's recovery is also indicated. In disorders of the hand such as arthritis, neuromuscular diseases, and Dupuytren's contracture an appropriate history should be recorded.

The patient's hand can be observed as the examiner is taking a history and measuring the upper portion of the limb. The general posture of the hand, the position of its various joints as active motion of the upper extremity is carried out, and the state of nutrition, color, moisture, swelling, or muscle weakness can be subtly checked without the patient's awareness.

Malingering or psychogenic overlay may make it difficult to obtain an accurate estimation of impairment. The patient whose complaints are not justified by objective findings or whose response to testing varies widely from time to time should put the examiner on guard. It may be impossible to identify the malingerer without the help of evidence gathered outside the examining room when the patient does not think he is being observed.

PHOTOGRAPHIC RECORD

Photographs are an important part of the record. A set of standard position photographs of the hand is essential for consistent and accurate interpretation of the hand disability. Suggested sequences should include views of the hand from various positions, carrying out flexion-extension of the fingers and the functions of grasp and pinch. Film sequences may also be used to evaluate the patient's adaptation to his needs of daily living. Manipulating buttons and safety pins, threading a needle, turning the screw-top lid of a jar, writing, picking up and releasing objects, and turning a nut on and off a bolt are but a few of the activities that are suitable for recording on film.

RADIOLOGIC EVALUATION

A standard series of roentgenograms including anterior, posterior, lateral, and oblique views of the hand and wrist should be part of the record. Films of the other joints of the upper extremity may also be included. The films should be taken without jewelry or other items about the extremity. The anatomic extended position is desired but must not be forced so that the degree of deformity can also be evaluated on the roentgenogram. Roentgenographic views should be less than 3 months old. Evaluation of the range of motion of the skeleton may also be aided by cineradiography, which can show the degree of movement of the digits and wrist.

ANATOMIC EVALUATION

The hand is primarily a grasping or prehensile organ. The action of the shoulder, elbow, and wrist joints enables the hand to be placed at almost any area of the body. The hand can be pulled toward or pushed away from the body through considerably more than a hemisphere. It is obvious, therefore, that every examination should include an evaluation of the entire limb.

The condition of all the structures of the extremity including skin and neurovascular structures, muscles, tendons, bones, and joints should be considered. Joint instability and ligamentous injury, deformities secondary to tendon loss, or imbalance are noted. Circumferential measurement of the extremity as compared to the opposite member should be recorded.

The skin covering the hand should be evaluated as to the presence of scars, loss of subcutaneous tissue, fixation, and adherence to deeper structures and their effect on hand function. The temperature, color, swelling, texture, and tenderness should be noted. Nail bed deformities should be described.

For each joint the presence and degree of synovitis, instability, subluxation, ankylosis, contracture, lateral deviation, and rotation should be recorded. Circumferential measurement of individual joints should be measured in centimeters, and angulation and rotation should be measured in degrees. The presence and severity of collapse deformities are noted for each digit. The status of the tendinous system is recorded by stating the presence of tendon ruptures, constrictive tenosynovitis, and extensor tendon subluxations. Description of the thumb should include length, mobility, stability, and capacity for placement to the rest of the hand. Flexibility and depth of the thumb web are noted.

Intrinsic tightness in the hand may be demonstrated by a test described by Bunnell.[3] Hyperextension of the metacarpophalangeal joint in a normal hand still allows passive flexion of the proximal interphalangeal joint. If the intrinsic muscles are tight or contracted, the available stretch of these muscles is taken up by the hyperextended position of the metacarpophalangeal joint, and passive flexion of the proximal interphalangeal joint will be difficult.

It is important to describe the posture of the hand as it relates to the normal arches. Any disturbance of the normal carpal and metacarpal transverse arches and the longitudinal arches of the digital rays should be noted. Collapse of these arches from joint instability, skeletal malalignment, or muscle imbalance contributes to the loss of function. The thumb ray on one side and the ring and little finger rays on the other side normally move widely around the firmly fixed, stable axis of the index and middle metacarpals. The normal longitudinal arch of the digit ray is especially necessary for small-object prehension.

A complete anatomic evaluation should also include measurement of the range of motion of individual joints, strength of pinch and grasp, muscle testing, sensory evaluation, and assessment of pain.

Some of the equipment necessary for evaluating the extremity is shown in Fig. 8-2. Important tools for a good examination include a goniometer, dynamometer, pinch meter, ruler, sensory testing devices, a two-point compass, familiar objects for tactile identification and the pickup test, and cylinders of various sizes to measure the effective grasp.

Prehension and strength measurements

One can make measurements of strength of pinch and grasp by comparing the force with that of the examiner and measuring the size of the arms, forearms, and hands for estimating atrophy; dynamometers are also used. The mechanical dynamometer may be too gross to measure the

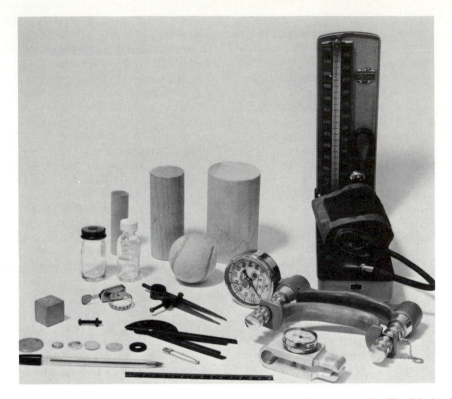

FIG. 8-2. Equipment suggested for evaluation of upper extremity. (From Swanson, A.B.: Flexible implant resection arthroplasty in the hand and extremities, St. Louis, 1973, The C.V. Mosby Co.)

TABLE 8-1. Average strength of grip (unsupported) listed by occupation (100 subjects)

	Unsupported grip (kg)			
	Male hand		Female hand	
Occupation	Major	Minor	Major	Minor
Skilled	47.0	45.4	26.8	24.4
Sedentary	47.2	44.1	23.1	21.1
Manual	48.5	44.6	24.2	22.0
Average	47.6	45.0	24.6	22.4

TABLE 8-2. Average strength of grip listed by age (100 subjects)

	Grip (kg)			
	Male hand		Female hand	
Age	Major	Minor	Major	Minor
20	45.2	42.6	23.8	22.8
20-30	48.5	46.2	24.6	22.7
30-40	49.2	44.5	30.8	28.0
40-50	49.0	47.3	23.4	21.5
50-60	45.9	43.5	22.3	18.2

TABLE 8-3. Average strength of chuck pinch by occupation (100 subjects)

	Chuck pinch (kg)			
	Male hand		Female hand	
Occupation	Major	Minor	Major	Minor
Skilled	7.3	7.2	5.4	4.6
Sedentary	8.4	7.3	4.2	4.0
Manual	8.5	7.6	6.1	5.6
Average	7.9	7.5	5.2	4.9

TABLE 8-4. Average strength of pulp pinch with separate digits (100 subjects)

	Pulp pinch (kg)			
	Male hand		Female hand	
Digit	Major	Minor	Major	Minor
II	5.3	4.8	3.6	3.3
III	5.6	5.7	3.8	3.4
IV	3.8	3.6	2.5	2.4
V	2.3	2.2	1.7	1.6

grasp in the weak arthritic hand. A sphygmomanometer may be used to record grips of lesser power. The blood pressure cuff is rolled to a 5 cm diameter and inflated to 50 mm Hg; the cuff is then squeezed and the change of millimeters of mercury from 50 mm is recorded as the power of grip. An electronic pinch meter based on the strain-gauge principle has been used by us for measuring the strength of pinch in pounds or kilograms of pressure. Other devices used for pinch or grasp measurement include a variety of mechanical pinch meters and the force-pressure measuring device of Mannerfelt.[8]

Many factors, including fatigue, handedness, time of day, age, state of nutrition, pain, and cooperation of the patient, influence the strength of the grip. It has been shown that tests repeated at intervals during the examination are reliable if there is less than a 20% variation in the reading. If there is more than 20%, one can assume that the patient is not exerting his full effort. The test is usually repeated three times with each hand at different times during the examination and then recorded and later compared.

Although strength is one of the important characteristics of a normal hand, this factor is not given enough attention in reconstructive surgery as compared to other parameters of motion and sensibility. A baseline of normal grip and pinch strength was studied in our clinic by testing a group of 100 healthy persons. As it is necessary to know the normal to appreciate the abnormal, a parallel evaluation of the disabled hand could further define the degree of impairment present. The strength of the normal hand was recorded as applied in basic hand patterns: grasp, chuck, pinch (three-digit pinch), pulp pinch with separate fingers, and lateral pinch. Measurements were expressed in kilograms of force units. The force of grip was recorded with a hydraulic dynamometer. The strength of chuck, pulp, and lateral pinch was tested with an electronic pinch meter based on the strain-gauge principle. However, similar findings were obtained with the standard pinch meter.

The strength of the grip was measured with the adjustable handle of a Jamar dynamometer spaced at 6 cm. Most subjects were comfortable at this breadth of grip and could apply maximal force when tested. The minimal and maximal strength of the grip measurement ranged from 30.4 to 70.4 kg in the male group, and 14 to 38.6 kg in the female group. Table 8-1 shows the average strength of grip listed by occupation, measured with the extremity unsupported. Table 8-2 shows the average strength of grip listed by age.

The majority of patients preferred chuck pinch to any other type of pinch for applying the most force. Table 8-3 shows the average strength of chuck pinch for the various groups examined. It is interesting to note that the interphalangeal joint of the thumb was hyperextended in most cases when maximal force of chuck pinch was applied.

The strength of pulp pinch with separate fingers was determined (Table 8-4). A tendency to hyperextend either the proximal interphalangeal or the distal interphalangeal joints was evident when maximal pinch force was applied. For the proximal interphalangeal joint, this tendency increased from the radial to the ulnar sides of the hand. Lateral pinch is a very strong type of pinch as noted in Table 8-5; it may be an important adaptation in the disabled hand and may pro-vide a very useful function when pulp pinch is lost.

In the comparison of major and minor hands, the major hand was usually stronger in heavy manual workers; however, the minor hand may be stronger in a significant percentage of other individuals tested. On the average, grip strength of the minor hand was found to be weaker in 5.4% of males and 8.9% of females. The strength of pinch in the minor hand was weaker by only 4% in males and 6% in females. The data obtained in our study indicated that there is less difference in strength of the major and minor hands than has generally been thought. It has been demonstrated that approximately 4 kg of force is needed for adequate grip to perform 90% of the activities of daily living. Patients can usually manipulate the objects of their environment like door handles and a variety of other objects if they have this degree of strength. The majority of simple activities can be accomplished with approximately 1 kg of pinch strength. However, an adequate examination of a person, as far as the necessity for strength of the hand is concerned, should include an evaluation of his personal environment and how his hand strength can help him.

Muscle testing

Muscle testing may be an important part of evaluating impairment in the hand disabled by paralysis or paresis resulting from a proximal or peripheral nerve lesion. Manual muscle testing is based on the ability to raise the distal part through its range of motion against gravity and holding the part against resistance. The determination of muscle strength impairment will be based on the therapist's or physician's interpretation as to whether the strength is (1) normal (no impairment of strength)—complete range of motion against gravity with full resistance; (2) good (1% to 25% impairment of strength)—complete range of motion against gravity with some resistance; (3) fair (26% to 50% impairment of strength)—range of motion against gravity; (4) poor (51% to 75% impairment of strength)—complete range of motion with gravity eliminated; (5) trace (76% to 99% impairment of strength)—evidence of slight contractility, no joint motion; and (6) zero (100% impairment of strength)—no evidence of contractility. When evaluating impairment for paralysis or paresis and associated sensory defects, it is not necessary to include impairment values for loss of motion or ankylosis of parts. This would result in a duplication of rating impairment.

TABLE 8-5. Average strength of lateral pinch by occupation (100 subjects)

| | Lateral pinch (kg) | | | |
| | Male hand | | Female hand | |
Occupation	Major	Minor	Major	Minor
Skilled	6.6	6.4	4.4	4.3
Sedentary	6.3	6.1	4.1	3.9
Manual	8.5	7.7	6.0	5.5
Average	7.5	7.1	4.9	4.7

Range of motion

The range of motion should be recorded on the principle that neutral position equals 0 degrees, as accepted by the American Academy of Orthopaedic Surgeons in 1975[1] (Fig. 8-3). In this method all motions of the joint are measured from defined zero as the starting position: The "extended anatomic position" of an extremity is therefore accepted as 0 rather than 180 degrees. Thus the degree of motion of a joint is added in the direction the joint moves from the zero starting position. Active motion is that motion obtained at the joints with full flexion or extension muscle force. Passive motion is the motion that is measured after normal soft tissue resistance to movement is overcome; in the finger joints this is approximately 0.5 kg of force.

A distinction should be made between the terms "extension" and "hyperextension." The term "extension" is used for motions opposite to that of flexion to the zero or neutral starting position. If motion opposite to flexion exceeds the zero or neutral starting position such as that seen at the finger joint, elbow, or knee, it may be referred to as "hyperextension." Motion of hyperextension is to be given a plus value. Incomplete motion of extension from a flexed position to zero starting position is reported as a negative or minus degree from zero. EXAMPLE: Finger joint flexion contracture of 15 degrees with flexion available to 45 degrees would be recorded as a range of motion of 30 degrees, in other words, − 15 to 45 degrees. This, therefore, refers to a lack of extension of 15 degrees to the zero position. A finger joint that has 15 degrees of hyperextension available to 45 degrees of flexion would be recorded as a joint motion of + 15 to 45 degrees.

The method of assigning the value of the angle within the sector of hyperextension as a "plus" or "minus" is a somewhat controversial subject. However, the method that we present employs the traditional terminology and is easily understood by most clinicians and therefore has the greatest validity.

Measurement of individual joints should be recorded in table form and expressed in degrees. Proximal joints should be in neutral or straight-line position when one is measuring the distal joints (Fig. 8-4, A to C). Ankylosis contractures and active motion should be noted. Digits are named rather than numbered, according to the terms thumb, index, middle (long), ring, and little fingers. Deformity of the fingers as to rotation and alignment should be noted. The spread of the fingers and the strength of the spreading can be measured.

The method, described by Boyes,[2] of measuring maximal finger flexion by noting the distance that the pulp of the finger lacks in touching the distal palmar crease should be included in the evaluating of finger flexion (Fig. 8-4, D). This is the most simple and informative basis for impairment evaluation. The range of motion of the individual joints of the digit should also be included for completeness of reporting and as an alternative method of evaluating impairment. Further description of the thumb should include a measurement of radial abduction, adduction, flexion, extension, opposition, anteposition (palmar abduction), and retroposition (Fig. 8-5).

The motion of the wrist in dorsal and palmar flexions and radial and ulnar deviations should be measured. Range of motion at the elbow in flexion, extension, pronation, and supination should be checked. Shoulder motion in flexion, extension, abduction, adduction, and internal and external rotation should also be measured.

Neurologic examination

The presence of neurologic disorders, brachial, radial, ulnar, and median nerve palsies, as they are evidenced by motor and sensory disturbances in the hand is noted. Digital nerve loss and the presence and localization of neuromas should be evaluated. Tenderness, sensitivity, and painful states such as the causalgias and other sympathetic dystrophies should be appraised. A complete sensory examination should be carried out.

The Ninhydrin test for sudomotor function can be a useful method for documenting the interruption of the digital nerves. However, it has limitations in evaluating the "re-

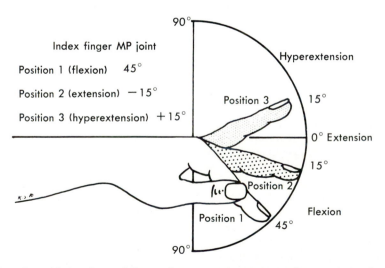

FIG. 8-3. Range of motion of index finger. Measure hyperextension as (+) value, extension lag as (−) value, and neutral position as 0 degrees, as suggested by the American Academy of Orthopaedic Surgeons.

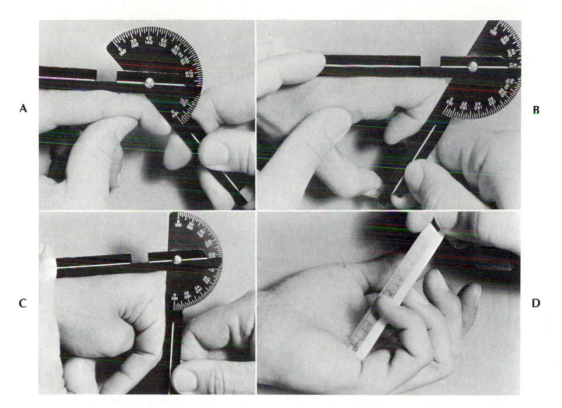

FIG. 8-4. Techniques of measurement of digital joints. **A,** Distal interphalangeal joint. **B,** Proximal interphalangeal joint. **C,** Metacarpophalangeal joint. **D,** Maximal flexion distance measured by Boyes' method as distance pulp of finger lack of touching distal palmar crease. (From Swanson, A.B.: Flexible implant resection arthroplasty in the hand and extremities, St. Louis, 1973, The C.V. Mosby Co.)

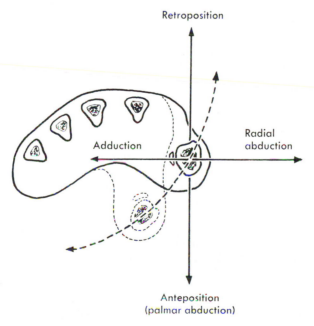

FIG. 8-5. Movements of thumb are adduction and radial abduction, anteposition or palmar abduction, and retroposition. Opposition, *dotted line,* is accomplished by movements of axial rotation, abduction, and flexion of all three joints of thumb, which result in rotation of thumb in position to present its palmar pad to pad of any finger. (Redrawn after Tubiana, R.: Surg. Clin. North Am. **48:**967-977, 1968.)

TABLE 8-6. Cosmetic result—example rating of a hand adding to a total of 11 of a possible 12 points

Examiner		Cosmetic improvement		Patient	
Rest	Activity			Rest	Activity
	2	Minimum	(1 point)		
		Moderate	(2 points)		
3		Marked	(3 points)	3	3

covering'' nerve, because there is not a direct relationship between return of sudomotor function and return of tactile gnosis. A two-point discrimination test can help determine functional loss of tactile gnosis. More than 18 to 20 mm in two-point discrimination testing is considered a total loss of this function. Functional isolation of the finger as noted in the blindfolded pickup test will aid the examiner in determining the presence or absence of any useful sensation in the digit.

Pain evaluation

Pain is difficult for the examiner to evaluate because it is a subjective symptom. Pain can be defined as ''a disagreeable sensation that has as its basis a highly variable complex made up of afferent nerve stimuli interacting with the emotional state of the individual and modified by his past experience, motivation, and state of mind.'' Pain may be verified and the intensity of pain may be evaluated in a thorough physical examination. Pretended pain may be detected by tests that confuse the patient into responding with signs that are contradictory to the usual clinical examination. Examination can further demonstrate whether the pain has an anatomic background or if it is associated with other signs of nerve dysfunction. Permanence of the loss of function because of pain or discomfort is described as a condition that exists after optimum physiologic adjustment and maximum medical rehabilitation have been administered. Subjective complaints of pain that cannot be substantiated along these lines should not be considered for impairment.

It is important to have an impairment classification for pain and discomfort in order to clarify subjective symptoms that interfere with the patient's activties. Such a classification must be set on arbitrary baselines. Pain associated with peripheral spinal nerve disorders can be classified according to how the pain interferes with the individual's performance of his activities: (1) Minimal—Is it annoying (0% to 25%)? (2) Slight—Does it interfere with activity (26% to 50%)? (3) Moderate—Does it prevent activity (51% to 75%)? (4) Severe—Does it prevent activity and also cause distress (76% to 100%)? The percentage of impairment of the part caused by pain or discomfort can be calculated the same as when one is evaluating for loss of sensation or amputation of the part (for example, in a severe causalgia there may be 100% loss of usefulness of the extremity). Partial impairment can be taken as a percentage of the whole part, by using the amputation tables to obtain the relative value of each part to the larger part.

COSMETIC EFFECT OF THE HAND

It should be remembered that the cosmetic effect of a hand implies both a passive and an active element: The *passive* cosmetic effect of the normal hand at rest may be simulated by certain artificial hands that are now available. They are made of plastic materials that closely resemble skin; however, the moment the patient moves the hand in space the normal postures and slight movements that a hand normally assumes are absent, and the hand loses some of its cosmetic effect. The *active* cosmetic effect concerns movements that are characteristic of the normal hand during performance. The movements provide a certain grace and elegance that gives a pleasing effect to the hand. These movements may compensate for other losses in the hand.

Our method of evaluating the cosmetic effect is described as follows: Evaluate the cosmetic result according to the general appearance of the hand at rest and on activity. Consider the aspect of the scar, the stiffness, residual joint imbalance, rotational deformities, and coordination. Using the cosmetic improvement ''point system,'' rate the number of points for the degree of cosmetic improvement at rest and on activity from both the patient's and the examiner's point of view. The maximum possible points are 12 (Table 8-6).

FUNCTIONAL EVALUATION AND MEASUREMENTS

Evaluation of an accurate profile of a patient's condition requires an appraisal of the resultant loss of function as it relates to activities of daily living and the more specialized hand activities common to all persons. In the evaluation of the functional capacity of a patient, it is important to determine his ambulatory status and his ability to perform certain basic activities in either an independent or an assisted fashion, or not at all. A special questionnaire is provided to rate his performance in dressing, personal hygiene, eating, communicating, opening doors and jars, and using aerosol cans as shown in Fig. 8-1, *A*.

The functional evaluation of the hand includes mainly the functional tests for activities of daily living and the motion-time-measurement method that is discussed later in this chapter.

The use of graduated sizes of cylinders and spheres to determine the ability to open the hand and to grasp and hold these objects can be a very useful method of measuring grasp functions. Recording the size of the sphere or cylinder grasped can give a picture of the patient's functional ability.

The end of the cylinder can be used to simulate the shape of the sphere. If the patient is cooperative, the use of these devices can be worthwhile in examining the disabled hand for strength and stability of the hand and wrist.

The examination should describe the ability of the patient to perform small and large grasp; pulp, tip, and lateral pinch; distal and proximal hook; and scoop functions. One should note whether further treatment is needed or further improvement will occur.

Functional evaluation systems

Most systems for evaluation of physical impairment attempt to establish a numerical deficit from normality by weighing factors such as missing or nonfunctional portions of the body. The resultant figure provides an index of anatomic impairment. However, this does not provide sophisticated insight into the effect the impairment will have or has had on the individual patient.

Most commonly, the physician is asked to judge physical impairment in order to permit a nonphysician or third-party judicial body to rate the patient's disability. Physical impairment, along with many other factors such as motivation, fatigue, and pain, is a most important factor in disability. In a way, the anatomic impairment evaluation is what the patient is able to put into a functional situation. The evaluation of disability should hinge to a certain degree on a measure of the patient's motor performance in accomplishment of functional activities.

Industrial engineers have been evaluating the motor performance of normal man in the industrial setting for many years. A person can be analyzed according to his ability to perform a given task composed of any given type of motion element and by matching his performance at a selected performance level. Therefore, from a synthetic test of performance ability, performance in an industrial setting may be predicted. A performance index may be described for specific tasks. An example of how a disabled person might perform certain activities would be a man who has lost his left upper extremity and is totally disabled as a pianist; however, he is very capable and essentially nondisabled as a radio announcer. Most injuries and vocational situations are less clear, however. It would be very useful to be able to indicate that an injured worker could perform 10% of normal on job A and 90% of normal on job B. It should also be possible to analyze job A to determine how that task could be altered to take advantage of the worker's abilities, while minimizing his disabilities and thereby improving his work performance.

The disability index should also be a measure of performance that could change from motivation, fatigue, pain, coordination, and strength. As only the output is measured, it could have an important place in the evaluation of the improvement of the patient's ability.

The system of analysis of motor performance, motion-time measurements, is concerned with the physical aspect of disability. It basically allows evaluation of general manual dexterity and helps predict specific skills. In the ideal evaluation there should be (1) a representation of all skills required by specific, available jobs and (2) a determination of all the significant manual skills possessed by the patient being tested. This method is contained in a predetermined motion-time system (PMTS) and is used widely in industry in the improvement, analysis, and timing of industrial work.

Sophisticated derivatives of motion-time study have been developed that are capable of (1) defining the subunits of the elements of motion that compose virtually any test performance, (2) timing the performance of these motion elements, and (3) relating the timed individual performance of these motion elements to the established "norms" of performance.

One of these systems is *methods-time-measurement (MTM)* system. MTM is a procedure that analyzes any manual operation or method into the basic motion elements required to perform it and assigns to each motion element a predetermined time standard that is determined by the nature of the motion and the conditions under which it is made. The system implies that the time involved in task performance is meaningless unless a manner of task performance is defined.

The principal elements employed in MTM are various degrees and purposes of reaching, grasping, moving, turning, applying pressure, and positioning. For complex analyses, there are guides for motion that can or cannot be performed simultaneously by two hands as well as eye-travel time, eye-focus time, principal gross body movements, walking, side-stepping, and so on.

An index of disability that will allow a numerical figure to compare the disabled person with a normal person can be obtained. The use of MTM elements should make it possible to evaluate the impaired hand from trauma or disease and to give it some index of impairment of function, which, combined with the physical impairment, can more fairly attest to the patient's true condition of disability. Further work and research are required in this area to develop the methods and personnel requirements to use the well-established MTM system in disability evaluation. We are now attempting to do this in our department.

PRINCIPLES AND METHODS OF IMPAIRMENT EVALUATION

The most practical and useful approach to the evaluation of digit impairment is through comparison of the loss of function found to be present with that resulting from amputation. Most schedules of evaluation consider the upper limb as a unit of the whole person and divide it into hand, wrist, elbow, and shoulder. The hand is further separated into digits and their parts.

Total loss of motion of a digit or total loss of sensation, or ankylosis and severe malposition that would render the digit essentially useless, are considered about the same as amputation of the part.

Ankylosis in the optimum functional position of joints is given the least disability on the charts. The great majority of functional activities of the hand require a 5 cm opening in the fingers and thumb, and therefore this degree of opening should be considered favorably in the impairment charts. The ability to flex the fingers to within 1 or 2 cm of the distal palmar crease is indicative of a useful range of motion and should also be considered favorably in the charts for impairment.

We will describe the methods for evaluation of amputation impairment, sensory impairment, finger range of motion, and ankylosis impairment. The principles for evaluating combined impairments of the entire extremity or a part will be defined. We will also present impairment charts for the fingers, thumb, wrist, elbow, and shoulder and describe the methods for their use.

AMPUTATION IMPAIRMENT EVALUATION

Amputation of the entire extremity of 100% loss of the limb is considered 60% impairment of the whole man. Amputations at levels below the elbow, distal to the biceps insertion and proximal to the metacarpophalangeal level are considered a 95% loss of the total limb (Fig. 8-6).

Prehension and sensation are, in essence, the sum of the roles played by the separate digits. Sensation and prehension of the palmar aspect of the palm and wrist are so gross that they are of no particular industrial use. Amputation of the fingers and thumb removes the most essential parts and is considered 100% impairment to the hand or 90% impairment to the total limb; since loss of the entire limb would equal 60% impairment to the whole person, 90% impairment of the limb would equal 54% impairment to the person. Using this principle of progressive multiplication of percentage values, the impairment of each digit or portion thereof can be related to the hand, the upper limb, and eventually to the whole man.

The digits represent five coordinated units into which all hand function is unequally divided. When evaluating the impaired function of the whole hand, one first has to evaluate each finger and the thumb separately according to the 100% scale in relation to the whole hand; each of these units is then weighed according to its respective value to the total hand as follows: thumb 40%, index and middle finger 20% each, and ring and little finger 10% each as shown in Fig. 8-6; any portion of the digit is taken as a percentage of the whole digit (Fig. 8-7). Amputation through the proximal interphalangeal joint equals 80% loss to the digit; amputation through the distal interphalangeal joint equals 45% loss to the digit, and amputation through the interphalangeal joint of the thumb equals 50% loss to the thumb. These values can be related to the whole hand; for example, amputation of the index finger equals 20% loss to the hand, amputation through the proximal interphalangeal joint represents 80% loss of the index finger, 80% × 20% loss to the hand or 16%. The values relating the loss of each part

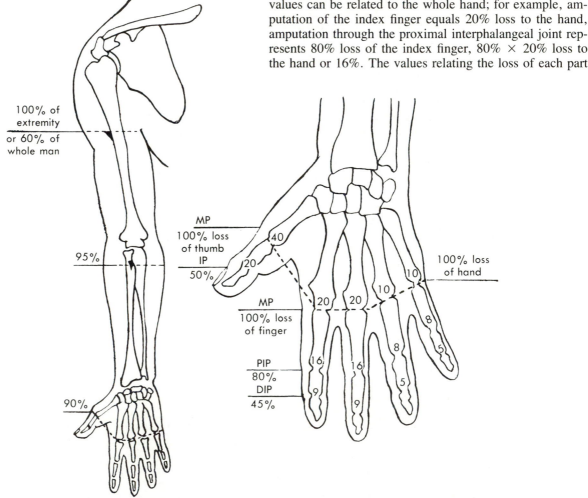

FIG. 8-6. Amputation impairment. Percentage of impairments related to whole man, extremity, hand, or finger. *MP*, Metacarpophalangeal; *IP*, interphalangeal; *PIP*, proximal interphalangeal; *DIP*, distal interphalangeal.

of each digit to the whole hand have been calculated as above and are shown in Fig. 8-6. Multiple digit losses are calculated as a sum of the parts and are related to the whole hand. For example, amputation of the entire thumb (40% loss to the hand) with amputation through the distal interphalangeal joint of the index finger (9% loss to the hand) equals 49% total impairment to the whole hand.

SENSORY IMPAIRMENT EVALUATION

Any loss resulting from sensory deficit, pain, or discomfort that contributes to permanent impairment must be unequivocal and permanent. Loss of sensation on the dorsal surface of the fingers is not considered disabling. Sensation on the palmar surface of the distal segment contributes to the function of the digit. Sensory loss on the least often opposed surfaces of the fingers and thumb should be given less value that the more important surfaces used in the usual pinch and grasp activities.

Complete loss of palmar sensation of the part is considered a 50% deficit of functional capacity. It is calculated, therefore, as 50% that of an amputation; for example, loss of both digital nerves of the thumb would be considered one half of an amputation loss, which equals half of 40%, or 20%, loss to the hand. Complete loss of sensation of the index or middle fingers would equal 10% loss to the hand each, and complete loss of sensation of the ring and little fingers would equal 5% loss to the hand each (Fig. 8-8).

Partial transverse sensory loss can be calculated as a percentage value of a portion of the digit; for example, sensory loss of the distal phalanx of the thumb equals one half of the value assigned for amputation through the interphalangeal joint, or 25% impairment to the thumb; the

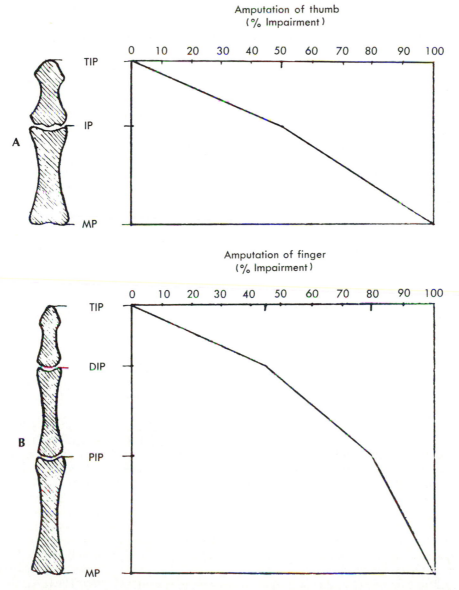

FIG. 8-7. Percentages of impairment to digit in amputation of, **A,** thumb or, **B,** finger.

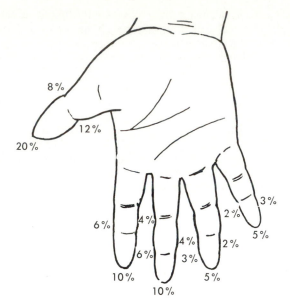

FIG. 8-8. Sensory impairment: relative value to whole hand for total sensory loss of digit and comparative loss of radial and ulnar sides. Sensory loss is calculated as 50% that of amputation.

loss to the whole hand would equal half of 20%, or 10%. The values for each transverse level of sensory loss can be easily calculated from the amputation values reported on Fig. 8-6.

Partial longitudinal loss is figured on the relative importance of the side of the digit for sensory function. Loss of sensibility of the radial half of the thumb is given 40% deficiency to the thumb, and loss of the ulnar half of the thumb is given 60% loss to the thumb. Sensory loss on the ulnar half of the fingers is given 40% deficiency to the digit except for the little finger where sensation on the ulnar border is more important. The impairment values for longitudinal sensory deficit as related to the whole hand can be easily calculated; for example, complete loss of sensation of the thumb equals 20% impairment to the hand, longitudinal loss of sensation on the ulnar side of the thumb equals 60% sensory loss to the thumb or 12% impairment to the hand. The values for radial and ulnar longitudinal sensory impairment to the hand for each digit and thumb are shown in Fig. 8-8.

FINGER MOTION IMPAIRMENT EVALUATION

There have been a variety of methods proposed for evaluation of flexor tendon repair. The method suggested by Boyes[2] of a *linear measurement* from the fingertip to the distal palmar crease has been used by many. Litchman and Paslay[7] have attempted to give values of impairment of the finger function as related to a linear distance from fingertip to distal palmar crease. Van't Hof and Heiple[11] proposed a method for evaluation of lack of extension as a linear measurement from the rim of the nail to the point to which the nail is expected to reach in case of full extension. White[12] used a numerical sum of the angles in maximum flexion of

the three finger joints. Swanson[9] in 1964 proposed a method for evaluating impairment caused by loss of flexion motion based on a *combined angular measurement principle*. The individual values for impairment of finger function caused by ankylosis and lack of flexion were obtained from the American Medical Association's "Guide for Evaluation of Permanent Impairment of the Extremities and Back."[6] A system based on the formula:

$$A\% + B\%(100\% - A\%) =$$
the combined values of $A\% + B\%$

was developed and used to add the combined values of impairment as is explained later in the text. Swanson also correlated the *combined angular measurement with the linear measurement of Boyes* and presented charts that could be used for everyday clinical practice[9] (Fig. 8-9). The Committee on Impairment Evaluation of the American Medical Association proposed the use of combining joint angles. Tubiana, Michon, and Thomine[10] have also proposed methods of evaluation of results after operations for Dupuytren's contracture.

Most impairment evaluations arbitrarily classify results as excellent, good, fair, and poor. We will not attempt to compare result evaluation according to the different methods, but we believe that arbitrary classifications that fail to consider joint motion in flexion and extension are incomplete and that the only reasonable approach to evaluation of finger function is to determine impaired motion in terms of percentage of impairment as this relates to the normal hand. Of course, hand function is very complex and depends not only on motion but sensibility, and strength, and coordination. The anatomic evaluation presented is a more important area of disability. However, the functional capacity must be also considered.

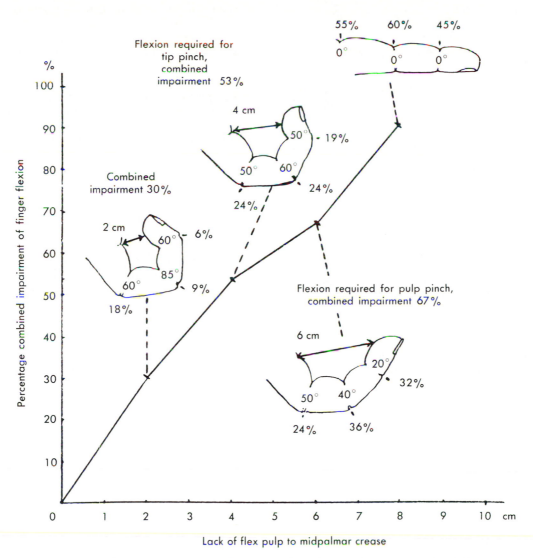

FIG. 8-9. Boyes' linear measurement of distance between finger pulp and middle palmar crease is simplest method for rating finger flexion capacity. Several common functional postures of fingers are noted. The impairment values to digit for loss of flexion of each joint in these positions are shown. Combined impairment values for each posture are also represented and were calculated from formula "A% + B% (100% − A%) = combined impairment value for finger." This figure correlates Boyes' linear measurements with combined angular measurement of finger flexion. For example, linear measurement of 6 cm lack of flexion from fingertip to palmar crease corresponds to 67% impairment according to Boyes' linear chart. For same position, ankylosis impairment can be obtained for each joint (MP at 50 degrees = 24%, PIP at 40 degrees = 36%, DIP at 20 degrees = 32%) and added according to above formula: 24% + 36% (100% − 24%) = 51%; 51% + 32% (100% − 51%) = 67%. Note that there is good correlation between linear and angular measurements of impairment. (From Swanson, A.B.: Surg. Clin. North Am. **44**:925-940, 1964.)

"A = E + F" METHOD FOR FINGER IMPAIRMENT EVALUATION

The evaluation of impaired joint motion that is presented here is based on the American Medical Association "Guide to the Evaluation of Permanent Impairment of the Extremities and Back"[6] and the work of Swanson,[9] which has been widely used. In these studies values for ankylosis and impaired flexion are calculated on the assumption that the normal extension for the metacarpophalangeal and interphalangeal joints is 0 degrees. Previously impairment values for lack of extension have not been adequately taken into consideration, and for that reason a method for evaluating the lack of extension impairment values has been worked out and is presented here.

The range of motion of a joint is the total number of degrees of movement traced by an arc from maximum ex-

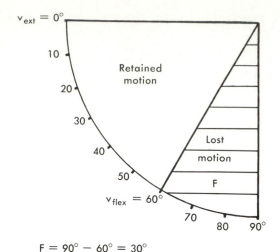

$$F = 90° - 60° = 30°$$

FIG. 8-10. Example of metacarpophalangeal joint presenting motion from 0 degrees extension to 60 degrees flexion; lost flexion, F, is equal to theoretically largest possible angle of flexion (90 degrees) minus measured flexion angle ($v_{flex} = 60$ degrees), or $F = 90$ degrees $- 60$ degrees $= 30$ degrees.

tension to maximum flexion. To determine the range of motion, one has to measure the two angles of extreme motion; they are represented by a small v. Flexion is the motion toward achieving the largest possible angle, and extension is the motion toward achieving the smallest possible angle. These values can be represented as follows:

Flexion v (v_{flex}) = largest possible angle to achieve by flexion
Extension v (v_{ext}) = smallest possible angle to achieve by extension

Assuming a metacarpophalangeal joint has a normal range of motion (ROM) from 0 degrees to 90 degrees, the largest possible angle to achieve by flexion is 90 degrees and the smallest possible angle to achieve by extension is 0 degrees. When $v_{flex} = 90$ degrees and $v_{ext} = 0$ degrees, there is no impairment of joint motion. Considerations for normal hyperextension of the metacarpophalangeal joints are discussed later.

Assuming a decrease of joint flexion from 90 degrees to 60 degrees while extension remains unchanged at 0 degrees, v_{flex} now equals 60 degrees and v_{ext} equals 0 degrees, as illustrated in Fig. 8-10. The lost flexion is represented by F and is equal to the theoretically largest v_{flex} minus the measured value of v_{flex}. For a metacarpophalangeal joint extending from 0 degrees to 60 degrees flexion, the lack of flexion can be expressed as follows:

$$F = 90°(v_{flex} \text{ largest}) - 60°(v_{flex} \text{ measured}) = 30°$$

Assuming there is a lack of extension of 20 degrees, v_{ext} equals 20 degrees, as illustrated in Fig. 8-11. The lost motion of extension is represented by E and is equal to the measured value of v_{ext} minus the theoretically smallest value of v_{ext}. For a metacarpophalangeal joint lacking 20 degrees of extension, the lost extension can be expressed as follows:

$$E = 20°(v_{ext} \text{ measured}) - 0°(v_{ext} \text{ smallest}) = 20°$$

With decreased flexion there is a decrease in v_{flex}, and with impaired extension there is an increase of v_{ext}; these two values will finally meet each other. In other words, v_{ext} and v_{flex} will be located at the same point of the arc or $v_{flex} = v_{ext}$. This situation is illustrated in Fig. 8-12. As can be seen, there is ankylosis. The total loss of joint motion is represented by A. This does *not refer to the angle of the arc of motion* at which a joint is ankylosed but to the *sum of the lack of extension (E) and the lack of flexion (F)* resulting from this ankylosis. The total loss of joint motion can be expressed as: $A = E + F$. If the joint is ankylosed at 40 degrees as shown in Fig. 8-12:

$v_{ext} = v_{flex} = 40°$
E (extension loss) $= 40°$
F (flexion loss) $= 90° - 40° = 50°$
A (total motion loss) $= 40° + 50° = 90°$

One should observe that the value A represents a total loss of joint motion and is always equal to the same number of degrees as the normal full range of motion of that joint. For a metacarpophalangeal joint, A always equals 90 degrees, no matter where in the arc of motion the ankylosis has occurred as long as v_{flex} equals v_{ext}.

Ankylosis at 30°: $A = 30°(E + 60°(F) = 90°$
Ankylosis at 80°: $A = 80°(E) + 10°(F) = 90°$

The above formula is of basic importance in the following discussion. Restricted joint motion will, of course, result in a certain degree of impaired function. Note that when we are referring to *lack of motion*, we are discussing *lack of function* and its evaluation. Impairment of finger function may be caused by lack of extension (E) with or without lack of flexion (F) or ankylosis (A). The restricted motion in terms of percentage impairment of finger function may then be called I_E, I_F, and I_A, respectively. These are functions of v, the angle measured at examination. More specifically, the percentage of impairment can be expressed in the following way:

I_E is a function of v_{ext} (smallest angle measured for extension) and goes to 0% when v_{ext} reaches its theoretically smallest value (for example, 0 degrees for the MP joint).
I_F is a function of v_{flex} (largest angle measured for flexion) and goes to 0% when v_{flex} reaches its theoretically largest value (for example, 90 degrees for the MP joint.)
I_A is a function of v when $v_{ext} = v_{flex}$ and similarly $I_A = I_E + I_F$

The function impairment is expressed in a percentage and relates to loss of function (or example, flexion) to the part affected (for example, the finger) on the 100% scale. From the AMA "Guide to the Evaluation of Permanent Impairment of the Extremities and Back."[6] we now have percentage values for impairment of finger function at the metacarpophalangeal joint from 0 degrees to 90 degrees because of lack of flexion, F, and ankylosis, A, called I_F and I_A, respectively. These values are shown on Tables 8-7 and 8-8 and can also be expressed as illustrated in Fig. 8-13, and 8-14. According to the formula previously described, $A = E + F$, which can also be written, $E = A - F$, we

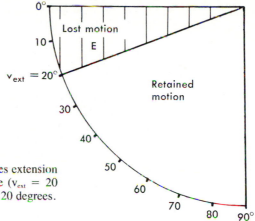

Fig. 8-11. Example of metacarpophalangeal joint presenting motion from 20 degrees extension lag to 90 degrees flexion; lost extension, *E,* is equal to measured extension angle (v_{ext} = 20 degrees) minus theoretically smallest possible extension angle (0 degrees), or E = 20 degrees.

$$E = 20° - 0° = 20°$$

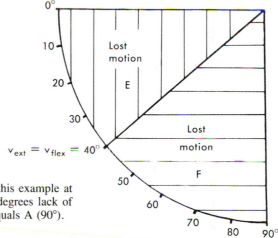

Fig. 8-12. When there is no motion retained in joint, we have ankylosis—in this example at 40 degrees. As can be seen, *total motion lost to ankylosis (A)* is equal to 40 degrees lack of extension, *E,* plus 50 degrees lack of flexion, *F;* sum of E (40°) and F (50°) equals A (90°).

TABLE 8-7. Impairment percentage* attributable to loss of flexion of the metacarpophalangeal joint from a neutral position (0°)

Flexion from 0° to	Degrees lost motion (F)	Percent impairment
0°	90	55
10°	80	49
20°	70	43
30°	60	37
40°	50	31
50°	40	24
60°	30	18
70°	20	12
80°	10	6
90°	0	0

*These figures are from the American Medical Association "Guide to the Evaluation of Permanent Impairment of the Extremities and Back."

TABLE 8-8. Impairment* attributable to metacarpophalangeal joint ankylosis

Degrees joint ankylosed	Percent impaired finger function
0	55
10	52
20	48
30	45
40	54
50	63
60	72
70	82
80	91
90	100

*These figures are from the American Medical Association "Guide to the Evaluation of Permanent Impairment of the Extremities and Back."

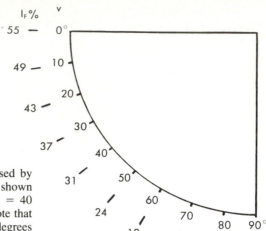

FIG. 8-13. Percentage impairment of finger function caused by lack of flexion (F) is expressed as I_F; here AMA values of I_F shown in Table 8-7 have been transposed to arc of motion. If $v_{flex} = 40$ degrees, F is 50 degrees and corresponds to $I_F = 31\%$. Note that I_F is function of v_{flex} and reaches 0% when v_{flex} equals 90 degrees or F goes to 0 degrees.

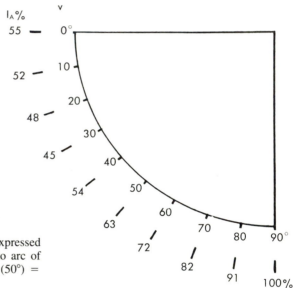

FIG. 8-14. Percentage impairment of finger function owing to ankylosis A is expressed as I_A. Here AMA values of I_A shown in Table 8-8 have been transposed to arc of motion. If joint is ankylosed at 40 degrees, A = E (40°) + F (50°) = 90° and $I_A = 54\%$.

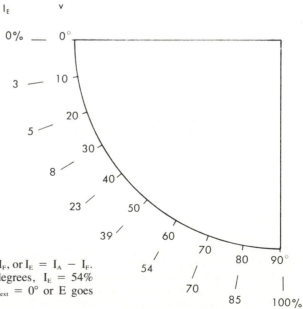

FIG. 8-15. Value of I_E can be derived for each angle from formula $I_A = I_E + I_F$, or $I_E = I_A - I_F$. When a metacarpophalangeal joint presents an extension lag of 40 degrees, $I_E = 54\%$ (I_A) − 31% (I_F) = 23%. I_E is a function of v_{ext} and reaches 0% when $v_{ext} = 0°$ or E goes to 0°.

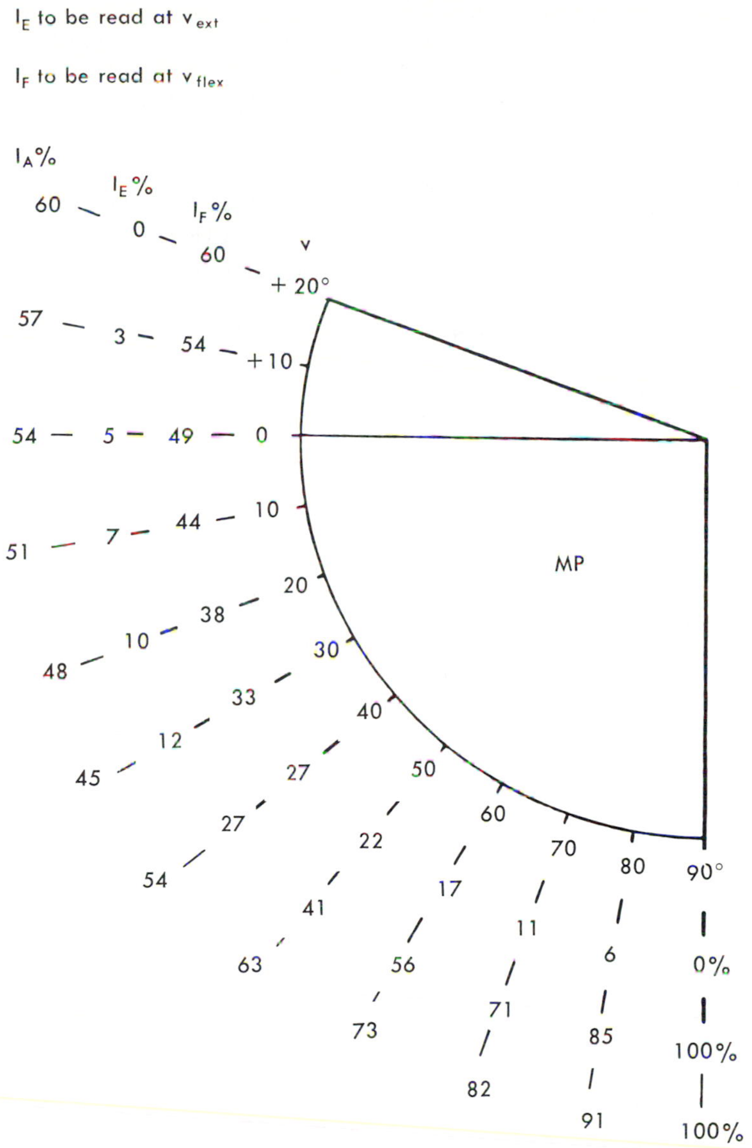

I_E to be read at v_ext

I_F to be read at v_flex

FIG. 8-16. Impairment of function for metacarpophalangeal joint (MP). I_A represents ankylosis impairment. I_F represents flexion impairment, and I_E represents extension impairment. Notice that position of function of MP joint having been established at 30 degrees, I_A is lowest or 45% at this angle. Impairment values for hyperextension deformities have been included in this chart.

can derive the value for extension impairment, I_E, at each given angle according to the following formula: $I_E = I_A - I_F$. For example, at an angle of 30 degrees, I_A equals 45% according to the presented AMA chart (Table 8-8), and I_F equals 37% (Table 8-7); the value of I_E can be derived according to the above formula and is found to be: 45% (I_A) − 37% (I_F) = 8% (I_E). This same process can be applied to each angle of the arc of motion from 0 degrees to 90 degrees to derive the values of I_E from the AMA percentage impairment values (Fig. 8-15). However, notice that the AMA guide has made no considerations for values of hyperextension; therefore we have slightly modified the values for I_F from the AMA guide (Table 8-7) to account for values of hyperextension of the metacarpophalangeal joint up to 20 degrees, which can be considered normal. The

modified values are represented for the metacarpophalangeal joint in Fig. 8-16. For an angle of ankylosis of 30 degrees, the I_E is calculated according to the usual formula, giving I_F a value of 33% instead of 37% as in the American Medical Association guide (Table 8-7):

$$I_E = I_A - I_F \text{ or } I_E = 45\% - 33\% = 12\%$$

The derivation of I_E is of fundamental importance for adequate evaluation of function impairment resulting from limitation of joint motion. This allows us to have values for both I_E and I_F to estimate the correct percentage of functional impairment relating not only to the degrees of lost movement but, most importantly, to the location of the impairment in the arc of finger motion.

By referring to Fig. 8-16 one can easily understand the

following examples. Assuming a situation where the metacarpophalangeal joint has 30 degrees of retained motion, one can see that this motion takes place between 10 degrees extension lag to 40 degrees flexion, the percentage of functional impairment is not so severe as it would be if the preserved motion occurred from 50 degrees extension lag to 80 degrees flexion. For a metacarpophalangeal joint extending from -10 degrees and flexing to 40 degrees $I_E = 7\%$, and $I_F = 27\%$, for a total impairment of $7\% + 27\% = 34\%$. For a metacarpophalangeal joint extending from 50 degrees to 80 degrees $I_E = 41\%$, and $I_F = 6\%$, for a total impairment of $41\% + 6\% = 47\%$. From Fig. 8-16 one can also see that ankylosis of the metacarpophalangeal joint at 30 degrees or the position of function would equal $12\% (I_E) + 33\% (I_F) = 45\%$ or the lowest value for I_A; it is also obvious that ankylosis at 80 degrees would represent a more severe degree of impairment $85\% (I_E) + 6\% (I_F) = 91\% (I_A)$.

The principles for evaluating impairment from ankylosis, loss of flexion, and/or loss of extension should now be clearly understood. Impairment tables for loss of function of the fingers, thumb, wrist, elbow, and shoulder have been derived from the basic formula discussed above and are presented.

IMPAIRMENT ESTIMATION FOR COMBINED VALUES

Disability present in each digit, whether attributable to decreased or lost motion, sensation, strength, or amputation, is evaluated adequately, and these separate evaluations are added and transposed into terms of the hand. The sum of impairments as related to the whole hand gives the total impairment. When multiple impairments may involve the whole finger, the principle of relating the smaller part to the next larger part to obtain a combined value is useful. In general, the method used to relate impairments is to give

TABLE 8-9. Combined values for impairment increments of 1%*

	1	2	3	4	5	6	7	8	9	10	11	12	13	14	15	16	17	18	19	20	21	22	23	24	25	26	27	28	29	30
1	2	3	4	5	6	7	8	9	10	11	12	13	14	15	16	17	18	19	20	21	22	23	24	25	26	27	28	29	30	31
2	3	4	5	6	7	8	9	10	11	12	13	14	15	16	17	18	19	20	21	22	23	24	25	26	27	27	28	29	30	31
3	4	5	6	7	8	9	10	11	12	13	14	15	16	17	18	19	19	29	21	22	23	24	25	26	27	28	29	30	31	32
4	5	6	7	8	9	10	11	12	13	14	15	16	16	17	18	19	20	21	22	23	24	25	26	27	28	29	30	31	32	33
5	6	7	8	9	10	11	12	13	14	15	15	16	17	18	19	20	21	22	23	24	25	26	27	28	29	30	31	32	33	34
6	7	8	9	10	11	12	13	14	14	15	16	17	18	19	20	21	22	23	24	25	26	27	28	29	30	30	31	32	33	34
7	8	9	10	11	12	13	14	14	15	16	17	18	29	20	21	22	23	24	25	26	27	27	28	29	30	31	32	33	34	35
8	9	10	11	12	13	14	14	15	16	17	18	19	20	21	22	23	24	25	25	26	27	28	29	30	31	32	33	34	35	36
9	10	11	12	13	14	14	15	16	17	18	19	29	21	22	23	24	24	25	26	27	28	29	30	31	32	33	34	34	35	36
10	11	12	13	14	15	15	16	17	18	19	20	21	22	23	24	24	25	26	27	28	29	30	31	32	33	33	34	35	36	37
11	12	13	14	15	15	16	17	18	19	20	21	22	23	23	24	25	26	27	28	29	30	31	31	32	33	34	35	36	37	38
12	13	14	15	16	16	17	18	19	20	21	22	23	23	24	25	26	27	28	29	30	30	31	32	33	34	35	36	37	38	38
13	14	15	16	16	17	18	19	20	21	22	23	23	24	25	26	27	28	29	30	30	31	32	33	34	35	36	36	37	38	39
14	15	16	17	17	18	19	20	21	22	23	23	24	25	26	27	28	29	29	30	31	32	33	34	35	36	36	37	38	39	40
15	16	17	18	18	19	20	21	22	23	24	24	25	26	27	28	29	29	30	31	32	33	34	35	35	36	37	38	39	40	41
16	17	18	19	19	20	21	22	23	24	24	25	26	27	28	29	29	30	31	32	33	34	34	35	36	37	38	39	40	40	41
17	18	19	19	20	21	22	23	24	24	25	26	27	28	29	29	30	31	32	33	34	34	35	36	37	38	39	39	40	41	42
18	19	20	20	21	22	23	24	25	25	26	27	28	29	29	30	31	32	33	34	34	35	36	37	38	39	39	40	41	42	43
19	20	21	21	22	23	24	25	25	26	27	28	29	30	30	31	32	33	34	34	35	36	37	38	38	39	40	41	42	42	43
20	21	22	22	23	24	25	26	26	27	28	29	30	30	31	32	33	34	34	35	36	37	38	38	39	40	41	42	42	43	44
21	22	23	23	24	25	26	27	27	28	29	30	30	31	32	33	34	34	35	36	37	38	38	39	40	41	42	42	43	44	45
22	23	24	24	25	26	27	27	28	29	30	31	31	32	33	34	34	35	36	37	38	38	39	40	41	42	42	43	44	45	45
23	24	25	25	26	27	28	28	29	30	31	31	32	33	34	35	35	36	37	38	38	39	40	41	41	42	43	44	45	45	46
24	25	26	26	27	28	29	29	30	31	32	32	33	34	35	35	36	37	38	38	39	40	41	41	42	43	44	45	45	46	47
25	26	27	27	28	29	30	30	31	32	33	33	34	35	36	36	37	38	39	39	40	41	42	42	43	44	45	45	46	47	48
26	27	27	28	29	30	30	31	32	33	33	34	35	36	36	37	38	39	39	40	41	42	42	43	44	45	45	46	47	47	48
27	28	28	29	30	31	31	32	33	34	34	35	36	36	37	38	39	39	40	41	42	42	43	44	45	45	46	47	47	48	49
28	29	29	30	31	32	32	33	34	34	35	36	37	37	38	39	40	40	41	42	42	43	44	45	45	46	47	47	48	49	50
29	30	30	31	32	33	33	34	35	35	36	37	38	38	39	40	40	41	42	42	43	44	45	45	46	47	47	48	49	50	50
30	31	31	32	33	34	34	35	36	36	37	38	38	39	40	41	41	42	43	43	44	45	45	46	47	48	48	49	50	50	51

*Based on the formula: $A\% + B\% (100\% - A\%)$ = the combined values of $A\% + B\%$. If three or more values are to be combined, two may be selected and their combined value found. This combined value and the third value are combined to give the total figure. This process can be repeated indefinitely, with the value obtained in each case being a combination of all the previous values. After having the two values, one enters the table at one value horizontally and at the other value vertically, and the combined value will be read at intersections. This combined value must then be combined with the third value to give a final combined value, for example, 30% impairment to DIP, 20% impairment to PIP, and 25% impairment to MP; this would add as follows on this chart: 30% DIP + 20% PIP = 44% to the digit. The following step is calculated on Table 8-8: 44% digit + 25% MP = 59% combined impairment to digit.

the percentage relationship of the smaller part to the next larger part in the appropriate impairment table. The process may be repeated successively so that any impairment may be expressed in terms of impairment of the whole man as already discussed.

The method generally employed to combine various impairments is based on the principle that each impairment acts not on the whole part (for example, the whole finger) but on the portion that remains (for example, the proximal interphalangeal joint and proximally) after the preceding impairment has acted (for example, on the distal interphalangeal joint). When there is more than one impairment to a given part, these impairments must be combined before the conversion to a larger part is made. The combined values determination is based on the formula:

$$A\% + B\%(100\% - A\%) =$$
the combined values of A% + B%

Individual parts are expressed in actual percentages unless it is a sole impairment; then it is rounded to the nearest 5%. The final impairment value is to be expressed in terms of the nearest 5% after all impairments have been computed and transposed to a common denominator. If three or more values are to be combined, two may be selected and their combined value found. This combined value and the third value are combined to give the total value. This procedure can be repeated indefinitely, with the value obtained in each case being a combination of all the previous values. Combined value tables for ease of determination are provided in Tables 8-9 and 8-10. Increments of 1% of impairment value are shown in Table 8-9 for values up to 30%; values greater than 30% are figured by increments of 5% such as shown in Table 8-10; combined values obtained represent the impairment to the total finger. This can then be related to the hand, the extremity, and the whole man.

For example, an index finger presents an amputation at the distal interphalangeal joint and ankylosis of the proximal interphalangeal joint at 90 degrees; the combined impairment to the index finger can be computed according to the formula as follows: amputation of the distal interphalangeal joint represents a 45% impairment to the index finger (Fig. 8-6), and ankylosis of the proximal interphalangeal joint at 90 degrees represents an 80% impairment to the index finger. These can be added:

$$45\% + 80\%(100\% - 45\%) =$$
$$45\% + 80\%(55\%) = 45\% + 44\% =$$
89% impairment to the index finger

TABLE 8-10. Combined impairment values representing increments of 5%

	5	10	15	20	25	30	35	40	45	50	55	60	65	70	75	80	85	90	95
5	10	15	19	24	29	34	48	43	48	52	57	62	67	72	76	81	86	91	95
10	15	19	24	28	33	37	42	46	51	55	60	64	69	73	78	82	87	91	96
15	19	24	28	32	36	41	45	49	53	58	62	66	70	75	79	83	87	92	96
20	24	28	32	36	40	44	48	52	56	60	64	68	72	76	80	84	88	92	96
25	29	33	36	40	44	48	51	55	59	63	66	70	73	78	81	85	89	93	96
30	34	37	41	44	48	51	55	58	62	65	69	72	76	79	83	86	90	93	97
35	38	42	45	48	51	55	58	61	64	68	71	74	77	81	84	87	90	94	97
40	43	46	49	52	55	58	61	64	67	70	73	76	79	82	85	88	91	94	97
45	48	51	53	56	59	62	64	67	70	73	75	78	81	84	86	89	92	95	97
50	52	55	58	60	63	65	68	70	73	75	78	80	83	85	88	90	93	95	98
55	57	60	62	64	66	69	71	73	75	78	80	82	84	87	89	91	93	96	98
60	62	64	66	68	70	72	74	76	78	80	82	84	86	88	90	92	94	96	98
65	67	69	70	72	73	76	77	79	81	83	84	86	88	90	91	93	95	97	98
70	72	73	75	76	78	79	81	82	84	85	87	88	90	91	93	94	96	97	99
75	76	78	79	80	81	83	84	85	86	88	89	90	91	93	94	95	96	98	99
80	81	82	83	84	85	86	87	88	89	90	91	92	93	94	95	96	97	98	99
85	86	87	87	88	89	90	90	91	92	93	93	94	95	96	96	97	98	99	99
90	91	91	92	92	93	93	94	94	95	95	96	96	97	97	98	98	99	99	100
95	95	96	96	96	96	97	97	97	97	98	98	98	98	99	99	99	99	100	100

The index finger represents 20% to the hand, and the above impairment would represent a 20% times 89% impairment to the hand, or 18%. The combined impairment value of the above example can also be found quickly in Table 8-10 at the intersection of the vertical and horizontal coordinates represented by 45% and 80%.

IMPAIRMENT EVALUATION TABLES AND HOW TO USE THEM
Finger impairment

Based on the previous discussion, the material for the evaluation of any finger joint is presented in Figs. 8-16 to 8-18 and shows the three different impaired functions (I_A, I_F, and I_E) for each one of the three finger joints (MP, PIP,

DIP). I_A gives the impairment of finger function attributable to ankylosis at any angle; I_E and I_F give the impairment of finger function attributable to lack of extension and lack of flexion, respectively. The positions of function in each joint are taken from the AMA guide, while hyperextension has been added to this material. This explains the slight differences in impairment values found when the values shown in Fig. 8-16 are compared with the AMA values shown in Table 8-7 (for example, $I_F = 55\%$ at 0° in Table 8-7, while $I_F = 49\%$ at 0° in Fig. 8-16). In a normal hand the metacarpophalangeal joint can usefully hyperextend to 20 degrees. A very small percentage of impairment has been assigned to loss of this normal hyperextension as seen on this chart: at 9 degrees extension of the metacarpophalangeal joint $I_E = 5\%$. Note that for the proximal interphalangeal and the distal interphalangeal joints, the normal functional extension is to 0°; consequently, $I_E = 0\%$ at 0° extension for these joints; the impairment values for the proximal interphalangeal and distal interphalangeal joints are given for lack of flexion and not for hyperextension. However, consideration for hyperextension angles now allows us to rate impairment of flexion when ankylosis in a hyperextended position occurs; for example, proximal interphalangeal joint ankylosis at +30° rated 80% impairment.

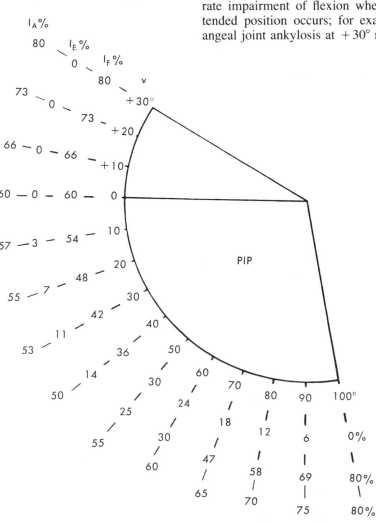

Fig. 8-17. Impairment of function for proximal interphalangeal joint (PIP). Notice that with position of function of PIP joint having been established at 40 degrees, I_A is lowest or 50% at this angle. Values for hyperextension deformities have been included in this chart.

Note that for each joint the percentage of impairment ankylosis, or I_A, is at the lowest at the angle of position of function; I_A at $30° = 45\%$ for the metacarpophalangeal joint, I_A at $40° = 50\%$ for the proximal interphalangeal joint, and I_A at $20° = 30\%$ for the distal interphalangeal joint.

These diagrams are used in the following way: measure the range of motion, for example, 20 degrees of extension lag to 60 degrees of flexion for the metacarpophalangeal joint. The impairment corresponding to this angle would be found in the row headed I_E or 10% extension impairment for 20 degrees extension lag, and the impairment corresponding to 60 degrees of flexion would be found under the row headed I_F or 17%. The impairment resulting from the above range of motion would total $10\% + 17\% = 27\%$.

Thumb impairment

The thumb represents 40% of the whole hand; in itself it may be considered to be three different functional units: (1) flexion-extension of the metacarpophalangeal and interphalangeal joints, (2) adduction-abduction, and (3) opposition. Adduction is measured as the distance of lack of adduction measured in centimeters from the flexor crease of the interphalangeal joint of the thumb to the distal palmar crease at the level of the fifth metacarpophalangeal joint. Opposition is measured in centimeters as the largest distance possible to achieve between the flexor crease at the interphalangeal joint of the thumb to the distal palmar crease at the third metacarpophalangeal joint.

The three different units contribute to the total thumb function in the following way; extension-flexion of the metacarpophalangeal and interphalangeal joints together are worth 20%, adduction 20%, and opposition 60%. The impairment values to adduction and opposition are shown in Figs. 8-19 and 8-20; these are values of impairment to the function described. The impairment value to the entire thumb function is obtained by relating the value percentage

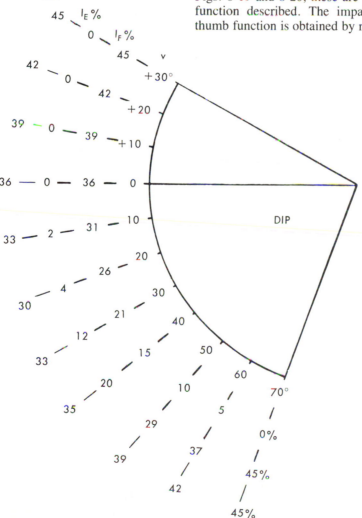

FIG. 8-18. Functional impairment of distal interphalangeal joint (DIP). Notice that with position of function of DIP having been established at 20 degrees, $I_A = 30\%$ or is lowest at this angle.

TABLE 8-11. Percentage of impairment of adduction to function of entire thumb*

Centimeters	Percent impairment of thumb
0	0
1	0
2	1
3	3
4	4
5	6
6	8
7	13
8	20

*Taking into consideration that adduction contributes to 20% of thumb function.

TABLE 8-12. Percentage of impairment of opposition to function of entire thumb*

Centimeters	Percent impairment of thumb
0	60
1	42
2	29
3	19
4	12
5	7
6	4
7	2
8	0

*Taking into consideration that opposition contributes to 60% of thumb function.

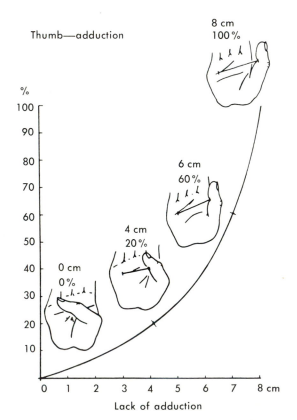

FIG. 8-19. Lack of adduction as impairment is derived as linear measurement as noted measuring from flexor crease of interphalangeal joint of thumb to distal palmar crease over metacarpophalangeal joint of fifth finger. Graph represents percentage value for lack of adduction relative to this function and not to whole thumb function. Adduction contributes to 20% of thumb function and impairments shown must be multiplied by 20% to obtain impairment percentage to entire thumb function such as shown in Table 8-10.

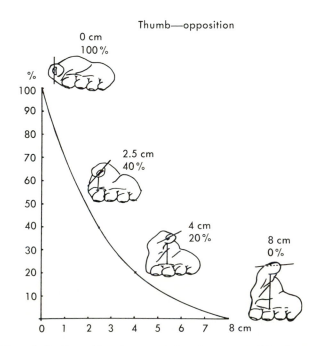

FIG. 8-20. Opposition is measured as largest possible distance from flexor crease of interphalangeal joint to distal palmar crease over third metacarpophalangeal joint. Impairment value curve for lack of opposition is shown relative to this function. Opposition contributes to 60% of entire thumb function, and values of impairment shown must be multiplied by 60% to obtain impairment percentage to entire thumb function such as shown in Table 8-11.

of each function to the entire thumb (Tables 8-11 and 8-12). For example, adduction at 4 cm represents a 20% impairment of adduction (Fig. 8-19), and since adduction is worth 20% of the thumb function, this impairment equals 20% × 20%, or 4% impairment to the entire thumb (Table 8-11).

The impairment percentages of the metacarpophalangeal and interphalangeal joints through loss of flexion or extension or ankylosis are shown in Figs. 8-21 and 8-22. Flexion and extension of the metacarpophalangeal and interphalangeal joints contribute to 20% of the total thumb function; this relative value has been taken into consideration in the impairment values to the total thumb as shown in these figures. Note that the functional position of the metacarpophalangeal and interphalangeal joints has been determined to 20 degrees, hence the I_A value is the lowest at these angles. For example, thumb metacarpophalangeal ankylosis at 20 degrees equals 7% impairment ankylosis (I_A), and interphalangeal ankylosis at 20 degrees equals 7% impairment ankylosis (I_A).

In practice, each unit may be evaluated according to Figs. 8-21 and 8-22 and Tables 8-11 and 8-12, giving each one its direct value contributing to the total thumb function. The values derived from each one of these figures and tables are then simply added numerically to get the impairment of the total thumb. The combined table is not used.

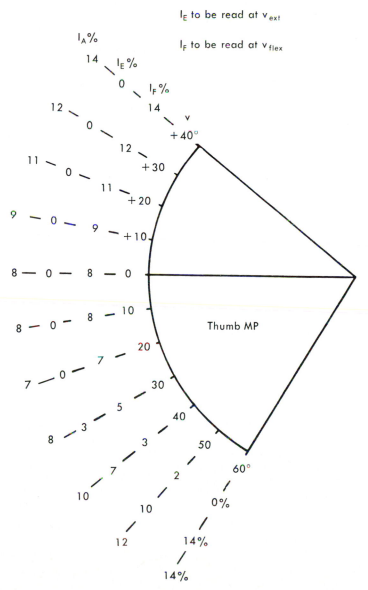

FIG. 8-21. Thumb metacarpophalangeal joint: impairment percentages to hand for loss of flexion and extension and for ankylosis of thumb metacarpophalangeal joint. Functional position has been established at 20 degrees.

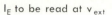

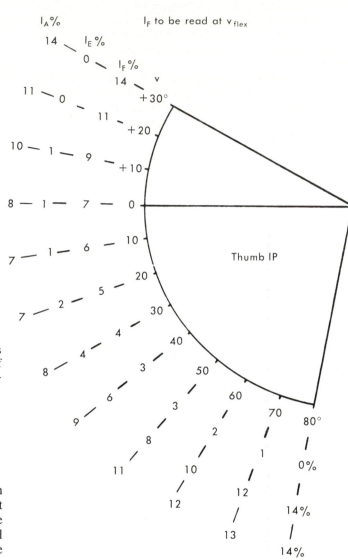

FIG. 8-22. Thumb interphalangeal joint: impairment percentages to hand for loss of flexion and extension and for ankylosis of thumb interphalangeal joint. Functional position has been established at 20 degrees.

Wrist, elbow, and shoulder impairment

The usefulness of the joints of the upper extremity in placing the hand in space for functional adaptations has great importance. The segments of the extremity have a value that may be calculated in terms of impairment to the total extremity and from that to the body. A definite percentage factor for impairment may be given to defects such as awkwardness, incapacity, disturbance of function, and necessary overactivity of the remaining joints resulting from total loss of function of one of the extremity segments. The shoulder segment is given 60% of the total extremity; the elbow, 70%; and the wrist, 60%.

Wrist joint. Evaluation of impairment of the wrist joint is reflected in loss of motion or ankylosis. Dorsal and palmar flexion are given a 70% value to the total range of joint motion, and radial and ulnar deviation are given a 30% value. The usual range of motion of the wrist is from 60 degrees dorsiflexion to 60 degrees palmar flexion; the position of function is from 10 degrees palmar flexion to 10 degrees dorsiflexion. The usual range of deviation of motion of the wrist is from 20 degrees of radial deviation to 30 degrees of ulnar deviation; the position of function in lateral deviation is from 0 to 10 degrees of ulnar deviation.

The impairment values for loss of motion in ankylosis, dorsiflexion, and palmar flexion are calculated from Fig. 8-23 and multiplied by 70%. The values for impairment of radial and ulnar deviation by ankylosis or restricted motion

are calculated from Fig. 8-24 and multiplied by 30%. These two factors are then added to give the total impairment of the wrist joint. The impairment to the total extremity can then be obtained by multiplying by the factor of 60% as follows:

Wrist with a range of motion of 50 degrees flexion to 30 degrees extension lag, and 10 degrees radial deviation (RD) with 5 degrees of ulnar deviation lag (UD)

From Fig. 8-23 one can find $I_F = 5\%$ and $I_E = 60\%$ for a total flexion-extension impairment of 65%. Impairment to the total wrist function is found by multiplication of 65% by the value of flexion-extension function, or 65% × 70% = 45.5%.

From Fig. 8-24 one can find $I_{RD} = 10\%$ and $I_{UD} = 45\%$ for a total radioulnar deviation impairment of 55%. Impairment to the total wrist function is found by multiplying 55% by the value of radioulnar deviation function, or 55% × 30% = 16.5%.

Wrist—flexion

Position of function from 10° palmar flexion to 10° dorsiflexion

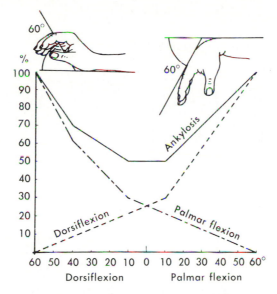

FIG. 8-23. Wrist flexion and extension impairment percentages: dorsal and palmar flexion are given 70% value of total wrist function. Figures shown are multiplied by 70% to obtain impairment percentage to total wrist function. Total loss of wrist function is considered 60% impairment to extremity. Calculated value of wrist impairment is multiplied by 60% to obtain wrist impairment percentage to entire extremity. Note that usual range of motion is from 60 degrees dorsiflexion to 60 degrees palmar flexion; position of function is from 10 degrees dorsiflexion to 10 degrees palmar flexion, and values for impairment ankylosis reach their lowest between these two angles, or $I_A = 50\%$.

Wrist—radial and ulnar deviation

Position of function from 0° to 10° ulnar deviation

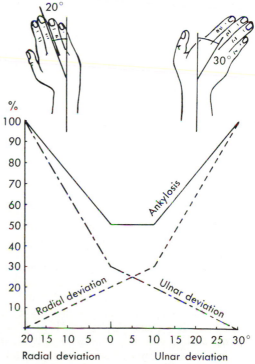

FIG. 8-24. Wrist radial and ulnar deviation impairment: radioulnar deviation is given 30% value of total wrist function. Figures shown are multiplied by 30% to obtain impairment percentage to total wrist function. Wrist relative values for impairment of flexion-extension and radioulnar deviations are added to obtain total wrist impairment value and then multiplied by 60% to obtain wrist impairment value to entire upper extremity. Note that usual range of motion is from 20 degrees radial deviation to 30 degrees ulnar deviation and that position of function is from 0 degrees to 10 degrees ulnar deviation. Ankylosis impairment values reach their lowest point between these angles or 50%.

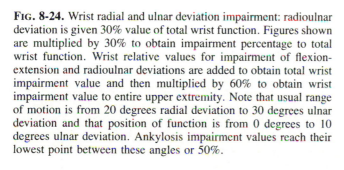

Elbow

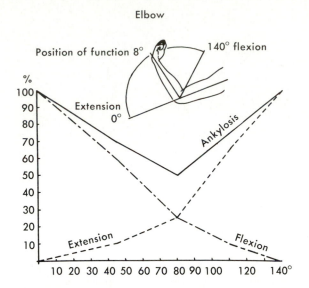

FIG. 8-25. Elbow flexion-extension impairment: elbow flexion-extension is given 60% of total elbow function value. Figures shown are multiplied by 60% to obtain impairment percentage to total elbow function. Total value of elbow impairment is multiplied by 70% to obtain impairment value to extremity. Range of motion of elbow is usually from 0 degrees extension to 140 degrees flexion, and position of function is 80 degrees flexion. Note that impairment ankylosis percentage is lowest for position of function, or 50%.

Rotation of the forearm

Position of function 20° pronation

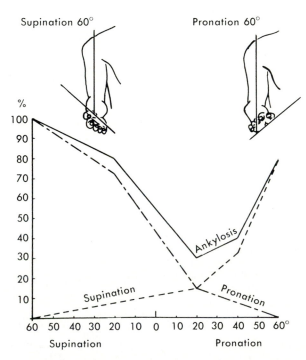

FIG. 8-26. Rotation of forearm impairment: forearm rotation motions are given 40% of total elbow function value. Figures shown are multiplied by 40% to obtain impairment percentage to total elbow function. Usual range of rotation is from 60 degrees supination to 60 degrees pronation, and position of function is considered to be 20 degrees pronation. Note that impairment-ankylosis percentage is lowest for position of function, or 30%.

The total wrist impairment percentage is calculated by adding the flexion-extension impairment value and the radioulnar deviation impairment value as follows:

$$(I_F + I_E)(70\%) + (I_{RD} + I_{UD})(30\%) =$$

Total wrist impairment

$$(5\% + 60\%)(70\%) + (10\% + 45\%)(30\%) = 45.5\% + 16.5\% = 62\% \text{ wrist impairment}$$

The wrist impairment value to the entire upper extremity is then derived as 62% (wrist impairment) times 60% (wrist value to the extremity) = 37%.

Elbow joint. Total loss of the elbow joint is considered to result in a 70% loss of the extremity's usefulness; elbow flexion is given 60% of this value and rotation is given 40%. The impairment values for restricted motion of the elbow may be calculated from Figs. 8-25 and 8-26. Evaluation of impaired flexion-extension and rotation are expressed in terms of percentage impairment of each function of the joint according to the 100% scale.

An average normal range of motion in the elbow is assumed to be from 0 to 140 degrees of flexion. The position of function is assumed to be 80 degrees of flexion. The most useful range of motion from the functional point of view is considered to be from 45 degrees to 110 degrees of flexion. Lack of extension less than 45 degrees and lack of flexion from 110 degrees to 140 degrees are therefore considered to give a relatively small impairment of function. The impairment values for restricted range of motion are calculated for flexion, extension, and ankylosis. These val-

ues are then added and multiplied by 60% to obtain the amount of impairment to the total elbow function.

The usual range of motion of rotation is from 60 degrees supination to 60 degrees pronation. The position of function is considered to be in 20 degrees of pronation. Impairment values for loss of rotation and ankylosis of the forearm are calculated from Fig. 8-26; this number is multiplied by 40% to obtain the percentage of impairment to the total elbow function from lack of rotation.

Elbow flexion and rotation impairments are then added and may be multiplied by 70% to obtain the total percentage impairment of the elbow to the extremity.

Shoulder joint. The loss of the shoulder segment is considered to be 60% impairment of the total extremity. Adduction and abduction are considered to contribute 50% of the total shoulder function. Extension and flexion are considered to contribute 30% of the total shoulder function. Internal and external rotation are considered to contribute 20% of the total shoulder function.

In each one of these three functions, the position of function has been chosen according to the recommendations in the literature concerning arthrodesis of the glenohumeral joint, even though motions of different joints are involved in each one of these three functions (glenohumeral joint, acromioclavicular joint, sternoclavicular joint, and the movement between the scapula and the chest wall). The restricted range-of-motion impairment is calculated for the three functions according to the 100% scale for each function as noted in Figs. 8-27 to 8-29. These figures are then added

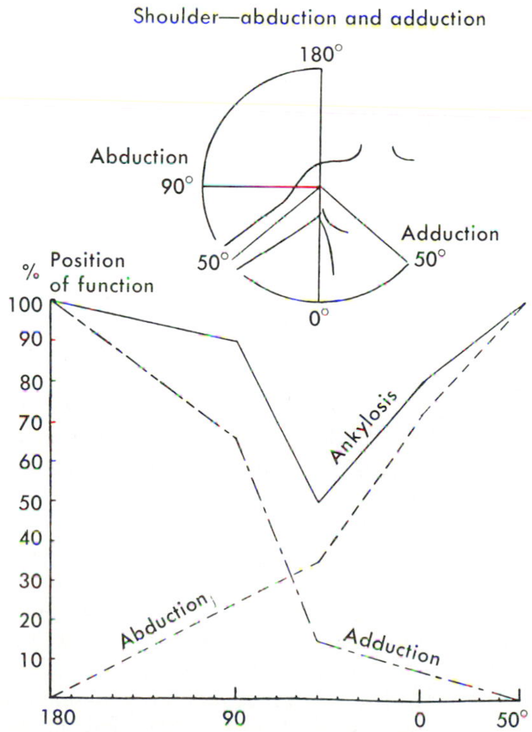

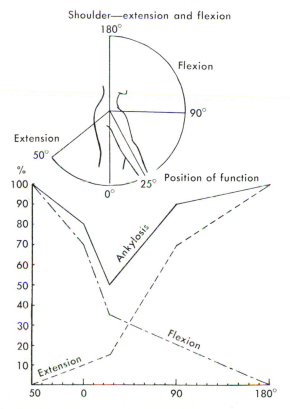

FIG. 8-27. Provides method of calculating restricted range of motion and ankylosis of shoulder for adduction and abduction, which are given 50% of shoulder value.

FIG. 8-28. Provides method of calculating restricted range of motion and ankylosis for extension and flexion of elbow, which are given 30% of shoulder value.

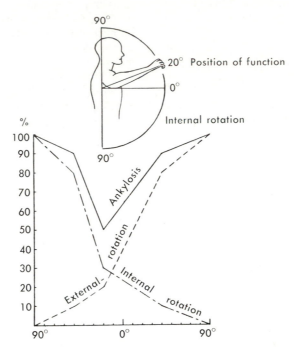

Shoulder—rotation

Fig. 8-29. Provides method of calculating restricted range of motion and ankylosis of shoulder for internal and external rotation, which are given 20% of shoulder value. Entire shoulder is given 60% of value of upper extremity.

and multiplied by the percentage factor as to the contribution of each function to the total shoulder function; when added together and multiplied by the factor of 60%, the impairment of the total shoulder for the extremity is found.

The diagram for evaluation of impaired shoulder function attributable to lack of *adduction-abduction* is represented in Fig. 8-27. An average normal range of motion is considered to be from 50 degrees of adduction to 180 degrees of abduction; the position of function being 50 degrees of abduction.[4,5] Ankylosis in the position of function (50% of abduction) gives 50% of impairment; ankylosis in 0 degrees abduction gives 80% of impairment, and ankylosis in 90 degrees of abduction gives 90% of impairment. Abduction from 0 degrees to the position of function (50 degrees of abduction) is considered to be the most important part of abduction with a decrease of impairment from 70% at a position of 0 degrees to 35% at the position of function (50 degrees of abduction). From there on the abduction curve goes relatively more flat to 0% of impairment at 180 degrees of abduction. The most important function of adduction is to bring the arm from 90 degrees of abduction down to the position of function with a decrease of the impairment from 65% at 90 degrees to 15% at 50 degrees. Adduction from the position of function to 50 degrees of adduction is considered to be of less importance, and the adduction-curve goes relatively flat within this range.

The diagram for evaluation of impaired shoulder function attributable to impairment of *extension and flexion* is shown in Fig. 8-28. An average normal range of motion is assumed to be from 50 degrees of extension to 180 degrees of flexion, the position of function being 25 degrees of flexion.[4,5] An-

kylosis in the position of function gives 50% impairment of function, ankylosis in 0 degrees gives 80% impairment, and ankylosis in 90 degrees of flexion gives 90% impairment. The most important range of flexion is from 0 degrees to the position of function with a decrease of impairment from 70% at 0 degrees to 35% at 25 degrees. From there on the flexion curve goes relatively more flat to end at 0% of impairment at 180 degrees of flexion. The most important range of extension is to bring the arm from 90 degrees of flexion to the position of function; the impairment consequently decreases from 70% at 90 degrees to 15% at 25 degrees. Extension from the position of function to 50 degrees is of less importance and the extension curve goes relatively flat within this range.

In Fig. 8-29 the diagram for evaluation of impaired shoulder function attributable to lack of *internal and external* rotation is presented. An average normal range of motion is assumed to be 90 degrees of internal rotation and 90 degrees of external rotation, the position of function being 20 degrees of external rotation.[4,5] Ankylosis in the position of function gives 50% impairment; ankylosis in 50 degrees of external rotation and 40 degrees of internal rotation gives the same impairment, or 90%. The most important range of external rotation is from 40 degrees of internal rotation to the position of function (20 degrees of external rotation), with a decrease of impairment from 80% to 20%. From there on the curve for external rotation goes more flat to 10% of impairment at 50 degrees of external rotation and finally still more flat for the last 40 degrees of external rotation with a decrease of only 10% of impairment within this range. The most important range of internal rotation is from 50 degrees of external rotation to the position of function, with a decrease of the impairment from 80% to 30%. From there on the curve for internal rotation goes relatively more flat to 10% of impairment at 40 degrees of internal rotation and for the last 50 degrees of internal rotation still more flat from 10% to 0% impairment.

DISCUSSION OF IMPAIRMENT EVALUATION METHODS

It is noted in the diagrams that the impairment has been given a linear configuration that is of practical benefit. It might have been of greater accuracy to note greater changes of impairment immediately around the positions of function for the various joints discussed. It should be observed that the angle of ankylosis has it lowest impairment at the position of function; we have used the recommendation of the American Medical Association of 30 degrees for the metacarpophalangeal joint, 40 degrees for the proximal interphalangeal joint, and 20 degrees for the distal interphalangeal joint in reference to their respective positions of function.

Values for hyperextension of the finger joints have been included in the charts presented here; these were not included in the American Medical Association guide or in our previous work. We consider about 20 degrees of hyperextension in the metacarpophalangeal joint to be normal and of some functional importance in order to open the hand completely. Lack of this hyperextension in the metacarpophalangeal joint is therefore considered to give some impairment. The linear function representing ankylosis, I_A, has simply been extended to include 20 degrees of hyperextension. Hyperextension is the proximal interphalangeal and distal interphalangeal joint is, however, considered unnatural, at least without importance functionally. Lack of hyperextension in these joints will therefore of course not give any impairment. Consequently, in the formula presented, $I_A = I_E + I_F$, I_A and I_F therefore are equal when I_E is 0 and so their functions coincide within the sector of hyperextension. We consider ankylosis or severely limited flexion within this sector, as in severe swan-neck deformity, to give a more pronounced impairment and have therefore drawn the functions more steeply within this sector.

For the evaluation of impairment of the basal joint of the thumb, two motions are measured, namely, thumb opposition and adduction. The difficulty in measuring the angles of the complex thumb movements make this simplified method logical.

SUMMARY

The responsibility of recording, evaluating, and assessing impairment of the upper extremity resulting from trauma and disease is a true medical entity. The method of measuring these defects, the mechanism of estimating impairment, and relating this physical loss of each anatomic segment to the body are presented. The mathematical principles of estimating incapacity are shown.

The common impairments are placed in table form for easier use. A new method of evaluating lack of extension and relating it to ankylosis and lack of flexion is described. A plea is made for the consideration of research into better functional evaluations, including the use of the motion-time-measurement method.

The principles presented and the methods outlined should aid the physician examiner as he attempts to assess impairment in the upper extremity and hand.

REFERENCES

1. American Academy of Orthopaedic Surgeons: Joint motion, method of measuring and recording, Chicago, 1965.
2. Boyes, J.H.: Bunnell's surgery of the hand, ed. 5, Philadelphia, 1970, J.B. Lippincott Co.
3. Bunnell, S.: The management of the non-functional hand—reconstruction vs. prosthesis, Artif. Limbs **4**:76-102, 1957.
4. Crenshaw, A.H., editor: Campbell's operative orthopaedics, ed. 5, St. Louis, 1971, The C.V. Mosby Co.
5. de Palma, A.: Surgery of the shoulder, ed. 2, Philadelphia, 1973, J.B. Lippincott Co.
6. Guide to the evaluation of permanent impairment of the extremities and back, J.A.M.A. **166**:February 16, 1958 (Special edition).
7. Litchman, H.M., and Paslay, P.R.: Determination of finger-motion impairment by linear measurement, J. Bone Joint. Surg. **56A**:85-91, 1974.
8. Mannerfelt, L.: Studies on the hand in ulnar nerve paralysis, Acta Orthop. Scand. (Suppl.) **87**:63, 1966.
9. Swanson, A.B.: Evaluation of impairment of function in the hand, Surg. Clin. North Am. **44**:925-940, 1964.
10. Tubiana, R., Michon, J., and Thomine, J.: Scheme for assessment of deformities of Dupuytren's disease, Surg. Clin. North Am. **48**:979-984, 1968.
11. Van't Hof, A., and Heiple, K.G.: Flexor tendon injuries of the fingers and thumb: a comparative study, J. Bone Joint Surg. **40A**:256-262, 1958.
12. White, W.: Personal communication, 1965, Pittsburgh.

BIBLIOGRAPHY

American Rheumatism Association: Primer on the rheumatic diseases, J.A.M.A. **171**:1205-1220, 1345-1356, 1680-1691, 1959.
American Society for Surgery of the Hand, Committee on Hand Evaluation, Richard Eaton, Chairman.
Bateman, J.E.: Disability evaluation about the shoulder, Surg. Clin. North Am. **43**:1721-1726, 1963.
Beasley, W.C.: Quantitative muscle testing: principles and applications to research and clinical services, Arch. Physiol. Med. **42**:398-425, 1961.
Bechtol, C.O.: Grip test, the use of a dynamometer with adjustable handle spacings, J. Bone Joint Surg. **36A**:820-824, 1954.
Bertelsen, A., and Capener, N.: Fingers, compensation and King Canute, J. Bone Joint Surg. **42B**:390-392, 1960.
Boyes, J.H.: Flexor tendon grafts in the fingers and thumb, J. Bone Joint Surg. **32A**:489-499, 1950.
Carroll, D.: A quantitative test of upper extremity function, J. Chron. Dis. **18**:479-491, 1965.
Flatt, A.E.: Rheumatoid Hand Research Project (Booklets), Department of Orthopaedics, University of Iowa, 1963.
Flatt, A.E.: The care of the rheumatoid hand, ed. 3, St. Louis, 1974, The C.V. Mosby Co.
Garrett, J.W.: The adult human hand; some anthropometric and biomechanic considerations, Hum. Factors **13**:117-131, 1971.
Guides to the evaluation of permanent impairment of the peripheral spinal nerves, American Medical Association Committee on Medical Rating of Physical Impairment, 1962.
Hamasaki, K.: The study of the hand, lost digit, Acta Med. Kyushu University, **31**:53-79, 1961.
Hollander, J.L.: Arthritis and allied conditions, a textbook of rheumatology, ed. 8, Philadelphia, 1972, Lea & Febiger.
Hunter, J.M., and Salisbury, R.E.: Flexor tendon reconstruction in severely damaged hands, J. Bone Joint Surg. **53A**:829-858, 1971.
Karger, D.W., and Bayha, F.H.: Engineered work measurement, ed. 2, New York, 1965, Industrial Press Inc.
Kirkpatrick, E.J.: Evaluation of grip loss, Calif. Med. **85**:314, 1956.
Kroemer, K.H.E., and Howard, J.M.: Towards standardization of muscle strength testing, Med. Sci. Sports **2**:224-230, 1970.
Lewey, F.H., Kuhn, W.G., and Juditski, J.T.: A standardized method for

assessing the strength of hand and foot muscles, Surg. Gynecol. Obstet. **85:**785-793, 1947.

Littler, J.W.: The physiology and dynamic function of the hand, Surg. Clin. North Am. **40:**259-266, 1960.

McBride, E.D.: Disability evaluation, ed. 6, Philadelphia, 1963, J.B. Lippincott Co.

McCormack, R.M.: Reconstructive surgery and immediate care of the badly injured hand, Clin. Orthop. **13:**78-83, 1959.

Moberg, E.: Objective methods for determining the functional value of sensibility in the hand, J. Bone Joint Surg. **40B:**454-476, 1958.

Moberg, E.: Dressings, splints and postoperative care in hand surgery, Surg. Clin. North Am. **44:**35, 941-949, 1964.

Parry, C.B.W.: Rehabilitation of the hand, ed. 2, London, 1966, Butterworth & Co. (Publishers) Ltd.

Patterson, H.McL.: Grip measurements as a part of the pre-placement evaluation, Ind. Med. Surg. **34:**555-557, 1965.

Rattner, I.N.: Injury ratings, New York, 1970, Crescent Publishing Co.

Slocum, D.B.: Amputations of the fingers and the hand, Clin. Orthop. **15:**35-39, 1959.

Slocum, D.B., and Pratt, D.R.: The principles of amputation of the fingers and hand, J. Bone Joint Surg. **26:**535-546, 1944.

Slocum, D.B., and Pratt, D.R.: Disability evaluation for the hand, J. Bone Joint Surg. **28:**491-495, 1946.

Smith, H.B.: Smith hand function evaluation, Am. J. Occup. Ther. **27:**244-251, 1973.

Smith, W.C.: Principles of disability evaluation, Philadelphia, 1959, J.B. Lippincott Co.

Stack, G., editor: Internal publication. International Federation of Societies for Surgery of the Hand, 1970.

Swanson, A.B.: Multiple finger amputations: concepts of treatment, J. Mich. Med. Soc. **61:**316-320, 1962.

Swanson, A.B.: Restoration of hand function by the use of partial or total prosthetic replacement, J. Bone Joint Surg. **45A:**276-288, 1963.

Swanson, A.B.: The Krukenberg procedure in the juvenile amputee, J. Bone Joint Surg. **46A**(7):1540-1549, 1964.

Swanson, A.B.: Surgery of the hand in cerebral palsy and the swan-neck deformity, J. Bone Joint Surg. **42A:**951-964, 1960.

Swanson, A.B.: Levels of amputation of fingers and hand: considerations for treatment, Surg. Clin. North Am. **44:**1115-1126, 1964.

Swanson, A.B., Mays, J.D., and Yamauchi, Y.: A rheumatoid arthritis evaluation record for the upper extremity, Surg. Clin. North Am. **48:**1003-1013, 1968.

Swanson, A.B., Matev, I.B., and deGroot, G.: The strength of the hand, Bull. Prosthet. Res., pp. 145-153, Fall, 1970. Swanson, A.B.: Flexible implant resection arthroplasty in the hand and extremities, St. Louis, 1973, The C.V. Mosby Co.

Taylor, C.L.: Biomechanics of the normal and the amputated upper extremity. In Klopsteg, P.E., and Wilson, P.D., editors: Human limbs and their substitutes, New York, 1954, McGraw-Hill Book Co.

Taylor, C.L., and Schwartz, R.J.: The anatomy and mechanics of the human hand, Artif. Limbs **2:**22-35, 1955.

Wechesser, E.C.: Reconstruction of a grasping mechanism following loss of digits, Clin. Orthop. **15:**69-73, 1959.

III
TRAUMA

9

Wound classification and management

WILLIAM E. BURKHALTER

All extremity wounds regardless of the wounding agent have three similarities and differ only in matter of degree. Host tissue injury, contamination by living organisms, and the presence of foreign bodies exist in all wounds. A cleanly incised wound secondary to a knife laceration in a relatively clean hand with a relatively clean knife has limited host injury and minimal contamination with foreign bodies and bacteria. A crush injury in a farmyard environment has widespread severe host injury with considerable foreign bodies and dangerous bacterial contamination. The term "tidy wound" has been applied to the first example, while the term "untidy" is definitely applicable to the second. These terms have definite therapeutic implications to the surgeon called upon to treat the wounds. The role of the surgeon in wound management is to obtain primary intention wound healing with minimal host tissue reaction.[1] In the tidy wound this sould be relatively easy, while in the more severe untidy wounds this could be quite complicated.

HISTORY OF INJURY

What tools are available to the surgeon to use in his desire to obtain wound healing with minimal reaction? First, there is the history of injury. A split in the skin of the finger without flexor tendon function may be secondary to a sharp laceration with a knife or secondary to a crush injury. In the first instance, the area of injury is in proximity to the wound tract, and the host injury is highly localized. In the crush injury, the finger has been split open from maximal compression of bone and soft tissue, and the host injury is widespread throughout the entire digit. Was the wound inflicted by a relatively clean knife in a kitchen or in an operating room or was it inflicted by the blade of a knife contaminated by a foreign body or many living organisms? The kitchen knife, though relatively free of pathogenic bacteria, may be contaminated by foreign protein from cutting raw pork or chicken. The blade of a rotary lawn mower is traveling at an extremely high velocity when the wound is inflicted and the wound has the same characteristics as a high-velocity bullet wound. In addition to the velocity of the injury, there is considerable conatmination of the wound by living soil organisms and foreign bodies from the ground. So, although the wound is a laceration, it is definitely an untidy wound and one that is prone to develop wound infection without proper management.

By history, then, the treating surgeon can determine to a large extent what he will find when he begins his initial wound management.

WOUND MANAGEMENT

Adequate light, instruments, assistants, and anesthesia are required for all wound management. Tetanus prophylaxis is mandatory and the use of antibiotics varies with the wound and the surgeon.

Wound management begins with the careful and meticulous preparation of the skin to reduce the foreign bodies and bacterial concentration in the area of the wound. Next, wound exploration under tourniquet ischemia determines the extent of the injury. "Débridement" is a word that means different things to different people, and its definitions vary. Nevertheless, the removal of anything in the wound that is detrimental to wound healing is functional débridement. This may include actual excision of necrotic muscle from a crush injury or a bullet wound; it may include the removal of a visible foreign body and wound irrigation to reduce both the foreign body and bacterial contamination. These are all part of wound débridement. Vital structures such as blood vessels, nerves, and tendons are obviously not excised no matter how badly contaminated but are superficially debrided surgically and copiously irrigated.

Débridement is usually felt to be complete when no visible foreign body or necrotic tissue is present within a wound. At this point, if the wound was secondary to a clean knife laceration with minimal foreign body and necrotic tissue and if only minimal débridement was necessary, the wound could be simply closed by sutures. Before this, however, repair of deep tissue may be carried out if there was damage. In this type of wound, tendon repairs, nerve repairs, and internal fixation of fractures can be carried out before actual closure of the wound; that is, wound débridement has been followed by repair of deep structures and primary closure of the wound. If, on the other hand, there has been widespread injury as occurs with a bullet wound, crush injury, or rotary lawn mower blade, the amount of host injury is great and located away from the actual wound tract. Widespread host injury plus high concentrations of foreign body and bacteria make the wound prone to infection. The surgery of débridement in this must be extensive, generally requiring additional incisions for exploration and the removal of necrotic tissue and foreign body. In this type of wound, the surgeon is frequently not able to say that his débridement is complete. He may be unable to state exactly what tissue is necrotic. In this situation, primary wound closures should not be carried out. The expectations of wound infection in primary closure of this type of wound is high. Even if frank suppuration does not occur, a highly reactive wound with considerable edema and redness will persist for many weeks. The wound closure should be delayed.

DELAYED WOUND CLOSURE

Immediately after débridement a dressing should be applied to the open wound and an occlusive hand dressing added to this. Clinically and experimentally it has been

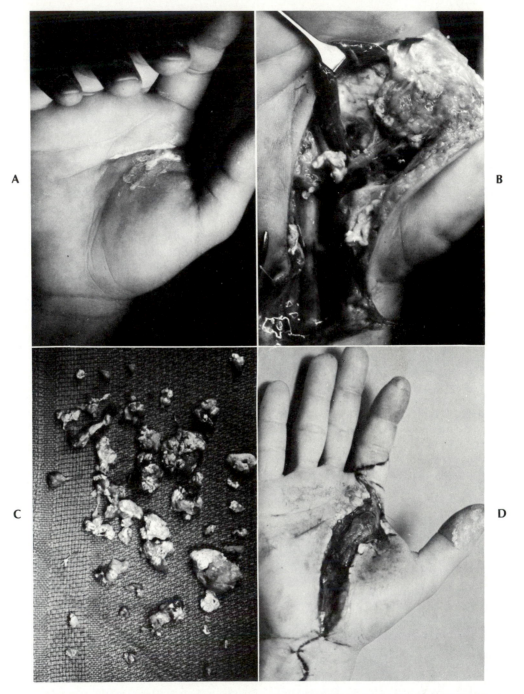

FIG. 9-1. Patient incurred paint-injection injury to radial aspect of index finger 3 hours before this initial photograph. **A,** Again note diffuse injury with foreign body exuding from injection site. **B,** At exploration and débridement additional incisions were required volarly and dorsally. **C,** Considerable foreign material was removed from palm and digit. **D,** It was believed that wound closure was not indication because of diffuse injury, residual foreign body, and bacterial contamination.

shown that delayed primary wound closure of contaminated wounds is more successful than primary closure. The optimum time of wound closure appears to be 4 or 5 days after initial wound surgery.[3,4] Thus 4 to 5 days after the initial wound surgery, the patient is returned to the operating room for wound exploration. At this time, removal of initially questionable tissue can be carried out, and if definite necrosis is seen, further wound irrigation and search for the foreign body are carried out. At this point, wound closure may be accomplished. However, remember that wound closure is an elective surgical operation that should be carried out only when all possible chances for success exist. This second look before wound closure allows the surgeon to evaluate the adequacy of the initial surgery and to redébride if necessary before wound closure. In addition, delayed primary repair of deep structures may also be carried out. Tendons and nerves may be repaired. Fractures may be internally fixed in an environment that has already demonstrated its freedom from necrotic tissue and foreign bodies. In this situation wound healing should occur with minimal tissue reaction.[2]

SECONDARY INTENTION HEALING

In certain wounds, generally the untidy type, wound closure may not be indicated for many days or perhaps it is believed that wound closure is not indicated at all. In this case wound closure occurs by secondary intention healing. Wounds in this category may include burns of the hand and wounds that occur after drainage and débridement of infections. In the latter cases healing by secondary intention is the usual method of management. Sometimes in elective surgery, wound closure by secondary intention healing is chosen by the surgeon. In Dupuytren's contracture, Mc-Cash[5] and many others have written extensively about the excision of the contracting band through transverse incisions in the palm. We have also used the same technique in the fingers with good success. In both cases wound healing by secondary intention is accepted. This is done so that the complications of skin slough, hematoma, and loss of motion are reduced. In all these situations—the hand burn, the postoperative hand infection, and the postoperative Dupuytren's contracture—wound healing occurs by secondary intention. The key to success in all these situations is active motion during wound healing. It has been said many times that allowing a wound of the hand to heal by secondary intention will give extreme stiffness and deformity. Certainly this may be true if there has been actual loss of skin and active motion cannot be instituted because of skeletal instability. However, with active motion, proper splinting, and proper explanation to the patient extremely functional hands can be regained from infections, burns, or Dupuytren's contracture with secondary intention wound healing (Figs. 9-1 and 9-2). Once again, wound closure is an elective procedure that should be carried out when the surgeon believes that the wound will accept closure. It should not be carried out on any rigid time schedule.

If secondary intention wound healing is deemed to be the safest for the patient as a method of obtaining a closed wound, we believe that function must be added as well. As stated before, to allow healing to occur without function is to invite disaster in the form of stiffness. Many times we have heard that immobilization must be maintained until solid wound healing is achieved. This is absolute nonsense and again courts stiffness. Here a question of timing arises.

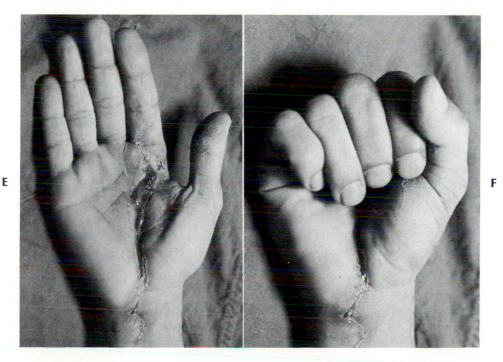

FIG. 9-1, cont'd. E and **F,** Wound gradually closed by secondary intention with active use of hand in a light dressing was allowed. Range of motion seen at 3 weeks.

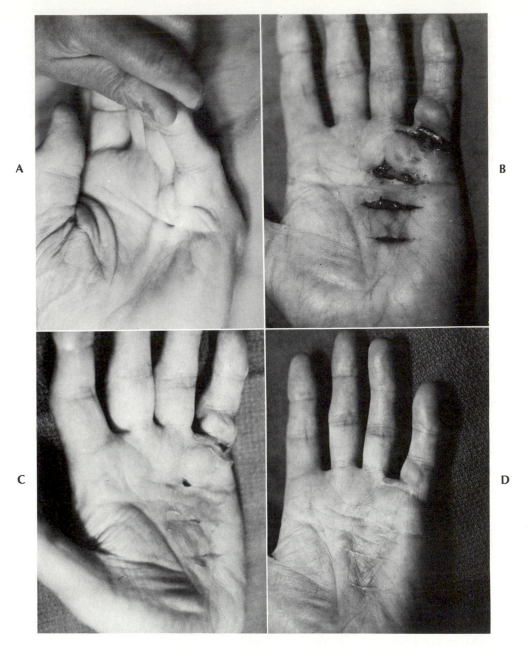

FIG. 9-2. Sixty-five-year-old patient with moderate Dupuytren's contracture, **A.** Treatment consisted of partial palmar fasciectomy without wound closure, **B.** Three days after surgery active motion of fingers was instituted with splinting of fingers in extension at night. At 3 weeks wounds are almost completely healed, and patient had a good range of active motion, **C.** Two years postoperatively the scars are well healed with good correction of the deformity maintained, **D.**

When is function instituted? How early is early function? In the case of the burn patient or the infection or the Dupuytren's patient that we have used before as examples of secondary intention wound healing, we believe that motion should be instituted within 24 to 48 hours of injury or operation. The undamaged structures in the hand will only deteriorate with immobilization and will be caught in the glue that accompanies injury without function. So then, early function is function within 1 to 2 days of accident or

surgical insult and this function must take precedence over wound closure. If wound closure and function can be instituted simultaneously, fine, but if the two are the last bit prejudicial, motion and function must be achieved before wound closure whether this be carried out by suture, skin graft, pedicle flap, or secondary intention healing.

Fig. 9-3 shows a dorsal infection of the hand treated by incision and drainage and active motion of the flexors and extensors within 24 hours. Notice that the patient initially

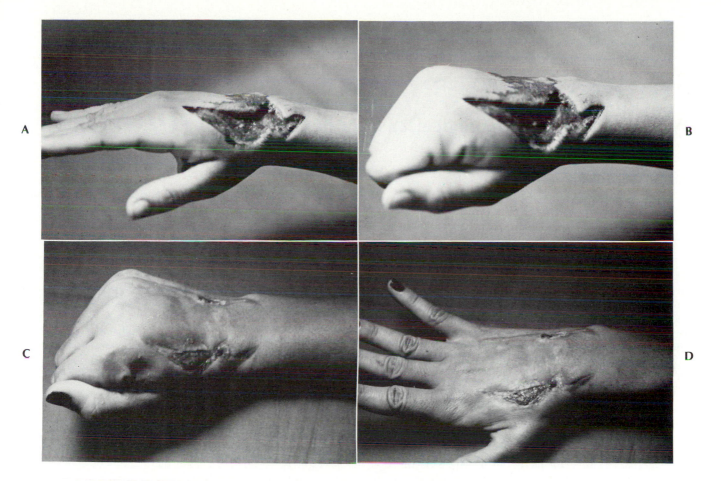

FIG. 9-3. A and **B,** Subcutaneous dorsal infection treated by débridement plus early motion. **C** and **D,** Healing progressed while the patient actively exercised the hand.

had an extensor lag but then gradually regained full motion. To wait for secondary intention wound healing before instituting function would have been to prejudice the ultimate functional recovery of this hand. As is seen, wound healing progressed as function continued to improve. Once again, wound closure is an elective procedure that should be carried out when the surgeon believes that the wound will accept closure. It should not be carried out on any rigid time schedule.

REFERENCES

1. Boyes, J.H.: A philosophy of care of the injured hand, Bull. Am. Coll. Surg. **50:**341, 1965.
2. Burkhalter, W., Butler, B., Metz, W., and Omer, G.: Experiences with delayed primary closure of war wounds of the hand in Viet Nam, J. Bone Joint Surg. **50A:**945, 1968.
3. DeMuth, W.E., Jr., and Smith, J.M.: High velocity bullet wounds of muscle and bone: the basis of rational early treatment, J. Trauma **6:**744, 1966.
4. Lowry, K.F., and Curtis, G.M.: Delayed suture in the management of wounds, analysis of 721 traumatic wounds illustrating the influence of time interval in wound repair, Am. J. Surg. **80:**280, 1950.
5. McCash, C.R.: The open palm technique in Dupuytren's contracture, Br. J. Plast. Surg. **17:**271, 1964.

10

Wound healing: the biological basis of hand surgery

JOHN W. MADDEN

In order to manipulate our environment effectively, the hand performs feats which, on superficial analysis, seem incompatible. The hand changes shape in thousands of subtle ways, adapting physical configuration to the requirements of the moment. Equally important, however, the hand becomes a stable transmitter of powerful forces on demand. This unique combination of strength, movement, and stability is inherent in the anatomic configurations of epidermal and mesenchymal tissues that comprise the hand. Almost all hand structures are dense connective tissues, the strongest of animal products. Movement is achieved by allowing architectural components to move relative to one another. Stability is obtained by arranging periarticular structures to allow movement in one plane and to resist movement in another, or by adding forces to create stability through active muscle contraction. Thus the key to normal hand function is the ability of strong, dense connective tissue structures to glide relative to one another.

Gliding depends on precise placement of blood vessels, fascial septa, areolar tissue, tendons, ligaments, and fascial sheaths. The physical properties of all normal hand structures are adapted to gliding. Any alteration in macroscopic anatomy that changes the physical characteristics or anatomic arrangement of tissues prevents relative gliding and reduces hand functions significantly. Because the basic reaction of tissue to injury alters physical properties by replacing normal structures with scar, a thorough understanding of wound healing reactions and scar formation forms the biologic foundation on which hand surgery rests.

SCAR FORMATION

The normal anatomic events occurring during the early phases of wound healing are familiar to most surgeons and will be reviewed only briefly. Within minutes after planned or accidental tissue disruption, the wound space fills with clotted blood. Within hours, a typical acute inflammatory response is well established: marked vasodilation occurs with accompanying local edema, white blood cells migrate through the walls of blood vessels, and fixed tissue macrophages become actively mobile. The initial cell population is predominantly polymorphonuclear leukocytes. Within a few days, however, monocytic macrophages become the most frequently encountered cell type. The removal of dead tissue fragments and foreign bodies, including bacteria, by phagocytic cells seems an obligatory part of the wound healing process. Recent data suggest that late stages of wound healing can be influenced significantly by the effectiveness of cellular phagocytosis.[28] If tissues are incised sharply and reapproximated quickly with minimal tissue damage, the inflammatory phase of wound healing is completed within a few days. If tissues are damaged significantly or if the wound becomes contaminated with bacteria, the inflammatory phase can last indefinitely.

As the inflammatory response evolves in the deeper portions of the wound, significant events occur at the wound surface. Epithelial cells along the margins of skin wounds begin to undergo dramatic changes within hours of injury. Fixed basal cells at the wound edge begin migrating down and across the surface, using fibrin strands as walkways.[50] Within 48 hours, cleanly incised, sutured wounds are completely epithelialized. Over several weeks, the epithelial surface becomes multilayered, thickens, and the restoration of the epithelial surface is obvious to the naked eye.

Within the first 72 hours, spindle-shaped cells associated with small blood vessels in the periphery of the wound begin to divide, and daughter cells invade the wound space.[49] By the end of the first week, this new cell type, the fibroblast, begins replacing the macrophage as the most frequent cell type. By the second week, the wound space is completely filled by these actively metabolizing cells. As fibroblasts migrate into the wound space, small blood vessels proximal to the area of injury begin to bud and growing capillaries follow the migration. Although collagen fibers comprise the majority of the mature scar, fibers cannot be visualized by the light microscope until the fourth or fifth day following injury. Once fibers appear, however, collagen accumulates in the wound rapidly. Thus, by the end of the second week, the wound is filled with a rich capillary network, large numbers of fibroblasts, and a moderate number of newly synthesized collagen fibers.

Morphological changes occurring during the early phases of healing are dramatic and rapid. From a physiologic point of view, changes occurring after the second or third week are equally dramatic, but morphology changes at a more leisurely pace. From the third to the sixth week after injury,

Reprinted with permission from *Clinics in Plastic Surgery*, vol. 3, No. 1, Jan. 1976. The author's work reported in this article supported by National Institute of Arthritis, Metabolism, and Digestive Diseases, Grant No. AM14047, National Institutes of Health, Bethesda, Maryland.

the number of fibroblasts and blood vessels within the wound space diminishes slowly. As the cell population decreases, scar collagen fibers increase. Gradually, the wound changes from predominantly cellular structure to a predominantly extracellular tissue. Because morphology changes so slowly during later stages, many biologists have been lulled into feeling that wound healing begins abruptly and ends within 1 month of injury. Nothing could be farther from the truth. Scars remain metabolically active for years, slowly changing in size, shape, color, texture, and strength.

Although wounds become stronger with time, gain in strength follows a sequence of time, gain in strength follows a sequence of physical changes not reflected precisely in macroscopic appearance. Because hand function ultimately depends on the physical properties of scar tissue, the kinetics of physical change is as important to the surgeon as morphology.

Within the first few days, cohesive forces between epithelial cells, fibroblasts, and endothelial cells add some strength to healing wounds.[51] Intercellular forces, however, are weak, and wounds may be disrupted with ease at this stage. When collagen fibers appear, wounds begin to gain strength rapidly. Although scars are composed of many chemical constituents, collagen fibers are responsible for the characteristic physical properties of scars.[1] Indeed, collagen is the basic structural protein of all animals, and the physical properties of mesenchymal tissues, from strong tendons to loose areolar tissues, depend upon the physical characteristics and weave of collagen fibers. By 3 weeks, the normal incised and sutured wound has less than 15 per cent of its ultimate tensile strength.[29] Strength of an incised wound increases linearly for at least 3 months in animals and probably much longer in man. Lacerated and repaired tendons gain strength at an even slower rate.[41] Factors responsible for this prolonged increase in strength will be discussed in a later section.

During the early phases of wound healing, the wound space is filled completely with cells and randomly oriented collagen fibers. Although surgeons attempt to compartmentalize wounds by carefully reapproximateing fascial layers, histologic study reveals that during the early phases of healing the scar is a single unit invading all areas of the wound space regardless of careful stitchwork.[43] Thus all injured tissues are bound together in a single unit by the newly synthesized scar tissue.

Rapidly uniting all injured tissues into a single strong mass has homeostatis advantages, reestablishing integrity and strength quickly and effectively. In some instances, a single massive scar produces an excellent functional outcome. As an example, the abdomen functions normally in the presence of a scar, welding peritoneum, muscle, fascia, subcutaneous tissue, and skin into a single unit. In the hand, however, scars of this nature are never satisfactory. The characteristic feature of hand architecture is strong collagenous structures moving freely relative to fixed units. Binding mobile and immobile units together limits function. For example, a wound binding skin, palmar fascia, lumbrical muscle, tendon, and bone into a single unit prevents active motion completely. In order to reestablish satisfactory function, cut tendon ends must be linked together by strong scar tissue, but the character of scar joining tendon with surrounding immobile structures must be altered to permit tendon gliding. During the later phases of wound healing, scars can and do change anatomic arrangement. This phenomenon, the remodeling of scar tissue, determines success or failure of reconstructive surgical procedures on the hand.

The "one wound" concept is useful in planning elective hand incisions or in routine tendon transfers and grafts. When a choice is possible, gliding structures must be placed next to tissues that also move. Tendon transfers and grafts should be placed in subcutaneous tissue away from skin incisions, old scars, or other fixed structures. If all injured tissues are free to move, less reliance need be placed on the remodeling process to restore normal function.

SCAR CHEMISTRY

Because collagen fibers determine the physical characteristics of scar tissue, an understanding of wound healing requires some familiarity with this unique protein. The collagen molecule is a long, straight, rigid, rodlike structure, measuring 3000 Å in length and 14 Å in width.[6] Individual molecules are composed of three polypeptide chains wound around each other in a helical fashion. The molecule is synthesized initially in precursor form. Individual chains, synthesized within fibroblasts on large polyribosomes, are composed of several sections. Chains come together within the cell to form the precursor molecule, procollagen. Procollagen has a large, nonhelical portion at the aminoterminal end, a long, rigid central section, and a small, nonhelical portion at the carboxy-terminal end.[7] After excretion into the extracellular space, the large, nonhelical portion of procollagen is deleted under enzymatic control, producing the typical helical molecules that comprise normal fibers.

Collagen is one of the few proteins synthesized by animal cells that is designed to become insoluble. When collagen molecules are brought together under physiologic conditions, even in the absence of cells, they aggregate quickly, forming a random mat of fibrils. Under normal physiologic conditions, collagen molecules aggregate in a three-dimensional array, overlapping each adjoining molecule by one quarter. Quarter staggering is responsible for the typical 640 Å band periodicity of collagen fibers seen in electron micrographs.

Initially, aggregated collagen molecules are held together by hydrogen bonds and other weak physical forces. New fibrils rupture easily when stressed. Within a matter of hours, however, fibrils demonstrate a marked increase in tensile strength. As fibrils mature, weak intermolecular forces are supplemented by the formation of strong covalent bonds.[25] Covalent bonding occurs between individual peptide chains within the molecule (intramolecular bonds) and between adjacent molecules (intermolecular bonds). Again, this process occurs even in the absence of living cells. Ultimately, collagen fibers become giant polymers, each molecule linked to neighbors by strong covalent bonds. Aggregation and covalent bonding produce a strong, flexible fiber that can be woven into many different tissue patterns.

The nature of covalent bonding between collagen molecules is still under intense investigation.[56] Although several types of bonding may be involved, the principal bond between adjacent molecules seems to be a reaction between aldehyde groups.[8] If crossbonding is prevented, collagen molecules aggregate, form fibrils, but fail to develop the characteristic strength of native collagen.[55] Thus, collagen synthesis, aggregation, and crossbonding are the chemical events that alter the physical properties of injured tissues. The quantity of scar collagen, the anatomic configuration of the fibers, and the density of covalent bonding determine the physical characteristics of the injured hand.

The collagen content of incised and sutured wounds increases rapidly during the first 3 weeks.[36] Following this initial rapid accumulation, however, total collagen content stabilizes and remains constant for long intervals. Histologically, the wound appears as a dynamic structure during the first 3 to 4 weeks, but undergoes few morphologic changes thereafter. How do wounds gain strength for prolonged intervals while maintaining a stable chemical and histologic appearance? Recent experiments on the kinetic chemistry of scar collagen have helped to resolve this paradox. Direct measurements of rate of new collagen deposition in primary and secondary wounds have demonstrated that scar collagen remains metabolically active for prolonged periods in spite of stable collagen content and histologic picture.[35,38] Fibroblasts within the wound area begin synthesizing collagen on the third day. The rate of new collagen deposition increased rapidly to a maximum between the second and fourth weeks, but remains elevated for prolonged intervals. Even 4 months after wounding, new collagen is being deposited at a significantly higher rate in the scar than in normal skin. Rapid collagen synthesis and deposition in the presence of stable amounts of scar collagen indicate simultaneous and rapid collagen destruction.[36] Thus, scar collagen content represents an equilibrium, the product of the destruction and removal of old collagen molecules and the synthesis and deposition of new molecules. The prolonged and rapid metabolic turnover of scar collagen provides the chemical mechanism responsible for scar remodeling and seems to account for a variety of abnormal wound healing reactions.[48]

In addition to collagen, scar tissue contains large amounts of glycosaminoglycans.[44] These large, sulphated mucopolysaccharides are synthesized locally within the wound space, presumably by fibroblasts. The precise role of the glycosaminoglycans in wound healing remains unknown. Under laboratory conditions, the size, weave, and physical characteristics of collagen fibers can be controlled, in part, by the character of the glycosaminoglycans in the environment. In all probability, glycosaminoglycans play a significant role in the organization of collagen molecules within normal and scarred tissues. Defining how the glycosaminoglycans influence wound healing and scar remodeling remains a significant challenge to interested investigators.

SCAR REMODELING

All wounds undergo remarkable changes in color, texture, firmness, and bulk with time. A well healed wound, 2 months following injury, bears little resemblance to the same wound 1 year later. As we have discussed, measurable physical properties of sutured wounds (tensile strength, burst strength, tear strength, etc.) change slowly for many months. Physical changes seem to be caused by alterations in the architecture of scar collagen fibers and by alterations in the density of covalent bonding between collagen molecules. Studies using the scanning electron microscope, in addition to the light microscopic observations, indicate that the organization of collagen fibers within the wound changes with time.[18,19]

Striking alterations in scar architecture occur in situations where gliding function is reestablished following injury. The randomly matted collagen fibrils uniting all injured structures during the early phases of healing become oriented in more specific ways with time.[43] Scar collagen between tendon ends becomes oriented in parallel bundles resembling normal tendon. Parallel organization establishes a strong union between tendon ends capable of transmitting powerful longitudinal forces. As a part of the same process, collagen fibers lying adjacent to gliding surfaces enlarge but retain their random orientation, creating a loose areolar configuration. Blood vessels present in the peritendinous scar become coiled and tortuous permitting movement without loss of vessel integrity. Over many months, scar tissue initially deposited in a random configuration becomes rewoven into structures that resemble the preinjury condition (parallel collagen bundles between tendon ends, peritenon-like structures surrounding gliding surfaces). In contrast, examining injured tendons that fail to regain gliding demonstrates an entirely different scar architecture. Instead of remodeling to resemble peritenon, scar tissue organizes into firm collagenous adhesions with parallel collagen fibers uniting the gliding surfaces firmly to fixed surrounding structures. The physical characteristics of these adhesions prevent tendon gliding completely.

Demonstrating prolonged and rapid metabolic turnover of scar collagen establishes the chemical mechanism responsible for the remodeling of scars but provides no clues as to why scar collagen in one wound remodels to permit gliding while scar in another becomes an ever stronger unit uniting mobile and immobile structures into an unyielding mass. Controlling the factors responsible for morphologic change in scar tissue seems to be the key to perfect restoration of the injured hand. If morphologic changes could be controlled precisely, all tendon repairs and grafts would be successful, all joint replacements would move freely, and all wounds would heal with minimal functional abnormalities.

Although factors controlling the morphogenic aspects of scar remodeling are poorly understood, certain biologic observations seem pertinent. Experimental and clinical evidence indicates that longitudinal and shearing stresses are responsible for the remodeling of bone.[3] The clinical behavior of scars supports the concept that physical forces play an equally important role in the remodeling of scar tissue. As an example, skin wounds placed across lines of changing dimension slowly but irrevocably hypertrophy. In contrast, scars placed along the midaxial line of a finger, or parallel to lines of changing dimension, become insignificant with time. Recently, the influence of tension on remodeling scar tissue has been demonstrated experimentally.[2] As yet, however, how the magnitude, rate of application, frequency, duration, and direction of stress application influence and ultimate size and physical properties of scar tissue remain unknown. Although every clinician uses the controlled application of stress to regain motion following tendon injury, treatment programs are empirical. If we knew precisely how to apply stresses, postoperative therapy could become more efficient and productive.

A variety of factors other than stress influence the remodeling of scars. The surfaces against which scar tissue is deposited influence the nature of remodeling. Scar deposited in the presence of cut tendon ends remodels to mimic the organization of tendon bundles; scar collagen adjacent to an uninjured tendon surface tends to remodel to resemble peritenon. How adjacent structures induce architectural changes is unknown.

Age seems to influence scar remodeling. Younger animals tend to remodel scar tissue more effectively than older animals. Although young children seem to produce more reactive scars than adults, remodeling is rapid and effective. An increase in the rate of metabolic turnover may be responsible for the excellent restoration of gliding seen in young patients undergoing tendon repair.

The total quantity of scar deposited seems to influence the remodeling process. The larger the scar, the less likelihood of effective restoration of physiologic function. Because the quantity of tissue deposited is related directly to the quantity of tissue injured, atraumatic surgical technique and careful débridement yield better restoration of function. Rough surgical technique and retained foreign bodies, including injured tissue, prolong the initial phases of healing and produce large amounts of scar tissue. In this case, remodeling reactions are insufficient to reestablish proper scar architecture.

These observations may provide a rationale for the excellent results reported in two stage flexor tendon grafts. Some authors claim that preliminary implantation of Silastic rod provides a smooth surface against which grafts may glide. Actually, the rod may serve only as a method of establishing tendon continuity with minimal tissue damage. At the first stage, extensive tissue dissection and injury initiate a normal wound healing response. After several months, the rate of new collagen deposition has slowed appreciably. At the second stage, only the tissues at either end of the tendon graft are disturbed. Restoration of the blood supply to the grafted tendon occurs in an environment in which fibrous protein synthesis is minimized. Without the extensive operative trauma and tissue damage, less new collagenous tissue is formed and remodeling occurs more effectively.

The presence of excessive quantities of old scar within a new wound has detrimental effects on remodeling. Although scar tissue remains metabolically active for years, the ability to change morphology is lost with time. Old scar, firmly bound to immobile structures, provides an unsatisfactory bed for subsequent gliding. To maximize remodeling potential, all old scar tissue should be excised prior to repairing gliding structures. In tendon transfers, old scars should be avoided and tendons placed in beds containing a minimal amount of scar tissue.

Finally, the biologic condition of tissues at the time of injury influences scar remodeling. Because wounds remain dynamic structures for prolonged periods, a second injury during this active metabolic period increases scar collagen synthesis.[38] Performing restorative procedures while the injured hand remains reactive produces unsatisfactory results. Although initial reconstructive procedures are often performed 6 to 8 weeks following injury, clinical and experimental evidence suggests that a much longer interval is advisable. The physical characteristics of injured tissues provide clues to their metabolic state. As long as wounds feel hard and immobile, attempts at secondary reconstruction should be avoided.

WOUND CONTRACTION

The biologic events described in the preceding sections are characteristic of sharply incised and primarily closed wounds. Open wounds, with or without tissue loss, present different clinical problems. Although the basic morphologic and the chemical processes operating in closed wounds participate, wound contraction becomes an important feature and epithelialization assumes a more prominent role.

Full-thickness defects in any mobile area of mammalian skin undergo dramatic changes in size and shape. After 1 2- or 3-day latent period, wounds begin to contract actively and by 2 or 3 weeks are less than 20 per cent of their original area.[4] In areas where skin is relatively loose and mobile structures are not nearby, wound contraction produces minimal deformity. In the hand, however, where no "extra skin" exists, wound contraction produces disastrous results. The forces of contraction act to close the wound until balanced by equal tension in the surrounding skin. Although tension in surrounding tissue may lessen with time, for all practical purposes a wound contracts until fixed tissues prevent further contraction. In the hand the mobility of the small joints permits open wounds to contract until joints become fixed in abnormal positions. For example, a 4 × 4 cm defect on the dorsum contracting to a 2 × 2 cm scar fixes the metacarpal phalangeal joints in extension. If joints are allowed to remain in abnormal positions for any length of time, secondary changes in the periarticular tissues produce permanent joint stiffness. Because of these potential disasters, minimizing wound contraction is critical to the proper management of open hand wounds.

Experimental data support the concept that living cells, rather than alterations in extracellular mesenchymal material, supply the force moving wound edges together.[57] Recently, Gabbiani and co-workers have identified a specific cell type in granulation tissue which may represent the contractile element.[22] This unique cell combines the ultrastructural features of the fibroblast and smooth muscle cell. Modified fibroblasts (myofibroblasts) have been identified in contracting tissues from several animal species and in a variety of human fibrocontractive diseases.[30,31] Although it is impossible to prove that atypical cells, identifiable by ultrastructural criteria alone, supply the motive force for wound contraction, a variety of data supports this interpretation. Biochemical measurements demonstrate that granulation tissue from contracting wounds contain as much actomyosin as uterus.[21] Human antismooth muscle sera label the cytoplasm of myofibroblasts.[23] Granulation tissue containing significant numbers of myofibroblasts contracts actively in vitro, behaving as vascular smooth muscle tissue.[40] Finally, topically applied antismooth muscle agents inhibit wound contraction completely.[34]

Although the use of smooth muscle antagonists or other methods of controlling the contraction process offer promise for the future, the only practical method of influencing contraction at the moment is the immediate replacement of missing skin with thick skin grafts or pedicle flaps. Contrary to popular opinion, epithelialization per se does not inhibit contraction.[53] Replacing missing tissue immediately does not prevent contraction, but the ultimate area of the defect is much larger following immediate coverage.[52] Once contraction has begun, however, replacing missing skin is less effective in inhibiting the process.[54] A combination of immediate coverage plus mechanical splinting, by skeletal structures in the area or by external devices, is the most effective method of minimizing wound contraction.[39] All open wounds of the hand must be covered as quickly as possible to prevent permanent residual deformities.

CONTROLLING THE WOUND HEALING PROCESS

Several novel solutions to the problems created by scar formation in the injured hand are being evaluated experimentally. Although all tissue injury produces scarring and potentially limits gliding, the location of newly deposited scar tissue can be controlled. As an example, the entire digital theca can be removed from cadavers and transplanted to animals as a single unit. Although the cellular components of the graft die and the extracellular components seem to be replaced by host protein, the architectural arrangement of the transplant is retained.[42] The blood supply to the tendinous structures is reestablished by connections between the local tissue and outer fibrous sheath. An intense wound healing reaction occurs but at the outer surface of the transplant protecting the gliding structures. The specialized mesenteric structures within the fibrous envelope and the gliding surfaces remain uninvolved in the scarring process. Several centers have reported encouraging long term results using allografts in human fingers.[20,24,46] Unfortunately, grafts are inconvenient to obtain. Attempts are being made to lyophilize human flexor mechanisms and produce a product that can be stored indefinitely and used conveniently.[9]

Another approach to the problem of healing and gliding involves fundamental manipulations of collagen chemistry. As we have discussed, the physical properties of collagen fibers, not the presence of scar tissue per se, prevent gliding in poorly remodeled wounds. The physical properties of individual collagen fibers are determined by their covalent bonding patterns. Inhibiting covalent bonding produces a fibril without significant tensile strength. A class of chemical compounds called osteolathyrogens specifically inhibit the enzyme responsible for intermolecular crosslinking.[55] Beta-aminoproprionitrile (BAPN), the most powerful known osteolathyrogen, reduces the tensile strength of experimental wounds, improves gliding following experimental tendon injury, prevents esophageal stenosis following lye burns, and restores esophageal diameter in fixed esophageal stenosis.[15,17,33,45] BAPN has been administered to human beings in clinical trials.[26,37,47] The agent causes significant bio-

chemical and physical effects on newly synthesized scar collagen. Whether or not lathyrogenic effects produce significant improvement in gliding, however, awaits further clinical investigation.

Inhibiting the synthesis and deposition of scar collagen specifically and selectively could control the healing process. The hydroxylation of proline is a unique and requisite step in collagen synthesis. The enzyme responsible for hydroxylation, peptidylproline hydroxylase, requires ferrous iron as a cofactor.[11] Chelating ferrous iron produces specific inhibition of collagen synthesis without effecting noncollagenous protein synthesis.[10,13] Although this technique has been used effectively in vitro, available chelators seem too toxic to be applied clinically.[14] Analogues of proline can also inhibit collagen synthesis specifically.[6] Several authors have claimed that administering proline analogues to animals inhibits collagen synthesis and improves tendon gliding.[5,16,27] The effects of proline analogues in vivo, however, are controversial and the effects in human beings remain unknown.[12,32]

Effective control of the healing process in man has not been achieved. However, experimental data suggest that clinical control of the healing process is feasible. Over the next decade, the development of clinically useful methods of controlling scar formation and wound contraction will be developed. Until these tools are in our possession, the skillful surgeon must utilize the biologic information covered in this article to regain maximum function in the injured hand. At the moment, we have no pharmacologic crutch to support poor wound management.

REFERENCES

1. Adamsons, R., Musco, F., and Enquist, I.: The relationship of collagen content to wound strength in normal and scorbutic animals. Surg. Gynec. Obstet., **119**:323, 1964.
2. Arem, A.J., and Madden, J.W.: Effects of stress on healing wounds: I. Intermittent noncyclical tension. J. Surg. Res. [**20**(2):93, 1976].
3. Bassett, C.A.: The effect of force on skeletal tissues. In Downey, J.A., and Darling, R.C., (eds.): Physiological Basis of Rehabilitation Medicine. Philadelphia, W.B. Saunders Co., 1971, p. 283.
4. Billingham, R.E., and Russell, P.S.: Studies on wound healing, with special reference to contracture in experimental wounds in rabbits' skin. Ann. Surg., **144**:961, 1956.
5. Bora, R.F., Jr., Lane, M.M., and Prockop, D.J.: Inhibitors of collagen biosynthesis as a means of controlling scar formation in tendon injury. J. Bone Joint Surg., **54A**:1501, 1972.
6. Bornstein, P.: The biosynthesis of collagen. Ann. Rev. Biochem., **43**:567, 1974.
7. Bornstein, P., Monson, J.M., Murphy, W.H., and Kruse, N.J.: Structure, synthesis and secretion of procollagen. In Slavkin, H.C., and Gruelich, R.C. (eds.): Extracellular Matrix Ingluences on Gene Expression. New York, Academic Press, 1975, p. 95.
8. Bornstein, P., and Piez, K.A.: The nature of the intramolecular crosslinks in collagen. The separation and characterization of peptides from the crosslink region of rat skin collagen. Biochemistry, **5**:3460, 1966.
9. Cameron, R.R., Contrad, R.N., and Latham, W.D.: Preserved composite tendon allografts. Acceptance and survival in the injured finger. Presented at the 49th Annual Meeting of the American Association of Plastic Surgeons, Colorado Springs, 1970.
10. Chvapil, M., Hurych, J., and Ehrlichova, E.: Effects of long term in vivo application of phenanthroline, penicillamine and further chelating agents on the synthesis of collagenous and noncollagenous proteins in fibrotic liver and wound granulation tissue. Hoppe Seyler Z. Physiol. Chem., **349**:218, 1968.
11. Chvapil, M., Hurych, J., Ehrlichova, E., and Tichy, M.: Mechanism of the action of chelating agents on proline hydroxylation and its

incorporation into collagenous and non-collagenous proteins. Europ. J. Beiochem., **2**:229, 1967.

12. Chvapil, M., Madden, J.W., Carlson, E.C., and Peacock, E.E., Jr.: Effect of cis-hydroxyproline on collagen and other proteins in skin wounds, granuloma tissue, and liver of mice and rats. Exper. Molec. Path., **20**:363, 1974.

13. Chvapil, M., McCarthy, D.W., Madden, J.W., and Peacock, E.E., Jr.: Invivo effect of 1,10-phenanthroline and desferrioxamine on peptidyl proline hydroxylase and hydroxylation of collagen in rats. Biochem. Pharmacol., **23**:2165, 1974.

14. Chvapil, M., Ryan, J.N., Madden, J.W., and Peacock, E.E., Jr.: Effect of chelating agents, proline analogs, and oxygen tension in in vivo and in vitro experiments on hydroxylation, transport, degradation, and accumulation of collagen. *In* Vogel, H.G. (ed.): Connective Tissue and Aging, Vol. I. International Congress Series, No. 264, Amsterdam, Excerpta Medica, 1973, p. 195.

15. Craver, J.M., Madden, J.W., and Peacock, E.E., Jr.: Biological control of physical properties of tendon adhesions. Effect of beta-aminoproprionitrile in chickens. Ann. Surg., **167**:697, 1968.

16. Daly, J.M., Steigher, E., Prockop, D.J., and Dudrick, S.J.: Inhibition of collagen synthesis by the proline analogue cis-4-hydroxyproline. J. Surg. Res., **14**:551, 1973.

17. Davis, W.M., Madden, J.W., and Peacock, E.E., Jr.: A new approach to the esophageal stenosis, Ann. Surg., **176**:469, 1972.

18. Forrester, J.C., Zederfeldt, B.H., Hayes, T.L., and Hunt, T.K.: Tape closed and sutured wounds: A comparison by tensiometry and scanning electron microscopy. Br. J. Surg., **57**:729, 1970.

19. Forrester, J.C., Zederfeldt, B.H., Hayes, T.L., and Hunt, T.K.: Wolff's law in relation to the healing skin wound. J. Trauma, **10**:770, 1970.

20. Furlow, L.T., Jr.: Homologous flexor mechanism replacement in four fingers of one hand. Plast. Reconstr. Surg., **43**:531, 1969.

21. Gabbiani, G., Hirschel, B.J., Ryan, G.B., Statkov, P.R., and Majno, G.: Granulation tissue as a contractile organ: A study of structure and function. J. Exp. Med., **135**:719, 1972.

22. Gabbiani, G., Ryan, G.B., and Majno, G.: Presence of modified fibroblasts in granulation tissue and their possible role in wound contraction. Experimentia, **27**:549, 1971.

23. Hirschel, B.J., Gabbiani, G., Ryan, G.B., and Majno, G.: Fibroblasts of granulation tissue: Immunofluorescent staining with anti-smooth muscle serum. Proc. Soc. Exp. Biol. Med., **138**:466, 1971.

24. Heuston, J.T., Hubble, B., and Rigg, B.R.: Homografts of the digital flexor tendon system. Aust. New Zeal. J. Surg., **36**:269, 1967.

25. Jackson, D.S., and Bentley, J.P.: On the significance of the extractable collagens. J. Biophys. Biochem. Cytol., **7**:37, 1960.

26. Keiser, H.R., and Sjoerdsma, A.: Studies on B-aminopropionitrile in patients with scleroderma. Clin. Pharm. Therap., **8**:593, 1967.

27. Lane, J.M., Bora, F.W., Prockop, D.J., Heppenstall, R.B., and Black, J.: Inhibition of scar formation by the proline analog cis-hydroxyproline. J. Surg. Res., **13**:135, 1972.

28. Leibovich, S.J., and Ross, R.: The role of the macrophage in wound repair. Am. J. Path., **78**:71, 1975.

29. Levenson, S.M., Geever, E.F., Crowley, I.V., Oates, J.F., Berard, C.W., and Rosen, H.: The healing of rat skin wounds. Ann. Surg., **161**:293, 1965.

30. Madden, J.W.: On "the contractile fibroblast." Plast. Reconstr. Surg., **52**:291, 1973.

31. Madden, J.W., Carlson, E.C., and Hines, J.: Presence of modified fibroblasts in ischemic contracture of intrinsic musculature of the hand. Surg. Gynec. Obstet., **140**:509, 1975.

32. Madden, J.W., Chvapil, M., Carlson, E., and Ryan, J.N.: Toxicity and metabolic effects of 3,4-dehydroproline in mice. J. Tox. Appl. Pharm., **26**:426, 1973.

33. Madden, J.W., Davis, W.M., Butler, C., II, and Peacock, E.E., Jr.: Experimental esophageal lye burns. 2. Correcting establishing strictures with beta-aminopropionitrile and bougienage. Ann. Surg., **178**:277, 1973.

34. Madden, J.W., Morton, D., Jr., and Peacock, E.E., Jr.: Contraction of experimental wounds. I. Inhibiting wound contraction by using a topical smooth muscle antagonist. Surgery, **76**:8, 1974.

35. Madden, J.W., and Peacock, E.E., Jr.: Studies on the biology of collagen during wound healing. I. Rate of collagen synthesis and deposition in cutaneous wounds of the rat. Surgery, **64**:288, 1968.

36. Madden, J.W., and Peacock, E.E., Jr.: Studies on the biology of collagen during wound healing. III. Dynamic metabolism of scar collagen and remodeling of dermal wounds. Ann. Surg., **174**:511, 1971.

37. Madden, J.W., Peacock, E.E., Jr., Boyer, J., and Parker, D.: Unpublished results, 1974.

38. Madden, J.W., and Smith, H.C.: Studies on the biology of collagen during wound healing. II. The rate of collagen synthesis and deposition in dehisced and resutured wounds. Surg. Gynec. Obstet., **130**:487, 1970.

39. Madden, J.W., and Stone, P.A.: Contraction of experimental wounds. IV. Effect of mechanical splinting on grafted wounds (in press).

40. Majno, G., Gabbiani, G., Hirschel, B.J., Ryan, G.B., and Statkov, P.R.: Contraction of granulation tissue in vitro: Similarity to smooth muscle. Science, **173**:548, 1971.

41. Mason, M.L., and Allen, H.S.: The rate of healing of tendons. Ann. Surg., **113**:424, 1941.

42. Peacock, E.E., Jr.: Restoration of finger flexion with homologous composite tissue tendon grafts. Am. Surg., **26**:564, 1960.

43. Peacock, E.E., Jr.: Fundamental aspects of wound healing relating to the restoration of gliding function after tendon repair. Surg. Gynec. Obstet., **119**:241, 1961.

44. Peacock, E.E., Jr.: Dynamic aspects of collagen biology. J. Surg. Res., **7**:433, 1967.

45. Peacock, E.E., Jr., and Madden, J.W.: Some studies on the effect of beta-aminoproprionitrile on collagen in healing wounds, Surgery, **60**:7, 1966.

46. Peacock, E.E., Jr., and Madden, J.W.: Human composite flexor tendon allografts. Ann. Surg. **166**:624, 1967.

47. Peacock, E.E., Jr., and Madden, J.W.: Some studies on the effects of beta-aminoproprionitrile in patients with injured flexor tendons. Surgery, **66**:215, 1969.

48. Peacock, E.E., Jr., Madden, J.W., and Trier, W.C.: Biologic basis for the treatment of keloids and hypertrophic scars. South. Med. J., **63**:755, 1970.

49. Ross, R.: The fibroblast and wound repair. Biol. Rev., **43**:51, 1968.

50. Ross, R., and Odland, G.: Fine structure observations in human skin wounds and fibrogenesis. *In* Dynphy, J.E., and Van Winkle, W. (eds.): Repair and Regeneration. New York, McGraw-Hill Book Co., 1969, p. 101.

51. Rovee, D.T., and Miller, C.A.: Epidermal role in the breaking strength of wounds, Arch. Surg., **96**:43, 1968.

52. Sawhney, C.P., and Monga, H.L.: Wound contraction in rabbits and the effectiveness of skin grafts in preventing it. Br. J. Plast. Surg., **23**:318, 1970.

53. Stone, P.A., and Madden, J.W.: Contraction of experimental wounds. II. The role of epithelialization (in press).

54. Stone, P.A., and Madden, J.W.: Contraction of experimental wounds. III. Effect of delayed vs. primary skin grafting (in press). [Cf. Surg. Forum **25**:41, 1974.]

55. Tanzer, M.L.: Experimental lathyrism. Int. Rev. Connect. Tissue Res., **3**:91, 1965.

56. Tanzer, M.L.: Cross-linking of collagen. Science, **180**:561, 1973.

57. Van Winkle, W., Jr.: Wound contraction. Surg. Gynec. Obstet., **125**:131, 1967.

11

Edema and bandaging

JAMES M. HUNTER and EVELYN J. MACKIN

Because it delays healing and causes pain and stiffness, thereby compromising functional results, the problem of edema should represent a constant challenge to concerned hand surgeons and hand therapists.

In the *normal* extremity mild edema of the hand may be produced in a few hours by immobilizing the upper extremity with the hand in a dependent position (sling). The addition of a dropped, unsplinted wrist and tight Ace bandage on the forearm can produce marked (balloonlike) swelling of the hand and fingers (Fig. 11-1). Edema produces bloating of the skin on the back of the hand, which results in flattening of the hand and loss of the longitudinal and transverse arches (Fig. 11-2).[2]

In the hand, afferent blood flow occurs on the volar surface controlled by arterial blood pressure. The major portion of the return blood flow takes place on the dorsal surface through the lymphatic and venous systems. The return systems require active movement of the hand to compress and produce retrograde venous and lymphatic flow by joint movement and compression of the fascial compartments. The dynamics of return flow are further augmented by motion of the elbow and shoulder.[7]

The picture of reduced dynamics becomes more alarming in chronic edema as soft tissues become fibrosed from foreign body tissue reaction. The greater the edema fluid and the longer it persists, the more extensive the scarring will be. All tissues—vessels, nerves, joints, and intrinsic muscles—become involved in a state of reduced nutrition and inelasticity. Although a certain amount of edema is reversible, fibrosis of moving tissue planes is not, and if edema is associated with injury and poor position, a "stiff" hand will result. *The prevention and treatment of edema are of paramount importance during all phases of management of the injured hand.*[2]

PREVENTION OF EDEMA

After severe injury the hand should be immobilized immediately in "the position of function"[4] and maintained in this position except for a few special exceptions. Postinjury dressings should be bulky and firm and evenly placed from fingertip to the upper forearm (Fig. 11-3). According to Boyes,[1] firm optimal pressure implies that the pressure has been applied with judgment and discrimination. The fingers should be separated. A splint should support the hand and wrist in the functional position, offering comfortable im-

mobilization. Volar or dorsal splints should be carefully padded to avoid pressure at bony prominences or over the dorsal venous system. The dressed, splinted hand should be elevated comfortably on pillows or in a canvas hand support. Cooling with ice bags will be helpful early if properly applied and arranged so that the weight of the bag is not carried on the hand. The initial dressing should remain undisturbed for the first 3 to 5 days, followed by débridement, daily open wound care, and skin grafting.[2]

The use of proteolytic enzymes given orally to reduce postoperative edema has not been effective in the controlled clinical situation. Hunter and Salisbury[3] studied 62 patients undergoing hand surgery who were given Orenzyme or a placebo in a double-blind study. No significant difference was noted in the postoperative course of edema or wound healing in the two groups.

Once established, edema should be approached with an active hand therapy program of supported elevation and supervised exercises, depending on the condition of the wound. The practice of making stab wounds or incisions over the dorsum of the hand to "drain the edema" is mentioned only to be condemned. Such techniques merely insult and open more tissue, provoking further inflammation and swelling.[2]

ASSESSMENT OF EDEMA

Observing changes in the amount of fluid in the patient's hand is of utmost importance in the management of edema. The volumeter* provides the hand therapist with a method to measure edema by submerging the patient's hand in a specifically designed water-filled container and measuring the water displacement (Fig. 11-4). Patients are assessed on their initial visit and checked routinely for changes in hand size from swelling and edema.

The concept of the volumeter to measure swelling by water displacement was designed by Dr. Paul Brand and Helen Wood, O.T.R., at the United States Public Health Service Hospital at Carville, Louisiana. The technique is as follows:

Purpose: To measure edema in the hand
Equipment needed
1. Plastic hand volumeter (Fig. 11-4, *A*)

---

*Volumeters Unlimited, 524 Double View Drive, P.O. Box 146, Idyllwild, Calif. 92349.

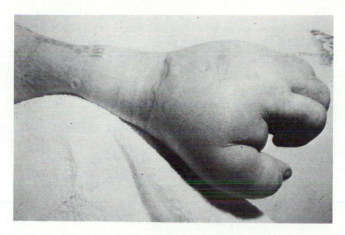

FIG. 11-1. "Balloon edema" of hand in 32-year-old man from chronic lymphatic and venous obstruction. This patient apparently, for purposes of secondary gain, methodically applied tight Ace bandage to midforearm over period of 3 to 4 months. Notice that healed incisions over dorsum of hand represent attempts to "drain edema."

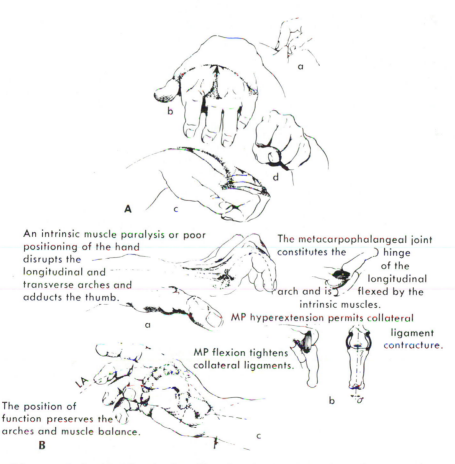

FIG. 11-2. A, *Edema* producing poor functional position, *b* and *c*, by obliterating soft tissue stretch on dorsum of hand. Functional use of hand, *d,* is in jeopardy. **B,** Loss of function of arches of hand by intrinsic paralysis, *a*. Contracture of relaxed collateral ligaments of joints produces fixed deformity. Objective of hand rehabilitation: a functioning hand, *c*. **A** from Littler, J.G.W.: In Converse, J.M.: Reconstructive plastic surgery, Philadelphia, 1977, W.B. Saunders Co.; **B** from Hunter, J.M.: Am. J. Surg. **92:**1427, 1956.

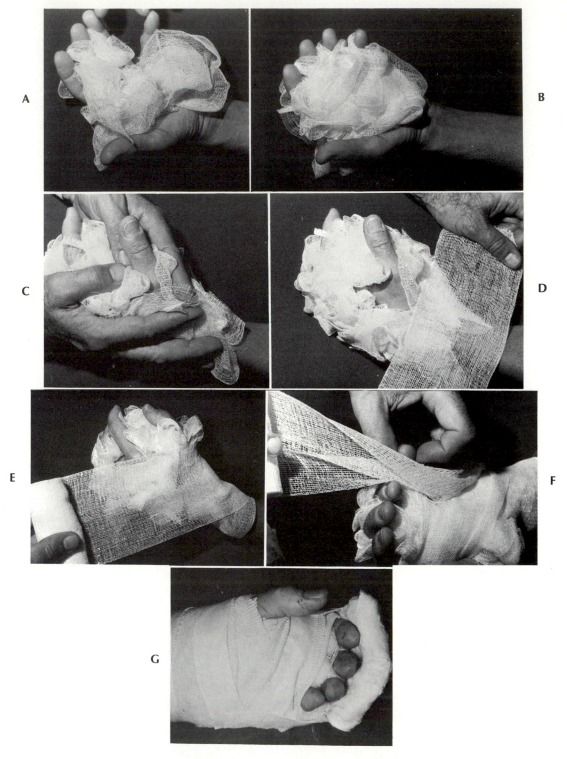

FIG. 11-3. Postinjury dressings. **A,** Light gauze fluffs pressed gently between fingers. **B,** Additional gauze fluffs placed in palm and thumb web. **C,** Fluffy gauze molded in palm and around thumb. **D,** Kling elastic gauze bandage (Johnson & Johnson, New Brunswick, N.J.) gently held in open position by ungloved hand. **E,** Bandage gently anchored at wrist and moved in oblique figure-of-eight manner throughout entire dressing. **F,** Bandage tension maintained by left hand as roll is flipped 180 degrees to compress bandage between each finger. **G,** Completed dressing should be comfortable, permitting light finger motion and unrestricted by splint or cast. Splint support for wrist is usually placed on dorsum.

FIG. 11-4. A, Plastic hand volumeter. All measurements are inside measurements. B, Patient is instructed to lower hand slowly so as not to spill water over rim of graduated cylinder. C, Hand should go down until stop dowel rests between web of middle and ring fingers.

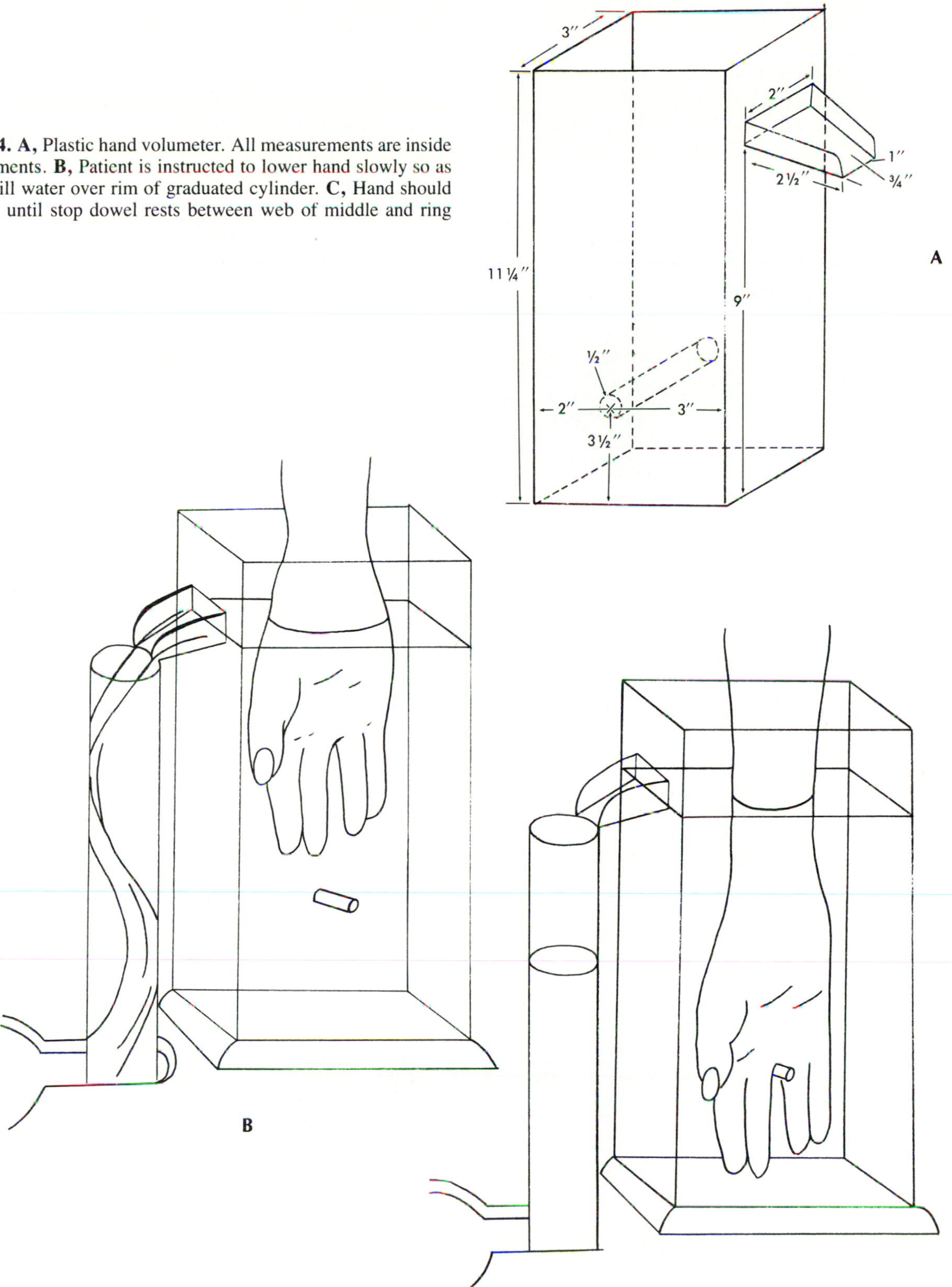

2. Graduated cylinder, 500 ml
3. Small bucket or container
4. Elevated wooden support for hand volumeter
5. Chair

Measurement procedure
1. The hand volumeter and graduated cylinder are properly positioned on the elevated wooden support, and water is poured into the hand volumeter from a small bucket or container until the water overflows and discontinues dripping into the graduated cylinder. Thoroughly empty the cylinder.
2. A chair is placed in a preset position at a height that easily allows the lowering of one third of the forearm into the plastic hand volumeter.
3. The patient is instructed to sit with the back well against the chair and the feet flat on the floor.

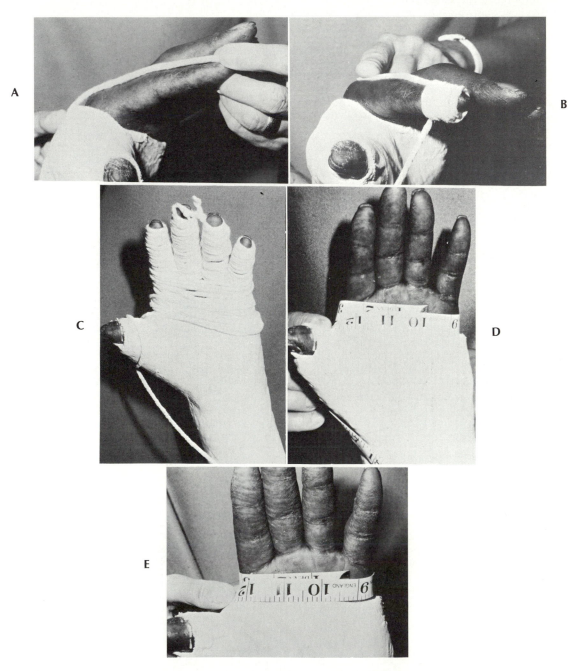

Fig. 11-5. **A,** String wrapping may be started while patient is in cast to begin early reduction of edema. **B,** Starting at distal end of index finger, cord is wrapped closely and firmly around finger. **C,** Patient's hand is placed in elevation. Cord remains on hand for 5 minutes. String wrapping is followed by active fist-making. **D** and **E,** Circumferential measurements taken before and after string wrapping indicate decrease in edema.

4. The hand is positioned with the palm in the anatomic position,* and the patient is instructed to lower the hand slowly so as not to spill water over the rim of the graduated cylinder (Fig. 11-4, *B*).

5. The hand should go down until the stop dowel rests between the web of the middle and ring fingers† (Fig. 11-4, *C*).

6. The hand is kept in this position until the water no longer flows from the spout.‡ The graduated cylinder is then removed and the patient is told to remove the hand from the water.§

7. Reading the water level in the graduated cylinder is accomplished on a flat surface that should be marked so that subsequent readings will always be taken at the same spot. Because of the water tension, it will appear that two lines are visible. Determine which line you will read and thereafter be consistent.

8. The chair is reversed and the same procedure is repeated for the opposite hand.

Another technique for measurement of edema is circumferential measurements of the hand and forearm. Measurements are taken with a tape measure before and after the treatment. To allow more valid comparison of sequential measurements, anatomic landmarks, such as the distal palmar crease or flexion crease, are used as reference points for placement of the tape.

TECHNIQUES FOR REDUCTION OF EDEMA

The therapist may use one or more of the following techniques in attempting to reduce edema and facilitate venous flow: (1) active motion, (2) elevation, (3) retrograde massage, (4) intermittent compression pump, (5) string wrapping, (6) surgical glove, and (7) Isotoner Glove.

Active motion

Active motion is effective in removing edema fluid because it assists return-flow circulation. Normal return-flow circulation is carried on to a large degree by muscle activity.[5] Fist making in elevation is encouraged when indicated. (Exceptions may be burns and infections.) Firm fist making pumps the hand and helps return flow circulation. Small wiggles or weak attempts at flexion will not do it. Active exercises should include full range of motion to the elbow and shoulder of the involved arm. The shoulder, elbow, and

hand of the uninvolved extremity should also be moved actively in a daily routine program.

For patients in a cast, reducing the edema and increasing the range of motion can be accomplished when the surgeon trims the cast so that maximum function is possible.

Elevation

For elevation to be effective, the distal part of the extremity must be above the proximal part, and the proximal part must be above the heart. This is sometimes difficult with the upper extremity. Elevation with the hand above the elbow and the elbow above the shoulder can be easily accomplished during the exercise program or at night in bed. Pillows may be used to elevate the arm and hand.[5] The patient should be informed about keeping the hand in as much elevation as possible during the day and not swinging it at his side. Patients should be informed as to what can happen if instructions are not followed. Circulation problems may be an exception if elevation causes ischemia of the extremity.

Retrograde massage

Probably the greatest single indication of massage is to overcome the swelling and induration that frequently occur after trauma. Retrograde massage asssits the return flow circulation of blood and lymph when the force of the massage stroke starts distally and progresses proximally. Therefore in the treatment of edema the stroke definitely should always be in a centripetal direction.[6]

Intermittent compression pump

An intermittent compression pump may be used to reduce edema. Intermittent mechanical compression is applied by a pneumatic sleeve that is inflated under pressure and then deflated. The pressure is applied for periods of 15 minutes to 2 hours. The intermittent pressure increases interstitial pressure, thereby driving lymphatic fluid back into the venous system.

Intermittent compression can be very beneficial in acute edema of after surgery or severe trauma. An edematous crushed hand may be placed in the arm pneumatic appliance as early as the first day after the trauma or surgery. The extremity is elevated on a table or pillows to an angle of 30 to 45 degrees to take advantage of the flow of gravity while the intermittent pressure is being applied.

The amount of pressure must be adjusted according to each patient's diagnosis and condition. Acute conditions, such as fractures, begin with a low amount of pressure and are supervised carefully by the therapist. Open wounds are not contraindicated so long as sterile dressings are used. Felt pads can be positioned around pins to prevent pressure on them.

The pressure at the initial treatment might be as low as 30 to 40 mm for 15 minutes. Time and pressure can be gradually increased when sufficient healing has occurred to allow the tissues to tolerate increased pressure.

After the mechanical massage by the intermittent compression unit, retrograde manual massage is applied by the therapist in a further attempt to push the extracellular fluid out of the hand.

---

*If the patient is unable to lower the hand into the hand volumeter in the anatomic position, he may reverse the position of the palm.

†If the patient has gross contractures or digits missing and cannot position the stop dowel on the web between the ring and middle fingers, a location between any finger will be acceptable if the test is done the same way at every reading.

‡If water continues to drip from the spout of the hand volumeter when the hand has reached the stop dowel, dry the spout thoroughly and spray a light coat of silicone on it.

§If it appears that a hand will measure more than 500 ml of water, have the patient stop lowering the hand in the hand volumeter before 500 ml is reached on the graduated cylinder. Raise the hand slightly and hold this position until the cylinder has been removed and the reading taken. Empty the water thoroughly and return the cylinder to its position. Instruct the patient to continue lowering the hand until the stop dowel is reached. Remove the cylinder and record the sum of the two readings. Each department should statistically analyze its own apparatus for error.

Some previously mentioned techniques may be initiated depending on the diagnosis, such as active fist making, gravitational exercises, and the Isotoner Glove. Ace bandaging of the entire extremity may be indicated.

String wrapping

An easy, inexpensive, and effective means to remove edema fluid is by string wrapping (Fig. 11-5, *A*). Soft cord may be used. Starting at the distal end of the index finger, the cord is wrapped closely and firmly around the finger (Fig. 11-5, *B*). It should be wrapped firmly enough to give good edema reduction. The string wrapping should progress distally to proximally until all the fingers and hand are wrapped proximally to the area of edema. The hand is then placed in elevation. The cord remains on the hand for 5 minutes (Fig. 11-5, *C*). When the cord is removed, the patient is instructed to make a fist 10 times. Most of the time the string wrapping produces the predicted results.

1. Circumferential measurements taken before (Fig. 11-5, *D*) and after (Fig. 11-5, *E*) the string wrapping indicate a decrease in edema.
2. The patient will find fist making easier.
3. Measurements taken of the patient's active range of motion will show an increase in active flexion of the finger pulp to the distal palmar crease.

The beneficial effects induced by the string wrapping may last only a short time at first. The treatment should be repeated three times a day for 5 minutes until return-flow circulation is restored adequately.

Use of surgical glove

The use of a surgical glove is another approach to the treatment of edema in the hand. The technique used at the Hand Rehabilitation Center in Philadelphia is one based on a paper written by Jan J. Perry, R.P.T., M.A.[8] She describes the treatment procedure as follows:

A simple readily available item that can be used to help reduce edema is a surgical glove. The glove is not used as a treatment in itself, but as an adjunct to other treatments such as massage, active exercise, or an intermittent compression unit.* The surgical glove is used to maintain the edema reduction obtained by other therapies and possibly to reduce edema even further. Surgical gloves are available in any hospital and come in a variety of sizes. A glove one or two sizes smaller than the patient would usually wear should be chosen. To make the glove easier to apply, either cornstarch or talcum powder can be put into the glove and a small hole made in the tip of each finger. The cornstarch or powder allows the glove to slip on the hand easily and it also absorbs perspiration. The hole in the tip eliminates air bubbles that may form at the fingertips of the glove. In putting on the glove, the patient may require assistance in eliminating wrinkles and getting his fingers all the way into the glove. After the glove is on, the patient can be given exercise or activities to do in an elevated position [Fig. 11-6]. Since the gloves are thin, sensitivity of the hand is not affected and the patient can carry out most activities. If edema continues to be a problem, a glove can be worn by the patient at home or at work. The patients at the Hand Rehabilitation Center have used these gloves with no problems or skin irritation. Since the glove is latex, however, the sweat produced on the hand cannot evap-

*Jobst, Box 653, Toledo, Ohio 43694.

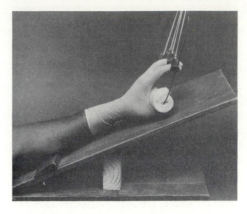

Fig. 11-6. Use of surgical glove with elevation and active exercise in decreasing edema. (From Perry, J.F.: Phys. Ther. **54:**498-499, 1974.)

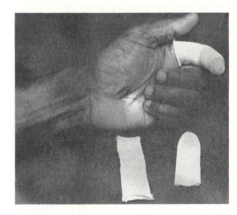

Fig. 11-7. Tubular gauze and single rubber glove finger for use in decreasing edema in single finger. Notice hole in tip of glove to eliminate formation of air bubble. (From Perry, J.F.: Phys. Ther. **54:**498-499, 1974.)

orate. To avoid maceration of the skin, the glove should be removed frequently and the hand allowed to dry thoroughly before the glove is reapplied.

Many patients have a problem with edema which involves only one or two fingers. Since an entire glove would be unnecessary for these patients, a finger of a glove can be cut off and the single finger applied to the patient's edematous finger. To avoid the problem of macerated skin, a piece of tubular gauze can be applied to the finger to serve as an absorbent layer between the skin and the latex glove [Fig. 11-7]. The gauze does not totally eliminate the need to remove the glove finger occasionally to allow the skin to dry. In applying the glove finger, a roll must not be allowed to form at the base of the finger, since the tourniquet effect caused by the roll would increase the problem of edema. As with a full glove, a small hole in the tip of the glove finger makes application easier.

The surgical glove or a finger of a surgical glove is a simple, readily available, and effective device to help decrease edema in the hand. Patients at the Hand Rehabilitation Center have used this without complications as an effective adjunct to other treatments.*

*Reprinted from *Physical Therapy* **54:**498-499, 1974, by permission of the American Physical Therapy Association.

Isotoner Glove

The Aris-Isotoner Glove* is another adjunctive measure that may be used in the treatment of edema. It is made of a washable blend of Antron-nylon-Lycra-Spandex. Inexpensive and readily available at department stores, the glove provides external compression to maintain the reduction of peripheral edema.

The patient wears the glove during his activities of daily living and through use of the glove will find hand discomfort minimized and hand function maximized most of the time.

USE OF PARAFFIN IN PRESENCE OF MILD EDEMA

It is generally believed that heat is contraindicated in edema; however, if the physiologic effects of heat and conforming pressure are desired and there are no open wounds, paraffin dips may be used if the edema is mild. Heat is transferred from the paraffin to the skin by conduction. G. Keith Stillwell[9] reported that by the addition of one part of light mineral oil to seven parts of paraffin, the melting point of the wax is lowered to about 52° C (125.6° F). Because its specific heat is only 0.5, the paraffin may be applied directly to the skin at this temperature if the circulation is normal. Patients with open wounds should never be given paraffin as a treatment. The advantage of paraffin is that it may be applied and then the extremity can be placed in elevation. The heat should be followed by massage with emphasis on distal to proximal stroking. Heat and massage should always be followed by active exercise.

Small paraffin baths such as the Therabath† are commercially available for home use. They are effective, safe, easy to use, and thermostatically controlled to hold the wax at a safe 126° to 130° F.

Patients unable to purchase a commercial unit may, with care, improvise a paraffin bath at home.

Materials required
Four pounds of paraffin
One cup of light mineral oil
Procedure
1. Place paraffin and light mineral oil in the top of a double boiler.
2. Heat slowly until the paraffin is completely melted.
3. Remove from heat and let the paraffin cool. *When a thin film forms on the top of the paraffin, it is a safe temperature for use (126° to 130° F). The temperature may be measured with a candy thermometer.*

*Aris-Isotoner Glove, Aris Gloves, Inc., 417 Fifth Avenue, New York, N.Y. 10016.
†Therabath, WR Medical Electronics Co., 19951 West County Rd. B-2, St. Paul, Minn. 55113.

4. Dip the hand quickly into the paraffin with the hand relaxed.
5. When the coat of paraffin hardens slightly, dip the hand again. Dip the hand about 12 times, until a layer of paraffin is built up.
6. Wrap the paraffin-covered hand with waxed paper and a towel.
7. Elevate the arm if the hand is swollen.
8. Exercise the fingers with the paraffin on.
9. When the paraffin has cooled (about 20 minutes), it may be removed and returned to the pan for reuse.
10. Treatment may be repeated twice a day.

SUMMARY

The prevention of edema is of vital importance in the care of the injured or surgical hand. Good early care should emphasize the principles of functional support dressing splints and elevation before surgery, atraumatic surgical techniques and skillfully applied postoperative dressings during surgery, and comfortable elevation and cooling with supervised early movement of uninjured parts after surgery. Once established, the assessment and application of techniques to reduce edema must be the prime concern of the surgeon and therapist in order to restore good hand function.

ACKNOWLEDGMENTS

Photographs by Earl Spangenberg, Audiovisual Department, Jefferson Medical College of Thomas Jefferson University, and Larry Kradle, Department of Orthopaedic Surgery, Jefferson Medical College of Thomas Jefferson University, Philadelphia, Pa.

REFERENCES

1. Boyes, J.H.: A philosophy of care of the injured hand, Bull. Am. Coll. Surgeons **50:**341, 1965.
2. Hunter, J.M.: Salvage of the burned hand, Surg. Clin. North Am. **47:**(5):1060-1061, 1967.
3. Hunter, J.M., and Salisbury, R.E.: Evaluation of oral trypsin-chymotrypsin for prevention of swelling after hand surgery, Plast. Reconstr. Surg. **49**(2):171-175, 1972.
4. Kanavel, A.B.: Infections of the hand, ed. 7, Philadelphia, 1943, Lea & Febiger.
5. Knapp, M.E.: Aftercare of fractures. In Krusen, F.H.: Handbook of physical medicine and rehabilitation, ed. 2, Philadelphia, 1971, W.B. Saunders Co., pp. 579-582.
6. Knapp, M.E.: Massage. In Krusen, F.H.: Handbook of physical medicine and rehabilitation, ed. 2, Philadelphia, 1971, W.B. Saunders Co., pp. 382-384.
7. Moberg, E.: Shoulder-hand finger syndrome, Surg. Clin. North Am. **40:**367, 1960.
8. Perry, J.F.: Use of a surgical glove in treatment of edema in the hand, J. Am. Phys. Ther. Assoc. **54**(5):498-499, 1974.
9. Stillwell, G.K.: Therapeutic heat and cold. In Krusen, F.H.: Handbook of physical medicine and rehabilitation, ed. 2, Philadelphia, 1971, W.B. Saunders Co., p. 264.

12

Management of the mutilated hand

ROBERT W. BEASLEY

The mutilated hand seems to present overwhelming problems, and it is easy to lose perspective and concentrate wrongly on the more dramatic but often more correctable aspects of the injury, such as long-bone fractures, rather than on the soft-tissue injuries. In no other situation is the dictum that primary care determines to a great extent the ultimate outcome more applicable. The principles of management are in fact the same for the mutilated hand as for less complex injuries.

As with other injuries of the hand the mandate is not to let the situation deteriorate through complications. Of the potential complications, stiffening of small joints, adhesions of tendons and gliding structures, and chronic pain problems are by far the most frequently encountered and, once established, often cannot satisfactorily be corrected secondarily.

PREVENTION OF SMALL JOINT STIFFENING AND TENDON ADHESIONS

The most important single long-term goal of management generally is to maintain mobility of the critical proximal interphalangeal joints. Stiffened metacarpophalangeal joints usually can be satisfactorily released, and the distal joints contribute so little to the digital flexion arc that their stiffening is not serious. Malaligned fractures usually can be secondarily corrected but rarely can the proximal interphalangeal joint fixed in acute flexion be relieved. So, much of the efforts of early treatment should focus on maintaining proximal interphalangeal joint mobility.

Small joint stiffening and also tendon adhesions develop rapidly when the three basic factors of edema, inflammation, and immobility are operating in a vicious cycle. Thus the approach to prevention is to deal with each of these as conditions allow.

EDEMA

The first step in minimizing edema is to check the dressings to be absolutely certain that they are not more tight proximally than distally, a condition that could cause obstruction to lymphatic and venous flow. The part should be elevated so that gravity can supplement proximal fluid movement and the point of reference for elevation is the right atrium of the heart. The hand in a sling at the waist is not elevated. It simply is less dependent than when it hangs at the side, whereas the hand placed anywhere over the trunk is elevated if the patient is reclining.

By far the most important factor in minimizing edema is to maintain as much *effective* muscle-pumping action as possible. With severe multilation the temptation to treat the dramatic roentgenograms should be resisted. The parts should be brought into the best possible alignment without additional tissue damage and splinted or internally stabilized with percutaneous pins so that active motion can be started promptly thereafter. The muscle activity must be vigorous to be effective in moving fluids. It is easily observed on one's own hand that wiggling the fingers does not empty the dorsal veins. Only with a tight fist is the skin blanched, veins and lymphatics are emptied, and fluids are propelled proximally.

Edema is obviously an inevitable part of the inflammatory reaction, but the steps just mentioned will go far to control it. Also, unless there are medical contraindications, the administration of systemic corticosteroids, initially in large doses, has proved to be very beneficial. This limits the inflammatory reaction, edema is less, pain is less, and active motion is greatly facilitated.

INFLAMMATION

Of the three factors leading rapidly to small-joint stiffening and tendon adhesions, inflammation is the most severe. Also it often requires the most time and is difficult to bring under control in the mutilated hand with extensive soft-tissue injuries. It is an unsuitable consequence of injury. As stated, corticosteroids minimize it and can be a helpful adjunct to treatment.

It is to minimize the inflammatory reaction that so much emphasis has appropriately been placed on the importance of primary wound healing. The premium factor in primary wound healing is adequacy of circulation. In fact, the only absolute emergencies in treating injuries of the hand are those cases in which there is vascular injury resulting in anoxia of otherwise salvageable parts. Obviously in such case immediate and definitive action to restore circulation is necessary, but with all other injuries there is time for organizing efforts, summoning experienced and skilled personnel, or even transferring the patient to a specialized unit if required to give optimal care. Initial care is critical to the ultimate outcome.

Infection is a disastrous complication of hand injuries and adequacy of circulation is of greatest importance to prevention of infection. Anoxic tissues are immunologically defenseless, and it is only a question of time before infection is established because contamination is always present. Infection is more a question of tissue vitality than wound contamination with rare and notable exceptions such as the human bite. Because hematoma is devitalized tissue and a most frequent cause of infections, meticulous attention to hemostasis and adequate drainage is of great importance. Foreign material like devitalized tissues is immunologically defenseless and careful débridement for removal of both is urgently required. Often immediately after injury one cannot judge the ultimate vitality of tissues, since those initially viable may subsequently be lost because of thrombosis. Therefore débridement may have to be done in several stages rather than being definitively accomplished as part of emergency care.

Primary wound healing may require tissue replacement for wound closure. This may be accomplished with skin grafts or may require application of a flap that provides not only full-thickness skin but also subcutaneous tissues. The simplest means of tissue replacement that meets the need is generally the best, and most often this will be split-thickness skin graft where the outer layer of skin is cut free and applied directly to the wound surface from which vessels grow into it to restore circulation essential to its survival. The more complicated flap procedures have the advantage that their circulation is maintained by vessels entering through their pedicle and is not even temporarily interrupted. Flaps are essentially indicated when the recipient wound bed is not suitable for rapid revascularization of a graft or when subcutaneous tissues and skin as well are required for repair.

IMMOBILIZATION

Early, active motion and reestablishment of effective muscular activity should be a constant goal in treating the multilated hand to minimize joint stiffening. Ideally this should be well along by a week after injury. As indicated, judicious use of anti-inflammatory medications (corticosteroids) can be enormously helpful toward this goal. It may be impossible to prevent tendon adhesions and joint stiffening when these parts have been directly injured, but understanding and determined efforts can greatly reduce these complications in minimally injured and uninjured parts.

Also experience bears out that the distressing late complications of dysesthesia, sympathetic dystrophies, and other chronic pain problems are rarely encountered among even badly injured patients whose injuries have been followed by primary wound healing and early active remobilization.

Roentgenograms of mutilated hands usually are dramatic and all too often cause one to focus unwisely on the fractures and lose perspective of the whole problem. In general fractures should be brought into reasonable alignment with special attention to rotational errors, but treatment requiring additional tissue damage such as open reduction or any procedure that will delay initiation of early motion should be avoided. Simple percutaneous pin fixation of fractures and dislocations greatly facilitates early active motion and causes no significant additional trauma.

As one gains experience in managing injuries of the hand, one comes to appreciate that it is the management of the soft-tissue injury that greatly determines the outcome of most hand injuries. Realization of this marks the maturity of the hand surgeon.

ROLE OF HAND THERAPY

Optimal care of the hand demands that surgical care be carefully coordinated in a single and continuous medical-surgical effort. It is absolutely wrong to look upon therapy as a separate and isolated effort independent of the surgical repairs as has generally been done in this country. Laboring under this traditional relationship with therapists but recognizing that early postoperative exercises and other therapy are essential for the best results of their surgical efforts, the most successful hand surgeons have for years endeavored to work personally with postoperative patients. However, it is being ever more clearly demonstrated that this essential role can be even better and more effectively filled by a therapist, provided that the therapist is given specialized training (just as the hand surgeon has specialized training) and works with the surgeon as an extension of the surgeon's effort to complete a unified team. It is essential that the surgeon and therapist work together, think alike through training and experience, understand clearly the goals and technical details of each effort, and communicate freely— all of which generally require daily contact. The potential benefits of coordinated medical-surgical care cannot be realized if the therapy unit is an isolated entity to which the patient is simply referred for postoperative care, regardless of the knowledge, experience, and qualifications of the therapist. A unified team working in a singular effort is essential.

13

Therapist's management of the mutilated hand

KAREN HULL PRENDERGAST

The functional result after a mutilating injury greatly depends on the postinjury management. This severe injury involves multiple-system trauma and always includes damage to the lymphovenous system. Wounds may be open or closed and may include any combination of fracture, joint disruption, nerve damage, tendon damage, or amputation of parts. Management is sequenced into three treatment phases dictated by biologic wound healing. Therapy management should begin within days after injury. This chapter addresses the time period when one can positively influence scar tissue remodeling and permanent fibrosis can still be averted.[27]

PRESERVATION PRIORITIES

Patient education is an essential component of management after a mutilating hand injury. The therapist is a teacher and guide who motivates the patient to take over responsibility for his progress. A written home program reinforces the idea that, in the end, it is the patient who must gain the recovery, not the therapist or the surgeon. The teaching plan includes a basic understanding of the structural anatomy of the hand, the injuries that exist, the inflammatory response, and the process of body repair. If the meaning of pain is discussed now, the patient will learn to sense the difference between the discomfort of mobilizing sore tissues and the burning perceived when tissue is dangerously abused. One will become recognized as acceptable discomfort, the other as a warning sign of impending tissue damage.

Edema control is essential in the early care of the mutilated hand (Fig. 13-1). A unique characteristic of a mutilating injury is massive pooling of edema promoted by the injury to lymphatics and veins. With inadequate drainage, arterial back pressure slows resolution of the inflammatory response. Massive deposition of collagen occurs—not isolated to the area of injury, but to the entire area of edema. Hence the more extensive the edema, the more extensive the area of potential disability. Edema control is a first priority in care.

Another priority is uncomplicated *wound closure*. The therapist and the patient must be aware of the signs of inflammation: edema, increased skin temperature, redness of surrounding tissues indicating vasodilatation, and wound drainage. The inflammatory exudate consists of fluids from the arterial vessels, destroyed blood cells, and bacteria. Inflammatory exudate does not necessarily mean that the

wound is infected; however, this can become the case. Under conditions where there is a decreased ability of a patient's blood cells to phagocytize bacteria, infection does become a threat. These conditions are an inadequate blood supply, high bacterial level or inadequate lymphovenous drainage, or all three. A bacterial level of 10^6 is defined as infection that can subsequently produce tissue necrosis.[28]

The therapist plays an essential role in wound care. After whirlpool therapy or during a dressing change, the therapist *debrides the extraneous tissue* on which harmful bacteria thrive. A whirlpool bath with antibacterial agents can *cleanse the wound*. The temperature should be adjusted so as not to further compromise the vascularity of the injured area that has a reduced arterial supply and depressed venous drainage. With the use of a skin-temperature probe, the area of coolest temperature is identified on the injured extremity and the water temperature is matched to protect the delicate vascular flow. This temperature is normally in the range of 86° to 94° F. After the whirlpool a *clean dressing* should be applied. The dressing should support and immobilize the delicate tissues, preventing further inflammatory response caused by friction from an insecure dressing.

All the joints and tissues in the area of the wound are subject to diffuse edema and fibrosis. If immobilization is necessary, the preferred position preserves the functional length of the tissues. The wrist is placed in 10 to 20 degrees of extension to balance the extrinsic tenodesis effect of the tendons. The thumb should be placed in full abduction to stretch the adductor pollicis muscle to prevent its contracture. If the metacarpophalangeal joints must be immobilized, 70 degrees of flexion would be optimal to take up redundancy of the collateral ligaments. When the slack is taken up, there is a limited amount of potential contracture possible. Most recently, Bowers[5] and associates recommended that the interphalangeal joints be placed at approximately 20 degrees of flexion to maintain the tautness of the collateral ligaments and the accessory collateral ligaments. If the hand must be immobilized, the arches must also be preserved. The volar splint approach would be recommended to mold and support both the transverse and longitudinal palmar arches. Wide diagonal straps are recommended to secure the splint.

The most effective way to preserve the anatomic structures is through active motion. Normal glide of the soft tissues and contraction of muscle maintains their excursion

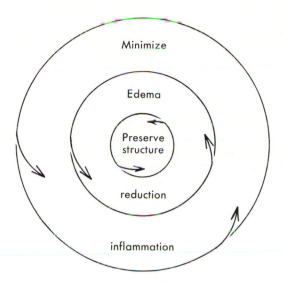

FIG. 13-1. Priorities in preservation of the structure within the mutilated hand.

and prevents adhesions. It preserves tissue nutrition, permits lymphovenous drainage, and reinforces the patient's personal management of the injury. The first approach to active mobilization of the severely traumatized hand is to begin with nonpainful joints. Start with shoulder elevation and rotational movements and then progress toward the injury to the elbow, forearm, and wrist. Exercise the extrinsic digital muscles last because their dynamic tendon excursion can cause soreness. Reinforce the patient's capabilities by incorporating a functional activity as a portion of the exercise regimen. Motions do not necessarily have to be painful to be effective. In this case pain is not gain. Keep in mind that any mobilization must be in accordance with the structural strength and stability of each injured part. Each digit and joint may have different capabilities and limitations, each requiring a specific regimen.

PHASE-ONE MANAGEMENT (1 TO 10 DAYS AFTER INJURY)

During the first treatment session, priorities are established according to absolute treatment necessity. Balance (1) the patient's energy and fatigue tolerance, (2) the time allotted for the treatment session, and (3) the physical environment. Treatment may take place at the hospital bedside or at an outpatient hand center. Each environment will have its own physical setup and conduciveness for the treatment session.

The initial therapy session is mostly educational. Discuss positioning the extremity for edema reduction and decreased pain. Hand elevation must be above the heart level. The higher the hand, the better. The venous pressure goes down the more the extremity is elevated in relation to the heart.[6] This should be demonstrated in both the sitting position and the supine. If the patient feels he must use an arm sling to permit him to move around adequately, proper wear should be discussed. The backstrap is diagonally positioned from the opposite shoulder across the scapula down to the elbow; the hand is positioned higher than the elbow on the chest.

This usually requires some alteration to the sling trough and the neck strap with safety pins or by a sewing machine. The hand itself should be supported within the trough of the sling; the wrist should not be dangling over the edge. Slings can be the reason for the typical shoulder adduction–internal rotation deformity that so often develops into a frozen shoulder, shoulder-hand syndrome, or cervical pain.

The patient should leave this initial session with a starter set of active exercises. Exercise level is also an important educational concept. There must be a strong enough muscular contraction to be effective though not done so overzealously as to create edema from an inflammatory response. Inflammation in response to this overuse stimulates macrophage migration, proliferation of fibroblasts, and therefore increased collagen deposition. The wound bed becomes more and more densely scarred.[6] The patient can learn to differentiate between expected soreness and tissue damage from overstress. The written exercise program should recommend the appropriate exercise level by time duration or number of repetitions.

During the initial therapy session, discuss the magnitude of the injury, both apparent and unseen. Explain the reason that the therapy will require sustained intensive effort. In communicating this in the first session, the therapist may avert the problem of the occasional patient who is lost to follow-up for lack of understanding of the severity of the injury. Now is the time to make the appropriate arrangements for transportation to the hand therapy center, for the financial commitment, and for child care during therapy sessions. Last, during the first therapy session the therapist should define the limitations that the patient has, if any, for activities of daily living and personal care. At times, the patient will believe that he can do more or do less than is truly possible.

Wound care is addressed in the first therapy session. Relaxed conversation during handling of the extremity may aid in promoting patient acceptance of the injury. This is also a forum for teaching techniques of bandaging for eventual patient takeover of wound-care duties. The first wound-care session may not be as lengthy as future sessions. This may be the patient's first visualization of the injury, and the response may be one of repulsion. Cold compresses and smelling salts are good to have available. The entire therapy session should not be taken up strictly with wound care; the time appropriation should reflect that the first priority in therapy is tissue preservation through elevation, exercise, and patient compliance.

First treatment session: checklist

☑ Elevation methods

☑ Patient responsibilities discussion

☑ One active shoulder-hand exercise

☑ Wound care

The acute phase includes the exudative stage of wound repair through initial fibroplasia. This would begin with the injury through approximately 10 days after the trauma. At this time the wound has very little strength. Only nonrepaired intact structures can be moved.

Especially within this first 10 days upper extremity elevation is primary. It is unrealistic to expect muscle contraction to bear the full burden of edema control. Gravity must be employed. Elevating the limb on a piece of furniture or on one's hand is perhaps one of the best and easiest methods of elevation.

If the joints are structurally stable as determined by the physician, active movement will preserve them and keep the joint surfaces lubricated. Splinting may be necessary to support or protect injured joints. Splints can be worn during rest periods between exercises or on a full-time basis, depending upon the surgeon's orders.

PHASE-TWO MANAGEMENT (10 DAYS TO 4 WEEKS AFTER INJURY)

The second management phase begins with early fibroplasia and lasts through the early remodeling stage of wound healing at approximately 4 weeks after injury. During this second phase, the fibroblasts deposit immature collagen into the entire wound bed. Toward the third week, this collagen synthesis will slow, but the process continues. At this time, the therapist and the patient may note that active motion may become more difficult as the complex of the wound becomes more densely packed with scar. If joint and tissue mobility is not accomplished, the stiff hand syndrome becomes more and more of a threat. Active exercise regimens are of prime importance.

Massage can improve circulation and elimination of waste products and can help restore elasticity to the skin. There are several types of massage that are beneficial to the severe mutilating hand injury. The first is graded *effleurage*. This is completed distally to proximally and should be done with the extremity in elevation. It is believed that evacuating the proximal part of the forearm first and then massaging to the distal structures aids in promoting an increased amount of drainage in the hand. Another variation is *effleurage for desensitization*. It is theorized that in completing this type of massage to hypersensitive tissues, there is an accommodation of the parts to the sensory input of the massage. It is believed that the disturbed sensory nerve endings when stimulated allow cortical reprogramming by the contact stimulus of the massage.[14] *Deep-friction massage* is believed to decrease the amount of edema surrounding the individual collagen fibers and therefore assist in favorable collagen remodeling.

Amputation sites are often immobile, edematous, and uncomfortable. Stump wrapping with elastic tape reduces the volume while shaping the site to prevent "dog ears." The tape requires practice to apply properly. The wrap should apply more pressure distally than proximally.

Joint mobilization is a skill that necessitates special care with mutilating injuries. Gentle grades of oscillation can help to mobilize stiff joints. The knowledgable hand therapist will know how to keep stress to a minimum to prevent further inflammation. In view of the delicacy of the lymphovenous system, hand placement to stabilize effectively the proximal and distal bones during mobilization is difficult. It is easy to block circulatory flow while gliding the joint. This is one form of therapy that should be reserved for those that are well trained in hand joint mobilization.

Therapeutic modalities

The modalities discussed below are appropriate to initiate during phase-two management and can be continued in phase-three management.

Therapeutic heat. Therapeutic heat is perhaps the most comfortable preexercise modality. The 10- to 20-minute application causes a local temperature increase. Metabolism increases with simultaneous arterial vasodilatation. This increased local circulatory flow speeds all processes, including phagocytosis, infiltration of leukocytes, antibodies, and flushing of metabolites or waste products from the wound area. There is also an increase of nutrients and oxygen delivery.[19]

Hot packs provide moist, high heat conducted directly to skin surfaces. They have the advantage of being able to be given with the extremity in elevation. There are contraindications, however, because the high heat will cause tissue necrosis and blistering if left over any prominence or area with insufficient subcutaneous covering. Any compromise of the peripheral circulation would be a contraindication to a hot-pack treatment. Insensible digits are not capable of interpreting tissue distress and therefore are extremely prone to tissue necrosis and blistering in response to the high heat. In the mutilated hand the hot pack is often given to a sore shoulder or forearm that is in spasm rather than to the injured hand itself.

A *paraffin bath* is another heat modality that can be useful. After submersion the hand can be elevated if edema is a problem. Joints can be positioned on a stretch to provide maximum benefit of the heat modality on contracting structures.[31] The oil in the wax provides lubrication to dry skin and improves tissue elasticity. Paraffin contours and heats all surfaces exposed so that one can obtain an even heating effect. There are disadvantages. This high heat of approximately 126° F can cause tissue damage as seen with the hot pack, especially in the face of vascular compromise. High heat can be noxious to patients with sensory disturbances, especially those patients with impending reflex dystrophy problems or regenerating sensory nerves. The paraffin bath cannot, of course, be used with patients who have open wounds or any skin condition that might be contagious or irritating to other patients. Exposed internal hardware such as Kirschner wires should not be immersed in the paraffin bath because of potential contamination. For these reasons many patients with mutilating injuries should not be immersed in the paraffin bath.

The *whirlpool bath* can be a modality of heat or neutrality because the temperature is readily adjustable. One can thus avoid compromising the vascularity of an injured part or damaging insensitive areas with extremes of heat or cold. The turbulence of the whirlpool bath creates a micromassage to the tissues by loosening extraneous matter and tissue and thus making débridement relatively easy. A clean whirlpool bath to a small area of open wound is believed to decrease the local bacterial count through the use of additives like chlorine.[3,25] A clean whirlpool bath without a disinfectant has not been shown through research to reduce the bacterial count in humans; therefore it is recommended that a disinfectant be used. The buoyancy of the water allows the patient to exercise the extremity easily during treatment. This is a nice advantage of the whirlpool bath over such heat modalities as the hot pack or paraffin bath.

The whirlpool bath also has a disadvantage: the extremity is dependent during the whirlpool treatment, and that position permits pooling of edema. I recommend that if a whirlpool treatment is utilized, it should be followed by a therapeutic exercise program completed in elevation to evacuate whatever extra edema might have accumulated during the whirlpool bath.

Fluidotherapy is a new form of therapeutic heat. High heat is delivered within a tank of particulate matter. It has been reported that the fluidotherapy can deliver an increased heat transfer to the tissues superior to a paraffin bath or therapeutic whirlpool bath.[4] In addition to the transfer of high heat by the fluidized solid particles, there is also a uniformity of temperature distribution within the tank. The limb can be in elevation and the patient can be completing active exercise during the treatment.

Microwave, diathermy, and infrared are ways of delivering local superficial dry heat. The area of application in the hand is small with many bony prominences. The structure of the hand makes delivery of radiant heat technically difficult. Alternate forms of therapeutic heat are therefore recommended.

Therapeutic cold. A 5-minute exposure to therapeutic cold has the local effect of vasoconstriction because of an increased muscle tone within the arteriole walls. This slows the metabolic processes in the area, including the response of the muscle spindles to stretch. There is a decrease in tone of large muscles. Cold may temporarily suppress the inflammatory response and therefore quiet a "hot" area. Another local effect of therapeutic cold is that of pain suppression. The cold is believed to elevate the pain threshold of the sensory nerve receptors, thereby decreasing the perceived pain.

Direct application of an *ice pack* for 5 minutes is one method of application. This 5-minute interval is normally all that a patient will tolerate and is sufficient time for vasoconstriction to occur. The other method of therapeutic cold is a *whirlpool bath* adjusted to a temperature below the skin temperature of the area. This will provide a relative cooling effect to the local tissues. In this case the whirlpool bath would be taken for a 10- to 20-minute period.

Therapeutic cold can be a good choice of modality for the patient with the mutilating hand injury. Guarding can be a problem with pain and muscle spasm in the proximal and distal parts of the extremity. Patients may prefer the effect of therapeutic cold to heat for the purpose of decreasing muscular spasm. Cold also helps to prevent edema pooling, which can be a problem with the vasodilatation created during or after a heat modality. On the other hand, patients may find the cold intolerable. Extremes of cold exposure result in the same consequences as those of overexposure to heat. Contraindications then would include any kind of

severe vascular difficulty that could allow the patient either not to preceive tissue damage or to have insufficient blood flow to withstand the stress on the distal circulation.[19]

Therapeutic ultrasound. Therapeutic ultrasound is a mode of treatment that has been used for many years in rehabilitation centers. There have been many claims as to the beneficial effects of ultrasound; however, the research has at best been confusing. The instruments found in the United States have a frequency of 1 megahertz (MHz) and are used in the intensity range of 0.5 to 1.5 watts per square centimeter (W/cm^2) for an approximate duration of treatment of about 5 minutes.[12] As a result of absorption, transmission, reflection, and refraction, physiologic effects both thermal and nonthermal are produced within the superficial layers of the extremity receiving treatment. The intensity, frequency, and duration of application affect these tissue responses. Thermal effects have been well documented in the literature at therapeutic dosages.[26]

Respected authors have tried to make an association between therapeutic ultrasound and its effect on wound healing. The majority of these research projects have been done on experimental models using rats as subjects. These experiments have also been conducted outside the range of therapeutic dosages. In the last reports by Dyson, the frequency used for the experiments was that of 2 to 2.5 MHz.[8-10] Other studies have tried to show a stimulation of protein synthesis as a result of ultrasound treatment. These studies have been in vitro, and one can only speculate on the effect of ultrasound in therapeutic dosages in vivo.[15] Shamberger and others[30] have stated that there are as yet no data to conclude that ultrasound stimulates wound healing.

A nonthermal effect of ultrasound is that of cavitation. This has been reported as justification for ultrasound treatments applied to scar tissue. Complete cavitation does not occur at a frequency of 1 MHz below an intensity of 4 W/cm^2 because there is little opportunity for the charge to build on the surface of the gas-filled cavities between the rarefaction phase and compression phase.[20] Therefore at therapeutic doses the cavitation effect of breaking of the scar tissue cannot be accomplished.

Another nonthermal effect of therapeutic ultrasound is that of increased membrane permeability.[22] This is independent of the temperature increase and is most useful in the therapeutic deliverance of medications with the ultrasound. This method of medicating is called *phonophoresis*. A threefold increase in cortisol levels in pig muscle tissue was reported when cortisol was driven into the tissues by ultrasound.[13] In 1975, Kleinkort and Wood reported that phonophoresis with a 1% solution of hydrocortisone was not so effective as using a 10% solution.[18] The 5% to 10% hydrocortisone solution in a petrolatum base is formulated by a pharmacist given a written prescription. This cream is applied directly to the skin surface. The medication is driven into the tissue in the usual manner with the ultrasound coupling medium applied on top of the cream. Either pulsed ultrasound using a stationary method of application or continuous ultrasound moving the soundhead is applied to the local area for approximately 5 minutes at an intensity of approximately 1 W/cm^2. This application method, of course, is modified by the extent of the surface area to be covered.

In the treatment of the mutilated hand, phonophoresis is not used on the wound area. However, its use on proximal inflamed joints is not contraindicated.

Electrostimulation. The use of therapeutic electrostimulation to innervated tissue can be an excellent adjunct to the management of this injury. For *innervated muscle* one can use either alternating current stimulation or high-voltage galvanic stimulation. It appears that one can achieve edema reduction by the use of this modality with an application of about 10 to 20 minutes. The pad electrodes are sandwiched about the edematous part, and the current is interrupted just enough to provide a rhythmic muscular contraction and relaxation about the area. The intensity of the contraction would be increased to the patient's tolerance. It is helpful to position the part in elevation during treatment. A distinct advantage of high-voltage galvanic stimulation is the ability to render the treatment under water. This method is of tremendous benefit to the patient with any kind of venous obstruction or if the part is very tender and painful because there is no need to strap down the electrodes.[24]

Mutilating injuries can induce muscle spasms and co-contraction. Electrostimulation to muscle tissue provides an awareness of relaxation and contraction phases of both the agonist and antagonist muscle groups. The electrostimulation initiates the contraction and can be an active assistive exercise when electrodes are placed on the agonist muscle belly and its tendon insertion. The agonist-antagonist relationship is gained when two sets of electrodes are used and their stimulation is reciprocated. A long-duration active assistive exercise session can be created. Ten minutes of low-intensity to tetanic contractions can usually provide the patient with a good workout. Any tissue that is not considered structurally strong enough to withstand active exercise, such as unstable fractures or early repaired tendons, would not be suitable for this form of therapy.

Research has shown that muscle atrophy cannot be prevented by direct-current stimulation, although muscle contraction does improve local exchange of nutrients and evacuation of waste products.[11]

Iontophoresis. During the application of direct current from one electrode pole to the other, positive ions flow toward the negative pole and negative ions toward the positive. Medications can be transported into the superficial layers of the skin along the lines of the electrical circuit toward the unlike-charged electrode. Iontophoresis can be an alternative to an injection or oral medication. This can be a nice mode of delivering a noninvasive medication about a joint capsule using a circumferential copper electrode. As with phonophoresis, this type of treatment requires frequent doses of at least three times a week to have a beneficial effect. Medicating by ion transfer or phonophoresis requires a physician's prescription and is rendered specific to problems encountered with the injury. Lists of chemicals used for iontophoresis and their concentrations are readily available.[17]

PHASE-THREE MANAGEMENT (4 TO 8 WEEKS AFTER INJURY)

Between 4 and 8 weeks after injury, remodeling of collagen is the dominant activity within the wound tissue. During the second month after injury the rate of collagen synthesis remains elevated. Simultaneously, strong covalent bonds are forming between the collagen fibers, rendering the structures strong but the adhesions unyielding. Some also believe that abnormal bonds are forming between polypeptide chains, causing inelasticity of tissue.[7] Equal amounts of collagen buildup and breakdown occur at a rapid rate during this phase. This rapid exchange makes it possible to influence the scar tissue to yield in a short period of time. It is hoped that with remodeling, full active joint range of motion and tendon glide may be achieved despite the expected scarring. Resisted muscular contraction with resisted tendon glide through the full excursion is the most beneficial exercise for functional collagen remodeling.[1]

Judgmental decisions as to progress will now depend on an objective picture of the patient's status. Base your decisions on the five following factors:

1. Volumetrics. This may be the first opportunity to do this evaluation because the wounds may have just closed or the Kirschner wires may have just been removed.
2. Goniometry. Total active motion (TAM) and total passive motion (TPM) should be used because the total arc of motion will indicate the state of the musculotendinous units in terms of adherence. Joint capsule problems will become apparent when one notices the difference between the TAM and the TPM.
3. Sensibility. Nerves are beginning to regenerate. Neurapraxias may now be resolving. Neuromas may be forming, and the first sign of dysesthesia can be evidenced. Sensory reeducation may be in order for this patient. Sensory testing will allow documentation of nerve recovery, and subtle disturbances can be detected by use of the Semmes-Weinstein monofilament test. Tinel signs help monitor nerve regeneration.
4. Reflex sympathetic dystrophy always being a threat with mutilating injuries. Our best defense against this problem thus far is early active movement and desensitization therapy. Aberrations in sudomotor function can be seen with a ninhydrin sweat test. This quick test using a qualitative filter paper and Ninsol spray gives objective proof of a disturbance or deficit in hydrosis.
5. Pain monitoring. At 1 month after injury various forms of depression may become apparent either subtly or in more glaring ways. Chronic pain cycles can take seed at this time. Visual analog scales are useful in showing progress and have proved to be reliable.[29] The patient indicates a point on a 10 cm line, one end representing the worst pain perceivable and one end representing no pain at all. One scale is used for pain intensity and a separate one for unpleasantness. The therapist uses new pain lines each visit and expresses pain on a scale of 1 to 10. Most patients genuinely desiring to recover will show an improvement, if only better coping behavior. Those patients that do not improve bear further investigation as candidates for sur-

gical intervention, psychologic counseling, or anti-depressive therapy or for litigation motives.

A work summary and history helps the therapist to assess if a patient "needs the injury." Sleep disturbances, medications taken, and dietary habits are cues to established problems.

An effective way of combating pain and depression is to begin a program of proper body conditioning such as walking or calisthenics. Nutrition should also be discussed because the patient's habits have been altered by the injury and now sedentary life-style.[2]

During the third management phase of treatment, the main thrust is directed toward strong resistive exercises to those parts that are determined to be structurally strong. All active and passive modes of therapy that have been of benefit in the second therapeutic phase should be carried over into the third phase. Written home-exercise programs should be upgraded frequently.

Graded-resistance exercise through a wide tendon excursion should be assigned. Begin gently "walking" the digits along a towel or picking up wood or stringing beads. Progress to more resistive putty molding and later upgrade the exercises to elastic resistance provided by a digital hand grip, commercially known as a Hand Helper.* Full upper extremity motions can be accomplished by the use of proprioceptive neuromuscular facilitation patterns. Diagonal patterns can be completed as home resistive exercise using a cuff weight strapped around the patient's wrist. The Delorme method of resisted power building is especially effective for building the forearm and wrist muscles. Dumbbell weights are beneficial if the patient can grasp. A wrist that is strong in extension is not only stable for function but also has improved grasp power. Progressive resistive exercises quickly restore the strength of the extensor carpi radialis brevis.[21]

Resistance can also be applied through *leisure* or *work activities*. The therapist can try to match the resistive activity with the patient's own likes and aptitudes by testing with the Leisure Activities Blank.[23] Two of the most practical and space-efficient resistive activities for the patient with a mutilating injury are *macramé* and *clay wedging*. If the patient has some form of prehension macramé can usually be worked. Knotting can be completed in an elevated position, which incorporates the patient's back and shoulders into the exercise. One should do clay wedging standing with a large wad of clay. It is a bilateral exercise and is effective in desensitizing the injured extremity. This activity is sloppy but can be creative for even the nonartistic patient. Woodworking, hammering, and leather tooling are sometimes too jarring to hypersensitive hands. If the patient has a strong interest in this type of activity, tool handles can be widened to grasp size and cushioned from impact.

At this time, the patient may be ready for some insightful questioning to determine his or her capacity to return to the original occupation. If the patient has a closed wound and the tissues are strong and structurally stable, endurance training is appropriate. Work simulation can either determine the feasibility of the patient's return to his occupation,

test his readiness, or build work tolerance. In those with severe loss of effective prehension, train to switch hand dominance.

Skill at personal care and activities of daily living are evaluated. In some patients with permanent disability, plans are drawn to adapt the home for safety, especially in the kitchen and bath. A steering-wheel knob is a consideration for some.

Some patients will find that this is a good time to enroll in classes to become proficient in a language, finish high school or college diplomas, or take a course for diversion. Others find this to be a time to have a discussion with an employer to see the possibility of adapting to a new job within the company. On some level, this third phase is an appropriate time for thoughts of the future.[16]

SUMMARY

The mutilating injury is a multifaceted management challenge. Injury to the lymphovenous system exacerbates the extent of the injury, and tissue fibrosis is the rule. Management is divided into three phases. The first-phase priority is tissue preservation through patient understanding, edema control, wound care, and active exercise. During the second phase, more aggressive active modes of treatment are introduced, including activities of daily living. Passive adjuncts such as therapeutic heat, cold, and electrostimulation are also added and when chosen wisely can be safe and effective in realizing treatment goals. During the third phase, vigorous resisted isotonic exercises and activities complement the passive modes of therapy. Detailed objective evaluation is an invaluable indicator of treatment effectiveness. Frequent modifications are necessary to allow the patient's hand to reach its full potential.

Each tissue and joint complex is evaluated for structural strength. Those deemed stable by the physician must be actively moved to preserve nutrition and full working length. Stable structures progress through the management phases as described, while unstable structures are immobilized to heal. The latter tissues join in the management sequence once they have been declared safe to move. Any delay in timely mobilization results in an automatic compromise in the functional potential of the mutilated hand. With full aggressive treatment it is possible to achieve as much function as the initial injury will allow.

REFERENCES

1. Arem, A.J., and Madden, J.W.: Effects of stress on human wounds. I. Intermittent noncyclical tension, J. Surg. Res. **20**:93, 1976.
2. Blumer, D., and Heilbronn, M.: Chronic pain as a variant of depression disease: the pain-prone disorder, J. Nerv. Ment. Dis. **170**:381, 1982.
3. Bohannon, R.W.: Whirlpool versus whirlpool and rinse for removal of bacteria from a venous stasis ulcer, Phys. Ther. **62**(3):304-308, 1982.
4. Borrell, R.M., Henley, E.J., Ho, P., et al.: Fluidotherapy: evaluation of a new heat modality, Arch. Phys. Med. Rehabil. **58**:69-71, 1977.
5. Bowers, W.H., Wolf, J.W., Jr., Nehil, J.L., and Bittinger, S.: The proximal interphalangeal joint volar plate. I. An anatomical and biomechanical study, J. Hand Surg. **5**(1):79-88, 1980.
6. Diegelmann, R.F., Cohen, I.K., and Kaplan, A.M.: Effect of macrophages on fibroblast DNA synthesis and proliferation, Proc. Soc. Exp. Biol. Med. **169**:445-451, 1982.
7. Donatelli, R., and Owens-Burkhardt, H.: Effects of immobilization

*Hand Helper, Medex Corp., P.O. Box 1352, Los Altos, Calif. 94022.

on the extensibility of periarticular connective tissue, J. Orthop. Sports Phys. Ther. **3**(2):67-72, 1981.

8. Dyson, M., and Pond, J.D.: The effect of pulse ultrasound on tissue regeneration, Physiotherapy **56**:136-142, 1970.

9. Dyson, M., and Suckling, J.: Stimulation of tissue repair by ultrasound: a survey of the mechanisms involved, Physiotherapy **64**(4):105-108, 1978.

10. Dyson, M., Pond, J.B., Joseph, J., et al.: The stimulation of tissue regeneration by means of ultrasound, Clin. Sci. **35**:273-285, 1968.

11. Fulford, G.E.: The treatment of severe upper limb paralysis: a general review, Physiotherapy **56**:282-288, 1970.

12. Griffin, J.E., and Karselis, P.: Physiological agents for physical therapists, Springfield, Il, 1978, Charles C Thomas, Publisher.

13. Griffin, J.E., and Touchstone, J.C.: The effects of ultrasonic frequency on phonophoresis of cortisol swine tissues, Phys. Ther. **51**(2):62-78, 1972.

14. Hardy, M.A., Moran, C.A., and Merritt, W.H.: Desensitization of the traumatized hand, Va. Med. **109**:134-137, 1982.

15. Harvey, W., Dyson, M., Pond, J.B., and Grahame, R.: The *in vitro* stimulation of protein synthesis in human fibroblasts by therapeutic levels of ultrasound, Proceedings of the second European Congress on Ultrasonics, May 1975.

16. Holland, J.L.: Making vocational choices: a theory of careers, Englewood Cliffs, NJ, 1973, Prentice-Hall, Inc.

17. Kahn, J.: Low volt technique, Syosset, NY, 1973, Joseph Kahn.

18. Kleinkort, J.A., and Wood, F.: Phonophoresis with one percent versus ten percent hydrocortisone, Phys. Ther. **55**(12):1320-1324, 1975.

19. Lehman, J.F., editor: Therapeutic heat and cold, Baltimore, 1982, The Williams & Wilkins Co.

20. Lehman, J., and Herrick, J.: Biological reactions to cavitations: a consideration for ultrasonic therapy, Arch. Phys. Med. Rehab. **34**:86-94, 1953.

21. Licht, S., editor: Therapeutic exercise, Baltimore, 1965, Waverly Press.

22. Lota, J., and Darling, R.: Changes in permeability of the red blood flow membranes in a homogenous ultrasonic field, Arch. Phys. Med. Rehabil. **36**:282, 1955.

23. McKechnie, J.E.: Leisure Activities Blank, Palo Alto, Calif., 1974, Consulting Psychologists Press, Inc.

24. Newton, R.: Personal communications, Richmond, Va., 1983.

25. Nieder, H., Stephanies, B.S., Stribley, R.F., and Koepke, J.H.: Reduction of skin bacterial load with use of the therapeutic whirlpool, Phys. Ther. **55**(5):482-486, 1975.

26. Payton, O., Lamb, R., and Kasey, M.: Effects of therapeutic ultrasound on bone marrow in dogs, Am. J. Phys. Ther. Assoc. **55**:20-27, 1975.

27. Peacock, E., and VanWinkle: Wound repair, Philadelphia, 1976, W.B. Saunders Co.

28. Robson, N.C.: Infection in the surgical patient: an imbalance in the normal equilibrium, Clin. Plast. Surg. **6**(4):493-503, 1979.

29. Scott, J., and Huskisson, E.: Visual pain analogue, Pain **2**:175-184, 1976.

30. Shamberger, R.C., Talbot, T.L., Tipton, H.W., et al.: The effect of ultrasonics and thermal treatment on wounds, Plast. Reconstr. Surg. **68**(6):860-870, 1981.

31. Warren, G.C., Leahmann, J.F., and Koblanski, J.N.: Heat and sweat procedures: an evaluation using rat tail tendons, Arch. Phys. Med. Rehabil. **57**:122-126, 1976.

IV
FRACTURES

14

Fractures and traumatic conditions of the wrist

GARY K. FRYKMAN and ELVERT F. NELSON

The wrist is a complex joint with 21 separate articulations and a network of ligaments. This unique joint complex produces flexion and extension, radial and ulnar deviation, and axial rotation. Powerful proximal forearm muscles are transmitted across this joint to move finger joints delicately and place the hand in an almost infinite number of spatial orientations. Nowhere else in the body are so many tendons, nerves, and vessels confined to such a concentrated area. A fall on the outstretched hand is so common that a large variety of wrist injuries can occur. A great deal of force must be absorbed by a very limited area, making the wrist vulnerable to injury. The frequency of wrist injuries, the variety of injury mechanisms, and confusing multiple roentgenographic patterns make exact diagnosis of traumatic wrist injuries sometimes difficult even for the experienced clinician.

Unlike many other conditions a careful history and physical examination on a patient with a wrist injury is not always helpful to the clinician attempting to make a diagnosis. Frequently the history is vague and incomplete and the physical examination may show diffuse swelling, generalized tenderness, and variable limitations in wrist motion. Deformity, shortening of the wrist, and point tenderness make the diagnosis easier. Usually one must rely primarily upon roentgenograms to make the exact diagnosis. Familiarity with normal bony anatomy and carpal alignment is essential if one expects to identify subtle malalignment and fractures with superimposed images (Figs. 14-1 and 14-2). The diagnosis of a wrist sprain must be made with extreme caution. When the wrist has sustained a significant injury, it must be treated as such in spite of normal roentgenograms. When serial clinical and roentgenographic follow-up has failed to demonstrate any serious condition, the wrist can be treated symptomatically.

It is helpful to be acquainted with the possible traumatic wrist conditions and the frequency of their occurrence. Large series of carpal injuries show the following breakdown: 60% to 70% scaphoid fractures, 10% carpal dislocations and fracture dislocations (traumatic carpal instability), 10% dorsal chip fractures, 3% lunate fractures, and 7% all other carpal fractures.[36]

PREVENTION OF COMPLICATIONS

A great deal can be done to prevent or minimize complications after wrist injuries. An accurate early diagnosis with adequate reduction and immobilization not only minimizes discomfort but also decreases swelling. Edema can be decreased by early cooling and elevation of the injured extremity. A well-molded cast avoiding the extreme positions, such as the cotton-loader position of palmar flexion, will help diminish compression of the median nerve in the carpal tunnel. Early active finger motion must be started. It is essential that the form of immobilization used allows full metacarpophalangeal flexion of the fingers (Fig. 14-3 and 14-4). The problem of neural or vascular compromise early in the course of injury can be avoided by use of a sugar-tong cast. When reduction is lost in comminuted or unstable distal radius fractures, prompt application of a self-contained traction apparatus will not only anatomically reduce the fracture but also allow unrestricted finger and thumb motion. Frequent follow-up and serial roentgenograms with remanipulation or operative intervention when indicated will minimize malunion and possible carpal instability.

Stiffness of the shoulder, elbow, and hand can usually be averted by proper education and avoidance of a sling. Although a sling has traditionally been used for patients with traumatic wrist conditions, it discourages movement of the entire extremity. The shoulder-hand-finger syndrome is believed to develop because of inadequate muscular activity with subsequent venous stasis.[33] It is the responsibility of the physician to educate the injured patient in frequent, regular active range-of-motion exercises to all the nonimmobilized joints in the upper extremity from the shoulder to the fingers. From the beginning the patient is taught to place his hand over his head at least 50 times a day and perform active range of motion of the fingers a thousand times a day. When watching television, he is told to move his fingers at least 10 times with each commercial. This kind of exaggeration will get the point across that we are serious about keeping the free joints moving actively and keeping the injured upper extremity elevated.

DISTAL RADIUS FRACTURES
Colles' fracture

The distal radius fracture is one of the most common fractures of the human skeleton. It was originally accurately described by an Irish surgeon, Abraham Colles, as a nonarticular fracture occurring 1½ inches proximally to the radiocarpal joint.[11] The eponym ''Colles' fracture'' is gen-

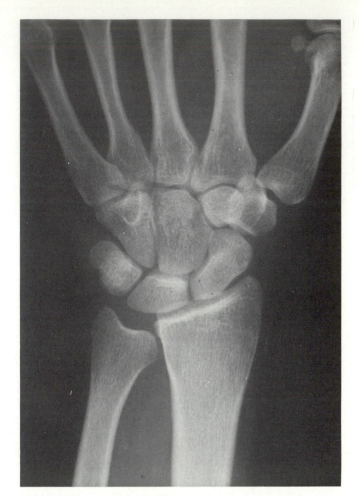

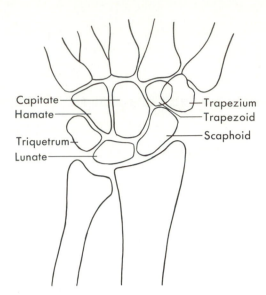

FIG. 14-1. Anteroposterior roentgenogram of a normal wrist. Radial styloid is distal to ulnar styloid with an ulnar-slope articular surface of distal radius. There is normally a wide space on roentgenogram between the distal ulna and the lunate and triquetrum. Scaphoid spans proximal and distal carpal row. There is an equal space between each carpal bone with overlapping of trapezium and trapezoid. Lunate is quadrilateral, and scaphoid is peanut or canoe shaped.

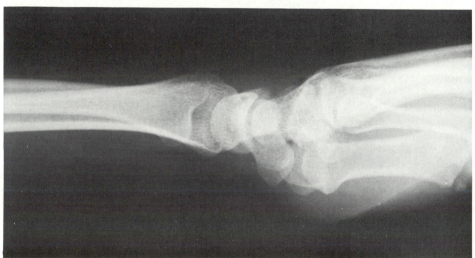

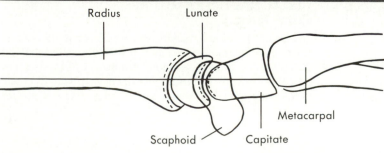

FIG. 14-2. Lateral roentgenogram of normal wrist. There is a slight volar tilt to distal radius articular surface. Since radial styloid extends distally, it is superimposed on lunate. Long axis of distal radius, lunate, capitate, and metacarpal bones are colinear. Articular surfaces of distal radius, lunate, and capitate fit together like multiple C's facing same direction.

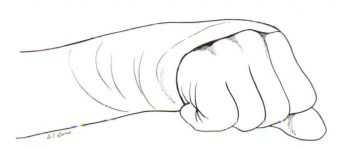

FIG. 14-3. Wrist immobilization. Volarly, cast or splint should extend only to distal palmar crease allowing full metacarpophalangeal flexion. This fitting not only keeps joint from getting stiff but also decreases finger edema by allowing active finger motion during wrist immobilization.

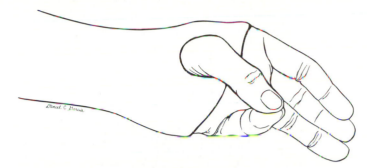

FIG. 14-4. Wrist immobilization. Except for injuries involving thumb axis or scaphoid, thumb should be free during wrist immobilization. Plaster and padding should not cover thumb metacarpal to allow full opposition.

erally used to describe any fracture involving the distal radius with dorsal displacement. It is caused by a fall on the outstretched hand, producing a variety of fracture patterns. A practical classification of these fractures is by Frykman,[15] who distinguished between extra-articular and intra-articular fractures and stressed the importance of the ulnar side of the wrist. The diagnosis is easily made when one finds a painful swollen wrist where the dorsally displaced distal radius gives the appearance of an upside-down dinner fork. Palpation reveals a tense tender wrist with a prominent ulnar styloid and frequently with the radial styloid at the same level as the distal ulna. Roentgenograms in two planes confirm the diagnosis (Fig. 14-5). Care must be exercised to avoid missing an associated carpal fracture, carpal dislocation, or subluxation of the distal radioulnar joint.

Treatment of Colles' fractures is considerably more difficult and controversial than its diagnosis. Over 85% of these fractures require some form of reduction.[22,31] General anesthesia, regional block anesthesia, or local anesthesia injected into the fracture hematoma are required before manipulation. Once radial length is restored by traction or manipulation, the dorsal angulation may be corrected by a palmar-directed manipulation of the distal radius. The reduction is then maintained by dorsal and palmar padded plaster splints molded so that three-point pressure is applied dorsally over the distal fragment and the midforearm and palmarly over the distal aspect of the proximal fragment.[12] The wrist is placed in slight palmar flexion and ulnar deviation. There is controversy whether the forearm should be immobilized in pronation[29] or supination.[39] We prefer the more pronated position because if forearm rotation is lost permanently it is more functional for the forearm to be in pronation. Successful noninvasive immobilization techniques include sugar-tong splints, short-arm casts, long-arm casts, and functional bracing. One method has not been shown to be statistically superior. Regardless of which form of immobilization is used, full finger motion must be permitted, avoidance of significant edema or neurologic symptoms, and frequent clinical follow-up is mandatory. Settling and displacement of the distal radius may occur during the

first 3 weeks.[35] Remanipulation during this time is sometimes necessary.

The exact clinical and roentgenographic criteria for an acceptable fracture reduction are not established. There is a good correlation between anatomic and functional results. Radial shortening is the most disabling deformity and must be corrected if possible.[15,17] It contributes to distal radioulnar problems and compromises hand mobility and power. Dorsal tilting is the most difficult deformity to correct but the least disabling, with up to 25 degrees of residual angulation associated with a good functional result.[29] If there has been no loss of reduction during the first 3 weeks, the elbow is freed by application of a short-arm cast for another 2 to 4 weeks. Immobilization is discontinued when there is no point tenderness at the fracture site and roentgenographic evidence of fracture consolidation.

The severely comminuted or intra-articular distal radius fractures are extremely difficult to hold with simple plaster immobilization. Various self-contained skeletal traction systems have been developed to hold the unstable fracture out to length (Fig. 14-6). Percutaneous pins are placed proximal and distal to the fracture site through the metacarpal and proximal forearm bones.[19] Fracture reduction can be maintained by incorporation of pins into the plaster of a short-arm cast. We have found that external fixation devices have been as effective as pins in plaster in maintaining reduction but also have the advantage of being lighter in weight and are less restrictive in allowing finger mobilization and seem to decrease edema formation more than pins in plaster. During the 8 weeks of immobilization that these fractures require, the elbow and fingers can be free to maintain their mobility. Pin-tract infections, pin breakage, and excessive overdistractions are complications that can easily be prevented with attention to detail.

Complications of Colles' fractures are common; they include the following:

Stiffness of finger, wrist, forearm, elbow, and shoulder
Carpal tunnel syndrome
Malunion
Weakness of grip

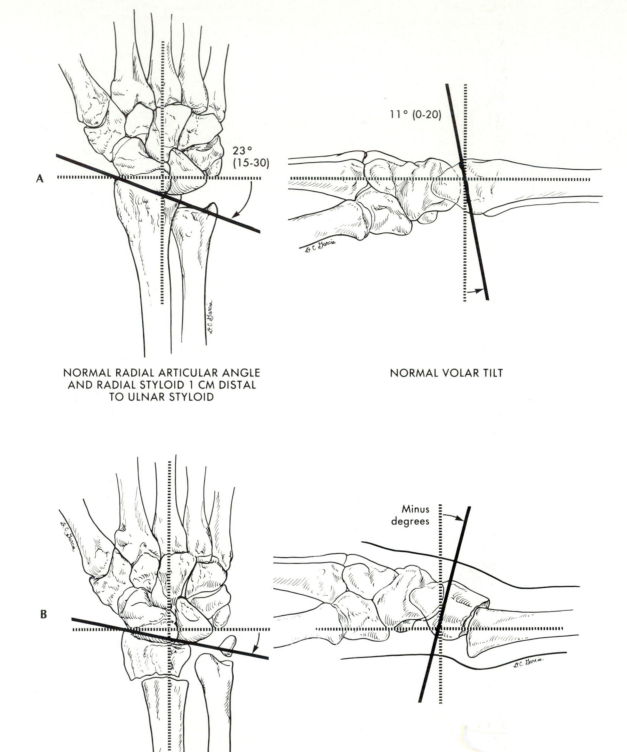

23°
(15-30)

NORMAL RADIAL ARTICULAR ANGLE
AND RADIAL STYLOID 1 CM DISTAL
TO ULNAR STYLOID

11° (0-20)

NORMAL VOLAR TILT

LOSS OF RADIAL ARTICULAR ANGLE
AND RADIAL LENGTH IN COLLES'
FRACTURE

Minus
degrees

DORSAL TILT OF COLLES' FRACTURE

FIG. 14-5. **A,** Normal wrist. Normal ulnar tilt of distal radius is 23 degrees to a line perpendicular to long axis of radius. Normal volar tilt is 11 degrees to a line perpendicular to long axis of radius. **B,** Colles' fracture.

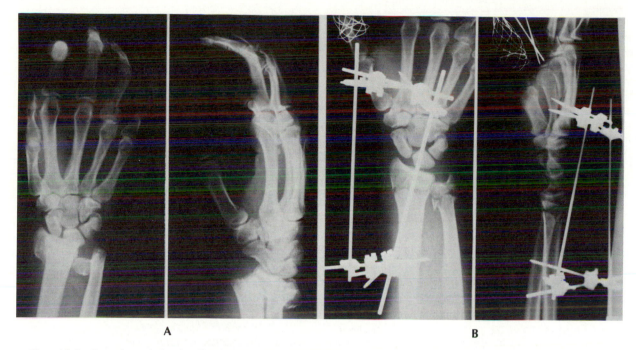

A   B

FIG. 14-6. Comminuted distal radius fracture. **A,** This severely comminuted distal radius and ulna fracture was not amenable to a closed reduction and plaster immobilization. **B,** Hoffman external fixator. Fracture was reduced and length reestablished with finger trap traction. External fixator system was applied to maintain the reduction, and distraction was released.

Radiocarpal arthritis
Distal radioulnar dysfunction
Extensor pollicis longus rupture
Posttraumatic reflex sympathetic dystrophy
Intrinsic contracture

Twenty percent of patients have residual symptoms and 10% have significant functional impairment.[29] Avoiding the extreme Cotton-Loder position of immobilization in extreme palmar flexion and ulnar deviation will decrease the risk of median nerve compression of the carpal tunnel. The last complication listed, intrinsic contracture, deserves additional comment. Although rarely mentioned in the literature as a complication of wrist fractures, we have found intrinsic tightness in most cases where there has been considerable swelling after wrist trauma. We hypothesize that this is a limited intrinsic ischemic contracture caused by excessive swelling and pressure in the interosseous compartments of the hand. It may be resistant to hand therapy and splinting and may require surgical release of the interossei.[9]

The poorest results can be expected if there is intra-articular involvement, pronounced initial displacement, severe comminution, and evidence of damage to the ulnar side of the wrist.[15] The young adult with vigorous functional demands who sustains a severe distal radius fracture has a guarded prognosis.

Smith's fracture

Smith's fracture of the distal radius is frequently called a ''reverse Colles' fracture.''[42] It occurs in a younger age group and is less frequent than the Colles' fracture. The

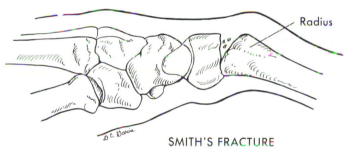

SMITH'S FRACTURE

FIG. 14-7. Smith's fracture.

mechanism of injury was classically believed to be a fall on the back of the hand. Other proposed mechanisms include a fall on the supinated wrist followed by pronation of the upper limb, and motorcycle injuries where the knuckles of the hand gripping the handlebar sustain a dorsal blow.

Three clinical types of Smith's fractures have been noted by Thomas based on the obliquity of the fracture line.[47] The patient presents with the hand and wrist palmarly displaced in reference to the forearm giving the appearance of a ''garden spade.'' Compared to Colles' fractures these injuries have dorsal displacement of the ulnar head and less noticeable subcutaneous crepitation. Lateral roentgenograms confirm the palmarly displaced distal radius (Fig. 14-7).

Treatment of Smith's fractures consists in longitudinal traction, manual manipulation with a dorsally direct force applied to the distal radius, and immobilization in supination and neutral wrist position. For many years the wrist was immobilized in dorsiflexion,[5] but recently it has been shown that this position placed the radiocarpal joint contact area volarly so that the deformity is increased,[47] and slight palmar flexion on the neutral position is recommended. Similar to Colles' fractures, loss of reduction or severe comminution requires remanipulation and possible self-contained traction. Uncomplicated Smith's fractures require long-arm plaster immobilization for 3 weeks followed by a short-arm cast for another 2 to 3 weeks. Complications of these palmarly displaced fractures are essentially similar to Colles' fractures. Median nerve injury is more common in Smith's fracture. Making up only 5% to 10% of distal radius fractures, these injuries are not regularly seen, and misinterpretation of the initial roentgenogram along with incomplete reduction is a problem leading to a worse prognosis compared to the Colles' fracture.[22,56]

Barton's fracture

John Barton described this injury as "a subluxation of the wrist consequent to a fracture through the articular surface of the carpal extremity of the radius."[1] This original description refers to dorsal and volar marginal articular fractures, but Barton believed the former was more common. Later, confusion arose as to whether a Barton's fracture involved the dorsal or volar articular surface, perhaps because the dorsal injury occurs less frequently.[4] The volar marginal fracture is actually a type III Smith's fracture described by Thomas.[47] Nevertheless, these injuries are called "dorsal Barton's" and "volar Barton's fractures" in current literature (Fig. 14-8).[48]

The mechanism of injury and the clinical presentation are similar to those of either the Colles' or Smith's fractures. The diagnosis can usually be confirmed with a lateral roentgenogram, but occasionally oblique films may be necessary to clarify the extent of articular involvement and displacement.

A common mistake is to treat the dorsal Barton's like a Colles' fracture. Immobilization of the wrist in *palmar flexion* allows the lunate to press against the unstable dorsal fragment and push it proximally and dorsally. The tendency

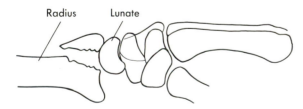

DORSAL BARTON'S FRACTURE

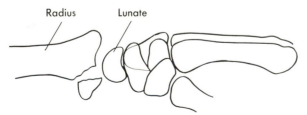

VOLAR BARTON'S FRACTURE

FIG. 14-8. Barton's fracture.

for redislocation after manipulative reduction is actually increased because the longitudinal axis of the carpus is directed into the fracture site creating instability.[48] This concept has been referred to as "Barton's enigma."

To achieve a stable reduction the wrist is immobilized toward the fracture. This places the lunate and the longitudinal axis of the carpus against the intact articular surface of the distal radius. The dorsal Barton's fracture is immobilized in slight dorsiflexion and the volar Barton's fracture is immobilized in slight palmar flexion. Open reduction and internal fixation are indicated in both fracture types if there is involvement of a large portion of the articular surface or inability to obtain and maintain satisfactory joint congruity after manipulative reduction.[13,36,48] Operative modalities include percutaneous pin fixation, bone screws, or T-plates. The joint can be explored, loose cartilaginous fragments removed, and anatomic reduction obtained. If good stability is achieved surgically, early active wrist motion can be started.

CARPAL FRACTURES
Scaphoid fractures

Carpal fractures are about one tenth as frequent as distal radius fractures. Scaphoid fractures account for over 60% of all carpal injuries.[4] The scaphoid or carpal navicular bone is canoe shaped with four of its six surfaces covered with articular cartilage. It spans the proximal and distal carpal row. It is the principle bone block to extreme wrist dorsiflexion, making it particularly vulnerable to injury. The blood supply to the scaphoid enters largely distally through dorsal and lateral volar vessels.[46] This diminished blood supply to the proximal scaphoid makes fractures in this area susceptible to avascular necrosis.

The mechanism of injury is similar to the mechanism of distal radius fractures. A fall on the outstretched hand forces the scaphoid between the dorsal lip of the distal radius and the palmar radiocapitate ligament. Point tenderness in the anatomic snuffbox is a constant and dependable physical finding in patients with scaphoid fractures. Swelling and limited wrist motion are nonspecific for scaphoid fractures. Negative roentgenographic findings do not exclude a scaphoid fracture. All patients with injury to the wrist and point tenderness in the scaphoid region should be treated as if they had a fracture until it has been disproved by negative roentgenograms and clinical findings at 2 and 4 weeks.[36]

Classification of scaphoid fractures is based on anatomic location. The four usual sites of fractures are distally through the tuberosity, the distal third, the waist (Fig. 14-9), and through the proximal pole. The waist fractures in the middle third are most common making up about 70% of all scaphoid fractures. Prognosis for healing is related to the site and obliquity of the fracture and promptness of diagnosis and treatment.

The more horizontal the fracture line in relation to the long axis of the scaphoid, the more rapidly healing will occur. There is a great variation in healing times between the anatomic location and the fracture types. The richly nourished distal tuberosity fractures heal in 5 to 6 weeks, while the relatively avascular proximal third fractures may require 20 weeks or longer to heal. The acute scaphoid fracture must be immobilized. The extent of support and position of immobilization is not uniform among those treating this injury. The most frequent type of support is the short-arm guantlet type of cast from the thumb proximal phalanx to the proximal forearm with the wrist in slight dorsiflexion and radial deviation.[37] There is no agreement whether the elbow or the entire thumb should be immobilized during fracture healing. The duration of immobilization is dependent on roentgenographic evidence of trabeculae across the fracture site and the absence of point tenderness in the scaphoid region. In spite of the well-recognized problems of scaphoid nonunions, 90% of these fractures heal without complications if treated early and casted properly.[30,32]

Scaphoid nonunion is the most frequent and disabling complication associated with scaphoid fractures. Differentiating between a delayed union and an established nonunion taxes even the most astute clinician. Roentgenographic evidence of delayed union includes absorption at the fracture line, cystic changes, and subchondral sclerosis[32] adjacent to the fracture. Many delayed unions will eventually heal if properly immobilized for a long enough interval. The scaphoid nonunion is a fracture that fails to show roentgenographic evidence of healing on three separate monthly examinations. Not all scaphoid nonunions are symptomatic or disabling. It is not uncommon to see an untreated ununited scaphoid fracture on an individual unaware of the problem.

Treatment depends on many factors including the patient's age, functional demands, disability, and degree of local degenerative changes. No uniform method has been universally accepted. Operative intervention with bone graft either through a dorsal or volar approach have been popular.[37] The need for internal fixation differs among those treating these injuries. An attractive new treatment modality is the use of electrical stimulation across the ununited fracture.[7] One method uses wire cathodes inserted transcuta-

neously into the scaphoid fracture site. Another uses a pulsating electromagnetic field generated from coils placed outside the cast. Preliminary studies with electrical treatment have shown healing rates of 71% to 85% in scaphoid nonunions.[16]

When local degenerative changes are present, different salvage procedures may be necessary. Radiocarpal or intercarpal fusion is usually reserved for the young patient with extreme functional demands. Scaphoid replacement arthroplasty is better suited to the older patient with limited wrist stress.[44] Other operative modalities include radial styloidectomy,[41] excision of one or both fragments,[36] and proximal row carpectomy.[22,23]

Triquetrum fractures

Fractures of the triquetrum are the second most common carpal fractures. Located on the ulnar side of the proximal carpal row the triquetrum forms one of the anchors of the wrist with strong volar and dorsal attachments. Excessive wrist dorsiflexion and ulnar deviation produce the common dorsal avulsion fracture when the hamate shears the posteroradial projection.[8] Pain and swelling on the dorsal ulnar aspect of the wrist help make the diagnosis, and a lateral roentgenogram of the wrist in flexion usually shows the avulsion fracture. It may be easily overlooked on the anteroposterior roentgenogram. The isolated ligamentous avulsions respond well to 4 to 6 weeks of immobilization with a short-arm cast in wrist dorsiflexion. If there is considerable displacement, some of these chip fractures do not heal and require excision and ligamentous repair. Rarer triquetral body fractures are caused by impingement or direct blows and are easily identifiable and heal with 6 weeks of immobilization.[2]

Lunate fractures

Accounting for about 7% of all carpal injuries, lunate fractures are the third most common carpal fractures. This half moon–shaped bone is well protected between both carpal rows and the distal radius and triangular fibrocartilage. A fall on the outstretched hand produces a translational compression force when the lunate is caught between the capitate and the dorsal aspect of the distal radius articular surface. If a dislocation does not occur, the lunate will fracture. Initial roentgenograms may be misinterpreted as normal unless one carefully searches for a thin lucent transverse line across the proximal pole of the lunate on the anteroposterior film. Numerous superimpositions in both planes make roentgenographic diagnosis difficult. If the diagnosis of lunate fractures can be made initially, immobilization in a short-arm cast until healing is well established in 6 to 8 weeks decreases the long-term morbidity.

All too frequently the lunate presents as a sclerotic collapsed painful bone better known as ''avascular necrosis'' or ''Kienböck's disease.''[25] There is no general agreement whether Kienböck's disease occurs from an acute fracture of repetitive trauma. Regardless of the exact mechanism there is definite interruption of the blood supply to a bone with a variable vascular pattern.[3,18,27]

Treatment of Kienböck's disease is quite similar to ununited scaphoid fractures. Early states of the disorder are

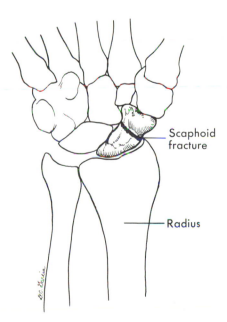

FIG. 14-9. Scaphoid fracture. This fracture is in waist.

Scaphoid fracture

Radius

treated with prolonged immobilization. When collapse is early without local degenerative changes, the ulnar variance may be treated with ulnar lengthening or radius shortening. In late stages of Kienböck's disease numerous salvage procedures are well established with decision making similar to that of late scaphoid nonunions.

Other carpal fractures

The remainder of carpal fractures are rare with the clinical and roentgenographic diagnosis difficult. Fractures of the trapezium are usually associated with fracture-dislocation of the thumb metacarpal base (Bennett's fracture). Capitate fractures are rare. The central position of this bone in the carpus protects it between the proximal carpal row and stable central metacarpal bones. Pisiform and hamate fractures may occur from a direct fall on the outstretched hand or a direct blow from the handle of rackets, golf clubs, or baseball bats.[6,50] Ulnar nerve symptoms may be present. The diagnosis may be missed, since routine roentgenograms are normal. Point tenderness over the pisiform or hook of the hamate and a carpal tunnel view will help make the diagnosis. Excision of the painful fragment may be necessary if casting does not help.[43]

The complications of these infrequent carpal injuries are usually preventable provided that diagnosis is made early and appropriate treatment is carried out.

CARPAL DISLOCATIONS

Before any discussion of carpal dislocation, a description of the normal complex intercarpal relationships is essential (Figs. 14-1 to 14-3). The most important film when examining suspected carpal dislocations is the lateral wrist roentgenogram.

Carpal instability depends on the maintenance of bony architecture interlaced with ligaments. The volar wrist ligaments (Fig. 14-10) are intracapsular, and more substantial than the dorsal ligaments. The scaphoid is supported proximally by the volar radioscaphoid and lunate-scaphoid ligaments and distally by the radial collateral, radiocapitate, and deltoid ligaments. The triquetrum is important in volar ulnar stability, with all ligaments converging on this bone like the spokes of a wheel from their origins in the lunate (lunotriquetral), the ulna (ulnotriquetral), and the capitate (deltoid ligament).[45] The general configuration of the volar ligaments is a double V-shaped structure with an area of potential weakness between them lying directly over the capitate-lunate articulation.[20] The dorsal wrist ligaments are weaker and less clearly defined.

Perilunate dislocations

Most carpal dislocations are of the dorsal perilunate type (Fig. 14-11). The lunate is the usual bone around which the remainder of the carpus dislocated. It, like most wrist injuries, occurs from violent hyperextension or dorsiflexion. There are rarely any physical findings that point to the diagnosis. Median nerve paresthesias may increase the index of suspicion.[10] Since dislocation occurs at the midcarpal joint, the scaphoid that bridges both must either sustain ligamentous disruption proximally and follow the capitate or fracture through its waist, producing the transscaphoid perilunate dislocation.[52]

If these injuries are seen within the first 3 weeks, closed reduction after adequate muscle relaxation can usually be accomplished by distraction of the carpus and gentle manipulation. Dorsally directed pressure on the palmarly dislocated lunate plus pressure directed palmarward on the

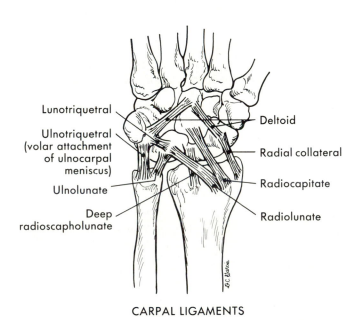

CARPAL LIGAMENTS

FIG. 14-10. Carpal wrist ligaments. This schematic representation of volar wrist ligaments show a proximal and distal V-shaped system. Majority of these intracapsular ligaments originate on radius laterally and triquetrum medially and insert on their adjacent carpal bones. (From Taleisnik, J.: J. Hand Surg. **1**:110, 1976.)

dorsally dislocated capitate is the maneuver needed to achieve reduction. If *anatomic reduction* is confirmed by good quality roentgenograms, the wrist is immobilized in a short-arm cast with slight palmar flexion from 6 to 8 weeks. If the reduction is not maintained by casting alone, percutaneous pinning is necessary. If reduction cannot be obtained, open reduction, internal fixation, and ligament repair are necessary.

Lunate dislocations

The volar lunate dislocations occur from the same mechanism as the perilunate dislocation. Many consider the lunate dislocation to be the end stage of a perilunate dislocation. Many variations are frequently seen between the two common dislocations making it easy to believe the injuries are different roentgenographic manifestations of the same injury.

Lunate dislocation frequently presents median nerve compression. On the anteroposterior roentgenogram the lunate appears triangular and there is a peculiar space between the scaphoid and the triquetrum. The appearance of this dislocation on the lateral roentgenogram is fairly typical (Fig. 14-12). Closed reduction can be achieved if the injury is seen early. Atraumatic closed reduction with muscle relaxation is attempted after a period of sustained traction. With the wrist in extension, digital pressure is exerted over the dislocated volar lunate. Once reduced, the wrist is brought into flexion and immobilized for 6 to 8 weeks.[54] Since there is a tendency for the reduction to be lost with time, percutaneous pinning of the lunate in its reduced position or open reduction may be necessary.

Posttraumatic instability of the wrist

When the normal carpal alignment is lost after a wrist injury, posttraumatic instability of the wrist occurs.[28] There is a range of ligamentous and bony injuries to the carpal bones causing malalignment. They may occur late and develop slowly or may be immediate and severe. Appreciation of normal carpal roentgenographic alignment is essential to understand these instability patterns. Dorsiflexion instability and palmar flexion instability are the most common instability patterns seen (Fig. 14-13).

Scapholunate dissociation is an instability pattern frequently seen after wrist injury. It is most commonly seen

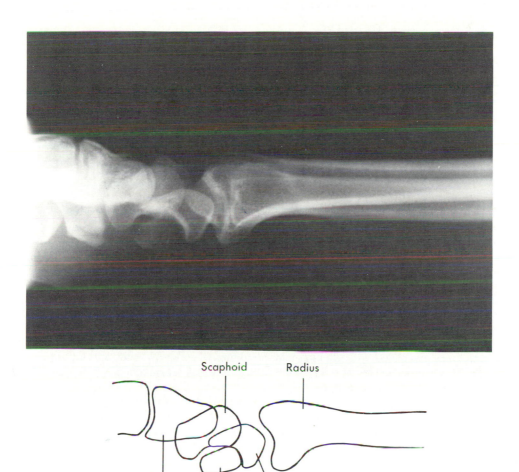

Scaphoid   Radius

Capitate   Pisiform   Lunate

FIG. 14-11. Dorsal perilunate dislocation. Lateral roentgenogram of this injury shows scaphoid and capitate displaced dorsally to lunate.

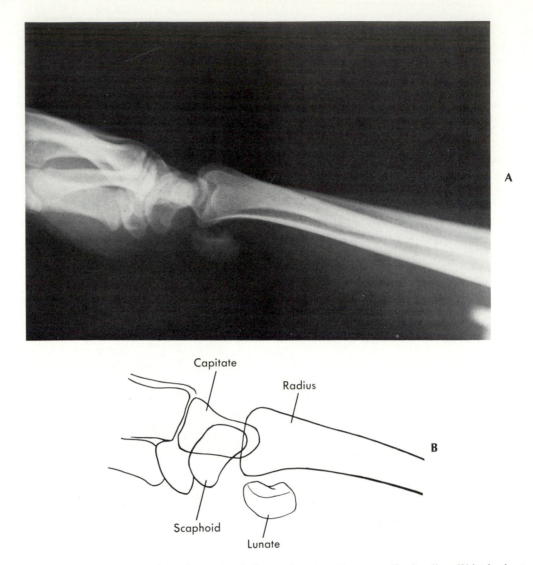

FIG. 14-12. Lunate dislocation. Lunate is displaced volarly to other carpal bones or distal radius. Wrist is shortened with capitate articulating with radius.

in combination with perilunate dislocations and dorsiflexion instability but may occur as an isolated phenomenon. Also known as rotatory subluxation of the scaphoid, it occurs when there is damage to the scapholunate and the volar radioscapholunate ligament allowing the proximal pole of the scaphoid to rotate dorsally. The symptoms are pain in the scaphoid area sometimes associated with clicking and no evidence of fracture on wrist roentgenograms. There are several key roentgenographic features that are unique to this injury (Fig. 14-14).

It may be necessary to obtain a series of roentgenograms to confirm the diagnosis if an instability pattern is suspected clinically. This includes a lateral roentgenogram with the wrist in the neutral position, anteroposterior in supination and in radial and ulnar deviation, and clenched fist positions.

The treatment of these complex instability patterns is based on reestablishing and maintaining normal intercarpal alignment. The acute injury must be differentiated from the chronic instability pattern. The degree of discomfort and

functional disability must be clearly defined. The presence of local degenerative changes and joint arthritis will profoundly affect the treatment recommendation.

The acute carpal dislocation is treated with a closed reduction after adequate relaxation. If the reduction is shown to be anatomic on good quality roentgenograms, plaster immobilization is used, and the injury is followed closely with weekly roentgenograms. Frequently a reduction cannot be achieved initially or cannot be maintained during the first several days after injury. Open reduction, internal fixation, and appropriate ligamentous repairs are strongly recommended in the acute situation.[43] The carpal bones are exposed through both volar and dorsal approach, and the dislocation is reduced anatomically under direct vision and held with Kirschner wires. Any ligamentous disruption is surgically repaired. Intraoperative roentgenograms confirm the reduction. When there is a paucity of ligamentous tissue available for repair, some have advocated ligamentous reinforcement, particularly between the scapholunate junction

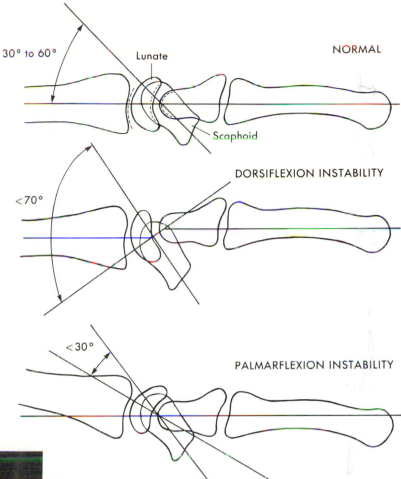

FIG. 14-13. Posttraumatic wrist instability patterns. When wrist is in neutral position on lateral roentgenogram, normal scapholunate angle is from 30 to 60 degrees. When lunate faces dorsally, scapholunate angle is greater than 60 degrees (usually about 100 degrees). This angle indicates a dorsiflexion instability pattern. When lunate faces palmarly and scapholunate angle is less than 30 degrees, palmar flexion instability pattern is demonstrated.

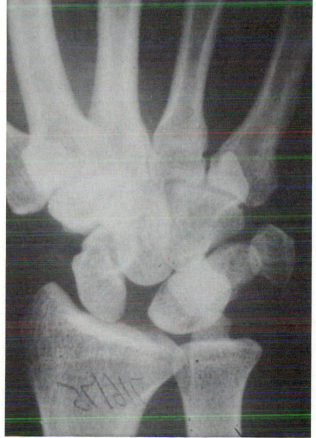

FIG. 14-14. Scapholunate dissociation. Scaphoid is tilted dorsally. It is oval in contour rather than having normal canoe shape. Since one is looking down long axis of scaphoid, there is a double density or cortical "ring" shadow of tuberosity. Scapholunate gap normally 2 mm or less is increased. This gap is popularly called "Terry-Thomas sign" and refers to the British actor with a wide gap between his front teeth.

using a slip of the extensor carpi radialis longus tendon.[14]

Treatment of chronic instability patterns is difficult with less uniform opinion regarding operative modalities.[14,34] Ligamentous reconstruction, although theoretically physiologic and effective early, has a tendency to fail with stretching out of the new ligament. Limited wrist arthrodesis, especially scaphotrapeziotrapezoid arthrodesis for scapholunate dissociation, has recently been shown to be effective, although long-term follow-up is lacking.[26,53] When local degenerative changes are present, the options are similar to those salvage procedures previously mentioned.

DISTAL RADIOULNAR INJURIES

Injury to the distal radioulnar joint and ulnocarpal region accompany almost every common distal radius fracture. Attention is directed toward restoring length and reducing the malalignment of the radial side of the wrist. Injuries to the ulnar side are often assumed to be minor and of secondary importance. Once the primary injury has healed, frequently there is pain and disability from injury and malalignment to the ulnar portion of the wrist.

There is a triangular flat band of fibrocartilage that originates on the ulnar aspect of the distal radius and inserts at the base of the ulnar styloid (Fig. 14-15). This articular disk separates the radiocarpal joint from the distal radioulnar joint.[51] There is a complex fibrous tissue formation on the ulnar carpal region providing stability, allowing motion, and connecting all local carpal bones. There is no contact between the distal ulna and the carpal joints. This absent ulnar carpal articulation filled with the articular disk and fibrocartilage permits range of motion in the form of ulnar deviation, pronation, and supination.[24]

There is frequently a history of a previous wrist or forearm fracture. There is pain and deformity after a twisting injury. There is a fullness in the ulnar aspect of the wrist with limited pronation and supination. Articular disk tears classically have point tenderness in the distal radioulnar area and a palpable click with certain rotation movements.

Lateral wrist roentgenograms may show the ulnar head either dorsal or volar to the radius, with proximal migration possible on the comparison anteroposterior film. Suspected

wrist disk tears are confirmed by a wrist arthrogram (Fig. 14-16). These are particularly relevant in the younger individual, since age-related degeneration may routinely occur in the normal population.[55]

Exploration and excision of a torn wrist disk is indicated only when a trial of immobilization has not helped and the diagnosis is confirmed with arthrography. Many torn disks are asymptomatic except for painless clicking with certain motions. Ligamentous reconstruction and resection of the distal ulna (Darrach) are salvage procedures for disabling distal radioulnar injuries.[21]

WRIST SPRAIN

The diagnosis of wrist sprain is incorrectly made all too frequently by those inexperienced with traumatic wrist conditions. There definitely are wrist sprains consisting of minor radiocarpal or intercarpal ligamentous tears. Basically the diagnosis of wrist sprain is one of exclusion. It can be accurately made only after careful exclusion of scaphoid or lunate fractures, dorsal chip carpal fractures, traumatic wrist instability patterns, and other carpal fractures. Frequently series repeat roentgenograms are required at weekly intervals after wrist immobilization to identify fractures suspected but only confirmed on initial roentgenographic evaluation. A history of minor trauma with mild generalized diffuse pain or swelling lasting 2 to 3 weeks with all other more serious conditions ruled out is the pattern required for an accurate diagonsis of a wrist sprain.

SECRETAN'S DISEASE

Secretan described a curious condition where minor trauma to the dorsum of the hand is followed by brawny nonpitting edema.[40,49] The extensor tendons become embedded in a mass of organizing fibrous tissue containing macrophages and hemosiderin. There is no bony injury or ecchymosis present. This chronic condition with an obscure cause is believed to be a self-inflicted entity producing prolonged disability in patients who have a possible claim for occupational injury. Since the condition is believed to be a form of reflex sympathetic dystrophy, treatment consists in benign neglect. Surgical intervention, heat, massage, and passive manipulations are not helpful.[38,49]

GENERAL PRINCIPLES FOR REHABILITATION OF WRIST INJURIES

All wrist injuries require some form of rehabilitation. Although there is a great variation in the type and severity of wrist injuries, the general principles of rehabilitation are the same. There are specific limitations for each injury. Good communication between the physician and the therapist can help incorporate these limitations into the rehabilitation plan. Pain is one limiting factor. It dictates the duration of immobilization yet limits exercises designed to mobilize and strengthen the wrist.

Edema of the injured wrist is always present to some degree. It involves the hand but may extend proximally to involve the entire upper extremity. Functional disuse of the hand in itself may result in edema. The required immobilization inhibits the pumping action of the muscles with subsequent venous stasis and edema. The most important

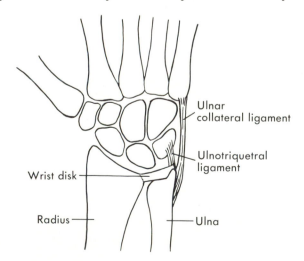

FIG. 14-15. Radioulnar carpal joint.

preventive measures are elevation and active motion of the uninjured joints. When in bed, the patient must elevate the injured wrist on pillows. The patient is taught to rest his elbow on the arm of a chair with the hand elevated above the elbow in the upright position and must avoid dependency. A comfortable sling or arm immobilizer is fitted to assist the patient in keeping the area of injury elevated. Active motion of uninjured joints must be done regularly and frequently. Exaggerated instructions are a good way to get the point across.

Chronic edema associated with traumatic wrist injuries is a difficult problem to treat. The Jobst Intermittent Compression Unit ''pumps'' the lymphedema out of the hand and arm. Alternating rest intervals allow for the lymph flow and venous return. The standard treatment consists in wearing the Jobst sleeve for 45 minutes with a pressure of 66 mm Hg in 60 second–30 second compression-rest intervals. Depending on the patient's tolerance, adjustments can be made in the duration of treatment, position of the hand during compression, pressure during compression, and the compression-rest interval.

Massage of the hand, another useful modality to treat chronic edema, assists venous and lymphatic circulation by its mechanical effects on the tissues. Massage should be performed with the patient comfortably seated and the arm resting in a softer surface with the hand elevated and the elbow extended. A skin lubricant is used to aid the long flowing strokes from a distal to proximal direction. The forearm is rotated frequently during massage.

The wrist is always stiff after immobilization for more than a few weeks. Mobilizing the stiff wrist cannot be started until the injured tissue has healed enough to provide some degree of stability. The longer the required immobilization, the greater the degree of wrist stiffness. The problem of wrist stiffness increases with age and the severity of the injury. If the type of immobilization used is properly applied and active exercises performed during the healing phase, joint stiffness proximal and distal to the wrist should not be a problem. Active wrist range of motion exercises should be started as soon as the cast is removed. The patient does not usually recognize that the wrist normally moves through both the dorsal palmar and the radial ulnar plane. They must be instructed to include these motions into their exercise program. Pronation and supination should not be overlooked. The elbow should be flexed 90 degrees and adducted close to the body during pronation-supination exercises to avoid shoulder abduction mimicking wrist pronation. Active assisted range-of-motion exercises should be started when the wrist motion is not increasing with active exercises. Pain is a guide when one is deciding how soon and how aggressive active assisted exercises should be started. The hand can be rested flat on a table and the wrist slowly bent forward and backward. Wrist dorsiflexion can be improved by putting both palms together in the praying position and moving the forearm to the horizontal position. Similarly palmar flexion can be assisted by putting the dorsum of each hand together. Turning a door handle against resistance or turning the hand over repeatedly in gloves with the fingers and palms sewn together are exercises to regain lost pronation and supination.

In most traumatic wrist injuries it is desirable to start mobilizing the joint before the bone and soft tissues are

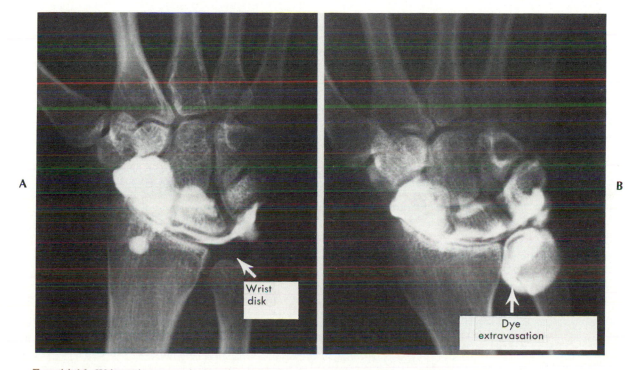

FIG. 14-16. Wrist arthrogram. **A,** Dye is confined to intercarpal area. Triangular fibrocartilage is clearly seen. **B,** A torn wrist disk with contrast material leaking into distal radioulnar joint.

completely healed. This requires the use of various splints to protect and support the wrist in its final stage of healing. A static wrist splint in the neutral or slightly dorsiflexed position is worn at night during the first few days or weeks after the cast is removed. During the day it is more desirable to fit the patient with a dynamic wrist splint. This increases the functional use of the wrist while stabilizing and strengthening it. The patient has the security of wrist support while attempting to regain motion.

Once the wrist is healed, edema controlled, and motion improved, the muscles crossing the wrist must be strengthened. Even vigorous athletic youths lose muscle mass quickly when immobilized for any length of time. One can best achieve strengthening by returning the patient to some type of functional activity. This may initially be the activities of daily living such as dressing, personal hygiene, or light housework. Before the patient is returned to his preinjury level of activity, progressive resistive exercises are necessary. The wrist flexors and extensors are actively contracted against maximum resistance through a full arc of motion. The hand is held over the edge of a table with a slight incline. Weights are attached to the hand. The supinated wrist is flexed to strengthen the wrist palmar flexors, and the pronated wrist is extended to strengthen the wrist dorsiflexors. Functional activities have the advantage of easy accessibility and usefulness and are less boring to the patient.

REFERENCES

1. Barton, J.R.: Views and treatment of an important injury to the wrist, Philadelphia Med. Exam. **1**:365, 1838.
2. Bartone, N.F., and Grieco, R.V.: Fractures of the triquetrum, J. Bone Joint Surg. **38A**:353, 1956.
3. Beckenbaugh, R.D., Shives, T.C., Dobyns, J.H., and Linscheid, R.L.: Kienböck's disease: the natural history of Kienböck's disease and consideration of lunate fractures, Clin. Orthop. **149**:98, 1980.
4. Bohler, L.: The treatment of fractures, ed. 4, Baltimore, 1942, William Wood & Co.
5. Bohler, L.: Treatment of fractures, Bristol, England, 1956, A. John Wright & Sons, Ltd.
6. Bowen, T.L.: Injuries to the hamate bone, Hand **5**:235, 1973.
7. Brighton, C.T.: Treatment of nonunion with constant direct current, Clin. Orthop. **124**:106, 1977.
8. Bryan, R., and Dobyns, J.H.: Fractures of the carpal bones other than the lunate and navicular, Clin. Orthop. **149**:107, 1980.
9. Bunnell, S.: Ischemic contracture, local in the hand, J. Bone Joint Surg. **35A**:88, 1953.
10. Campbell, R.D., Lance, E.M., and Yeoh, C.B.: Lunate and perilunate dislocations, J. Bone Joint Surg. **46B**:55, 1964.
11. Colles, A.: On the fractures of the carpal extremity of the radius, Edinb. Med. Surg. J. **10**:182, 1814.
12. Charnley, J.: The closed treatment of common fractures, ed. 3, Baltimore, 1961, Williams & Wilkins Co.
13. DeOliveira, J.C.: Barton's fracture, J. Bone Joint Surg. **55A**:586, 1973.
14. Dobyns, J.H., Linscheid, R.L., Chao, E.S., Weber, R.R., and Swanson, G.E.: Traumatic instability of the wrist, American Academy of Orthopedic Surgeons: Instructional course lectures, vol. 24, St. Louis, 1975, The C.V. Mosby Co.
15. Frykman, G.: Fracture of the distal radius including sequelae-shoulder-hand-finger syndrome, disturbance in the distal radioulnar joint, and impairment of nerve function: a clinical and experimental study, Acta Orthop. Scand. Suppl. **108**:1, 1967.
16. Frykman, G.K., Helal, B., Kaufman, R., Peters, G., and Taleisnik, J.: Pulsing electromagnetic field treatment of ununited scaphoid fractures. Read at annual meeting of American Society for Surgery of the Hand, New Orleans, Jan. 19, 1982.
17. Gartland, J.J., Jr., and Werley, C.W.: Evaluation of healed Colles' fractures, J. Bone Joint Surg. **43B**:245, 1961.
18. Gelberman, R.M., Salamon, P.B., Jurist, J.M., and Posch, J.L.: Ulnar variance in Kienböck's disease, J. Bone Joint Surg. **57A**:674, 1975.
19. Green, D.P.: Pins and plaster treatment of comminuted fractures of the distal end of the radius, J. Bone Joint Surg. **57A**:304, 1975.
20. Green, D.P., and O'Brien, E.T.: Classification and management of carpal dislocations, Clin. Orthop. **149**:55, 1980.
21. Hartz, C.R., and Beckenbaugh, R.D.: Long-term results of resection of the distal ulna for post-traumatic conditions, J. Trauma **19**:4, 1979.
22. Heppenstall, R.B.: Fracture treatment and healing, Philadelphia, 1980, W.B. Saunders Co.
23. Inglis, A.E., and Jones, E.C.: Proximal row carpectomy for disease of the proximal row, J. Bone Joint Surg. **59A**:460, 1977.
24. Kauer, J.M.G.: Functional anatomy of the wrist, Clin. Orthop. **149**:15, 1980.
25. Kienböck, R.: The classic concerning traumatic malacia of the lunate and its consequences: degenerative and compression fractures, Clin. Orthop. **149**:4, 1980.
26. Kleinman, W.B., Steichen, J.B., and Strickland, J.W.: Management of chronic rotatory subluxation of the scaphoid by scapho-trapezio-trapezoid arthrodesis, J. Hand Surg. **7**:125, 1982.
27. Lee, M.L.H.: Interosseous arterial pattern of the carpal lunate bone and its relationship to avascular necrosis, Acta Orthop. Scand. **33**:43, 1963.
28. Linscheid, R.L., Dobyns, J.H., Beabout, J.W., and others: Traumatic instability of the wrist: diagnosis, classification and pathomechanics, J. Bone Joint Surg. **54A**:1612, 1972.
29. Lidstrom, A.: Fractures of the distal end of the radius: a clinical and statistical study of end results, Acta Orthop. Scand. Suppl. **41**:1, 1959.
30. London, P.S.: The broken scaphoid bones: the case against pessimism, J. Bone Joint Surg. **42B**:237, 1961.
31. Mayer, J.H.: Colles' fractures, Br. J. Surg. **27**:629, 1940.
32. Mazet, R., and Hohl, M.: Fractures of the carpal navicular: analysis of 91 cases and review of the literature, J. Bone Joint Surg. **45A**:82, 1967.
33. Moberg, E.: The shoulder-hand-finger syndrome, Surg. Clin. North Am. **40**:367, 1960.
34. Palmar, A.K., Dobyns, J.H., and Linscheid, R.L.: Management of posttraumatic instability of the wrist secondary to ligament rupture, J. Hand Surg. **3**:507, 1978.
35. Parisen, S.: Settling in Colles' fracture: a review of the literature, Bull. Hosp. Joint Dis. **34**:117, 1973.
36. Rockwood, C.A., and Green, D.P.: Fractures, Philadelphia, 1975, J.B. Lippincott Co.
37. Russe, O.: Fracture of the carpal navicular, J. Bone Joint Surg. **42A**:759, 1960.
38. Saferin, E.H.: Secretan's disease, Plast. Reconstr. Surg. **58**:703, 1976.
39. Sarmiento, A.: The brachioradialis as a deforming force in Colles' fractures, Clin. Orthop. **38**:86, 1965.
40. Secretan, H.: Hard edema and traumatic hyperplasia of the dorsum of metacarpus, Rev. Med. Suisse Romande **21**:409, 1901.
41. Smith, L., and Friedman, B.: Treatment of ununited fractures of the scaphoid by styloidectomy of the radius, J. Bone Joint Surg. **38A**:368, 1956.
42. Smith, R.W.: A treatise on fractures in the vicinity of joints, and on certain forms of accidental and congenital dislocations, Dublin, 1854, Hodges & Smith.
43. Stark, H.H., Jobe, F.W., Boyes, J.H., and Ashworth, C.R.: Fractures of the hamate in athletics, J. Bone Joint Surg. **59A**:575, 1977.
44. Swanson, A.B.: Silicone rubber implants for replacement of the carpal scaphoid and lunate bone, Orthop. Clin. North Am. **1**:299, 1970.
45. Taleisnik, J.: The ligaments of the wrist, J. Hand Surg. **1**:110, 1976.
46. Taleisnik, J., and Kelly, P.J.: The extraosseous and intraosseous blood supply to the scaphoid bone, J. Bone Joint Surg. **48A**:1126, 1966.
47. Thomas, F.B.: Reduction of Smith's fractures, J. Bone Joint Surg. **39B**:463, 1959.

48. Thompson, G.H.: Barton's fractures—reverse Barton's fractures, Clin. Orthop. **122:**210, 1977.
49. Van Demark, R.E.: Peritendinous fibrosis of the dorsum of the hand, J. Bone Joint Surg. **30A:**284, 1948.
50. Vasilas, A., Gireco, R.V., and Baritone, N.F.: Roentgen aspects of injuries to the pisiform bone and pisotriquetral joint, J. Bone Joint Surg. **42A:**1317, 1960.
51. Vesely, D.G.: The distal radioulnar joint, Clin. Orthop. **51:**75, 1967.
52. Wagner, C.J.: Fracture-dislocation of the wrist, Clin. Orthop. **15:**181, 1959.
53. Watson, H.K., and Hempton, R.F.: Limited wrist arthrodesis, I. The triscaphoid joint, J. Hand Surg. **5:**320, 1980.
54. Watson-Jones, R.: Fractures and joint injuries, ed. 5, Edinburgh, 1976, E. & S. Livingstone.
55. Weigl, K., and Spira, E.: The triangular fibrocartilage of the wrist joint, Reconstr. Surg. Traumatol. **11:**139, 1969.
56. Woodyard, J.E.: Review of Smith's fractures, J. Bone Joint Surg. **51B:**324, 1969.

15

Management of hand fractures

ROBERT LEE WILSON and MARGARET S. CARTER

While fractures in the hand occur more frequently than in any other location, their significance is often underestimated. When hand fractures are incorrectly managed or associated with injuries to other tissues, stiffness, pain, or contracture may result and produce a loss of normal hand function. The two factors that most influence the end result after a digital fracture are the severity of the initial injury and the method of primary treatment. While the seriousness of some injuries precludes a perfect result, our goal should be to recover maximal function in every injured hand.

More than one half of all hand fractures are sustained at work. Fractures occur with less frequency from motor vehicle accidents, recreational activities, and household mishaps. The location of fractures within the hand has been reviewed by several authors. Distal phalanx fractures are the most common (45% to 50%), followed by metacarpal (30% to 35%), proximal phalanx (15% to 20%), and lastly middle phalanx fractures (8% to 12%).

In evaluating digital fractures, one must first consider the force that produced the injury and the extent of soft tissue involvement. The hand is examined for rotational deformities of the fingers as well as angulation and fracture displacement. X-ray evaluation should include three views (anteroposterior, oblique, and a true lateral) of the digit. Lastly, the stability of the fracture must be assessed to determine the exact immobilization needed to obtain bony union.

The first principle in the treatment of hand fractures is *accurate fracture reduction*. As little as 5 degrees lateral angulation may create overlapping of the fingers. While immobilization of the injured finger may be necessary to ensure union, the *uninvolved fingers must be actively moved* to prevent stiffness. *Elevation of the extremity* at all times is the best method to limit edema.

The fingers that are *immobilized should be placed in the "clam-digger" or, intrinsic-positive position:* the wrist in 30 to 60 degrees extension, the metacarpophalangeal joints in 60 to 70 degrees flexion, and the interphalangeal joints in neutral to 10 degrees flexion. This position maintains the ligaments of the digital joints under maximal tension, hopefully preventing the most serious joint contractures. Immobilization of the wrist in extension produces synergistic flexion of the metacarpophalangeal joints and overcomes the pain reflex position (wrist flexion and metacarpophalangeal joint extension with clawed fingers). However, the clam-digger position invites intrinsic contracture, and in-

trinsic tendon stretching exercises should be initiated early (Fig. 15-1).

Early mobilization of the injured finger is necessary to prevent stiffness and should be started as soon as local pain and fracture healing permit. Motion prevents adherence of the tendons at the fracture site, diminishes edema by pumping fluid from the finger, and decreases ligament contracture (Fig. 15-2).

An *exercise program must be directed toward the particular problems* that are characteristic of each individual fracture. The *most important joint in the hand is the proximal interphalangeal joint,* and many of the exercises will be aimed at preventing stiffness and preserving function in this most important articulation.

The treatment of specific hand fractures is adequately described in several texts.[1,3] In the remainder of this chapter, fracture treatment will be discussed for only the more common injuries, with an emphasis on the cause of the fracture deformities and the treatment of specific fracture problems that may occur following reduction or internal fixation.

DISTAL PHALANX FRACTURES

Fractures of the distal phalanx occur more frequently than any others in the hand and present themselves most commonly in the middle finger and thumb. A crushing force such as a punch press usually causes these fractures, and associated skin loss and nail injuries are frequent. The extreme pain following distal phalanx trama results from swelling and hematoma formation within the septated compartments of the fingertip. Chronic pain after such an injury is produced by a secondary fibrosis. Several types of fracture can occur (Fig. 15-3). Comminuted tuft fractures do not become displaced, however, as no tendon pull is exerted beyond the distal phalanx base.

Treatment of distal phalanx fractures should be directed toward the soft tissues, much as in a fingertip injury. Fracture immobilization is rarely necessary; a short splint, however, will prevent the digit from reinjury and more discomfort. Two fractures deserve special attention. Open displaced distal phalanx fractures that lose soft tissue control of the fragments and displaced transverse basilar fractures may require reduction and pin stabilization for 3 to 4 weeks to achieve rapid union.

Articular fractures of the distal phalanx usually involve the dorsal surface and can be classified with the mallet or

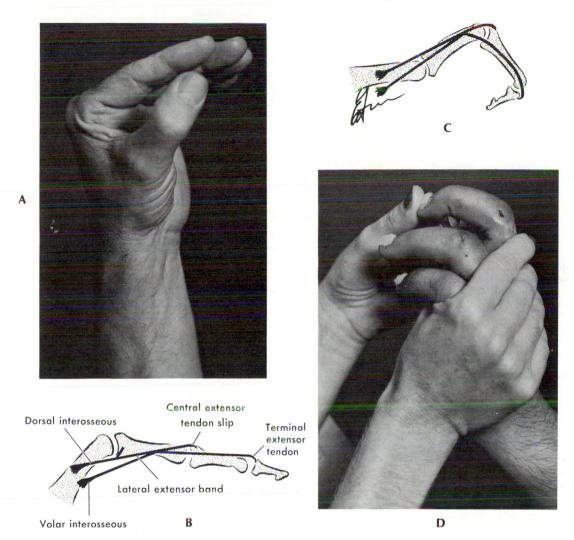

Dorsal interosseous

Central extensor
tendon slip

Terminal
extensor
tendon

Lateral extensor band

Volar interosseous

A   **B**   **C**   **D**

FIG. 15-1. While "clam-digger" position, **A,** prevents joint contractures, intrinsic tendons are being maintained at their shortest length, **B.** To prevent intrinsic contracture, these tendons must be stretched, **C** and **D.**

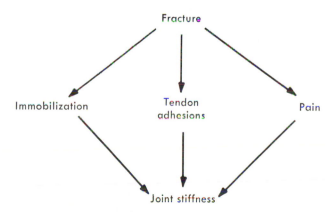

Fracture

Immobilization   Tendon
adhesions   Pain

Joint stiffness

FIG. 15-2. Causes of joint stiffness.

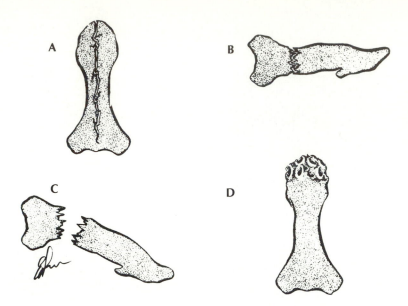

FIG. 15-3. Distal phalanx fractures may be, **A,** longitudinal, **B,** impacted, **C,** displaced transverse basilar, or **D,** tuft. The last is most common.

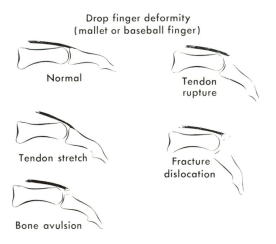

FIG. 15-4. Drop-finger deformity (mallet or baseball finger).

drop-finger deformity (Fig. 15-4). The most common injury producing this deformity is stretching of the terminal extensor tendon. The patient is first seen with a 20- to 35-degree extension lag at the distal joint, but some weak active extension remains. With complete tendon rupture, the tip is dropped 45 degrees. Occasionally, a fragment of bone from the site of extensor insertion is avulsed. On x-ray film the distance the tendon has retracted is indicated by the displacement of the bone chip. Fragments that are minimally displaced (3 mm or less) or extremely small should be treated nonoperatively. A fracture involving one third or more of the articular surface can lead to dislocation of the distal joint, particularly with vigorous splinting into the hyperextended position.

Nonoperative treatment of mallet injuries consists of continuous distal joint immobilization in 10 degrees hyperextension for 6 weeks. Splints may be applied dorsally or volarly (Fig. 15-5). The proximal interphalangeal joint is not immobilized but should be exercised to prevent stiffness. Splinting at night is needed for an additional 2 or 3 weeks should an extensor lag occur.

One final distal phalanx injury to keep in mind is the "football jersey injury." This injury occurs when a football player accidentally grabs his opponent's jersey while missing a tackle, and his finger is forced into the extended position as the runner breaks away. The contracted profundus tendon becomes avulsed from the distal phalanx, often with a piece of bone. Profundus avulsion occurs most commonly in the ring finger and produces tremendous reaction within the tendon sheath. A lateral x-ray film of the digit may reveal a distal phalanx volar avulsion fracture that has retracted with the tendon (Fig. 15-6). Tendon reattachment within the first 2 weeks should restore nearly normal motion.

Therapy program

As soon as the distal phalanx can be mobilized, exercises should be directed toward regaining distal interphalangeal motion and desensitizing the tip area. The more proximal joints of the finger are blocked to isolate flexor profundus and terminal extensor tendon activity. Desensitization of the tip is achieved through progressive activities that begin with rubbing and tapping and proceed to resistive pinching and grasping activities. A painful fingertip will not be incorporated in normal prehension patterns.

PROXIMAL AND MIDDLE PHALANX FRACTURES

Fractures of the proximal and middle phalanges are more difficult to treat than metacarpal or distal phalanx fractures, because of the frequent association of serious tendon and skin injuries as well as instability resulting from lack of soft tissue support. Fracture displacement and angulation are determined by the mechanism of injury and the deforming forces of various tendons attached to each bone fragment.

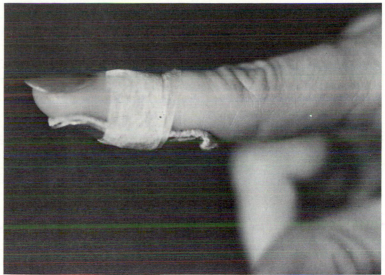

FIG. 15-5. Volar padded metal splint bent to maintain slight distal joint extension can be simply applied and maintained.

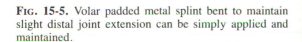

A

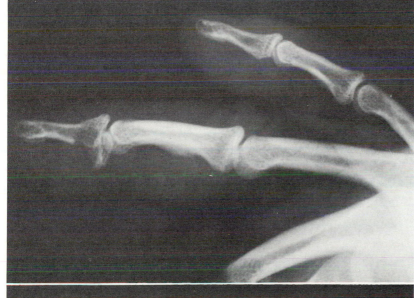

B

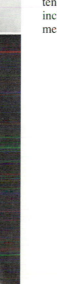

FIG. 15-6. Fractures of distal phalanx volar base can be associated with profundus avulsion, **A.** Sometimes bone fragment becomes displaced with tendon marking distance of retraction. Treatment includes fracture reduction with tendon advancement, **B.**

For instance, a direct blow to a digit may produce a transverse or comminuted fracture, while a twisting force results in an oblique or spiral fracture.

Proximal phalanx fractures occur most commonly on the radial side of the hand (thumb and index finger) and are usually located in a proximal or midshaft area. Such fractures are produced either by a fall or by a direct blunt injury. The characteristic deformity is volar angulation, the interossei flexing the proximal fragment and the central extensor tendon slip extending the distal portion (Fig. 15-7).

The major problem in the management of proximal phalanx fractures is the preservation of proximal interphalangeal joint motion. Stiffness of this joint occurs rapidly as the adjacent tendons become adherent to the fracture callus. A volar collapsed deformity will compound any potential flexion contracture as the extensor and intrinsic tendons are functionally lengthened, preventing full active proximal interphalangeal joint extension. Splint immobilization of the digit eliminates early motion and adds to the stiffness.

Middle phalanx fractures occur with the least frequency of all hand fractures. A crushing injury is the most common cause and the fracture is usually located in the distal portion of the shaft. Fractures of the middle phalanx are displaced by the central slip attachment to the proximal fragment and the broad volar superficialis insertion. Thus a distal fracture will angulate volarly, while a fracture near the phalanx base will have dorsal angulation. The major problem is to obtain

union in a fracture that is frequently comminuted and open while maintaining proximal interphalangeal joint motion.

Before the appropriate treatment is selected, fracture stability must be assessed. The angle of the fracture is an important factor in determining this stability. Transverse fractures are frequently stable, while oblique fractures are inherently unstable. It is also important to know whether the fracture has been impacted or displaced and what deforming forces are acting on it. If there is any question of the fracture's stability, the digit is anesthetized and stress is applied. More than one half of all digital fractures are stable—that is, longitudinal fracture lines in the proximal phalanx (Fig. 15-8). *Such fractures should be started on early protected motion* as soon as pain subsides (within the first 3 to 5 days). Protection is provided by taping the injured finger to the adjacent digit (Fig. 15-9)—a form of dynamic splinting. It may be necessary to rest the finger intermittently in a metal or plaster splint to prevent reinjury while the patient is working or performing heavy activities.

A type of fracture that is potentially unstable is an oblique but nondisplaced proximal phalanx fracture (Fig. 15-10). Early movement may well displace such a fracture, and the finger is best immobilized for 10 to 14 days. Then the digit should be reexamined and radiographed again, and a motion program should be started.

Many displaced fractures become converted to stable fractures after reduction. With sufficient anesthesia, the fracture

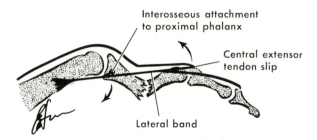

FIG. 15-7. Proximal phalanx fractures angulate volarly, interossei attached to proximal fragment flexing this portion. Central slip extends distal portion.

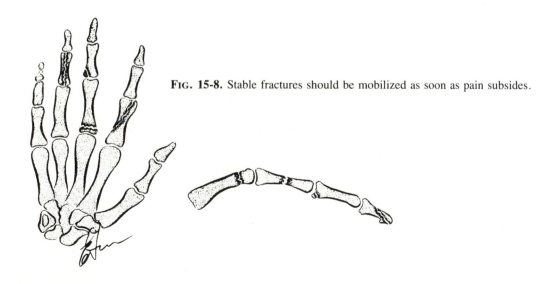

FIG. 15-8. Stable fractures should be mobilized as soon as pain subsides.

is manipulated and the controllable distal fragment aligned with the proximal fragment. A splint is applied after reduction to stabilize and maintain this position. One form of immobilization is a plaster gutter that includes the adjacent noninjured finger for support and alignment and to judge rotation. The fingers are placed in the clam-digger position with the least amount of proximal interphalangeal flexion necessary to maintain reduction. A second technique is to incorporate a metal splint or padded bent wire into plaster and tape the finger to this splint. The advantage of this latter method is that the finger can be easily observed and radiographed for any shift of the fracture, since no plaster intervenes (Fig. 15-11).

Several other treatment techniques previously recommended have been discarded owing to the complications encountered. Traction is now indicated only when bone loss or severe comminution is being treated. Skin traction has been known to produce circulatory compromise and pulp traction necrosis, while nail traction often results in loss of the nail. Banjo splints, gauze rolls placed in the palm, and various commercial splints have been discredited.

Unstable fractures will require supplemental fixation, usually with a Kirschner wire or pin, to maintain the correct position. Closed reduction of some fractures is possible with pins inserted percutaneously to provide stabilization. Such a technique allows early motion and prevents the adhesions inherent with open reduction, when the extensor mechanism must be split and the periosteum reflected. Percutaneous pinning is best applied to proximal phalanx fractures. Pins may be started proximally at the wide metaphyseal flares

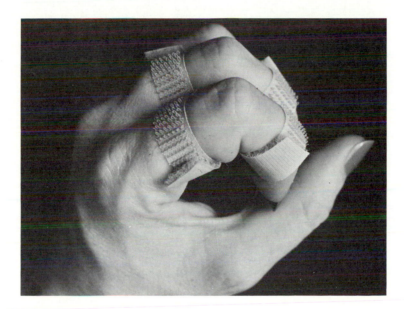

FIG. 15-9. Adjacent digit taping encourages motion while providing protection.

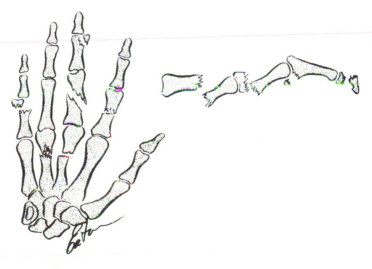

FIG. 15-10. Unstable fractures require reduction and immobilization. Pin fixation may be needed.

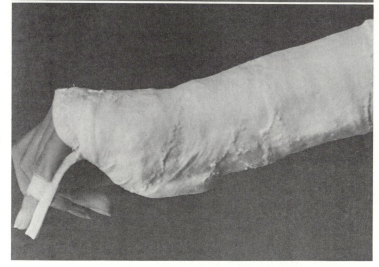

FIG. 15-11. Plaster gutter splint, **A,** can maintain reduction with adjacent finger for support and to control alignment. Metal splint, **B,** incorporated into plaster requires tape to maintain fracture position. X-ray reevaluation is more easily achieved.

and advanced distally across the fracture site. Transverse fractures are difficult to treat using a percutaneous technique, and such treatment is contraindicated for comminuted or displaced intra-articular fractures (Fig. 15-12).

Open reduction is indicated in certain problem fractures, the most common being unstable fractures not amenable to closed reduction and splinting or percutaneous pinning (see list). In the proximal phalanx, this frequently includes basilar fractures with volar angulation greater than 25 degrees, displaced transverse shaft fractures, oblique fractures, and neck fractures. Displaced articular fractures (greater than 2 mm) and those that involve a single condyle with rotation will require internal fixation. Fractures incompletely reduced or with fragments poorly positioned such that malunion is likely need to undergo open reduction.

Hand fractures for which open reduction and fixation are indicated
Unstable fractures
Inadequately reduced fractures
Open fractures
Associated soft tissue problems
Multiple fractures
Articular fractures
Bone loss

Open fractures occur frequently (25% to 35%). If they are unstable or if tendon injuries or serious soft tissue management problems coexist, internal fixation is indicated. The presence of an open fracture in the hand is not a contraindication to pin or wire fixation as it might be with large-bone fractures. The fracture stabilization that can be provided by internal fixation will make treatment of a tendon injury easier. Attention may be directed toward the restoration of tendon gliding without fear of displacing the fracture. The management of soft tissue injuries such as a potential skin slough following a crush injury is only compounded by trying to maintain the fracture position with a plaster cast rather than utilizing pin fixation. Delayed closure is indicated in wounds with contamination or questionable tissue viability.

Multiple fractures in the hand occur more frequently (9%) than one might expect. Unless aggressively treated, stiffness of many digits will result. Pin or wire stabilization of fractures that are amenable to such treatment will greatly facilitate an early motion program.

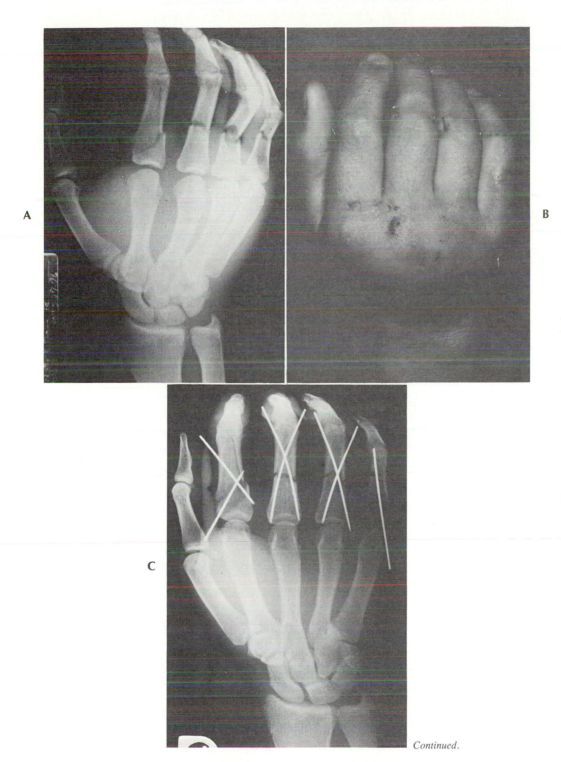

Continued.

FIG. 15-12. M.H., 19-year-old male, sustained crush injury to right hand in hamburger machine with displaced unstable transverse proximal phalanx fractures in all fingers, **A.** Closed reduction and percutaneous pin fixation, **B** and **C,** was followed by early (1-week) exercise program and splint protection. At 9 weeks patient had regained near normal motion and returned to work, **D** to **H.**

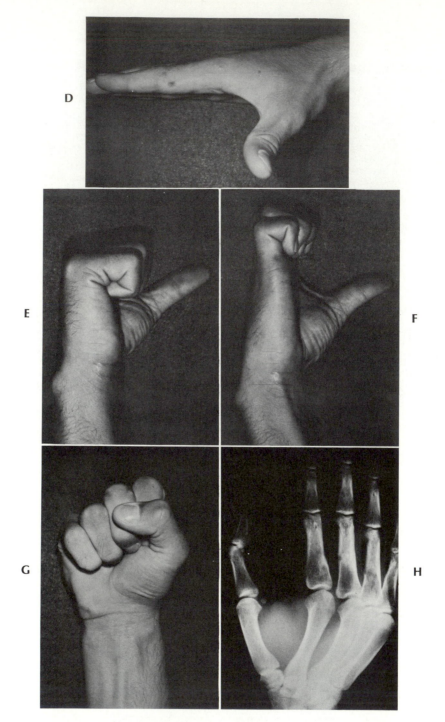

FIG. 15-12, cont'd. For legend see p. 187.

Bone loss in the hand, such as is caused by gunshot wounds, is a subject that has received insufficient attention. When a portion of a metacarpal is lost, temporary pin stabilization and delayed bone grafting are indicated. In the finger such reconstruction should be undertaken only when reasonably good eventual function can be anticipated. The goal of internal fixation is to achieve sufficient stabilization of fracture fragments to allow early protective motion.

The questions most frequently asked regarding fractures are: how long does it take to heal, when can motion be started, and how much splinting is necessary (and for how long)? The average time for a phalangeal fracture to show complete bone union on radiographs is 5 months, with a range of 1 to 14 months. The question is better phrased: when is a fracture solid enough to allow unprotected motion? For most closed nondisplaced fractures, motion should commence in the first 21 days, depending on stability. Immobilization for longer than 3 weeks will lead to stiffness and

Fracture consolidation time

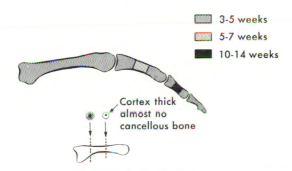

FIG. 15-13. Fracture consolidation varies within each segment of hand and is slowest where ratio of cortical to cancellous bone is highest (after Moberg).

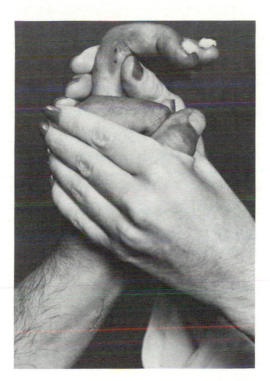

FIG. 15-14. Manual support of proximal phalanx fracture is provided by therapist while encouraging active proximal interphalangeal flexion by patient.

loss of hand function. Fractures of the tapered midshaft region of the phalanges, however, require a longer time to become consolidated (Fig. 15-13). In this area the cortical bone is thick, with minimal cancellous bone. Protection in the form of intermittent splinting for midshaft proximal phalanx fractures is needed for 5 to 7 weeks and in the middle phalanx for 10 to 14 weeks. Gentle motion protecting the fracture site is initiated at 3 weeks. The presence of pins stabilizing a fracture should not prevent an exercise program. Comminuted fractures and those requiring open reduction will take longer to become solid, and prolonged protection is necessary.

Therapy program

If internal fixation has provided satisfactory fracture stabilization, the patient is mobilized as soon as pain permits (5 to 15 days). Stable fractures or ones that have been splinted 3 weeks may be treated in a similar manner.

The goal in the treatment of proximal phalanx fractures is to attain maximal proximal interphalangeal joint motion while preventing a flexion contracture. Tendon adhesions at the fracture site are the main cause of joint stiffness. The therapist provides additional manual support at the level of the fracture while encouraging active proximal interphalangeal flexion and extension (Fig. 15-14). The injured digit is immobilized in the clam-digger position when not undergoing exercise, until the fracture is consolidated. Intrinsic stretching is mandatory to prevent contracture (Fig. 15-1). While the dorsal and lateral tendons frequently adhere, the fibro-osseous flexor sheath must be violated by the bone for flexor tendon adhesions to occur (Fig. 15-15). Thus the therapist, exercising a nondisplaced fracture, will encounter little difficulty in having the tendons glide by the fracture, while the converse is true of a markedly displaced fracture.

The most serious complication following a proximal phalanx fracture is a proximal interphalangeal joint flexion contracture. At rest, the hand assumes a position of proximal interphalangeal joint flexion, and this position can become fixed. The proximal interphalangeal joint must be splinted at neutral or as close to neutral as possible until the likelihood of a contracture ceases (usually by 5 weeks). When the fracture is considered solid (Fig. 15-13), a dynamic splinting program can commence, alternating dynamic flexion (flexion cuff) with extension (reverse finger knuckle bender or Capener splint).

The primary objective with middle phalanx fractures is to achieve full motion in the two more proximal joints, the metacarpophalangeal and proximal interphalangeal joints. The goal is to achieve a ''superficialis hand.'' If prolonged splinting includes the proximal phalanx, the proximal interphalangeal joint will become stiff. Thus fractures of the middle phalanx that will require longer than 3 weeks to consolidate should have pin stabilization to allow early motion. Later the distal joint will be exercised and the oblique retinacular ligament stretched to overcome contracture (Fig. 15-16).

METACARPAL FRACTURES

Fractures of the metacarpals can be classified for treatment by their location (head, neck, shaft, base). The event leading to a fracture in this area is usually a fight or a fall. Metacarpal fractures generally are more stable than phalangeal fractures because of the support provided the bones by the intrinsic musculature. Flexor and extensor tendons are not in close contact with the bone and become adherent less frequently. However, an intrinsic contracture can occur easily from swelling and direct trauma to the intrinsic muscles. The metacarpophalangeal joint, unless carefully splinted, can develop an extension contracture.

The most common metacarpal fractures involve the neck, where the bone is weakest. Comminution of the volar cortex allows collapse into the flexed position. Reduction should be attempted by flexing the metacarpophalangeal and proximal interphalangeal joints 90 degrees and pushing the metacarpal head into position. The proximal interphalangeal joint should never be left in this fixed position, since a flexion contracture may develop. It should be held with a plaster gutter or cast in the clam-digger position. Motion is begun at 2 to 3 weeks after removal of the splint, with further protection for 2 more weeks. With severe angulation of the fracture, clawing may result from collapse of the tendon system and will require fixation of the reduced fracture. Hunter has shown, however, that as much as 70 degrees volar angulation is acceptable as long as no malrotation is present.[2]

Transverse metacarpal shaft fractures develop dorsal angulation and are usually caused by a direct blow (Fig. 15-

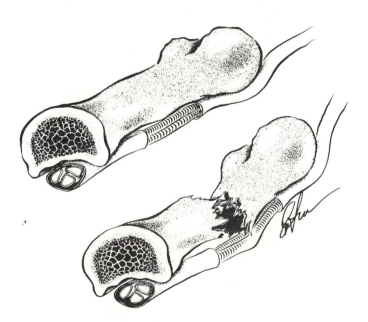

FIG. 15-15. Fracture disruption of fibro-osseous flexor tendon sheath will encourage tendon adherence at fracture site.

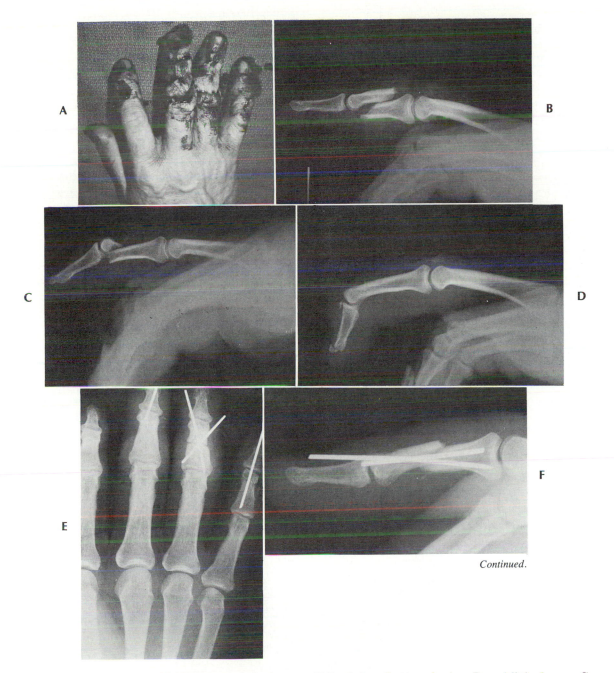

Continued.

FIG. 15-16. C.F., 35-year-old machinist, sustained open middle phalanx fractures in ring, **B,** and little fingers, **C,** and extensor tendon disruption in middle finger, **A** and **D.** Fracture reduction (ring and little), **F** and **G,** and distal joint stabilization with extensor repair (middle), **H,** was followed with early (10 days) mobilization, **E.** At 3 weeks good proximal interphalangeal flexion was attained, **I** and **J,** and by 12 weeks patient had regained sufficient motion and strength to return to work, **K** to **M.**

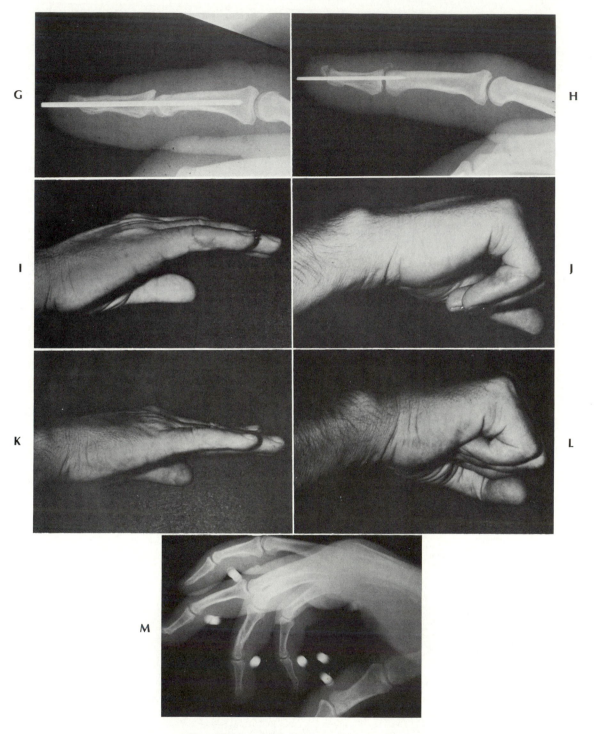

Fig. 15-16, cont'd. For legend see p. 191.

17). Fractures in the midshaft of the third and fourth metacarpals frequently occur simultaneously and will disrupt the transverse arch unless correctly reduced. Reduction of the fracture can be maintained with pin fixation. Stabilization should be attempted percutaneously with a longitudinal wire to control angulation and possibly a transverse pin to prevent malrotation.

Oblique metacarpal fractures are caused by a torque force with the finger acting as a lever arm. The result will be shortening and rotation but no angulation. The third and fourth metacarpals shorten least, owing to the tethering effect of the interossei and the transverse metacarpal ligament. Two to three millimeters of shortening is acceptable, but anything further requires internal fixation.

Comminuted metacarpal fractures are produced by crush injuries, such as those that occur in punch-press accidents. Sometimes such fractures are minimally displaced and can be treated with a gutter splint for 3 weeks, followed by gentle motion and 3 more weeks protection. Displaced or unstable fractures can be easily controlled with transverse pins.

Metacarpal bone loss, such as in a gunshot wound, will usually have an associated soft tissue problem that will command primary attention. Transverse and possibly longitudinal pins will control the fracture, and secondary bone grafting will make up for the bone loss.

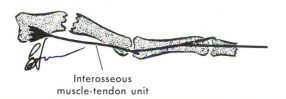

Interosseous
muscle-tendon unit

FIG. 15-17. Metacarpal fractures angulate dorsally as intrinsic muscles lie palmarward and tendons pass volar to axis of metacarpophalangeal joint.

Therapy program

The objectives of treatment in metacarpal fractures are elimination of edema, maintenance of architectural integrity, and prevention of contractures.

Excessive dorsal edema characterizes metacarpal fractures. Initially, constant elevation can lessen the swelling. Motion, massage, and intermittent compression will also reduce edema later in the therapy program.

With second- and third-metacarpal fractures, the transverse arch of the hand must be supported by the therapist during exercising and with a splint when the hand is at rest. After a fracture of the first metacarpal, the thumb web space must be protected with a splint to prevent contracture (Fig. 15-18).

Extension contractures of the metacarpophalangeal joints can easily occur unless these joints are immobilized in 60 to 70 degrees flexion. This may require frequent fabrication of a new clam-digger splints as edema diminishes.

SUMMARY

Many of the serious complications that can occur after hand fractures (see list) may be prevented by observing a few basic principles. The safe position for immobilizing a fractured hand is the clam-digger, or intrinsic-positive, position. Early protective motion is the best means of preventing joint stiffness or contracture.

Complications following hand fractures
Joint stiffness
Joint contractures, especially flexion contractures
Pain
Weakness
Intrinsic contractures
Chronic edema
Tendon adherence
Malrotation
Associated injuries (for example, soft tissue loss, nerve, vascular)
Reflex asympathetic dystrophy
Infection
Nonunion

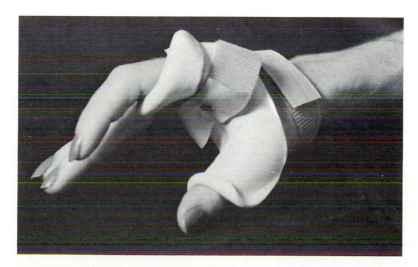

FIG. 15-18. Thumb web-space contracture can occur after any injury producing significant dorsal edema (that is, burn, crush, fracture). Resting splint can protect against such an occurrence.

REFERENCES

1. Flynn, J.E.: Hand surgery, ed. 2, Philadelphia, 1975, The Williams & Wilkins Co.
2. Hunter, J.M., and Cowen, N.J.: Fifth metacarpal fractures in a compensation clinic population, J. Bone Joint Surg. **52A:**1159-1165, 1970.
3. Rockwood, C.A., and Green, D.P.: Fractures, Philadelphia, 1975, J.B. Lippincott Co.

BIBLIOGRAPHY

Barton, N.: Fractures of the phalanges of the hand, Hand **9:**1-10, 1977.

Bloem, J.J.A.M.: The treatment and prognosis of uncomplicated dislocated fractures of the metacarpals and phalanges, Arch. Chir. Neerl. **23:**55-65, 1971.

Borgeskov, S.: Conservative therapy for fractures of the phalanges and metacarpals, Acta Chir. Scand. **133:**123-130, 1967.

Burton, R.I., and Eaton, R.G.: Common hand injuries in the athlete, Orthop. Clin. North Am. **4:**809-839, 1973.

Butt, W.D.: Fractures of the hand. I. Description, Can. Med. Assoc. J. **86:**731-735, 1962.

Butt, W.D.: Fractures of the hand. II. Statistical review, Can. Med. Assoc. J. **86:**775-779, 1962.

Butt, W.D.: Fractures of the hand. III. Treatment and results, Can. Med. Assoc. J. **86:**815-822, 1962.

Carroll, R.E., and Match, R.M.: Avulsion of the flexor profundus tendon insertion, J. Trauma **10:**1109-1118, 1970.

Clinkscales, G.S., Jr.: Complications in the management of fractures in hand injuries, South. Med. J. **63:**704-707, 1970.

Coonrad, R.W., and Pohlman, M.H.: Impacted fractures in the proximal portion of the proximal phalanx of the finger, J. Bone Joint Surg. **51A:**1291-1296, 1969.

Crawford, G.P.: Screw fixation for certain fractures of the phalanges and metacarpals, J. Bone Joint Surg. **58A:**487-492, 1976.

Dobyns, J.H.: Articular fractures of the hand, J. Bone Joint Surg. **48A:**610, 1966.

Flatt, A.E.: The care of minor hand injuries, ed. 4, St. Louis, 1979, The C.V. Mosby Co.

Green, D.P., and Anderson, J.R.: Closed reduction and percutaneous pin fixation of the fractured phalanges, J. Bone Joint Surg. **55A:**1651-1654, 1973.

Howard, L.D., Jr.: Fractures of the small hand bones, Plast. Reconstr. Surg. **29:**334-335, 1962.

James, J.I.P.: Fractures of the proximal and middle phalanges of the fingers, Acta Orthop. Scand. **32:**401-412, 1962.

James, J.I.P.: Common, simple errors in the management of hand injuries, Proc. R. Soc. Med. **63:**69-71, 1970.

Kilbourne, B.C.: Management of complicated hand fractures, Surg. Clin. North Am. **48:**201-213, 1968.

Lipscomb, P.R.: Management of fractures of the hand, Am. Surg. **29:**277-282, 1963.

Milford, L.: The hand. In Edmonson, A.S., and Crenshaw, A.H., editors: Campbell's operative orthopedics, ed. 6, St. Louis, 1980, The C.V. Mosby Co.

Moberg, E.: Emergency surgery of the hand, Edinburgh, 1968, E & S Livingstone.

Peacock, E.E.: Management of conditions of the hand requiring immobilization, Surg. Clin. North Am. **33:**1297-1309, 1953.

Riordan, D.C.: Fractures about the hand, South. Med. J. **50:**637-640, 1957.

Ruedi, T.P., Burri, C., and Pfeiffer, K.M.: Stable internal fixation of fractures of the hand, J. Trauma **11:**381-389, 1971.

Smith, F.L., and Rider, D.L.: A study of the healing of one hundred consecutive phalangeal fractures, J. Bone Joint Surg. **17:**91-109, 1935.

Stark, H.H.: Troublesome fractures and dislocations of the hand. In AAOS: Instructional course lectures, vol. 19, St. Louis, 1970, The C.V. Mosby Co. pp. 130-149.

Sutro, C.J.: Fracture of metacarpal bones and proximal manual phalanges: treatment with emphasis on the prevention of rotational deformities, Am. J. Surg. **81:**327-332, 1951.

Swanson, A.B.: Fractures involving the digits of the hand, Orthop. Clin. North Am. **1:**261-274, 1970.

Watson-Jones, R.: Fractures and joint injuries, ed. 3, Edinburgh, 1943, E & S Livingstone.

Weeks, P.M., and Wray, R.C.: Management of acute hand injuries: a biological approach, ed. 2, St. Louis, 1978, The C.V. Mosby Co.

Wright, T.A.: Early mobilization in fractures of the metacarpals and phalanges, Can. J. Surg. **11:**491-498, 1968.

16

Joint injuries in the hand: preservation of proximal interphalangeal joint function

ROBERT LEE WILSON and MARGARET S. CARTER

Trauma to the small joints in the hand is frequently treated as a trivial injury. However, the stiffness, pain, and occasional instability that may occur in these joints after injury or prolonged immobilization may seriously restrict hand function. The most important small hand joints are the proximal interphalangeal joints. This chapter will deal with trauma to this most critical articulation. Other sources provide a comprehensive view of injuries to the remaining joints in the hand.[2,3,5] First, to better understand the pathomechanics of proximal interphalangeal joint injuries, we review the anatomic features of this joint.

ANATOMY

The proximal interphalangeal joint is hinged in the sagittal plane and has considerable stability as contrasted to the metacarpophalangeal joint.[6,7] Lateral stability is provided by the bicondylar head of the proximal phalanx with its convex condyles and intercondylar groove, which articulate with the concave condyles and intercondylar ridge of the middle phalanx base. These articular surfaces are only slightly incongruous allowing minimal lateral and torsional movements.[8] The width of this joint is twice the vertical height. The collateral ligaments enclose both sides of the joint arising from the proximal phalanx condyles and attach to the volar base of the middle phalanx and volar plate. The proximal interphalangeal collateral ligaments are under constant tension throughout the entire arc of motion in contrast to those of the metacarpophalangeal joint, which are relaxed in extension and tightened in flexion. The accessory collateral ligament, a more anterior continuation, attaches to and suspends the volar plate and flexor tendon sheath. The accessory ligament is more flexible and folds during maximal joint flexion. The fibrocartilaginous volar plate surrounds the anterior aspect of the proximal interphalangeal joint acting as a gliding surface for the proximal phalanx condyles on one side and the flexor tendons on the other. The proximal lateral portion of the volar plate is thickened and attached to the proximal phalanx to check or prevent joint hyperextension. Synovial recesses are present both dorsally and volarly. Prolonged joint immobilization particularly in the flexed position will obliterate these spaces with volar plate and collateral ligament adherence. Although the dorsal capsule may also become adherent, contracture

in this more pliable dorsal tissue takes longer to develop. Therefore the recommended position for immobilization of the proximal interphalangeal joint is 0 to 15 degrees of flexion (Fig. 16-1).

The stability provided by this capsular-ligamentous structure is supplemented by several tendons passing around the joint. The central slip of the long extensor tendon inserts into the dorsal tubercle of the middle phalanx and extends the proximal interphalangeal joint. The lateral bands, receiving contributions from the intrinsic and the extrinsic extensor tendons, pass laterally about both sides of the joint and lie dorsal to the proximal interphalangeal joint axis. The transverse retinacular ligament runs from the anterior border of the lateral band to the flexor sheath at the level of the joint and prevents dorsal displacement of the lateral bands. Landsmeer's oblique retinacular ligament begins at the flexor sheath over the proximal phalanx, lies volar to the axis of motion of the proximal interphalangeal joint, and attaches to the terminal extensor tendon. With proximal interphalangeal joint extension the oblique retinacular ligament tightens, pulling the terminal extensor tendon proximally and preventing passive distal joint flexion. This ligament also prevents proximal interphalangeal joint hyperextension (Fig. 16-2).

Thus a number of factors contribute to proximal interphalangeal joint stability, the most important being the base of the middle phalanx, the volar plate, and the collateral ligaments. The key point is where these three structures intersect. To dislocate the proximal interphalangeal joint, at least one and sometimes all three of these structures must be damaged.

However, it is the stability of the proximal interphalangeal joint that makes it susceptible to injury. The metacarpophalangeal joint is anatomically dissimilar, having lateral movement as well as flexion and extension. Thus, when the finger is struck at the tip such as with a baseball, the force is dissipated at the metacarpophalangeal joint because of the mobility but concentrated at the proximal interphalangeal joint.

EVALUATION

The first step in examining the patient who has sustained an injury about the proximal interphalangeal joint is to de-

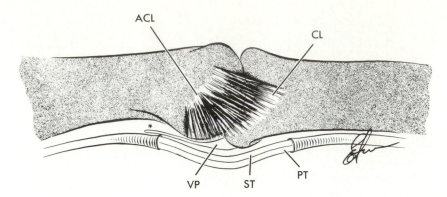

FIG. 16-1. Proximal interphalangeal joint in lateral view showing collateral, *CL,* and accessory collateral ligaments, *ACL,* attaching to middle phalanx and volar plate, *VP.* Flexor tendon sheath containing superficialis, *ST,* and profundus tendons, *PT,* is closely attached to periosteum of phalanges and volar plate. Recess (*) is present between volar plate and phalanx.

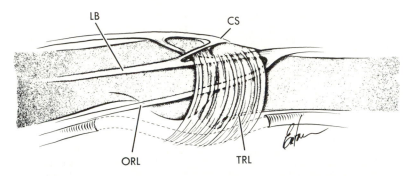

FIG. 16-2. Diagram of proximal interphalangeal joint, emphasizing digital extensor mechanism. Central extensor tendon slip, *CS,* extends proximal interphalangeal joint. Lateral bands, *LB,* are supported by transverse retinacular ligament, *TRL,* and along with oblique retinacular ligament, *ORL,* provide coordinated distal joint extension.

termine the mechanism of injury (hyperextension, lateral dislocation, and so on). The area about the proximal interphalangeal joint should be carefully palpated, especially over each collateral ligament and the volar plate, to localize any area of tenderness and tissue damage. Note that the radial collateral ligament is injured more frequently than the ulnar. A digital nerve block should be performed before one stresses the joint if the injured finger is painful. Each collateral ligament should be stressed, and confirmatory roentgenograms should be taken if there is any question of joint stability. Next, active flexion and extension of the injured digit by the patient will determine if joint stability is present throughout the full flexion arc. Frequently after hyperextension injuries, the joint will redislocate in the last 20 degrees of extension. If dislocation occurs with active motion, the joint is considered functionally unstable.

In the following discussion, injuries about the proximal interphalangeal joint have been arranged arbitrarily into six categories (see list). Although they are discussed individually, one must remember that these joint injuries can occur in combination.

Proximal interphalangeal joint injuries
1. Collateral ligaments
2. Dorsal dislocations

   a. Acute
   b. Chronic
3. Volar dislocations
4. Articular fractures
5. Boutonnière deformities
6. Pseudoboutonnière deformities

COLLATERAL LIGAMENT INJURIES

Unilateral stress to the extended finger can produce a collateral ligament injury. The injuries are of varying degrees of severity, from complete disruption to sprains (functionally intact ligament but with diffuse individual fiber disruption). Although stress testing will reveal the relatively infrequent complete ligament rupture, no clinical test can differentiate between minimal ligament injury and almost complete ligament disruption. Ligaments are notoriously slow to heal, and symptoms vary with the extent of ligament damage, persisting for many months.

Ligament sprains that are stable to stress and active motion testing are immobilized until the acute discomfort subsides—usually from 3 to 10 days. The joint and ligament are further protected when the injured finger is taped to the adjacent digit (Fig. 16-3). Easily adjustable Velcro loops may be substituted for adhesive tape. This protection may

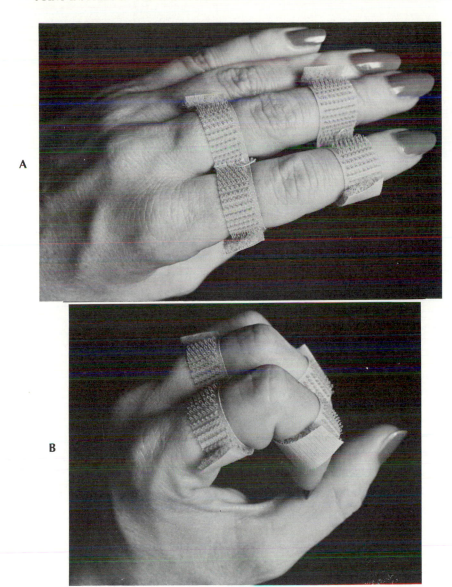

FIG. 16-3. Adjacent digit taping (seen here with Velcro loops) provides protection by keeping fingers together in extension, **A**, as well as flexion, *B*.

need to be continued for months to prevent minor reinjuries that can prolong the healing period and disability.

Partial or almost complete ligament tears may require immobilization up to 3 weeks. With any collateral ligament injury, the adjacent lateral band may adhere to the ligament (Fig. 16-4). For prevention of this adherence from becoming a contracture, intrinsic stretching must be incorporated into the exercise program.

Lateral dislocations are produced by shear stress. The collateral ligament is ruptured at the proximal phalangeal achment and often is displaced into the joint. Incomplete transverse tears into the volar plate are associated with this injury. Treatment of complete ligament rupture remains controversial, with some authors recommending splinting of the reduced joint for 3 weeks whereas immediate surgical repair is advised by others.[12-14] Joints that are grossly unstable (that is, an additional 25 degrees or more of lateral

deviation on stress testing) should be explored, and the extent of damage assessed. Volar plate repair and collateral ligament reattachment may be necessary. After surgery, the joint is immobilized for 3 weeks in the extended position and then gradually mobilized. Further splinting is usually necessary.

Therapy considerations

Successful management of collateral ligament injuries is largely the result of patient education. The principle objectives in a therapy program are mobilization of the joint to overcome stiffness, prevention of proximal interphalangeal flexion contractures, and protection from recurrent injuries. Patients are placed on a treatment program of specific exercises and splinting. Counseling as to the potential seriousness of the injury and the length of time required for ligament healing must be provided early and reinforced fre-

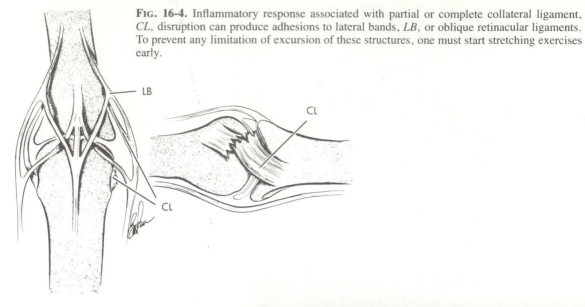

FIG. 16-4. Inflammatory response associated with partial or complete collateral ligament, *CL,* disruption can produce adhesions to lateral bands, *LB,* or oblique retinacular ligaments. To prevent any limitation of excursion of these structures, one must start stretching exercises early.

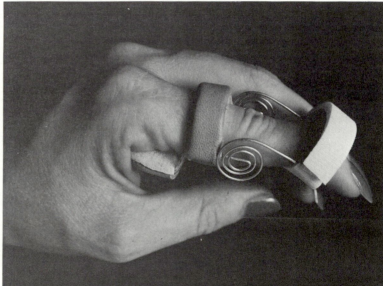

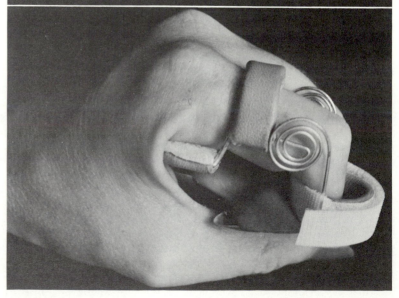

FIG. 16-5. Capener splint provides dynamic extension assist, with wires closely paralleling collateral ligaments in extension, **A,** and in flexion, **B.**

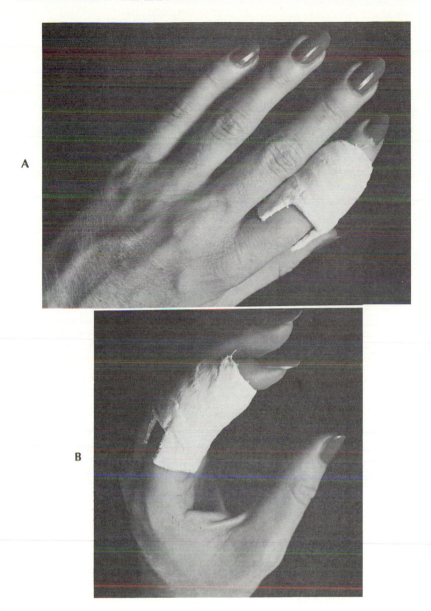

FIG. 16-6. Plaster finger casts are cut out dorsally, **A,** in order to slip past an enlarged joint. Proximal interphalangeal joint is thus statically maintained in maximal extension, **B,** to combat any tendency for increasing flexion contracture.

quently during the many months of healing. Reevaluation of joint motion and circumference measurements are made frequently, and the exercise program is altered accordingly. A directed exercise program includes stretching of the intrinsic tendons and retinacular ligaments, isolated intrinsic exercises, and a graduated progressive resistive exercise program to increase grip and pinch strength. Significant weakness of grip frequently accompanies ligament injuries.

All exercises are performed for 3 to 5 minutes and repeated every hour over the course of the day to prevent further joint swelling. Antiinflammatory agents (phenylbutazone, oxyphenbutazone) may decrease joint swelling but should only be used for a short course. When persistent pain or swelling becomes localized to one area, an injection of a cortisone type of drug is frequently beneficial. Edema

of the digit and hand can be controlled through the use of the Jobst Intermittent Compression Unit, elevation, heat, and retrograde massage. A splinting regime must provide protection, prevent flexion contractures, and increase active flexion and extension.

Dynamic daytime splinting besides the digital taping or Velcro loops might include a Capener splint (Fig. 16-5) because it provides ideal protection with the lateral wires adjacent to the collateral ligaments. The digital taping must be altered with a dynamic extension splint such as a reverse knuckle bender is a flexion contracture is noted.

Static night splinting with either a metal splint or serial finger cast (Fig. 16-6) cut out proximally and dorsally to accommodate joint swelling will rest the finger in an optimal position. Night splinting should be instituted with the appearance of any flexion contractures. To establish maximal proximal interphalangeal motion, one has the constant dilemma with either exercising or splinting of attaining full joint flexion while preventing a flexion deformity.

DORSAL DISLOCATIONS

Dorsal displacement of the proximal interphalangeal joint is the most common acute dislocation. This injury may occur in association with a mallet finger injury. Proximal interphalangeal dorsal dislocations can be produced by a longitudinal force on the extended finger, as when a baseball strikes the digit's tip with the interphalangeal joints in extension. The proximal phalangeal head divides the volar plate insertion at the middle phalangeal base. This injury may include an avulsion of the volar plate, a collateral ligament tear, or a middle phalangeal fracture. After x-ray evaluation and digital nerve block, the dislocation is reduced by traction and flexion. After postreduction roentgenograms, lateral stress testing determines collateral ligament integrity. Then joint stability through a full arc of flexion is assessed (see boxed material).

If the dislocation after reduction is stable and has no fracture, the proximal interphalangeal joint is splinted in 25 degrees flexion for 3 weeks to allow soft tissue healing. If the middle phalangeal base is fractured, but on postreduction roentgenograms the fracture fragment is not displaced and the joint is stable through an active range of motion, immobilization for 3 weeks should be sufficient. Fractures involving less than one quarter of the middle phalangeal base are usually stable.

The proximal interphalangeal joint that is unstable, redislocating with active extension but demonstrating no fracture, has disruption of both the volar plate and collateral ligaments. In the nonsurgical approach to this problem, a dorsal metal splint is incorporated in a plaster cast immobilizing the hand and wrist. The dorsal metal splint is bent so as to limit the last 25 degrees of proximal interphalangeal extension, thus blocking dorsal dislocation (Fig. 16-7). This splint should be continued for 5 weeks with the joint exercised by active flexion. This same program is also applicable to the stable injuries previously mentioned.

Unstable dorsal dislocations with displaced fractures require open reduction. The joint is best approached through a volar zigzag incision. Large fracture fragments are reattached to the middle of the phalanx with Kirschner wires. If multiple small fragments are present, these are excised and the volar plate is advanced into the middle phalangeal defect with a pullout wire. If the injury is old or the treatment is delayed, first the adherent dorsal capsule and extensor tendon must be released and then the contracted collateral ligaments divided to allow reduction (Fig. 16-8).

Volar plate advancement will prevent redislocation; the transarticular wire holds the joint surfaces in the reduced position. Three weeks after surgery this pin is removed, and the patient is started on active and active assisted proximal interphalangeal flexion exercises. By 5 weeks a dynamic flexion splint can usually be added, and at 7 weeks extension splinting is begun (Fig. 16-9).

A chronic dorsal subluxation or dislocation may occur if a middle phalangeal base fracture is unrecognized or untreated. If, at exploration, collapse of the middle phalanx is encountered and the amount of joint damage minimal, an opening wedge osteotomy can reestablish the volar buttress. Frequently, the amount of articular damage is so severe that fragment excision and volar plate advancement arthroplasty are necessary.[1]

A common sequela of untreated proximal interphalangeal hyperextension injuries is the swan-neck deformity, which occurs from damage to the volar plate and collateral and retinacular ligaments. Surgery to correct this established deformity is indicated if the joint becomes locked in the hyperextended position. Pain produced by damage to the articular surface is a surgical contraindication to soft-tissue reconstruction alone. Numerous surgical procedures have been advocated. Curtis[2] recommends dividing one slip of the superficialis and attaching it to the proximal phalanx, producing a tenodesis effect. Littler[9] reconstructs the oblique retinacular ligament using a portion of the lateral band, which has been detached proximally, tunneled volarly to Cleland's ligament, and attached to the flexor tendon sheath over the proximal phalanx to prevent proximal interphalangeal hyperextension.

If painful partial ankylosis of the dislocated proximal interphalangeal joint is present, arthrodesis or implant arthroplasty may be indicated.

VOLAR DISLOCATIONS

Volar or anterior proximal interphalangeal joint dislocations are infrequent injuries. Experiments in which stress was applied to cadaver joints revealed that two forces are necessary to produce volar displacement. An angular or lateral force produced collateral ligament avulsion and a tear that extended through the transverse retinacular ligament

---

Treatment: acute dorsal dislocations

1. Stable: no fractures	Splint 25 degrees flexion—3 weeks
2. Stable: fracture nondisplaced	Splint 25 degrees flexion—3 weeks
3. Unstable: no fracture	Dorsal block—5 weeks
4. Unstable: fracture displaced	Open reduction or dorsal block
5. Comminuted fracture	Volar plate advancement

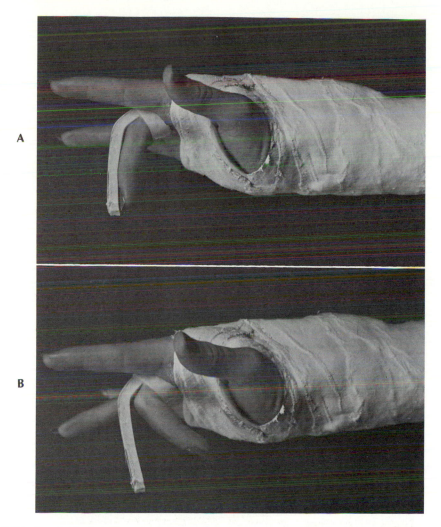

FIG. 16-7. With dorsal block splint, proximal phalanx is taped to splint, limiting extension, **A,** while allowing flexion, *B*.

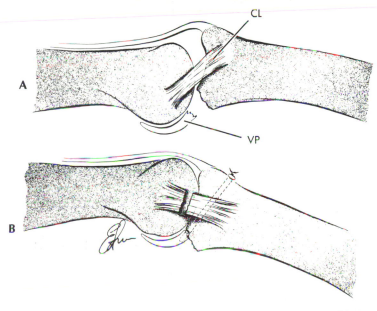

FIG. 16-8. To reduce dorsal dislocation, **A,** any dorsal capsule adhesions or collateral ligament, *CL,* contractures must be released. Small fracture fragments are removed and volar plate, *VP,* is advanced into defect with wire suture, **B.**

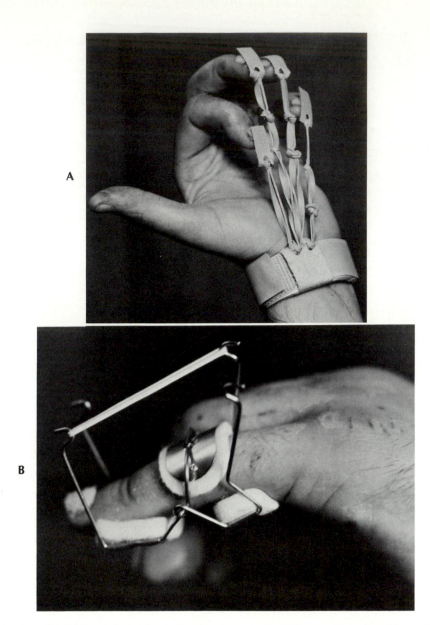

Fig. 16-9. Direction of pull of each finger should be toward scaphoid, **A.** Reverse finger knuckle bender, **B,** or Capener splint can give dynamic extension.

and volar plate. A volarly or anteriorly directed force ruptured the central extensor tendon attachment to the middle phalanx and produced a boutonnière deformity.

Anterior or lateral dislocations may be irreducible with either the lateral band interposed or the proximal phalanx forced through the extensor mechanism and trapped. If this dislocation is capable of being reduced and the joint is congruent on follow-up examination with an extensor lag of 30 degrees or less, splinting the proximal interphalangeal joint in the extended position is the recommended treatment. More frequently, open reduction with repair of all injured structures will be necessary. Treatment for chronic anterior dislocation requires reconstruction of the collateral ligament and central tendon plus release of the tight retinacular ligaments. Thus what appears to be a straightforward bouton-

nière deformity may be a more complex injury with multiple structures damaged. Testing the collateral ligament and volar plate integrity may confirm this severe injury.

FRACTURES

Articular fractures can involve the proximal interphalangeal joint, the head of the proximal phalanx being the most common location (Fig. 16-10). To evaluate fully any injury to a small joint in the hand, one should take three roentgenograms (anteroposterior, lateral, and oblique) to rule out an obscure but potentially dangerous fracture. Joint fractures are classified by their stability, displacement, and amount of joint involvement. Stable, minimally displaced fractures should be immobilized for 3 weeks and then begun on gentle motion with further protection by splinting for 3

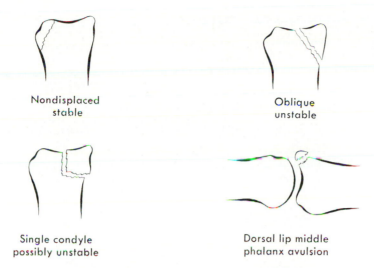

Nondisplaced
stable

Oblique
unstable

Single condyle
possibly unstable

Dorsal lip middle
phalanx avulsion

FIG. 16-10. Articular fractures of proximal interphalangeal joint can be nondisplaced, unstable, involve single condyle with rotation, or avulse central slip at middle phalanx base dorsally.

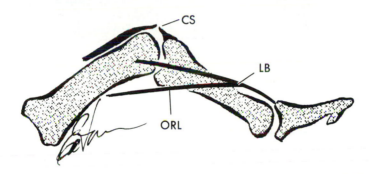

FIG. 16-11. In boutonnière deformity, lateral bands, *LB*, are displaced below axis of proximal interphalangeal joint. Any repair must recenter these bands and release any retinacular ligament, *ORL*, contracture. *CS*, Central extensor tendon slip.

additional weeks. Unstable or displaced fractures are usually oblique; angulation and rotation can occur. Such a fracture will require open reduction through a dorsal approach, which divides the dorsal apparatus between the central tendon and the lateral band on the side of the fracture. After reduction the fracture is transfixed with small wires or a screw and protected for 10 to 14 days in the extended position before motion is begun. The extensor tendon must be protected by splinting for an additional 2 to 4 weeks.

Fractures involving a single condyle must be carefully evaluated because rotation can occur. A dorsal midphalangeal fracture requires open reduction and stabilization with a wire or suture, with the proximal interphalangeal joint maintained in extension for 4 weeks before flexion is begun.

BOUTONNIÈRE DEFORMITY

The boutonnière deformity results from rupture or attenuation of the central extensor tendon over the proximal interphalangeal joint; the digit assumes a position of proximal interphalangeal flexion and distal joint extension (Fig. 16-11). The lateral bands slide volarly to the proximal in-

terphalangeal joint axis, concentrating their extensor forces at the distal interphalangeal joint. This inability to flex the distal joint is the most disabling aspect of the boutonnière deformity and will become fixed with time.

Closed boutonnière injuries are the most common and frequently occur when the digit's tip is struck with a ball. Treatment includes splinting of the proximal interphalangeal joint in the extended position; the distal joint is left free for flexion exercises for prevention of lateral band adherence and retinacular ligament contracture. Open injuries (tendon lacerations) require suture of the extensor tendon with immobilization of the proximal interphalangeal joint in extension for 4 weeks.

Many different reconstructive procedures have been suggested to repair the established boutonnière deformity.[4,10,15] The purpose of any of these operations is to rebalance the extensor mechanism either by directly repairing the central tendon or reinforcing it with at least one lateral band. Before any surgery, full passive extension of the proximal interphalangeal joint should be obtained. This can be accomplished by splinting if necessary. The extensor tendon at the level of the proximal interphalangeal joint, whether repaired

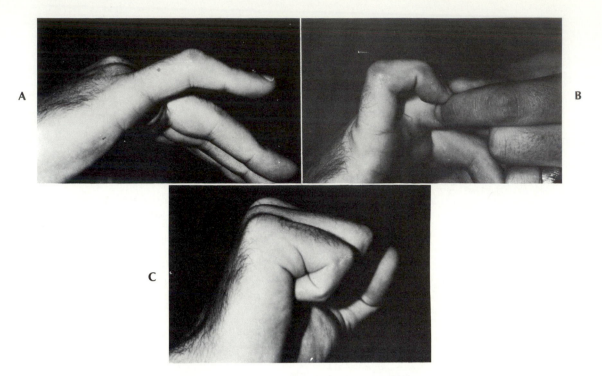

Fig. 16-12. Pseudoboutonnière deformity is seen as proximal interphalangeal flexion contracture, **A,** but with good passive, **B,** and active, **C,** flexion of distal joint.

or reconstructed, must be immobilized for at least 4 weeks and then gradually moved with protection against an extensor lag for the total of 8 weeks.

PSEUDOBOUTONNIÈRE DEFORMITY

The term "pseudoboutonnière" has been suggested for a group of proximal interphalangeal hyperextension injuries, which present a boutonnière-like appearance (Fig. 16-12).[11] On examination a proximal interphalangeal flexion contracture is found, but the distal joint while positioned in extension is flexible. The extensor mechanism has not been damaged, but the volar plate's proximal attachment has been avulsed with subsequent scarring in the flexed position. It can be differentiated from the true boutonnière deformity by complete active and passive distal joint flexion. Flexion deformities of the proximal interphalangeal joint greater than 45 degrees may require surgical release.

In summary, proper management of injuries of the proximal interphalangeal joint can significantly reduce the stiffness and impairment all too often seen when a patient is uninformed and unsupervised in his treatment. A thorough knowledge of the anatomy and understanding of all the injuries to this most important joint are required before one begins such treatment. In mobilizing the proximal interphalangeal joint, a gentle progressive exercise program should be closely monitored to prevent possible complications (that is, flexion contractures and increasing stiffness).

REFERENCES

1. Adams, J.P.: Correction of chronic dorsal subluxation of the proximal interphalangeal joint by means of a cross-cross volar graft, J. Bone Joint Surg. **41A:**111-115, 1959.
2. Curtis, R.M.: Injuries to joints. In Flynn, J.E., editor: Hand surgery, ed. 2, Baltimore, 1975, The Williams & Wilkins Co., pp. 225-239.
3. Eaton, R.G.: Joint injuries of the hand, Springfield, Ill., 1971, Charles C Thomas, Publisher.
4. Elliott, R.A.: Boutonnière deformity. In Cramer, I.M., and Chase, R.A., editors: Symposium on the hand, vol. 3, St. Louis, 1971, The C.V. Mosby Co., pp. 42-56.
5. Green, D.P., and Rowland, S.A.: Fractures and dislocations in the hand. In Rockwood, C.A., Jr., and Green, D.P., editors: Fractures, Philadelphia, 1975, J.B. Lippincott Co., pp. 310-319.
6. Kuczynski, K.: The PIP joint: anatomy and causes of stiffness in the fingers, J. Bone Joint Surg. **50B:**656-663, 1968.
7. Kuczynski, K.: Less-known aspects of the proximal interphalangeal joint of the human hand, Hand **7:**31-33, 1975.
8. Landsmeer, J.M.F.: The proximal interphalangeal joint, Hand **7:**30, 1975.
9. Littler, J.W., and Cooley, S.G.: Restoration of the retinacular system in hyperextension deformity of the proximal interphalangeal joint, J. Bone Joint Surg. **47A:**637, 1965.
10. Littler, J.W., and Eaton, R.G.: Redistribution of forces in the correction of boutonnière deformity, J. Bone Joint Surg. **49A:**1267, 1967.
11. McCue, F.C., Honner, R., Gleck, J.H., and others: A pseudoboutonnière deformity, Hand **7:**166-170, 1975.
12. Moberg, E.: Fracture and ligamentous injuries of the thumb and fingers, Surg. Clin. North Am. **40:**297-309, 1960.
13. Moberg, E., and Stener, B.: Injuries to the ligaments of the thumb and fingers, diagnosis, treatment and prognosis, Acta Chir. Scand. **106:**166-186, 1953.
14. Redler, L., and Williams, J.T.: Rupture of a collateral ligament of

the proximal interphalangeal joint of the fingers, analysis of eighteen cases, J. Bone Joint Surg. **49A:**322-326, 1967.

15. Souter, W.A.: The problem of boutonnière deformity, Clin. Orthop. **104:**116-133, 1974.

BIBLIOGRAPHY

Aufranco, O.E., Jones, W.N., and Bierbaum, B.E.: Fracture dislocation of the proximal interphalangeal joint of the finger, J.A.M.A. **204:**815-819, 1968.

Bate, J.T.: An operation for the correction of locking of the proximal interphalangeal joint of finger in hyperextension, J. Bone Joint Surg. **27:**142-144, 1945.

Brunelli, G., Morelli, E., and Salvi, V.: Traumatic lesions of tendons and ligaments of the proximal interphalangeal joint, Hand **7:**43-45, 1975.

Howard, L.D.: Treatment of posttraumatic recurvation deformity of the proximal interphalangeal joint with occasional locking but with other free joint mobility. In Cramer, L.M., and Chase, R.A., editors: Symposium on the hand, vol. 3, St. Louis, 1971, The C.V. Mosby Co., pp. 33-41.

Johnson, F.G., and Greene, M.H.: Another cause of irreducible dislocation of the proximal interphalangeal joint of a finger, J. Bone Joint Surg. **48A:**542-544, 1966.

Kleinert, H.E., and Kasdan, M.L.: Reconstruction of chronically subluxed PIP finger joint, J. Bone Joint Surg. **47A:**958-964, 1965.

Lee, M.L.H.: Intra-articular and peri-articular fractures of the phalanges, J. Bone Joint Surg. **45B:**103, 1963.

London, P.S.: Sprain and fractures involving the interphalangeal joints, Hand **3:**155, 1971.

McCue, F.C., Honner, R., Johnson, M., and others: Athletic injuries of the proximal interphalangeal joint requiring surgical treatment, J. Bone Joint Surg. **52A:**937-956, 1970.

McElfresh, E.C., Dobyns, J., and O'Brien, E.T.: Management of fracture-dislocation of the proximal interphalangeal joints by extension-block splinting, J. Bone Joint Surg. **54A:**1705-1711, 1972.

Neviaser, R.J., and Wilson, J.N.: Interposition of the extensor tendon resulting in persistent subluxation of the proximal interphalangeal joint of the finger, Clin. Orthop. **83:**118-120, 1972.

Portis, R.B.: Hyperextensibility of the proximal interphalangeal joint of the finger following trauma, J. Bone Joint Surg. **36A:**1141-1146, 1954.

Robertson, R.C., Cawley, J.J., and Faris, A.M.: Treatment of fracture-dislocation of the interphalangeal joints of the hand, J. Bone Joint Surg. **28:**68-70, 1946.

Shrewsbury, M.M., and Johnson, R.K.: A systematic study of the oblique retinacular ligament of the human finger: its structure and function, J. Hand Surg. **2:**194-199, 1977.

Spinner, M., and Choi, B.Y.: Anterior dislocation of the proximal interphalangeal joint, J. Bone Joint Surg. **52A:**1329-1336, 1970.

Stark, H.H.: Troublesome fractures and dislocations of the hand. In A.A.O.S.: Instructional course lectures, vol. 19, St. Louis, 1970, The C.V. Mosby Co., pp. 130-149.

Thompson, J.S., and Eaton, R.G.: Volar dislocations of the proximal interphalangeal joint, Orthop. Trans. **1:**5, 1977.

Trojan, E.: Fracture dislocation of the bases of the proximal and middle phalanges of the fingers, Hand **4:**60-61, 1972.

Van Der Meulen: The treatment of prolapse and collapse of the proximal interphalangeal joint, Hand **4:**154-162, 1972.

Wiley, A.M.: Instability of the proximal interphalangeal joint following dislocation and fracture dislocation: surgical repair, Hand **2:**185-191, 1970.

Wilson, J.N., and Rowland, S.A.: Fracture-dislocation of the proximal interphalangeal joint of the finger, J. Bone Joint Surg. **48A:**493-503, 1966.

V

THE STIFF HAND

17

Management of the stiff hand

RAYMOND M. CURTIS

The joints of the hand are the means by which the power of the muscles moving the bones of the hand bring about useful function. When these joints are stiffened by fibrosis, destroyed by disease, or deformed by dislocation or fracture, the function of the hand is impaired or even destroyed. This alteration in function may occur despite all our efforts; however, it more frequently occurs because of improper methods of treatment.

CAUSES OF JOINT STIFFENING IN THE HAND

The primary factors behind stiffening of the hand are (1) edema, (2) fibrosis, (3) collagen alteration,[17] (4) anatomic factors, and (5) disease. The patient with rheumatoid arthritis or dermatomyositis has a primary disease that leads to stiffness.

To prevent stiffness of the hand, the following principles should be followed: (1) elevation of the injured extremity, (2) mild compression dressing, (3) elimination of pain, (4) prevention of hematomas, (5) prevention of infection, and (6) understanding of the underlying emotional factors that occur with hand injuries.

Bunnell[2] has stated that all uninjured parts should be kept unrestrained and free to move. This is the functional treatment of fractures as described by Bohler[1] and Watson-Jones.[22] Moberg and Stener[15] have emphasized that contraction of the muscles pumps the tissue fluids through the limb, preventing edema and stasis and keeping the tissues nourished. Bunnell[2] has stated that ''one should be alert to recognize early those cases that will go on to the edematous, immobile osteoporotic hand, by recognizing the signs of tropic disturbance and the disposition on the part of the patient to hold his hand completely immobile.''

A pressure point produced by the dressing or cast will lead to edema and swelling of the injured or postoperative hand. For this reason, the dressing should be checked 12 to 24 hours after surgery and released at least along one border, much as one would do in splitting a cast. Any point where the patient complains abnormally about pressure and pain should also be checked.

Peacock[17] has stated on the basis of his clinical and experimental studies that the stiffness that follows simple immobilization is attributable to fixation of the joint ligaments to bone in areas normally meant to be free from such fixation and shortening of the ligaments by new collagen synthesis.

It is possible that with injury we may have an imbalance between fibrin formation and lysis of fibrin.

CONSERVATIVE METHODS OF TREATING STIFFENED JOINTS

Elevation. Elevation of the injured part is important in that it minimizes the degree of swelling. This should be used immediately after all surgery on the hand, and one should be sure that the patient, when ambulatory, keeps the hand elevated as well.

Elastic splints and elastic traction. Elastic splints and traction should be used early and continuously; the amount of tension used should not produce swelling.[18]

Molded plaster splints or casts. Molded plaster splints or casts can be applied and changed at regular intervals (daily is possible) to gradually stretch the finger joints or wrist joint into flexion or extension.

Intermittent compression unit. Intermittent compression therapy (with the Jobst Intermittent Compression Unit) has been very helpful in reducing swelling in the posttraumatic and postoperative hand and in mobilizing the stiff interphalangeal joints. The hand is placed in the sleeve with the fingers in extension for 10 minutes, under pressure, and then in flexion for 10 minutes. The amount of pressure that can be easily tolerated by the patient is used, with the time in the pneumatic sleeve being gradually increased from 30 minutes to 1 hour, one or more times a day, and with the pressure (in mm Hg) in the sleeve also being gradually increased.

The fact that the extracellular fluid is pressed out of the hand by the intermittent pressure and that the tight capsular ligaments are stretched first into extension and then into flexion makes it possible to mobilize some joints where splinting and other methods of treatment have failed.

Local heat therapy. Physiotherapy in the form of warm water soaks or whirlpool bath is helpful, as is hot wax therapy.

Stellate ganglion blocks and local nerve blocks. The local nerve blocks, or blocks with local anesthesia of the painful trigger areas, are very helpful. When indicated in sympathetic dystrophy, the stellate ganglion block or sympathectomy can be an aid in relieving pain and decreasing edema.

Active exercise. The need for active use of the hand in mobilizing stiff joints cannot be overemphasized.

Passive exercise. Passive exercises can be used to improve the range of motion in the stiff joints of the hand. The force applied must not increase the swelling or pain in the joints that are stiff.

Medical treatment. There are various drugs available for systemic use that may be helpful. Two of the most effective are phenylbutazone (Butazolidin) and prednisone. Triamcinolone may also be used in an amount of 2 mg injected intra-articularly into the small finger joints. Some tranquilizers seem to aid in the patient's recovery.

METACARPOPHALANGEAL JOINTS
Anatomy

The metacarpophalangeal joints of the four fingers can be flexed and extended. When the hand is open in extension, the fingers can also be abducted and adducted; thus they perform the four movements that make up circumduction and are called ''condyloid joints.'' Grant[8] indicates that if it were not for the presence of ligaments, these joints would be ball-and-socket joints. When the joints are completely flexed, neither abduction nor adduction is possible. The reason is that the heads of the metacarpals, though rounded at their ends, are flattened in the front. Another reason is that the collateral ligaments, though slack on extension, are taut on flexion because of their eccentric attachments to the sides of the heads of the metacarpals and because the metacarpal head is broader volarly.

The collateral ligament is attached to a pit in front of the eccentrically placed tubercle on the head of the metacarpal; it is composed of two parts: a dorsally placed portion or ''cord'' ligament and a fan-shaped volar portion, the accessory collateral ligament, which extends from the metacarpal to the sides of the palmar or volar plate.

For allowance of flexion and extension, the anterior and posterior parts of the capsule must be lax. Dorsally there are no ligaments to these joints. Here the extensor or dorsal expansion of the extensor tendons effectively serves the part. The synovium of the joint closes the joint dorsally.

Anteriorly the capsule is replaced by a fibrocartilaginous plate, the palmar ligament or ''volar accessory ligament.'' This plate is firmly united to the front edge of the phalanx and loosely attached to the metacarpal by areolar tissue.

Consequently, if a finger is wrenched off the hand, the platelike palmar ligament will part from the metacarpal and remain attached to the phalanx. Fibers of the collateral ligaments radiate to the sides of this plate and keep it firmly applied to the front of the head of its metacarpal, visor fashion.

The palmar or volar ligaments of the fingers are united to each other by three ligamentous bands, the deep transverse ligaments of the palm, which help to prevent the metacarpals from spreading.

Ankylosis

Anatomic structures that limit metacarpophalangeal joint flexion are (1) adhesions of the extensor tendons over the dorsum of the hand or adhesions of the extensor hood mechanism over the metacarpophalangeal joints, (2) thickening of the dorsal capsule of the metacarpophalangeal joints, (3) contracture of the collateral ligament (cordlike portion), (4) insufficient skin coverage of scar of the skin over the dorsum of the hand, as in a burn, and (5) bony block within the joint.

Immobility of the metacarpophalangeal joints for whatever reason, particularly if there is swelling with the deposition of edema fluid in the ligamentous tissue, leads to adhesions of the extensor mechanism, contracture and adhesions of the collateral ligaments, thickening of the entire capsular ligamentous structure, and the ankylosis so commonly seen in the metacarpophalangeal joints.

This immobility is seen in hands in which there has been infection, trauma of all types, burns of the hand with burn-scar contracture over the dorsum of the hand, congenital aplasia of the metacarpophalangeal joints, and certain systemic diseases such as rheumatoid arthritis and dermatomyositis.

The prevention of this very disabling abnormality is of primary importance. It can best be prevented by (1) early motion of the metacarpophalangeal joints, (2) elevation of the injured extremity with prevention of edema, (3) elimination of plaster casts or splints, which immobilize the metacarpophalangeal joint, and (4) early elastic band traction in patients who are developing this clinical entity.

Treatment by splinting and physiotherapy

In patients seen early after injury, attempts should be made to carry out rubber-band traction along with the use of a small volar plaster splint, worn 12 to 24 hours a day, or the practical Bunnell knuckle-bender splint, to determine what can be achieved with such conservative treatment.

This type of therapy can be coupled with various forms of physiotherapy. Alternating positive pressure with a compression unit can be of great help in reducing edema of the hand and mobilizing the joints. In addition, active exercise should be carried out.

If one is making progress with this form of treatment, the operative release should be delayed. If after several months of this type of conservative treatment there is no progress in the range of active or passive motion in the metacarpophalangeal joints, then there is an indication for surgical release of the metacarpophalangeal joints.

It is important to point out that in most normal hands the metacarpophalangeal joints passively flex to a 90-degree angle. However, when one flexes the fingers for grasp, as in a closed fist, the index finger actively flexes 75 degrees, the middle finger flexes 75 degrees, the ring finger flexes 80 degrees, and the little finger flexes 80 to 85 degrees. It is not necessary to achieve 90 degrees of active flexion in the metacarpophalangeal joints to have a useful hand.

These ranges of motion should be remembered, for in a given hand it must be decided whether to proceed with surgical release in the patient who can flex somewhat at the metacarpophalangeal joint. If the patient has no flexion at the metacarpophalangeal joint but does have an intrinsically good joint, one can expect to achieve a good result from the release of the tight capsular ligaments and extensor tendon mechanism. If 75 degrees of active motion are ap-

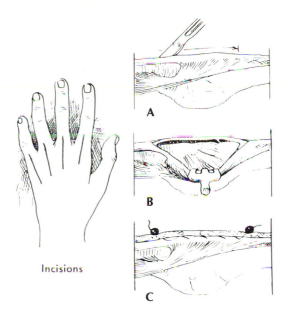

FIG. 17-1. Incisions for exposure of capsular ligaments of metacarpophalangeal joints of fingers for capsulectomy. **A,** Splitting extensor tendon. **B,** Retraction of extensor hood to expose capsular ligament. **C,** Closure of extensor tendon with running 4-0 stainless-steel wire (redrawn from Bunnell). (From Curtis, R.M., as reported in Flynn, J.E.: Hand surgery, Baltimore, 1966, The Williams & Wilkins Co.)

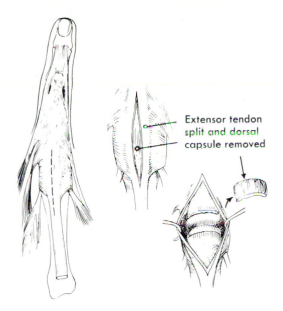

FIG. 17-2. Exposure of joint by dorsal approach through extensor tendon, with excision of thickened synovium that forms dorsal part of capsule. (From Curtis, R.M., as reported in Flynn, J.E.: Hand surgery, Baltimore, 1966, The Williams & Wilkins Co.)

proached in the metacarpophalangeal joint, there is less indication for surgical intervention.

I do not perform capsulectomies on the metacarpophalangeal joints if the patient flexes as much as 65 degrees in these joints. This patient should continue physiotherapy and special splinting. In patients whose hands are fixed in full extension or have a range of motion less than 65 degrees of flexion, sufficient improvement in the range of motion can be expected to warrant operative intervention.

Bunnell[2] has stated that the essentials for the success of capsulectomy are the presence of good surrounding tissue, good nerve supply and nutrition, redundant dorsal skin, good working muscles about the joints, and free extensor and intrinsic muscles or some correction for them to furnish strong flexion.

The choice between arthroplasty or capsulectomy in a given situation where there is an ankylosis in the metacarpophalangeal joint will depend on the appearance of the metacarpal head and the base of the phalanx in the roentgenogram. Frequently, it is possible to salvage a good range of motion in the metacarpophalangeal joint even in instances where by roentgenogram there has been considerable joint destruction.

Capsulectomy

Operative technique (Figs. 17-1 to 17-3). The extensor tendons are exposed by four straight longitudinal incisions over the metacarpals. The extensor tendon is then split longitudinally for a distance of approximately 2.5 cm on either side of the metacarpophalangeal joint.[11] The aponeurotic hood, or extensor hood, is then retracted to either side, and

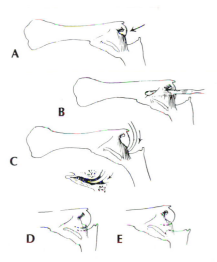

FIG. 17-3. Technique for capsulectomy with release of "cord" portion of ligament. Continuity is maintained between distal portion of "cord" ligament and accessory collateral ligament to prevent ulnar deviation even when small wedge of "cord" portion of ligament is excised. **A,** Dorsal capsule excised and "cord" portion released at point of attachment to metacarpal; accessory collateral ligament still intact. **B,** Elevator frees adhesions between ligament and head of metacarpal. **C,** Elevator releases adherent volar capsule and recreates normal pouch beneath metacarpal head. **D,** Proper relation of phalanx to metacarpal. **E,** With inadequate release of volar capsule, phalanx does not rest beneath head of metacarpal. (From Curtis, R.M., as reported in Flynn, J.E.: Hand surgery, Baltimore, 1966, The Williams & Wilkins Co.)

the attachments of the extensor tendon to the base of the proximal phalanx are severed when they are present. The synovium, which forms the dorsal part of the capsule of the joint between the base of the phalanx and the head of the metacarpal, is excised, for this may be greatly thickened in severe cases. This dorsal capsule is excised from one collateral ligament across to the opposite collateral ligament over the dorsum of the joint.

Since the cordlike portion of the collateral ligament limits flexion, this can be released from its attachment just beneath the tubercle on either side of the head of the metacarpal, leaving it attached to the accessory collateral ligament, but freeing any adhesions that may have formed between the cord portion of the collateral ligament and the head of the metacarpal.[6] Pressure against the base of the proximal phalanx will then carry the proximal phalanx into flexion beneath the head of the metacarpal.

In those patients with much thickening in the collateral ligament, a section of the cordlike portion of the ligament should be removed near the tubercle on either side of the head of the metacarpal. The remainder of the cordlike portion of the collateral ligament should be left attached to the accessory collateral ligament. This will prevent ulnar deviation of the finger, which is seen when too much of the cord portion of the collateral ligament and its accessory ligament are removed.

This deviation is likely to occur in the patient with ulnar nerve palsy. One must also take care not to sever the attachment of the interosseous tendon into the base of the phalanx just distal to the attachment of the collateral ligament to the phalanx, since this may also lead to ulnar deviation of the fingers.

If the phalanx does not drop into flexion beneath the head of the metacarpal, a curved periosteal elevator should be inserted around the head of the metacarpal to recreate the volar pouch beneath the head of the metacarpal, because in long-standing cases this pouch becomes obliterated when the volar plate becomes adherent to the metacarpal head.

The excursion of the extensor tendons over the dorsum of the hand should be checked. If these are not gliding freely, they should be tendolyzed over the dorsum of the hand and, if necessary, over the dorsum of the wrist and into the forearm. In addition, it may be necessary to free the extensor hood well onto either side of the metacarpophalangeal joint.

I prefer to place 2 mg of triamcinolone acetonide (Kenalog) into each joint before closing the extensor tendon and distribute another 10 mg beneath the extensor tendons on the dorsum of the hand if they have been tendolyzed.

The extensor tendon is closed with a running suture of 4-0 stainless steel wire. The hand is dressed in a pressure dressing with the metacarpophalangeal joints in moderate flexion—however, not in such a severe degree of flexion as to cause the extensor tendons to open over the metacarpophalangeal joint. This pressure dressing is left in place for 72 hours, at which time it is removed and a volar plaster splint applied so that one may begin rubber-band traction by leather loops about the proximal phalanges for flexion.

The elastic splinting must be continued as long as necessary, both day and night. After 4 to 6 weeks, a Bunnell

knuckle-bender splint may be used. During the period of elastic splinting some active extension is allowed as well. If the patient has a problem with finger extension, a dynamic splint for extension is alternated with one for flexion.

Complications. Certain complications may occur after the operative procedure of capsulectomy.

1. Ulnar deviation of the fingers as a result of a too radical resection of the collateral ligament on the radial side, particularly in the presence of ulnar nerve palsy, may occur. Also, if one inadequately releases the collateral ligament on the ulnar side of the joint, ulnar deviation may result.

2. Disruption of the extensor tendons over the metacarpophalangeal joint may occur in those patients in whom one has not adequately tendolyzed the extensor tendons. It may also occur in those patients in whom there has been considerable shortening of the extensor muscles themselves. This latter complication can usually be prevented if the metacarpophalangeal joints are not forced into full flexion immediately postoperatively instead of flexing with rubber-band traction as the tight extensor tendons gradually loosen.

3. Recurrence of the ankylosis may occur where the abnormality was inadequately corrected at surgery or where adequate rubber band traction was not maintained after surgery. If a good result is not obtained, the procedure can be repeated after 4 to 6 months.

Arthroplasty

Arthroplasty with the use of a joint prosthesis may be the procedure of choice for patients who have such severe destruction of the metacarpal head or the base of the proximal phalanx that release of the capsular ligament may not provide a satisfactory range of motion.[7] It is indicated in the rheumatoid arthritic patient, where there has been such severe destruction of the metacarpal head that satisfactory stabilization cannot be accomplished in the metacarpophalangeal joint by the usual imbrication of the extensor hood and reconstruction of the collateral ligaments.[21] In addition, it is used in osteoarthritic patients, in whom there is pronounced deformity in this joint, and in destruction of the joint after trauma.

The best arthroplasty result is obtained by the use of a joint prosthesis interposed between the metacarpal and the proximal phalanx.

PROXIMAL INTERPHALANGEAL JOINTS

When the surgeon treats a crippled hand, he is confronted frequently with a hand that fails to function properly because of limitation of flexion or extension in the interphalangeal joints. Bunnell[2] noted that it is the narrow joint space present in the interphalangeal joints that produces limitation of motion when there is even the slightest shortening of the capsular ligaments as might be produced by nonuse or edema of the ligaments and subsequent fibrosis.

This shortening, with limitation in motion, may occur despite the most rigid attention to proper splinting and physical and occupational therapy, with proper reduction of fractures or dislocations. However, it more often follows he improper use of these methods of treatment.[17]

Anatomy

The proximal interphalangeal joint is constructed on essentially the same plan as the metacarpophalangeal joint. It possesses collateral ligaments, a palmar fibrocartilage, and a loose dorsal capsule or synovial tissue guarded by an extensor expansion. This is considered a hinge joint, since movements are restricted to flexion and extension by the anteroposterior flattening of the ends of the bones.

An important fascial structure covers the collateral ligaments on either side of the joint. This has been described in detail by Landsmeer[13] as being composed of a transverse portion extending from the extensor tendon dorsally to the lateral border of the volar plate. The oblique portion of the ligament passes from the proximal phalanx to the extensor tendon over the middle phalanx. Stack[20] believes that this ligament is really a portion of the extensor tendon mechanism. Kaplan[12] has described this as a deep fascial cuff.

Sprains

Sprains may occur with varying amounts of injury to the capsular ligaments about the joint, from minute tears of the ligament to more extensive damage. The usual history is that of a patient having twisted or jammed the finger. There may be a hemarthrosis associated with the ligament injury. After the injury, there may be months of painful swelling of the joint, with stiffness on both flexion and extension.[16]

These injuries should receive careful attention in the acute stage; they should be splinted in slight flexion for 2 to 3 weeks. If possible, the splint should be removed periodically with careful flexion and extension, guarding against forced flexion and extension.

Local injection of the joint with triamcinolone acetonide (Kenalog) may be helpful in relieving pain in chronic cases and aid in mobilizing the joint.

In those cases seen late, with thickened capsular ligaments and stiffness on flexion and extension, the most careful splinting will be required to stretch the joint into full flexion and extension. For a severely ankylosed joint in extension or flexion a capsulectomy may be needed to restore function.

Ankylosis in extension

The surgeon about to correct a limitation of flexion of the proximal interphalangeal joint must have in mind the various anatomic structures in the finger that may limit this motion. These structures are (1) scar contracture of the skin over the dorsum of the finger, (2) contracted long extensor muscle or adherent extensor tendon, (3) contracted interosseous muscle or adherent interosseous tendon, (4) contracted capsular ligament, particularly the collateral ligament, (5) retinacular ligament adherent to capsular ligament, (6) bone block or exostosis, and (7) adherence of the flexor tendons within the finger.

Before surgically correcting the lack of flexion of the interphalangeal joint, it is important to determine first by clinical examination and roentgenogram just which anatomic structures are limiting flexion and to be certain that a true ankylosis or bony fusion is not present. Bunnell, Doherty, and Curtis[3] have described various test positions of the hand and fingers to determine which structures are to blame.

Operative technique. (Fig. 17-4). The proximal inter-

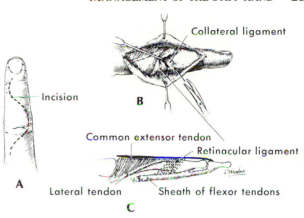

FIG. 17-4. Capsulectomy of proximal interphalangeal joint. **A,** Dorsal excision; dorsal skin is elevated and retracted. **B,** Retracted skin, with elevation of retinacular ligament exposes the collateral ligament, which is totally excised. **C,** Relationship of retinacular ligament to joint capsule and flexor and extensor tendons. (A from Curtis, R.M., first published in Adams, J.P., editor: Current practice in orthopaedic surgery, St. Louis, 1965, The C.V. Mosby Co.)

phalangeal joint is approached by a dorsal curvilinear incision.[4] The incision is deepened through the skin and subcutaneous tissue to expose the transverse retinacular ligament.[13]

In some long-standing cases, the volar synovial pouch will have become obliterated and must be reformed with a small, curved elevator or by forcing of the base of the middle phalanx into flexion. When there is an associated contracture of the interosseous muscle, the interosseous tendon is lengthened by tenotomy at the point where the longitudinal fibers join the middle slip of the extensor tendon, allowed to slide proximally, and then resutured to the extensor aponeurosis. One can also overcome this interosseous contracture by excision of a triangle including the longitudinal fibers from the interosseous and lumbrical muscles, as recommended by Littler[14] in the Littler release procedure (see Harris and Riordan[9]).

If there is severe contracture of the interosseous muscle with flexion deformity at the metacarpophalangeal joint as well, it may be necessary to tenotomize this tendon proximally to the metacarpophalangeal joint and divide the volar capsular ligament of the metacarpophalangeal joint. If necessary, the extensor tendon mechanism should be freed over the dorsum of the finger. The dissection and the freeing of all contracted tissues must continue until there is a free range of motion of the middle phalanx about the distal end of the proximal phalanx. This may necessitate freeing of the extensor tendon from the phalanx, opening of the dorsal synovium of the joint, resection of the collateral ligaments, and a release of the contracted interosseous tendon mechanism.

One may elect to place 2 mg of triamcinolone acetonide (Kenalog) into the interphalangeal joint after this procedure.

The hand is placed in a dorsal plaster splint, using mechanics' waste and mild compression, with the fingers in moderate flexion at the proximal interphalangeal joints. Within 48 to 72 hours rubber-band traction is begun either by leather loops over the finger tips or by traction through the nail, pulling the fingers gradually into the flexed position. It may be necessary to alternate between rubber-band traction for flexion at the interphalangeal joints and rubber-band traction for extension of the fingers together with active exercise. Elastic splinting is continued until the patient is able to maintain by active and passive exercise the range of motion obtained at surgery. In some cases this necessitates part-time splinting for 3 or 4 months.

When the proximal interphalangeal joint may be actively flexed to 75 degrees or more, it is better judgment to rely on conservative measures such as physiotherapy and special splinting to achieve further flexion. In that group of patients who have a lesser degree of flexion, even in those whose fingers are held in rigid extension but without bony ankylosis, one can expect to improve flexion by this operative procedure. This was true in a series of patients even though capsulectomy had to be combined with other operative procedures when other anatomic structures were limiting flexion.

The results seem to indicate that the more anatomic structures there are involved in the limitation of motion, the poorer is the result.[4]

If the only limiting factor for flexion in the interphalangeal joint was a capsular ligament, capsulectomy of the collateral ligaments would produce a good result for both flexion and extension. However, if it was necessary to free the extensor tendon over the proximal phalanx to perform a tenotomy of the interosseous tendons and a capsulectomy of the collateral ligaments to obtain flexion of the proximal interphalangeal joint, the result achieved by surgery was not so successful. This was particularly true of the finger bound by cicatrix. In some of these patients the increase in motion was only 20 to 30 degrees, while in others there was an increase in motion as much as 80 degrees beyond what existed before the operation. In many of these patients this increase meant the difference between a hand that could be used for work and one that could not. It cannot be expected that function will be restored completely by this procedure, but is can be expected to improve.

This approach is applicable to a joint stiff in extension, whether secondary to trauma or rheumatoid arthritis or whatever cause, if the joint surfaces are not too badly destroyed. In cases where there is extensive joint surface damage, an arthroplasty with a joint prosthesis is the procedure of choice.

Sprague[19] and Harrison[10] reported their results of the surgical treatment of the stiff proximal interphalangeal joint. Harrison recommends division only of the main collateral ligament and the dorsal capsule for the joint stiff in extension.

Ankylosis in flexion

The anatomic structure that limits extension of a finger at the proximal interphalangeal joint may be caused by these structures: (1) scar of the skin over the volar surface of the finger, (2) contraction of the superficial fascia in the finger, as in Dupuytren's contracture, (3) contracture of the flexor tendon sheath within the finger, (4) contracted flexor muscle or adherent flexor tendon, (5) contraction of the volar plate of the capsular ligament, (6) adherence of the retinacular ligaments of Landsmeer to the collateral ligaments, (7) adherence of the collateral ligaments with the finger in the

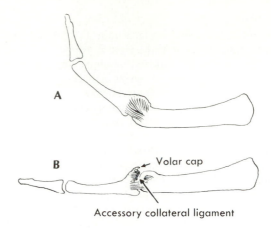

FIG. 17-5. Capsulectomy for release of flexion contracture of finger. **A,** Fixed flexion contracture. **B,** Excision of portion of volar capsule and release of accessory collateral ligament, with cord portion being left to maintain stability of joint. (From Curtis, R.M., as reported in Flynn, J.E.: Hand surgery, Baltimore, 1966, The Williams & Wilkins Co.)

flexed position, and (8) bony block or exostosis. Frequently, more than one structure is involved in this flexion contracture.

In congenital flexion contracture of the finger, all tissues from the skin to the joint capsule, and even the joint itself, may be involved. There may be an absence of interosseous function. Abnormal insertions of the lumbrical muscles have been reported.

Similarly, in the patient with Dupuytren's contracture that has existed for a long period of time and in whom there is pronounced flexion contracture of the proximal interphalangeal joints, the skin is contracted, there is a thick strand of contracted superficial fascia, the flexor superficialis tendon may be contracted, and the volar capsule and accessory collateral ligaments shorten in such a way as to prevent extension.

Operative technique. (Fig. 17-5). Operative release of the finger in an acutely flexed position is usually through a midlateral incision that is deepened to expose the flexor tendon sheath and the joint itself. (A Z-plasty on the flexor surface of the finger may be preferable in Dupuytren's contracture and congenital flexion contracture.) My initial approach is to excise a portion of the flexor tendon sheath distal to the A_2 pulley and see whether this simple excision will allow any extension. In some instances, it may be the only structure that is contracted.

This excision is then followed by checking of the flexor tendons to see whether they are adherent over the proximal phalanx or whether they are contracted. If they are severely contracted, it may be necessary to tenotomize and lengthen the flexor tendons in the forearm.

The retinacular ligament is freed from the lateral capsular ligament, and the volar capsule is then excised from the proximal interphalangeal joint. When necessary, the accessory collateral ligament is incised on either side of the proximal interphalangeal joint. Subluxation of the middle phalanx may occur if the cord portion of the lateral ligament is completely severed. In some instances, it will be necessary to divide the retinacular ligament of Landsmeer as well. The surgical release of the contracted structures will then allow extension of the proximal interphalangeal joint. The joint is fixed in moderate extension by a Kirschner wire across the proximal interphalanageal joint. The Kirschner wire is removed in 1 week, and active motion for flexion and extension is begun with rubber-band traction to improve the degree of extension and maintain the gain that was achieved operatively.

If a Dupuytren's contracture is present, a partial volar capsulectomy is performed with excision of the accessory collateral ligaments when excision of the thickened fascial band does not achieve complete extension of the joint.[5]

REFERENCES

1. Bohler, L.: The treatment of fractures, Baltimore, 1932, William Wood & Co.
2. Bunnell, S.: Surgery of the Hand, ed. 3, Philadelphia, 1948, J.B. Lippincott Co.
3. Bunnell, S., Doherty, E.W., and Curtis, R.M.: Ischemic contracture, local, in the hand, Plast. Reconstruct. Surg. 3:424-433, 1948.
4. Curtis, R.M.: Capsulectomy of the interphalangeal joints of the fingers, J. Bone Joint Surg. 36A:1219-1232, 1954.
5. Curtis, R.M.: Volar capsulectomy in Dupuytren's contracture. In Tubiana, R., and Hueston, J.T., editors: Les Monographies Du Groupe D'Etude de la Main, Paris, 1972, Expansion Scientifique Française, pp. 165-167.
6. Curtis, R.M.: Joints of the hand. In Flynn, J.E., Editor: Hand surgery, ed. 2, Baltimore, 1975, The Williams & Wilkins Co.
7. Fowler, S.B.: Mobilization of metacarpophalangeal joint, arthroplasty and capsulotomy, J. Bone Joint Surg. 29:193-202, 1947.
8. Grant, J.C.B.: A method of anatomy, ed. 4, Baltimore, 1948, The Williams & Wilkins Co.
9. Harris, C., Jr., and Riordan, D.C.: Intrinsic contracture in the hand and its surgical treatment, J. Bone Joint Surg. 36A:10, 1954.
10. Harrison, D.H.: The stiff interphalanged joint, The Hand 9:102, 1977.
11. Howard, L.D.: Cited by S. Bunnell in Surgery of the hand, ed. 2, Philadelphia, 1948, J.B. Lippincott Co., p. 301.
12. Kaplan, E.B.: Functional and surgical anatomy of the hand, Philadelphia, 1953, J.B. Lippincott Co.
13. Landsmeer, J.M.F.: The anatomy of the dorsal aponeurosis of the human finger and its functional significance, Anat. Rec. 104:31, 1949.
14. Littler, J.W., and Howorth, M.B.: A textbook of orthopedics, Philadelphia, 1952, W.B. Saunders Co., p. 251.
15. Moberg, E., and Stener, B.: Injuries to the ligaments of the thumb and fingers: diagnosis, treatment, and prognosis, Acta Chir. Scand. 106:166-186, 1953.
16. Peacock, E.E., Jr.: Preservation of interphalangeal joint function: a basis for the early care of injured hands, South. Med. J. 56:56-63, 1962.
17. Peacock, E.E., Jr.: Some biochemical and biophysical aspects of joint stiffness: role of collagen synthesis as opposed to altered molecular their treatment, Trauma 16:259, 1976.
18. Pratt, D.R.: Joints of the hand and fingers—their stiffness, splinting and surgery, Calif. Med. 66:22-24, 1947.
19. Sprague, B.L.: The proximal interphalangeal joint contractures and their treatment, Trauma 16:259, 1976.
20. Stack, H.G.: Muscle function in the fingers, J. Bone Joint Surg. 44B:899-909, 1962.
21. Vainio, K., and Pulkki, T.: Surgical treatment of arthritis mutilans, Ann. Chir. et Gynaecol. Fenniae 48:361-367, 1959.
22. Watson-Jones, R.: Fractures and other bone and joint injuries, Baltimore, 1940, The Williams & Wilkins Co.

18

Therapist's management of the stiff hand

PAMELA M. McENTEE

Prevention of the stiff hand presents a challenge to the therapist, the surgeon, and the patient. An acutely stiff hand, characterized by pitting edema, pain, and decreased range of motion, can follow trauma to the hand whether minor or severe (Fig. 18-1). If left untreated, it can progress to a chronically stiff hand, characterized by brawny edema, soft-tissue fibrosis, and serious loss of hand function (Fig. 18-2). Early intervention by trained occupational and physical therapists is essential in remediation of the acutely stiff hand and prevention of the chronically stiff hand. The primary goal of treatment of the stiff hand is restoration of hand function. Evaluation, patient education, edema control, therapeutic exercise, therapeutic activities, and splinting are all avenues that lead to this goal (Fig. 18-3). The purpose of this chapter is to discuss the management of the stiff hand in both the acute and the chronic stages.

THE ACUTELY STIFF HAND

An acutely stiff hand is often seen after injuries such as a blow to the dorsum of the hand or a crush injury. The importance of early treatment for the acutely stiff hand cannot be overemphasized. A patient is often anxious about the condition of such a hand, because he fears it may restrict his ability to work or carry out activities of daily living. He has a natural inclination to protect the injured hand by complete immobilization. It is the responsibility of the therapist to assure the patient that early motion is essential for a quick recovery.

Evaluation

A thorough evaluation is essential before the initiation of treatment. It enables the therapist to formulate an innovative treatment plan to fit the individual patient's needs. Follow-up evaluations determine progress and the need for changes in the treatment program.

History. The evaluation begins with a detailed history, including the patient's age, occupation, hand dominance, description of injury, diagnosis, and previous surgeries. Pertinent psychosocial information, such as the patient's transportation and financial status, aids the therapist in determining the length and frequency of therapy visits.

Inspection. The patient's hand is closely examined for color, infection, and the presence of pain and edema. If edema is present, its area and extent are recorded before and after treatment. One method to measure edema objectively is to use a tape measure to compare the circumferences of the involved and uninvolved hands or fingers (Fig. 18-4). For tape measurements to be accurate, the same anatomic reference point is used for each sequential measurement. The volumeter[4] provides another method to evaluate edema. The patient's hand is submerged in a specifically designed water-filled container, and the amount of water displaced by the submerged hand is measured (Fig. 18-5). Measurements before and after a therapy visit are often useful to teach the patient the beneficial effect of the elevation, massage, and active range of motion carried out in therapy.

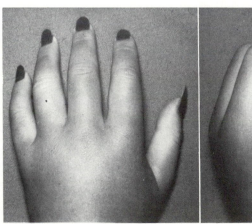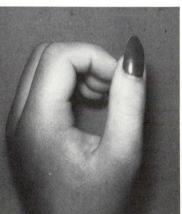

FIG. 18-1. A, "Pitting" edema in an acutely stiff hand. B, Pain and edema restrict active range of motion.

216

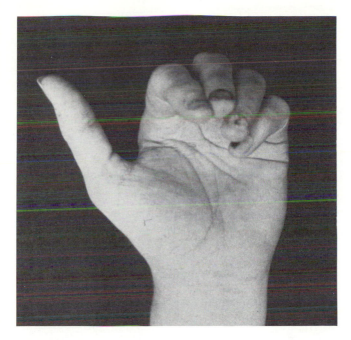

FIG. 18-2. In this chronically stiff hand, active flexion is restricted by malrotation of the fingers, joint contractures, and tendon adhesions.

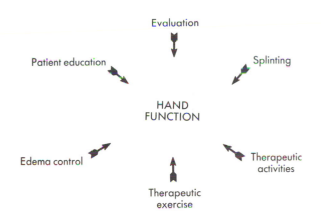

FIG. 18-3. Restoration of hand function is the primary goal in management of the stiff hand.

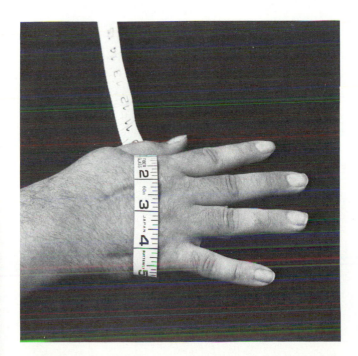

FIG. 18-4. Circumferential measurements are used as an indicator of edema.

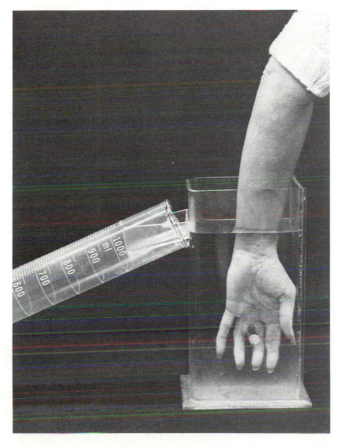

FIG. 18-5. The volumeter is used to measure edema in the stiff hand.

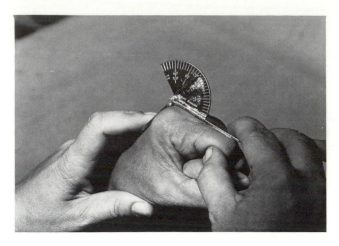

FIG. 18-6. Active range-of-motion measurements are taken using a finger goniometer.

Range of motion. The emphasis of the range-of-motion assessment in the acutely stiff hand is on active motion, because improvement in active motion will be the best indicator of progress in treatment. Active motion is measured by use of a finger goniometer, with the wrist positioned in neutral (Fig. 18-6).

Treatment guidelines

Edema control. A primary goal of treating the acutely stiff hand is the reduction of edema, because its presence can result in stiff and painful joints that lead to further loss of active motion. Elevation of the hand above the level of the heart allows gravity to assist in the reduction of the edema. This, along with active range of motion, is the most effective way to manage edema in the early stages. String wrapping of the hand distally to proximally for a period of 5 minutes (Fig. 18-7), followed by a retrograde massage and active fist making, is also an effective technique when pitting edema is present. Other techniques that can be used include an intermittent pressure pump, Aris Isotoner

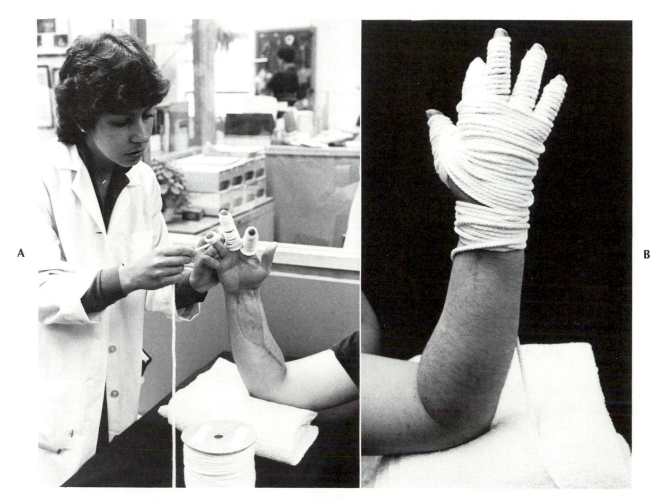

FIG. 18-7. A, Patient's hand is wrapped with string distal to proximal. **B,** Hand is then elevated for a period of 5 minutes.

Glove,* and elastic tape for wrapping of individual fingers (refer to the discussion of edema and bandaging, Chapter 11).

Therapeutic exercise. Active exercises within the patient's pain tolerance should always follow whatever edema control technique is utilized. Active exercises, such as fist making, produce a milking action in the deep veins of the hand. Active exercise of the hand is accompanied by gentle active range of motion of the shoulder, elbow, and wrist when severe swelling is present. Graded resistive exercises are begun at the therapist's discretion, but they must not cause an increase in pain or edema. They include activities such as using a foam squeeze, squeezing putty, or using the Hand Helper.† In some cases, active exercise and edema control will reverse the cycle of immobilization and no further treatment will be needed.

Therapeutic activities. It is essential in the early stage of treatment that the patient begin using his hand even for

---

*Aris Isotoner Glove, 10 E. 38th Street, New York, N.Y. 10016.
†Hand Helper, Medex Corporation, P.O. Box 1352, Los Altos, Calif. 94022.

the simplest activities. Prehension tasks (Fig. 18-8) such as light pick-ups, macramé, and light sanding are examples of activities that can be done in elevation and encourage range-of-motion exercise of all joints of the involved extremity.

Splinting. Supportive static splinting may be indicated to prevent strain of a severely swollen and painful hand. A functional resting splint worn at night or a wrist cockup splint worn during functional activities are two examples of splints that are used during the early stages of recovery. These splints are secured with a figure-of-eight elastic wrap when severe edema is present, so that pressure is distributed over a large area (Fig. 18-9). Static splinting can lead to greater stiffness, and therefore splints must be removed frequently to allow for range-of-motion exercises. Uncontrolled pitting edema is a contraindication for dynamic splinting.

Patient education. Each patient must be instructed on a home program that carries out the treatment techniques utilized during the therapy session. Exercises should be performed at least 4 times daily, with each exercise being repeated 10 times. Therapeutic activities such as macramé are carried out for three to five sessions daily according to the patient's tolerance. The patient must be cautioned to follow the home program exactly as prescribed. Overzealous patients, who believe it is best to exercise constantly, may suffer an increase in pain and edema of their hand. Contrary to this, patients who are fearful that active exercise will be harmful to the hand will not perform their exercise program with the amount of frequency that is necessary to restore function. Home programs are written and reviewed at each therapy session. Illustrations of exercises are given to help clarify written instructions (Fig. 18-10).

Ongoing evaluation. In the treatment of an acutely stiff hand, a significant decrease in edema and an increase in active range of motion should be seen during the first week of treatment. If improvement is not noted, check to see if the patient is performing his home therapy program correctly. If he is, the initial treatment plan must be reevaluated

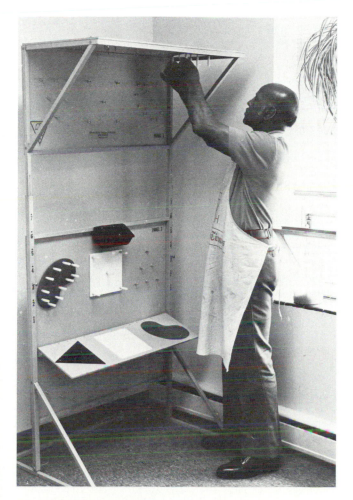

FIG. 18-8. Prehension activities performed with the extremity in elevation help reduce edema.

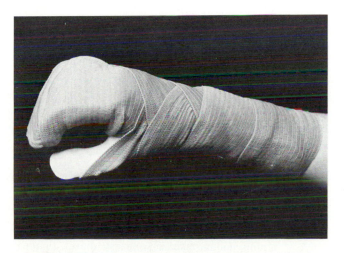

FIG. 18-9. A functional resting splint is secured with a figure-of-eight elastic wrap when severe edema is present, to help distribute pressure over a wide area.

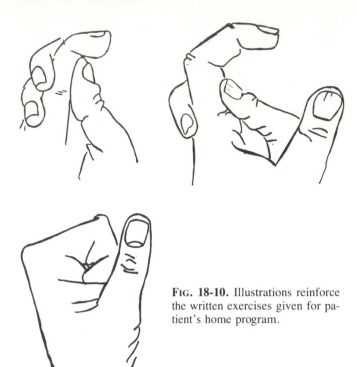

FIG. 18-10. Illustrations reinforce the written exercises given for patient's home program.

and the patient's surgeon notified. After a discussion with the patient's surgeon, appropriate changes in the treatment program are made.

THE CHRONICALLY STIFF HAND

The patient with the chronically stiff hand requires a comprehensive therapy program in which there is ongoing communication between the patient, the therapist, and the surgeon. Examples of problems that commonly lead to a chronically stiff hand are fractures of the wrist or fingers, serious crush injuries, and acutely injured hands that were left untreated. The initial treatment session begins with an explanation about what has caused the patient's stiff hand and what must be done to restore function to it. The patient must understand that progress will be slow and strongly dependent on how motivated he is in consistently carrying out his therapy program.

Evaluation

Evaluation of the chronically stiff hand is more in-depth than that of the acutely stiff hand. As with the acutely stiff hand, a thorough history and a thorough hand inspection are done. Assessment of range of motion, strength, sensibility, and the patient's ability to perform activities of daily living completes the evaluation.

Range of motion. Knowledge of the causes of joint stiffness is essential before evaluation of the range of motion of the chronically stiff hand. Tests for skin tightness, joint range of motion, and intrinsic and extrinsic muscle tightness are routinely done.

Joint motion may be limited by tight skin around a joint or by a scar that crosses a joint. To evaluate this con-

dition, one puts the joints adjacent to the joint being evaluated on slack before a passive stretch is applied. If blanching of the skin or scar occurs during passive motion of the joint, stretch to these structures should be incorporated in the treatment program. If the skin puckers when a stretch is applied, it indicates adherence to the underlying structures.

Active range of motion is measured by means of standard methods for measuring and recording, as described by the American Academy of Orthopaedic Surgeons.[1] If joint stiffness is present, closely examine the "end feel" of each joint before measuring passive range of motion with a goniometer. To do this, move the finger gently in the direction in which the joint motion is limited. If the joint comes to a slow stop and has a springy feel, the prognosis for improvement is good. However, if the joint moves freely to a certain point and then stops abruptly, the prognosis for conservative treatment is poor (see Chapter 76). To measure passive joint motion with a finger goniometer, place the adjacent joints in whatever position is necessary to allow for maximum motion of the joint being measured, to eliminate influence from adherent tendons.

To complete the evaluation for range of motion, tests for intrinsic and extrinsic muscle tightness must be done. Intrinsic tightness exists if the proximal and distal interphalangeal joints can be passively flexed with the metacarpophalangeal joint in flexion (Fig. 18-11, A) but cannot be fully flexed when the metacarpophalangeal joint is extended[2] (Fig. 18-11, B). Extrinsic extensor tightness is present if the proximal and distal interphalangeal joints will passively flex when the metacarpophalangeal joint is extended (Fig. 18-12, A) but cannot be fully flexed when the metacarpophalangeal joint is flexed[2] (Fig. 18-12, B). Extrinsic flexor tightness is present if the proximal and distal interphalangeal joints will passively extend with the metacarpophalangeal joint flexed (Fig. 18-13, A) but cannot be fully extended when the metacarpophalangeal joint is extended (Fig. 18-13, B).

Strength. Pinch and grip strength are measured on both extremities and compared. Grip strength is measured on all five handle positions of the adjustable Jamar* dynamometer (Fig. 18-14). Lateral, tip, and pulp pinch are measured on a pinch meter (Fig. 18-15). Individual muscle testing is done on selected patients to determine the motor function of a particular nerve and the relative strengths of the involved muscles.

Sensibility. When indicated, tests for light touch and two-point discrimination are administered to determine the sensory function of a particular nerve.

Activities of daily living. An interview and the Jebson Hand Function Test[8] are used to determine the patient's ability to perform activities of daily living independently. The Jebson Hand Function Test assesses a person's ability to write, manage eating utensils, manipulate small objects, and manipulate both light and heavy objects.

---

*Jamar dynamometer, Asimow Engineering Co., 1414 So. Beverly Glen Blvd., Los Angeles, Calif. 90024.

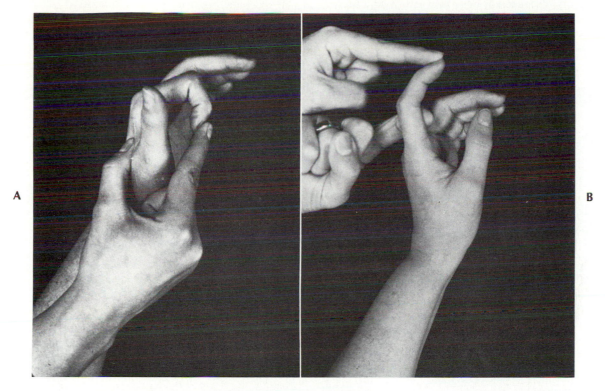

FIG. 18-11. Intrinsic tightness exists if the proximal and distal interphalangeal joints can be passively flexed with the metacarpophalangeal joint in flexion (**A**) but cannot be fully flexed when the metacarpophalangeal joint is extended (**B**).

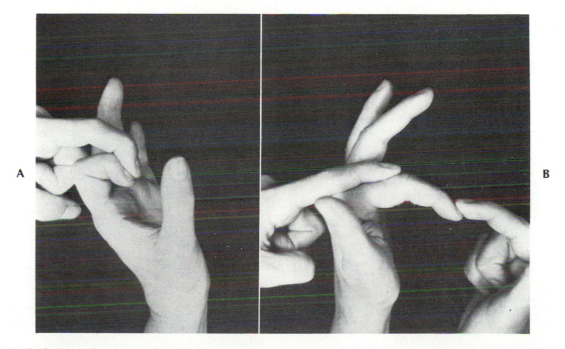

FIG. 18-12. Extrinsic extensor tightness is present if the proximal and distal interphalangeal joints can be passively flexed when the metacarpophalangeal joint is extended (**A**) but cannot be fully flexed when the metacarpophalangeal joint is flexed (**B**).

Treatment guidelines

Edema control. In the chronically stiff hand, pitting edema has usually disappeared, but it leaves behind a brawny type of edema that is much more difficult to treat. Treatment for this brawny edema includes retrograde massage, exercise, elasticized gloves, and functional activities.

Massage done firmly in a retrograde manner is used in an attempt to mobilize edema and adherent tissues. Massage of the patient's hand by the therapist is an ideal way to begin the therapist-patient relationship. It gives the therapist an opportunity to transmit feelings of caring and understanding to the patient and at the same time allows the patient

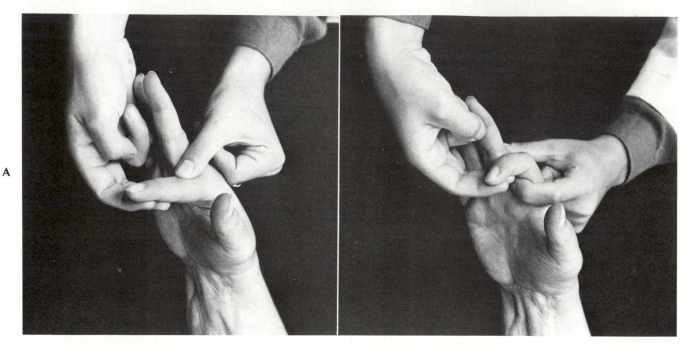

A   B

FIG. 18-13. Extrinsic flexor tightness is present if the proximal and distal interphalangeal joints can be passively extended with the metacarpophalangeal joint flexed (**A**) but cannot be extended as fully when the metacarpophalangeal joint is extended (**B**).

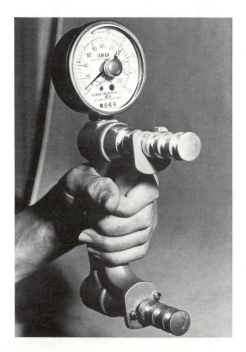

FIG. 18-14. The adjustable Jamar dynamometer is used to evaluate grip strength on five handle positions.

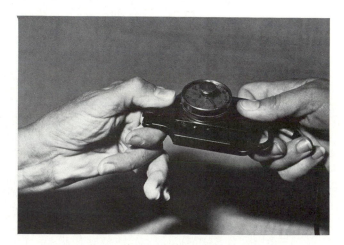

FIG. 18-15. Lateral, tip, and pulp pinch are measured on a pinch meter.

to become more relaxed and able to discuss any problems related to his hand injury. After massage, exercises that encourage full tendon excursion are performed.

An Aris Isotoner Glove may be used to provide external compression to a chronically swollen hand and can be effective in reducing dorsal edema. The patient wears the glove while performing activities of daily living and prehension tasks such as macramé and leather work.

Therapeutic exercise.

Passive range-of-motion exercises. Passive range-of-motion exercises are helpful before one begins active motion.

*Coban, Medical Products Division, Minnesota Mining & Manufacturing Co., St. Paul, Minn. 55144.

In order for the effects of passive range-of-motion exercises to be of lasting benefit, they should be done for a prolonged period of time with a low to moderate amount of tension.[3,5,6,8] Sapega and co-workers have proposed that stretching be combined with a rise in tissue temperature. In vitro studies suggest that a prolonged stretch, accompanied by an elevated tissue temperature, assists lengthening of connective tissue.[9] The therapist can incorporate the principle of combining heat and stretch to a stiff hand in the following way. Using an elasticized tape, such as Coban,* apply a stretch to the involved finger or fingers in the direction in which you wish to increase motion. Once the hand is stretched with the tape, dip it in paraffin, and place it under a hot pack for approximately 30 minutes (Fig. 18-16). Cau-

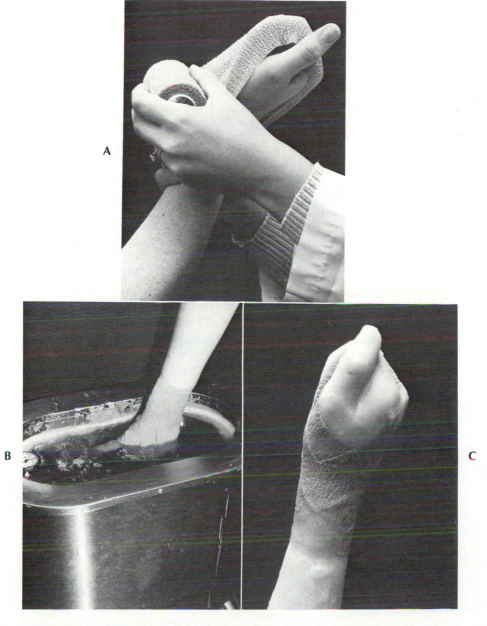

FIG. 18-16. A, Elasticized tape is used to gently stretch the fingers into flexion. **B** and **C,** Hand is then dipped in paraffin and placed in elevation under a hot pack for 30 minutes.

tion must be taken when applying heat to areas with decreased sensibility or poor skin quality. Active exercise should immediately be done after this procedure.

As an adjunct to prolonged stretch, manual passive range-of-motion exercises can be performed. To administer passive range-of-motion exercises, ask the patient to relax his hand, and place both of your hands close to the axis of the joint being mobilized. Gently distract the joints to avoid compression of the segments being mobilized, and move the joint in the direction desired (Fig. 18-17) until a slight resistance is felt; hold the joint in that position of stretch for several seconds, and then relax the joint and repeat. During the performance of passive range-of-motion exercises, it is important to teach the patient to distinguish between the sensation of pain and the sensation of stretch. Forceful manipulations are always contraindicated because they result in pain and swelling around the involved joints.

Active range-of-motion exercises. The patient's active exercise program includes motion of all joints of the involved extremity, because uninvolved joints quickly become stiff after trauma to the hand. The following exercises are always included:

1. Blocking of the distal interphalangeal and proximal interphalangeal joints of each finger to encourage isolated motion of the flexor digitorum profundus (Fig. 18-18, *A*) and flexor digitorum superficialis (Fig. 18-18, *B*)
2. Fist making
3. Extension of the fingers
4. Abduction and adduction of the fingers
5. Opposition, abduction, flexion, and extension of the thumb
6. Blocking of the interphalangeal joint of the thumb to encourage isolated flexor pollicis longus action
7. Wrist flexion, extension, and ulnar and radial deviation

When one is instructing patients in active range-of-motion exercises, they must be taught to perform the correct pattern of motion. For example, excessive attempts at finger flexion often result in simultaneous wrist flexion. To correct this problem, the patient is instructed to hold his wrist in slight extension when performing finger flexion. If the patient is unable to support voluntarily his wrist with finger flexion,

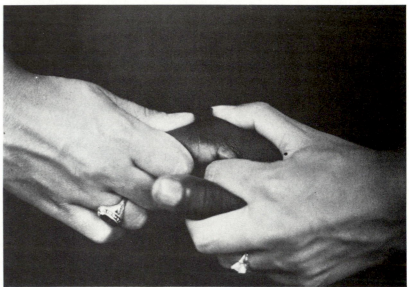

FIG. 18-17. To perform passive range-of-motion exercises, gently distract the joint being mobilized before flexing or extending it.

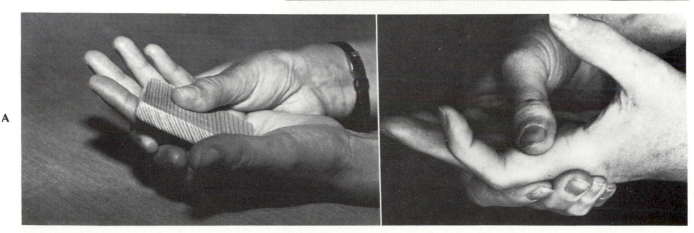

A   B

FIG. 18-18. A wood block (**A**) or finger blocking (**B**) is used to facilitate isolated pull-through of the long flexor tendons.

an external wrist support is used for exercise until finger flexion is strengthened. Also, if the goal of exercise is to improve active motion of the long flexors, the patient must be taught to support the metacarpophalangeal joint in extension while flexing the distal joints, thereby eliminating the action of the intrinsic muscles.

It should be stressed to the patient that the correct motion is more important than the strength of motion. Often a paitent will try so hard to perform a motion that he will co-contract the agonist and antagonistic muscles. The patient is taught to prevent co-contraction by relaxing the opposing muscles. Biofeedback can be used for this purpose by placing three surface electrodes on the opposing muscles and setting the machine to pick up the unwanted muscle activity. If the patient co-contracts his muscles, the machine will give off an auditory signal telling the patient he has performed the motion incorrectly (Fig. 18-19). Patients using biofeedback can work independently on their exercise programs.

Resistive exercises. For patients who have little or no pull-through of the flexor or extensor tendons because of adhesions or weakness, resistive exercises must be initiated immediately. Graded resistive activities progressing from a foam squeeze, putty, or the Hand Helper* to progressive resistive weights, ceramics, and woodworking are some of the many activities selected to help increase strength of the hand.

Therapeutic activities. Therapeutic activities are used to help increase active motion, strength, and endurance of a

---

*Hand Helper available from Meddev Corp., P.O. Box 1352, Los Altos, Calif., 94022.

chronically stiff hand. They are an integral part of the therapy program, since they encourage patients to again consider their hands as functional and working parts of their bodies. When a patient's dominant hand is injured, he is encouraged to write, dress, and eat with it, even if it requires the use of a piece of adaptive equipment such as a built-up handle. Activities such as macramé and light pickups are used for patients who are not ready for heavy resistance. These activities can be done in elevation in the case of a swollen hand. Leatherwork and ceramics provide active motion and moderate resistance to a stiff hand, while woodworking and woodcarving are used to provide heavy resistance. It is important when the patient is performing his activities that the handle on the working tools be built up to the point where the fingers are able to maintain a sustained grip around them (Fig. 18-20). The patient's endurance for whatever activity he is performing is increased daily if the therapist has him perform the activity for longer periods of time each day.

Splinting. Dynamic splinting is the most effective modality that can be used to apply a low-to-moderate amount of tension to a stiff joint over a prolonged period of time. If evaluation reveals that limitation in the range of motion is strictly related to soft-tissue contracture around a particular joint, a splint must be designed to apply traction to that specific joint. Fig. 18-21 shows an example of a splint that is being used to apply passive flexion to a proximal interphalangeal joint stiff in extension. When evaluation reveals that restrictions in active range of motion are attributable to a combination of joint contracture and muscle tightness, a two-stage splinting program is required. Initially a splint is designed to increase the passive range of motion of the

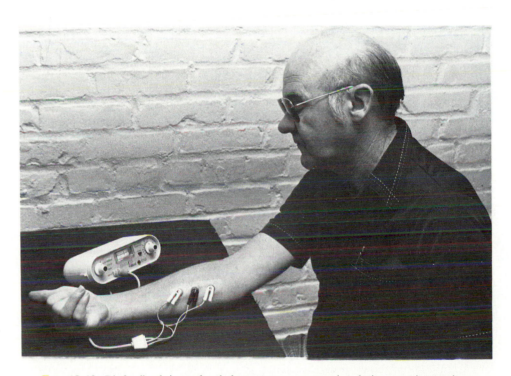

FIG. 18-19. Biofeedback is used to help prevent co-contraction during exercise sessions.

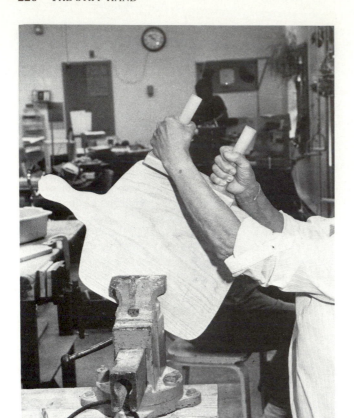

FIG. 18-20. Sustained-grip activities such as wood sanding are used to strengthen weakened muscles in the stiff hand.

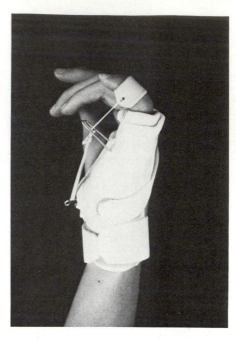

FIG. 18-21. A dynamic, hand-based splint is used to improve flexion of the proximal interphalangeal joint.

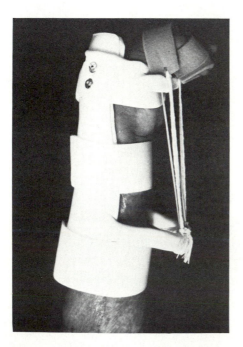

FIG. 18-22. An extrinsic extension stretching splint holds the metacarpophalangeal joints flexed with string while dynamic flexion is applied to the interphalangeal joints.

involved joint. Once this has been achieved, the splinting program is directed at providing a stretch to the involved intrinsic or extrinsic musculature. Fig. 18-22 demonstrates a splint designed to apply traction to an adherent extrinsic extensor mechanism. In the following chapter, Colditz provides a full review of the principles and methods of splinting the stiff hand.

''Quick splints'' are named for the fact that they can be quickly and inexpensively fabricated. Situations may arise in which one or both of these factors necessitates the use of a quick splint. It is important to remember that they are not the answer to every splinting problem. The following are descriptions of the more commonly used quick splints.

1. Web strap. The web strap (Fig. 18-23) provides a passive stretch necessary to improve the range of motion from the finger pulp to the palmar crease. It is most effective in gaining the final degrees of proximal interphalangeal flexion. This strap is worn over the proximal interphalangeal joint and behind the metacarpophalangeal joint. The strap is fabricated from a 1-inch-wide lamb wick and a 1-inch-wide buckle.

2. Combination web strap. The combination web strap (Fig. 18-24) is effective when all joints of one or two fingers are stiff in extension. It is comfortable and easily adjusted and can be worn as a night splint. One should keep in mind that the combination web strap

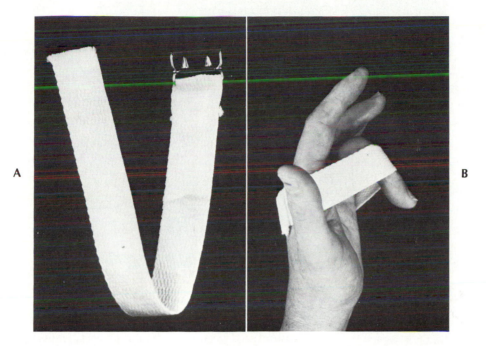

FIG. 18-23. The web strap is used to improve passive range of motion of the proximal interphalangeal joint.

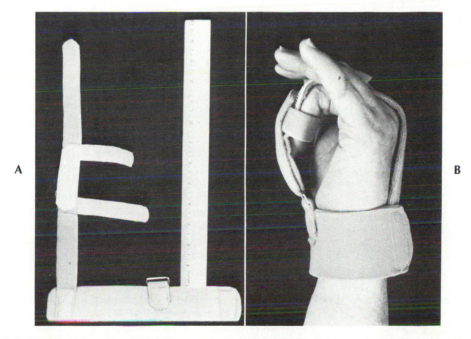

FIG. 18-24. A Combination web strap. **B** This strap is used when all joints of one or two fingers are stiff in extension, but it exerts its force most effectively at the least stiff joint.

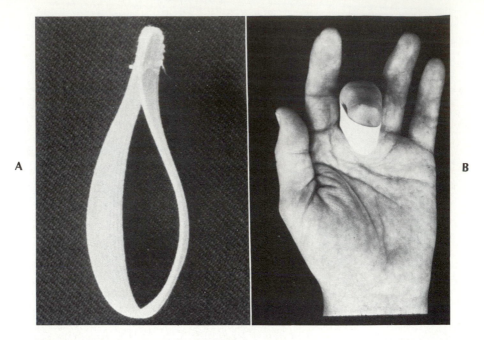

FIG. 18-25. To improve passive range of motion of the distal interphalangeal joint, an elastic strap is worn periodically during the day over the interphalangeal joints.

will be most effective on the joints that are least restricted. The combination web strap is not effective in gaining the final degrees of proximal interphalangeal or distal interphalangeal joint motion. The materials necessary to construct the combination web strap are a 1-inch-wide buckle, a Velcro* hook and loop, and a 1-inch-wide D ring.

3. Elastic flexion strap. The elastic flexion strap (Fig. 18-25) is used to obtain primarily distal interphalangeal motion and, to a lesser extent, proximal interphalangeal motion of a stiff finger. The elastic flexion strap is worn over the distal and proximal interphalangeal joints. To construct the strap, a piece of elastic with a width of a half an inch and a length of 4 inches is fitted around the patient's interphalangeal joints while they are held in maximum flexion. A mark is made on the elastic at the point where the two ends of the elastic meet on the proximal phalanx, and the elastic is sewn together on that mark. At night, the elastic strap is replaced by a retaining splint that is similar in design to the elastic strap but, because its tension can be adjusted, is more comfortable to wear during sleep (Fig. 18-26).

Patient education. Restoration of hand function to a chronically stiff hand is strongly dependent on the patient's level of motivation. Therapeutic exercises and activities must be performed consistently at home. The patient must understand that any splint that has been prescribed will only be effective if it is worn for a long period of time with a low-to-moderate amount of tension. The home program should be written and reviewed at each therapy session.

Ongoing evaluation. Evaluation is an integral part of the

_____
*Velcro USA, Inc., 681 Fifth Avenue, New York, N.Y. 10022.

treatment program. Ongoing evaluations assist the therapist in determining when changes in the treatment program are necessary and provide information as to when the patient has plateaued in his therapy program. When the patient's progress has plateaued for a significant period of time, the surgeon must then determine if the patient has achieved maximum function or if surgical intervention is indicated. Surgical procedures that might be performed on a stiff hand include tenolysis, joint capsulectomies, and joint arthroplasties.

Case study: The chronically stiff hand

The following case study demonstrates the principles of treating the chronically stiff hand. The patient is a 46-year-old, right-handed housewife who injured her left shoulder in a fall 1 year before referral to the Hand Rehabilitation Center in Philadelphia. The patient initially sustained a tear to her rotator cuff muscles and underwent surgical repair 3 months after injury. The patient's shoulder was immobilized for six weeks, and she reported that during that time she developed severe swelling and limitation in the range of motion of her hand. The patient attended therapy at a local hospital for 6 months and stated that she received painful therapy to her shoulder and hand. The patient was referred to the Hand Therapy Department at the Hand Rehabilitation Center 1 year after injury for rehabilitation of her left upper extremity. Evaluation revealed a painful, sensitive extremity with severe limitations in hand-and-shoulder range of motion and strength. Intrinsic muscle tightness and mild extrinsic extensor tightness were noted. The patient reported that she was only able to use her hand to assist in light activities of daily living.

Most of the first treatment session was used to help establish a trusting relationship. Once the patient realized that

FIG.18-26. The elastic strap is replaced at night with an adjustable distal-interphalangeal flexion strap, fabricated from leather and Velcro, to maintain gains made during the day.

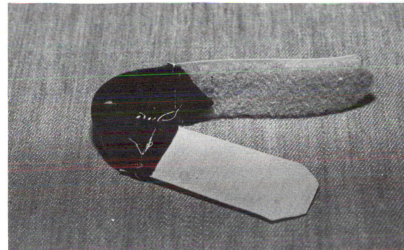

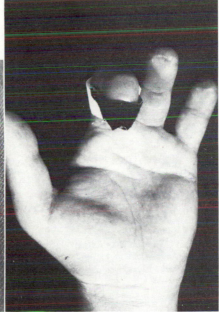

the philosophy of treatment stressed nonpainful therapy, she became more willing to participate actively in the program. The patient was given an Isotoner glove to help alleviate the internal pressure from brawny edema that she felt in her hand. Before exercise, the patient's hand was wrapped in an elasticized tape, pulling her fingers into flexion. The patient's hand was then dipped in paraffin and placed under a hot pack to retain the heat for a period of 30 minutes. Active range-of-motion exercise of all joints of the extremity was encouraged through the use of specific exercises and therapeutic activities. The patient was begun on macramé and light pick-ups to help increase shoulder-and-hand range of motion. In 1 month she progressed to a resistive weight program, woodworking, and the potter's wheel for strength and endurance.

A splinting program was initiated at the patient's second visit. Since the patient had severe intrinsic tightness, a splint was fabricated to stretch the intrinsics by holding the metacarpophalangeal joints in extension and applying moderate tension that pulled the proximal and distal interphalangeal joints into flexion (Fig. 18-27). A timetable for a home program of exercise, functional use, and splinting was discussed with the patient and designed to fit her individual needs.

This patient attended therapy three times weekly for half-day sessions for a total of 6 months. At that time, the patient had regained the full range of motion of her hand. Shoulder range of motion, though occasionally painful, had improved significantly and was within functional limits. Grip strength of the involved hand, measured by the Jamar dynamometer, was 70% of that of the uninvolved hand.

SUMMARY

A patient with an acutely swollen, stiff hand who receives the proper treatment immediately after injury will not require long-term care. Once edema and pain have stabilized and

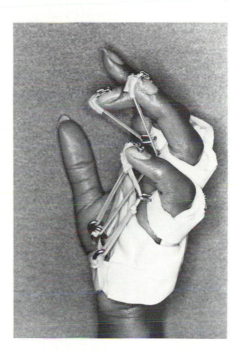

FIG. 18-27. An intrinsic stretching splint positions the metacarpophalangeal joints in extension while flexing the interphalangeal joints.

active range of motion has been restored, the patient should be able to resume his normal activities. An acutely stiff hand, left untreated, will progress to a chronically stiff hand, with serious loss of hand function. Treatment of the chronically stiff hand may be long term and will require innovative problem solving by the therapist. Evaluation techniques and treatment guidelines described in this chapter are intended to aid the therapist in designing a treatment program that fits the individual needs of each patient.

REFERENCES

1. American Academy of Orthopedic Surgeons: Joint motion, Chicago, 1965, the Academy.
2. American Society for Surgery of the Hand: The Hand: examination and diagnosis, Aurora, Colo. 1978, The Society.
3. Becker, A.H.: Traction for knee-flexion contractures, Phys. Ther. **59:**1114, Sept. 1979.
4. Brand, P.W., and Wood, H.: Hand volumeter instruction sheet, United States Public Health Service Hospital, Carville, La.
5. Glazer, R.M.: Rehabilitation. In Happenstal, R.B., editor: Fracture treatment in healing, Philadelphia, 1980, W.B. Saunders Co., pp. 1041-1068.
6. Jackman, R.V.: Device to stretch the achilles tendon, J. Am. Phys. Ther. Assoc. **43:**729, Oct. 1963.
7. Jebson, R.H., Taylor, N., Trieschman, R.B., Trotter, M.J., and Howard, L.A.: An objective and standardized test of hand function, Arch. Phys. Med. Rehabil. **50:**311-319, 1969.
8. Kottke, F.J., Pauley, D.L., and Ptak, K.A.: The rationale for prolonged stretching for correction of shortening of connective tissue, Arch. Phys. Med. Rehabil. **47:**345-354, June 1966.
9. Sapega, A.A., Quedenfeld, T.C., Moyer, R.A., and Butler, R.A.: Physiological factors in range-of-motion exercise, Physician in Sports Med. **G:**57, Dec. 1981.

BIBLIOGRAPHY

Beasley, R.W.: Hand injuries, Philadelphia, 1981, W.B. Saunders Co.
Curtis, R.M.: Joints of the hand. In Flynn, J.E., editor: Hand surgery, ed. 2, Baltimore, 1975, The Williams & Wilkins Co.
Harrison, D.H.: The stiff proximal interphalangeal joint, Hand **9**(2):102, 1977.
Peacock, E.E., Jr.: Preservation of interphalangeal joint function: a basis for the early care of injured hands, South. Med. J. **56:**56-63, 1962.
Peacock, E.E., Jr.: Some biochemical and biophysical aspects of joint stiffness: role of collagen synthesis as opposed to ultra-molecular binding, Ann. Surg. **164:**1-6, 1966.
Pratt, D.R.: Joints of the hand and fingers—their stiffness, splinting and surgery, California Med. **66:**22-24, 1947.

19

Dynamic splinting of the stiff hand

JUDY C. COLDITZ

SPLINTING RATIONALE
Physiology of stiffness

Dynamic splinting of the injured hand is well accepted as a treatment modality in hand rehabilitation.[7,8,12,13,16] The unavoidable response to injury of edema production within the finely balanced tissues of the hand often demands a modality beyond pure active motion in order to regain the balance of motion. To understand the rationale of dynamic splinting, one must understand the physiology of stiffness. No one has stated it better than Sterling Bunnell in 1946: "Hands are particular in that they are prone to become stiffened—evidently because the joint surfaces are so accurately approximated, and there are more close fitting, gliding parts than elsewhere in the body. Joint ligaments are just long enough, but not too long. If, from any cause, a hand remains swollen and immobile, the serum-soaked ligaments become short and thick, binding the joints. From the fluid of oedema, fibrin settles between the movable tissues and within them—muscles, tendons, and joints alike. Fibroblasts invade; the whole becomes organized and shrinks; and the hand becomes congealed."[7]

This process may be seen most vividly in the crushed hand with multiple tissue injuries, but stiffness secondary to immobility and edema production may also be demonstrated in a hand with minor trauma that has been immobilized excessively. In either case the combination of edema and immobilization has altered the balance of motion. Thus, dynamic splinting to stretch the tightness and reestablish the balance is frequently an appropriate tool of the therapist.

Splinting frequently may be a replacement for surgery.[13,15] For what can be quickly altered by the scalpel can often be slowly altered by the stress applied by a dynamic splint. Surgery to regain motion reestablishes the vicious cycle of edema and pain and requires again a period of initial immobilization to promote wound healing. Conservative means of gaining motion by dynamic splinting allows increasing strength and tissue glide while gaining motion and thus avoids the stimulation of edema production. One must emphasize that dynamic splinting is only part of a comprehensive rehabilitation of the hand.[14,18] The splint helps gain passive motion by the stress applied, but only active and active resistive motion can reestablish a balance of power and glide. Dynamic splinting imposes immobility on the hand, since only one direction of motion can be gained at a time. Periods out of the splint must allow for other motions.

Static versus dynamic splinting

Dynamic splints create motion. Static splints prevent motion. It is therefore appropriate that static splints be reserved for the healing phase of injury and dynamic splints be applied to gain motion after the initial healing stage. Static splints used for serial splinting are helpful in gaining motion when they are based on the same principle as dynamic splinting, in that the tissue is stressed to a new length each time. Static splints may also provide the appropriate input for a hand with nerve palsy, supplying a substitution for muscle action. Except for the few cases in which positive pressure is useful for retaining a flattening of scar, static splinting tends to extend the period of immobilization initially used immediately after injury. In the majority of cases the use of dynamic splinting is clearly the choice over static splinting when one attempts to gain joint motion in the injured hand.[1,4-6,17]

Static splints that position the whole hand and are meant to stretch a tight joint frequently position the tightest structure the poorest. The great advantage of dynamic splinting is the ability to provide a specific force to specific tightness, be it joint tightness, tendon adhesions, skin tightness, muscle-tendon unit tightness, or any combination. Forces applied by a dynamic splint are translated easily to the loose joints of a paralyzed hand, but in the stiff hand application of force needs to be more specific.

Tissue response to splinting

The effectiveness of dynamic splinting is based on a sound physiologic theory: a long period of applied tension alters cell proliferation.[19-20] The tension must be of such low magnitude so as not to tear or force the tissues and thus stimulate the inflammatory response, causing more edema and then more fibrosis. It must be applied for a long enough period to alter the way in which new tissue is synthesized. This can be achieved by serial casting, in which a new tension is applied daily and the tissues accommodate to it, or by a dynamic splint, which accomplishes the same goal and can provide a more constant tension over a longer period of time. It must be clear to the patient that the goal is not to tolerate increasing amounts of tension on the rubber band, but rather to tolerate it for increasing periods of time. The hand may need an initial period of adjustment to the tension applied, but the time should slowly increase so that the patient is comfortable with the splint for hours at a time.

The patient should be aware of a sensation of stretching, but it should not be painful.

Human tissue is viscoelastic; that is, it responds to the stress applied. The immediate response of the tissues is one of elasticity; tissue stretched will return to its original shape and length. Only with a period of prolonged stretch will one achieve a viscous or plastic response, in that the tissues now take on the shape to which they have been deformed by the force applied.[4] Thus it is the prolonged quality of the stretch that mobilizes stiffness. The analogy of a stretched rubber band is helpful when this phenomenon is described to patients: quickly stretch a rubber band and when you let it go it will return to its original length, but hold the rubber band stretched for a day and it will not contract to its original resting length and will then go the stretched distance with greater ease. This phenomenon is the principle of prolonged stretch, which mobilizes stiffness. Patients should report that the dynamic splint relieves a sense of tightness in the hand, which they are otherwise unable to affect, and they should demonstrate a certain eagerness about the splint in that wearing it relieves the internal tension. If this is not the case, the splint is ill fitting or the tension too great.

Like rubber, scar when inactive (cool) is tight and nonelastic. Heat (created by stretch or friction) allows it to become more elastic, and tension within the scar is decreased. This explains the phenomenon of morning stiffness, since the tissues have been immobile during sleep. For this reason, gentle prolonged stretch at night to produce motion in the direction with the greatest deficit is encouraged. After there has been a prolonged stretch at night, the plastic response (that is, changing shape) allows easier elastic response (that is, stretching the distance) during the day, and the potential for active motion is maximized. Extension splinting is generally more easily tolerated at night because flexion splinting may be somewhat constrictive. Therefore any flexion splinting at night needs to be of a lesser force than that applied during the day. This decreased force is true of all-night splinting, since distracting events during the day allow tension to be easily tolerated, but the lack of stimuli at night causes one to become much more aware of the stress. Additionally, during periods of rest and inactivity, the natural pumping assistance of active muscles is removed from the extremity, again clearly pointing up the need for a lesser tension so as not to constrict blood flow.

Because of the constant activity of cell multiplication and proliferation within a healing area, the use of a dynamic splint must be not only for long periods at a time but also over a long span of time. Many patients are encouraged by the rapid gains of motion from the fitting of a dynamic splint only to become discouraged when they remove the splint and the deformity reccurs. When fitting a splint, one would be wise to instruct the patient that when he removes the splint for any long period he will be unable to retain what the splint has gained. It is only when he has worn the splint long enough to encourage cell proliferation in the direction and of the length needed that he can retain the motion without the splint. Explaining this at the time of splint fitting prevents the patient from being unnecessarily discouraged and increases compliance with the long-term need for splinting.

SPLINTMAKING
History

The art and science of splintmaking as we know it today is relatively new, but the word "splint" has its origin in the Middle Ages. Splints were the triangular parts of armor that allowed motion at the joints but offered protection from arrows and other missiles. Although the modern use of the word frequently refers to static immobilization, it is useful to remember that the original device allowed motion.

Many early devices for splintage of the upper extremity were reminiscent of armor design, undoubtedly fashioned by the village blacksmith. Although there are numerous isolated original splint designs published both before and after World War II, there is little written about the rationale for splinting except for the original work of Bunnell.[1,5,7,8] He was instrumental in organizing hand treatment centers within the United States military medical system and did much to document and standardize surgical treatment, immobilization, and rehabilitation techniques. Although the army had issued a manual on hand splints in 1917, it was Bunnell's chapter on splints in the *Orthopaedic Appliance Atlas* in 1952 that began the standardization of splint design.[1] In his first edition of *Surgery of the Hand* there is a chapter devoted to splints, splintmaking, and current materials.[8]

Many early splints had a somewhat homemade appearance, since there were no special materials available. Plaster of paris was often the material choice for the splint base, since one could achieve a close-fitting mold with the hand. Ingenuity often replaced the sophisticated materials and during World War II aluminum salvaged from wrecked airplanes were used, as were corset spring steel strips. Bunnell illustrates a splint with clock springs,[7] and Capener in England used window curtain springs.[11] The army hand centers frequently used brass wire as an outrigger incorporated into a plaster base, as described by Peacock.[16]

The orthotist who was trained in materials and construction techniques executed beautiful orthoses for the hand, but the construction time required for these permanent devices did not allow immediate fit. Fitting of the splint was a process removed from therapy. Adjustments of these permanent devices were then hardly encouraged. The metal and high-temperature plastics did not lend themselves to the intricate plasticity of the hand shape, and often these splints forced the hand into position rather than the hand dictating the splint needed. Capener described this problem well: "Surgical appliance making has been in the past and still is in the hands of the commercial craftsmen who have done a splendid work, yet who are often divorced from adequate medical guidance."[11]

In an attempt to standardize hand surgery and treatment many of Bunnell's original designs were made commercially available and still are widely used today. Unfortunately, the metal and felt used for commercial production did not offer a custom device. The era of polio influenced the thinking about upper extremity orthotics, and to standardize the language, splints were defined by the components in the splint system: lumbrical bar, C-bar, palmar bar, and so on. Unfortunately, the component system that effectively harnesses a hand with muscular imbalance has often become confused with the outrigger systems needed to stretch tight internal structures.

Advent of splinting materials

As hand surgery continued to establish itself as a specialty, it became clear that the fitting of the splint should be incorporated into the therapy treatment to avoid some of the problems above. A number of high-temperature plastics became available (Lucite, Nyloplex, Plexiglas, and Royalite), but these materials required such high temperatures to become workable that it required making a positive plaster mold from which to work. Thus construction time and easy adjustability remained a problem. These materials and the traditional plaster and metal did not encourage a timely response to a changing hand.

The advent of low-temperature materials designed specifically for splinting needs (such as Orthoplast, Polyform, K-splint, and Aquaplast) allowed dynamic splinting to become a more active part of hand therapy. Therapists now could quickly cut, mold, and finish even a complicated splint that was appropriate for use early in treatment and even with open wounds. With these new materials alteration to accommodate increased motion, relieve a pressure area, or adjust tension could be immediate. The thermoplastic materials were responsive to the hand, instead of the hand being forced to respond to the material.

With the strong influence of commercial splints, the process of custom splinting of the hand has been poorly documented for indications, timing of applying splints, and design choices. It is now often the dilemma of the hand therapist to evaluate critically whether the time-saving fitting of a commercial splint or the application of a custom-made splint is the better treatment for the hand in question. Only as the hand therapist develops better skills at design and application of splints within the total framework of hand rehabilitation will this decision become clear.

READINESS FOR SPLINTING
Use of splint

The trained hand therapist must be thoroughly knowledgeable about many treatment modalities in order to effect improvement in the injured hand. Dynamic splinting is only one of these. The use of the splint should complement the gains made during therapy visits. It not only prevents loss of motion because of contraction of the constantly tightening tissues, but it can also make passive gains beyond what is achieved during therapy. Therapy visits should concentrate on active pull-through and strengthening, thus reinforcing the passive gains made by the splint. Only very mild deformities, such as the slight proximal interphalangeal joint flexion contracture resulting from a sprain of the collateral ligaments, respond to splinting without a strong complementary exercise program.

Edema control

The natural phenomenon of edema production discussed earlier is often the key to understanding the appropriate timing for splinting application.[14] The amount of edema produced varies depending on both the severity of the injury and the individual response the body makes to the injury.

Because of these variations, there is no clear rule as to the time to begin dynamic splinting after injury. Edema of the hand can be compared to the sausage skin stuffed full of sausage. Just as the sausage is difficult to bend, so are the joints of the hand until some of the "stuffing" is removed. Although the goal of early dynamic splinting is to prevent chronic stiffness, which requires more long-term treatment, the decision for application of the splint must be based on a state of good control of post-injury edema and on the absence of gross fluctuations of the edema. Otherwise the constricting forces of the splint stimulate even more accumulation of edema in the hand. The dilemma of splinting for increased motion at the expense of aggravating edema is always the early problem. The acutely injured hand, with pitting edema, red swollen joints, and pain with motion, is a hand to be treated gently, elevated, and moved primarily with active motion. At this stage the goal of edema and pain reduction far exceed any splinting goals. Any dynamic splint, no matter how well constructed, will by virtue of the force it is applying be a constrictive force to the already borderline circulatory and drainage status of the injured hand.

Tolerance to stretch

In addition to the hand demonstrating a reduction of edema, it is ready for dynamic splinting when there is a tolerance to both active motion and gentle prolonged passive stretch. Rarely is it appropriate to dynamically splint the injured hand immediately out of the surgical dressing. A few days in therapy of gaining active pull-through, monitoring edema levels, and allowing the tissues to gain a tolerance to the stress of active and very gentle passive motion readies the hand to be very tolerant of a splinting program. Unfortunately, the few days of therapy may stretch into a longer period for those patients who demonstrate a hyperactive inflammatory response to injury.

In the evaluation of a hand for dynamic splinting it is helpful to gain a feel for the springiness of the tight tissues. Manual evaluation of the resistance within the tissues will indicate to the therapist whether splint gains will be rapid or long term. A hand that responds well to a gentle passive stretch may not need the help of a splint, and a short period of active therapy may be appropriate before there is a final decision about splinting. On the contrary, a joint that has almost full range of motion but demonstrates significant resistance to stretch in the end ranges is an excellent candidate for splinting. It is the prolonged stretch at the end of the range that gives the patient full, easy joint motion. The more acutely one is able to apply the splint, the less the tension and the shorter the period of time the patient will need the splint. Patients seen late who present with fibrotic stiffness often need months of splinting, and because the tissues are more organized, one must apply greater tension to effect reorganization of collagen. The longer the time after injury that one is able to institute splinting, generally the longer the patient will need to wear the splint.

Goniometric measurements

Accurate goniometric measurements are helpful in determining both the readiness for splinting and the indications for altering the splinting routine. Whenever full passive range of motion is not present, it is appropriate to consider splinting. However, if there is a large discrepancy between the active and passive range of motion, the emphasis should lie on active pull-through, with splinting being the secondary goal. If the active and passive range of motion is equal, concentration on the splinting program will allow passive gains to be made so that the potential for active motion is greater. The final result can only be as good as the passive potential.

One may also see early rapid improvements of joint motion with other clinical modalities, but one joint may plateau in its improvement, thus an indication of the appropriateness for splinting. Careful and frequent monitoring of goniometric measurements often give precise direction for the splinting program.

PRINCIPLES OF SPLINTING
Positioning

Basic principles of splinting often refer to the "position of function,"[7] which is slight wrist extension (usually 30 degrees) accompanied by metacarpophalangeal flexion and slight interphalangeal flexion and thumb abduction. It was not Bunnell's intent that this "position of function" be a rule for all splinting, but he advocated this as a position to be used during the period of initial immobilization and healing. The balance of motion could be maintained more easily than when the wrist was allowed to fall into a position of flexion creating the typical clawhand. Although it is good to maintain this basic position whenever possible, the goal of dynamic splinting is to stretch the tight motions. This may mean that appropriately the wrist may need to be in flexion as when one flexes the fingers to stretch extrinsic extensor adherence proximal to the wrist or when one protects a newly repaired flexor tendon. Dynamic splints are not permanent devices but are intermittent, applying a specific force, and thus must position the hand as demanded by the specific tightness.[16]

Palmar bars are routinely designed to end proximally to the proximal palmar crease to allow full metacarpophalangeal flexion. But if the goal of the splint is to gain proximal interphalangeal joint flexion with the metacarpophalangeal joints stabilized, it may be appropriate to end the splint distally to the crease for better stability of the metacarpophalangeal joint (Fig. 19-1). When blocking a proximal joint to stretch a more distal joint into flexion, one must stop the block well proximally to the skin creases, thus allowing for folding of the volar tissues.

This is only one example of the way in which dynamic splint designs may differ from basic principles of static splinting. Dynamic splints are supplying a specific force, and the splint must thus provide a specific good that outweighs the general constriction and immobility it demands.[3] Dynamic splints should be applied to effect the tightest structures, and this often demands an awkward position in the splint. The intermittent nature of the splinting allows these awkward positions to be tolerated, and the active therapy combines with the splinting program to regain the balance of motion.

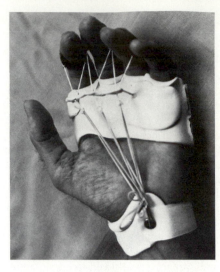

FIG. 19-1. Palmar bar is extended beyond to palmar crease to provide stability to metacarpophalangeal joints during dynamic flexion stretch to proximal interphalangeal joints.

Goal of dynamic splinting

A dynamic splint can only effectively achieve one motion at a time, although it may be able to achieve different motions on different fingers concurrently. For example, if one attempts concurrent flexion of the metacarpophalangeal joints and extension of the interphalangeal joints, the effectiveness of the force will cancel itself. A splint may indeed be multipurpose in that one splint base can provide multiple outriggers so that joints can be stretched alternately in opposite directions or concurrently in the same direction. For example, one may continue to achieve a dynamic flexion force for metacarpophalangeal tightness while stretching the interphalangeal joints into flexion, reducing extrinsic tightness (Fig. 19-2). The splint must be constructed with sound mechanical principles in order to be effective.

Frequently one sees badly traumatized hands that have stiffness in multiple planes, and it is difficult to rate the splinting needs by priority. After a clinical assessment of the motion present it is reasonable to splint the motion that has the most resistance to passive stretch for this is the least likely motion to gain with only active and intermittent passive stretching. Additionally it is helpful to remember the naturally weaker kinesiologic patterns of wrist extension, metacarpophalangeal flexion, and interphalangeal extension, favoring these weaker motions. An example is the proximal interphalangeal joint, which lacks full flexion and extension. Because of the great mechanical advantage of the flexors arising from the ability to transmit power through the efficient pulley system, one expects the potential for gaining flexion to be greater than that for gaining extension through the inefficient and weaker extensor hood mechanism. One may begin a splinting program with this as a baseline approach, but the constantly changing balance of motion may indicate a change of splinting priorities.

Evaluation for splinting

Proper splinting demands that the splint objective be based on the specific evaluation of impaired function.[10] Being

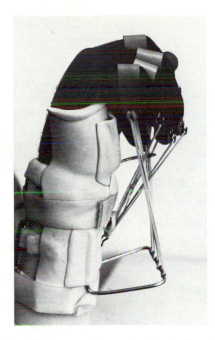

FIG. 19-2. Use of concurrent forces stretches both metacarpophalangeal joints and interphalangeal joints, thus effectively reducing metacarpophalangeal joint tightness and extrinsic extensor tightness.

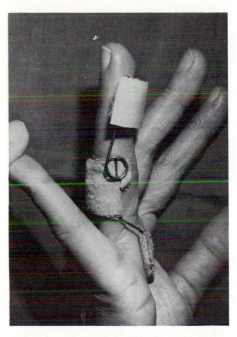

FIG. 19-3. Spring-wire splint (Capener design) for isolated tightness of proximal interphalangeal joint.

able to determine whether there is a need for changing (1) skin tightness, (2) joint tightness, (3) tendon adherence, or (4) muscle-tendon unit tightness is of basic importance. Frequently the splint must be adapted for a combination of these problems.

One may determine skin tightness by applying a stretch to the area and observing blanching or palpable tightness of the scar line or skin graft and local immobility of the tissue bed. When the skin is placed in its shortest length, it should allow increased joint motion proximally or distally. This range of joint motion is diminished as the proximal joint is positioned so as to place a stretch on the skin. Any splinting program to stretch a tight scar or shortened skin must also position the joints at the proximal and distal ends of the tightness in order to allow elongation of the tissue. It is not the scar that is stretched so much as it is the normal skin at the end of the scar that accommodates to the stress of the stretched position. Unlike the other areas discussed below where tightness can frequently be best stretched by dynamic forces, pure skin tightness is best altered by a static splint that holds the skin at maximum length as it simultaneously provides direct position pressure to the scar.

One best evaluates joint tightness by determining the easy passive range of the joint and then evaluating if this passive range changes as proximal and distal joint positions are changed. If the range of the joint motion does not change, there is isolated joint tightness, indicating the appropriateness of a splint that goes only proximally and distally to that specific joint (Fig. 19-3). In dynamic splinting one wishes to immobilize only the minimum number of joints possible.

Tendon adherence and muscle-tendon unit tightness are

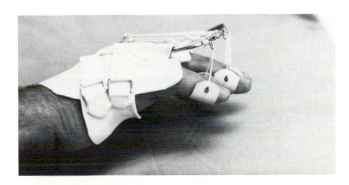

FIG. 19-4. Splint to stretch interphalangeal joints into extension without immobilization of wrist.

both demonstrated by a distinct difference in the ease of distal joint motion when the proximal joints are positioned in either flexion or extension. Adherence may be present anywhere along the course of the muscle-tendon unit where there has been direct trauma, and therefore a difference in tightness is seen only distally to this point, requiring a splint only from this point distally. A good example is a flexor tendon lacerated within the middle portion of the flexor tendon sheath. If it is adherent within this sheath, limiting extension, the splint needs to come only proximally to the metacarpophalangeal joint and not proximally to the wrist (Fig. 19-4). This can be proved by positioning the wrist in flexion and extension and demonstrating that there is no difference of the tightness within the finger.

When evaluating muscle-tendon unit tightness (which may or may not have an element of tendon adherence),

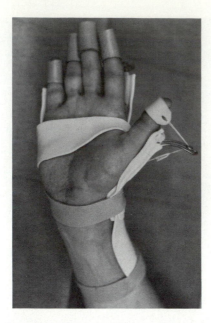

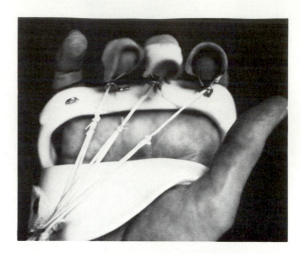

FIG. 19-5. Dynamic splint that positions wrist in extension while extending fingers and thumb in order to stretch adherence of flexor tendons proximal to wrist.

FIG. 19-6. Splint to stabilize metacarpophalangeal joints in extension while dynamically flexing interphalangeal joints, thus effectively stretching intrinsic muscle tightness.

one must evaluate the tightness of the unit from origin to insertion. The most proximal joint crossed by the unit is the key in determining tightness. With tightness of the extrinsic extensors the fingers will be unable to flex as far with the wrist in flexion as with the wrist in extension. Therefore a splint to stretch this tightness must include the wrist and position it in flexion. The opposite is true of extrinsic flexors in that with wrist extension finger extension is limited by the shortness of the unit, but when the wrist is dropped, the fingers can extend. To achieve an effective stretch to the extrinsic flexors, the wrist must be held in extension by the splint while the fingers are being dynamically extended (Fig. 19-5). The same principle holds true for the intrinsics of the hand, with the position of the metacarpophalangeal joint being the key for determining tightness. Since the intrinsic tendons run volarly to the axis of the metacarpophalangeal joint and dorsally to the axis of the proximal interphalangeal joint, the maximum stretch of this muscle-tendon unit occurs with the metacarpophalangeal joints are held in maximum extension and the interphalangeal joints are flexed. If the range of interphalanageal joint flexion is less and demonstrably tighter when the metacarpophalangeal joint is held in extension, the intrinsic muscles are tight. A splint to stretch this tightness thus need not include the wrist (Fig. 19-6).

PRINCIPLES FOR DESIGN
Analysis of forces

Analyzing the deficit in an injured hand and translating that need into a splint design is a critical skill for any hand therapist. Each and every splint should be approached as a unique device, and even though the splints will often fall into standard groups, it is a pitfall of the insecure therapist to try to fit the hand into a type of splint rather than design

the splint totally based on the clinical evaluation of the hand. One of the easiest ways to determine a splint design is to simply hold the hand and apply a passive stretch to the tight area. Analyze the specific joint positions and the points at where the therapist's hands are applying stabilizing pressure and where they are applying stretching pressure. Translation of these forces into the splint design is the goal.

The hand is a three-dimensional structure, and frequently it is difficult for the therapist to position the hand on paper, mark the landmarks, and then draw a shape that will translate into a three-dimensional shape. The method of applying a rubber glove to the patient's hand and drawing on the glove allows one to draw the hand in three dimensions and then to reduce the drawing to the two-dimensional sheet splinting material. Taking care and time to achieve a good basic splint pattern provides a specific, well-fitted device and saves material usage. Since one is applying a force with a dynamic splint, it is a basic requirement that the splint base be well designed so that it provides a stable base for attachment of outriggers. Force applied to a stiff joint will easily be transmitted to a poorly stabilized proximal joint with normal flexibility. Heating the splinting material so that it drapes to the true shape of the hand and paying attention that the splint achieves total contact are also basic requirements. No other aspect of hand therapy so well combines the elements of art and science as does splintmaking. Just as one can learn to be a skilled dressmaker by studying sewing principles, one can become an effective splintmaker by studying mechanical principles.

Effectiveness of splinting

Making a splint a comfortable device is of paramount importance if the splint is to be effective.[12] All details must be attended to, and pressure must be distributed over as large an area as possible. Listen to the patient; some minor detail may be the limiting factor for comfort, and the patient can easily point out what changes are needed. Making a device as streamline as possible so as to interfere minimally with daily function and devising the splint so that it is easy to apply and remove aid in the patient's integration of the splint into a home therapy routine.[1,16]

As previously described, the usefulness of splinting is based on a prolonged stretch of the tissues. Rubber bands have long been the accepted means of applying this force.[9,16] Although therapists have begun to measure the amount of force applied by the rubber-band tension, there is still no proved rationale for any specific amount of tension. Weeks and Wray describe the present problem well: "... we do not know the optimal amount of stress, the optimal length of time of application of stress, or the optimal method of application to bring about the most rapid favorable modification of scar tissue."[18] Brand clarifies for us that the critical question is not the amount of force we are applying but rather the pressure exerted on the skin where we are applying the force and this often becomes the limiting factor.[3] Although one can measure how much pressure can be tolerated before skin necrosis occurs, this is only indirectly of value, since dynamic splints allow motion and the force can be applied on an intermittent basis. Brand states that the pressure becomes relatively unimportant in the presence of intermittent application.[3]

Therapists should measure the amount of force applied by the rubber-band traction to standardize their approach, but at the present time clinical observation is the only guideline to determine appropriate tension. A well-made splint that effectively stretches a tight area should not be painful. The patient may be aware of a pulling sensation, but he can clearly distinguish between the pull and a painful sensation. Tearing of fibrotic adhesions is not the goal. Patients often exhibit an eagerness about their dynamic splint in that it relieves a sensation of tightness they cannot otherwise effect. Rather than prescribing a specific hourly routine for splinting, instruct the patient to remove the splint when it reaches maximum tolerance. This period may be realistically short as one starts the splinting program, but if the patient cannot quickly increase splinting tolerance to 1 or 2 hours, the tension should be decreased.

Make it clear to the patient that the goal is to be able to tolerate the splint for longer periods of time and not at increasing tensions. If a patient cannot increase the splinting time, it is the result of a splint being ill fitted, applied too early or exerting too great a force.

To achieve increased motion, one must execute a good design and be keenly aware of the need for constant monitoring of the splint. The patient must understand the specific goals of the splint and should see splint changes as a reflection of improvement. Since the goal is to provide a 90-degree angle pull, the line of pull must be adjusted frequently to maintain the correct directional pull as the joint motion increases. Reminding patients to bring their splint to each therapy session encourages ease of adjustment. A good approach is to begin the therapy session frequently with a trying on of the spoint, asking the patient if any area is uncomfortable, how long it can be worn continuously, and if he feels any adjustments would be helpful to increase tolerance.

CLINICAL APPLICATION
Design choice

The variety of splint designs is as limitless as human imagination. Simplicity of design and effective material utilization is of vital importance. In observing the normal hand one is able to use the normal kinesiologic and anatomic parameters as guidelines for splinting designs to approach specific tightness. Barr states: "It must be emphasized that the design of any sort of splint stems from the patient's own problems and has no other valid identity."[2]

In effecting joint motion it is the goal of the splint to provide a line of pull at a 90-degree angle to the axis of the long bone of the joint in question (Fig. 19-7). It is of utmost importance that the splint be designed so that this 90-degree line of pull is achieved and easily maintained. Application

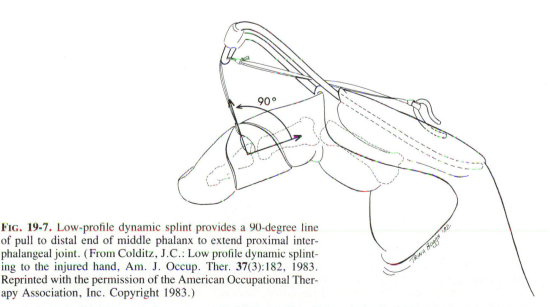

FIG. 19-7. Low-profile dynamic splint provides a 90-degree line of pull to distal end of middle phalanx to extend proximal interphalangeal joint. (From Colditz, J.C.: Low profile dynamic splinting to the injured hand, Am. J. Occup. Ther. **37**(3):182, 1983. Reprinted with the permission of the American Occupational Therapy Association, Inc. Copyright 1983.)

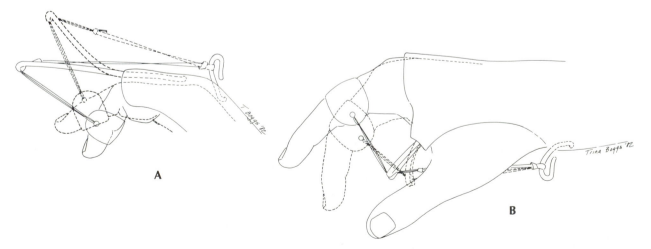

FIG. 19-8. Low-profile design splint for interphalangeal joint extension, with wrist and metacarpophalangeal joints stabilized.

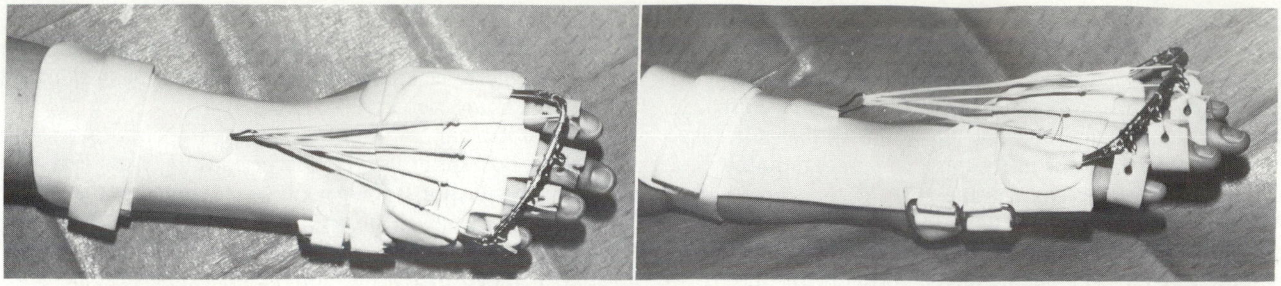

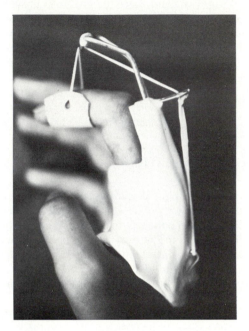

FIG. 19-9. Use of low-profile system allows redirection of line of pull and avoids large bulky outrigger arms when one attempts to extend a severe proximal interphalangeal joint flexion contracture.

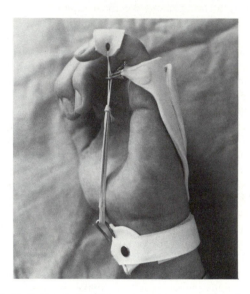

FIG. 19-10. Splint designed to gain last ranges of proximal interphalangeal joint flexion by blocking metacarpophalangeal joint flexion and directing line of pull by use of wire-loop pulley.

FIG. 19-11. Ease of adjustment of low-profile wire outrigger system is accomplished by simple bend of wire outrigger. This allows maintenance of 90-degree line of pull when either extension, **A,** or flexion, **B,** is accomplished. (From Colditz, J.C.: Low profile dynamic splinting to the injured hand, Am. J. Occup. Ther. **37**(3):182, 1983. Reprinted with the permission of the American Occupational Therapy Association, Inc. Copyright 1983.)

of the force at the end of the bone (that is, maximum length of lever arm) allows efficiency for the force. Although it can be argued that application of the finger loop at maximum distance from the joint can supply a compressive force to the joint, this appears insignificant because of the intermittent nature of dynamic splinting. Normally dynamic splints are not used as exercise splints, since pulling against the force strengthens the opposite motion. A carefully supervised program of active and active resistive motion is mandatory to compliment the splinting program, which only increases the passive potential.

Low-profile designs

Use of a low-profile splint design where the line of pull is redirected by means of a pulley system and then carried parallel to the splint base is an effective means of applying the 90-degree line of pull without large bulky outrigger arms (Fig. 19-8). This system is particularly helpful with a severe flexion contracture of the proximal interphalangeal joint where a long outrigger arm would normally be required (Fig. 19-9). In this case the line of pull may be redirected more than once; thus the device is kept as small as possible and patient compliance is particularly encouraged in climates where outer layers of clothing are frequently applied and removed.

Equally efficient is the use of the low-profile pulley system for the last ranges of proximal interphalangeal joint flexion (Fig. 19-10). The small pulley on the proximal phalanx ''ring'' allows specific direction of the line of pull on the middle phalanx and allows use of a long rubber band when the band is attached to the splint base at the wrist. Use of the pulley system is the only way to provide a force for the last ranges of proximal interphalangeal joint flexion, since there is no room in the palm for a traditional outrigger for rubber band attachment.

Use of wire (brass welding rod) as the outrigger base is perhaps the greatest advantage to a low-profile splinting system, since the correct line of pull may be maintained by a simple bend of the wire (Fig. 19-11). In the case of an increased extension range the wire is easily bent dorsally and proximally, maintaining the correct angle of pull. Conversely, a gain in the range of flexion may also be adjusted when the wire is bent more volarly and proximally.

The ease with which one can stabilize a proximal bone and apply force to the distal bone allows for minimum immobilization of the uninvolved joints. As with isolated metacarpophalangeal joint flexion it is not necessary to immobilize the wrist, thumb, or other metacarpophalangeal joints in the splint; thus there is increasing patient compliance as the cumbersomeness of the splint is decreased (Fig. 19-12).

The system of pulleys is additionally useful for providing to the patient a specific feedback of gains of motion. A small mark on the string as it slides over the outrigger pulley provides a visual indication as the joint gains motion. If one desires, one may also harness active motion and provide visual feedback as the mark moves away from the pulley. In this case one must provide enough length of the string beyond the outrigger to allow sliding of the string without the knot where the rubber band is attached hanging on the pulley.

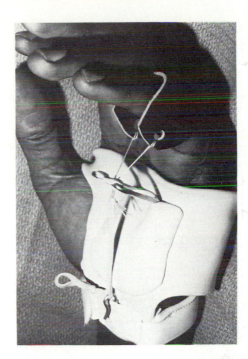

FIG. 19-12. Splint to stretch isolated metacarpophalangeal joint tightness. No other joints are immobilized with low-profile technique.

CONCLUSION

Splintmaking is truly the ultimate combination of art and science. Effective dynamic splinting requires both the scientific knowledge of wound physiology and mechanical design and the creative ability to construct a splint based on these principles. It is a skilled hand therapist who can effectively assess to the injured hand, establish priorities for treatment, and then create a splint that is an effective tool in reestablishing motion. As hand surgery and hand therapy continue to develop as a well-recognized medical speciality, every hand therapist should continue to face the challenge of being accountable for effective splinting of the stiff hand.

REFERENCES

1. American Academy of Orthopaedic Surgeons (Office of the Surgeon General of the Army and Veteran's Administration): Orthopaedic appliance atlas, Ann Arbor, Mich., 1952, J.W. Edwards Co.
2. Barr, N.: The hand: principles and techniques of simple splintmaking in rehabilitation, Sevenoaks, Kent, 1975, Butterworth & Co. (Pubs), Ltd., p. xiii.
3. Brand, P.: The forces of dynamic splinting: ten questions before applying a dynamic splint to the hand. In Hunter, J.M., Schneider, L.H., Mackin, E.J., and Bell, J.A., editor: Rehabilitation of the hand, St. Louis, 1978, The C.V. Mosby Co., pp. 591-598.
4. Bunch, W.H., and Keagy, R.D.: Principles of orthotic treatment, St. Louis, 1976, The C.V. Mosby Co.
5. Bunnell, S., ed.: Hand surgery in World War II, Washington, D.C., 1955, U.S. Surgeon General's Office.
6. Bunnell, S.: Spring splint to supinate or pronate the hand, J. Bone Joint Surg. **31A:**664, 1949.
7. Bunnell, S.: Active splinting of the hand, J. Bone Joint Surg. **28:**732, 1946.
8. Bunnell, S.: Surgery of the hand, Philadelphia, 1944, J.B. Lippincott Co.
9. Bunnell, S., and Howard L.D.: Additional elastic hand splints, J. Bone Joint Surg. **32A:**226, 1950.

10. Cailliet, R.: Hand pain and impairment, Philadelphia, 1971, F.A. Davis Co.

11. Capener, N.: Physiological rest, Br. Med. J. **2:**761, 1946.

12. Fess, E.E., Gettle, K., and Strickland, J.: Hand splinting: principles and methods, St. Louis, 1981, The C.V. Mosby Co.

13. Littler, J.W.: Dynamic splinting and immobilization. In Littler, J.W., editor: Reconstructive plastic surgery, Philadelphia, 1964, W.B. Saunders, vol. IV, pp. 1569-1573.

14. Littler, J.W.: Tendon transfers and arthodesis in combined median and ulnar nerve paralysis, J. Bone Joint Surg. **31A:**225, 1949.

15. Nachlas, I.W.: A splint for the correction of extension contractures of the metacarpophalangeal joints, J. Bone Joint Surg. **27:**507, 1945.

16. Peacock, E.E., Jr.: Dynamic splinting for the prevention and correction of hand deformities, J. Bone Joint Surg. **34A:**789, 1952.

17. Pearson, S.O.: Dynamic splinting. In Hunter, J.M., Schneider, L.H., Mackin, E.J., and Bell, J.A., editors: Rehabilitation of the hand, St. Louis, 1978, The C.V. Mosby Co.

18. Weeks, P., and Wray, R.C.: Management of acute hand injuries, St. Louis, 1973, The C.V. Mosby Co.

19. Wynn Parry, C.B.: Stretching. In Rogoff, J.B., editor: Manipulation, traction and massage, ed. 2, Baltimore, 1980, The Williams & Wilkins Co.

20. Wynn Parry, C.B.: Rehabilitation of the hand, ed. 3, Sevenoaks, Kent, 1978, Butterworth & Co. (Pubs.), Ltd.

20

Splinting for mobilization of the thumb

ELAINE EWING FESS

The thumb is a multiarticular open kinematic chain that moves through the three motion planes and combinations thereof. The distal segment of the chain is allowed a high degree of freedom of movement as the result of the summation of the participating joints. This arrangement helps minimize the disabling effect of the restriction of loss of motion of individual joints as the result of trauma or disease.

Severely limiting the functional capacity of the hand, a thumb that has been disabled by injury or disease assumes a posture of adduction, flexion, and external rotation, which if untreated may result in fixed deformity. Direct trauma to the tissues of the first web space, trauma to adjacent parts of the hand or extremity, nerve paralysis, ischemia, infection, or disease processes such a rheumatoid arthritis are potential causative agents for contractures of the first web space. The specific pathomechanics of thumb-adduction deformities are complicated, often involving the combination of immobility and edema from tissue reaction to injury or loss of balance of the thumb musculature from denervation. Normally, superficial venous and lymphatic drainage from the palm and digits flows around the medial and lateral borders of the hand and digits to the dorsum of the hand. In the injured state, tissue reaction to trauma results in considerable distention of the dorsal cutaneous surface of the entire hand (Fig. 20-1). This interstitial fluid accumulation between the dorsal fascial planes pulls the thumb into an adducted position, and when such accumulation is unattended, as the process of wound healing progresses, scar formation occurs, producing adhesions of soft-tissue structures, shortening of lax carpometacarpal joint ligaments, first metacarpal immobility, and potential myostatic contracture of the thumb adductor.

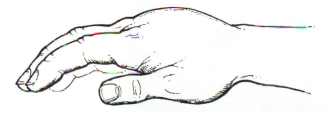

FIG. 20-1. Dorsal swelling promotes a posture of thumb adduction, which when unattended may result in a fixed contracture of first web space.

Muscle imbalance from median nerve or combined median and ulnar nerve disruption may also lead to thumb-adduction deformities. Depending on the level of injury, median nerve lacerations result in loss or weakening of thumb abduction, opposition, and flexion. The primary and secondary thumb adductors, the adductor pollicis and the extensor pollicis longus, innervated by the ulnar and radial nerves respectively, remain functional, creating muscle imbalance and the potential for contracture of the first web space. The combination of median and ulnar nerve lesions magnifies the chances of developing thumb-adduction deformities. Active motion is further diminished, and the resultant posturing of the hand and thumb contributes significantly to creating a stiff hand with concomitant contracture of the first web space.

Since optimal effectiveness of the thumb is contingent on its mobility, preservation or restoration of the various degrees of freedom of motion of the three joints is paramount in the rehabilitation process. Splinting and active range-of-motion exercise, combined with purposeful activity, are the cornerstones of this process. Passive range of motion of the involved joints must be acquired and maintained before full active range of motion can be expected or before surgical procedures may be attempted. Splinting is generally accepted as the most effective nonsurgical tool for achieving an improved passive range of motion. In this chapter the concepts of utilizing splinting for the maintenance or acquisition of thumb motion are discussed.

CARPOMETACARPAL LEVEL

The problem of a limited arc of motion of the first metacarpal bone and the resulting narrowing of the first web space occurs primarily at the carpometacarpal level. Any splint designed to maintain or increase the passive range of carpometacarpal motion must have the site of force application on the first metacarpal. Practically speaking, however, this is difficult because of the intervening soft tissue of the first web space. Many ill-conceived splints fitted with the intent of increasing the carpometacarpal range of motion actually apply most of the rotatory force to the proximal phalanx, resulting in stretching of the ulnar collateral ligament of the metacarpophalangeal joint, radial deviation of the proximal phalanx, pressure over the radial metacarpal condyle, and instability of the thumb (Fig. 20-2). Care, then, must be taken to ensure that as much of the distal aspect of the first metacarpal is included in the splint as feasible and that the application site of the rotatory force is on the first metacarpal. To decrease the amount of pressure on the first metacarpal, one can widen the area of force application to include the proximal phalanx, but this addition must not jeopardize the stability of the metacarpophalangeal joint by exerting a stretching force on the ulnar collateral ligament, and in most instances it need not be extended distally beyond the interphalangeal flexion crease, thus allowing full motion of the distal phalanx. The splint should also be fitted proximally to the distal palmar flexion crease, to permit full metacarpophalangeal flexion of the adjacent digits.

Since the carpometacarpal joint of the thumb is a triaxial saddle articulation and possesses two degrees of freedom of motion, the position of the first metacarpal should be altered from full extension to full abduction to minimize the possibility of shortening of the five carpometacarpal articular ligaments as described by Haines and Napier. Depending on the severity of stiffness, this may be accomplished through a carefully supervised exercise routine or through a combination of splinting and exercise. The construction of two splints, one in full extension and the second in abduction, which are worn alternatively, facilitates acquisition or maintenance of full passive motion.

A carpometacarpal maintenance splint (Fig. 20-3) is an example of one of the many splints that can be used to preserve the range of motion of the thumb carpometacarpal joint.

If full passive range of motion is not present at the carpometacarpal joint, slow, progressive inelastic traction may be applied through the use of serial carpometacarpal mobilization splints (web spacers) (Fig. 20-4), which are changed and widened every 3 or 4 days. Progressive wedging of the thumb is continued until the passive measurements of abduction and extension duplicate those of the normal thumb, or until the passive motion remains unchanged for three or four consecutive splint changes. Surgical intervention may be considered when the latter occurs. In my experience, inelastic traction is more effective than elastic traction splinting for increasing thumb carpometacarpal passive range of motion.

METACARPOPHALANGEAL LEVEL

The metacarpophalangeal joint of the thumb, unlike the metacarpophalangeal joints of the fingers, tends to be more nearly of the ginglymoid or hinge type. In mobilizing this joint of the thumb, care should be taken to apply the rotatory force perpendicularly to the center of the axis of rotation of the metacarpophalangeal joint. If this concept is disregarded, stretching of either the metacarpophalangeal ulnar or radial collateral ligament may occur with resulting deviation of the proximal phalanx and metacarpophalangeal joint instability. The force angle of approach should also be at 90 degrees to the proximal phalanx.

A simple metacarpophalangeal flexion splint (Fig. 20-5) is one of the least complicated means of facilitating thumb metacarpophalangeal flexion. Of importance to note is the concept that this splint affects motion at the thumb carpometacarpal joint in addition to the metacarpophalangeal joint. Becuase of this, an incorrect force angle of approach may cause medial or lateral rotation of the first metacarpal with stretching of the carpometacarpal ligaments and intraarticular pressure, as well as undue stressing of the metacarpophalangeal collateral ligaments and joint surfaces.

Application of the full magnitude of the rotatory force to the metacarpophalangeal joint may be accomplished by stabilization of the thumb carpometacarpal joint (Fig. 20-6).

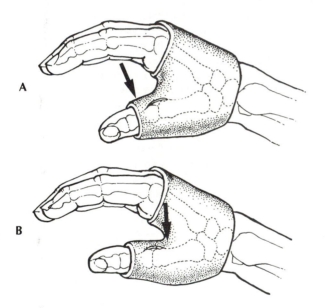

FIG. 20-2. Attempts to mobilize thumb carpometacarpal joint frequently result in improper placement of rotary force on proximal phalanx, causing attenuation of ulnar collateral ligament of metacarpophalangeal joint. **A,** Incorrect. **B,** Correct.

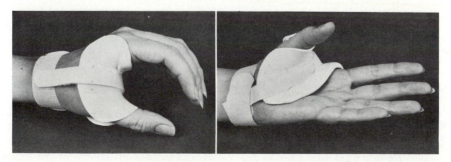

FIG. 20-3. Maintenance splint allows full range of motion of adjacent metacarpophalangeal joints and gives purchase against distal aspect of first metacarpal. Straps are designed to minimize distal migration of splint.

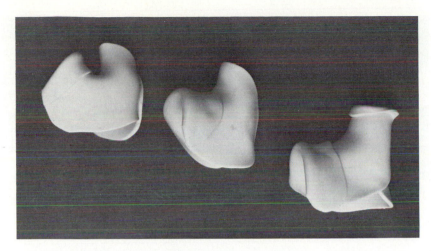

FIG. 20-4. Serial carpometacarpal mobilization splints (web spaces) are widened every 3 to 4 days.

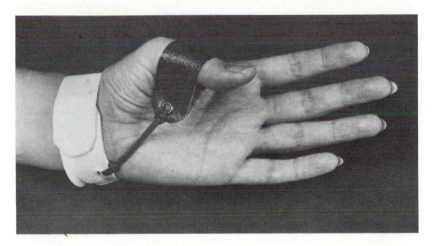

FIG. 20-5. In this simple thumb metacarpophalangeal flexion splint, the rigid, low-temperature plaster component of band is closely fitted around ulnar border of wrist to prevent splint rotation as elastic traction is applied to metacarpophalangeal joint.

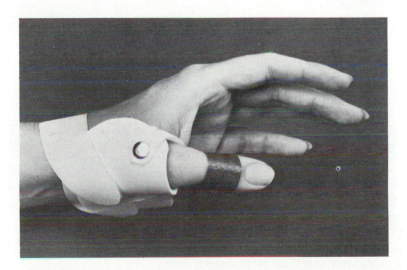

FIG. 20-6. Compound thumb metacarpophalangeal flexion splint designed by Karan Harmon, O.T.R.

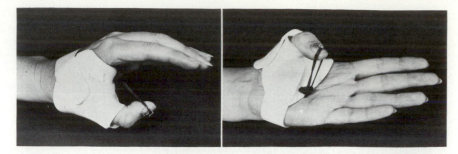

FIG. 20-7. Compound interphalangeal flexion splint with fingernail clip allows application of dynamic traction to thumb interphalangeal joint as the carpometacarpal and metacarpophalangeal joints are stabilized. Clip, a dressmaker's No. 2 hook, is attached with ethyl cyanoacrylate glue.

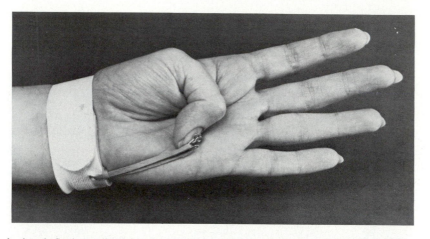

FIG. 20-8. Simple thumb flexion splint with rigid ulnar component and fingernail clip enhances simultaneous passive flexion of carpometacarpal, metacarpophalangeal, and interphalangeal joints of thumb.

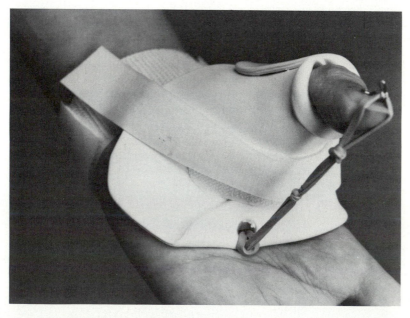

FIG. 20-9. Combination of thumb carpometacarpal mobilization (web spacer) and fingernail clip allows for simultaneous force application to the carpometacarpal and interphalangeal joints.

Once again, attention must be directed toward ensuring that the force angle of approach is directed 90 degrees to the proximal phalanx and perpendicularly to the axis for rotation of the metacarpophalangeal joint.

INTERPHALANGEAL LEVEL

Since the interphalangeal joint of the thumb is a true uniaxial hinge articulation, the principles of mechanical theory previously mentioned regarding mobilization of the thumb metacarpophalangeal joint are applicable to the mobilization of the interphalangeal joint: for optimum results the angle of approach should be 90 degrees to the distal phalanx of the thumb and perpendicular to the axis of rotation of the interphalangeal joint.

A compound thumb interphalangeal flexion splint (Fig. 20-7) may be utilized to stabilize the carpometacarpal and metacarpophalangeal joints of the thumb, thus allowing for increased magnitude and accuracy of the application of the rotatory force at the interphalangeal joint by means of a fingernail clip. To decrease the amount of pressure incurred by inhibiting motion at the carpometacarpal and metacarpophalangeal joints, the thumb post should be extended as far distally as possible along the proximal phalanx without interfering with full interphalangeal flexion. Complete flexion of the adjacent metacarpophalangeal joints of the fingers and support of the transverse metacarpal arch should also be present.

The fingernail clip should be attached to the center and proximal aspect of the thumbnail to eliminate the possibility of transverse rotation of the distal phalanx and to minimize the leverage effect of the nail on the proximal nail bed. Problems of detachment of the nail from the nail bed are rare.

MULTIPLE JOINTS

The techniques discussed in this chapter for splinting individual joints may be combined effectively for the simultaneous mobilization of multiple joints of the thumb.

A simple thumb flexion splint consisting of a wrist band and a fingernail clip (Fig. 20-8) mobilize the carpometacarpal, metacarpophalangeal, and interphalangeal joints of the thumb. When fitting this splint, one must take care to check the angle of force application. The incorporation of all three joints of the thumb into the splint leaves little room for error and may tend to cause or accentuate deformity because of the multiple lever arms. The angle of approach of the rubber band must be perpendicular to the axis of rotation of the metacarpophalangeal and interphalangeal joints without causing transverse rotation of the first metacarpal.

A carpometacarpal mobilization splint, combined with a fingernail clip (Fig. 20-9), facilitates motion at both the carpometacarpal and interphalangeal joints. In designing and fitting this splint one needs to be certain that the plastic fully extends around the proximal phalanx of the thumb, thus rendering the metacarpophalangeal joint immobile and diminishing the pressure on the volar aspect of the phalanx. Once again, the angle of approach of the rubber band should be at a 90-degree angle to the distal phalanx and perpen-

dicular to the center of the axis of rotation of the interphalangeal joint. The metacarpophalangeal joints of the fingers should also be permitted full range of motion into flexion.

EXERCISE

Splinting should be routinely augmented with active and passive range-of-motion exercises and purposeful activity. Generally, patients are instructed to remove their splints, inspect the skin under the splint, and exercise the involved joints for 15 minutes a minimum of every 2 hours. The presence of additional circumstances such as skin grafts, unstable fractures, and tendon, nerve, or vascular repairs may change the splinting and exercise programs considerably.

CONCLUSION

In conclusion, it is of utmost importance that splints be designed to meet the specific needs of individual patients in accordance with basic anatomic and mechanical construction and fit principles. If done properly, the combination of splinting, exercise, and purposeful activity may enhance the results of surgery and help to minimize the disabling effect of disease and trauma to the thumb.

BIBLIOGRAPHY

Barr, N.: The hand, principles and techniques of simple splintmaking in rehabilitation, Reading, Mass., 1975, Butterworth Inc.

Beasley, R.: Hand injuries, Philadelphia, 1981, W.B. Saunders Co.

Boyes, J.: Bunnell's surgery of the hand, ed. 4, Philadelphia, 1964, J.B. Lippincott Co.

Brumstrom, S.: Clinical kinesiology, ed. 3, Philadelphia, 1972, F.A. Davis Co.

Fess, E., Gettle, K., and Strickland, J.: Hand splinting principles and methods, St. Louis, 1981, The C.V. Mosby Co.

Flatt, A.: The care of minor hand injuries, ed. 4, St. Louis, 1982, The C.V. Mosby Co.

Haines, R.: The mechanism of rotation at the first carpometacarpal joint, J. Anat. **78:**44, 1944.

Hollinshead, W.: Anatomy for surgeons, ed. 2, New York, 1969, Harper & Row, Publishers, vol. 3.

Kuczynski, K.: General anatomy. In Lamb, D., and Kuczynski, K.: The practice of hand surgery, Boston, 1981, Blackwell Scientific Publications.

Littler, J.: The prevention and correction of adduction contracture of the thumb, Clin. Orthop. **13:**182, 1959.

Milford, L.: The hand, ed. 2, St. Louis, 1982, The C.V. Mosby Co.

Napier, J.: The form and function of the carpometacarpal joint of the thumb, J. Anat. **89:**362, 1955.

Phelps, P., and Weeks, P.: Management of the thumb-index web space contracture, Am. J. Occup. Ther. **30:**543, 1977.

Rasch, P., and Burke, R.: Kinesiology and applied anatomy, ed. 5, Philadelphia, 1974, Lea & Febiger.

Strickland, J.: Reconstruction of the contracted first web space. In Strickland, J., and Steichen, J., editors: Difficult problems in hand surgery, St. Louis, 1982, The C.V. Mosby Co.

Strickland, J.: Restoration of thumb function after partial or total amputation. In Hunter, J., Schneider, L., Mackin, E., and Bell, J., editors: Rehabilitation of the hand, ed. 2, St. Louis, 1984, The C.V. Mosby Co.

Weeks, P., and Wray, C.: Management of acute hand injuries, ed. 2, St. Louis, 1978, The C.V. Mosby Co.

Williams, M., and Lissner, H.: Biomechanics of human motion, Philadelphia, 1962, W.B. Saunders Co.

Wynn-Parry, C., Salter, M., and Millar, D.: Rehabilitation of the hand, ed. 3, London, 1973, Butterworth and Co. (Publishers) Ltd.

21

Postoperative management of capsulectomies

GEORGIANN F. LASETER

Capsulectomy of the metacarpophalangeal and the proximal interphalangeal joints is performed to improve motion in stiff joints with normal articular surfaces and is necessitated by the failure of conservative procedures, such as exercises and splinting, to improve motion.

The therapist's role in the management of the postoperative capsulectomy patient begins before the surgery. Many times the patient undergoes therapy before the decision to perform a capsulectomy is made. It is the result of that therapy program that can actually be the determining factor as to whether the patient needs a capsulectomy. Once tissue equilibrium has been reached and the decision has been made to perform the capsulectomy, the therapist's important function before surgery is to educate the patient about what will be expected of him after the capsulectomy and why his postoperative performance is critical in obtaining optimum motion and function.

The therapist must have a good knowledge of hand anatomy and a keen appreciation for the physiology of wound healing and tissue reaction to injury that causes and prolongs stiffness. Multiple variables in the results of capsulectomy are involved, and as more supplementary procedures are added to the capsulectomy, poorer results and even complications may be anticipated.[4] For this reason, it is important that the therapist obtain a copy of the operative report to have information regarding exactly what structures in the capsulectomy procedure were surgically involved.

COMPARISON OF TREATMENT NEEDS IN ACUTE INJURIES AND THOSE AFTER CAPSULECTOMY

The general needs of treatment applicable to the acutely injured patient closely correlate with the needs of treatment applicable to postcapsulectomy patients and include the following:

1. Pain control
2. Edema reduction
3. Exercises
4. Splinting
5. Functional activities

Control of pain and reduction of edema postoperatively are of paramount importance in the management of the patient who has undergone a capsulectomy procedure.

Pain

The amount and duration of pain vary considerably among patients with hand injuries. Some patients may have minimal and transient discomfort, whereas in others pain is the major problem with the hand.[13] Many patients who undergo capsulectomies have had significant difficulties with pain and reflex sympathetic dystrophy before the capsulectomy. Gould and Nicholson[6] reported in their series that patients with quiescent reflex sympathetic dystrophy who underwent capulectomy tended to have poor results despite sympathetic blockades performed during and after the operations. In many cases, their reflex sympathetic dystrophy symptoms recurred in various degrees after the capsulectomy.

Useful methods of controlling pain after a capsulectomy may be the use of a transcutaneous nerve stimulator and/or elevation to decrease edema. In addition, modalities producing either heat or cold can be interspersed with other treatment techniques to improve circulation and help the hand relax. Massage and the use of goal-directed activities are also useful in assisting the patient to work through his pain.

Edema

The need to control edema is obvious when the effects of this condition are reviewed. Swelling around a joint causes stretching of the skin and soft tissue in that area, which in turn produces limited motion and ultimately increased scarring about the joint.[13]. Elevation is the primary treatment for edema, and the proper position is with the wrist higher than the elbow and the elbow higher than the shoulder at all times, regardless of whether the patient is lying, sitting, or standing. Just exactly what is meant by elevating the hand is subject to broad interpretation by the patient unless it is specifically spelled out and constantly reinforced until the edema is gone.

Lying down, the patient can properly elevate the hand by positioning two to three pillows at his side (Fig. 21-1) or with the use of a commercial arm-elevation device.

When sitting, the patient should sit next to a table and place a stack of magazines or pillows under the elbow (Fig. 21-2).

When standing or walking, the patient should place his hand on top of his head (Fig. 21-3). Doing so will properly elevate the hand and is not so fatiguing for the upper extremity as just attempting to ''salute the ceiling'' with the hand.

Elevation is of prime importance in decreasing pain, especially in immediate postoperative situations, and this should be stressed to the patient. As healing progresses and reaction decreases, the hand may still swell intermittently. The patient is instructed that when the hand does swell he should resume strict elevation until this again subsides.

In addition to elevation of the hand during treatment, active exercises,[1,8] massage in a distal-to-proximal direction,[7] and other measures such as the use of elastic compression garments and gloves and an intermittent compression unit[5] may be helpful to eliminate excess fluid in the hand.

Clinically the measurement of edema can be accomplished by the use of a commercially available water-displacement device (Fig. 21-4) or by recording of the circumferential measurements at certain landmarks on the hand and wrist, with care being taken to record the exact way in which the measurements are performed so that they can be repeated consistently upon reevaluation.

Exercises

Active exercises are carried out entirely by the patient's own muscle power in the affected limb under varying degrees of encouragement by the therapist. Passive exercises are produced by a force other than normal contraction of the muscle—for example, by the therapist or by the patient using his unaffected hand to exercise his affected hand.

Active range-of-motion exercise is the only therapy of permanent benefit.[1] In active movement, the blood flow in the limb varies directly with the degree of activity in the muscle. Passive range-of-motion exercise produces very little change in the blood flow of the limb, but it does tend to prevent adhesions between muscle planes and to maintain range of motion of the joints.[2]

Both passive and active exercises are important in improving motion after a capsulectomy. In attempting to decide what type of exercise program should be emphasized, determine whether passive motion exceeds active motion at a particular joint. If the passive motion exceeds the active motion, an active exercise program to overcome tendon weakness or adherence proximal to that site is necessary. If the passive motion does *not* exceed active motion, passive exercises to assist in overcoming the restriction in joint range of motion should *augment* the active exercise program.

The patient must learn that all active and passive exercises must be gentle enough to avoid tissue reaction, but frequent enough to gently stretch, but not tear, adhesions. The patient can usually be taught to apply the appropriate force for short periods of time, many times per day. The key to such self-

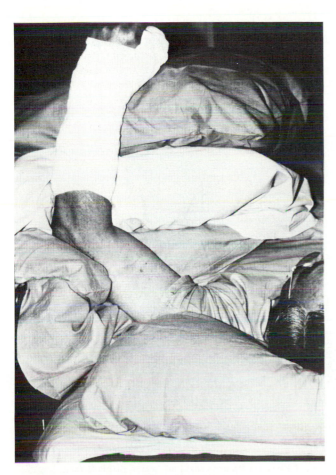

FIG. 21-1. Position of elevation while patient is supine.

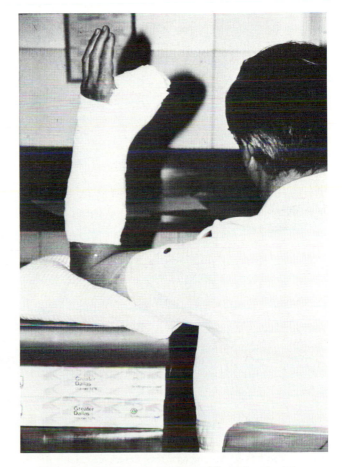

FIG. 21-2. Position of elevation while patient is sitting.

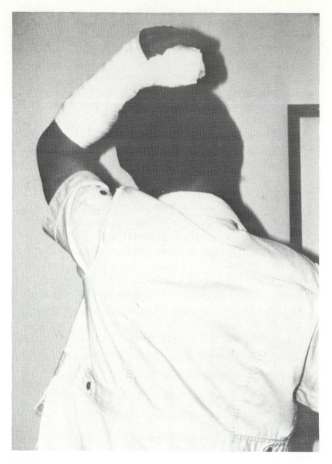

Fig. 21-3. Position of elevation while patient is standing.

treatment is the appreciation of the difference between discomfort and pain. The discomfort of a properly applied force is beneficial and should be tolerated, since the tissues will gradually yield to such treatment. The amount of force and direction of its application must be reduced until the discomfort is tolerable and the tissue reaction is not excessive.

The patient should be instructed in the specific reasons for and the correct way to perform the individual exercise programs. The exercises are best done in small amounts, frequently throughout the day, and for a certain number of repetitions. For example, the patient could be told to sustain each exercise effort for 10 seconds, and repeat it five times on the hour while awake.

Splinting

Splinting is an important part of the postoperative rehabilitation of capsulectomies. A static progressive splint fitted while the parts to be splinted are being stretched allows the splint to conform to this forced fixed position and is useful in that the stresses developed in the tissues are transmitted to the offending scar.[13] When the scar matures and loosens, another splint is fitted to progressively increase the position desired. Thus a static progressive splint is helpful for night wear in that it helps the patient keep the gains he has made during the day with his exercises. In the early stages after his surgery, a static splint is safer for wear at night than a dynamic splint because of the edema and the possibility of circulatory constriction.

The use of dynamic splints is important for daytime wear as an adjunct to the patient's exercise program. When not exercising or performing skin care, the patient must be splinted in the desired position to maintain and improve the surgical correction.

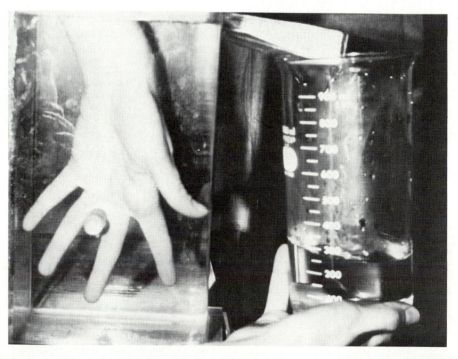

Fig. 21-4. Volumeter. This device calculates the degree of hand edema by measurement of water displacement. Measurements should be made bilaterally as a basis for comparison.

It is extremely important that the patient's splints are very closely monitored, and it may be necessary to change them daily. The patient needs to be given very detailed wearing instructions and precautions, and every step must be taken to ensure that the splints are as comfortable as possible.

Functional activities

Along with the specific exercises and splinting, it is beneficial to involve the patient in performance of some type of functional activity. It is not enough to regain a certain number of degrees in range of motion. This must be combined with the actual functional use of the hand by performance of some type of purposeful activity with tools and materials.[9] The use of functional activities is also helpful in retraining the patient in the way in which he uses his hands and in showing him that the improvement in motion that he has gained from his capsulectomy has also upgraded the function of his hand.

• • •

Now that the general principles have been discussed, the specifics of treatment for patients who have undergone capsulectomies at the metacarpophalangeal joint or at the proximal interphalangeal joint can be detailed. Most capsulectomy patients start their postoperative programs anywhere from the first to the third day after surgery (Fig. 21-5). The sutures remain in place from 14 to 21 days postoperatively. The patient must be taught skin care to avoid reactivity about the sutures or infection. These patients need to be closely monitored for 3 to 6 weeks after surgery. Maximum improvement from a capsulectomy may be expected 3 to 5 months postoperatively.[3]

METACARPOPHALANGEAL JOINTS

Metacarpophalangeal joint capsulectomies are performed to improve flexion. Exercise and dynamic splinting are the primary means of maintaining and increasing the metacarpophalangeal joint flexion gained through surgery.[13]

The patient should be carefully instructed in the passive and active exercises necessary. The metacarpals should be firmly stabilized before force is applied to the proximal phalanx. It is extremely important to observe the patient's response to passive stretching and to be aware of his pain tolerance. Although some degree of discomfort is experienced during passive exercise, the patient should be taught that this should subside shortly after completion of the passive stretching. Active exercises are beneficial in decreasing edema and in preventing the joint surfaces from adhering during this edematous phase. Active exercise is necessary to maintain the gains made by the passive stretching. In general, the patient should perform both passive and active exercises after capsulectomy three to five times every 30 minutes to 1 hour while awake, depending on the edema and tissue reactivity.

Many patients undergoing metacarpophalangeal joint capsulectomy have been using their digital extensors to extend their wrists for a long period of time, as is seen in patients who have had a Colles' fracture (Fig. 21-6). This substitution pattern has actually contributed to metacarpophalangeal joint stiffness in extension or hyperextension. Preoperatively, it is important to recognize this pattern and attempt to reeducate and strengthen the wrist extensors in extending the wrist without the use of the digital extensors.[12] Patient reeducation and strengthening of the wrist extensors must continue postoperatively because if not watched

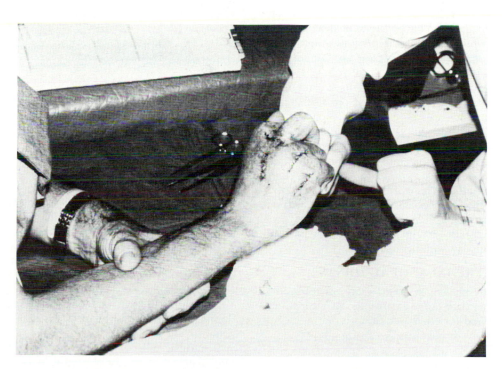

FIG. 21-5. Exercise program is usually started 1 to 3 days postoperatively.

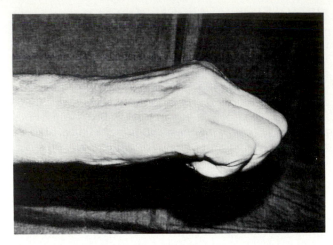

FIG. 21-6. Attempted wrist extension with digital extensors. This substitution pattern is counterproductive to finger flexion and must be overcome to develop range of motion in flexion and to develop grip strength.

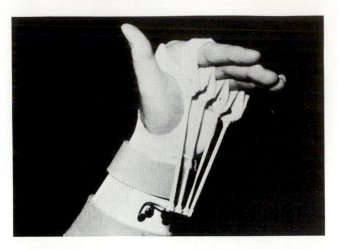

FIG. 21-7. Dorsal splint with dynamic metacarpophalangeal joint flexion slings: This splint adequately stabilizes the wrist, supports the metacarpal arch, and flexes the metacarpophalangeal joints. This is worn during the day, following metacarpophalangeal joint capsulectomies.

closely the patient will again be attempting to extend his wrist with his digital extensors, and so his efforts will be counterproductive to metacarpophalangeal joint flexion.

Flexion splints for the metacarpophalangeal joints can be fabricated to include either a volar or a dorsal forearm splint. The volar splint covers the forearm and palm to the distal palmar crease to provide stability of the wrist, but unfortunately, when dynamic traction is applied, the splint slips distally and flexion of the metacarpophalangeal joints is blocked by the displaced edge of the splint.[13]

The use of a dorsal splint can avoid this problem. The outrigger arises from a volar forearm piece to provide the proper angle of 90 degrees on the proximal phalanges (Fig. 21-7). To ensure stability, this dorsal splint must include a properly fitting metacarpal bar, which should be thin, rounded, and positioned proximally to the distal palmar crease. When the proper force of the splint is established and there is no evidence of decreased circulation or pressure areas, the patient gradually increases the amount of time that the splint is worn during the day.[11]

In the early stages after surgery, when edema is still a problem, the wearing of the patient's dynamic splint may aggravate the edema or produce pressure areas. Therefore a progressive static splint to be worn at night to extend the wrist and flex the metacarpophalangeal joints is made, of either plaster or thermoplastic material (Fig. 21-8), and is preferable in assisting the patient to keep the gains that he has made during the day with his exercises.

PROXIMAL INTERPHALANGEAL JOINTS

The proximal interphalangeal joints more often become fixed in flexion than they do in extension, but a capsulectomy may be required for either condition.

Extension contracture

Initially, the exercise program includes passive flexion and extension of the proximal interphalangeal joint and ac-

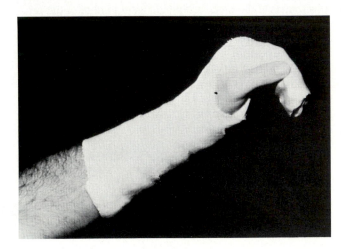

FIG. 21-8. Progressive static splint. For night wear after a metacarpophalangeal joint capsulectomy, this splint keeps the wrist in extension and the metacarpophalangeal joints in maximum flexion. Use of a stockinette to secure the splint in place is preferable to elastic wraps, which have a greater chance of causing edema and circulatory constriction.

tive blocked flexion and extension exercises. The patient is instructed to do these exercises three to five times on the half-hour or every hour while awake.

He is splinted alternately in flexion and extension in a dynamic splint during the day. According to how he progresses, it may be necessary to splint the patient alternately each night in flexion and extension or only in flexion.

Alternating the dynamic action can keep the joint mobile during the period of fibrous tissue deposition and organization.

If intrinsic releases are performed with the proximal interphalangeal joint capsulectomy, it is necessary to splint the patient in the position of intrinsic stretch—with the

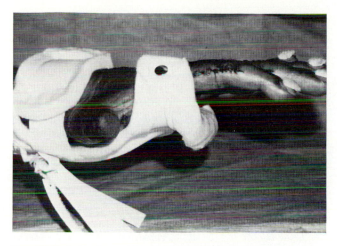

FIG. 21-9. Intrinsic stretch position splinting. When intrinsic releases are carried out with proximal interphalangeal joint capsulectomies, the hand needs to be splinted with the metacarpophalangeal joints extended and the proximal interphalangeal joints flexed.

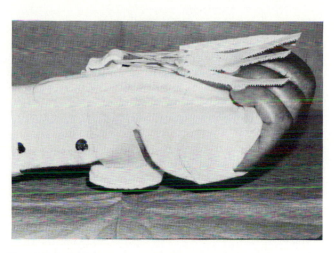

FIG. 21-10. Intrinsic stretch exercise. Holding the metacarpophalangeal joint in maximum extension and then attempting to flex the proximal interphalangeal joint puts the intrinsic muscle on a stretch.

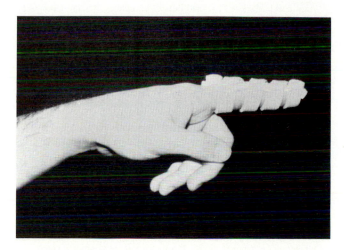

FIG. 21-11. Static finger extension splint. This is used after a proximal interphalangeal joint capsulectomy for a flexion contracture. The splint is padded and has soft strapping for comfort and ease of application and removal for exercises.

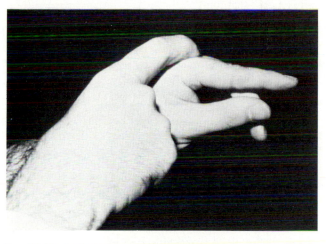

FIG. 21-12. Active extension of the proximal interphalangeal joint can be encouraged by holding the metacarpophalangeal joint in flexion while actively attempting to extend the proximal interphalangeal joint. This technique transfers the power of the extrinsic extensors and enhances the contribution of the intrinsics in extending the proximal interphalangeal joint.

metacarpophalangeal joints extended and the proximal interphalangeal joints flexed (Fig. 21-9). Intrinsic stretch exercises (Fig. 21-10) should be part of the postoperative exercise regimen.

Flexion contracture

Depending on the severity of the flexion contracture to be corrected and the preferred method of the surgeon, the proximal interphalangeal joint may be pinned in extension after a capsulectomy. Proximal interphalangeal joint exercises and splinting for capsulectomies performed to release flexion contractures in the proximal interphalangeal joints are initiated after the pins are removed. The patient is then fitted with a static finger-extension splint after the removal

of the pin (Fig. 21-11). Extension is emphasized and maintained by the use of the splint because the extensor tendon has become so stretched as a result of the flexion contracture that it needs to be protected.[10] Failure to splint the finger constantly in extension after this procedure, except during exercise or skin care, will result in a recurrence of the flexion contracture.

The exercise program should include passive and active extension and active flexion exercises. One can encourage extension at the proximal interphalangeal joint by having the patient passively flex the metacarpophalangal joint while he attempts to extend the proximal interphalangeal joint actively (Fig. 21-12). In this manner, the power of the extrinsic extensors is transferred to the proximal interpha-

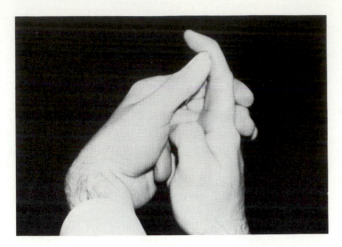

FIG. 21-13. Oblique retinacular ligament stretching is performed by stabilizing the proximal interphalangeal joint in maximum extension and then actively flexing the distal interphalangeal joint.

langeal joint and enhances the contribution of the intrinsics in extending that joint.

When the swelling diminishes, a dynamic proximal interphalangeal joint extension splint may be introduced and may be alternated with the use of a dynamic flexion splint during the day and a static extension splint at night, depending on the patient's progress.

If the oblique retinacular ligaments at the distal interphalangeal joint have become tight because of a prolonged flexion contracture in the proximal interphalangeal joint, it is necessary to institute oblique retinacular ligament stretching exercises postoperatively (Fig. 21-13). During the finger flexion exercises, it is important for the patient to maintain wrist extension actively or passively so that the flexor tendons are working through their optimal range of motion.

CONCLUSION

The management of patients who have undergone either metacarpophalangeal or proximal interphalangeal joint capsulectomy correlates closely with the management of acute hand injuries. Patient education before the surgery and the control of pain and edema after the surgery are critical factors in the success of the exercise and splinting programs in the patient after capsulectomy. The home exercise and splinting programs must be reviewed often and changed as the patient progresses.

Initially these patients are encouraged to begin using the postsurgical hand for light, everyday activities. A patient progresses to more dextrous activities and heavier tasks as the hand function improves. Skillful observation, accurate reevaluation, and adaptation on the part of the therapist in managing the patient's postoperative program, as well as the motivation and follow-through of the patient, are the keys to gaining and retaining improved range of motion and function after a capsulectomy procedure.

REFERENCES

1. Beasley, R.W.: Principles of managing acute hand injuries. In Converse, J., McCarthy, J., and Littler, J.W., editors: Reconstructive Plastic Surgery, ed. 2, vol. 6, Philadelphia, 1977, W.B. Saunders Co., p. 3000.
2. Boyes, J.H.: Bunnell's surgery of the hand, ed. 5, Philadelphia, 1970, J.B. Lippincott Co., p. 287.
3. Carter, P.R.: Personal communication, Dallas.
4. Curtis, R.M.: Capsulectomy of the interphalangeal joints of the fingers, J. Bone Joint Surg. **36:**1219, 1954.
5. Curtis, R.M.: Management of the stiff hand. In Hunter, J.M., Schneider, L.H., Mackin, E.J., and Bell, J.A., editors: Rehabilitation of the hand, St. Louis, 1978, The C.V. Mosby Company.
6. Gould, J., and Nicholson, B.: Capsulectomy of the metacarpophalangeal and proximal interphalangeal joints, J. Hand Surg. **4**(5):482, Sept. 1979.
7. Knapp, M.E.: Massage. In Kottke, F., Stillwell, G.K., and Lehmann, J.F., editors: Krusen's handbook of physical medicine and rehabilitation, ed. 3, Philadelphia, 1982, W.B. Saunders Co. p. 386.
8. Kottke, F.J.: Therapeutic exercise to maintain mobility. In Kottke, F.J., Stillwell, G.K., and Lehmann, J.F., editors: Krusen's handbook of physical medicine and rehabilitation, ed. 3, Philadelphia, 1982, W.B. Saunders Co., p. 389.
9. Lankford, L.L., Carter, P.R., and Magnenat, G.F.: The value of a hand therapy unit in rehabilitation of the disabled hand. Unpublished paper, Dallas, 1977.
10. Littler, J.W.: Principles of reconstructive surgery of the hand. In Converse, J., McCarthy, J., and Littler, J.W., editors: Reconstructive plastic surgery, ed. 2, vol. 6. Philadelphia, 1977, W.B. Saunders Co., p. 3103.
11. Malick, M.H.: Manual on dynamic hand splinting with thermoplastic materials, Pittsburgh, 1974, Harmarville Rehabilitation Center, p. 2.
12. Rosenthal, E.A.: The extensor tendons. In Hunter, J.M., Schneider, L.H., Mackin, E.J., and Bell, J.A., editors: Rehabilitation of the hand. St. Louis, 1978, The C.V. Mosby Company.
13. Weeks, P.M., and Wray, R.C.: Management of the stiff hand. In Management of acute hand injuries, St. Louis, 1978, The C.V. Mosby Co., p. 329.

VI
TENDONS

22

Nutritional aspects of tendon healing

PETER C. AMADIO, SCOTT H. JAEGER, and JAMES M. HUNTER

Controversy over nutritional and healing pathways in tendons has existed since well before the start of the twentieth century. In 1852, Sir James Paget studied the healing of Achilles tendons in rabbits and concluded that the "nucleated blastema" that formed derived from the cut tendon ends rather than the sheath of surrounding soft tissue. William Adams, studying the same animal model 2 years later, came to the opposite conclusion. Over 100 years later there is still discussion as to whether tendon as a tissue has the potential to heal an injury, and the extent to which such "intrinsic" healing occurs in actual clinical practice is still unknown.

Recently a great deal of information has become available to shed new light on the field of tendon nutrition and metabolism. By correlating data from anatomic, biochemical, physiologic, and clinical research conducted over the past decade, we hope to achieve a perspective for better understanding of this crucial problem for the hand surgeon and the hand therapist.

ANATOMIC DATA

Careful injection studies of flexor tendons have delineated the pattern of vascular anatomy by tendon and by digit. Outside the digital sheath, tendons have an excellent blood supply, arriving through circumferential mesotendineal vessels. A preputial infolding of this mesotendineum allows this type of vascular nutrition to extend into the proximal portion of the digital sheath as well. Within the sheath, blood is carried to the tendon through a series of vincula, whose number varies from digit to digit and which decrease in extent with age. Between the vascular domains of the vincula, relatively avascular watershed zones are seen (Fig. 22-1).

The vincula are known to be fed by constant branches of the digital arteries, which take their origin roughly at the level of the metacarpophalangeal and interphalangeal joints. These branches are in jeopardy during surgical dissection to expose the neurovascular bundles or the lateral margins of the pulley system.

The flexor pulley system has been well described by Doyle, who provided the currently accepted nomenclature of annular and cruciate pulleys (Fig. 22-2). The importance of the fibrous pulleys in controlling active motion by prevention of bowstringing is well known. More recently, attention has been focused on the nutritional role the pulleys might play in providing a firm opposing surface to the volar, avascular areas of tendon, allowing for contact lubrication and pumping of nutrients into the interstitium in a manner similar to that in articular cartilage. Lundborg has shown that tenocytes in the volar avascular areas reside in lacuna-like structures, as chondrocytes do. Recent biochemical and physiologic data suggest that the volar tendon and cartilage analogy extends beyond microscopic appearance, as discussed later in this chapter.

BIOCHEMICAL DATA

Research in tendon biochemistry has focused on two areas: intracellular mechanisms and extracellular matrix composition.

Tenocyte systems have been used by biochemists for many years in the study of collagen metabolism and its regulation. These cells have been shown to be very active metabolically, with the ability to divide, migrate, and alter the mechanical properties of tendon in response to a variety of stimuli. In both cell and tissue culture, tenocytes synthesize large amounts of type I collagen, and smaller amounts of a number of glycosaminoglycans (GAG). All the respiratory enzymes needed for aerobic and anaerobic metabolism are present in tenocytes.

In the presence of serum, tenocytes, even of mature animals, will divide; a series of recent experiments by Graham and others has shown that a serum clot encasing a plug of rabbit tendon provides sufficient nutrition for cell division and, if fibrin is added to the system, the tenocytes will migrate out of the plug along the fibrin strands.

Both the number and organization of collagen fibrils in tendon are under tenocyte control. When experimental animals are exercised, the stressed tendons hypertrophy, with increases in both collagen content and tensile strenth. Cells grown on a pulsating membrane not only synthesize collagen, but also orient the fibers parallel to the lines of tension.

In living tendon the collagen fibers are oriented longitudinally and consist of a bimodal population of very large and more numerous small fibrils. The large fibrils have great tensile strength and increase in number with exercise. The smaller fibrils, with high surface-to-volume ratios, bind extensively to each other and to the larger fibrils, giving excellent resistance to creep deformation (that is, "stretching out"). A given quantity of collagen then might have very

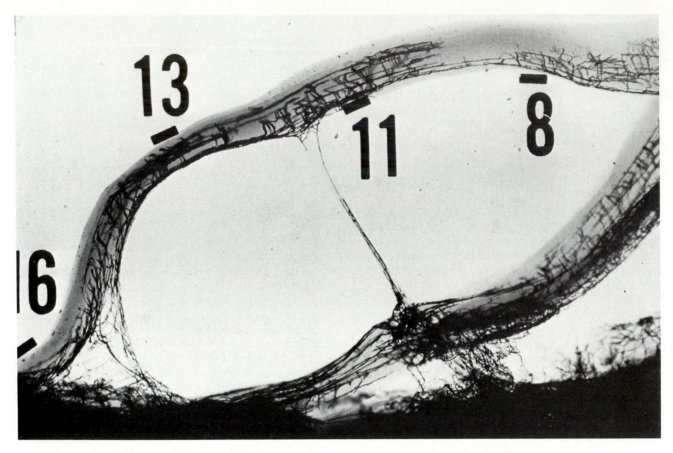

FIG. 22-1. Injection study showing the typical vascular pattern in human flexor tendons. Note the volar avascular area between marker 8 and marker 11.

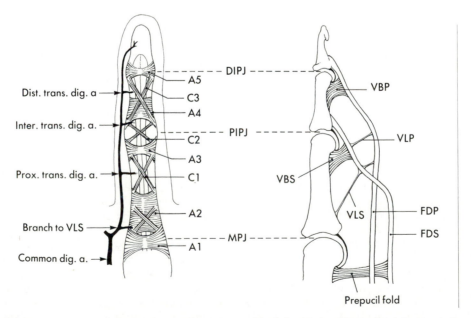

FIG. 22-2. The annular (A) and cruciate (C) pulleys, along with their relationship to the joints and the transverse branches of the digital artery, which nourish the tendon sheath and the vincula.

different mechanical properties, depending on the fibrillar organization.

The regulation of fibril size in tendon has been studied in experimental animals. The critical factor appears to be the type of GAG that the cells synthesize. It is known that the presence of chondroitin sulfate in culture medium promotes rapid growth of small collagen fibrils and that dermatan sulfate promotes slower growth, but of larger fibrils. Chondroitin sulfate interacts with hyaluronic acid, another GAG found in tendon, to form a fairly rigid structure not directly bound to collagen, thus separating the fibrils and inhibiting their growth. Dermatan sulfate binds directly to the collagen fibrils, allowing closer packing of large fibrils around a dermatan sulfate core.

In the absence of tension, collagen organization is significantly disturbed. Beckham treated chick embryos with curare and found that development of tendon and tendon sheath was completely arrested in the absence of movement.

Where tendons pass through a fibro-osseous sheath, the areas of the tendon directly beneath the fibrous pulley experience compressive forces. This area of the tendon has been shown to be rich in chondroitin sulfate, measuring about 3.5% of the dry weight. On the opposite side or the tension surface of the tendon, the GAG is much less, only about 0.5%, and it is almost all dermatan sulfate. (GAG is about 9% of the dry weight of articular cartilage.) The compression side has a higher percentage of smaller fibrils than the tension side, consistent with the hypothesis that, with less tensile stress, fewer large "tensile" fibrils would

be made. Gillard performed an experiment in which he transposed the tendon away from the pulley, eliminating the "compression side." Biochemical analysis of the transposed tendon showed a decrease in total GAG toward 0.5% and the conversion of GAG type to dermatan sulfate, a trend that was reversed when the tendon was relocated beneath the pulley.

It is interesting to speculate on the possible nutritional relevance of the data just presented. The volar, avascular areas of human tendon are exposed to compressive forces; increased chondroitin sulfate in this area would, by dispersing the collagen fibrils, provide a better milieu for diffusion of nutrients from the synovial fluid into the tendon. Weber has recently demonstrated that this volar area does indeed have increased diffusional capability, and that this capacity was increased by tendon motion, suggesting a milking action similar to that seen in articular cartilage. The work of Salter has demonstrated the benefit of early passive movement in the healing of cartilage injury. One wonders whether this therapy may apply to analogous areas within tendon.

PHYSIOLOGIC DATA

The relative contribution of synovial and vascular nutritional pathways to tendon inside the digital sheath has been the subject of considerable debate. This point has clinical relevance, since frequently tendon injury includes some damage to the vincular system. The resulting avascular areas can be extensive (Fig. 22-3). If synovial nutrition plays a

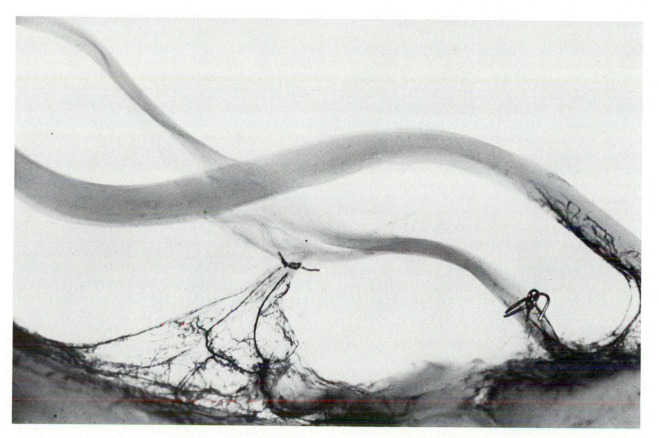

FIG. 22-3. Injection study as in Fig. 22-1, but with the two vincula to the superficialis ligated, showing loss of intratendinous circulation not only in the superficialis but also in the profundus.

TABLE 22-1. Relative frequency of triggering versus distribution of vincula

Finger	Relative frequency of triggering (%)*	Absent vinculum longus superficialis (%)†	Absent vinculum longus profundus (%)†
Index	10	10	0
Middle	39	40	12
Ring	39	55	10
Little	12	10	3

*Data from Lipscomb, P.R.: Surg. Clin. North Am. **24**:780-797, 1944.
†Data from Ochiai, N., Matsui, T., Miyaji, N., and others: J. Hand Surg. **4**:321-330, 1979.

small role, such injuries would be practically doomed to adhesions and a poor result. If synovial nutrition is significant, even avascular tendons might survive to heal without restricting adhesions.

Manske has reported a series of experiments comparing the relative contribution of synovial and vascular routes in nutrition in metabolic studies of hydrogen washout and amino acid uptake. His work shows a much greater and more rapid uptake of nutrient by the synovial fluid pathway. Lundborg developed an experimental model in which segments of rabbit tendon were encased in dialysis tubing (to prevent cellular migration from synovium) and implanted within the knee joint as a "tissue culture in situ." He showed not only preservation of viability in this system, but also attempts at healing of experimental wounds to the implanted tendon. In this model, the healing cells appeared to arise from both the epitenon and tenocytes themselves. These studies indicate an important role for synovial fluid in tendon nutrition.

No discussion of the physiology of tendon healing would be complete without mention of the classic work of Potenza. In his dog model, experimental tendon injuries were repaired within the flexor sheath and treated, in the then-standard way for humans as well as for uncooperative laboratory animals, by immobilization. This work repeatedly demonstrated a lack of intrinsic response within the tendon, with all healing arriving from the sheath and surrounding soft tissue by way of adhesions. This work also showed that more extensive soft-tissue injury such as resection of sheath, or of superficialis tendon in the case of profundus repair, caused much greater adhesions. Even forceps marks on the tendons stimulated adhesion formation. For many years, the well-documented evidence from this study was used to claim that there was no potential for intrinsic healing in any injured tendon within a fibro-osseous sheath. Subsequent work by McDowell and Synder, however, demonstrated that even with a dog model this might not be the case. First, they pointed out that since the vincular system is poorly developed in the dog, the only potential for tendon nutrition within the sheath is by diffusion of synovial fluid. Because the Potenza model calls for complete tendon immobilization, the pumping mechanism is lost, this route is blocked, and the tendon is left with inadequate nutrition.

Salter has shown that avascular cartilage heals experimental wounds much better if motion, and therefore active diffusion, occurs. The same may be true for the analogous avascualr areas in tendons. In the McDowell model, the sheath is not disturbed, a partial injury is creased in the tendon, and no immobilization occurs, thus allowing continued free synovial nutrition. Uniformly, these dog tendons were able to heal without adhesions. More recent work by Schepel, in a primate model perhaps more similar to the human case, was again able to demonstrate adhesion-free tendon healing when vincula and synovial relationships were not disturbed.

Twenty years ago, Ellis showed that ischemia was the major cause of adhesions. When experimental conditions can be created, as in the McDowel and Schepel models, which avoid ischemia, adhesion-free tendon healing can apparently occur.

The careful control evident in laboratory experiments unfortunately cannot be brought into the clinical situation completely, not only because of variables related to the type of injury, but also because of patient variables such as number and location of vincula and quality of synovial fluid nutrition. Matthews has shown by injection studies that in cases of experimental injury to rabbit flexor tendons, adhesions formed only when the experimental injury had caused a loss of vascularity to the cut tendon end. This varied with the level of injury. This line of evidence would suggest that although synovial nutrition is sufficient for homeostasis and limited healing, in tendon systems in which a vincular system is well developed, both routes may be required for healing of major tendon injury.

A clinical demonstration of the importance of blood supply to tendon healing may exist in the case of the common trigger finger. Histologic evaluation of trigger tendons shows similar degenerative changes to those found in other collagenous structures where hypovascularity and attrition take their toll, such as the rotator cuff of the shoulder. Light and electron microscopy have shown similar pathologic features, including calcification, in both conditions. When the relative frequency of triggering by digit is compared with the known distribution of vincula as calculated by Ochiai and associates,[26] an interesting cooorespondence is noted (Table 22-1). The anatomic location of tendon swelling and degeneration in trigger fingers is usually in the hypovascular watershed areas of the flexor profundus and superficialis; perhaps it represents a hypertrophy because of a relative lack of nutrient flow.

A COMPOSITE PICTURE

Sufficient data has accumulated over the past decade to confirm that tendon is vital, dynamic tissue. Tenocytes re-

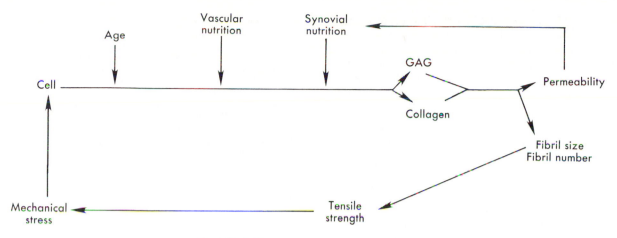

FIG. 22-4. The tenocyte and its environment.

spond to mechanical stimuli to modify their intercellular matrix strength and permeability. Nutrition arrives through both synovial and vascular sources; where both are present, both are important. Given adequate nutrition, tenocytes can divide and migrate and have been shown now in several different experimental models to be capable of adhesion-free healing.

Fig. 22-4 outlines our current concept of the self-regulation of tendon structures. Tenocytes respond to changes in mechanical stress by altering the type and amount of glycosaminoglyan synthesized and thereby the spacing and amount of collagen fibrils, thus altering tendon strength. Permeability to nutrients, important in maintaining the higher metabolic level required at increased synthetic rates, is also changed. The changes in matrix strength then modify the perceived stress on the cell, completing the self-regulatory loop. The entire process is modified by tissue age and available base-line vascular nutrition. When the system fails, degenerative changes such as triggering can occur and the response to injury is modified.

CLINICAL APPLICATION

These concepts of tendon healing can be applied in the approach to the patient with flexor tendon injury. The goal is to restore the best possible environment for tendon healing and to maintain it throughout the recovery period. As a first step, it is important to obtain a better understanding of the anatomy of the injury. To this end, a record should be made not only of the level of injury on the skin with relation to the flexion creases, as described by many authors, but also of the level with regard to tendon and vincular anatomy. Bleeding of tendon ends is evaluated before repair. All lacerated tendons are repaired with a volar, nonhemostatic, minimally reactive nonabsorbable suture. Careful handling of the tendon is emphasized, since the work of Potenza has clearly shown that all areas of forcep or clamp violation of epitenon serve as foci for adhesions. For similar reasons, a circumferential repair at the tendon juncture is used to invert tendon fibers and present a smooth surface to facilitate rapid reestablishment of epitenon continuity. Finally, the tendon sheath is repaired to restore the potential for synovial fluid

nutrition. Secondarily, sheath closure may also help prevent triggering of the tendon juncture as it glides through the pulley system.

Postoperatively, early mobilization techniques are employed to apply controlled tension to the repair site, to stimulate tenocyte synthesis, and to promote the milking action of sheath or synovial fluid penetration of the tendon. We have used a combination of the methods described by Kleinert and by Duran and Houser to provide differential gliding of profundus and superficialis and also the dynamic effects of active extension with passive flexion, and to provide positioning of the wrist and metacarpophalangeal joints to further control the maximum possible tensile stress exerted on the repair.

One may assess the duration of the postoperative protection by the type of healing that is occurring. In a patient with more severe vincular or sheath damage or in the older person, more extrinsic adhesions are expected, and earlier release from immobilization and protection might be advised. The reasons are that we believe healing by extrinsic means is quicker than by the intrinsic route and also there is a desire to stretch the adhesions as soon as possible. On the other hand, in the younger patient with intact vinculums and a well-repaired sheath, a good potential for intrinsic tendon healing is anticipated. These patients might be protected longer, particularly if they rapidly develop a full active range of motion when voluntary flexion is initiated.

THE FUTURE

Increased knowledge of tendon nutrition and tendon biology will further our understanding of the metabolic processes called into play after tendon injury and the cells responsible for them. Whether the healing cells arise from within the tendon or from the surface of the tendon, float freely across the synovial space, or are some combination of the three is ultimately less important than the concern that they do their job without physically binding tendon to sheath with adhesions. We now know that such adhesion-free healing can occur. In the future, it will be necessary for us to use our growing understanding to select more precisely those patients in whom such healing is possible and preserve this fragile capability through appropriate repair and rehabilitation. In those patients in whom such healing is not possible, alternative forms of hand rehabilitation must be pursued. Our ultimate goal is to provide for each patient with flexor tendon injury an individually tailored solution that will result in a predictably successful outcome.

REFERENCES

1. Adams, W.: On the reparative process in human tendons. 1; also a series of experiments on rabbits, London, 1860, Churchill.
2. Amadio, P.C., Frasca, P., and Hunter, J.M.: Histology and SEM and flexor tendons in trigger fingers, Trans. Orthop. Res. Soc. **7**:345, 1982.
3. Beckham, C., Dimond, R., and Greenlee, T.K., Jr.: The role of movement in the development of a digital flexor tendon, Am. J. Anat. **150**:443-460, 1978.
4. Doyle, J.R., and Blythe, W.: The finger flexor tendon sheath and pulleys. In American Academy of Orthopaedic Surgeons: Symposium on tendon surgery in the hand, St. Louis, 1975, The C.V. Mosby Co.
5. Duran, R.J., and Houser, R.G.: Controlled passive motion following flexor tendon repair in zones 2 and 3. In American Academy of Orthopaedic Surgeons: Symposium on tendon surgery in the hand, St. Louis, 1975, The C.V. Mosby Co.
6. Eiken, O., Hagberg, L., and Lunborg, G.: Evolving biologic concepts as applied to tendon surgery, Clin. Plast. Surg. **8**:1-11, 1981.
7. Fahey, J.J., and Bollinger, J.A.: Trigger finger in adults and children, Jand. Bone Joint Surg. **36A**:1200-1218, 1954.
8. Gillard, G.C., Reilly, H.C., Bell-Booth, P.G., and Flint, M.H.: The influence of mechanical forces on the glycosaminoglycan content of the rabbit flexor digitorum profundus tendon, Connect. Tissue Res. **7**:37-46, 1979.
9. Gillard, G.C., Merriless, J.J., Bell-Booth, P.G., Reilly, H.C., and Flint, M.H.: The proteoglycan content and axial periodicity of collagen in tendon, Biochem. J. **163**:145-151, 1977.
10. Graham, M.D., Becker, H., Cohen, K., and Diegelman, R.: Intrinsic tendon healing documentation by vitro studies, Presented at the American Society for Surgery of the Hand annual meeting, New Orleans, 1982.
11. Hansson, H.A., Lundborg, G., and Rydevik, B.: Restoration of superficially damaged flexor tendons in synovial environment, Scand. J. Plast. Reconstr. Surg. **14**:109-114, 1980.
12. Jósza, L., Bálint, J.B., Réffy, A., and Demel, Z.: Histochemical and ultrastructural study of adult human tendon, Acta Histochem. **65**:250-257, 1979.
13. Ketchum, L.D.: Primary tendon healing: a review, J. Hand Surg. **2**:428-435, 1977.
14. Kleinert, H.E., Schepel, S., and Gill, T.: Flexor tendon injuries, Surg. Clinic. North Am. **61**:267-286, 1981.
15. Leung, D.Y., Glagov, S., and Mathews, M.B.: Cyclic stretching stimulates synthesis of matrix components, Science **191**:475, 1979.
16. Lipscomb, P.R.: Chronic nonspecific tenosynovitis and peritendinitis, Surg. Clin. North Am. **24**:780-797, 1944.
17. Lundborg, G., and Rank, F.: Experimental intrinsic healing of flexor tendons based upon synovial fluid nutrition, J. Hand Surg. **3**:21-31, 1978.
18. Lundborg, G., and Rank, F.: Experimental studies on cellular mechanisms involved in healing of animal and human flexor tendon in synovial environment, Hand **12**:3-11, 1980.
19. Lundborg, G., Holm, S., and Myrhage, R.: The role of the synovial fluid and tendon sheath for flexor tendon nutrition, Scand. J. Plast. Reconstr. Surg. **14**:99-107, 1980.
20. Lundborg, G., Myrhage R., and Rydevik, B.: The vascularization of human flexor tendons within the digital synovial sheath region: structural and functional aspects, J. Hand Surg. **2**:417-427, 1977.
21. Manske, P.R., Whiteside, L.A., and Lesker, P.A.: Nutrient pathways to flexor tendons, J. Hand Surg. **3**:32-36, 1978.
22. Matsui, T., Miyagi, N., Merklin, R.J., and Hunter, J.M.: Vascular anatomy of flexor tendons, part II, J. Jpn. Orthop. Assoc. **53**:307-320, 1979.
23. McDowell, C.L., and Synder, D.M.: Tendon healing: an experimental model in the dog, J. Hand Surg. **2**:122-126, 1977.
24. Matthews, P.: The pathology of flexor tendon repair, Hand **11**:233-242, 1979.
25. Matthews, J.P.: Vascular changes in flexor tendons after injury and repair: an experimental study, Injury **8**:227-233, 1979.
26. Ochiai, N., Matsui, T., Miyaji, N., Merklin, R.J., and Hunter, J.M.: Vascular anatomy of flexor tendons. I. Vincular system and blood supply of the profundus tendon in the digital sheath, J. Hand Surg. **4**:321-330, 1979.
27. Page, J.: Lectures on surgical pathology, **1**:266-269, London, 1853.
28. Parry, D.A.D., Barnes, G.G., and Craig, A.S.: A comparison of the size distribution of collagen fibrils in connective tissues a a function of age and a possible relation between fibril size distribution and mechanical properties, Proc. R. Soc. Lond. **203**:305-321, 1978.
29. Parry, D.A.D., Craig, A.S., and Barnes, G.R.G. Tendon and ligament from the horse; an ultrastructural study of collagen fibrils and elastic fibers and elastic fibers as a function of age. Proc. R. Soc. Lond. [Biol.] **203**:293-303, 1978.
30. Potenza, A.D.: Effect of associated trauma on healing of divided tendons, J. Trauma **2**:173-183, 1962.
31. Potenza, A.D.: Prevention of adhesions to healing digital flexor tendons, J.A.M.A. **187**:187-191, 1964.
32. Potenza, A.D.: Tendon healing with the flexor digital sheath in the dog, J. Bone Joint Surg. **44A**:49-64, 1962.
33. Salter, R.B., Simmonds, D.F., Malcolm, B.W., Rumble, E.J., MacMichael, D., and Clements, N.: The effect of continuous passive motion on healing of full thickness degects in articular cartilage, J. Bone Joint Surg. **62A**:1232-1244, 1980.
34. Scott, J.E.: Proteoglycan-collagen arrangements in developing rat tail tendon, Biochem. J. **195**:573-581, 1981.
35. Van Der Meulen, J.C., and Leistikow, P.A.: Tendon healing, Clin. Plast. Surg. **4**:439-458, 1977.
36. Videman, T., Eronen, I., and Candolin, T.: Effects of Motion load changes on tendon tissues and articular cartilage, Scand. J. Work Environ. Health **5**(suppl. 3): 55-67, 1979.
37. Weber, E.R., Hardin, G., and Haynes, D.: Synovial fluid nutrition of flexor tendon, Presented at 36th annual meeting of the American Society for Surgery of the Hand, Las Vegas, 1981.
38. Woo, S.L.-Y., Ritter, M.A., Amiel, D., and others: The biomechanical and biochemical properties of swine tendons: long term effects of exercise on the digital extensors, Connect. Tissue Res. **7**:177-183, 1980.

23

Primary care of flexor tendon injuries

SCOTT H. JAEGER and EVELYN J. MACKIN

Flexor tendon injuries can result in severe limitations of hand function. The proper early care of these injuries is essential, because delayed tendon reconstruction can be extremely costly and time consuming. However, to undertake a primary tendon repair, one must consider a number of important factors.

GENERAL CONSIDERATIONS
Surgeon and hand therapist

Flexor tendon lacerations are major injuries and should be treated by a surgeon who has had specific training and ongoing experience in surgery of the hand. The surgery should be performed in a well-equipped operating room with anesthesia that will provide muscle relaxation. The surgery should be considered by both the surgeon and the patient as only the initial phase of a treatment plan that will require at least 8 to 12 weeks of effort. The rehabilitation phase is essential to the result. A surgeon should not undertake the surgery unless he or she is committed to provide the necessary postoperative care either personally or through an experienced hand therapist.

Wound and timing considerations

In cases involving tidy wounds, primary repair of the flexor tendon laceration is indicated along with the repair of all other injured structures. If primary repair cannot be performed under the correct circumstances, a delayed primary repair is indicated. A delayed primary repair can be performed during the period of 3 to 10 days after injury. In tidy lacerations the skin should be closed immediately in all cases.

Delayed primary repair is especially useful in cases of some untidy wounds. Here wound care can be completed, and the untidy wound can be converted to a tidy one before the tendon repair.

If there are untidy wounds that cannot be converted to tidy wounds in a limited amount of time, during which a delayed primary repair can be performed, or if skin coverage is not sufficient, then primary repair should be abandoned and plans made for secondary tendon reconstruction.

Associated injuries

Early controlled mobilization is the key to success in most cases of flexor tendon lacerations. Any associated injury that can interfere with the early controlled motion program may detract from the quality of the result of the flexor tendon repair. The best examples are fractures that can be stabilized enough to allow early controlled motion of the flexor tendon, and lacerations of the extensor tendon, which must be protected. Replantation at the digital level is the extreme example. The surgeon must repair associated injuries in such a way that they will not be disrupted by a program of early controlled motion. If it is impossible to obtain adequate stabilization, it may be prudent to abandon primary repair of the flexor tendon and allow complete healing of skin, bone, extensor tendon, and other associated injuries before flexor tendon reconstruction. Here primary passive tendon implants are of value as an acute preparation for secondary flexor tendon reconstruction.

Retinacular pulley injuries

An adequate retinacular pulley system is essential to obtainment of a good result from a flexor tendon injury. It is necessary that if retinacular pulley reconstruction is required the reconstruction be performed in such a way that the reconstructed pulley is able to withstand the stresses of an early controlled motion program for the lacerated flexor tendon.

The A_2 and A_4 pulleys are the most important segments of the retinacular system. They can be reconstructed by use of either a slip of tendon or dorsal retinaculum. The reconstruction should involve the threading of the material either through or around bone. This will ensure the greatest possible strength of the reconstruction. In the rehabilitation phase, external prosthetic rings can be used to splint and protect the reconstructed pulley during the controlled motion of the repaired tendon.

Partial flexor tendon lacerations

There is much controversy with regard to partial lacerations of flexor tendons. There are some overall considerations. All wounds that may involve possible laceration of flexor tendons should be explored. The presence or absence of a significant tendon laceration should not be assumed on clinical examination alone. Whenever a partial laceration is noted, whether it is repaired or not, the tendon should be protected for at least 4 weeks with a program of early controlled motion.

Repair should be performed if the laceration involves greater than 50% of the tendon. Repair is indicated in lacerations that are less than 50% when the laceration creates a "trap door" or other mechanical obstruction to tendon excursion. Partial lacerations of flexor tendons involving less than 50% of the tendon and offering no mechanical obstruction can be treated with early controlled motion.

General technical considerations

In general, the better condition of the digit, the better is the chance of a successful result of a primary tendon repair. The skin, joints, bones, nerves, vessels, extensor mechanism, and retinacular pulley systems should be preserved, repaired, and protected.

With regard to the tendon repair, some important technical considerations include the adherence to strict atraumatic technique. The tendons should only be handled at these cut ends if possible. Nonreactive suture materials should be employed, and the suture technique should be strong but not adversely affect the intrinsic vascularity of the tendon. These techniques are discussed specifically later.

Level of tendon laceration

Assuming that the above considerations indicate a primary repair of a flexor tendon laceration, the most important parameter to determine the treatment plan is the level of the laceration. It is essential that the site of the laceration be identified by direct vision with the finger extended. The site of the skin laceration is nearly always erroneous as an indicator for the site of the laceration on the flexor tendon. A methodical exploration of the wound is essential.

The best incision for this purpose is the Brunner zigzag type. The incision is planned to include the original skin laceration and to allow extension for exposure either distally or proximally. At first, only the central legs of the incision are dissected down to the retinacular pulley system. The true level of tendon laceration is determined by visualization of the distal stump of the tendon and by passive flexion and extension of the digit. Once this identification is made, the incision can be extended either proximally or distally to repair the laceration. In addition, by knowing the true site of tendon laceration, one can choose the appropriate treatment plan.

ZONE 1
Definition

Zone 1 refers to that portion of the flexor digitorum profundus tendon distal to the insertion of the flexor digitorum superficialis. There are two mechanisms of injury that are most common: sharp laceration and avulsion of insertion during a hyperextension injury of the distal interphalangeal joint. The avulsion injury may be associated with a fracture of the distal phalanx. With either injury, proximal retraction of the flexor digitorum profundus tendon may occur. The retraction may be limited by preservation of the vinculum breve profundum. However, if this vinculum is also ruptured, the flexor digitorum profundus can retract further and block the action of the flexor digitorum superficialis or more seriously cause intrinsic tightness through tension applied through the lumbrical muscle by its origin from the flexor digitorum profundus.

Operative treatment

In the case of the avulsion injury, the preferred treatment is retrieval of the tendon through a Brunner incision and reinsertion of the tendon to the distal phalanx. This can be done acutely or as late as 14 weeks after injury. A flap composed of periosteum and any remnant of tendon stump is dissected, and the tendon is secured to the bone by a suture that is secured by a button on the nail. A monofilament suture of either nylon or stainless steel is preferred, and it should be either 3-0 or 2-0 in size. A 5-0 Dacron polyester suture is used to secure the flap to the tendon.

If the injury is of the sharp laceration type and 1.5 cm or less from the insertion of the tendon, the tendon can be advanced by the same technique used in the avulsion injury. If the laceration is greater than 1.5 cm from the insertion, end-to-end repair is indicated. The repair is extremely difficult to perform because of space limitations under the A_4 pulley. It may be necessary to open a window in the A_4 pulley to accomplish the repair, but this should be done judiciously because bow stringing and triggering may occur. The technique of end-to-end tendon repair is discussed in the section on zone 2.

Postoperative management

The technique of early controlled motion (ECM) is employed after repair of injuries in zone 1.

In the cases of advancement, the repair is protected by a splint and rubber-band traction for 4 weeks. A cuff with rubber-band traction is used for an additional 2 weeks. At 6 weeks, the button and suture are removed. In the cases of end-to-end repair, the postoperative management is the same repair in zone 2 and will be discussed in that section.

Alternative treatment regimens

Although the results of the avulsion injuries and those lacerations treated by advancement are usually quite good, the results of the end-to-end repairs can be less gratifying. In addition an end-to-end repair may be technically impossible. Therefore alternative treatment plans are necessary. If the digit has an intact and functioning flexor digitorum superficialis tendon, tenodesis, capsulodesis, or arthrodesis of the distal interphalangeal joint may be indicated. If there is no function of the flexor digitorum superficialis tendon or the patient requires active flexion of the distal interphalangeal joint, a primary tendon graft may be indicated.

ZONE 2
Definition

Zone 2 refers to those portions of the flexor digitorum profundus and superficialis tendons from the proximal edge of the A_1 pulley to the A_4 pulley. This area was referred to by Bunnell as "no-man's-land" because of the extreme difficulty in obtaining a good result with primary repair of tendon lacerations in this area. He advocated primary tendon grafting rather than primary repair for these injuries. His clinical observations were confirmed in the laboratory by Potenza. Using dogs, Potenza demonstrated that flexor tendons were not capable of intrinsic healing and help from surrounding tissues in the form of adhesions was required for flexor tendon union. The need for extrinsic healing along with mechanical factors such as the presence of two tendons in a tight fibrosseous tunnel and independent excursion of the tendons that is required for functions contributed to the poor success rate.

However in the 1950s, Duran, Kleinert, and Verdan reported success with primary repairs of flexor tendons; "no-man's-land" soon became known as zone 2. Recent laboratory evidence in a variety of animal models, including primates, has demonstrated that flexor tendons are capable of intrinsic healing and this property will allow success of primary repairs. The chapter on the nutritional aspects of tendon healing deals in depth with this subject.

In clinical practice, flexor tendons heal by a combination of both the extrinsic and intrinsic mechanisms. To obtain a good result from a primary repair in Zone 2, one should direct the operative and rehabilitative treatment toward an attempt to increase the ratio in favor of the intrinsic mechanism. This is accomplished by atraumatic surgical technique by use of nonreactive suture material and nonhemostatic suture methods. The vinculums to both tendons should be preserved. The flexor digitorum superficialis should never be sacrificed because it provides the vascular nutrition to a large segment of the flexor digitorum profundus. Care should be taken to preserve the synovial sheath and all defects in the sheath should be repaired watertight. The key

to success is the hand rehabilitation that is directed to a well-supervised program of early controlled motion. The time required for the development of tension strength is longer when a tendon heals intrinsically, but the results are much better.

Operative treatment

The Brunner zigzag approach is the preferred incision because it allows for extension both proximally and distally and, along with providing good exposure, does not interfere with the intrinsic vascular supply to the tendons and synovial sheath (Fig. 23-1, *A*). The tendon stumps are approached through transverse incisions in the retinacular pulley and synovial sheath systems (Fig. 23-1, *B*). The tendons are manipulated at their cut ends, and a modified Kessler suture is placed in each round tendon stump. Horizontal mattress sutures are placed in flat portions of the superficialis tendons. A 3-0 or 4-0 Dacron polyester suture is adequate for these purposes (Fig. 23-1, *C*). Once the tendon stumps are controlled with the sutures, a Swanson suture passer is used to retrieve the sutures through the synovial sheath and out through a transverse incision in the sheath (Fig. 23-1, *D*). The sutures should be delivered at a site where both tendon stumps can be brought out with little tension. A Keith needle can be used to implate and immobilize the tendons and the sheath if the tendons tend to retract. The sutures are tied

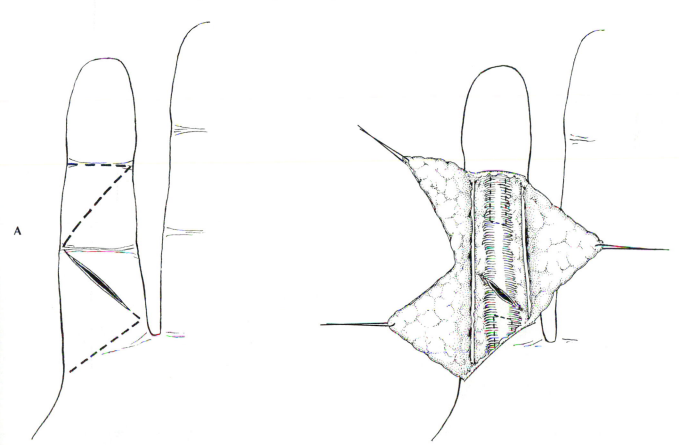

A

FIG. 23-1. Technique for primary tendon repair. **A,** Brunner zigzag approach is preferred incision because it allows for extension both proximally and distally and along with providing good exposure it does not interfere with the intrinsic vascular supply to tendons and synovial sheath.

Continued.

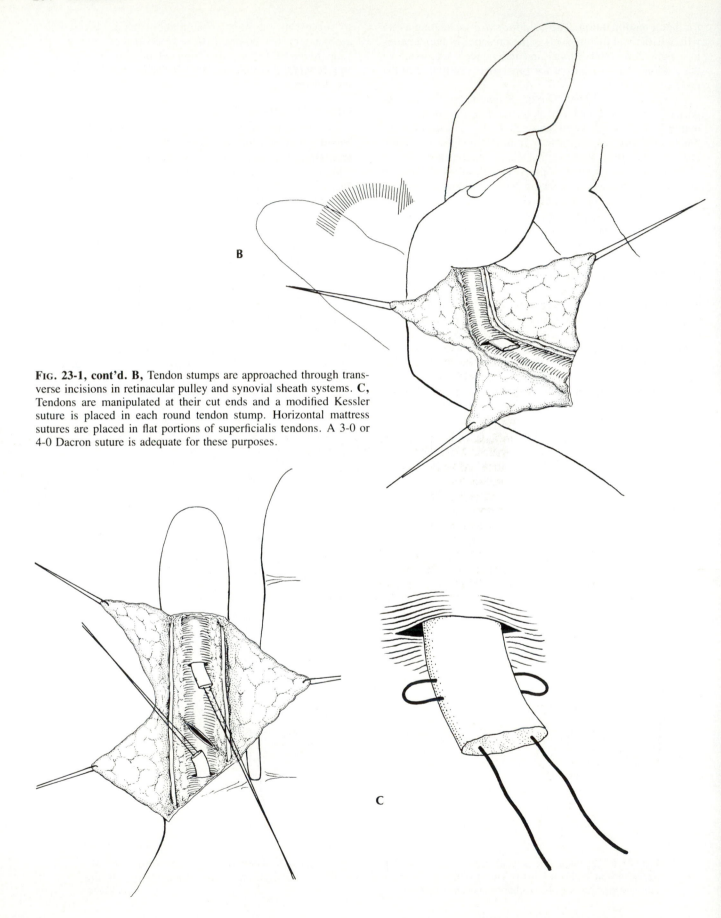

B

FIG. 23-1, cont'd. B, Tendon stumps are approached through transverse incisions in retinacular pulley and synovial sheath systems. C, Tendons are manipulated at their cut ends and a modified Kessler suture is placed in each round tendon stump. Horizontal mattress sutures are placed in flat portions of superficialis tendons. A 3-0 or 4-0 Dacron suture is adequate for these purposes.

C

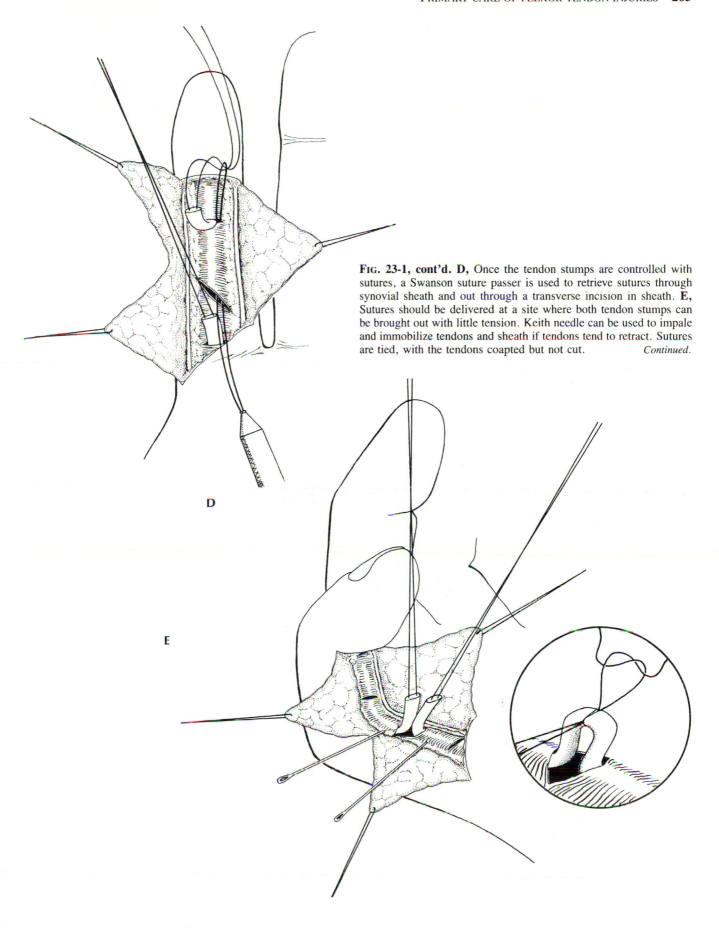

FIG. 23-1, cont'd. D, Once the tendon stumps are controlled with sutures, a Swanson suture passer is used to retrieve sutures through synovial sheath and out through a transverse incision in sheath. **E,** Sutures should be delivered at a site where both tendon stumps can be brought out with little tension. Keith needle can be used to impale and immobilize tendons and sheath if tendons tend to retract. Sutures are tied, with the tendons coapted but not cut. *Continued.*

D

E

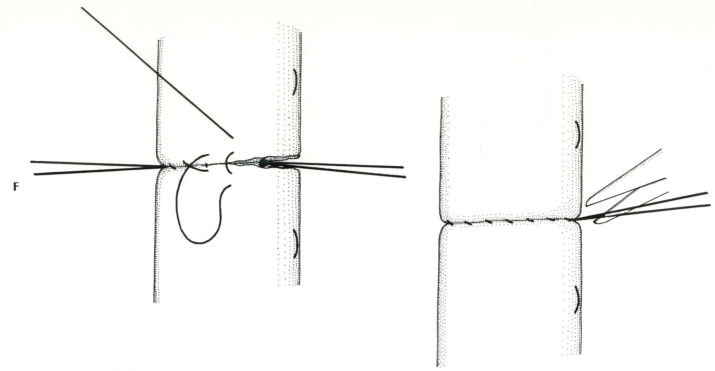

F

FIG.23-1, cont'd. **F,** Long suture ends are used to control tendons while a running circumferential finishing suture of 6-0 Dacron is used to smooth the edges of tendon juncture. **G,** All sutures are cut, and tendon is allowed to retract into synovial sheath. Suture of 6-0 absorbable material is used to repair all defects in synovial sheath so that it is watertight.

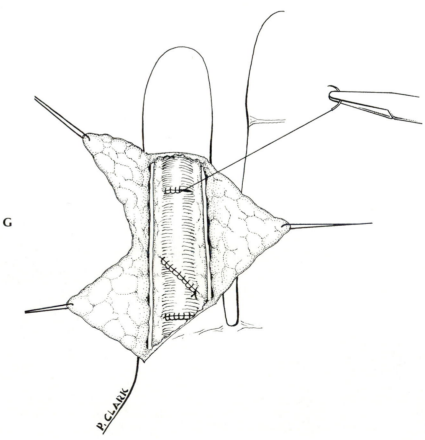

G

P. CLARK

with the tendons coapted but not cut (Fig. 23-1, *E*). The long suture ends are used to control the tendons while a running circumferential finishing suture of 6-0 Dacron is used to smooth the edges of the tendon juncture (Fig. 23-1, *F*). All sutures are cut, and the tendon is allowed to retract into the synovial sheath. A suture of 6-0 absorbable material is used to repair all defects in the synovial sheath so that it is watertight (Fig. 23-1, *G*). This serves two purposes: the synovial fluid provides nutrition for the healing tendon, and the repaired sheath does not present any irregular edges for the swollen juncture site to catch upon and lead to possible rupture. The finger should be put through a gentle passive range of motion to ensure smooth gliding before skin closure. A 2-0 monofilament nylon suture is placed in the fingernail for fixation of the rubber-band traction.

The postoperative dressing is of extreme importance. It should be composed of a volar slab of plaster to the distal palmar flexion crease and a dorsal slab that extends 3 cm beyond the fingertips. Padding should be kept at a minimum, approximately six or seven layers of cotton bandage. The wrist should be flexed at 45 degrees, and the metacarpophalangeal joints at 45 degrees. It is extremely important that the splint allows full extension of the proximal and distal interphalangeal joints.

Postoperative hand therapy

One to 4½ weeks after surgery. The patient is seen by the hand therapist the first postoperative day. The surgeon during a brief session with the therapist explains in detail the surgical procedure. A thorough knowledge of the structures repaired is vital before initiation of early mobilization, that is, flexor tendons repaired, sheath repaired, nerves repaired, and pulleys repaired, as well as the zone of injury. Rubber-band traction is indicated in repairs in all zones, with some variations in the standard dynamic traction or timing depending on the surgical procedure.

The patient's hand is maintained in the dorsal splint applied at surgery. Compressive dressings that might restrict motion are removed from the fingers, so that passive flexion to the palm is possible within the confines of the splint. If dressings are removed, the splint may not fit as securely and the hand may slide proximally in the splint thereby altering the wrist and finger position. In that case, adhesive tape should be applied across the forearm, wrist, and palm to ensure a snug fit with the wrist and digits in proper position.

An elastic band is placed 3 to 4 inches proximally to the wrist crease on the volar aspect of the forearm dressing with the finger in its normal alignment. The tension should be adjusted so that the elastic band pulls the finger into flexion (Fig. 23-2, *A*) when the finger is resting with only slight tension on the band and yet the band permits the antagonist muscles to completely extend the finger (Fig. 23-2, *B*) within the limits of the dorsal splint. This full extension is vital. Failure to completely extend the interphalangeal joints can result in flexion contractures.

One advantage of elastic band traction is that it facilitates tendon and joint movement without requiring active pull on the flexor tendon. Another advantage is protection against sudden injury. Should the patient slip or fall, the elastic band will protect the juncture from stress of active flexion.

Although the suture is put in the free border of the fingernail at surgery, we prefer to wait until the first day when the patient comes to therapy, to apply the elastic band so that the quality, positioning, and tension of the elastic band can be accurately established. As earlier stated, the tension of the elastic band requires careful attention. It must hold the finger in the appropriate flexion at rest and allow the patient to extend his finger to the full limit of the dorsal splint. This full extension is vital. A failure to extend the proximal and distal interphalangeal joints completely by the fifth postoperative day may result in flexion contractures. Elastic thread* best suits our needs. Initially a single strand may be used, and as the patient's active extension becomes

---

*Elastic thread, no. 7034 AliMed, 68 Harrison Avenue, Boston, MA 02111.

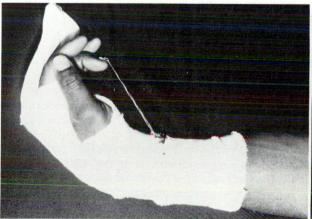
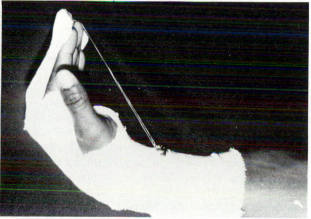

A   B

FIG. 23-2. A, Elastic band traction. Adhesive tape applied across forearm, wrist, and palm to ensure a snug fit. Elastic band pulls the fingers into flexion at rest with slight tension on the band. **B,** Antagonist muscles completely extend interphalangeal joints within limit of dorsal splint.

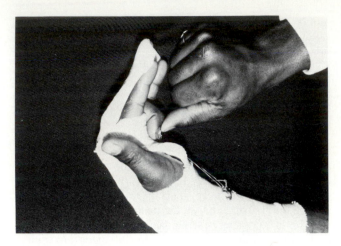

FIG. 23-3. Gentle passive flexion of distal interphalangeal joint.

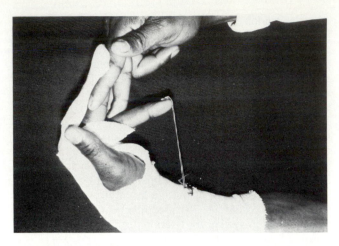

FIG. 23-4. Full extension can be facilitated by passive flexion of metacarpophalangeal joint and then active extention of interphalangeal joint.

stronger, the strands may be doubled, thereby increasing the tension. The patient is checked by the hand therapist twice a week to ensure proper tension of the elastic traction. Readjustment of the elastic traction is frequently required because the bands lost their tension.

Positioned in the splint and with light tension on the elastic band, the patient may actively extend the finger and permit the elastic band to flex the finger passively 10 times each hour. This exercise begins on the first day and continues until the elastic-band traction is removed. In addition, four times a day gentle passive flexion of the proximal and distal joints is carried out 10 times.

The distal interphalangeal joint must be gently passively flexed to the distal palmar crease (Fig. 23-3). Because of the position of the elastic band on the volar forearm, the proximal interphalangeal joint is pulled into full flexion, but not the distal interphalangeal joint. To obtain more joint motion at the distal interphalangeal joint, the therapist can apply downward pressure to the elastic band on the patient's finger to pull the distal interphalangeal joint into full flexion. Then, as the patient extends the finger, he obtains more motion of the interphalangeal joints and the underlying tissues.

Particular attention must be paid to initial signs of a flexion contracture. If the patient is unable to achieve full extension of the interphalangeal joints within the splint, full extension can be facilitated by having him first passively flex the metacarpophalangeal joint of the involved finger and then actively extend the interphalangeal joints (Fig. 23-4). The passive metacarpophalangeal flexion will facilitate full interphalangeal joint extension.

When the therapist is alerted to interphalangeal joint contractures developing, passive extension of the interphalangeal joints may be begun as early as the first week. No "tendon-tension" passive extension may be initiated. Tension is taken off the tendon when the adjacent joint is flexed. With the dorsal splint supporting the wrist and metacarpophalangeal joints in flexion, the therapist may support the metacarpophalangeal joint in flexion and gently passively extend the proximal interphalangeal joint to improve exten-

sion. If the distal interphalangeal joint shows a beginning contracture, the therapist may support the metacarpophalangeal and proximal interphalangeal joints in flexion and gently passively extend the distal interphalangeal joint. Passive extension done by this technique decreases the tension at the tendon juncture. These passive extension exercises should be included in the patient's home program.

Persistent flexion contractures may require a proximal joint wedge or a proximal or distal interphalangeal extension splint (see Fig. 28-11). These devices should be worn intermittently during the daytime. The exact schedule will depend on the "feel" of the contractures, that is, whether it will quickly or slowly respond to stretching. With this technique of passively stretching we have found our problems with flexion contractures to be minimal, and overall tendon function is enhanced.

Four and a half weeks after surgery. The surgeon may elect to remove the dorsal splint at 4½ weeks postoperatively. The patient's hand is then maintained in a wristlet with elastic-band traction. The purpose of the wristlet is to permit full active extension of the interphalangeal and metacarpophalangeal joints with the wrist in neutral (Fig. 23-5, *A*). At rest, the elastic band pulls the fingers into flexion (Fig. 23-5, *B*). Wrist dorsiflexion is permitted with the fingers resting in flexion.

Six weeks after surgery. At 6 weeks the wristlet is removed, and the patient may begin active flexion, including differential tendon-gliding exercises. The patient rests the dorsum of his hand on a flat surface and performs the following exercise sequence: flexion and extension of the interphalangeal joints while the metacarpophalangeal joints are maintained in full extension; flexion and extension of the interphalangeal joints with the metacarpophalangeal joints in full extension, followed by full metacarpophalangeal flexion to make a full fist; and finally after fist making, full extension of the fingers followed by flexion of the proximal interphalangeal joints and the metacarpophalangeal joints for superfiscialis function. Ten repetitions of this exercise may be performed each hour (Fig. 23-6).

Eight to 10 weeks after surgery. Mild resistive exercise

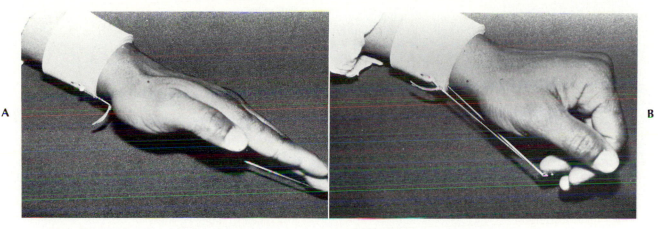

FIG. 23-5. Four and a half weeks postoperatively, dorsal splint is removed and patient's hand is maintained in a wristlet with elastic-band traction. **A,** Wristlet permits extension of interphalangeal and metacarpophalangeal joints, with wrist in neutral. **B,** Wrist dorsiflexion is permitted with the fingers resting in flexion.

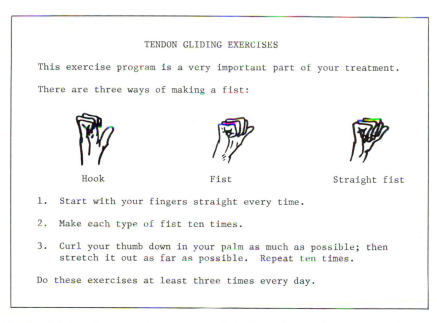

```
                    TENDON GLIDING EXERCISES

    This exercise program is a very important part of your treatment.

    There are three ways of making a fist:


         Hook            Fist            Straight fist

    1.  Start with your fingers straight every time.

    2.  Make each type of fist ten times.

    3.  Curl your thumb down in your palm as much as possible; then
        stretch it out as far as possible.  Repeat ten times.

    Do these exercises at least three times every day.
```

FIG. 23-6 A direction sheet showing the tendon-gliding exercise is given to the patient.

may be initiated at 8 weeks postoperatively beginning with newspaper crumbling and increasing to putty (Fig. 23-7) and light sustained grip activities (sanding, filing) by the tenth week.

Twelve weeks after surgery. Heavy resistive exercise and return to heavy labor activities are usually permitted at 3 months in most cases.

Summary. One must remember that the juncture is more vulnerable to rupture in the tendon that is moved early than in the tendon repair that is immobilized for 3 weeks with its firmer wound adhesions. Therapists who work with tendon repair must have a feeling for tendons and their patient. The athlete or laborer who has excellent flexion at 6 weeks is likely to be just the person who if removed from all protective splinting will go home and do push-ups or move furniture and rupture the repair. The patient must be told when he is removed from the cast at 4½ weeks and the

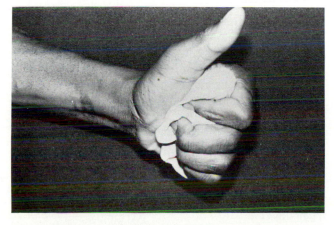

FIG. 23-7. Eight to 10 weeks postoperatively, mild resistive exercise is initiated.

wristlet at 6 weeks that if he picks up something heavy he will rupture the repair. The patients who glide and slide and demonstrate early smooth pain-free motion should be protected 1 to 2 weeks longer, since the development of adhesions is apparently limited and intratendinous healing may require additional time for consolidation. There could be a later rupture in this type of patient. In such a patient, a profundus repair may rupture after mild trauma 8 to 10 weeks after repair.

If the tendon is moved in a controlled fashion, that is, with elastic-band traction, during healing, we end up with greater mobility of the tendon repair ultimately; however, these patients must be supervised closely. It is vital to remember that if we move tendons early we have to control and protect them longer.

Alternative treatment regimens

If the injury and conditions contraindicate a primary or delayed primary repair, alternative treatment plans may be necessary. If the retinacular pulley system is intact, a free tendon graft is indicated. If these are associated injuries such as fractures or the retinacular pulley system requires significant reconstruction, a passive tendon implant may be indicated.

Another alternative that may be indicated in some patients is tenodesis, capsulodesis, or arthrodesis of the distal interphalangeal joint, and all operative and rehabilitative efforts are directed toward a regaining of function of the flexor digitorum superficialis tendon and the proximal interphalangeal joint.

ZONE 3
Definition

Zone 3 refers to the portion of the flexor digitorum profundus and superficialis tendons between the distal edge of the carpal ligament and the proxinal edge of the A_1 pulley. Repairs in this zone yield very good results because the tendon nutrition is good and the bed is forgiving when adhesions with the surrounding tissues result. Repairs that fall in the proximal portion of zone 2 can be converted to zone 3 repairs by release of a portion of the A_1 pulley. This is worthwhile because of the significantly better results obtained from zone 3 injuries.

Operative treatment

The incision should incorporate the original laceration if possible, but, more important, the incision should be planned so that it can be extended proximally and distally with ease. The tendons are easily retrieved because the origin of the lumbrical muscle on the flexor digitorum profundus tethers this tendon. Retrieval of this tendon often delivers its accompanying flexor digitorum superficialis tendon. The modified Kessler suture is employed, and both tendons are repaired.

Postoperative management

The postoperative hand rehabilitation is similar to that of repairs in zone 2.

ZONE 4
Definition

Zone 4 refers to that portion of the flexor digitorum profundus and superficialis tendons beneath the carpal ligament. Tendon lacerations in this area are uncommon secondary to wounds in the carpal ligament region, but lacerations at the wrist with the fingers flexed can cause retraction of the distal stumps when fingers are extended.

Operative treatment

Release of the carpal ligament is usually required to expose the lacerated tendons, and it will prevent postoperative median-nerve compression resulting from swelling and hematoma. It is not necessary to repair the ligament; at most a loose repair of the overlying palmar aponeurosis is all that is required on wound closure. The repaired skin and palmar fascia are all that is required to contain the tendons in the carpal canal. Modified Kessler sutures are used to repair all tendons that are lacerated.

Postoperative management

The postoperative dressings and hand therapy are the same as those discussed for zone 2.

ZONE 5
Definition

Zone 5 refers to the volar forearm proximal to the proximal carpal ligament. Here tendons, musculotendinous junctions, and muscles may be involved. The results from repairs in this area are uniformly excellent.

Operative treatment

A curvilinear incision incorporating the original wound is preferred. A meticulous dissection is necessary for identification of all lacerated structures. All injured structures including wrist flexors, finger flexors, arteries, and nerves should be repaired. A modified Kessler suture is indicated for all tendons.

Postoperative management

The postoperative dressings and hand therapy for zone 5 repairs are the same as those for zone 2.

FLEXOR POLLICIS LONGUS
Definition

The flexor pollicis longus tendon can be divided into five zones for treatment purposes. Zone 1 is distal to the interphalangeal joint. Zone 2 is distal to the metacarpophalangeal joint. Zone 3 is from the distal edge of the carpal ligament to the proximal edge of the A_1 pulley. Zone 4 is beneath the carpal ligament, and zone 5 is proximal to the carpal ligament. The treatment considerations for lacerations of this tendon correspond to those for lacerations in the fingers at the same zones.

Operative treatment

A Brunner zigzag incision incorporating the original wound is preferred. The ability to extend the incision proximally is very important because this tendon will often retract all the way into the forearm even if the laceration occurs in zone 1 or 2. If this is the case, the proximal stump can be identified in the forearm and tagged with one half of a modified Kessler suture. A Brand tendon passer can then be used to deliver the tendon into the thumb, without exposure of the carpal canal and thenar muscles. Otherwise the operative technique is the same as in finger tendon lacerations.

Postoperative management

The postoperative management and dressings are the same as in finger tendon lacerations except for the positioning of the rubber-band traction. The origin of the rubber band should be 10 cm proximal to the wrist and over the ulna.

CONCLUSION

Flexor tendon lacerations are major injuries. A good result requires that the surgeon and the hand therapist have a thorough understanding of flexor tendon physiology and biomechanics. In addition, it requires a commitment on the part of the surgeon, the hand therapist and the patient to understand the gravity of the injury and to work together to regain the hand function.

REFERENCES

1. Becker, H., Orak, F., and Duponselle, E.: Early active motion following a beveled technique of flexor tendon repair: report on fifty cases, J. Hand Surg. **4**:454-460, 1979.
2. Bergljung, L.: Vascular reactions after tendon suture and tendon transplantation: a stereo-microangiographic study on the calcaneal tendon of the rabbit, Scand. J. Plast. Reconstr. Surg. **4**(suppl.):7, 1968.
3. Bergljung, L.: Vascular reactions in tendon healing, Angiology **21**:375, 1970.
4. Bohler, J.: Cited in Carroll, R.E., and Match, R.M.: Avulsion of the flexor profundus tendon insertion, J. Trauma **10**:1109, 1970.
5. Bowers, W.H., and Hurst, L.C.: Chronic mallet finger: the use of Fowler's central slip release, J. Hand Surg. **3**(4):373-376, 1978.
6. Boyes, J.H.: Flexor tendon grafts in the fingers and thumb: an evaluation of end results, J. Bone Joint Surg. **32A**:489, 1950.
7. Boyes, J.H.: Selection of a donor muscle for tendon transfers, Bull. Hosp. Joint Dis. **23**:1, 1962.
8. Boyes, J.H.: Discussion. In Cramer, L.M., and Chase, R.A., editors: Symposium on the hand, vol. 3, St. Louis, 1971, The C.V. Mosby Co.
9. Boyes, J.H., and Stark, H.H.: Flexor tendon grafts in the fingers and thumb, J. Bone Joint Surg. **53A**:1332, 1971.
10. Bruner, J.M.: The zig-zag volar-digital incision for flexor tendon surgery, Plast. Reconstr. Surg. **40**:471, 1967.
11. Bruner, J.M.: Surgical exposure of flexor tendons in the hand, Ann. R. Coll. Surg. Engl. **53**:84, 1973.
12. Bunnell, S.: Repair of tendons in the fingers, Surg. Gynecol. Obstet. **35**:88, 1922.
13. Bunnell, S.: Tendon transfers in the hand and forearm. In American Academy of Orthopaedic Surgeons: Instructional course lectures, vol. 6, Ann Arbor, Mich., 1949, J.W. Edwards.
14. Bunnell, S.: Surgery of the hand, ed. 4, Philadelphia, 1964 J.B. Lippincott Co.
15. Dolphin, J.A.: Extensor tenotomy for chronic boutonnière deformity of the finger: report of two cases, J. Bone Joint Surg. **47A**:161, 1965.
16. Eiken, O., Lundborg, G., and Rank, F.: The role of the digital synovial sheath in tendon grafting, Scand. J. Plast. Reconstr. Surg. **9**:182, 1975.
17. Eiken, O., and Rank, F.: Experimental restoration of the digital synovial sheath, Scand. J. Plast. Reconstr. Surg. **11**:213, 1977.
18. Flynn, J.E., and Graham, J.H.: Healing following tendon suture and tendon suture and tendon transplants, Surg. Gynecol. Obstet. **115**:467, 1962.
19. Flynn, J.E., and Graham, J.H.: Healing of tendon wounds, Am. J. Surg. **109**:315, 1965.
20. Green, D.P., and Rowland, S.A.: Fractures and dislocations in the hand. In Rockwood, C.A., and Green, D.P., editors: Philadelphia, 1975, J.B. Lippincott Co.
21. Kessler, F.B.: Use of a pedicled tendon transfer with a silicone rod in complicated secondary flexor tendon repairs, Plast. Reconstr. Surg. **49**:439, 1972.
22. Kessler, I.: The grasping technique for tendon repair, Hand **5**:253, 1973.
23. Kessler, I., and Missim, F.: Primary repair without immobilization of flexor tendon division within the flexor tendon sheath: an experimental and clinical study, Acta Orthop. Scand. **40**:587, 1969.
24. Ketchum, L.D.: The effects of triamcinolone on tendon healing and function, Plast. Reconstr. Surg. **47**:471, 1971.
25. Ketchum, L.D.: Primary tendon healing: a review, J. Hand Surg. **2**:428, 1977.
26. Kleinert, H.E., and Bennett, J.B.: Digital pulley reconstruction employing the always present rim of the previous pulley, J. Hand Surg. **3**:297, 1978.
27. Kleinert, H.E., Kutz, J.E., and Cohen, M.J.: Primary repair of zone 2 flexor tendon lacerations. In American Academy of Orthopaedic Surgeons: Symposium on tendon surgery of the hand, St. Louis, 1975, The C.V. Mosby Co.
28. Kleinert, H.E., Kutz, J.E., Ashbell, T.S., and Martinez, E.: Abstract: Primary repair of lacerated flexor tendons in "no-man's land," J. Bone Joint Surg. **49A**:577, 1967.
29. Kleinert, H.E., Kutz, J.E., Atasoy, E., and Stormo, A.: Primary repair of flexor tendons, Orthop. Clin. North Am. **4**:865, 1973.
30. Lister, G.D., Kleinert, H.E., Kutz, J.E., and Atasoy, E.: Primary flexor tendon repair followed by immediate controlled mobilization, J. Hand Surg. **2**:441, 1977.
31. Lundborg, G.: Experimental flexor tendon healing without adhesion formation—a new concept of tendon nutrition and intrinsic healing mechanisms: a preliminary report, Hand **8**:235, 1976.
32. Lundborg, G., and Myrhage, R. The vascularization and structure of the human digital tendon sheath as related to flexor tendon function, Scand. J. Plast. Reconstr. Surg. **11**:195, 1977.
33. Lundborg, G., Myrhage, R., and Rydevik, B. The vascularization of human flexor tendons within the digital synovial sheath region: structural and functional aspects, J. Hand Surg. **2**:417, 1977.
34. Mason, M.L., and Sheron, C.G.: The process of tendon repair, Arch. Surg. **25**:615, 1932.
35. Matsui, T., Miyaji, N., Merklin, R., and Hunter, J.M.: A study of vascularization of the flexor tendons of the hand, Orthopedics (Japanese) **28**(13):1315-1318, 1977.
36. Mayer, L., The physiological method of tendon transplantation, Surg. Gynecol. Obstet. **22**:298, 1916.
37. Mayer, L., and Ransohoff, N.: Reconstruction of the digital tendon sheath: a contribution to the physiological method of repair of damaged finger tendons, J. Bone Joint Surg. **18**:607, 1936.
38. O'Brien, B.McC., MacLeod, A.N., and Morrison, W.A.: Microvascular frog flap transfer, Orthop. Clin. North Am. **8**:349, 1977.
39. Peacock, E.E.: A study of the circulation in normal tendons and healing grafts, Ann. Surg. **149**:415, 1959.
40. Peacock, E.E.: Biological principles in the healing of long tendons, Surg. Clin. North. Am. **45**:461, 1965.
41. Potenza, A.D.: Tendon healing within the flexor digital sheath in the dog, J. Bone Joint Surg. **44A**:49, 1962.
42. Potenza, A.D.: Critical evaluation of flexor tendon healing and adhesion formation within artificial digital sheath, J. Bone Joint Surg. **45A**:1217, 1963.
43. Potenza, A.D.: The healing of autogenous tendon grafts within the flexor digital sheath in dogs, J. Bone Joint Surg. **46A**:1462, 1964.
44. Pulvertaft, R.C.: Tendon grafts for flexor tendon injuries in the fingers and thumb: a study of technique and results, J. Bone Joint Surg. **38B**:175, 1956.
45. Reynolds, B., Wray, R., and Weeks, P.M.: Should an incompletely severed tendon be sutured? Plast. Reconstr. Surg. **57**(1):36, 1976.

46. Robins, P.R., and Dobyns, J.H.: Avulsion of the insertion of the flexor digitorum profundus tendon associated with fracture of the distal phalanx: a brief review, In American Academy of Orthopaedic Surgeons: Symposium on tendon surgery in the hand, St. Louis, 1975, The C.V. Mosby Co.

47. Rowland, S.A.: Palmar finger tip use of silicone rubber followed by free tendon grafting. In American Academy of Orthopaedic Surgeons: Symposium on tendon surgery in the hand, St. Louis, 1975, The C.V. Mosby Co.

48. Stark, H.H., Boyes, J.H., and Wilson, J.N.: Mallet finger, J. Bone Joint Surg. **44A:**1061-1068, 1962.

49. Tubiana, R.: The hand, vol. 1, Philadelphia, 1980, W.B. Saunders Co.

50. Urbaniak, J.R., Cahill, J.D., and Mortenson, R.A.: Tendon suturing methods: analysis of tensile strengths. In American Academy of Orthopaedic Surgeons: Symposium on tendon surgery in the hand, St. Louis, 1975, The C.V. Mosby Co.

51. Urbaniak, J.R., Bright, D.S., Gill, L.H., and Goldner, J.L.: Vascularization and gliding mechanism of free flexor tendon grafts inserted by the silicone rod method, J. Bone Joint Surg. **56A:**473, 1974.

52. Verdan, C.: Primary repair of flexor tendons, J. Bone Joint Surg. **42A:**647, 1960.

53. Verdan, C.: Half a century of flexor tendon surgery, J. Bone Joint Surg. **54A:**472, 1972.

54. Verdan, C., and Crawford, G.: Flexor tendon suture in the digital canal, Proceedings of the fifth International Congress of Plastic Surgeons, Melbourne, Feb. 22-25, 1971.

24

Management of flexor tendon lacerations in zone 2 using controlled passive motion postoperatively

ROBERT J. DURAN, ROBERT G. HOUSER, CARL R. COLEMAN, and MARY G. STOVER

Our purpose in this chapter is to present the technique of repair and the postoperative management and rehabilitation of flexor tendon injuries in zone 2.

As previously reported, Duran and Houser[1] have found that 3 to 5 mm of extension motion of the tendon anastomosis in a passive exercise program is sufficient to prevent firm adherence of a repaired flexor tendon in zone 2 of the hand. We have chosen the term "controlled passive motion" to best describe the postoperative exercise program. The experimental work of Gelberman and co-workers[2] and the clinical studies of Strickland and Glogovac[3] have been supportive of this method of management of flexor tendon lacerations in zone 2.

SURGICAL TECHNIQUE

It is important to repair the flexor digitorum superficialis and the flexor digitorum profundus as well. If the joint capsule, nerves, and arteries are severed, they are also repaired. The flexor tendons are retrieved as gently as possible. We prefer to control the tendons with traction sutures at the periphery of their cut ends.

Tenorrhaphy is achieved by a modified Bunnell or a Kessler-Mason-Allen suture of 5-0 nonabsorbable synthetic material. This is supported by peripheral 6-0 mattress sutures. Because the flexor digitorum superficialis becomes thin near its insertion, mattress sutures alone are used.

Considerable attention is given to the flexor tendon sheath. It may be necessary to release the sheath laterally for a few millimeters to permit the tendon anastomosis to move distally for 5 mm; otherwise the anastomosis may not clear the damaged area and could actually impinge on the annulus distally, increasing the risk of tendon separation. Closing the sheath is desirable if it does not interfere with the extension motion of 3 to 5 mm.

After repairs are completed, the wrist is placed in 20 degrees of flexion. The metacarpophalangeal joint of the finger is maintained in its normal balanced position throughout the controlled passive motion program. Only the distal interphalangeal and proximal interphalangeal joints are moved during the postoperative passive motion exercises.

In surgery under direct vision, the distal phalanx is moved enough in extension so that one can see the anastomosis of the flexor digitorum profundus glide distally 3 to 5 mm (Fig. 24-1, *A* and *B*). Motion is at the distal interphalangeal joint only during this exercise. To be certain of moving the anastomosis, the movement of the digit *must* be a motion of *extension*. This motion of extension has assured us that the anastomosis of the flexor digitorum profundus has been moved, not only away from fixed structures that may have been damaged in the area (sheath, capsule), but also away from the repair of the flexor digitorum superficialis.

Continuing under direct vision in surgery, one grasps and extends the middle phalanx until both anastomoses glide distally 3 to 5 mm (Fig. 24-1, *C* and *D*). Motion is at the proximal interphalangeal joint only during this exercise. This motion is essential for the flexor digitorum superficialis anastomosis. Both anastomoses have moved distally away from fixed, damaged structures. Actually measuring the range of the distal interphalangeal joint and proximal interphalangeal joint may be helpful as a guide later in the passive motion exercises (Fig. 24-2). We suggest using these measurements particularly when the surgeon does not have experience with this technique. This allows precision in the number of degrees required at distal interphalangeal and proximal interphalangeal joints to give 3 to 5 mm of motion of the anastomosis.

A dorsal splint extending distally to the level of the proximal interphalangeal joints is used for wrist immobilization, with the wrist maintained in a flexed position at 20 degrees (Fig. 24-3). A removable inclined sponge wedge beneath the hand may be helpful in managing the index finger, since the flexed wrist places it in considerable extension at the distal interphalangeal joint, creating difficulty with the extension exercises in some cases (Fig. 24-4). During exercises, the wedge can be removed and the wrist allowed to be a neutral position. The wedge is replaced after passive exercises are completed. This has not been a problem in the long, ring, and little fingers, and the wrist may remain in 20 degrees of flexion during the exercises.

At the end of the procedure, a hole is placed in the free border of the fingernail and a nylon suture is placed through it, tied and connected to a rubber band. The rubber band is secured with a safety pin to the volar aspect of the forearm dressing under light tension. Alternatively, a corset hook may be glued to the nail and elastic traction applied. The

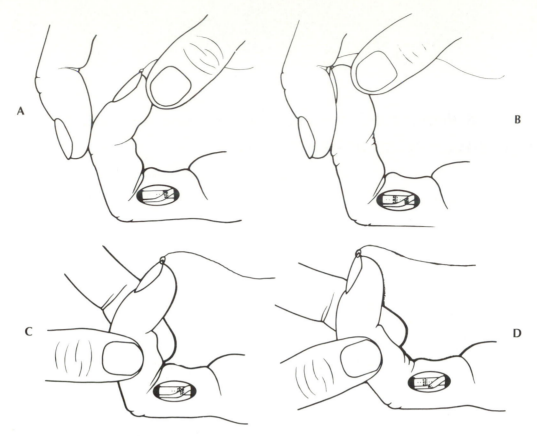

Fig. 24-1. A, Diagram of controlled passive motion exercise. Metacarpophalangeal joint should remain in normal balanced position. Extension of distal interphalangeal joint sufficient to move anastomosis 3 to 5 mm. Only distal interphalangeal joint moves during this exercise. **B,** Note distal migration of anastomosis of flexor digitorum profundus tendon away from that of flexor digitorum superficialis tendon. **C,** When middle phalanx is extended, both anastomoses glide distally. Only the proximal interphalangeal joint moves during this exercise. **D,** Anastomoses are thus moved away from fixed structures that may have been injured. Elastic traction returns finger to original position.

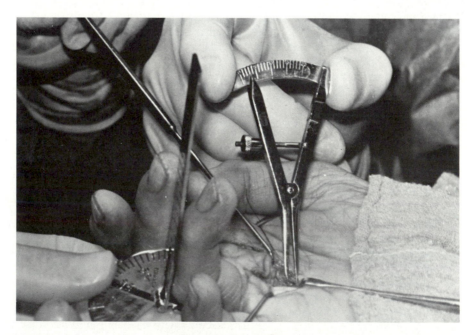

Fig. 24-2. Evaluation of degrees of extension of proximal interphalangeal and distal interphalangeal joints is necessary to have 3 to 5 mm of extension motion of anastomoses. A helpful aid in precise postoperative passive exercises.

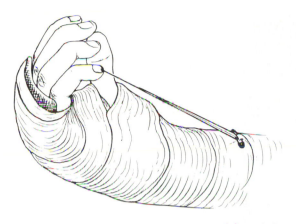

FIG. 24-3. Dorsal splint extending to proximal interphalangeal joints with wrist in approximately 20 degrees flexion. Metacarpophalangeal joints remain in normal balanced position.

elastic traction acts to return the distal interphalangeal and proximal interphalangeal joints to their original position after the passive extension exercises are completed.

POSTOPERATIVE MANAGEMENT

Exercises are started *immediately,* the first having been carried out during direct vision of the anastomosis in surgery, as described previously (Fig. 24-1). Our routine is to carry out the exercises twice daily, once in the morning and once in the evening, with six to eight motions for each tendon per session. Between exercises the fingers are covered securely with a stockinette (Fig. 24-5). This prevents impulsive grasping. Uninvolved fingers are actively or passively exercised at each session and more often if necessary. Training of the patient or parents is essential for success of the procedure. Instruction is begun immediately, with the patient observing during the first session and then carrying

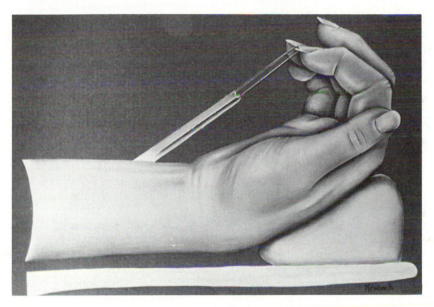

FIG. 24-4. Removable inclined sponge wedge to be used in tendon lacerations of index finger.

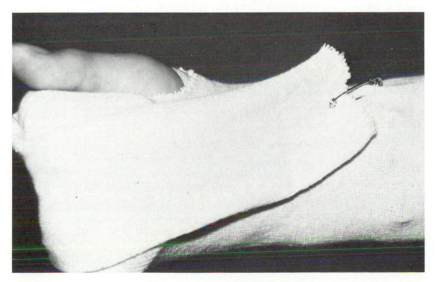

FIG. 24-5. Fingers are covered securely with stockinette between exercises. This provides additional protection to fingers. In this case flexor tendons in three fingers are involved.

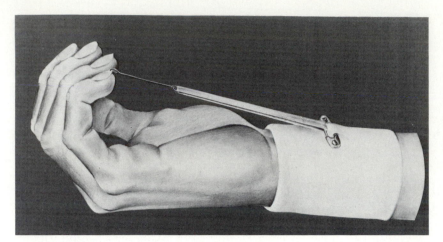

FIG. 24-6. Dorsal splint removed and wrist band applied at 4½ weeks with nail suture and rubber band traction. Passive motion exercises continued an additional week along with gentle active extension exercises.

out the exercises when both surgeon and patient are confident.

Controlled passive motion alone is continued for 4½ weeks. The dorsal splint is then removed and the rubber band traction is attached to a wrist band (Fig. 24-6). Passive motion exercises are continued along with gentle active extension exercises. One week later the wrist band and nail suture are removed.

Active flexion is now started for the first time since the tendon repair. The flexor digitorum profundus tendon is exercised actively by stabilizing the middle phalanx and gently, actively flexing and extending the distal phalanx 10 to 12 times. The flexor digitorum superficialis is then exercised by holding the uninvolved fingers in extension and actively flexing and extending the proximal interphalangeal joint 10 to 12 times. After this, all fingers are flexed and extended approximately 10 to 12 times as in normal grasping and extension. Gentle passive stretching for joint mobilization is initiated. Each joint is gently, passively flexed. To increase proximal interphalangeal and distal interphalangeal joint range of motion in extension, the metacarpophalangeal joint is fully flexed, and then the proximal interphalangeal joint or distal interphalangeal joint is gently extended. Metacarpophalangeal joint flexion during this exercise is necessary to prevent undue tension on the repaired flexor tendons. These exercises are repeated each hour. Active extension is gradually increased. The finger is protected from resistive flexion during the next 2 weeks, that is, until 7½ weeks have elapsed form the time of tendon repair.

Occasionally, it is necessary to use a dynamic splint to correct a proximal interphalangeal joint contracture whether it is related to primary joint injury or secondary contracture. If splinting is necessary, it is used 6 weeks after tendon repair. For the next 2 weeks it is used gently, and then the tension is gradually increased as needed.

Approximately 7½ to 8 weeks after tendon repair, gentle resistive flexion exercises are introduced, first using a rubber sponge and then advancing to a soft-grade therapy putty. Light grasping is allowed, but excessive force to the injured finger is avoided for 2 to 4 weeks. Active flexor digitorum profundus and flexor digitorum superficialis exercises and joint mobilization are continued. Generally most of the gain in flexion and extension has been achieved by 3 months after surgery.

COMPLICATIONS

Early in our clinical experience with the controlled passive motion program, we experienced tendon ruptures in two cases. In one patient an excellent result was present at 6 weeks postoperatively; however, at that time because the patient lifted many bales of hay, a rupture of the flexor digitorum profundus tendon resulted. In the second case the flexor digitorum profundus and flexor digitorum superficialis tendons ruptured in an uncooperative child who was not a candidate for this procedure at that time.

As a result of our experience, we believe there are six prerequisites that must be followed to prevent tendon rupture if this technique is to be used:

1. Controlled passive motion
2. If necessary, released tendon sheath to allow unrestricted extension
3. Protective stockinette to prevent impulsive active flexion
4. *No* active flexion for 5½ weeks
5. Protected anastomosis for 2 additional weeks
6. Cooperative patient

It is our opinion that tendon ruptures should not occur if the details of the surgical procedure and postoperative program are carefully followed. Distal zone 2 injuries frequently involved the proximal interphalangeal joint, and some loss of extension was not unusual.

CONCLUSION

A method of controlled passive motion after primary flexor tendon repair in zone 2 has been presented. The tendon ruptures that occurred early have been studied, and by our present techniques and safeguards they should be preventable.

REFERENCES

1. Duran, R.J., and Houser, R.G.: Controlled passive motion following flexor tendon repair in zones 2 and 3, In American Academy of Orthopaedic Surgeons: Symposium on tendon surgery in the hand, St. Louis, 1975, The C.V. Mosby Co.
2. Gelberman, R.H., Woo, S.L.-Y., Lothringer, K., Akeson, W.H., and Amiel, D.: Effects of early intermittent passive mobilization on healing canine flexor tendons, J. Hand Surg. **7:**170-175, 1982.
3. Strickland, J.W., and Glogovac, S.V.: Digital function following flexor tendon repair in zone 2: a comparison of immobilization and controlled passive motion techniques, J. Hand Surg. **5:**537-543, 1980.

25

Indications for tendon grafting

R. GUY PULVERTAFT

A tendon divided by injury, destroyed by disease or infection, or absent through congenital fault may under favorable circumstances be replaced successfully by a tendon taken from elsewhere in the body. A tendon transferred to serve a different purpose may be lengthened by a tendon graft to reach a new attachment.

The use of tendon grafts stems from the teaching of Bunnell, whose first publications on this subject appeared in 1918[3] and 1922.[4] The earliest mention of the successful use of a free tendon graft was by Robson in 1889,[18] who restored an extensor tendon by using a flexor tendon taken from a severely injured finger of the same hand.

Over the years many investigations have been made into the nature of tendon healing. We now know that when the ends of a divided tendon are held in apposition, healing takes place by cells arising from the tendon itself[9-11] as well as by the proliferation of cells from the surrounding synovium or paratenon.[14] The same process occurs at the junction of tendon and graft. It has been demonstrated that two sections of tendon, isolated within the synovial cavity of a joint and devoid of blood supply, will heal by cells from their epitenon and are nourished by the synovial fluid of the joint.[9,10] Surgical technique needs to be gentle and precise in order to limit the cellular ingrowth from the surrounding tissue, which is attracted to the tendon-graft junction and to any damaged areas on the graft surface. It is these links that are the precursors of adhesions.

Successful results from tendon grafting depend on (1) a mobile digit with minimal scarring and at least one digital nerve intact, (2) a meticulous surgical technique, (3) a cooperative patient, and (4) carefully graduated mobilization. If the digital unit is not in satisfactory overall condition, consideration should be given to a two-stage procedure.[7] At the first operation scars are excised, contractures are corrected, the damaged tendons are removed and new pulleys constructed if necessary, and injured nerves are repaired. A flexible silicone rubber rod is placed in the tendon bed; it is attached securely to the distal phalanx, while its proximal end is left free to glide in the tissue planes above the wrist. The digit is exercised by passive motion, causing the development of a sheathlike tunnel into which a tendon graft is inserted to replace the rod a few months later (see Chapter 26).

The most common cause of failure is adhesion between tendon or graft and the surrounding tissues. In an effort to overcome this problem specialized forms of grafting have been used, including pedicle grafts[12] and homografts of the complete flexor system.[6,13] Permanent artificial "tendons" have also been used.[7,19] The generally accepted practice today is secondary autogenous grafting according to established techniques, with recourse to two-stage grafting when necessary.

There is rarely any lack of autogenous tendons for use as grafts, the most suitable being plantaris, palmaris longus, and extensor digitorum longus. The choice depends on their availability and the nature of the case. The plantaris is the longest tendon and makes an excellent graft. It is my first choice. Its slimness is an advantage, particularly when one is restoring profundus in the presence of a normal superficialis. Palmaris will reach from the distal phalanx to the proximal palm but, except for the thumb, will not reach above the wrist, and this can sometimes be a disadvantage. Plantaris and palmaris, which are occasionally absent, are removed by use of a distal and proximal exposure; the tendon is freed through the distal wound and drawn out through the proximal wound, so that the use of a tendon stripper is avoided. In this manner the tendons are removed with the minimum of paratenon. The toe extensor tendons cannot be slipped out in the same fashion, owing to linkage with the adjacent tendons, which necessitates open dissection. The flexor digitorum superficialis is a convenient tendon, when it is divided, to bridge a gap in the profundus tendon divided in the central and proximal palm and at the wrist.

It has become accepted practice to encourage controlled movements within a day or two of performing a direct suture of flexor tendons injured within the digital theca. My own experience leads me to believe that after grafting operations it is wiser to keep the hand at rest for 3 weeks before allowing movement.[15]

The graft enlarges with the stimulus of work and becomes capable of withstanding normal strains. I have not seen a rupture or detachment later than 10 weeks after operation. There is ample evidence that a graft performed in childhood increases in length with the growth of the hand.

INJURY
Flexor profundus division

Division of the flexor profundus tendon beyond the insertion of the flexor superficialis is normally treated by immediate suture when wound conditions permit. If the profundus is cut more proximally but the superficialis is intact (a not uncommon injury), it has been my practice to ignore the tendon injury with the intention of elective treatment later because the results of suture were not dependable. However, improved techniques now offer a good prospect of success by direct suture in this difficult zone. If the profundus injury was overlooked or deliberately ignored, the choice of later treatment depends on several factors. Secondary suture may be possible in the distal part of the finger, but if this cannot be done because of retraction and for the proximal divisions, the ideal treatment is the replacement of profundus by a graft, with the superficialis being left intact.[16] This operation is one of some magnitude for a comparatively small defect, and it should be advised only when the patient is determined to seek perfection or when the patient is a child with an unknown future occupation. The possibility of increasing the disability by failed surgery exists, and the surgeon should therefore be experienced in tendon grafting. The choice, which should be fully discussed with the patient, lies between tendon grafting, arthrodesis or tenodesis of the distal joint, or acceptance of the disability.

Flexor profundus and superficialis division

The arguments in favor of primary, or secondary, suture versus secondary grafting when both tendons are cut in the distal palm or in the finger have strengthened in recent years. The use of magnification and the improvements in technique are leading surgeons to perform direct suture and obtain a high level of success.[8] I believe it is fair comment to say that these results are attributable to the wise selection of cases and superb craftsmanship. There are surgeons called upon to treat these difficult injuries who do not have a wide experience of hand surgery, and there remains a case for skin suture only to be followed by grafting later by a surgeon qualified to do so. Secondary grafting under favorable circumstances has a success rate of 70% to 80%.[1,15] Minimal requirement for ''success'' is defined as flexion to within 2.5 cm or less of the distal palmar crease, with extension restricted by less than a sum total of 40 degrees at the interphalangeal joints.

Flexor pollicis longus division

Division of the flexor pollicis longus tendon distal to the metacarpophalangeal joint is normally treated by suture. Division of the tendon deep to the thenar muscles may also be sutured at the emergency operation, but one should not forget that the tendon lies in close relationship to the digital sensory nerves and the motor nerve to the thenar muscles and that these structures are at risk. In replacement of the flexor pollicis longus by a tendon graft it is important that the graft should reach from the distal phalanx to above the wrist. In my experience it is a reliable operation that rarely fails to give an adequate flexion range.

Division of flexor tendons in palm and wrist

The best results are obtained by primary suture. It may prove impossible to perform a secondary suture, owing to retraction of the proximal part, without causing undue tension. This retraction is most pronounced when the injury has been in or proximal to the carpal tunnel. Under these circumstances, continuity can be restored when the gap in the profundus is bridged by a short graft taken from he superficialis. Apart from divisions in the distal palm, which should be regarded as being within the finger, there is rarely any need to perform complete graft replacement for these injuries.

Extensor tendon divisions

Tendon divisions on the dorsal surface of the hand and wrist under suitable conditions of wounding are well treated by primary suture. Secondary end-to-end suture may be possible, but, in late cases, attachment to an adjacent intact tendon or transfer of a tendon such as the extensor indicis proprius may be indicated. Tendon grafting is more likely to be required after severe wounds where there has been extensive skin damage and subsequent scarring. Since free tendon grafts should not be placed in scar tissue, it is necessary to these cases to replace the scar by a skin flap as a preliminary procedure.

Tendon grafting after long delay

A patient may be seen several years after a tendon injury has been sustained, either because treatment has not been given or because previous surgery has failed. These neglected cases are usually encountered after divisions within the digital theca. Tendon grafting can restore function, provided that there is good passive movement of the digit and there is acceptable sensibility. Surprisingly, in my own series of 42 patients suffering from profundus and superficialis divisions with an average delay of 5 years, the overall results were slightly better than those of the regular series.[17] In all the delay cases one of the muscles of the affected digit was used as a motor. On reflection, it would have been wiser in some of the cases to have transferred a superficialis tendon, prolonged if necessary by a free graft, from an adjacent finger.

A stricter selection for operative suitability in the delay series probably accounts for the better results. The lesson I have learned from this experience is that delay does not worsen the prognosis and it is safe and advisable to wait for some months to permit the tissues to make a full recovery from the initial trauma. One should bear this in mind when treating children under 4 years of age, who are unlikely to cooperate well in the aftercare. No harm will come from delaying the operation for a year or two.

Rheumatoid disease

Tendon rupture in rheumatoid disease occurs as a complication in rheumatoid nodules within the tendon, disease of the synovium and the tendon sheaths, and attrition against sharp edges of eroded bone. Tendon suture is usually impossible because of actual loss of tendon substance and retraction. Linkage to an unaffected adjacent tendon or tendon transfer is usually the best method of repair for extensor tendons. Occasionally it is necessary to extend a transferred tendon by a free graft. Standard methods of grafting are sometimes indicated for flexor tendon restoration, but the prognosis is less favorable than in nonrheumatoid patients.

INFECTION

Sometimes one sees a patient in whom the flexor tendons have become adherent or destroyed within the digital sheath after septic tenosynovitis but the finger has retained good passive mobility. A tendon grafting operation offers a chance of restoring function, and a two-stage procedure should be considered.

A guarded prognosis should be given.

CONGENITAL ABSENCE OF TENDONS

Provided that there is an adequate joint motion and a suitable muscle available, a free tendon graft can be used successfully to provide active movement. Pulleys may need to be set up and use made of the two-stage method.

PARALYSIS

Loss of function caused by irreparable lesions of the spinal cord and peripheral nerves can be restored in many instances by transference of expendable active muscles. The tendons of these muscles may need to be lengthened by tendon grafts. Leprosy is the most common cause of peripheral nerve lesions; in the upper limb the effects are seen in the ulnar nerve at the elbow and in the median nerve at the wrist, producing partial or total intrinsic paralysis of the hand. Given suitable conditions and effective aftercare, consistently good results can be obtained from operations for the clawed fingers and thumb of the intrinsic-minus hand, by use of some adaptation of the Stiles-Bunnell principle.[2] The muscle chosen to provide power may be a superficialis, which is divided into four slips to reach the wing tendons of the extensor tendon complex without an intervening graft, or extensor carpi radialis brevis prolonged by grafts taken from plantaris tendon[2] or fascia lata.[5]

SUMMARY

Autogenous tendon grafting is widely used in the restoration of tendon defects and paralysis in the hand. Success depends on careful selection of the case, a gentle and precise surgical technique, and efficient aftercare.

REFERENCES

1. Boyes, J.H., and Stark, H.H.: Flexor-tendon grafts in the fingers and thumb, J. Bone Joint Surg. **53A:**1332, 1971.
2. Brand, P.W.: Tendon transfers in the forearm. In Flynn, J.E., editor: Hand surgery, ed. 3, Baltimore, 1982, The Williams & Wilkins Co.
3. Bunnell, S.: Repair of tendons in the fingers and description of two new instruments, Surg. Gynecol. Obstet. **26:**103, 1918.
4. Bunnell, S.: Repair of tendons in the fingers, Surg. Gynecol. Obstet. **35:**88, 1922.
5. Fritschi, E.P.: Reconstructive surgery in leprosy, Bristol, 1971, John Wright & Sons, Ltd.
6. Hueston, J.T., Hubble, B., and Rigg, B.R.: Homografts of the digital flexor tendon system, Aust. N.Z. J. Surg. **36:**269, 1967.
7. Hunter, J.M., and Aulicino, P.L.: Salvage of the scarred tendon systems, utilizing the Hunter tendon implant. In Flynn, J.E., editor: Hand surgery, ed. 3, Baltimore, 1982, The Williams & Wilkins Co.
8. Lister, G.D., Kleinert, H.E., Kutz, J.E., and Atasoy, E.: Primary flexor tendon repair followed by immediate controlled mobilization, J. Hand Surg. **2:**441, 1977.
9. Lundborg, G., and Rank, F.: Experimental intrinsic healing of flexor tendon based upon synovial fluid nutrition, J. Hand Surg. **3:**21, 1978.
10. Lundborg, G., Hansson, H.-A., Rank, F., and Sydevik, B.: Superficial repair of severed flexor tendon in synovial environment, J. Hand Surg. **5:**451, 1980.
11. Matthews, P., and Richards, H.: The repair potential of digital flexor tendons, J. Bone Joint Surg. **56B:**618, 1974.
12. Paneva-Holevich, E.: Two-stage tenoplasty in injury of the flexor tendons of the hand, J. Bone Joint Surg. **51A:**21, 1969.
13. Peacock, E.E., Jr., and Madden, J.W.: Human composite flexor tendon allografts, Ann. Surg. **166:**624, 1967.
14. Potenza, A.D.: Concepts of tendon healing and repair. In American Academy of Orthopaedic Surgeons: Symposium on tendon surgery in the hand, St. Louis, 1975, The C.V. Mosby Co.
15. Pulvertaft, R.G.: Tendon grafts for flexor tendon injuries in the fingers and thumb, J. Bone Joint Surg. **38B:**175, 1956.
16. Pulvertaft, R.G.: The treatment of profundus division by free tendon graft, J. Bone Joint Surg. **42A:**1363, 1960.
17. Pulvertaft, R.G.: Flexor tendon grafting after long delay. In Tubiana, R., editor: The hand, vol. 2, Philadelphia, W.B. Saunders Co. (In press.)
18. Robson, A.W.M.: A case of tendon grafting, Trans. Clin. Soc. London **22:**289, 1889.
19. Sarkin, T.L.: The plastic replacement of severed flexor tendons of the fingers, Br. J. Surg. **44:**232, 1956.

26

Tenolysis: dynamic approach to surgery and therapy

LAWRENCE H. SCHNEIDER and EVELYN J. MACKIN

The surgical release of nongliding adhesions that form along the surface of a tendon after injury or repair is a useful procedure in the salvage of tendon function.[9] Tendon adhesions occur whenever the surface of a tendon is damaged either through the injury itself, be it laceration or crush, or by surgical manipulation.[5] At any point on the surface of a tendon where violation occurs an adhesion will form in the healing period.[6] Whenever these adhesions cannot be mobilized by therapy techniques, tenolysis should be considered. This procedure is as demanding as tendon repair itself and cannot be undertaken lightly. It represents another surgical onslaught in an area of previous trauma and surgery. If the procedure is unsuccessful, the patient's hand may show no improvement or even be worse. The risk of further decreasing the circulatory supply and innervation to a borderline finger is a real one. Rupture of the lysed tendon, a disastrous complications, is another hazard of tenolysis.

PREOPERATIVE EVALUATION FOR TENOLYSIS

Patient selection is a vital aspect in successful tenolysis. The patient should have been in an adequate therapy program combining active motion techniques with gentle passive motion exercises for approximately 3 months and progress should be at a standstill. This time interval allows for wound healing and maturation while the patient is trying to stretch the adhesions that have formed. The patient's level of cooperation in a postoperative program can also be evaluated during this interval. A patient unable to put himself fully into the program should be rejected for lysis.

At 3 months, if the range of movement attained is regarded by patient and surgeon as inadequate, discussion is entered into regarding the risks and rewards of lysis in view of the functional demands and needs of the patient. A realistic picture must be drawn. A cold, insensate finger will not be improved even if a full range of motion could be regained. The decision to perform tenlysis is often subjective. For example, 50% of a normal range of motion may be reasonable to accept, especially in an aged person or one who has concurrent joint surface injury or degenerative arthritis. Adequate skin cover should be present as another prerequisite for this surgery.

Ideally, the patient who would be best would be one whose repaired tendon had a localized adhesion that limited gliding. On release a full range of motion is regained. This,

however, is the uncommon situation. More frequently, the adhesions involve a long segment of the involved tendon and require extensive exposure for release. Joint contracture, which can occur secondary to the tendon fixation, may also require correction and further complicates the surgery and the patient's recovery.

TECHNIQUE

Once the patient meets the criteria established, lysis is performed on an inpatient basis under local anesthesia to allow full evaluation during the procedure itself.[4] It is through this technique that one can determine whether release of the offending tendon-system adhesions is adequate to restore motion or the patient also requires surgical release of the joints. At times it is necessary to turn the hand over and release the opposing tendon system also. This situation is not uncommon in crushing injuries, especially if there are associated phalangeal fractures. All patients for flexor lysis have been prepared for the possibility of staged tendon reconstruction if a reasonable flexor mechanism cannot be salvaged.[3]

The local anesthesia used in 1% or 2% lidocaine infiltrated locally in the skin or as a digital block at the metacarpal level. Nerve blocks at the wrist can also be used but, with resultant paralysis of the intrinsic muscles, some benefits of this technique are sacrificed.

The administration of intravenous medication relieves anxiety and alleviates tourniquet pain. The use of a fentanyl-droperidol mixture marketed as Innovar* has proved useful. The anesthesia technique has been modified slightly in that less of the combination is now used for induction. First, 0.5 to 1 ml of fentanyl-droperidol is given intravenously, and then a second and third dose of a similar amount of fentanyl alone is added at intervals of 4 to 5 minutes for induction. Only fentanyl is then added as required for the patient's comfort and allowed by the vital signs.

Monitoring of the vital signs by experienced anesthesia personnel in an operating room environment is necessary. Careful titration of the medication is also necessary. Overuse depresses the patient's function and his ability to cooperate. With proper dosage, the tourniquet has been tolerated for as long as 1 hour. The dissection proceeds rapidly and the patient's range of motion is constantly reevaluated until

---

*Innovar, McNeil Co., Ft. Washington, Pa.

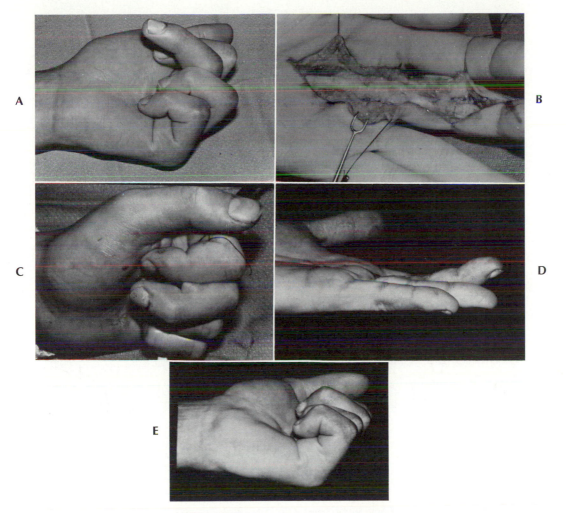

Fig. 26-1. Flexor lysis: a 17-year-old boy severed both flexor tendons in his left long finger. After primary repair of his flexor digitorum profundus, he had minimal pull-through of his flexor system at 4 months after repair. **A,** Attempted flexion of left long finger. **B,** At tenolysis, repair site was found to be involved with massive adhesions. **C,** After lysis under local-sedation technique, he obtained excellent active flexion on table. **D** and **E,** Through active therapy program he maintained gains made at surgery. Photographs taken at 3 months after surgery in extension and flexion.

tourniquet paralysis intervenes at between 20 and 25 minutes. If further dissection is needed, it is continued as necessary and evaluation is carried out after the tourniquet is released and hemostasis is obtained. If further surgery is deemed necessary, reinflation can be carried out and dissection continued until completed. The surgeon can directly determine whether the tendon motor actually is effective and flexor pulleys are adequate. He can also tell whether the lysed tendon appears healthy or a tendon graft in one or two stages is advisable. When lysis is successful and the range of motion actively attained appears acceptable, the wounds are closed and a dressing is applied, so that an early postoperative motion program is allowed.

Summary of surgical technique

Flexor lysis[7] (Fig. 26-1)
1. Zigzag incision; if necessary, be prepared to expose the entire course of the tendon.

2. Preserve pulleys as possible.
3. Release joints if significant contractures exist.
4. Be prepared to create a tendon out of scar in a heavily involved repair site.
5. Prepare patient for possibility of staged tendon reconstruction if lysis by this technique appears unfeasible.

Flexor lysis after failed direct repair has been more successful than after failed tendon graft, a finding that leads us to prefer direct repair, early, in flexor injuries when wound conditions allow.[8]

Extensor lysis (Fig. 26-2)
1. Curvilinear incision over adherent area is utilized.
2. Joint releases; dorsal capsulotomies are often needed.
3. Try to preserve dorsal retinaculum at wrist.

When both flexor and extensor tendons are involved in adhesions, the prognosis is notably poorer but occasionally finger salvage can be achieved (Fig. 26-3).

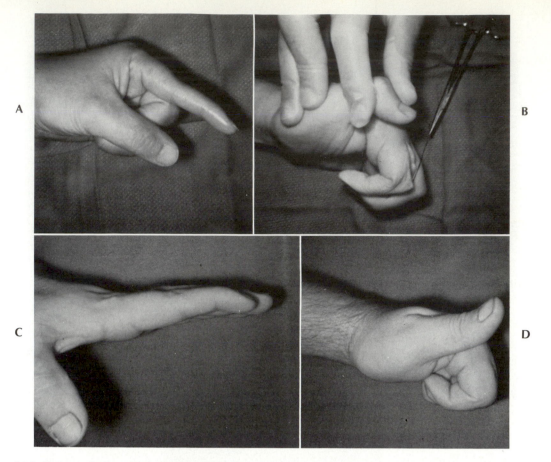

FIG. 26-2. Extensor lysis: a 42-year-old man severed his extensor mechanism over proximal interphalangeal joint of his left index finger. After repair, extension contracture persisted despite active exercise program. A, Fixed extension posture of finger before lysis. B, On operating table, after lysis of tendon adhesions and release of dorsal capsule of proximal interphalangeal joint, he could flex actively to 90 degrees. C and D, Range of motion retained in therapy shown at 3 months after tenolysis.

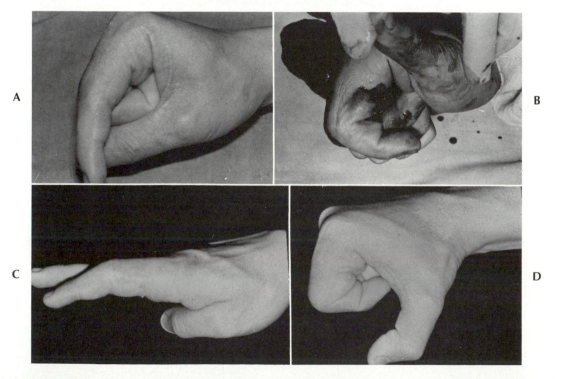

FIG. 26-3. Combined extensor and flexor lysis: a 35-year-old man sustained crush injury to his right index finger. His extensor system was primarily involved. His finger became contracted in extension and he had only 20 degrees of flexion from straight position at proximal interphalangeal joint. A, Maximum active flexion at proximal interphalangeal joint. B, Lysis of extensor tendon system with release of proximal interphalangeal joint dorsal capsule returned passive flexion, but active flexion was not regained until volar exposure revealed adhesions of flexor tendons. With release of these adhesions, he regained active flexion as shown here. C, Active extension maintained at 4 months. D, Active flexion possible at 4 months.

POSTOPERATIVE MANAGEMENT

The procedures surrounding the tenolysis operation are as vital as the lysis itself. The main thrust of the postoperative program is to get the patient to pull the tendon actively through the lysed area in an effort to maintain the gains made at surgery. The postoperative dressing is debulked to allow for active exercises at the time of hospital discharge 24 hours after surgery. The patient is given a prescription for analgesic medication and instruction in gentle active motion as limited by pain. He is then seen by the surgeon and hand therapist on the first postoperative day. The surgeon informs the therapist of the findings at surgery, the intraoperative range of motion, and the prognosis.

The dressing applied at surgery is changed and specific active range-of-motion exercises are performed under the supervision of the hand therapist. The therapist must encourage the patient to pull through actively with his lysed tendon despite the discomfort and swelling associated with a fresh wound. Gentle passive motion is also performed by the therapist and patient to keep the joints mobile. Pain and swelling are limiting factors in this exercise program. The patient must expect some discomfort; however, it is vital that the patient work through the "soreness" of the early postoperative days if the range-of-motion potential attained at surgery is to be maintained. Forceful passive motion of the joints is not indicated. Such motion is painful and only increases pain and edema. When pain becomes intolerable, therapy will not succeed. The patient's hand is maintained in a dorsal resting splint. The dressing applied to the finger or fingers must not restrict the patient's exercise program. Most often full active and passive range-of-motion exercises can be carried out within the confines of the dorsal splint. Elevation of the extremity is important. When not exercising, the patient's hand is maintained in a sling, hand-over-heart position, during the first week after surgery to minimize the degree of swelling. During sleep the hand should be elevated on pillows. The patient is seen daily by the therapist during the first postoperative week. Goniometric measurements of range of motion are recorded during the initial visit to therapy and checked routinely by the therapist. Whirlpool treatment is not permitted for at least 2 weeks.

The active and passive exercise program generally would include the following:

1. Active flexion and extension of the interphalangeal and metacarpophalangeal joints.
2. Gentle passive flexion and extension of the interphalangeal joints.
3. Finger blocking (distal interphalangeal joint flexion with the proximal interphalangeal joint supported and proximal interphalanageal joint flexion with the metacarpophalangeal joint supported).
4. *Full* flexion of the interphalangeal joints with the metacarpophalangeal joint in *full* extension followed by metacarpophalangeal flexion to make a fist (Fig. 26-4).
5. Passive fist-making. (Patient rolls involved hand into a tight fist with the uninvolved hand. Then the hand is released, and the patient tries to retain the fist with his own muscle power [Fig. 26-5].)

The home exercise program is carried out within the splint. Special emphasis is on exercises 4 and 5 from the above list; these are performed five to 10 times each hour depending on the level of discomfort. Five to 10 repetitions of the other exercises are performed three times a day.

Joint flexion contractures corrected through lysis require immediate post-operative splinting in extension in order to maintain the extension achieved in the operating room. The splint may be applied as early as the first day depending on

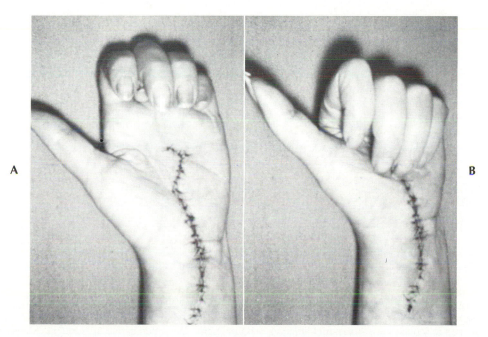

FIG. 26-4. Tendon-gliding exercise. **A,** Full flexion of interphalangeal joints with metacarpal joints in full extension. *Maintain full flexion* of interphalangeal joints and roll fingers in to make a tight fist, **B.**

the quality of the tendon and the surgeon's orders. The plaster dorsal resting splint applied at surgery is replaced with an aluminum extension splint if one digit is involved or else with a thermoplastic extension splint. The splint is worn day and night and is removed only for exercise. At 2 weeks, if full extension or the intraoperative extension has been achieved, the splint may be removed during the day for activities of daily living and strengthening activities. However, the extension splint may need to be worn at night for several months to prevent recurrence of the contracture.

Joint extension contractures corrected through lysis may also require immediate postoperative splinting intermittently during the day and all night. A web strap or distal interphalangeal stretcher (Chapter 16) may be used. A distal interphalangeal stretcher fabricated from leather and Velcro (Chapter 16) or the web strap may be worn at night to maintain and perhaps increase flexion gains made at surgery.

Postoperative management using local anesthesia

A technique that has been useful in helping a patient get through the difficult first week after lysis employs an indwelling polyethylene catheter[2] inserted after the surgical procedure in the area of the tenolysis (Fig. 26-6). Before closure of the wound the catheter is laid proximally to the site of surgery over the sensory nerve branches. This catheter is used to instill small amounts (1 or 2 ml) of local anesthetic into the operated area to allay pain during the exercise periods. The catheter is left in place for 5 to 7 days, during which time the patient is on a regime of systemic antibiotics.

Postoperative therapy begins a few hours after surgery in the patient's hospital room, assisted by the nursing staff and the surgeon. The patient is shown how to self-administer the anesthesic slowly into the wound. Rapid instillation produces pain. Active assistive exercise is encouraged.

When the patient is seen by the therapist on the first postoperative day, the dressing applied at surgery is removed. The petrolatum gauze covering the incision line is left on as a protective covering for a few days. To protect the catheter entrance site and surgical incision from contamination, the therapist places the patient's hand on a sterile field during the exercise session (Fig. 26-7, A). The therapist wears sterile gloves during the treatment (Fig. 26-7, B). The exercise program is the same as that previously described.

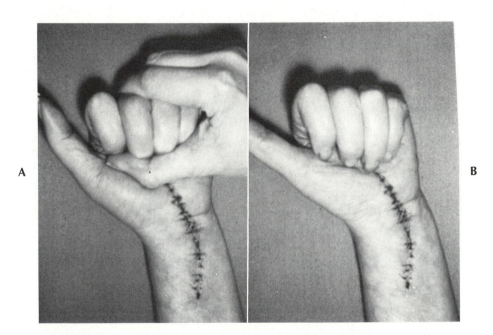

A   B

FIG. 26-5. Passive fist-making. **A,** Patient presses involved hand into a tight fist with uninvolved hand. **B,** Then involved hand is released, and patient tries to retain fist with his muscle power.

FIG. 26-6. Extensor lysis. Patient lacerated his extensor tendon over dorsum of proximal phalanx. **A,** Passive flexion of finger 2 years after repair. Preoparative range of motion: MP 0°/90°, PIP 20°/20°, DIP 0°/45°. **B,** After extensor tenolysis and proximal interphalangeal joint capsulectomy under local-sedation technique, patient obtained excellent flexion. Intraoperative active range of motion: MP 0°/90°, PIP 0°/90°, DIP 0°/60°. Flexion ½ inch to DPC. **C,** Before closure of wound a soft Jackson-Pratt catheter is laid proximally to site of surgery over sensory-nerve branches. **D,** Active flexion. **E,** Syringe (20 ml) containing the local anesthetic is taped to forearm dressing. **F,** Sterile dressing applied to wound must not restrict home exercise program, and so full active flexion and extension can be carried out within the confines of splint. **G,** Three months after tenolysis procedure. Patient exceeded range of motion gained intraoperatively: MP 0°/90°, PIP 0°/95°, DIP 0°/60°. Full flexion to the DPC. **H,** Extension.

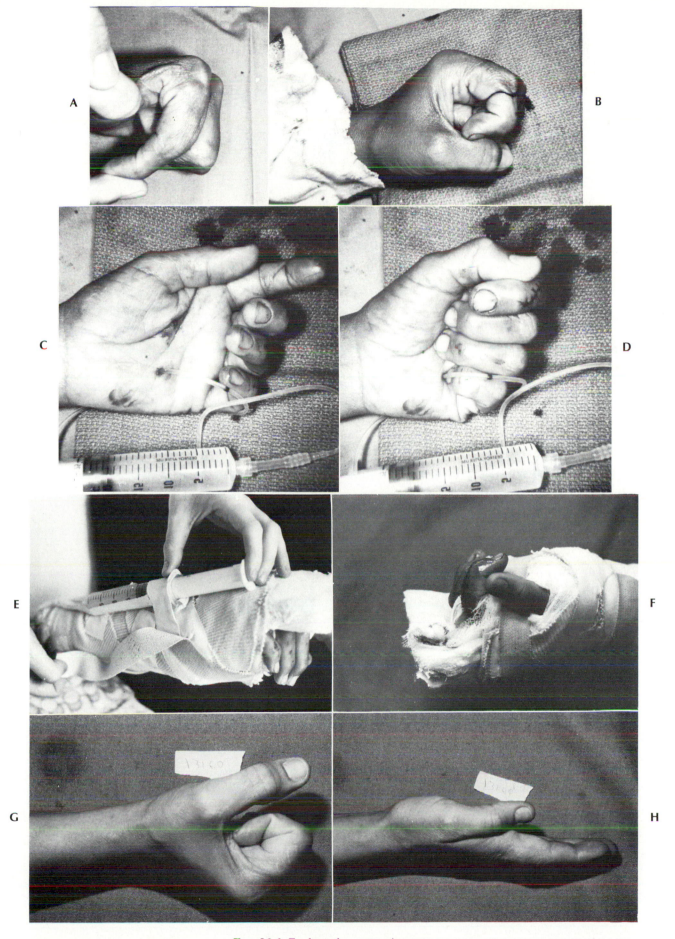

FIG. 26-6. For legend see opposite page.

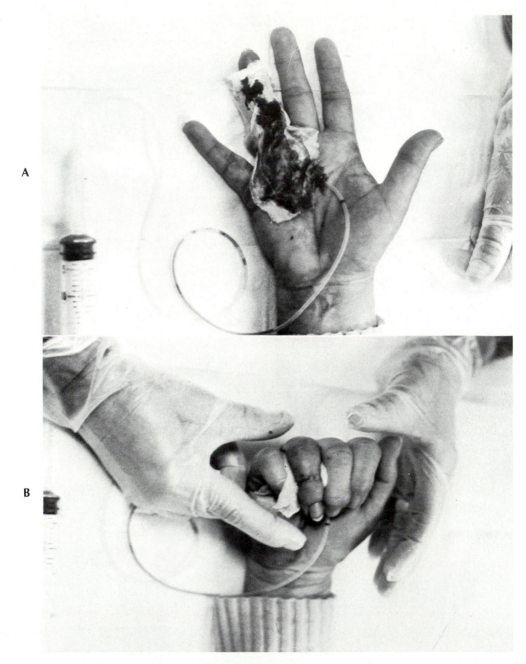

FIG. 26-7. A, Postoperative therapy is carried out in as clean an environment as possible. Patient's hand is placed on a sterile field. Petrolatum gauze covering incision line is left on as a protective covering for a few days. **B,** Therapist wears sterile gloves during treatment.

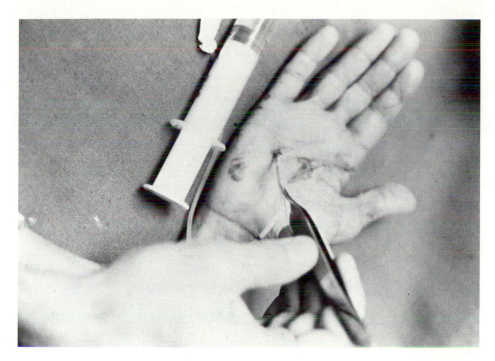

FIG. 26-8. Catheter is removed on approximately fifth postoperative day. Skin suture holding catheter in place is cut and catheter is easily removed. Antibiotic ointment is applied to catheter entrance site.

At the end of the exercise session, an antibiotic ointment is applied to the catheter entrance site and along the incision line. Dry sterile dressings are then applied and are not removed until the treatment session on the following day.

The goal is to achieve the active range of motion obtained at surgery by the time the catheter is removed at 5 to 7 days.

The catheter is removed on approximately the fifth postoperative day. The skin suture holding the catheter in place is cut, and the catheter is easily removed (Fig. 26-8). Antibiotic ointment is applied to the catheter entrance site. A whirlpool bath is not permitted until the wound has completely healed.

Light activities of daily living may be begun at 2 to 3 weeks along with an increased exercise program using wood blocks and dowels.

Graded grip-strengthening activities are begun at 3 to 4 weeks, for example, beginning with putty and the Hand Helper and progressing to woodworking, ceramics, progressive resistive exercises, and pulleys. The goal during this phase of therapy is to maintain the active range of motion gained in the early postoperative days and to increase strength within that range. Heavy resistive exercise is generally begun at the eighth postoperative week. The goal is to return the patient to full work at 8 to 12 weeks after tenolysis (depending on the job description).

Through the judicious use of tenolysis, a surgical procedure of such magnitude that it should not be underestimated, salvage of tendon function is attainable in patients whose results after tendon injuries are unsatisfactory. Close cooperation between patient, surgeon, and therapist is necessary to make this procedure worthwhile.

REFERENCES

1. Fetrow, K.O.: Tenolysis in the hand and wrist, J. Bone Joint Surg. **49A:**667-684, 1967.
2. Hunter, J.M., Seinshimer, F., and Mackin, E.J.: Tenolysis: pain control and rehabilitation. In Strickland, J., and Steichen, J., editors: Difficult problems in hand surgery, St. Louis, 1982, The C.V. Mosby Co.
3. Hunter, J.M., and Salisbury, R.E.: Flexor tendon reconstruction in severely damaged hands, J. Bone Joint Surg. **53A:**829-858, 1971.
4. Hunter, J.M., Schneider, L.H., Dumont, J., and Erickson, J.C.: A dynamic approach to problems of hand function, Clin. Orthop. **104:**112-115, 1974.
5. Lindsay, W.K., and Thomson, H.G.: Digital flexor tendons: an experimental study, Br. J. Plast. Surg. **12:**289-316, 1960.
6. Potenza, A.D.: Critical evaluation of flexor tendon healing and adhesion formation within artificial digital sheaths, J. Bone Joint Surg. **45A:**1217-1233, 1963.
7. Schneider, L.H., and Hunter, J.M.: Flexor tenolysis. In American Academy of Orthopaedic Surgeons: Symposium on tendon surgery in the hand, St. Louis, 1975, The C.V. Mosby Co.
8. Schneider, L.H., Hunter, J.M., Norris, T.R., and Nadeau, P.O.: Delayed primary flexor tendon repair in no man's land, Orthop. Trans. **1**(1):2, 1977.
9. Verdan, C.E., Crawford, G.P., and Martini-Benkeddache, Y.: The valuable role of tenolysis in the digits. In Cramer, L.M., and Chase, R.A., editors: Symposium on the hand, vol. 3, St. Louis, 1971, The C.V. Mosby Co.

27

Staged flexor tendon reconstruction

JAMES M. HUNTER

The objective of the two-staged flexor tendon method is to improve the predictability of final results in difficult problems dealing with tendon reconstruction. The surgeon who is capable of achieving a good result with flexor tendon grafting in a tendon bed with minimal scarring may achieve better results in the poorer grade of cases by using the two-stage method. Patients who are considered suitable candidates for flexor tenolysis should also be considered candidates for reconstruction, because the preoperative assessment may prove inaccurate at the time of surgery. Only at the time of surgery can the surgeon make a true estimate of the extent of scarring and injury to the tendon gliding bed and retinacular pulley system.

The transformation of the stiff, scarred, and functionless tendon complex to its gliding, pliable preinjury state can be accomplished by the two-stage tendon graft method utilizing at stage I the Hunter silastic tendon implant.* Restoration of the fibro-osseous canal by reconstruction of pulleys and fibrous sheath around the tendon implant has resulted in good gliding biomechanics and a fluid nutrition system that can nourish the subsequent stage II tendon graft without adhesions, resulting in a useful finger.

This chapter highlights the indications and technique of the two-stage tendon graft utilizing the Hunter gliding tendon implant.

INDICATIONS FOR STAGED TENDON RECONSTRUCTION

A tendon implant is indicated in the following situations: (1) as a temporary segmental spacer in selected primary injuries where tendon repair is not possible (when the conditions are favorable, a primary flexor tendon repair is the procedure of choice); (2) scarred tendon beds where a one-stage tendon graft can be predicted to fail; and (3) salvage situations where despite predicted degrees of stiffness, scarred tendon bed, and reduced nutrition, useful function

can be returned. This procedure has been successfully utilized in extensor tendon reconstruction, reconstruction of the severely mutilated hand, and construction of tendon systems in congenital anomalies with deficient tendon systems.[15] Any tendon transfer that would have to traverse a suboptimal bed is also a candidate for this procedure (Fig. 27-1). This procedure may also be indicated for grafting of a profundus tendon through an intact sublimis when the profundus tendon bed is scarred.[16]

In acute trauma, the tendon implant may also be utilized, provided that the wounds have been adequately debrided and rendered surgically clean. When the injury requires simultaneous fracture fixation as well as flexor and extensor tendon repair, one should consider the use of a tendon implant in the flexor system.

The most recent indication for a two-stage procedure has been in replantation surgery. In multiple digital amputations the use of the implant in the flexor system at the time of replantation may significantly simplify the postoperative rehabilitation. A full-length implant or even a short spacer can maintain the fibro-osseous canal and regenerate a flexor sheath in damaged areas after the fracture or fusion has healed and the neurovascular status is stabilized. The passive flexion and active extension have helped rehabilitate both the flexor and extensor systems simultaneously and have significantly improved the function of replanted digits. If the replantation is proximal to zone 2 or at wrist level, it is reasonable to repair the flexor tendons primarily and place extensor implants dorsally, since the wrist is usually flexed to protect the neurovascular repairs. Again the postoperative rehabilitation is simplified.

Acute infection, of course, is an absolute contraindication to this procedure. Appropriate surgical and antimicrobial treatment and subsequent wound healing will allow the procedure to be carried out at a later date without complication. A digit that has borderline nutrition, bilateral digital nerve injuries, and severe joint stiffness, may better be treated by amputation rather than reconstruction.

Before tendon surgery, all patients should be placed on a hand therapy program designed to mobilize stiff joints and improve to the maximum the condition of the soft tissue (Fig. 27-2). The timing of stage I tendon surgery should combine the judgments of the surgeon and the hand therapist, for patient input and motivation are the keys to the successful result.

Portions of this chapter are paraphrased from Hunter, J.M.: Two-stage tendon reconstruction using gliding tendon implants. In Pulvertaft, R.G.: Hand, ed. 3, Sevenoaks, Kent, 1977, Butterworth & Co. (Publishers), Ltd., and Hunter, J.M., and Aulicino, P.L.: Salvage of the scarred tendon systems utilizing the Hunter tendon implant. In Flynn, J.E.: Hand surgery, ed. 3, Baltimore, 1981, The Williams & Wilkins Co.
*Hunter tendon implant, Holter-Hausner International, P.O. Box 1, Bridgeport, Pa. 19405.

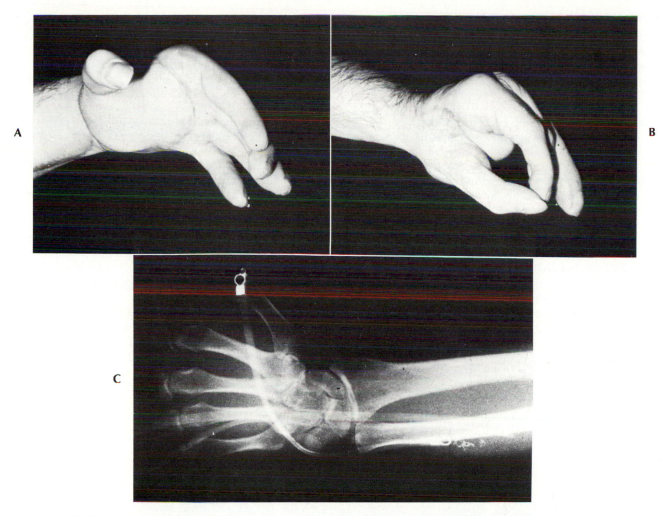

FIG. 27-1. A, Opponensplasty utilizing an active tendon implant. This can also be performed with passive implant. The motor is the flexor digitorum superficialis of the long finger. **A,** Thumb extension. This patient lost all thenar muscles and flexor pollicis longus tendon in a hamburger press. Following débridement, metacarpophalangeal arthrodesis, and pedicle skin grafting, first-stage active tendon was used to restore opposition. **B,** Thumb in opposition. **C,** Roentgenogram of patient shown in **A** and **B.** Excursion was approximately 2.5 to 3 cm.

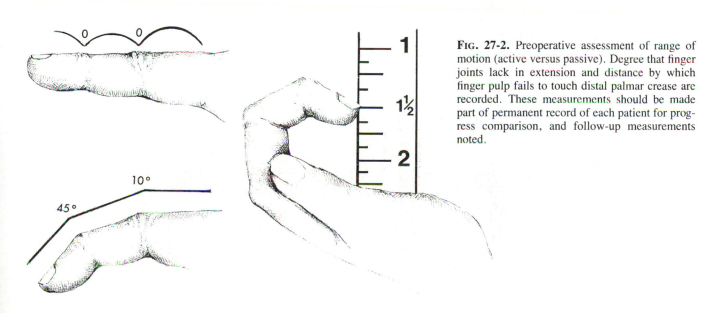

FIG. 27-2. Preoperative assessment of range of motion (active versus passive). Degree that finger joints lack in extension and distance by which finger pulp fails to touch distal palmar crease are recorded. These measurements should be made part of permanent record of each patient for progress comparison, and follow-up measurements noted.

TYPES OF IMPLANTS

Four types of Hunter tendon implants have evolved from the experience gained in experimental and clinical trials during the past 22 years: two passive implants and two active implants (Fig. 27-3).

The active gliding concept in its early stage (1960) had been the designing of an artificial tendon or prosthesis. Limited success was achieved, and I published a report about it in 1965.[5] However, because of terminal juncture separation under stress, the method was later converted to passive gliding until more advanced research could produce proximal and distal attachments that was reliable for an extended period.[7]

Currently, active implants are in the field clinical investigational stage.[9] All the implants have a woven or braided Dacron core that is pressure molded into a radiopaque silicone rubber. The surface finish is smooth and the cross-sectional design is ovoid to aid optimal tendon sheath development (Fig. 27-4).

The passive gliding program implies that the distal end of the implant is fixed securely to bone or tendon while the proximal end glides freely in the proximal palm or forearm. Movement of the implant is produced by active extension and passive flexion of the digit. A new biologic sheath begins to form around the implant rather quickly during the period of gliding that follows stage I surgery. The new sheath progresses through a 4-week phase of biologic maturity and develops a fluid system that supports gliding after stage I and nutrition gliding for the tendon graft after stage II. In approximately 3 to 4 months after stage I surgery the implant can be electively replaced by a tendon graft.

The implant incorporates design characteristics of firmness and flexibility to permit secure distal suture fixation and minimize the buckling effect during the passive push phase of gliding. The implant is available commercially.

The two passive tendon implants differ only in their distal juncture. One implant (Fig. 27-5) has a stainless steel distal component that is attached to the distal phalanx with a screw fixation metal end plate. It provides excellent fixation to bone, and we have had few problems with loosening of the screw and subsequent proximal migration of the implant, the principal cause of sheath synovitis.

It also provides the added benefit in shortening the second-stage procedure. The screw hole in the distal phalanx acts as a guide hole that is further enlarged in an oblique fashion for the acceptance of the tendon graft. The Woodruff 2 mm bone screws* are available in various sizes and are self-tapping. The length of the screw is determined from the preoperative roentgenogram. A pilot hole is drilled (Fig. 27-6, *A*) at a 15- to 20-degree angle with a 0.035-inch Kirschner wire, and the screw is advanced to a finger tightness. The length should be sufficient to engage the dorsal

---

*Zimmer-Rodewalt Associates, Inc., R.D. #4, Box 163A, Woodbury Glassboro Rd., Sewell, N.J. 08080.

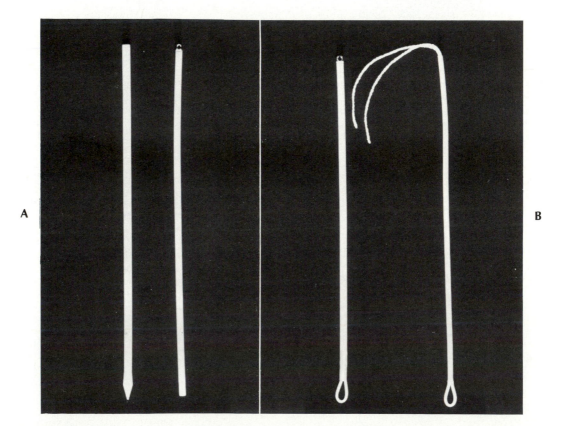

FIG. 27-3. A, Passive gliding tendon implants. **B,** Active gliding tendon implants. *Left,* Metal end screw fixation and loop system a fixed length. *Right,* Dacron braid interlacing and loop system with adjustable length design.

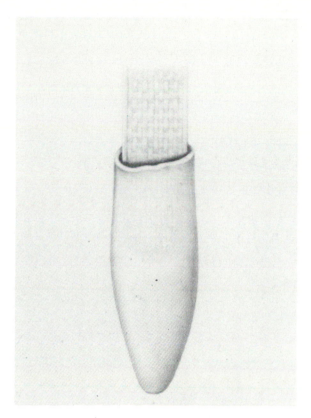

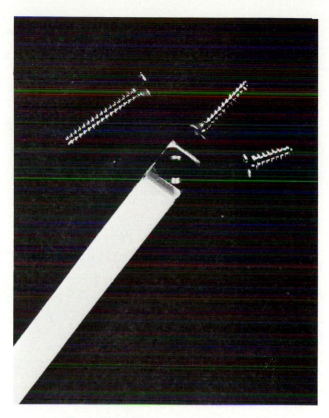

FIG. 27-4. Implant. Silicone rubber has been cut away to show Dacron woven tape added to give body to implant.

FIG. 27-5. Distal juncture with screw fixation metal end plate.

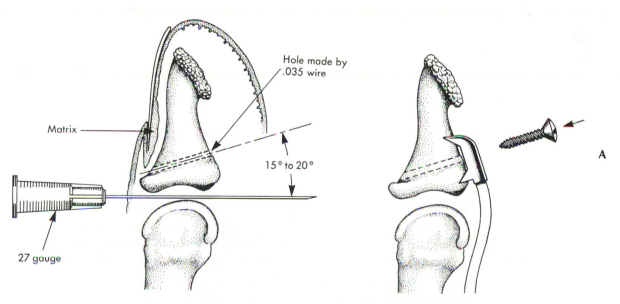

FIG. 27-6. A, Distal plate fixation plan for Hunter tendon implant.

Continued.

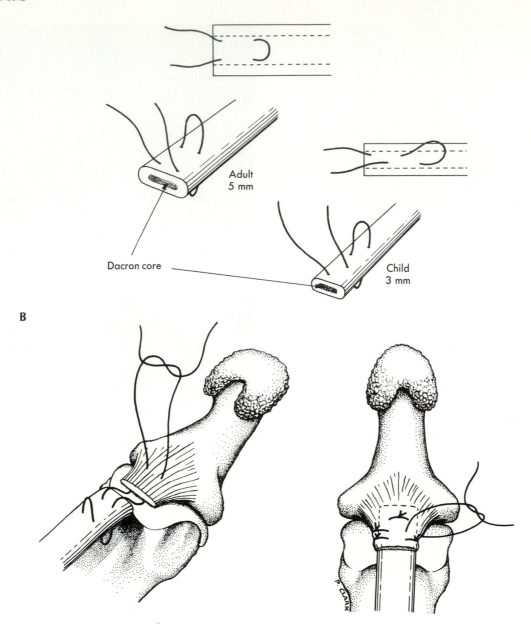

B

FIG. 27-6, cont'd. **B,** Fixation of reinforced tendon implant (rod) without metal plate.

cortex of the phalanx but not pass beyond it because this may result in a painful area dorsally. It should also be proximal to the germinal matrix of the nail. This implant is available in 6, 5, 4, and 3 mm diameters. The lengths are either 23 or 25 cm. These implants can be trimmed proximally to the appropriate length.

The passive tendon implant without a screw fixation terminal device is held in place when a 4-0 monofilament stainless steel wire or a 4-0 Dacron polyester suture is woven through the distal end of the implant and this end is secured under the profundus stump (Fig. 27-6, *B*).

Care must be taken to place the wire through the central Dacron core. If the wire is placed too peripherally, it may possibly pull through the silicone coating and allow the tendon implant to migrate proximally. The distal juncture is also reinforced with two lateral sutures, which may be

of wire or Dacron. This implant is available in the following sizes: 3 mm × 23 cm, 4 mm × 23 cm, 5 mm × 25 cm, and 6 mm × 25 cm. This implant can also be shortened and should be trimmed at the distal end.

A molded radiopaque silicone rod (Swanson-Hunter design) is available from the Dow Corning Company. It also comes in 6, 5, 4, and 3 mm diameters and may be cut to the appropriate length (Fig. 27-7).

The 1983 active tendon implants for temporary total tendon replacement are reinforced by Dacron braid that terminates proximally in a loop coated with silicone, through which the proximal tendon motor is woven (Fig. 27-8). Autoclave preparation for surgery requires special care (Fig. 27-9). The active implants also have two types of distal juncture: the previously described screw-plate juncture and a special impacter and wire guide (Fig. 27-10), or two

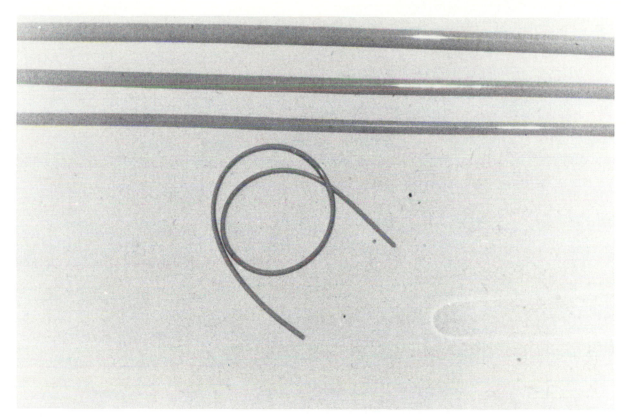

FIG. 27-7. Molded unreinforced silicone rods. Notice flexibility of implant without Dacron core. (Dow Corning Corp., Midland, Mich.)

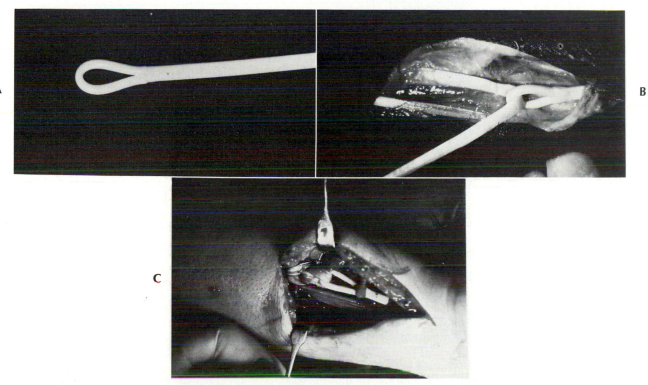

FIG. 27-8. A, Active-implant proximal silicone-coated Dacron loop for motor tendon unit juncture. **B,** Appropriate motor is chosen and pulled through loop to set tension. **C,** Completed juncture of active tendon implant and proximal motor tendon.

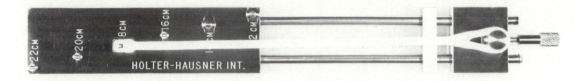

FIG. 27-9. Active tendon autoclave instrument maintains tendon length integrity and permits touch-free handling during surgery.

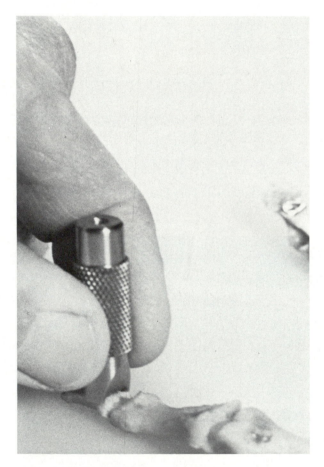

FIG. 27-10. Distal plate impacter and wire guide for Hunter Mark II Active Tendon Implant. (Holter-Hausner International, Bridgeport, Pa.)

molded Dacron cords that can be placed through drill holes in the bone. The distal profundus stump may also be woven through a preformed loop and back through itself and then sutured (a future implant design) (Fig. 27-11). The tensile strength of the distal metal juncture to tendon shaft has been rated at more than 100 pounds. The active implants remain in a clinical testing phase, with research and manufacturing programs aimed toward a permanent implant. They are not yet available for general distribution. These implants are to be used as temporary extended tendon prostheses. The benefit of this type of implant has been the ability to select a motor before stage II and to have this motor "tuned," in that it is actively moving the finger. It also serves to test the pulleys that have been reconstructed during the first stage. The proximal motor juncture is easily identified in the second stage, and the fibrous sheath motor tendon unit is kept intact and the graft slipped through the healed tendon complex. The tension is set and the graft is sutured.

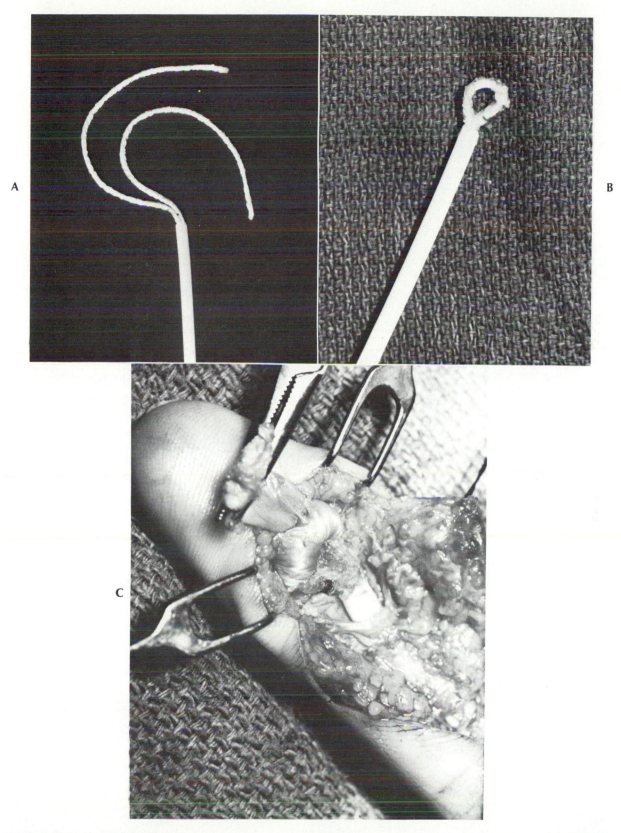

FIG. 27-11. A, Distal braided Dacron cords. **B,** Loop fashioned and sutured with Dacron. **C,** Profundus tendon woven through the loops and itself and sutured in place.

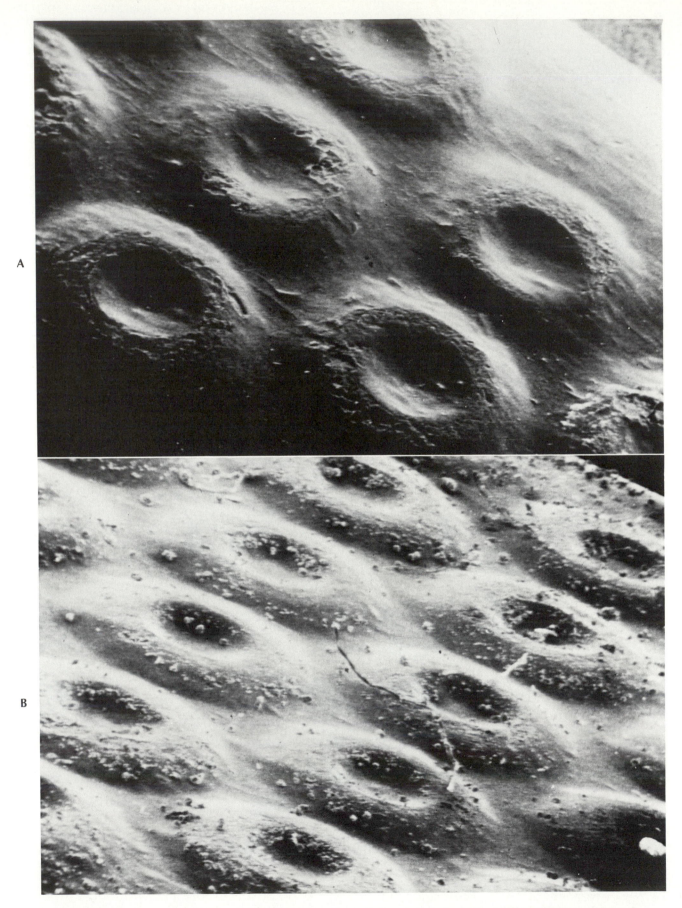

FIG. 27-12. A, Scanning electron micrograph of surface of clean and sterile implant before handling. (40×.) **B,** Scanning electron micrograph of implant after handling with dry gloves. Notice surface contaminants. (40×.)

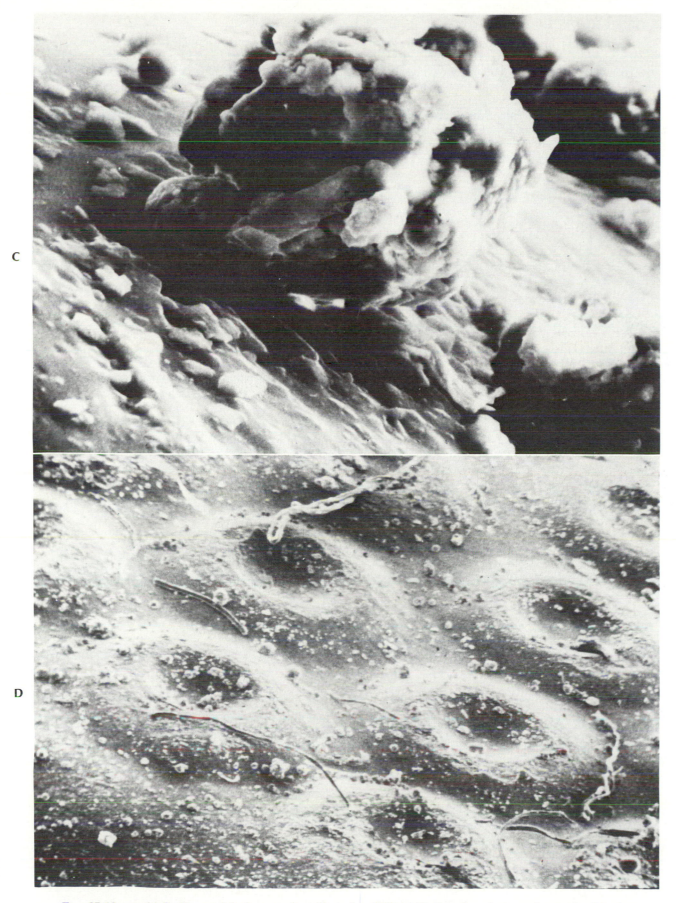

FIG. 27-12, cont'd C, One particle from previous illustration (800×.) **D,** Scanning electron micrograph of implant after handling with dry gloves and placing on a towel. Notice large increase in surface contaminants. One can avoid contamination by keeping the implant and gloves moist at all times. (40×.)

CARE OF SILICONE RUBBER

Silicone rubber is highly electrostatic, and as a result it attracts airborne particles and surface contaminants (Fig. 27-12). Once the implants are removed from the sterile package, they must be kept moist at all times. They should be placed in a sterile solution of saline, Ringer's lactate, or triple antibiotic irrigant. Gloves and sponges coming into contact with the tendon implant should always be wet. Attention to these details will prevent the development of a synovitis, which could interfere with the subsequent development of the neosheath.

ANESTHESIA

If a passive tendon implant is to be performed, this is done under axillary block or general anesthesia. If patient participation is required to determine function—that is, tenolysis versus implant or an active tendon implant—we prefer to use local anesthesia (1% lidocaine infiltration)[4] and tourniquet control augmented by intravenous analgesia such as Innovar (droperidol and fentanyl) or titrated intravenous Demerol (meperidine) and Valium (diazepam). This will allow patient compliance for assessment of function of the lysis or help in establishment of the appropriate tension in the active tendon implant. Selected second stage procedures have also been done in this manner. This allows appropriate tension of the graft to be set.

To perform these complicated procedures under local anesthesia, one needs to have a qualified anesthesiologist with the patient and to keep the patient sufficiently sedated to allow the tolerance of the tourniquet. The patient should, however, be arousable when his compliance is required. Adequate premedication and a good rapport between the anesthesia personnel and the patient are mandatory. Patients have tolerated the tourniquet for sequence periods up to 1 hour in this manner. The tourniquet is deflated intermittently (approximately every 30 minutes) to avoid tourniquet paralysis, and function is tested. If the patient cannot tolerate this procedure, the anesthesiologist can provide a general anesthetic. Most patients do not recall the surgical procedure postoperatively. This anesthetic technique has been utilized in some procedures lasting for as long as 4 hours.

STAGE I SURGERY

In the finger the volar zigzag incision popularized by Julian Brunner, is the incision of choice (Fig. 27-13). This incision spares the deep vascular connections to the tendon bed and permits a complete exposure of the tendon bed. The incision begins at the tip of the finger and proximally enters the palm. The incision must reach the distal extent of the transverse carpal ligament to facilitate the subsequent passage of the implant. The skin flaps should be of full thickness, with the corners lying over the neurovascular bundles to prevent marginal skin necrosis. The digital neu-

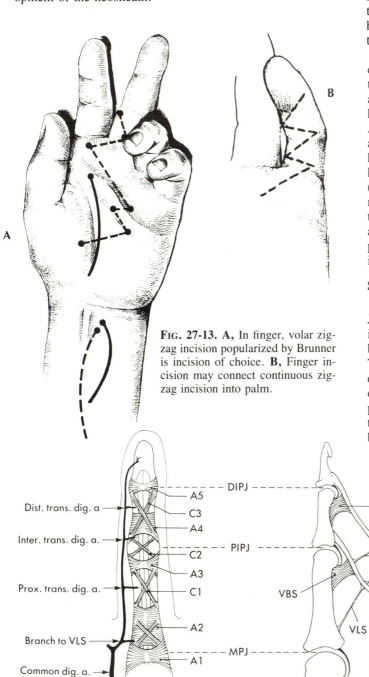

FIG. 27-13. **A,** In finger, volar zigzag incision popularized by Brunner is incision of choice. **B,** Finger incision may connect continuous zigzag incision into palm.

FIG. 27-14. Diagram of pulley system and relationship of digital artery branches and vinculum system.

rovascular bundles must be identified and protected. All the undamaged segments of the fibro-osseous pulley system are spared. After the entire fibro-osseous canal has been exposed, an isolated, curved incision is made proximally to the wrist crease. This incision is usually based on the ulnar aspect of the forearm. The ulnar artery and nerve and median nerve are identified and protected. The plane between the sublimi and profundi is identified and enlarged with blunt finger dissection. By making transverse window incisions in the flexor canal between A_1 and A_2, the cruciates, and mid-A_2 pulley levels, one carefully excises the scarred tendons. At the levels of the cruciate pulleys, the proper digital arteries give four transverse tributaries that supply the synovial bed and the vincular system. If possible, these arterial branches are spared (Fig. 27-14).

The excision of damaged tendons will often be time consuming. The surgeon must carefully excise scarred and adherent tendons while preserving uninjured portions of the sheath retinaculum. A generous segment of the distal profundus tendon, at least 1 cm, is preserved, and the joint capsule is left intact. It will probably be necessary to sacrifice the A_5 pulley to perform this adequately. The metacarpophalangeal and distal and proximal interphalangeal joints should be left undisturbed if all contractures can be released by tendon removal and by incision of the contracted cutaneous skin ligaments of Cleland or the oblique retinacular ligament of Landsmeer. The contracted finger will often require shifting or advancement of the full-thickness skin flaps. The V to Y techniques may be applied to gain extension and release skin tension (Fig. 27-15). One may

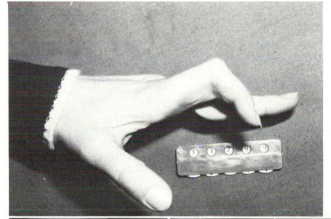

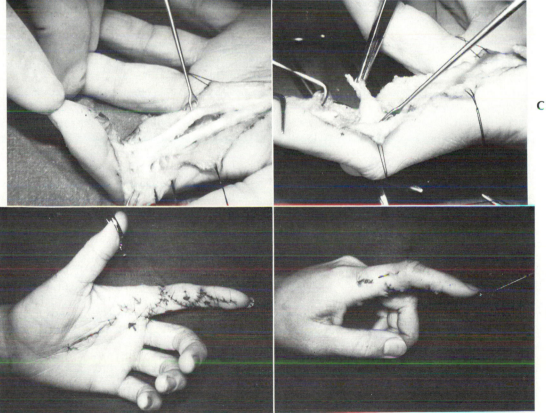

FIG. 27-15. **A,** Preoperative photograph of patient with a flexion contracture at the proximal interphalangeal joint and bowstringing of tendons caused by absence of pulleys. **B,** Scarred tendons are exposed through zigzag incision. Note absence of pulley system and scar underneath bowed tendons. **C,** Scarred tendons are excised and contractures are released. **D,** After implant has been inserted and pulleys have been reconstructed, V to Y technique is applied to zigzag incision to gain extension and release skin tension. **E,** Postoperative stage I. Notice absence of bowing across proximal interphalangeal joint after contracture release, pulley reconstruction and skin advancement. Proximal interphalangeal joint is temporarily pinned in extension.

best salvage severe contractures with skin loss by shifting skin flaps proximally in the finger and skin grafting the distal defects. A compromise in ultimate function may become a necessary and reasonable way to proceed, by creating a "sublimis finger."[11] The implant covered by viable skin flaps is fixed to the base of the middle phalanx, and the distal joint is arthrodesed.

If the superficialis tendon bed has not been injured, it is left intact over the proximal interphalangeal joint. Scarring of the tendons at the proximal interphalangeal joint level is often responsible for a flexion contracture. Meticulous dissection of mature scar at this level will permit increased ranges of motion and minimize flexion contracture after stage II.

The profundus and superficialis tendons are removed from the proximal pulley and sharply divided in the proximal palm. Scarred or shortened lumbrical muscle is resected to prevent the problem of a "lumbrical-plus" finger. If the palm is uninjured, the lumbrical and profundus complex with surrounding mesotenon is carefully preserved for stage II juncture. If more than one implant is to be used and crowding is observed in the carpal canal, the sublimi may be pulled through the carpal canal and excised in the forearm.

If resection of scarred tendons fails to release the contracture, scarring of the joint capsule or skin ligaments should be suspected. Capsulotomy of the volar plate will release contracture if confined to the joint only. The cord portion of the joint ligament is preserved for stability. Scarring of skin and of the ligament complex on either side of the finger, will maintain a contracture and may require opening by V and Y incision or shifting the skin flap and skin grafting. The joint should be mobilized postoperatively with a Kirschner wire for 10 days and then by controlled intermittent splinting. These procedures will be most effective if the neurovascular bundle on only one side of the finger is damaged. In all instances of release, the tourniquet should be deflated and the vascularity of the finger inspected frequently. In poor situations, arthrodesis or amputation may be indicated.

Pulley reconstruction

The basic anatomy of the flexor pulley system is a precise biomechanical design that permits lubricated gliding of two tendons while transmitting the power of the forearm musculature to the bones of the fingers (Figs. 27-14 and 27-16). After stage I, the functional arc of motion for grip, cannot be restored despite good hand-therapy programs.

The pulley retinaculum is preserved when possible and some collapsed sections may be dilated by instrumentation. If the pulley segments are of insufficient size to carry the implant, they should be excised, with a flap of the base portion in the periosteum being left for suture during tendon graft pulley reconstruction. The pulleys are then dilated with a hemostat and tested for strength and integrity. If the A_1, A_2, and A_4 pulleys appear weak or are absent, they are reconstructed. Four pulleys are preferred: one proximal to each of the three finger joints and one at the base of the proximal phalanx (Fig. 27-17).

Tendon material (flexor digitorum superficialis or pro-

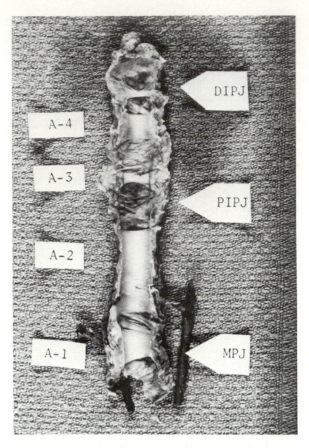

FIG. 27-16. Anatomic dissection of flexor canal viewed from within.

fundus) to be discarded is excellent for pulley building. Several techniques may be applied, depending on location of injury and the surgeon's preference. We prefer to wrap it extraperiosteally and under the extensor apparatus. It is wrapped twice around the phalanx and sutured to itself or to the rim of the fibro-osseous canal (Fig. 27-18). This is performed over a sizer implant to prevent making the pulley too tight. The pulley should be as broad as possible, and an implant should be used that fills the tendon bed but does not bind on glide testing. The average-sized implant generally has been 3 to 4 mm and in men 4 to 5 mm (Fig. 27-19). The pulleys must not be unduly bulky or too close to the joint, or they may act as a mechanical block to flexion by abutting on one another.

Tendon implant sizers are passed through the pulley system. The finger is held flat on the table, and the implant is *moistened* and pulled gently back and forth. A malleable blunt tendon instrument is passed deep through the carpal tunnel to present in the forearm deep to the superficialis and superficial to the profundus. The instrument is passed gently when one is seeking the soft mesotenon spaces. Implant binding will occur most often at the narrow, flat distal (A_4) annulus requiring tendon-graft pulley reconstruction. The length of the implant is determined so that on full extension of the finger the proximal end can be seen 1 to 2 inches proximal to the wrist crease. The implant is then secured to the distal phalanx as previously described. One tests pas-

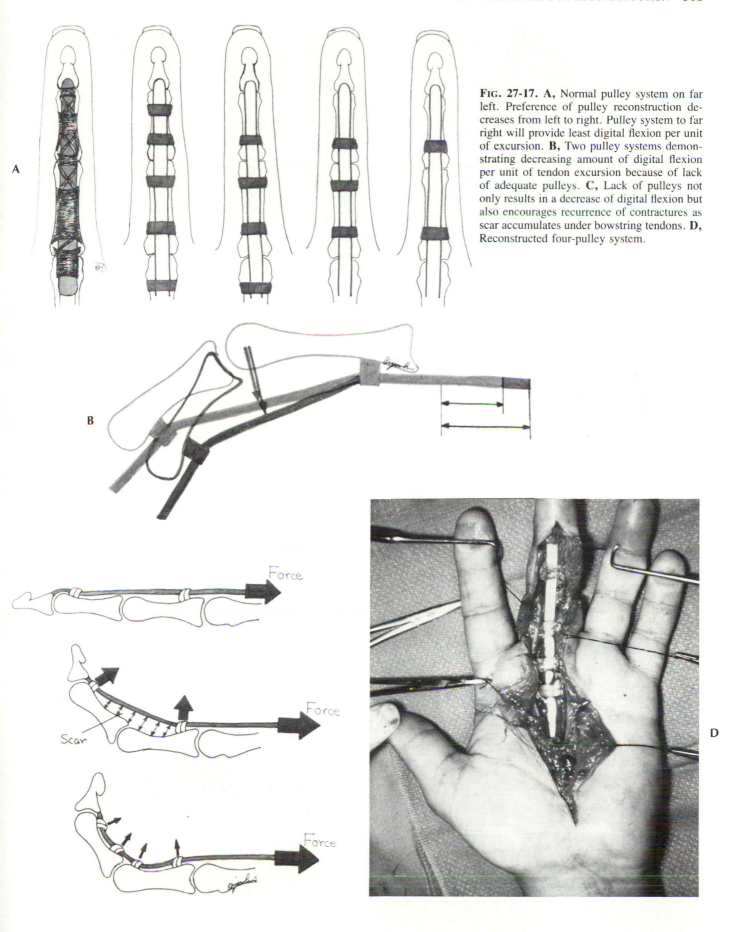

FIG. 27-17. A, Normal pulley system on far left. Preference of pulley reconstruction decreases from left to right. Pulley system to far right will provide least digital flexion per unit of excursion. **B,** Two pulley systems demonstrating decreasing amount of digital flexion per unit of tendon excursion because of lack of adequate pulleys. **C,** Lack of pulleys not only results in a decrease of digital flexion but also encourages recurrence of contractures as scar accumulates under bowstring tendons. **D,** Reconstructed four-pulley system.

FIG. 27-18. **A,** Sublimis remnant is wrapped under extensor apparatus and over implant to reconstruct the A_2 pulley. **B,** After tendon is wrapped around twice, it is sewn to itself and rim of fibro-osseous canal. Pulley should be as wide as possible without blocking motion itself.

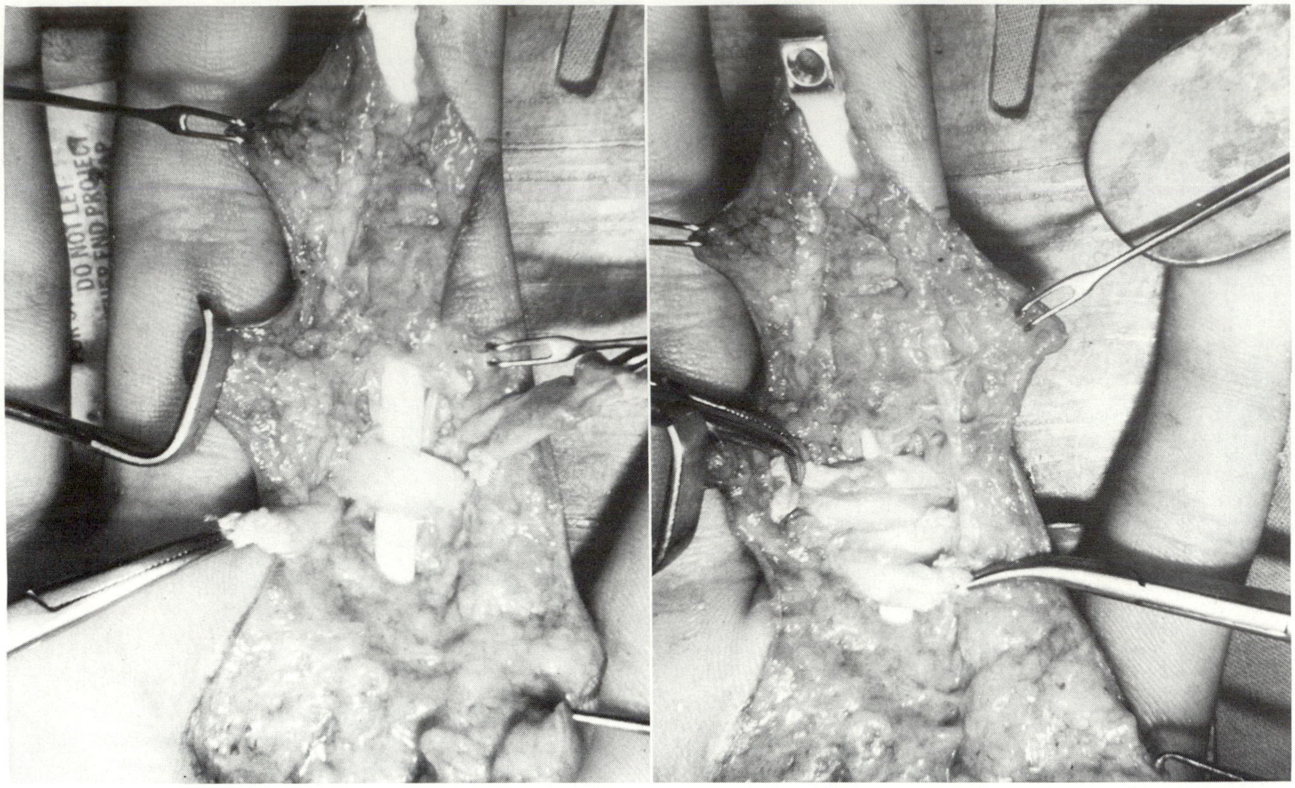

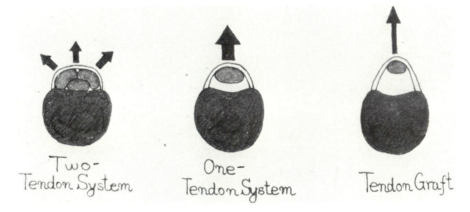

FIG. 27-19. The practice of replacing the anatomical two-tendon system with a small tendon graft causes a basic failure in the biomechanics of gliding. At stage I the pulley should be snug, and at stage II the tendon graft should closely represent the size of the new synovial space to enhance *good* flexion. Normal cannot be achieved; it was lost at injury.

sive gliding of the implant by moistening the implant bed with saline solution, holding the wrist and digit in neutral flexion while passively flexing and extending the finger. Motion should be free, with a measured range of motion between 3 and 4 cm at the proximal end. Buckling of the implant may occur distally to the tight pulley and, if present, must be corrected by free grafting before closure or a synovitis may develop between stage I and

stage II and adversely affect the development of the neosheath.

Testing the pulley system and recording range of motion constitute the important last maneuver of stage I before wound closure. The free proximal end of the implant is grasped and pulled, with the finger being brought from extension to maximum flexion. The following are recorded: (1) the predicted active range of motion versus the passive

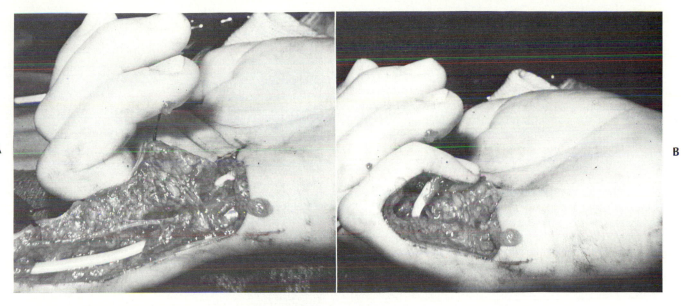

FIG. 27-20. A, Digital extension with implant in flexor canal. Notice lack of pulleys around proximal interphalangeal joint. **B,** Tension is placed on implant, and digital flexion is recorded. Notice deficient flexion because of lack of pulleys. Pulley reconstruction is indicated to maximize digital flexion.

range of motion; (2) the measured distance of the proximal end necessary to produce the active function (this will assist in selection of the stage II motor tendon); (3) the attitude of the finger in relation to the pulley system (if this maneuver does not produce full flexion or produces a pulley rupture, it may be necessary to modify the pulley system [Fig. 27-20]); and (4) the security of the distal end attachment of the tendon implant should be carefully checked. The implant is then placed in the interval between the flexor superficialis and flexor profundus. This interval must allow the implant to glide proximally without kinking when the metacarpophalangeal joints and wrist are flexed.

The wound is then closed distally to proximally, and finally the soft-tissue recess for the implant in the forearm is checked with a moistened gloved finger and passive gliding is reviewed. The hand is positioned with the wrist in 30 degrees of flexion, the metacarpophalangeal joints in 60 to 70 degrees of flexion, and the interphalangeal joints extended for closure and final dressing. This position after stage I permits the proximal sheath to form in the long position.

Postoperative therapy

During the first 3 weeks, the patient is kept in a dorsal extension-block plaster splint with the wrist flexed to 30 degrees, the metacarpophalangeal joint to 70 degrees, and the interphalangeal joints in extension. This position of flexion allows the neosheath to form deep into the forearm at the level where the subsequent motor will be close.[8] A roentgenogram of the hand is taken during the first and sixth weeks postoperatively for documentation of the excursion of the tendon with passive motion and for ascertainment of the integrity of the distal juncture.

The hand therapist and the surgeon confer with the patient during the first postoperative week. Gentle passive motion of all joints is started gradually during the first week. If a contracture was present preoperatively, extension splinting will be started in the splint between exercise sessions during the first weeks. Programmed activity and passive flexion devices are initiated at 3 weeks. Splinting for persistent flexion contractures will continue intermittently during the day and night (refer to Chapter 28). Usually by the sixth week there is a functional range of passive motion. During this time the hand should be examined regularly for evidence of synovitis in the new sheath. If this has not developed within the first 6 weeks, it is not likely to occur and the patient may resume normal activities, including going back to work, until he is ready for the second stage. If synovitis develops, as evidenced by swelling, the finger and wrist should be immobilized promptly. The cause of the synovitis should be sought and corrected. Overzealous therapy may be the cause, and rest of the digit will remedy this problem.

Joint range of motion should be recorded regularly between stages I and II, the movement and position of the implant in full extension and full flexion should be checked by roentgenograms. This should be done early when motion is started and later just before stage II surgery.

The timing between stages I and II can vary depending on the condition and biologic state of the hand. The sheath system theoretically could carry a tendon graft at 4 weeks, but the primary objective is a soft hand with maximal joint movements. Therefore most stage II surgery will be best planned at 3 to 4 months. The results of our research programs indicate that the well-balanced, compatible stage I implant could remain in place indefinitely without compromising the result of stage II tendon grafting. This is an important fact to remember as clinical research progresses with the active tendon prosthesis.

Complications

Complications are rare if the procedure has been performed meticulously with careful handling of the soft tissues and the implant. Proper postoperative therapy and careful monitoring of the patient's progress also help prevent any complications. The reported complications are synovitis infection and loosening of the distal juncture with proximal migration of the implant.

Synovitis is characterized by discomfort in the operated digit, swelling along the volar aspect of the finger, decreased motion, swelling at the incision site in the forearm, and lack of signs of systemic illness. Synovitis may result from improper handling of the implant at the time of insertion. Silicone rubber attracts free particles of lint or glove powder. This problem is best treated by prevention. As previously stated, the implant should be kept moist at all times and wet gloves should be used to handle the implant. Buckling of the implant under tight pulleys will also result in a synovitis. This also is easily prevented, by attention to detail at the time of pulley reconstruction. Overzealous therapy has also caused synovitis. However, this should resolve within 5 to 7 days of immobilization followed by gradual resumption of activity. Rupture of the distal juncture of the implant, the most common problem, and its subsequent proximal migration will result in a synovitis (Fig. 27-21). One should obtain a good distal juncture intraoperatively and follow up with roentgenographic observation at 1 and 6 weeks and before stage II. If the prosthesis becomes dislodged after stage I, one should rest the hand and proceed with the second-stage tendon graft.

If synovitis from all the above causes is not remedied by rest and immobilization, the stage II procedure should be performed earlier and the thickened synovium excised in the region of the proximal anastomosis. Continued mobilization of the digit in the face of a synovitis results in a thickened sheath, and the result will be a recurrence of contractures and loss of motion.

Infection is very rare and will usually manifest itself in the early postoperative period. Pain, fusiform swelling, lymphadenopathy, elevated temperature, and increased white blood count are the classic symptoms. The patient is systemically ill, and treatment should be immediate. Removal of the implant, immobilization, adequate irrigation, débridement, and appropriate antibiotics will resolve the problem. After the soft tissue is healed and the infection is resolved, there is no contraindication to performing the stage I procedure again. It is our practice to place the patient on perioperative antibiotics, as is done with most other orthopedic implants.

STAGE II SURGERY

As previously stated, the compliance of the patient in setting the tension in stage II greatly facilitates the outcome of this procedure. The anesthesia employed may be local and intravenous sedation (Innovar) in selected cases, or one can use routine general anesthesia.

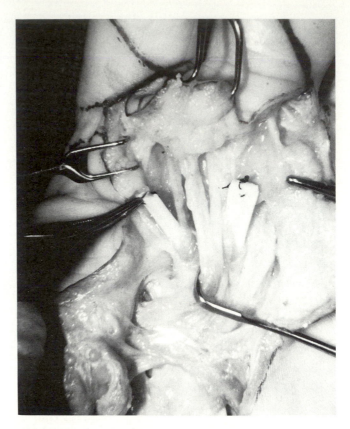

FIG. 27-21. Synovitis caused by rupture of distal juncture and proximal migration of implants into palm. Improper suture technique of the implant to profundus stump resulted in this avoidable complication.

On the operating table the passive range-of-motion improvements are frequently under tourniquet control, noted after stage I hand therapy. Distal and proximal incisions are made over the previous incisions for identification of the sheath and implant.

The exposure of the distal juncture should be adequate; however, it does not have to extend across the proximal interphalangeal joint. Care is taken not to injure the neosheath. After the distal juncture has been exposed, it is left intact and the proximal juncture is exposed. Proximally the implant is grasped with an instrument (rubber-shod forceps), and the sheath at the site of juncture is carefully examined. Portions of soft sheath may be retained at the surgeon's discretion. However, if synovitis has been present, the thickened sheath must be completely removed at the proximal juncture site to the wrist flexion crease. The active potential range of motion of the finger and the excursion necessary to produce it are determined by laying the hand and finger flat on the table and then firmly pulling the implant proximally. The surgeon should note (1) the excursion of the implant to produce the range of motion from maximum extension to maximum flexion (Fig. 27-22), (2) the distance the finger pulp rests from the distal palmar crease, (3) joints with restricted motion, and (4) the easy gliding of the implant and the fluid lubrication system of the tendon bed.

The motor tendon (flexor digitorum superficialis or flexor

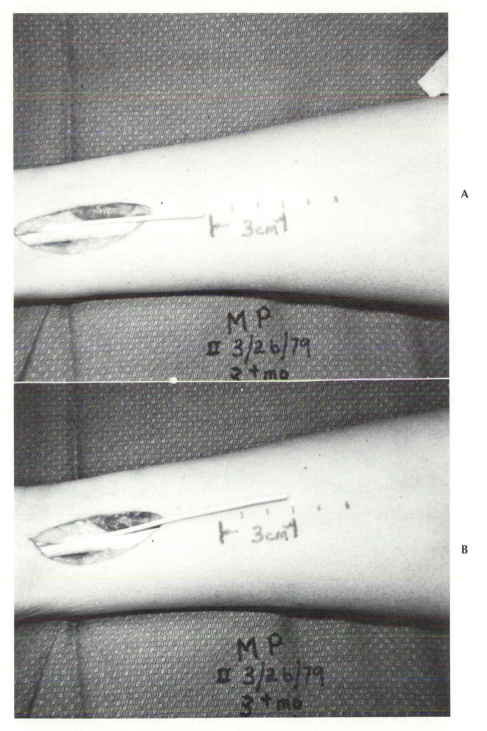

FIG. 27-22. A, Implant is exposed in forearm. **B,** Excursion of implant is 3 cm.

digitorum profundus) is selected and grasped with a small hemostat. The hand is elevated and the tourniquet released while the lower leg is prepared to remove a long plantaris tendon graft. The plantaris tendon is preferred because it is larger in size and usually approaches the size of the implant that is being removed, that is, approximately 3 mm. If the plantaris tendon is absent, a long toe extensor is harvested. Brand tendon stripper is utilized to harvest the grafts.[1,17]

I have frequently used a long toe extensor tendon when the plantaris is absent. This technique employs the Brand tendon stripper. If a toe extensor is utilized, it is usually necessary to make three or four transverse incisions to prevent injury to the graft. One incision is made at the metatarsophalangeal joint of the toe, the next just distal to the retinaculum of the ankle, and a third just proximal to the retinaculum. The tendon is stripped and passed through each

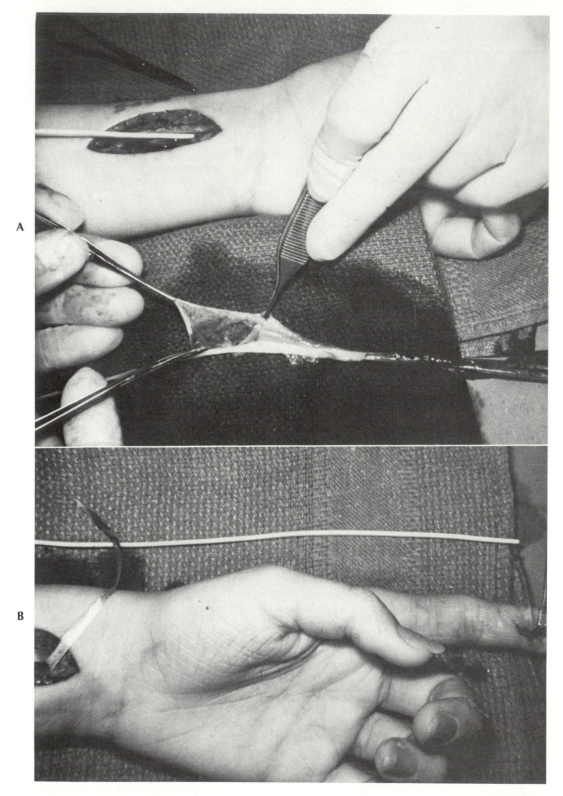

FIG. 27-23. A, Peritenon is carefully removed from tendon graft. **B,** Tendon graft has been sutured to proximal aspect of implant and then pulled into new tendon bed from proximal to distal position.

incision until the musculotendinous juncture is reached. The fifth toe should not be used because it usually has only one toe extensor. Shorter tendon grafts, palmaris longus, extensor indicis, extensor digiti minimi, and segments of superficialis are removed by standard technique and may be used for (1) thumb, little finger, and sublimis fingers with an attachment to the middle phalanx or (2) index, long, and ring fingers with an attachment to a tendon juncture in the uninjured palm.

The tendon graft, carefully stripped of all paratenon, is sutured to the proximal end of the implant and pulled through the new tendon bed (Fig. 27-23). The implant is detached from the distal phalanx and discarded.

A Bunnell type of weave is placed through the distal end of the graft with monofilament stainless steel, 4.0 wire.[2,3] A pull-out wire is no longer utilized. An oblique hole is made in the distal phalanx under the profundus stump remnant and enlarged with a curette. A Keith needle is drilled through the distal phalanx and exits dorsally in the middle of the nail. The wire suture is then pulled through the distal phalanx by threading of it through the Keith needle. As the Keith needle is advanced through the tip of the finger, one must watch the graft being pulled into the drill hole on the volar side of the finger. This tendon-to-bone juncture is most important and, when healed, will prevent any distal ruptures

of the graft. The wire is tied over a button on the dorsum of the fingernail (Fig. 27-24). Reinforcing sutures of 3-0 Mersilene polyester on either side of the graft will help anchor the distal juncture. After this is completed, the distal juncture is closed. If a sublimis finger is being performed, the same procedure is followed; however, the drill hole is placed at the base of the middle phalanx (Fig. 27-25).

Proximal juncture

The final phase of the stage II technique is directed toward completion of the proximal juncture. The motor is selected, and the graft is placed through the tendon motor temporarily and fixed with either wire or Mersilene fiber. The attitude of the finger with the wrist in neutral should be one of slightly more flexion than the adjacent digit (Fig. 27-26). At this point, the patient's compliance is enhanced if the patient is under leptoanalgesia, alleviating the quesswork in setting the tension of the graft. The patient is asked to flex and extend his fingers, and the tension of the graft is then adjusted accordingly. The selected tendon motor must supply the same excursion or better if a good result is to be achieved. When the tension is correct, the graft is woven through the motor tendon and sutured into place using the technique described by Pulvertaft (Fig. 27-27).

The Pulvertaft end-weave technique is preferred for a

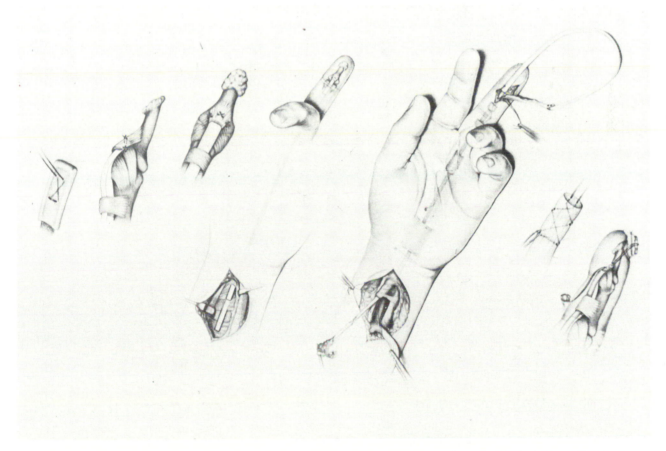

FIG. 27-24. Diagram of stage I procedure, the four figures on left, and of stage II, the three figures on right. (From Hunter, J.M., and Salisbury, R.E.: J. Bone Joint Surg. **53A**:836, 1971.)

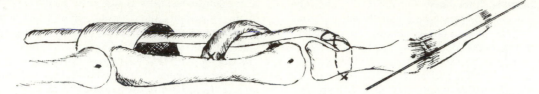

FIG. 27-25. Stage I. Sublimis finger. Implant is carried to base of middle phalanx and fixed in place by wire suture passed through two small drill holes. Reinforcing sutures are added. Distal phalanx is either tenodesed or arthrodesed.

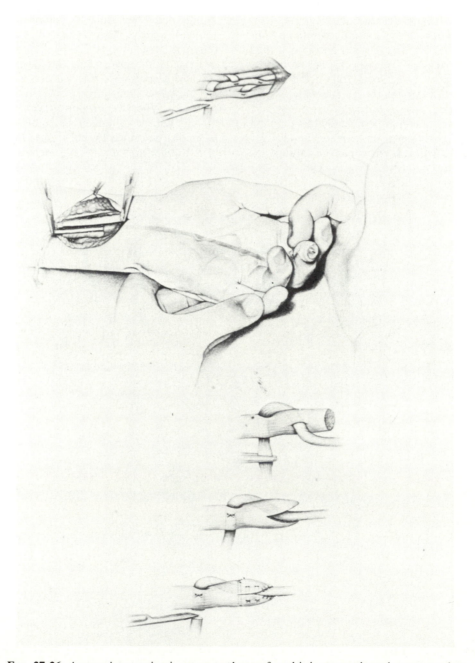

FIG. 27-26. Appropriate tension is set on tendon graft and it is woven through motor tendon.

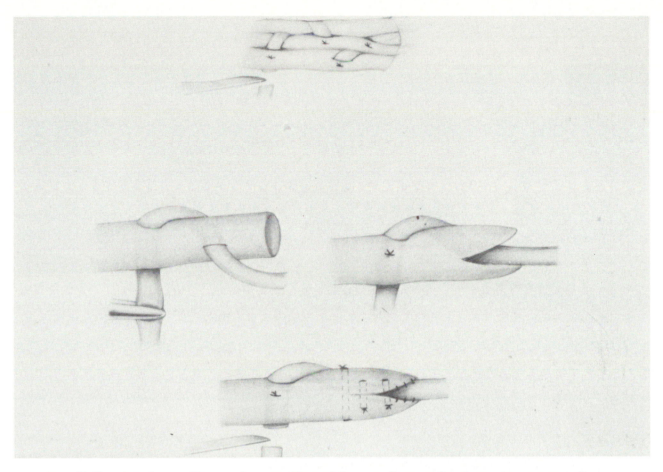

FIG. 27-27. Pulvertaft type of weave of motor tendon graft juncture. Care must be taken to assure passage of sutures through donor and recipient tendons to avoid complication of proximal anastomosis rupture.

single tendon juncture, that is, profundus of the index, flexor pollicis, or superficialis. The multiple end weave is preferred for a profundus, long, ring, or little finger juncture. It is extremely important to make sure that the suture passes through the graft and into the motor to prevent subsequent slipping of the proximal juncture. One must also be sure that the neosheath does not impede excursion of the tendon graft juncture, and, if necessary, more of the proximal sheath should be excised to permit full extension.

After repeated manipulations of the finger, it remains in slightly more flexion than normal. The juncture is completed by a second interweave and suture fixation, and the wound is closed. The postoperative plaster splint dressing fits securely with the wrist in 30 degrees of flexion, metacarpophalangeal joints in 70 degrees of flexion, and interphalangeal joints extended.

Superficialis finger

An alternative technique for the serious salvage situation is a superficialis finger. This useful technique is indicated in contracted fingers with poor nutrition, multiple-finger situations, and fingers with mallet deformities or poor distal interphalangeal joint function. By eliminating distal interphalangeal motion (tenodesis or arthrodesis) the surgery-therapy team can concentrate on metacarpophalangeal and

proximal interphalangeal motion only. This arc of motion represents approximately 85% of the normal need for grip, thereby simplifying postoperative training.

At stage I the implant is carried to the base of the middle phalanx and fixed in place by a wire suture passed through two small drill holes. Reinforcing sutures are added. The distal phalanx is either tenodesed or arthrodesed (Fig. 27-25). At stage II, reconstruction for the superficialis finger follows the same procedure as described for tendon grafting to the distal phalanx. If the range of motion at the metacarpophalangeal and proximal interphalangeal joints is good, the superficialis finger is a very acceptable salvage technique. A possible complication after stage II tendon grafting is pulley rupture, distal or proximal to the proximal interphalangeal joint, resulting in a bowed finger. A useful result may be salvaged by detachment of the tendon graft distally and attachment of the graft to the base of the middle phalanx. Tenodesis or arthrodesis of the dorsal interphalangeal joint completes this procedure.

Postoperative therapy

Postoperative therapy of stage II begins in the operating room. The application of the padded dorsal splint prevents sudden forceful extension, which may rupture the graft. The wrist should be in 30 degrees of flexion, the metacarpo-

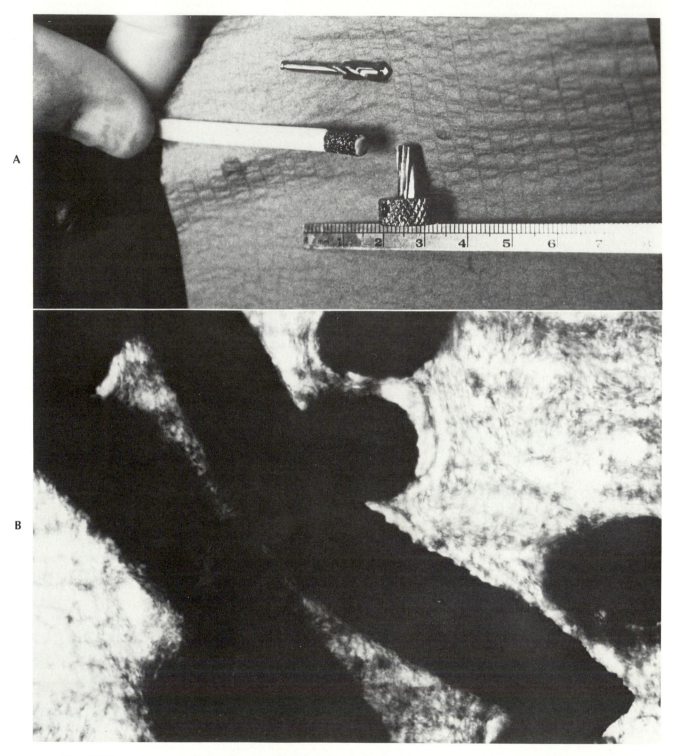

FIG. 27-28. A, Porous-titanium distal juncture on active tendon prosthesis and drill bits used to implant prosthesis into terminal phalanx. **B,** High-power microscopic appearance of distal juncture in terminal phalanx at 4 weeks. Dark areas are titanium fibers; light areas are woven bone.

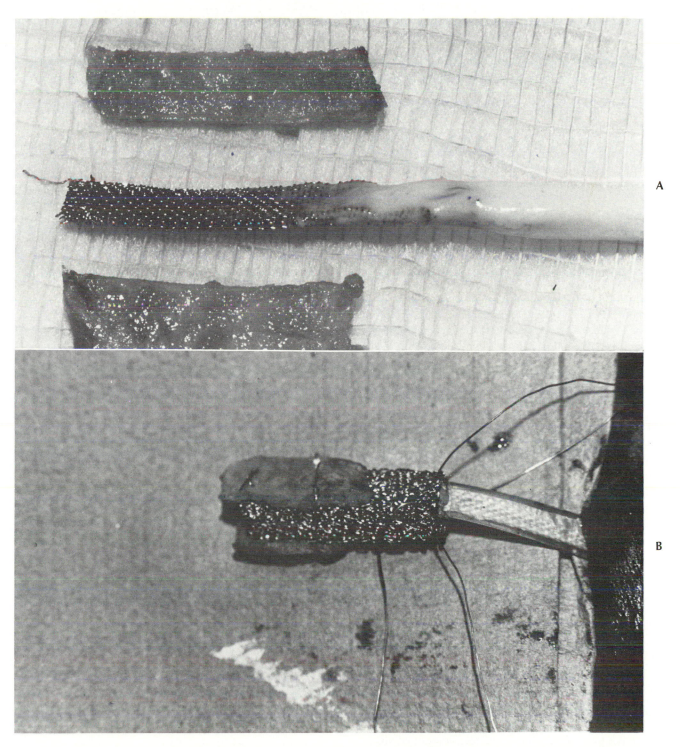

FIG. 27-29. A, Proximal porous-titanium juncture and cortical bone grafts. **B,** Unit prepared for implantation into motor unit.

phalangeal joints in 70 degrees of flexion, and the interphalangeal joints in extension. The splint should not block full extension of the proximal interphalangeal joints. The splint should be secured at the wrist with tape to prevent any slipping that could result in undue tension on the graft junctures. Elastic traction is applied in the operating room on the first day or within the first postoperative week when the patient is allowed to extend the finger actively while in the splint and the elastic band will then flex the finger passively. Particular attention should be paid to the distal and proximal interphalangeal joints for prevention of flexion contractures. (Refer to Chapter 28.)

At 5 to 6 weeks, the pull-out button is removed, and by 6 to 8 weeks, the extension block splint is also discarded. Hydrotherapy and gentle active and passive flexion of the wrist and the finger joints are begun. By 8 weeks, light resistive exercises are begun. Heavy resistive exercises are not utilized until 12 weeks postoperatively.

Complications

There are two complications after stage II tendon grafting that deserve discussion: (1) adhesions along the tendon graft or at the proximal anastomosis and (2) rupture around the anastomosis of the tendon graft. Restrictive adhesions may occur anywhere along the course of the graft; however, they are most common at the anastomosis. They are also prone to occur in areas where there is poor graft gliding and thus an inadequate fluid nutrition system. This may happen in areas where the pulleys are too tight or there has been dense scar. If these adhesions significantly restrict motion, a tenolysis procedure should be performed.

If *tenolysis* is necessary for adhesions, it is performed 4 to 6 months after stage II using local anesthesia, Innovar analgesia, and a tourniquet control.[4,12] The region of the proximal anastomosis should be explored first, with attention directed initially to the junction of the new tendon sheath and the tendon graft, then to the proximal anastomosis, and last to the tendon graft within the new sheath. Only adhesions that actually restrict motion should be treated.

After surgery, immediate active motion of the lysed tendon graft is necessary to preserve the increased ranges of motion. Many of these patients will return to therapy with an indwelling Jackson-Pratt catheter placed next to the digital nerves and 0.5% marcaine is injected every 4 to 6 hours postoperatively to minimize pain and maximize active movement. The catheter can be left in place up to 5 days. All these patients will require a most carefully coordinated management program directed by surgeon and therapist. (Refer to Chapter 26.)

Rupture of the graft can occur at either end and is usually attributable to faulty operative technique. One must be sure that the tendon is drawn into the bone at the distal juncture. If there is a good tendon-bone interface, rupture at this area is highly unlikely once healing has occurred. Rupture early at the proximal juncture is usually the result of missing the tendon graft with the suture when one is performing the Pulvertaft weave.[13,14] If care is directed at suture placement, from distal tendon stump laxity and fibrous gap and usually is an operative technical problem.

Late tendon rupture is unusual but may occur if extreme force is applied. Immediate exploration is indicated, for it is often possible to reattach the graft, particularly in instances where the patient had a good gliding situation before rupture.

THE FUTURE

Presently, the procedure of two-stage tendon grafting utilizing the passive Hunter tendon implant has proved to be a consistently reliable method of salvaging the scarred tendon systems. The active tendon system will be available commercially in the future. These active implants offer the opportunity of ''tuning'' the tendon motor unit while the neosheath is forming. Both these implants at this time require two surgical procedures. The future will, one would hope, yield a permanent tendon prosthesis, which would eliminate the need for any subsequent operative procedure. The previous attempts at active tendon prosthesis have failed because of the lack of strength and durability of the proximal and distal junctures.

This problem of juncture strength is being studied experimentally by use of a porous titanium distal juncture that is implanted into a drill hole in the distal phalanx (Fig. 27-28). Within 4 weeks, woven bone ingrowth occurs into the titanium plug resulting in a strong and durable interface. The proximal juncture is bonded to the muscle by interposition of cortical grafts between the porous titanium and the muscle. The bone grows into the titanium, and the muscle heals to bone. This graded interface results in a strong durable attachment (Fig. 27-29). This prototypic active tendon prosthesis has been successfully implanted into adult chimpanzees. Clinical studies are progressing, and it is hoped that a permanent active tendon prosthesis will be available in the near future.

SUMMARY

The two-stage tendon graft technique utilizing the Hunter tendon implant has been clinically proved to be a consistently reliable technique of salvaging scarred tendon systems.[6,10] The production of a neosheath provides the fluid nutrition system for nourishment of the subsequent tendon graft. This fluid nutrition system, combined with early protected gliding of the graft, has resulted in a significant reduction of postoperative adhesions. The release of contractures and the reconstruction of pulleys of the proper size, location, and quantity, combined with a supervised therapy program, result in maximal postoperative digital motion.

Meticulous, well-planned surgery, preceded and followed by appropriate supervised therapy, is the key to a successful two-stage procedure.

REFERENCES

1. Brand, P.: Principles of free tendon grafting, including a new method of tendon suture, J. Bone Joint Surg. **41B:**208, 1959.
2. Bunnell, S., editor: Hand surgery in World War II, Medical Department of the United States Army, Office of the Surgeon General, Department of the Army, Washington, D.C., 1955, p. 49.
3. Bunnell, S.: Bunnell's surgery of the hand, ed. 4, revised by J.H. Boyes, Philadelphia, 1964, J.B. Lippincott Co.
4. Erickson, J.C., III, Hunter, J.M., and Schneider, L.H.: Neuroleptanalgesia and local anesthesia for a dynamic approach to surgery of the

hand, video tape narrative description, scientific exhibit, American Academy of Orthopaedic Surgeons, April 11-14, 1976, Philadelphia, Pa.

5. Hunter, J.M.: Artificial tendons: early development and application, Am. J. Surg. **109**:325, 1965.

6. Hunter, J.M., and Aulicino, P.L.: Salvage of the scarred tendon systems utilizing the Hunter tendon implant. In Flynn, J.E., editor: Hand surgery, ed. 3, Baltimore, 1981, The Williams & Wilkins Co.

7. Hunter, J.M., and Jaeger, S.H.: The active gliding tendon prosthesis: progress. In American Academy of Orthpaedic Surgeons: Symposium on tendon surgery in the hand, St. Louis, 1975, The C.V. Mosby Co.

8. Hunter, J.M., and Jaeger, S.H.: Tendon implants: primary and secondary usage, Orthop. Clin. North Am. **8**(2):473-489, 1977.

9. Hunter, J.M., and Jaeger, S.H.: Flexor tendon implants and prostheses. In Rubin, L.R., editor: Biomaterials in reconstructive surgery, St. Louis, 1983, The C.V. Mosby Co.

10. Hunter, J.M., and Jaeger, S.H.: Staged tendon grafting using tendon implants. In Tubiana, R., editor: The hand, Philadelphia, W.B. Saunders Co., vol. 3, Ch. 29. (In press.)

11. Hunter, J.M., Schneider, L.H., and Fietti, V.G.: Reconstruction of the sublimis finger, Orthop. Trans. **3**:321-322, 1979.

12. Hunter, J.M., Schneider, L.H., Dumont, J., and Erickson, J.C., III.: A dynamic approach to problems of hand function: using local anesthesia supplemented by intravenous fentanyl-droperidol, Clin. Orthop. **104**:112-115, 1974.

13. Pulvertaft, R.G.: Tendon grafts for flexor tendon injuries in the fingers and thumb: a study of technique and results, J. Bone Joint Surg. **38B**:175-194, 1956.

14. Pulvertaft, R.G.: Experiences in flexor tendon grafting in the hand, J. Bone Joint Surg. **41B**:629-630, 1959.

15. Tubiana, R.: Greffes des tendons fléchisseurs des doigts et du pouce: technique et résultats, Rev. Chir. Orthop. **46**:191-214, 1960.

16. Verdan, C.E.: Primary and secondary repair of flexor and extensor tendon injuries. In Flynn, J.E., editor: Hand surgery, Baltimore, 1966, The Williams & Wilkins Co., pp. 220-275.

17. White, W.L.: Secondary restoration of finger flexion by digital tendon grafts: an evaluation of seventy-six cases, Am. J. Surg. **91**:662-668, 1956.

BIBLIOGRAPHY

Brand, P.: Principles of free tendon grafting, including a new method of tendon suture, J. Bone Joint Surg. **41B**:208, 1959.

Bruner, J.M.: The zig-zag volar digital incision for flexor tendon surgery, Plast. Reconstr. Surg. **40**:571-574, 1967.

Doyle, J.R., and Blythe, W.: The finger flexor tendon sheath and pulleys: anatomy and reconstruction. In American Academy of Orthopaedic Surgeons: Symposium on tendon surgery in the hand, St. Louis, 1975, The C.V. Mosby Co.

Hunter, J.M., and Salisbury, R.E.: Use of gliding artificial implants to produce tendon sheaths: techniques and results in children, Plast. Reconstr. Surg. **45**:564, 1970.

Hunter, J.M., and Salisbury, R.E.: Flexor tendon reconstruction in severely damaged hands, J. Bone Joint Surg. **53A**:829, 1971.

Hunter, J.M., Subin, D., Minkow, F., and Konikoff, J.: Sheath formation in response to limited active gliding implants (animals), J. Biomed. Mater. Res. **5**(1):163, 1974.

Hunter, J.M., Steindel, C., Salisbury, R., and Hughes, D.: Study of early sheath development using static non-gliding implants, J. Biomed. Mater. Res. **5**(1):155, 1974.

Hunter, J.M.: Artificial tendons: early development and application, Am. J. Surg. **109**:325-338, 1965.

Hunter, J.M.: Artificial tendons: their early development and application, J. Bone Joint Surg. **47A**:631-632, 1965.

Hunter, J.M.: Two-stage tendon reconstruction using gliding tendon implants. In Rob, C., and Smith, R.: Operative surgery, Sevenoaks, Kent, 1978, Butterworth & Co. (Pubs), Ltd., pp. 601-616.

Hunter, J.M., and Jaeger, S.H.: Tendon implants: primary and secondary usage, Orthop. Clin. North Am. **8**(2):473-489, 1977.

Hunter, J.M., and Jaeger, S.H.: The active gliding tendon prosthesis: progress. In American Academy of Orthopaedic Surgeons: Symposium on tendon surgery in the hand, St. Louis, 1975, The C.V. Mosby Co.

Hunter, J.M., Salem, A.W., Steindel, C.R., and Salisbury, R.E.: The use of gliding artificial tendon implants to form new tendon beds, J. Bone Joint Surg. **51A**:790, 1969.

Pulvertaft, R.G.: Tendon grafts for flexor tendon injuries in the fingers and thumb: a study of technique and results, J. Bone Joint Surg. **38B**:175, 1956.

Pulvertaft, R.G.: Experiences in flexor tendon grafting in the hand, J. Bone Joint Surg. **41B**:629, 1959.

Rayner, C.R.W.: The origin and nature of pseudo-synovium appearing around implanted Silastic rods: an experimental study, Hand **8**:101, 1976.

Urbaniak, J.R., Bright, D.S., Gill, L.H., and Goldner, J.L.: Vascularization and the gliding mechanism of free flexor-tendon grafts inserted by the silicone-rod method, J. Bone Joint Surg. **56A**:473, 1974.

28

Therapist's management of staged flexor tendon reconstruction

EVELYN J. MACKIN

After trauma to the hand, tendons not severed or severely crushed may be activated again by supervised motion programs. Often, however, in spite of careful primary treatment, the tendon and the tendon sliding bed have been so damaged that a healing complex of scar develops and tendon function is lost. If this is the case, a two-stage tendon graft procedure using a silicone-Dacron reinforced gliding implant to assist organization of a new tendon bed may be indicated. The implant is inserted as the first stage of the two-stage tendon reconstruction. The implant stimulates the formation of a sheath that provides a smooth gliding surface and a nutritional mechanism. The tendon implant is removed at approximately 3 months for stage II tendon grafting.[1-6]

When the surgeon has determined that the patient is a candidate for two-stage tendon procedure, the patient is referred to the hand therapist for orientation, evaluation, and a therapy program. The orientation should cover the entire therapy program, from before stage I surgery to after stage II surgery, emphasizing the role of the patient as a member of the hand rehabilitation team. An anatomic model of the hand with the tendon implant in place can be useful in explaining the purpose of the implant to the patient.

STAGE I
Preoperative therapy

Preoperative therapy is necessary in that the condition of a very poor finger, such as one with joint stiffness, limitation of passive motion, or flexion contracture, can be improved before stage I surgery. Preoperative therapy includes whirlpool bath, massage, active and passive exercise, and splinting.

The whirlpool bath, providing heat and relaxation of muscles, is an excellent preliminary to massage. Lanolin or cocoa butter massage softens tissues.

The patient who cannot actively flex his finger because of the loss of the flexor tendon system (Fig. 28-1) is shown how to trap the involved finger into flexion with the adjacent finger to increase its pliability. The Velcro trapper (Fig. 28-2) is an aid for incorporating the finger without a flexor tendon system into useful function. The injured finger and the adjacent normal finger are strapped together to simulate active flexion. Whenever the adjacent finger is used, the involved finger must also come into play. The trapper pro-

vides a means for the patient to carry out his activities of daily living and in many instances permits him to return to his employment between stage I surgery and stage II surgery. The use of the trapper aids in the conditioning of the finger, preventing further stiffness and aiding in venous return.

Web straps and the passive flexion glove as described in Chapter 18 provide a means to increase passive finger flexion. Ideally the patient should be able to passively touch the distal palmar crease before stage I. The better the range of motion, the better the final result. If a patient is to be able to actively flex to the distal palmar crease after stage II surgery, he must attain the passive potential preoperatively. Measurements are taken and recorded.

Splinting to correct flexion contractures begins before stage I surgery and continues through stage I and stage II. It must be emphasized that a flexion contracture before stage I can become a worse problem after stage II. Splinting to correct and prevent further contractures must be integrated into the patient's daily regimen during the entire tendon reconstruction procedure. In patients who have a deep cicatrix resulting from previous injury or previous surgery, or who form scar tissue easily, it may be necessary to continue night-extension splinting for 6 months after stage II.

A variety of splinting techniques may be used to correct flexion contractures. Extension splints may be fabricated from a thermoplastic material or a strip of aluminum padded with foam.

When passive flexion of the finger is limited and full extension of the proximal interphalangeal joint is limited, the patient should alternate the extension splint with the flexion device; that is, the web strap is worn intermittently during the day and the extension splint worn at night. Whatever the plan, correction of flexion deformities and maximum passive flexion of the finger are essential before stage I surgery.

Surgery

When the surgeon is satisfied with the preoperative condition of the hand, the patient is scheduled for stage I surgery. At surgery the implant is placed in the distal part of the forearm, through the palm, and under the pulleys, and secured distally to the profundus stump or to the distal phalanx (Fig. 28-3). No proximal juncture is made. This is a passive gliding implant. An alernate method uses the Hunt-

314

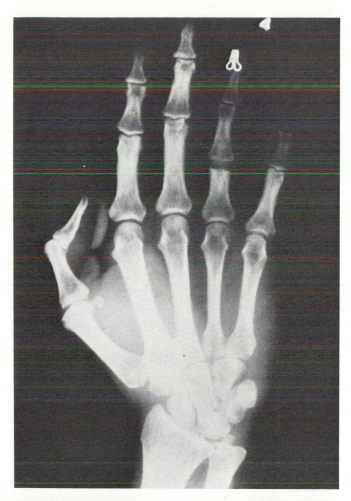

FIG. 28-1. Microsurgical replantation of the ring finger with insertion of a Swanson Silastic implant in the proximal interphalangeal joint. The patient, a 49-year-old right-handed welder, had sustained a band saw amputation of the left ring finger at the proximal interphalangeal joint, with partial amputation of the small finger at the distal interphalangeal joint. The patient suffered a myocardial infarction 3 days after discharge from hospital. There was no previous cardiac history or any indication of cardiac distress while in the hospital. As a result, therapy was not initiated until 7 weeks after replantation. At that time the wound had healed; however, the delay in beginning therapy, because of his cardiac problems, resulted in an adhered flexor tendon system in the ring finger limiting active flexion. He became a candidate for staged tendon reconstruction. Figs. 28-2 to 28-14 also illustrate this patient's case.

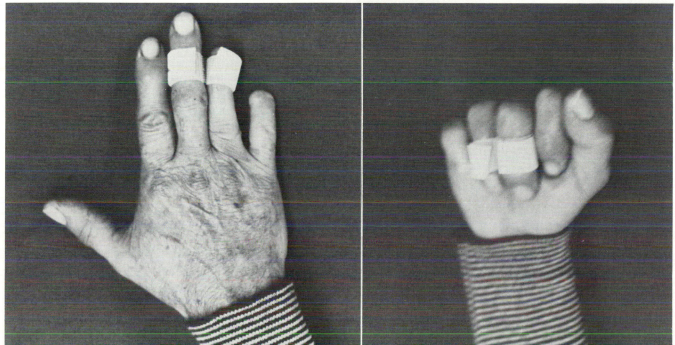

A   B

FIG. 28-2. Joint stiffness and limitation of passive motion can be improved with the use of a Velcro trapper. **A,** Extension. **B,** Flexion.

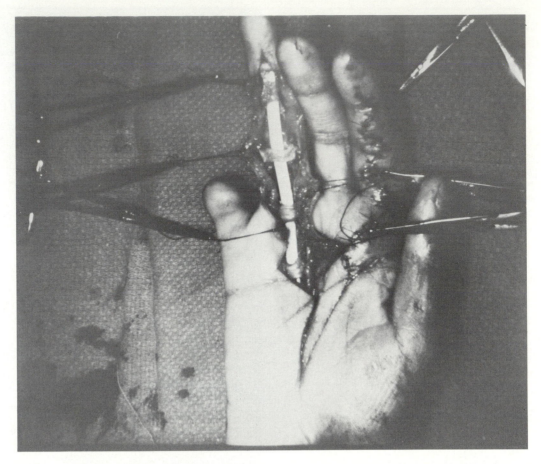

FIG. 28-3. Scarred flexor digitorum profundus and flexor digitorum superficialis resected. Tendon implant inserted under four reconstructed pulleys and secured to distal phalanx.

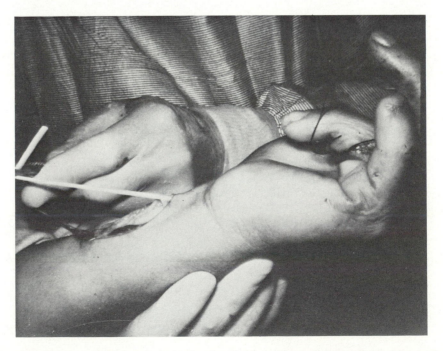

FIG. 28-4. Free proximal end of implant is grasped and pulled by surgeon, bringing finger into maximum flexion.

er-Hausner Passive Tendon Implant,* in which the distal attachment is securely fixed to the bone using a metal end device and screw. This permits forceful flexion of the finger at surgery—the only real opportunity for assessment of the mechanics of the finger pulley system before therapy training of the tendon-grafted finger after stage II. The implant is grasped at the proximal end by the surgeon and several kilograms of force are put on the pulley system as the finger flexes (Fig. 28-4). Weak pulleys that rupture or attenuate will require reconstruction as described in Chapter 27. As the surgeon grasps the tendon and the finger flexes to the distal palmar crease, he or she also gets an active potential prediction.[4-6]

---

*Hunter-Hausner Passive Tendon Implant, Holter-Hausner International, P.O. Box 1, Bridgeport, Pa. 19405.

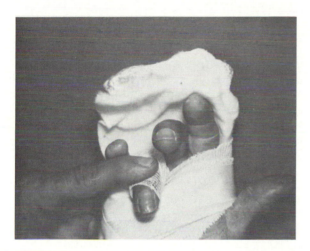

FIG. 28-5. Gentle passive motion is initiated the first week after stage I surgery.

It is helpful for the therapist to understand the pulley system of the finger. Every effort is made by the surgeon to reconstruct weakened or destroyed pulleys. If this is not done, a weak pulley may rupture during a training session with the therapist. An absent pulley means an alteration in tendon function. When this occurs, the patient will never achieve his full flexion despite the best therapy efforts.

Postoperative therapy

Postoperatively the hand is placed in a plaster splint for 3 weeks to permit organization of the new sheath around the implant. The wrist is positioned in 30-degree flexion, the metacarpal joints in 60- to 70-degree flexion, and the interphalangeal joints in extension. Light protected function is started in the first week. It consists of gentle passive flexion (Fig. 28-5) and light finger trapping.

When a proximal interphalangeal or distal interphalangeal flexion contracture was present before stage I surgery, it is very likely to recur after stage I. The therapist must be alert to a beginning flexion contracture as early as the first day. If the patient is not able to extend his proximal or distal joints fully, splinting will be initiated. An aluminum metacarpophalangeal block splint, as described in Chapter 23, will be fabricated and worn within the dorsal splint. It will be worn day and night and removed only for exercise.

The protective dorsal splint is removed 3 weeks postoperatively, and programmed activity is begun. Whirlpool bath and massage are initiated. The patient continues with finger trapping (Fig. 28-6) and progresses to the use of the Velcro trapper. Splinting for stubborn flexion contractures will continue intermittently during the day and at night.

Patients are carefully observed for the presence of synovitis. Synovitis may occur when a zealous patient or therapist overexercises the finger, resulting in a painful, shiny, swollen finger. Synovitis often responds to rest in a dorsal

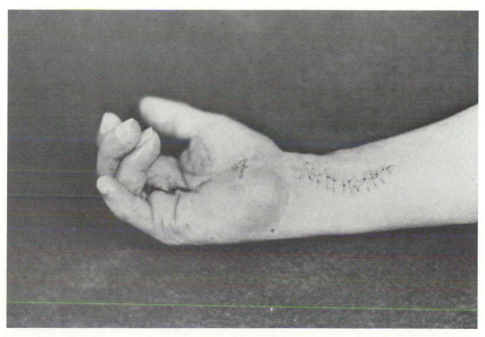

FIG. 28-6. Finger trapping.

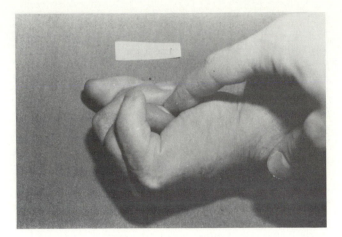

FIG. 28-7. Condition of patient's finger improved; finger supple with good skin condition; active potential of 1.5 cm achieved (1.5 cm at stage I surgery); Tinel sign to fingertip; x-ray film revealed good excursion of the tendon implant.

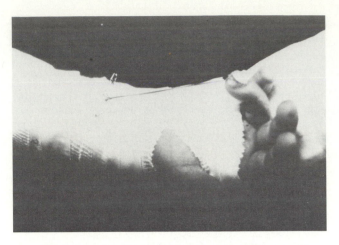

FIG. 28-8. Dynamic splinting initiated first day after stage II surgery. Active extension and passive flexion with elastic band attached to fingernail.

splint. Synovitis may also be caused by a mechanical problem of the implant, such as juncture disruption or buckling, or it may be due to irritants on the implant. If it cannot be controlled, the surgeon will perform the second stage of surgery early.

Usually by the sixth week, gliding of the implant should take place without complication, as evidenced by full passive flexion and extension. The patient can often return to work, depending on his job requirements, until he is scheduled for the second stage.

About 3 months is allotted between stage I and stage II to allow for optimal healing, softening of the tissues, and mobilization of the joints. The patient's hand should be upgraded to its maximum potential before stage II; ideally that means passive flexion of the finger pulp to the distal palmar crease (Fig. 28-7) and correction of flexion contracture. Roentgenograms to visualize the location of the tendon implant and demonstrate its gliding with passive flexion are taken before stage II surgery.

STAGE II
Surgery

At stage II surgery the patient's active potential is measured. The implant is pulled firmly, and the distance between the finger pulp and the distal palmar crease is recorded. If the patient's active potential is 1 cm from the distal palmar crease at stage II surgery, active flexion to within 1 cm of the distal palmar crease as a final result will be the goal.

The implant is replaced with a tendon graft. A plantaris or long toe extensor tendon graft may be used. The distal end is attached to the distal phalanx by use of standard techniques such as the Bunnell method of fixation with a button and pull-out wire. The proximal juncture might be made to superficialis or profundus tendon in the distal part of the forearm and palm.[4,5] A carefully fitted dorsal splint is applied to the patient's hand at surgery, with the wrist in 30-degree flexion, the metacarpophalangeal joints in 70-degree flexion, and the interphalangeal joints in 0-degree flexion.

One to 6 weeks after surgery

The patient is seen by the hand therapist on the first postoperative day. Constant supervision and encouragement by the surgeon and the hand therapist are vital. The surgeon relates to the therapist how much tension the tendon, the pulleys, and the juncture will tolerate. Only a complete understanding of the tendon graft procedure will give the therapist a safe guide to the postoperative phase of early motion. Patients should be seen by the surgeon once a week and by the therapist two or three times a week.

The patient's hand is maintained in the dorsal splint applied at surgery. The dressing applied to the fingers is partially removed so that passive flexion to the palm is possible within the confines of the splint. After partial removal of the dressing from the fingers the splint may not fit as securely as before. Adhesive tape should be applied across the forearm, wrist, and palm to ensure that the patient's hand will not slip back into the splint and put tension on the newly sutured junctures.

In selected cases of two-stage tendon reconstruction the surgeon may opt to incorporate elastic-band traction (Fig. 28-8) into the postoperative program. One advantage of the elastic-band traction is that it facilitates tendon and joint movement without requiring active pull on the flexor tendon. Another advantage is protection against sudden injury. Should the patient jerk the hand during sleep, or fall, the rubber band will protect the juncture from the stress of active flexion.

At surgery a nylon suture is put in the tip of the fingernail so that an elastic-band active training program may be initiated early in the postoperative period. It is preferable to wait until the first day after surgery, when the patient comes to therapy, so that the quality, positioning, and tension of the elastic band can be accurately established. The elastic band must be placed 3 to 4 inches proximally to the wrist crease on the volar aspect of the forearm dressing with the finger in its normal alignment. The tension should be adjusted so that the elastic band pulls the finger into flexion when resting and yet permits the antagonist muscles to com-

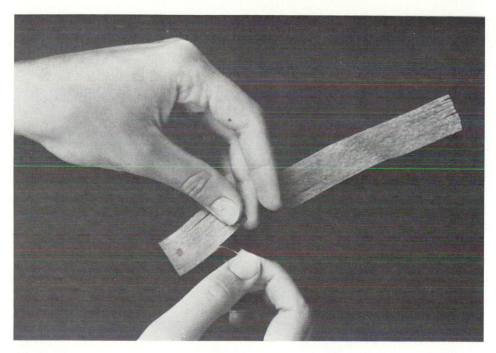

FIG. 28-9. Elastic thread.

pletely extend the finger within the limits of the dorsal splint so that flexion contractures will not develop.

The tension of the elastic band is very important. We have found that the commercially available graded rubber bands are never quite right. If such a rubber band holds the finger in the appropriate flexion at rest, it very often does not allow the patient to extend his finger fully against the tension of the rubber band. A failure to extend completely the proximal and distal interphalangeal joints will result in flexion contractures. We have found that the elastic that best suits our purpose is elastic thread.* It may be used as a single strand, and as the patient becomes stronger, the strands may be doubled to increase the tension (Fig. 28-9).

When the finger is flexed and at rest, there should be very little tension on the elastic band. Carefully positioned in the splint and with light tension on the elastic band, the patient may actively extend the finger and permit the elastic band to flex the finger passively five to 10 times each hour. In addition, gentle passive flexion of the proximal interphalangeal and distal interphalangeal joints is carried out for 10 repetitions three or four times a day.

Early attention to beginning flexion contractures is of primary importance because those patients who have difficulty with contractures before stages I and II are likely to develop recurrent contractures. If the dorsal splint does not allow full extension of the proximal interphalangeal joint, the patient must be instructed to flex passively the metacarpophalangeal joint of the involved finger to facilitate active extension of the interphalangeal joints. If the patient is able to extend fully his proximal interphalangeal joint in the described manner, further passive stretching will not be necessary.

When the therapist is alerted to interphalangeal joint contractures developing, passive extension of the interphalangeal joints may be begun as early as the first week. No "tendon-tension" passive extension may be initiated. Tension is taken off the tendon by flexion of the adjacent joint. With the dorsal splint supporting the wrist and the metacarpophalangeal joints in flexion, the therapist may support the metacarpophalangeal joint in flexion and gently passively extend the proximal interphalangeal joint to improve extension. If the distal interphalangeal joint shows a beginning contracture, the therapist may support the metacarpophalangeal and proximal interphalangeal joints in flexion and gently passively extend the distal interphalangeal joint (Fig. 28-10). Passive extension done by this technique decreases the tension at the tendon juncture. These passive extension exercises should be included in the patient's home program.

Despite all efforts to maintain full extension of the interphalangeal joints, persistent flexion contractures may require splinting as early as the first postoperative week. To correct this problem, gentle, prolonged, passive extension of the contracted joint is required. An AlumaFoam* splint that positions the metacarpophalangeal joint in greater flexion and gently pulls the contracted interphalangeal joint into extension is custom-fitted within the dorsal splint (Fig. 28-11). These should be worn intermittently during the daytime. The exact schedule will depend on the "feel" of the contractures, that is, whether they will quickly or slowly respond to stretching. With this technique of passive stretching, problems with flexion contractures can be minimized and overall tendon function enhanced.

*Elastic thread #7034, AliMed, 68 Harrison Ave., Boston, Mass. 02111.

*AlumaFoam, Conco Medical Co., Bridgeport, Conn. 06610.

When full excursion of the tendon graft occurs within the first 3 to 4 weeks postoperatively, it indicates the formation of minimal adhesions. In such a case the tendon junctures are under greater risk of rupture if stressed. If the tendon graft is sliding well, the measurements taken by the surgeon and the therapist indicate rapid improvement weekly in active flexion to the distal palmar crease, the patient will be maintained in the dorsal splint for 6 weeks. The button suture is removed at 5 to 6 weeks.

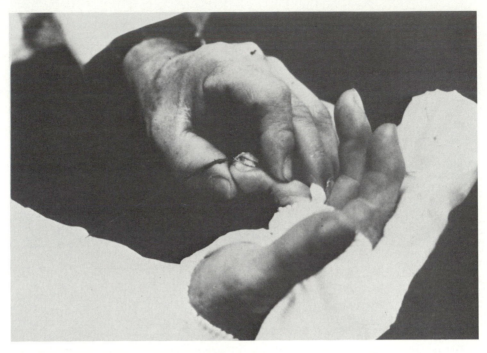

FIG. 28-10. Gentle passive extension of distal interphalangeal joint. Metacarpophalangeal and proximal interphalangeal joint flexion decreases tension at the tendon juncture.

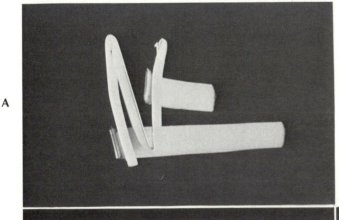

A

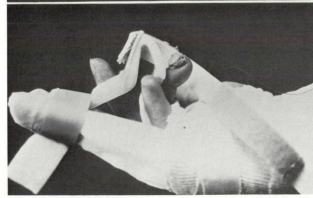

B

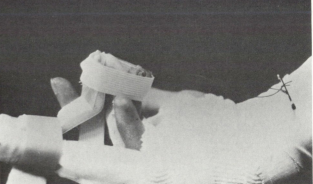

C

FIG. 28-11. A, AlumaFoam interphalangeal passive extension splint. **B,** AlumaFoam distal splint fitted within dorsal splint. Metacarpophalangeal and proximal interphalangeal joints are positioned in maximum flexion. **C,** Distal interphalangeal joint pulled gently into extension with Velcro strap.

Six to 12 weeks after surgery

As a further protection when the dorsal splint is removed, the patient's hand is maintained in a wristlet with elastic band traction, as described in Chapter 23. The purpose of the wristlet is to permit full active extension of the interphalangeal and metacarpophalangeal joints with the wrist in neutral. Wrist dorsiflexion may be done with the fingers resting in flexion.

At 8 to 10 weeks the wristlet is removed and the patient begins active flexion exercises, including finger blocking.

Exercises with putty may be initiated at this time. The whirlpool bath may be started again. Fingers that have shown stiffness before stage I may require softening with lanolin massage.

At 10 weeks, the patient may begin light supervised woodworking (such as sanding or filing) (Fig. 28-12). Progressive weight resistance exercise (Fig. 28-13) and heavy resistive exercises are not permitted until 3 months postoperatively (Fig. 28-14).

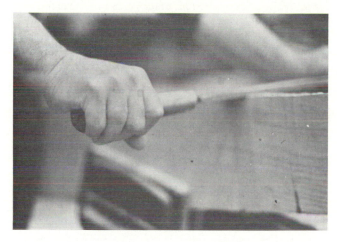

FIG. 28-12. Tendon and joint reconstruction enables patient to use ring finger as a stabilizer when using a tool in a sustained grip activity.

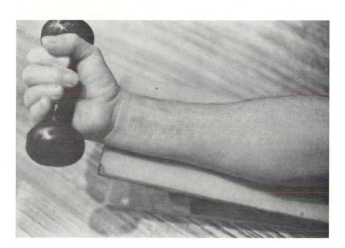

FIG. 28-13. Grip strengthening at 3 months.

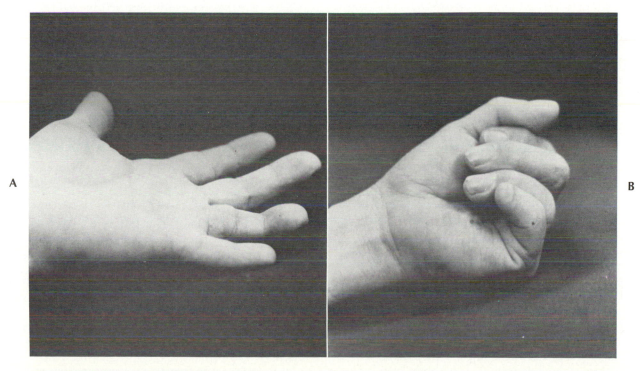

FIG. 28-14. When one considers the severe nature of this patient's amputating injury, with subsequent tissue ischemia and the unique problems of establishing adequate circulation to the replanted part, as well as the development of a new functionally adapted fibrous capsule for the Swanson Silastic implant, and tendon gliding following the two-stage tendon reconstruction using a Hunter tendon implant, and in addition the myocardial infarction, this patient at 12 weeks after surgery had come a long way. **A,** Extension. **B,** Flexion.

SPECIAL CONSIDERATIONS
Pulley reconstruction

At stage I surgery the surgeon may have to rebuild ruptured pulleys. He also will apply traction to the implant where pulleys seem to be satisfactory, to determine the active potential. If the finger cannot be fully flexed to the distal palmar crease, it may be necessary for the surgeon to modify the pulley system or to accept the reduced active potential as a final result after stage II.[4,5] This predicted potential is measured and recorded. Stage I postoperative therapy follows the same procedure as stage I without pulley reconstruction. Since this is a passive gliding implant, there is no tension on the pulley. When the A_2 pulley has been reconstructed after late stage II rupture or after tenolysis, it is essential to protect the pulley during active flexion for 6 weeks postoperatively. A thermoplastic ring may be fabricated (Fig. 28-15). Pulleys may also be supported by a finger from the patient's uninvolved hand during active flexion. With support, the patient may begin early active motion without stressing the pulley (Fig. 28-16).

Moleskin sling

When a nylon suture has not been attached to the tip of the fingernail at surgery, a sling of moleskin may be used to provide elastic-band traction around the button and pull-out wire (Fig. 28-17). A segment of moleskin about 3 inches long and ½ inch wide is folded in half, and an eyelet is punched through at the folded end of the moleskin. An S hook, made from a paper clip, is hooked through the eyelet opening and an elastic band is attached from it to a safety pin on the volar surface of the forearm dressing or (when the protective splint is no longer required) to a wrist cuff. Tincture of benzoin applied to the finger will help make the moleskin adhere.

Adhesions

Remember that each patient is an individual and that postoperative treatment must always be modified and changed according to the patient's progress. If active flexion improves steadily each week of reevaluation by the surgeon and the therapist, the program is not changed. If the formation of adhesions is limiting active motion, the dorsal splint will be discarded at 4 weeks and a more active exercise program will be initiated earlier, beginning with finger blocking and then progressing to resistive exercise with the Bunnell wood block (Chapter 18) and putty exercises at 5 weeks. Light sustained-grip activities, such as woodworking, would be instituted at 6 weeks, progressing to heavy-resistance exercise by the twelfth postoperative week.

Superficialis finger

In the case of severely injured fingers with stiffness, borderline circulation, and nerve defects, a superficialis finger implant and a later graft to the base of the middle phalanx and distal arthrodesis constitute a good solution. At stage I the implant is securely fixed to the base of the middle phalanx by suture or a screw fixation device. The distal phalanx is either tenodesed or arthrodesed. At stage II reconstruction the superficialis finger follows the same procedures as tendon grafting to the distal phalanx. Postoperative therapy is directed to the proximal interphalangeal joints, with good results. The training program becomes simplified and the result more predictable.[4,5]

EARLY ACTIVE MOTION
One to 6 weeks after stage II surgery

One to 6 weeks postoperatively active flexion may be initiated without the use of an elastic band. The method of distal fixation becomes very important if this method of early mobilization is utilized. Suture material and techniques must be strong enough to stand the stress. With this method of fixation, active flexion is initiated as early as the first day postoperatively within the dorsal splint applied at surgery. The same guidelines for this method of early motion are followed as were discussed for early motion utilizing elastic-band traction; for example, the dressing applied at surgery is partially pulled away from the fingers so that passive flexion is possible, and adhesive tape is applied across the palm, wrist, and forearm to secure the splint firmly.

The patient gently actively flexes the interphalangeal joints with the metacarpophalangeal joints in as much extension as is allowed by the dorsal splint, several times each hour. Passive flexion of the interphalangeal joints to the palm is also carried out, with 10 repetitions three or four times a day.

Passive fist-making may also be initiated early. The patient gently flexes his involved fingers into his palm with his uninvolved hand. He then releases the uninvolved hand, retaining the fist with his own muscle power. The force required to retain the fist in this manner is less than the force required to actively pull the fingers into flexion. Several repetitions of this exercise at full flexion and partial flexion may be performed several times a day.

If flexion contracture develops, a splinting program would be initiated with use of an aluminum passive extension splint, as previously described in this chapter.

Six to 12 weeks after stage II surgery

When the tendon junctures are strong, the surgeon may permit the patient to discard the dorsal splint and begin light active exercise at 6 weeks and light resistance at 8 weeks, progressing to heavy resistance by 3 months.

SUMMARY

Therapists who work with tendon reconstruction must have a feeling for tendons. Although there are time frames for moving the patient through the postoperative period, the therapist must consider each patient individually. The muscular man whose tendon graft slides and glides at 6 weeks is just the person who if removed from all protective splinting at that time is likely to go home and do push-ups and rupture an excellent result. Patients who demonstrate early excellent tendon gliding must be protected longer.

Postoperative management of staged tendon reconstruction must always be tailored to the surgical procedure. Each procedure has its own specific goals that lead to maximum hand function.

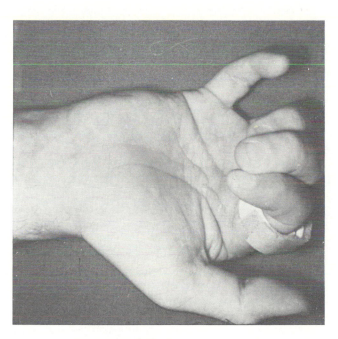

FIG. 28-15. Thermoplastic pulley ring.

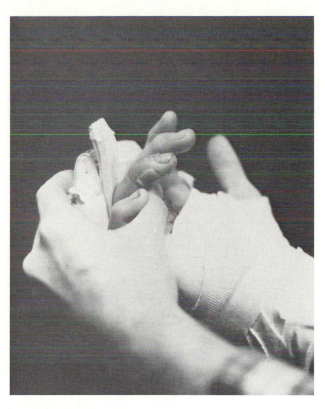

FIG. 28-16. Pulley supported with finger during active flexion.

A

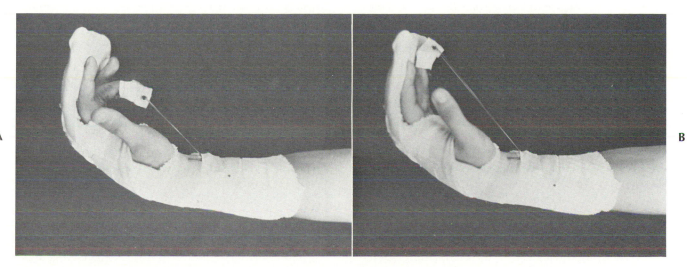

B

FIG. 28-17. Moleskin sling may be used to provide elastic-band traction. **A,** Passive flexion. **B,** Active extension.

REFERENCES

1. Mackin, E.J., and Hunter, J.M.: Pre- and post-operative hand therapy program for patients with staged gliding tendon prosthesis (Hunter design), Philadelphia, 1983, Hand Rehabilitation Foundation.
2. Boyes, J.H.: Flexor tendon grafts in the fingers and thumb—an evaluation of end results, J. Bone Joint Surg. **32A:**489, 1950.
3. Boyes, J.H.: Evaluation of results of digital flexor tendon grafts, Am. J. Surg. **89:**116-119, 1955.
4. Hunter, J.M.: Two-stage tendon reconstruction using gliding tendon implants. In Operative surgery—the hand, ed. 3, London, 1977, Butterworth & Co. (Publishers), Ltd., pp. 134-148.
5. Hunter, J.M., and Aulicino, P.L.: Salvage of the scarred tendon systems utilizing the Hunter tendon implant. In Flynn, J.E.: Hand surgery, ed. 3, Baltimore, 1981, The Williams & Wilkins Co.
6. Schneider, L.H.: Staged flexor tendon reconstruction using the method of Hunter, Clin. Orthop. **171:**164-171, 1982.

29

The extensor tendons

ERIK A. ROSENTHAL

Normal hand function mirrors the integrity of the extensor tendons. Their contribution to the balance, power, dexterity, and range of hand activities is critical, and any restraint upon them will be reflected in a proportional loss of function. The impact of an injury upon the extensor tendons is often regarded less seriously then a flexor tendon insult. The treatment and rehabilitation of the injury are often believed to be less intricate, less time consuming, and associated with a relatively favorable prognosis compared with flexor tendon injuries. The truth of experience, however, is that injuries to the extensor tendons can be equally complex, time consuming, frustrating, and disappointing. The extensor muscles are relatively weaker than their flexor antagonists. Their amplitude of glide is less, yet they require a latitude of motion that is not necessary for flexor function. The extensor tendons are relatively thin, broad structures that present a disproportionally large surface for injury and formation of restraining scar. The complex interrelationships in the intricately designed extensor tendons of the digits increase their susceptibility to injury and functional disarray. Virtually any interference with the extensor tendons or their investments is reflected in a functional deficiency.

WRIST EXTENSOR TENDONS

The wrist extensor tendons are the key to balanced hand function and the success of rehabilitation after an injury. Positional grip depends on the selective stabilizing forces of the three wrist extensor tendons. The digital extensor tendons, in the absence of the wrist extensor tendons, can secondarily induce wrist extension. Their substitution, however, lacks normal power and is devoid of flexibility in spatial positioning of the hand. Wrist extension is then the obliged follower of finger extension.

The stations of the extensor carpi radialis longus and brevis and the extensor carpi ulnaris are fixed relative to the axis of wrist motion at the level of the distal radius by the septa that partition the fibro-osseous tunnels beneath the dorsal carpal ligament (Fig. 29-1). The three wrist extensors differ in muscle mass (strength) and distance from the axis of wrist motion (moment arm).[15] These differences are reflected in their individual variations in performance and impact on wrist motion.

The extensor carpi radialis brevis has the longest moment arm relative to the axis of wrist flexion and extension; the

extensor carpi ulnaris has the shortest. The radial wrist extensors have an amplitude of 37 mm during wrist flexion and extension; the extensor carpi ulnaris has only 18 mm.[3] The extensor carpi ulnaris has the longest moment arm for ulnar deviation; the extensor carpi radialis brevis has the shortest. Summarily, the extensor carpi radialis longus has the greatest muscle mass (strength), the extensor carpi radialis brevis the most efficient position (moment arm) for wrist extension, and the extensor carpi ulnaris the greatest moment arm (leverage) for ulnar deviation of the wrist. These three muscles with varied endowments are cerebrally integrated to balance wrist extension, flexion, and ulnar and radial deviation.

The extensor carpi ulnaris is unique among the wrist extensor tendons. It exhibits some degree of contraction during all phases of wrist motion. Its variable potential for wrist extension depends on the position of forearm rotation. In pronation the normal tendon rests on the medial side of the ulnar head and stabilizes the wrist. In this position it is a strong ulnar deviator and balances the tension of all tendons radial to the axis of wrist motion, which lies in the proximal end of the capitate. It becomes a stronger wrist extensor when the forearm is supinated.

The tendon of the extensor carpi ulnaris is firmly stabilized in its groove on the ulnar head by a strong collar of synovium-lined deep fascia, which is distinct from the overlying dorsal carpal ligament[33] (Fig. 29-2). Supination increases the angulation of the tendon as it courses to insert on the base of the fifth metacarpal. Flexion and ulnar deviation during supination may rupture the deep fascial yoke of the extensor carpi ulnaris tendon in its groove, producing a painful subluxation during forearm rotation.[6] The condition reflects a specific anatomic lesion and is amenable to reconstruction with a radially based flap from the dorsal carpal ligament.[5]

Deterioration of wrist extensor function often occurs after an injury to the hand or wrist without direct trauma to the wrist extensor tendons. A wrist drop occurs, and a substitution pattern implementing the digital extensors is adopted to extend the wrist. This centrally mediated inhibition of the wrist extensor tendons should be detected early, and supportive splinting initiated. The wrist is supported in slight extension, permitting digital flexion and extension while the wrist extensors are being retrained. Extending the wrist against resistance while the digits are fully flexed is helpful in this pursuit. The natural synergy between the wrist extensors and digital flexors facilitates recovery (Fig. 29-3).

Laceration of the extensor carpi ulnaris may introduce a significant imbalance in some patients. The inability to balance the tension of the radial wrist extensors produces persistent radial deviation of the wrist. Extension in ulnar deviation is precluded, grip is weak, and most functions are

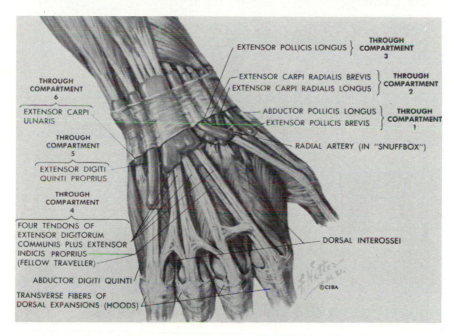

FIG. 29-1. Extensor tendon anatomy. (Reprinted from Lampe, E.W.: Surgical anatomy of the hand, Summit, N.J., 1969, by permission CIBA Pharmaceutical Co.).

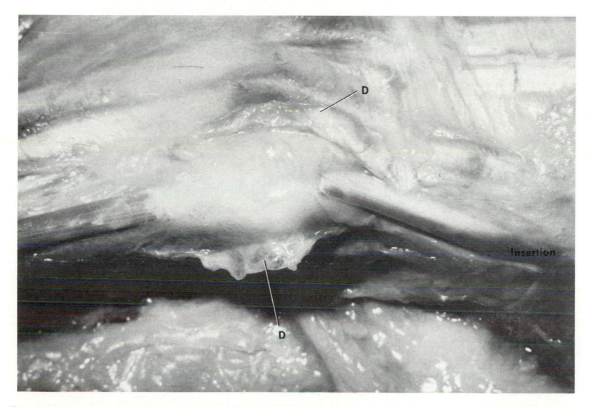

FIG. 29-2. Fascial anatomy of extensor carpi ulnaris tendon. Dorsal carpal ligament is seen reflected. Tendon secured in groove of ulnar head by collar of deep fascia. Angulation of tendon increases during supination. Insertion of tendon to right. *D,* Dorsal carpal ligament.

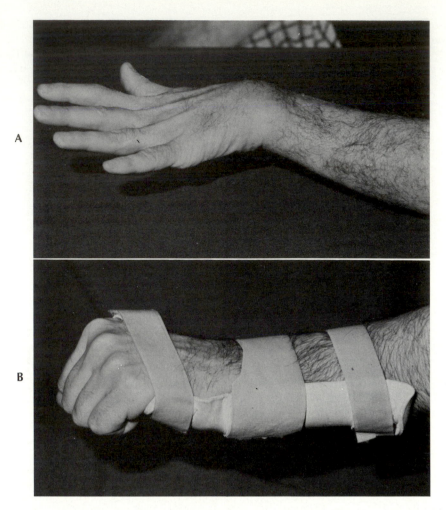

FIG. 29-3. Loss of wrist extensor function after trauma. There was no direct insult to wrist extensors. **A,** Substitution pattern employing digital extensors to extend wrist. **B,** Early splinting and reeducation of wrist extensors are necessary.

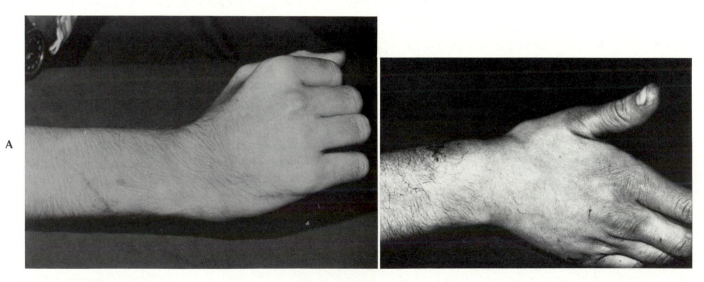

FIG. 29-4. A, Interruption of extensor carpi ulnaris introduces imbalance of wrist extensors. Therapy after repair requires awareness of multiple facets of normal extensor carpi ulnaris function. **B,** Laceration of radial wrist extensor tendons. Inability to deviate wrist radially introduces major deficiency in spatial positioning of hand and grip strength.

awkwardly performed. (Fig. 29-4, *A*). Laceration of the radial wrist extensors, too, can significantly interfere with the balance of spatial positioning of the hand and the dexterity of grip (Fig. 29-4, *B*). All the wrist extensor tendons contribute significantely to normal function, and each should be repaired after injury.

DORSAL FASCIA

An appreciation of the fascial anatomy of the dorsum of the hand is helpful in the designing of surgical procedures and in the modification of hand therapy after an injury. The skin over the dorsum of the hand is pliable, lacking the fascial septa that characterize the stable palmar skin. The skin redundancy associated with digital extension is erased during grip. This tightening of the dorsal skin compresses the underlying dorsal veins and lymphatics, providing an efficient venous and lymphatic pump.

The superficial fascia is composed of a variable fatty layer and a deeper membranous layer and contains the large dorsal veins, superficial lymphatics, and sensory branches of the radial and ulnar nerves. The superficial fascia is loosely attached to the deep fascia, with the interface representing a potential space. Dorsal subcutaneous bleeding and lymphedema distend this reservoir, tethering the fingers in extension and the thumb in supination. The pump mechanism is hampered, swelling increases, and the grip becomes further restrained. Dorsal cicatrix similarly blocks the normal mechanics of grip. The penalty for uncontrolled dorsal swelling is secondary joint stiffness, collateral ligament, and thumbweb fascial tightness (Fig. 29-5).

The dressing applied after repair of a wound or operative procedure should contribute to the control of dorsal edema and discourage hematoma formation. Sterile Dacron batting,* immersed in saline solution and applied wet about the wound, affords gentle compression of the hand and serves to diffuse expressed blood away from the wound. This has proved comfortable for patients and is a useful technique (Fig. 29-6).

---

*Manufactured as Mountain Mist by Stearns & Foster, Cincinnati, Ohio.

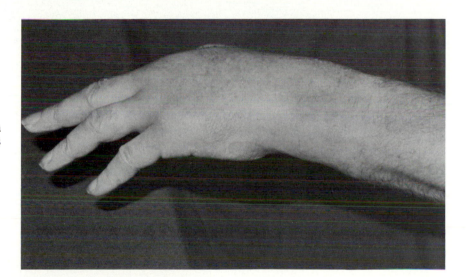

FIG. 29-5. Distention of dorsal skin and fascia reverses transverse metacarpal arch and tethers digits in extension.

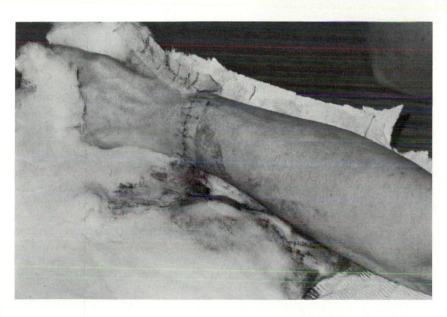

FIG. 29-6. Wet polyester batting makes comfortable, gently compressive dressing and disperses blood away from wound.

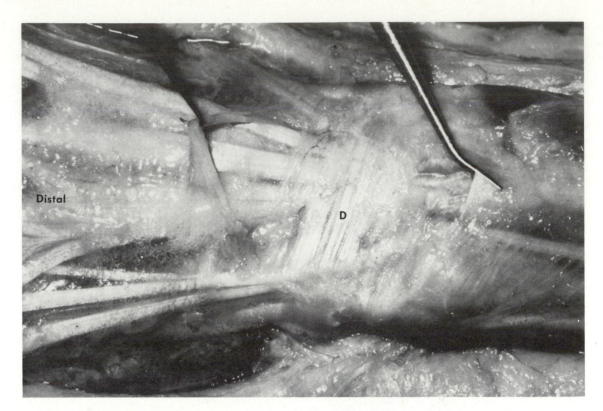

FIG. 29-7. Anatomy of deep dorsal fascia. Probe elevates deep fascia proximally and hook holds deep fascia distally to transverse fibers of dorsal carpal ligament. Areolar peritendinous fascia, the paratenon, envelops extensor tendons beyond dorsal carpal ligament. Fascia contributes to efficiency of tendon excursion and intrinsic tendon circulation. *D*, Dorsal carpal ligament.

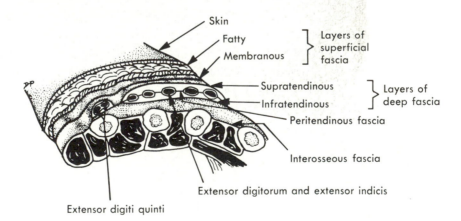

FIG. 29-8. Dorsal fascia of hand. (Redrawn from Anson, B.J., et al.: Surg. Gynecol. Obstet. **81**:327, 1945.)

The deep fascia of the extensor surface of the forearm is reinforced over the axis of wrist motion as the dorsal carpal ligament and continues distally as the superficial layer of the deep fascia over the dorsum of the hand (Fig. 29-7). Vertical septa beneath the dorsal carpal ligament attach to the radius and ulna, defining fibro-osseous tunnels that contain the extensor tendons and their synovial sheaths. These septa position and maintain the extensor tendons relative to the axis of wrist motion located in the proximal pole of the capitate. Distally to the dorsal carpal ligament the deep fascia is composed of two layers, a dorsal supratendinous

layer and a volar infratendinous layer. They define a closed fascial space bordered by the synovial sheaths of the extensor tendons, the index and fifth metacarpals, and the metacarpal heads. The flattened finger extensor tendons course between these two layers of the deep fascia, invested in a vascularized film of peritendinous fascia, the paratenon. The infratendinous layer of the deep fascia rests on the interosseous fascia (Fig. 29-8).

The peritendinous fascia is represented in the embryonic hand and is believed to give rise to the extensor tendons. Anatomic variations in the extensor tendons may reflect

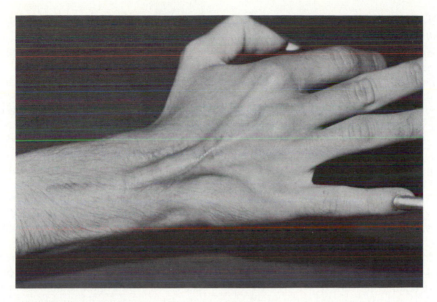

FIG. 29-9. Dorsal bowing and reduced effective extensor excursion as result of removal of dorsal retaining layers. Segments must remain to preserve function and avoid disfigurement.

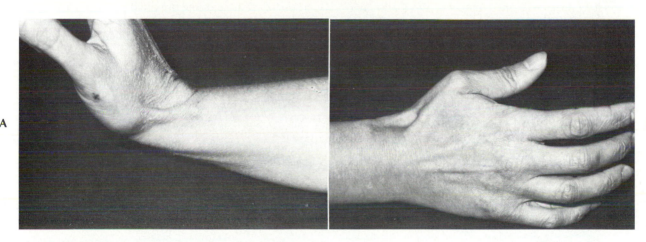

FIG. 29-10. Thumb imbalance reflecting removal of dorsal carpal ligament and deep fascia retaining abductor pollicis longus and extensor pollicis brevis. **A,** Increased excursion of tendons with wrist extension-flexion with bowing. **B,** Exaggerated extension of first metacarpal with extensor lag at metacarpophalangeal joint resulting from alteration of moment arms and effective excursions of these tendons.

developmental variations in the precursor of adult paratenon.[11] This transparent vascular membrane permits gliding of the extensor tendons within the small tolerances of the two layers of the deep fascia. Its response to certain traumatic situations demonstrates a prodigious capacity for generating scar tissue and adhesions.

The extensor tendons receive their blood supply through vascular mesenteries, mesotendons, which are analogous to the vincula of the flexor tendons. Branches of the radial and ulnar arteries, perforating dorsal branches of the anterior interosseous artery, and vessels originating in the deep palmar arch are carried to the tendons in these flexible folds of delicate fascia. The mesotendons are longer and adapted to a longer tendon excursion while the extensor tendons are synovial beneath the dorsal carpal ligament and are significantly shorter within the deep fascial pocket over the meta-

carpals.[39] The intratendinous vascular architecture of the extensor tendons is similar throughout.[36]

The deep layers of the dorsal fascia contribute a dual function to the extensor tendons. The supratendinous layer represents a dorsal pulley, essential for an efficient implementation of the inherent strength and amplitude of each of the muscles. Selective removal of portions of the dorsal fascia is compatible with retained function. Excessive removal, however, results in unsightly bowing and altered extensor kinetics (Fig. 29-9). Fasciectomy can also introduce thumb imbalance with extensor tendon deficiencies (Fig. 29-10). The contribution of the deep fascia to the intrinsic circulation of the tendons is speculative but may parallel that of the skin and superficial fascia, contributing to the venous and lymphatic circulations.

FINGER EXTENSOR TENDONS
Proximal to metacarpophalangeal joints

The extensor tendons of the metacarpophalangeal joints of the fingers are the extensor digitorum, extensor indicis, and the extensor digiti minimi. The tendons of the extensor digitorum pass beneath the dorsal carpal ligament within synovial sheaths. They flatten distally between the layers of the deep fascia. The extensor digitorum contributes substantial tendons to the index, long, and ring fingers, giving a variable slip to the small finger (Fig. 29-11). Extension of the metacarpophalangeal joints is dependent on the position of the adjacent fingers; independent extension is lacking. The long-finger extensor has less autonomy, the ring-finger extensor the least. This reflects fibrous connecting bands within the muscle belly of the extensor digitorum in the forearm.[13]

The extensor indicis and extensor digiti minimi have independent muscles that allow independent function. Extension of these fingers is readily performed, irrespective of the flexed position of the other fingers (Fig. 29-12).

The juncturae tendinum are broad intertendinous connections that diverge from the ring-finger extensor tendon. These bands connect with the tendons of the long, small, and, variably, the index-finger extensor tendons (Fig. 29-11). These bands transfer extension forces during extension and thereby assist adjacent connected fingers. They may therefore superficially disguise a lacerated proximal tendon.

Demonstration of a full range of potential motion and direct inspection of the integrity of the tendons are therefore required to eliminate the possibility of a lacerated tendon (Fig. 29-13).

The juncturae tendinum develop increased tension with a relatively transverse orientation as they glide distally with finger flexion. This distal migration with active finger flexion dynamically stabilizes the fingers by transmitting forces to the radial sagittal bands of the index and long fingers and to the ulnar sagittal bands of the ring and small fingers. Active grip thus contributes to the stability of the transverse metacarpal arch as well as the central station of the extensor tendons over the dorsum of the metacarpophalangeal joints.[1]

The extensor tendons to the small finger have significant anatomic features.[27] An oblique junctura from the ring finger will permit continued extension of the small finger after interruption of the extensor digiti minimi more proximally. The patient is frequently unaware of any deficit unless the decreased power and lost autonomy are demonstrated. This situation is frequently encounterd in treatment of patients with rheumatoid arthritis (Fig. 29-14).

The extensor digiti minimi inserts into the abductor tubercle of the base of the proximal phalanx together with the abductor digiti quinti (Fig. 29-15). Some patients with an ulnar palsy, who are incapable of hyperextension of the metacarpophalangeal joints and do not develop a claw deformity, acquire an abduction deformity of the small finger

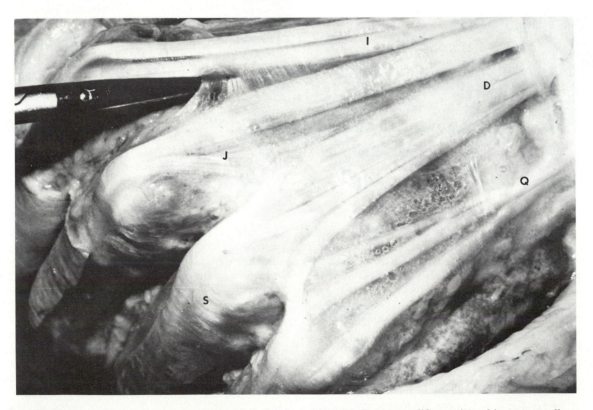

FIG. 29-11. Extensor tendon anatomy. Deep fascia has been removed. Instrument lifts vestige of junctura tendinum to index extensor tendons. *D*, Extensor digitorum; *I*, extensor indices; *Q*, extensor digiti minimi; *J*, junctura tendinum; *S*, sagittal bands over ring metacarpophalangeal joint. Juncturae tendinum dynamically stabilize extensor tendons during grip.

(Wartenburg's sign) from paralysis of the third palmar interosseous muscle. The abducted small finger is associated with an oblique junctura from the ring finger, a weak biomechanical link. The extensor digiti minimi thus is relatively unopposed in abducting the small finger. Patients who do not acquire this deformity have been found to have a transverse orientation of the juntura, a biomechanically forceful link that opposes the deformity.[2]

Recognition of the functional contributions of the juncturae is given when one is reconstructing tendon ruptures by suturing the distal ends of the ruptured tendons to adjacent intact tendons. This is commonly performed in rheumatoid patients. The tension at the tendon junction is adjusted with the fingers fully flexed. This ensures a sufficiently oblique angle for transmission of extension forces and prevents a blocking tenodesis with active flexion.

Secretan's disease. The condition of hard, brawny edema involving the dorsum of the hand has created controversy since it was described in 1901.[29] The condition follows trauma to the dorsum of the hand, often pursues a protracted course, and has been implicated with an unfavorable prog-

nosis after surgery.[26] It has been considered synonymous with factitious, or self-induced, edema.[23,31] Monetary gain from a compensation award has been afforded weighty consideration as a causative factor. The anatomy of the dorsum of the hand and the clinical observations at surgery support the contention that there is a specific pathologic entity involving peritendinous fibrosis about the extensor tendons and juncturae tendinum within the confines of the layers of the deep fascia, which is amenable to isolation, removal, and rehabilitation.[24,25] The form and distribution of the fibrosis conform to the fascial anatomy already described[12] and are supported by our clinical experience. The inelastic peritendinous scar restricts excursion of the finger extensor tendons and their juncturae. The effect is a mechanical blockage of longitudinal and transverse tendon glide, which is essential for the mechanics of normal grip.

Distal to metacarpophalangeal joints

The form and complexity of the extensor tendons abruptly change at the level of the metacarpophalangeal joints of the fingers. From this level the extensor tendons are represented

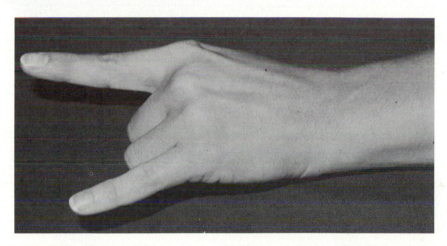

FIG. 29-12. Extensor indicis and extensor digiti minimi have independence of function from separate muscles. No distal tenodesis exists with flexion of other fingers.

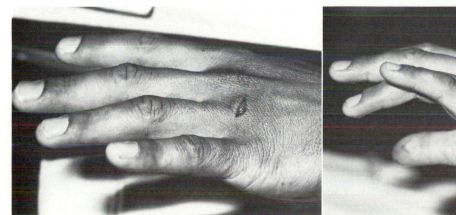 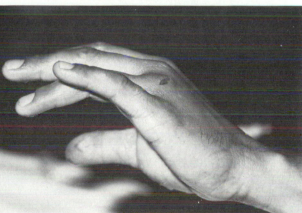

A   B

FIG. 29-13. Laceration of extensor tendon to ring finger. **A,** No apparent deficit with wrist in neutral. Metacarpophalangeal extension accomplished through fascial connections. **B,** Deficit apparent when function was tested with combined wrist and finger extension.

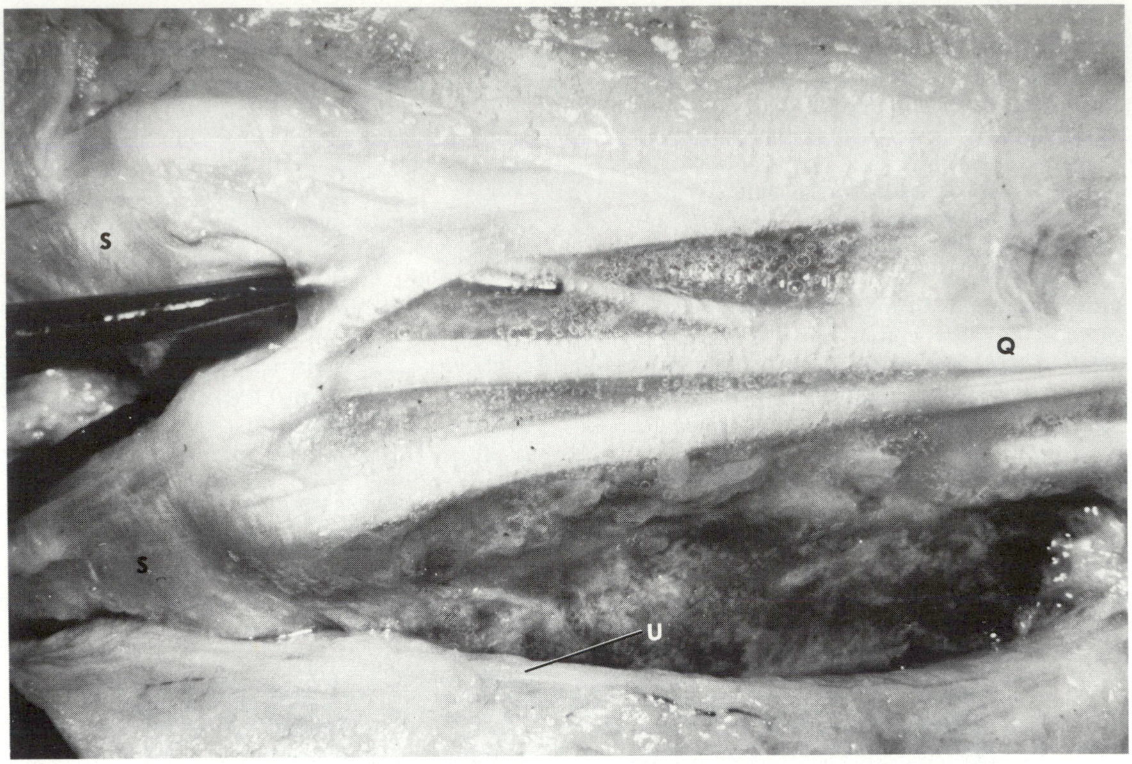

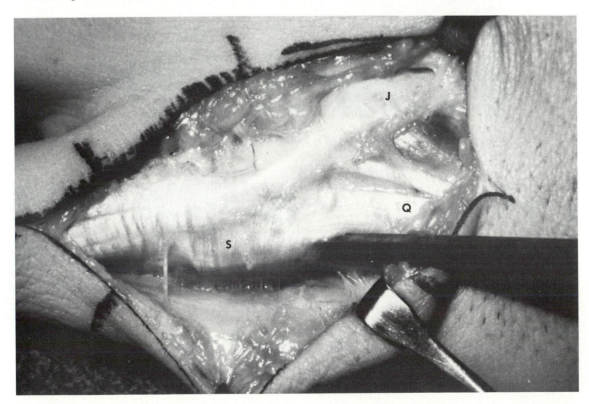

FIG. 29-14. Extensor tendons to the small finger. Deep fascia has been removed. Instrument lifts oblique junctura to small finger. This oblique connection may disguise rupture of the extensor digiti minimi proximally, *Q*, Extensor digiti minimi; *S*, sagittal bands; *U*, dorsal sensory branch of ulnar nerve.

FIG. 29-15. Extensor tendon insertion at metacarpophalangeal joint of small finger. Extensor tendon inserts on lateral tubercle of proximal phalanx. This produces an abduction deformity of small finger in some patients with ulnar nerve palsy. *J*, Junctura tendinum; *Q*, extensor digiti minimi; *S*, sagittal bands.

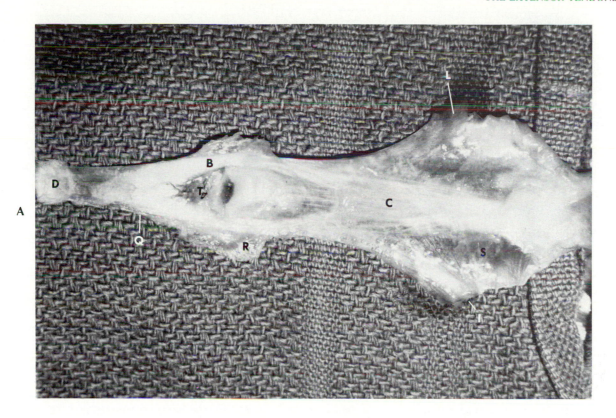

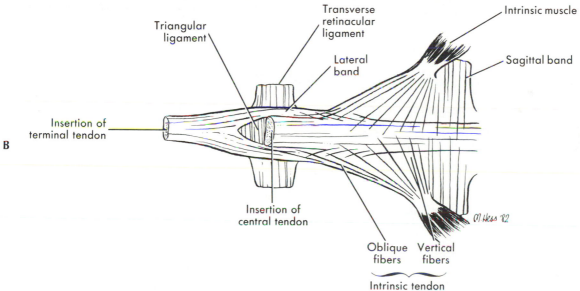

FIG. 29-16. Extensor tendons in fingers are represented by a continuous sheet of specialized fibers and are stabilized by retinacular ligaments. **A,** Deep side of extensor tendon complex. Terminal tendon is to left. **B,** Schematic drawing of **A.** *S,* Sagittal bands; *I,* interosseous muscle; *L,* lumbrical muscle; *C,* central tendon; *R,* transverse retinacular ligament; *Q,* oblique retinacular ligament; *T,* triangular ligament; *B,* lateral band; *D,* terminal tendon.

by a continuous sheet of functionally oriented fibers that can precisely transmit tension (Fig. 29-16). This array of functional fibers closely wraps the finger skeleton in the form of a bisected cone. It is composed of a tendon system, transmitting tension and producing motion, and a retinacular system, stabilizing the tendon system. An imbalance in the linkage of the three phalanges of the fingers alters the nor-

mally adjusted forces of the tendon systems and permits the retinacular system to foreshorten.[17] Whereas the imbalance permits the tendon system to establish the deformities, the tightening of the retinacular system can fix deformities and resist correction.

The extensor tendons have no significant insertion on the base of the proximal phalanx.[37] Extension of the metacar-

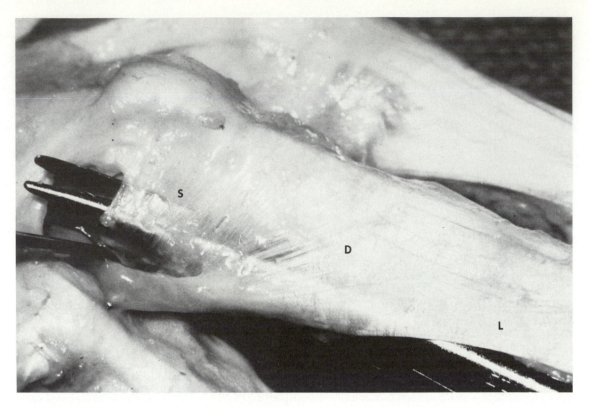

Fig. 29-17. Dorsal apparatus of finger. Hook retracts interosseous muscle. Sagittal bands separate intrinsic muscles from metacarpophalangeal joint capsule. Sagittal bands and oblique fibers of intrinsic tendon transmit extension forces. Vertical fibers of intrinsic tendons transmit flexion forces. Delicate fibers are vulnerable to interference by scar. *S*, Sagittal bands; *D*, vertical fibers of intrinsic tendon; *L*, oblique fibers of intrinsic tendon.

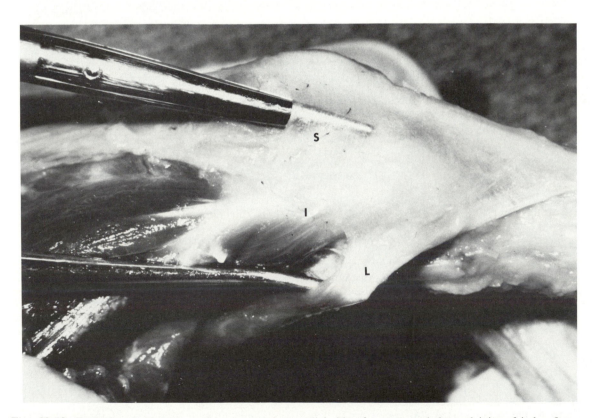

Fig. 29-18. Extrinsic and intrinsic tendons merge about radial side of metacarpophalangeal joint of index finger. Sagittal bands transmit metacarpophalangeal extension, interosseous muscles transmit metacarpophalangeal flexion, and lumbrical muscle transmits tension through lateral bands for interphalangeal extension. *S*, Sagittal bands; *I*, interosseous tendon; *L*, lumbrical tendon.

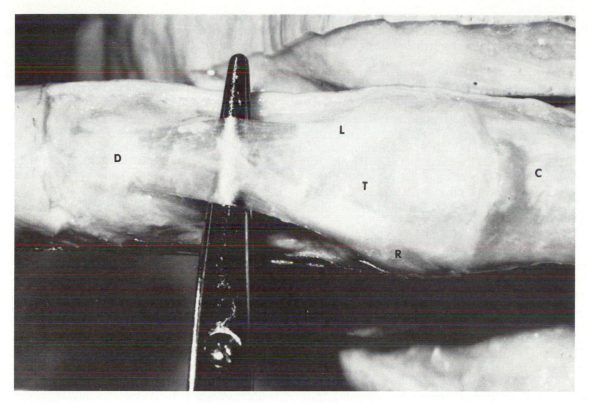

FIG. 29-19. Extensor tendon anatomy about proximal interphalangeal joint and middle phalanx. Connections between oblique retinacular ligaments and merged lateral bands have been torn to demonstrate tendon anatomy. Dissection of extensor tendon over middle phalanx during repair of mallet injuries invites scarring and restricted distal interphalangeal joint motion. *C,* Central tendon; *L,* lateral band; *R,* transverse retinacular ligament; *D,* terminal tendon; *T,* triangular ligament.

pophalangeal joints is achieved by the sagittal bands, vertically oriented fibers that shroud the capsule and collateral ligaments, connecting the extensor tendons with the volar plate and proximal phalanx on both sides of the joint.[10] These broad bands constitute a functional sling that separates the joint capsule from the intrinsic muscles (Fig. 29-17). They hood the axis of joint motion during extension and pass distally to the axis of motion during flexion. During flexion, they contribute to stabilizing the central tendons over the dorsum of the metacarpophalanageal joints, augmenting the juncturae tendinum.[38]

Fibers of the sagittal bands pass over the dorsum of the extensor tendons at the level of the metacarpophalangeal joint—except in the long finger, in which the tendon is attached to the underlying sagittal bands by a relatively weak layer of connective tissue.[16]

Lacerations or closed rupture of the sagittal bands disrupts the stability of the extensor tendons over the metacarpophalangeal joints. Rupture usually involves the radial bands, resulting in ulnar displacement during flexion. Before contractures develop, the extensor tendon translates to the ulnar side of the joint during flexion. Active extension produces ulnar angulation of the metacarpophalangeal joint with supination of the finger. The act of extension may be heralded by a painful snap as the tendon relocates dorsally.

Acute closed injuries with significant ecchymosis, swelling, and evident tendon dysfunction deserve open reconstruction of the interrupted lateral band. Closed injuries with

edema, mild subluxation, and evidently less tissue damage are successfully treated with 3 weeks of immobilization, with positioning of the wrist and metacarpophalnageal joints in a neutral position. Interphalangeal motion is permitted during the period of immobilization. The long-finger tendon is particularly vulnerable to rupture because of its fragile attachment to the underlying sagittal bands.[16]

Distal to the sagittal bands the lumbrical and interosseous muscles contribute proximal vertical and distal oblique fibers to the extensor tendon over the proximal phalanx (Fig. 29-18). The vertical fibers transmit flexor forces to the proximal phalanx, flexing rhe metacarpophalangeal joint. The oblique fibers transmit extension forces to the proximal and distal interphalangeal joints. This combination of extrinsic and intrinsic tendon fibers over the proximal phalanx is more appropriately termed the ''dorsal apparatus,'' reflecting its contribution to both flexion and extension.[32]

The extensor tendon continues as the central tendon to insert on the dorsal base of the middle phalanx. The lateral bands represent the continuation of the oblique fibers of the intrinsic tendons, supplemented by fibers from the central extensor tendon. The lateral bands insert a small medial tendon on the base of the middle phalanx adjacent to the central tendon and then continue distally, converging over the middle phalanx as a single terminal tendon that inserts on the dorsal base of the distal phalanx (Fig. 29-19).

The functional composite of extrinsic and intrinsic tendons in the fingers thus transmits extension and flexion forces. The extrinsic extensor tendons are primarily extensors of the metacarpophalangeal joints, secondarily capable of extending the interphalangeal joints only if hyperextension of the metacarpophalangeal joints is prevented. The intrinsic tendons flex the metacarpophalangeal joints and extend the interphalangeal joints.[19]

The lateral bands normally lie dorsally to the axis of motion of the proximal interphalangeal joint during extension. They shift volarly during flexion, approximating the axis of motion. This shift of the lateral bands compensates for the difference between the radii of the proximal and distal interphalangeal joints, permitting synchronized motion of both joints. Without this shift, the smaller distal interphalangeal joint would respond to a given tendon excursion with a greater range of motion.[32]

The connection between the central tendon and the lateral bands represents a crisscrossing of fibers in separate layers, with those from the central tendon passing superficial to those from the intrinsic lateral bands. Descent of the lateral bands during flexion is accompanied by an increase in the longitudinal angle between these fibers. This shift in geometric form is analogous to the expansion of a taut mesh.[28] The delicacy of this fiber interface emphasizes the vulnerability of the extensor tendons in the fingers to the restraints of scar.

The retinacular system consists of the transverse retinacular ligament and the oblique retinacular ligament. The transverse retinacular ligament is the homolog of the sagittal bands. Its fibers encircle the finger adjacent to the proximal interphalangeal joint, connecting the lateral bands with the fibro-osseous sheath of the flexor tendons. Its dorsal transverse fibers distal to the insertion of the central tendon constitute the triangular ligament; its fibers restrain the volar descent of the lateral bands during flexion. The volar fibers of the transverse retinacular ligament contribute to the stability of the proximal interphalangeal joint and restrain dorsal displacement of the lateral bands during extension.[38] They can execute extension of the proximal interphalangeal joint as the sagittal bands extend the proximal phalanx. Their contribution to deformities associated with extensor tendon injuries at the proximal and distal interphalangeal joints is significant (see Figs. 29-26 and 29-36). The oblique retinacular ligament connects the flexor fibro-osseous sheath at the proximal phalanx with the terminal extensor tendon passing volarly to the axis of motion of the proximal interphalangeal joint.[9] Its fibers interdigitate with those of the terminal tendon before inserting on the lateral base of the distal phalanx adjacent to the terminal tendon,[38] an important anatomic feature reflecting on the clinical presentation of the mallet tendon lesion[34] (Fig. 29-31). The oblique retinacular ligament probably contributes little to the extensor mechanism in the normal finger.[10,30] It can potentially extend the distal interphalangeal joint by means of a dynamic tenodesis with active extension of the proximal interphalangeal joint. This ligament can significantly contribute to deformities in the imbalanced finger (Fig. 29-27).

THUMB EXTENSOR TENDONS

The extensor pollicis longus is the most mobile of the digital extensor tendons. Its 58-mm longitudinal excursion exceeds that of the other digital extensor tendons. A 13-mm mediolateral translation accompanies thumb adduction and abduction. The extensor pollicis longus supinates and adducts the first ray, extends the metacarpophalangeal joint, and is capable of hyperextending the interphalangeal joint.

The abductor pollicis longus and extensor pollicis brevis tendons are secured over the lateral border of the radius in the first dorsal fibro-osseous compartment. Distal to the transverse carpal ligament they are contained beneath the superficial layer of the deep fascia. Liberal fasciotomy distal to the transverse carpal ligament may alter the balance of the thumb. Radial bowing of the abductor translates their moment arms, producing an exaggerated extension of the first metacarpal with an extensor lag at the metacarpophalangeal joint (Fig. 29-10).

The extensor tendon anatomy at the metacarpophalangeal joint level resembles that of the finger proximal interphalangeal joint. Transverse fibers, the homolog of the transverse retinacular ligaments, shroud the capsule, reaching the flexor fibro-osseous sheath.[20] The adductor pollicis on the ulnar side and the abductor pollicis on the radial side contribute dorsal expansions, which transmit additional stability to the extensor tendons and transfer extension forces to the interphalangeal joint (Fig. 29-20). The thumb intrinsics are thus able to extend the interphalangeal joint but are incapable of hyperextension.

The extensor pollicis brevis usually inserts on the dorsal base of the proximal phalanx but commonly continues to the distal phalanx.[14] It extends the first metacarpal and the metacarpophalangeal joint. Interruption of the extensor pollicis brevis introduces extension weakness at the base of the proximal phalanx. As the metacarpophalangeal joint flexes, increased tension through the extensor pollicis longus hyperextends the interphalangeal joint (Fig. 29-21).

The extensor pollicis longus can extend the metacarpophalangeal joint by means of the fibers of the dorsal apparatus. Diastasis or rupture of these fibers permits volar displacement of the tendon. Below the axis of joint motion, the displaced tendon flexes the metacarpophalangeal joint and exaggerates extension forces at the interphalangeal joint. This extrinsic-minus deformity is analogous to the boutonnière deformity of the finger.

The extensor pollicis longus usually ruptures at the level of the distal radius. Rheumatoid synovitis and fractures of the distal radius, often undisplaced, are predisposing conditions. The cause of the rupture is believed to be segmental ischemia of a segment of the tendon that is already poorly vascularized. Microangiographic studies suggest that the pressure of the effusion that accompanies a fracture or synovitis jeopardizes the blood flow in this portion of the tendon, which is already poorly prefused.[8] The most disabling impairment after rupture of the extensor pollicis longus is loss of extension at the metacarpophalangeal joint (Fig. 29-22).

EXTENSOR TENDON INJURIES AT THE PROXIMAL INTERPHALANGEAL JOINT

Interruption of the extensor tendons at the proximal interphalageal joint may result from lacerations, closed trauma, burns, rheumatoid arthritis, or tightly applied casts and

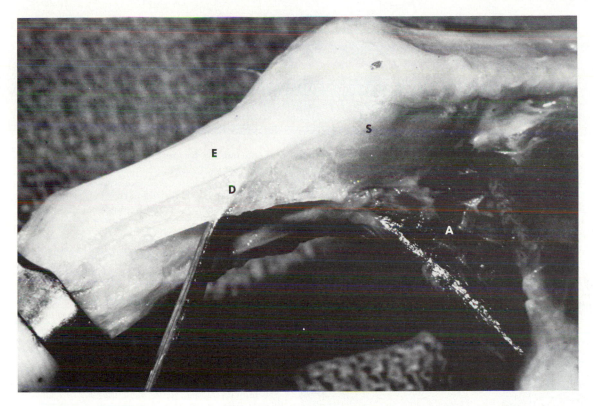

FIG. 29-20. Extensor apparatus of thumb. Adductor pollicis contributes to expansion of dorsal apparatus and assists extension of interphalangeal joint. Vertical fibers about metacarpophalangeal joint are homolog of transverse retinacular ligament of fingers. *A*, Adductor pollicis muscle; *S*, Fibers representing homolog of transverse retinacular ligament; *D*, dorsal apparatus; *E*, extensor pollicis longus tendon over proximal phalanx.

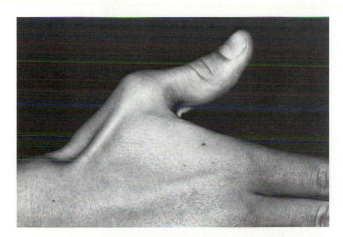

FIG. 29-21. Rupture of extensor pollicis brevis and dorsal fibers of extensor apparatus produces loss of metacarpophalangeal extension. Displacement of extensor pollicis longus may accentuate flexion of metacarpophalangeal joint and contributes to hyperextension of interphalangeal joint. Extensor pollicis longus tendon is clearly identified.

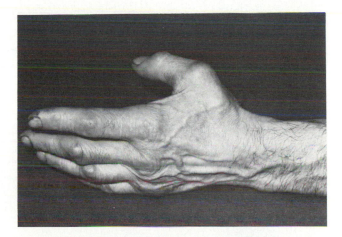

FIG. 29-22. Rupture of extensor pollicis longus at level of Lister's tubercle. Tendon is not clinically apparent. Loss of metacarpophalangeal extension is most significant functional loss. Demonstrated extension of interphalangeal joint is by intrinsic muscles through their contribution to dorsal apparatus.

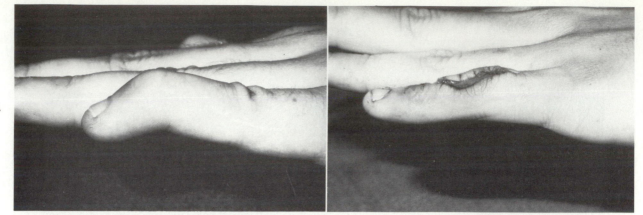

FIG. 29-23. Selective tenotomy of central tendon insertion on middle phalanx for treatment of selected patients with mallet deformity. Tenotomy permits readjustment of tensions through extensor tendons, reversing extensor deficiency at distal interphalangeal joint and lessening forces at proximal interphalangeal joint, **A,** Preoperative view in case of patient with history of two previous surgical attempts at anatomic reconstruction, and three ruptures of the terminal tendon when patient was playing football. **B,** Active extension after tenotomy of central tendon with tenolysis over middle phalanx. Both transverse retinacular ligaments were spared.

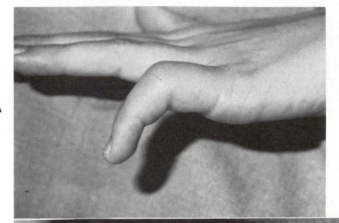

FIG. 29-24. Closed rupture of extensor tendon about proximal interphalangeal joint. Active and passive extension of proximal interphalangeal joint were limited. There was no resistence to flexion of distal joint. **A,** Clinical posture of injured finger. **B,** Operative findings. Rupture of central tendon, with herniation of head of proximal phalanx. Triangular ligament was preserved, with radial lateral band trapped beneath condyle of head of proximal phalanx. Inability to passively extend proximal interphalangeal joint is indication for primary surgical intervention in extensor tendon injuries at this level. *T,* Triangular ligament; *U,* ulnar lateral band.

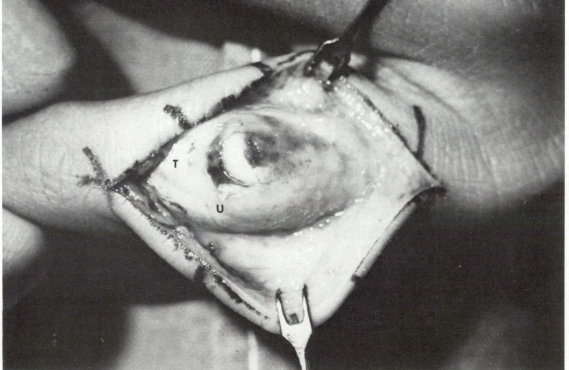

splints. The deformities that develop reflect a distortion of the forces normally balanced by the tendon and retinacular systems. Early deformities can usually be reversed; others require surgery. The longer a deformity persists, however, the more resistant it becomes.

Selective interruption of the central tendon may not interfere with extension of the proximal interphalangeal joint if the transverse retinacular ligaments remain intact. Extension forces are transmitted to the middle phalanx by means of the transverse retinacular ligaments, which lift the middle phalanx as the sagittal bands lift the proximal phalanx during extension of the metacarpophalangeal joint. Release of the attachment of the central tendon permits the entire finger extensor mechanism to slide proximally. This increases the forces transmitted to the middle phalanx through the transverse retinacular ligament and to the distal phalanx through the conjoined lateral bands and terminal tendon. Hyperextension of the proximal interphalangeal joint is opposed by the volar fibers of the transverse retinacular ligament, which restrain dorsal displacement of the lateral bands during extension. The volar plate also stabilizes the joint during extension. These functional observations provide the rationale for surgical tenotomy of the central tendon in the treatment of selected patients with a mallet deformity[21] (Fig. 29-23).

Interruption of the central tendon insertion and a tear of the dorsal fibers of the transverse retinacular ligament (triangular ligament) introduce an extension deficiency to the extensor tendons at the proximal interphalangeal joint. Partial tears of the triangular ligament may preserve sufficient integrity of the ligament to allow them to regulate the volar shift of the lateral bands during flexion, thus permitting active flexion and extension to continue. Partial tears, however, are prone to extending if unprotected motion continues after an injury.[22] A completely torn triangular ligament superimposed upon interruption of the triangular ligament significantly impairs extensor tendon function. Initiation of extension of the flexed joint is then opposed by the lateral bands, which have shifted volarly to the axis of motion of the proximal interphalangeal joint and maintain flexion. When the joint is passively extended, however, the lateral

bands relocate and the injured extensor mechanism may be capable of maintaining extension against resistance. Active *and* passive extension of the proximal interphalangeal joint is blocked if a lateral band becomes trapped beneath the condylar flare of the proximal phalanx after a tear of the triangular ligament (Fig. 29-24).

Development of boutonnière deformity

The boutonnière deformity develops from an injury to the extensor mechanism and specifically denotes flexion of the proximal interphalangeal joint associated with hyperextension of the distal interphalangeal joint (Fig. 29-25). The head of the proximal phalanx herniates through a structural defect in the extensor mechanism after rupture of the central tendon and dorsal fibers of the transverse retinacular ligament (triangular ligament).[7] An analogous situation occurs in the thumb, with metacarpophalnageal flexion and interphalangeal hyperextension. The mechanisms of closed injuries include the involuntary forceful flexion of an actively extended digit, blunt trauma to the dorsum of the joint, and dislocation of the joint with an associated tear of the extensor tendon and stabilizing ligaments.

Interruption of the central tendon and triangular ligament permits proximal slide of the extensor mechanism and volar shift of the lateral bands. The unopposed flexor digitorum superficialis pulls the proximal interphalangeal joint into flexion. The extrinsic extensor, detached from the middle phalanx, transfers forces through the sagittal bands to augment extension of the metacarpophalangeal joint. The extrinsic and intrinsic muscles transmit exaggerated forces through the conjoined lateral bands that extend the distal interphalangeal joint. Early in the evolution of the deformity the transverse retinacular ligament, oblique retinacular ligament, and check ligaments of the volar plate of the proximal interphalangeal joint are loose (Fig. 29-26, *A* and *B*). The test for retinacular tightness is negative, and passive reversal of the deformity can be easily accomplished (Fig. 29-27, *A*).

In the established deformity, the transverse retinacular ligament, oblique retinacular ligament, and volar plate lig-

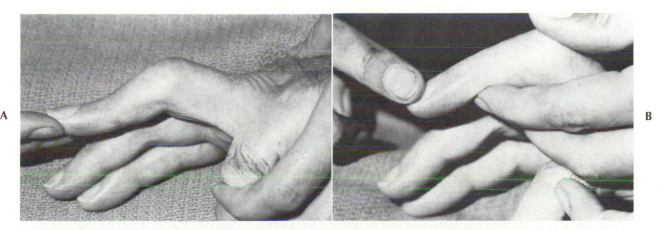

FIG. 29-25. Established boutonnière deformity. **A,** Fixed flexion deformity of proximal interphalangeal joint with hyperextension of distal interphalangeal joint. **B,** Resistent passive flexion of distal interphalangeal joint with attempted extension of proximal interphalangeal joint discloses retinacular tightness with implied tightness of extensor tendons through displaced lateral bands.

aments have shortened; their contractions oppose passive correction (Fig. 29-26, *C*). The retinacular tightness test is then positive (Fig. 29-27, *B*).

Nonoperative treatment

Closed injuries to the extensor tendons about the proximal interphalangeal joint must be monitored. Partial tears of the dorsal fibers of the transverse retinacular ligament may ex-

tend unless the injured digit is protected. Swelling and tenderness over the dorsum of the proximal interphalangeal joint should be regarded as signifying an injury of the underlying extensor tendons. The proximal interphalangeal joint is splinted in extension, and the digit reassessed in 1 week. Distal interphalangeal joint motion is permitted during this period. The continued ability of the patient to actively initiate and maintain extension with good power

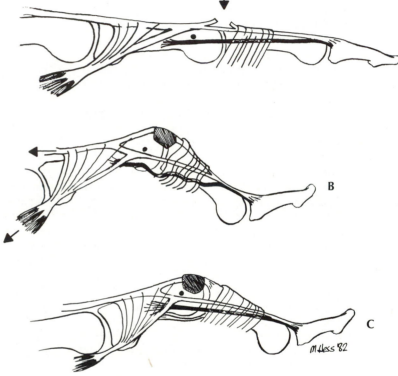

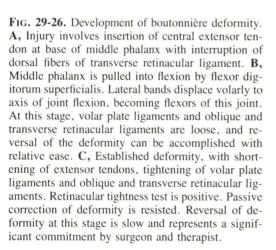

FIG. 29-26. Development of boutonnière deformity. **A,** Injury involves insertion of central extensor tendon at base of middle phalanx with interruption of dorsal fibers of transverse retinacular ligament. **B,** Middle phalanx is pulled into flexion by flexor digitorum superficialis. Lateral bands displace volarly to axis of joint flexion, becoming flexors of this joint. At this stage, volar plate ligaments and oblique and transverse retinacular ligaments are loose, and reversal of the deformity can be accomplished with relative ease. **C,** Established deformity, with shortening of extensor tendons, tightening of volar plate ligaments and oblique and transverse retinacular ligaments. Retinacular tightness test is positive. Passive correction of deformity is resisted. Reversal of deformity at this stage is slow and represents a significant commitment by surgeon and therapist.

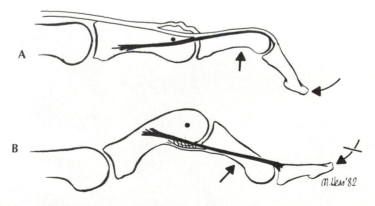

FIG. 29-27. Testing for tightness of oblique retinacular ligament. **A,** Passive extension of middle phalanx with passive flexion of distal phalanx is performed without resistence in normal finger, a negative test. **B,** Contracture of oblique retinacular ligament, with resistant flexion of proximal interphalangeal joint and hyperextension of distal interphalangeal joint. Distal joint cannot be passively flexed when extension of proximal interphalangeal joint is passively increased, a positive test.

would imply functional integrity of the extensor mechanism. If swelling, tenderness, or echymosis is noted on reexamination, however, splinting should be continued for an additional 2 weeks. Splinting is discontinued after 3 weeks if the patient continues to demonstrate integrity of the extensor tendons, and no deformity has developed.

Splinting or digital casting positions the proximal interphalangeal joints in extension, permitting continued active flexion of the distal interphalangeal joint. Active flexor digitorum profundus flexion produces a distal slide of 3 to 4 mm by the retracted extensor tendon by synergistic relaxing of the intrinsic and extrinsic extensor muscles and by directly transmitted forces initiated through the terminal tendon. This continued motion also exercises the oblique retinacular ligament.

The dynamic splinting program recommended for treatment of the established boutonnière deformity should be tailored to meet the tissue requirements of the patient. The physician and the therapist should be familiar with the anatomy of the extensor mechanism and the pathomechanics of the deformity being treated. Initial splinting supports the proximal interphalangeal joint in neutral, permitting active flexion of the distal interphalangeal joint. This is continued for 6 weeks. Carefully monitored flexion of the proximal interphalangeal joint is then begun. The proximal interphalangeal joint is supported in extension for an additional 2 to 4 weeks whenever active motion is not being pursued. The need for continued support of the proximal interphalangeal joint reflects the postural stability of the finger. If the proximal interphalangeal joint develops an extensor lag, or the boutonnière posture recurs, proximal joint splinting is continued. If proximal joint extension can be sustained and no deterioration is noted on subsequent visits, then splinting is recommended only at night.

The time required for rehabilitation of the boutonnière deformity by splinting can be prolonged. Resistant cases can require attention and supervision for 6 to 9 months after injury. Realization of the full functional potential of the finger may not be achieved for a full year (Fig. 29-28).

Surgery

The principal functional handicap with an established boutonnière deformity reflects loss of flexion of the distal interphalangeal joint. The impact of the flexed proximal

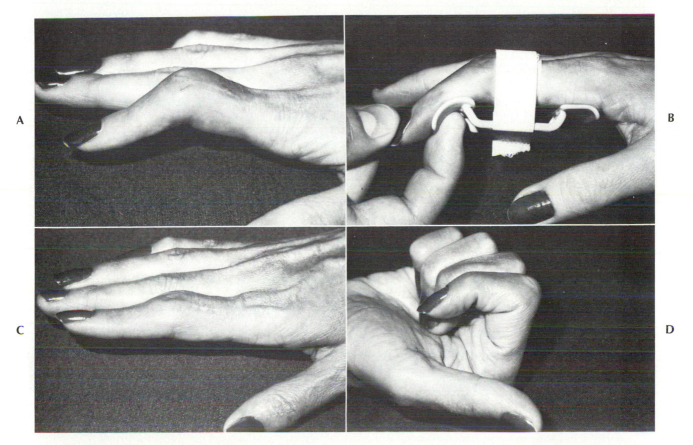

FIG. 29-28. Conservative treatment of boutonnière deformity. Laceration of extensor tendons with delayed primary treatment and wound infection. **A,** Fixed deformity with resistent flexion of proximal interphalangeal joint and extension of distal joint. **B,** Supervised dynamic splinting, designed to reestablish extension of proximal and flexion of distal deformed joints. (Marketed as New Extension Finger Splint in six sizes by Christensen Orthopedic Supply Company [COSCO], Hermosa Beach, Calif.) **C,** Five months after program was instituted, active extension with normal power was present. Tissue softening is evident. Dorsal bump presents a cosmetic disfigurement. **D,** Active flexion was still improving. Time frame for treatment of boutonnière deformities may require 6 to 9 months for maximum improvement.

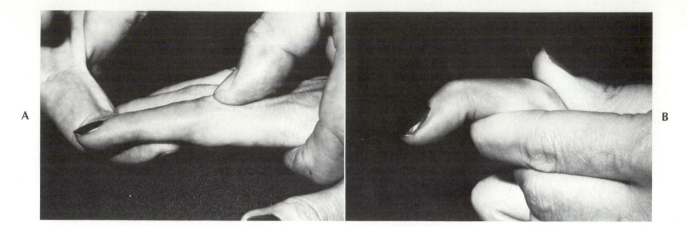

FIG. 29-29. Passive correction of deformity before surgery is done improves prognosis. **A,** Reversal of flexion deformity of proximal interphalangeal joint. **B,** Active flexion of distal interphalangeal joint with associated passive extension of proximal interphalangeal joint verifies sufficient lengthening of extensor tendons and retinacular ligaments for proper timing of surgery.

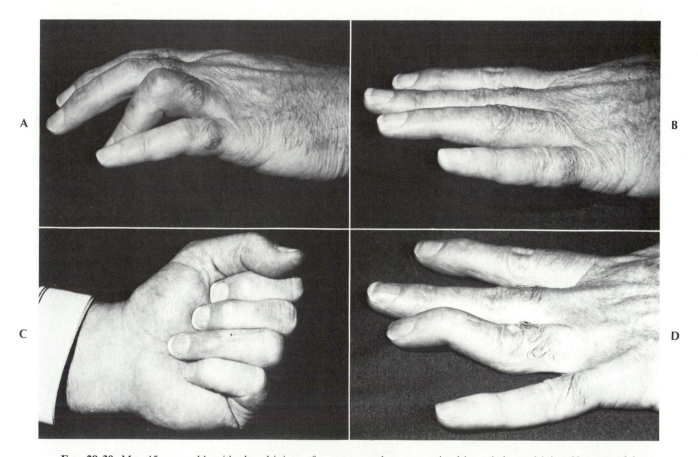

FIG. 29-30. Man 45 years old, with closed injury of extensor tendons at proximal interphalangeal joint. Unsuccessful surgery performed 3 months after injury for uncorrected boutonnière deformity. Surgery included dorsal suturing of lateral bands and tenotomy of terminal tendon. **A,** Fixed deformity when first seen 4 months after surgery. **B,** Clinical extension 6 months after anatomic reconstruction, with volar plate release and resection of accessory collateral ligaments of proximal interphalangeal joint. No invasion of extensor tendon over middle phalanx was made. **C,** Active flexion 6 months after surgery. There is minimal flexion of distal interphalangeal joint. **D,** Posture 9 years after reconstruction. A reversal of boutonnière deformity with swan-neck deformity has evolved, reflecting instability of proximal interphalangeal joint. Distal interphalangeal joint actively flexes. Mature scar retains some capacity for remodeling when subjected to chronic tensions. Extensive surgical releases introduce a potential for imbalances beyond those of original deformity.

interphalangeal joint has wide individual variation and may not significantly interfere with grasp or finger function. The unsightly bump over the dorsum of the proximal interphalangeal joint is often disliked by patients but, in itself, is usually not sufficient reason to recommend surgical reconstruction. A comfortable and useful range of active flexion of both interphalangeal joints provides excellent function, even though a slight flexion deformity of the proximal interphalangeal joint persists.

Candidates for surgery should be carefully selected. Their selection implies a willingness to participate in a closely supervised, often prolonged, rehabilitation program after surgery.

Reversal of the proximal interphalangeal flexion and active distal interphalangeal joint flexion should be achieved before surgery (Fig. 29-29). The results from surgery are generally better when joint deformities are corrected preoperatively. Fingers that cannot be corrected by means of splinting and supervised therapy require extensive surgical releases, which can introduce additional imbalances and a potential for further deformity. Mature, hard, resistant scar occasionally demonstrates a surprising plasticity when subjected to tensions for long periods of time (Fig. 29-30).

Surgery, too, projects a long-term commitment to a rehabilitative program. The Kirchner wire stabilizing the proximal interphalangeal joint is usually removed 5 to 6 weeks after operation. Mobilization is then pursued as already discussed for nonoperative treatment. Realization of the full potential from a surgical reconstruction may require 9 to 12 months of supervised care.[7]

EXTENSOR TENDON INJURIES AT THE DISTAL INTERPHALANGEAL JOINT

Mallet finger is synonymous with interruption of the extensor tendon mechanism at the level of the distal interphalangeal joint. The term is not descriptive but has gained universal acceptance for the deformity that results (Fig. 29-31).

The terminal extensor tendon represents the distal extension of the merged lateral bands that insert on the dorsal base of the distal phalanx. The more central fibers of the tendon are bordered by the distal extensions of the oblique retinacular ligaments that insert on the lateral base of the distal phalanx adjacent to the terminal tendon.[38] There is an interweaving of tendon and ligament fibers before their insertion, which has significant bearing upon the treatment of some injuries at this level.

Patterns of injury

The pathomechanics of the varieties of injuries at this level differ. The treatment depends on the type of injury.

Closed injuries reflect the position of the distal interphalangeal joint at the time of injury. A blow to the dorsum of the distal phalanx in less the 45 degrees of flexion is opposed only by tension transmitted through the terminal tendon. The oblique retinacular ligaments are relaxed in this range of flexion in the normal finger. The result is fraying of the central portion of the terminal tendon over the trochlea of the head of the middle phalanx.[34] The oblique retinacular ligament, not under tension, remains intact (Fig. 29-32). The interweaving between the tendon and border ligaments preserves some anatomic continuity, which continues to transfer extension forces to the lateral bases of the distal phalanx. These patients are able to perform some active extension, reflecting the contribution of the oblique retinacular ligaments, but they lack the final 45 degrees of active extension (Fig. 29-33). This is a pure tendon lesion.

When the dorsum of the distal phalanx is struck while the distal interphalangeal joint is flexed greater than 45 degrees, both the terminal tendon and the oblique retinacular ligaments are under tension. This produces a small dorsal avulsion fracture from the base of the distal phalanx with

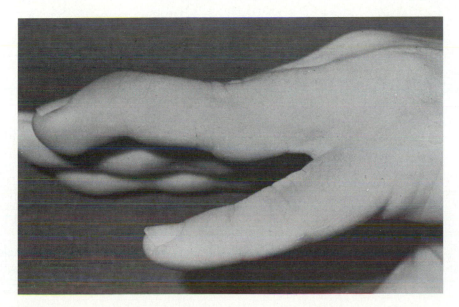

FIG. 29-31. Mallet finger with hyperextension deformity of proximal interphalangeal joint. Interruption of terminal tendon concentrates extension forces of extrinsic and intrinsic tendons at middle phalanx through central tendon and transverse retinacular ligaments, producing hyperextension.

total functional interruption in the continuity of the extensor mechanism[35] (Fig. 29-34).

An impaction injury to the distal interphalangeal joint positioned in extension produces a large articular fracture of the base of the distal phalanx (Fig. 29-35, *A*). The significance of this injury is the damage to the joint. The impact upon extensor tendon function is often small, with little evident deformity. Patients are often inclined to dismiss the injury as trivial and may not seek early treatment.

The large fracture fragment retains the collateral ligament attachments from the middle phalanx. The distal phalanx is unstable and develops volar subluxation from persistent tension through the flexor digitorum profundus (Fig. 29-35, *B*). Large articular fractures do not represent tendon lesions but require open reduction with accurate approximation of the fracture fragments.[35]

Development of deformity

Interruption of the distal insertion of the extensor tendon permits retraction of the proximal tendon stump. This transfers tension to the conjoined lateral bands and the central tendon. The central tendon, through its bony insertion, and the lateral bands, through the transverse retinacular ligaments, concentrate extension forces on the middle phalanx. The initial attitude of the proximal interphalangeal joint reflects the inherent stability of the volar plate. The oblique retinacular ligament is initially loose. As the volar plate becomes attenuated, a hyperextension or swan-neck deformity develops. The oblique retinacular ligaments may become displaced dorsally to the axis of the proximal interphalangeal joint and shorten. The tight ligaments are unable to traverse the condylar flares of the proximal phalanx during early flexion. This alters the mechanics of synchronized interphalangeal flexion (Fig. 29-36).

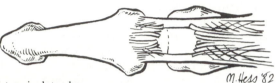

FIG. 29-32. Mallet tendon lesion. Rupture of terminal tendon occurs proximally to its insertion over the trochlea of head of middle phalanx. Continuity of extensions of oblique retinacular ligaments are preserved, maintaining some continuity of extensor tendon mechanism with distal phalanx. There is normally interweaving of fibers between tendon and retinacular ligaments.

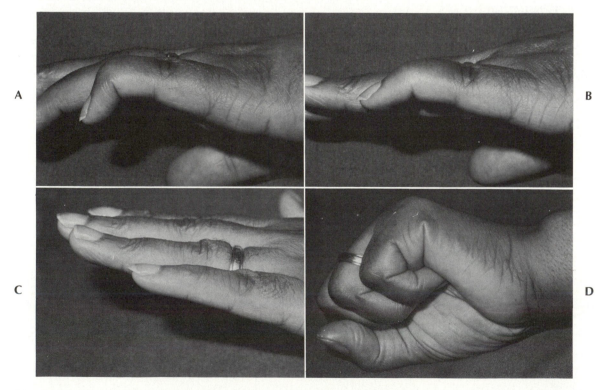

FIG. 29-33. Chronic mallet deformity from blunt injury in 54-year-old female. **A,** Resting attitude of 70 degrees. **B,** Active extension to 55 degrees, indicating potential benefit of splinting. **C,** Active extension after 7 weeks of uninterrupted splinting and 4 additional weeks of night splinting. **D,** Active flexion.

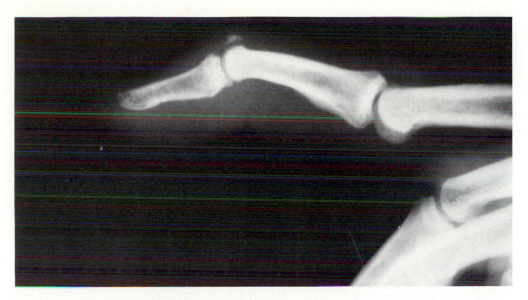

FIG. 29-34. Total interruption of terminal insertion of extensor tendon and adjacent oblique retinacular ligaments is usually associated with a small dorsal avulsion fracture. This produces a mallet deformity with virtually no retained capacity for extension of distal interphalangeal joint.

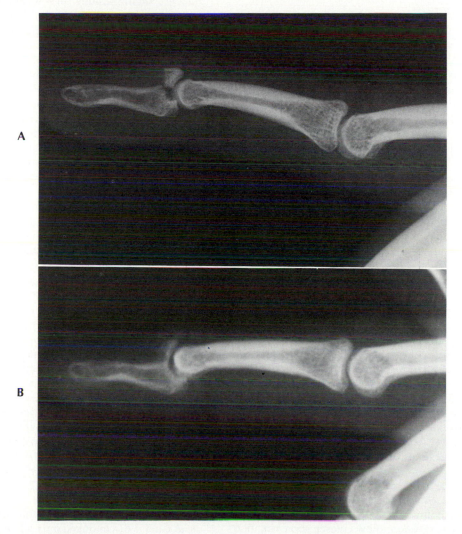

FIG. 29-35. Impaction injury produces a major articular fracture with instability of distal interphalangeal joint, but usually without a mallet deformity. A, Roentgenogram at time of injury. Patient was treated with digital casting for 3 weeks followed by 3 weeks of splinting. B, Roentgenogram 3 months after injury. Major articular fractures represent an unstable situation with a threat to integrity of joint and require operative reduction with internal stabilization.

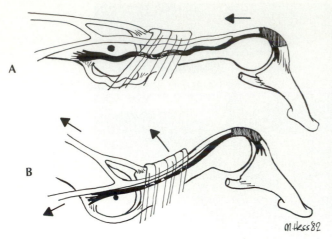

FIG. 29-36. Development of mallet deformity. **A,** Interruption of extensor tendon over distal interphalangeal joint permits unopposed flexion of joint by flexor digitorum profundus tendon. Loss of distal restraint permits proximal slide of entire extensor mechanism. Oblique retinacular ligaments and lateral bands become slack. Integrity of volar plate resists extension at proximal interphalangeal joint. **B,** Concentration of extension forces from extrinsic and intrinsic muscles transmitted through central tendon, lateral bands, and transverse retinacular ligament produces hyperextension at the proximal interphalangeal joint. As volar plate yields, extension increases. Lateral bands and tightened oblique retinacular ligaments, transposed dorsally to axis of motion of proximal interphalangeal joint, then preclude flexion until forced over flare of head of proximal phalanx after extreme flexion of distal joint by flexor profundus.

Treatment

Lacerations of the terminal tendon should be approximated. Pinning the distal interphalangeal joint with an intramedullary Kirschner wire in slight extension will coapt the tendon ends in tidy wounds, making tendon suture unnecessary. Divided tendons requiring sutures should be approximated with fine 5-0 or 6-0 synthetic sutures. The distal joint is still pinned, since primary security of the repaired tendon rests with the Kirschner wire. Motion is begun after 6 weeks. The distal joint is supported by splinting between active motion sessions for an additional 2 weeks. Evidence of an extensor lag indicates the need for further splinting.

The mallet tendon lesion without fracture should be treated with uninterrupted splinting of the distal interphalangeal joint in slight extension for 6 weeks. Hyperextension may produce blanching with obvious ischemia of the dorsal skin. The safe position for splinting is individualized. Some patients require changing the attitude of the splinted joint as the swelling of injury resolves and further extension is tolerated.

Dorsal splinting of the distal interphalangeal joint with a foam-padded aluminum splint does not encroach on the tactile volar surface of the finger and avoids localized pressure over the injury site (Fig. 29-37). Thinning of the foam of commercially available splints permits better fitting. A layer of cloth adhesive between the foam and the skin reduces maceration. The splint may be changed periodically by an insightful patient; some patients require weekly visits to the physician or therapist for this.

Active motion of the proximal interphalangeal joint in continued throughout the period of splinting. Flexion of the proximal joint reduces tension at the injury site.

The most frequently observed limitation after treatment of the mallet lesion with splinting is loss of active extension, an extensor lag. The elongated scar constitutes a functional lengthening of the terminal tendon. Positioning the distal joint in slight hyperextension allows closer approximation of the ends of the injured tendon. Splinting must be continuous. Night splinting for 4 weeks after institution of motion, begun 6 weeks after the injury, supports the elastic tendon scar and is necessary. Full-time splinting should be reinstituted if clinical regression occurs when active flexion of the distal interphalangeal joint is begun (Fig. 29-33).

Treatment of the distal avulsion fracture is the same as that for a pure tendon lesion. Positioning the distal joint in slight extension returns the distal phalanx to the small proximal fragment. The success of the positioning can be monitored by comparison roentgenograms before and after splinting. Calcification of the bridging scar frequently creates a small dorsal beak. This, nonetheless, represents functional continuity of the extensor tendon and is not usually a problem.

The most frequent limitation after open reduction of an articular fracture of the distal phalanx is loss of distal interphalangeal joint flexion, reflecting scarring of the extensor tendon and oblique retinacular ligaments over the middle phalanx. The original lesion is purely intra-articular. Repositioning can be accomplished through a localized transverse incision over the fracture site, without disturbing the vulnerable tendon-ligament complex proximally. The distal phalanx is brought to the proximal fragment without dissection of the proximal tendon. This is a delicate and challenging reconstruction, which may be difficult. Respect for the integrity of the delicate joint capsule, however, will reward care with return to distal joint motion. An oblique buttress wire compresses the fracture site and prevents proximal retraction of the terminal tendon.[18] The volar edge of the fracture fragment can be rongeured to accommodate the Kirschner wire. The fundamental aim is to return the distal phalanx to the proximal fragment without intruding upon the vulnerable extensor tendon over the middle phalanx (Fig. 29-38).

The wires are removed after 6 weeks, and supervised therapy is begun. Night splinting is continued for 2 to 4 weeks and is discontinued only when absence of an extensor lag from adhesions is assured.

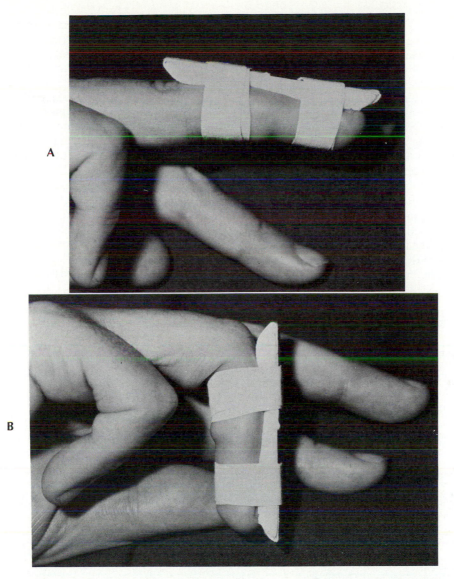

FIG. 29-37. Dorsal splint for mallet finger. **A,** Splint maintains distal joint in slight hyperextension. **B,** Proximal interphalangeal joint motion is preserved. Flexion is encouraged during the 6 weeks of recommended splinting for initial treatment of mallet finger. This relaxes extension forces at injury site.

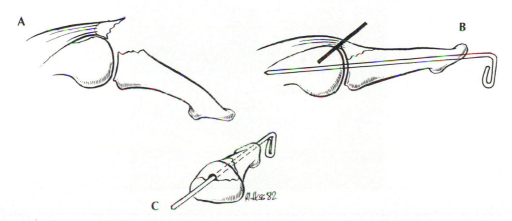

FIG. 29-38. Operative method for major articular fracture of distal interphalangeal joint. **A,** Injury represents significant interruption of articular surface, with potential instability. There may be insignificant impact upon extensor tendons. **B,** Accurate reduction of fracture fragments. Longitudinal wire stabilizes distal joint in neutral or slight extension. Oblique buttress wire compresses fracture site and prevents proximal retraction of extensor tendon. **C,** Volar surface of fracture fragment may be furrowed to accommodate Kirschner wire.

REHABILITATION

The extensor tendons are vulnerable to scar formation and may be difficult to rehabilitate. They are less powerful than their flexor antagonists. Their amplitude of glide is relatively small, and their surface area disproportionly large. The entire system of extensor tendons distal to the synovial sheaths beneath the dorsal carpal ligament is wrapped in delicate paratenon, a biologically active tissue with significant capacity for generating scar tissue after trauma. It is advantageous, therefore, to localize areas of scar restraint and to concentrate therapeutic efforts accordingly.

Motion of a joint distal to an injured or adherent tendon will stretch adhesions and reestablish gliding. Active motion automatically relaxes antagonistic muscles by central pathways. The efficiency of active motion reflects the work capacity and excursion of the muscle-tendon unit. The work capacity of the extensor muscles is approximately half that of their flexor counterparts,[3] as shown here:

Extensor digitorum	1.7 m-kg (meter-kilograms)
Extensor carpi radialis brevis	0.9 m-kg
Extensor carpi radialis longus	1.1 m-kg
Flexor carpi ulnaris	2.0 m-kg
Flexor digitorum profundus	4.5 m-kg

Each wrist extensor tendon has a potential excursion of about 33 mm. Each finger extensor tendon has a total excursion of about 50 mm. Combined wrist-metacarpophalangeal-interphalangeal motion imparts the full 50 mm of tendon glide. Isolated wrist motion, however, transmits only 31 mm of glide to the finger extensor tendons proximally.

Isolated metacarpophalangeal joint motion can impart 16 mm of glide to the finger extensors proximal to this level. Proximal interphalangeal joint motion transmits only 3 mm of glide to the extensor tendons over the proximal phalanx. The terminal tendon glides 3 to 5 mm during flexion-extension of the distal interphalangeal joint.[3]

The extensor pollicis longus has a total excursion of 58 mm. Wrist flexion-extension transmits 35 mm of glide, but metacarpophalangeal flexion-extension transmits only 15 mm, and interphalangeal joint motion only 8 mm of tendon motion.[3]

Comparison between active and passive ranges of joint motion can localize sites of tendon adhesions. Skin adherence, focal induration, and dimpling with active motion are other useful signs in the detection of sites of restraining scar. The following discussions concern the extensor tendons and their retinacular systems. The principles presented are invalid unless the joints are passively mobile.

PATTERNS OF SCAR RESTRAINT
Proximal to dorsal carpal ligament

Scar or adhesions proximal to the dorsal carpal ligament restrain combined wrist-finger flexion when the finger extensor tendons are involved, and wrist flexion alone when only the wrist extensor tendons are involved. Passive wrist flexion invokes a tenodesis that passively extends the fingers. Finger flexion passively extends the wrist. Wrist extension permits the fingers to flex by shortening the distance between the site of scar restraint and the insertions of the extensor tendons. (Fig. 29-39).

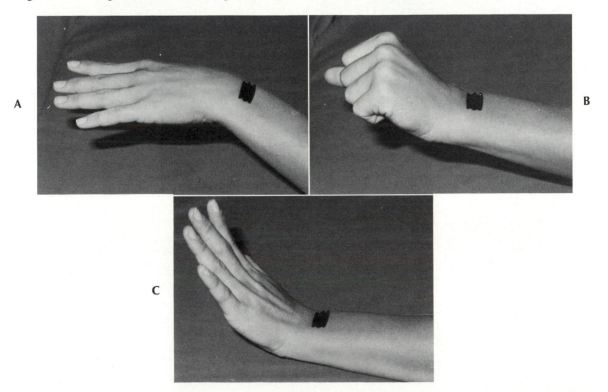

FIG. 29-39. Tendon restraint proximal to dorsal carpal ligament. **A,** Wrist flexion prematurely extends digits because of extensor tenodesis. **B,** Active digital flexion passively extends wrist. **C,** Active combined wrist and digital extension may be preserved, reflecting unobstructed proximal glide.

Distal to dorsal carpal ligament

Active and passive motion of the wrist is not impaired. The patterns of scar restraint at this level depend on whether the scar glides, such as a bulky tendon repair, or is anchored to the deep fascia. Gliding scar limits motion by its inability to glide beneath the dorsal carpal ligament. This restricts combined wrist and finger extension. One may increase wrist extension by first flexing the fingers. This pulls the bulky scar distally, further from the distal edge of the dorsal carpal ligament, and allows a greater proximal excursion with wrist extension before the scar is again obstructed by the dorsal carpal ligament (Fig. 29-40).

Scar fixing the finger or thumb extensor tendons to the deep fascia produces an extensor-plus phenomenon. This is a tenodesis whereby the interphalangeal joints of the digits are passively extended as the metacarpophalangeal joints are flexed. Combined flexion of the metacarpophalangeal and interphalangeal joints is prevented. As the interphalangeal joints are flexed, the tenodesis is transferred proximally and the metacarpophalangeal joints extend. Active and passive reciprocity exists between the metacarpophalangeal and interphalangeal joints (Fig. 29-41).

Intrinsic tightness versus tendon scarring

Tightness of the intrinsic muscles and adhesions of the fibers of the dorsal apparatus can both interfere with the

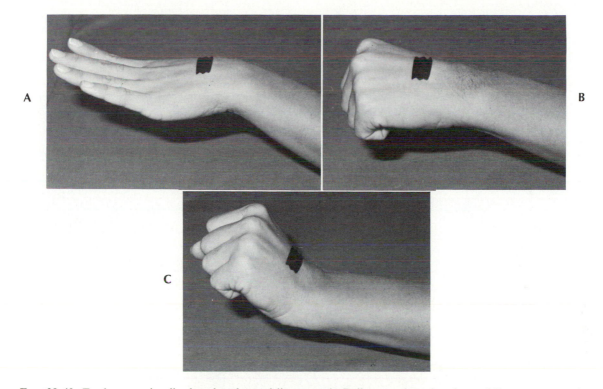

FIG. 29-40. Tendon restraint distal to dorsal carpal ligament. **A,** Bulky scar abuts dorsal carpal ligament preventing simultaneous wrist and digital extension, **B,** Digital flexion before wrist extension increases potential for wrist extension. **C,** Wrist and digital flexion may not be impaired.

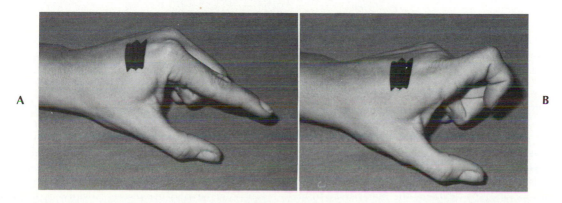

FIG. 29-41. Extensor-plus finger condition caused by extensor tendon restrained proximal to metacarpophalangeal joints. **A,** Active and passive flexion of metacarpophalangeal joint produces tenodesis with passive extension of interphalangeal joints. **B,** Active or passive interphalangeal flexion passively extends metacarpophalangeal joints.

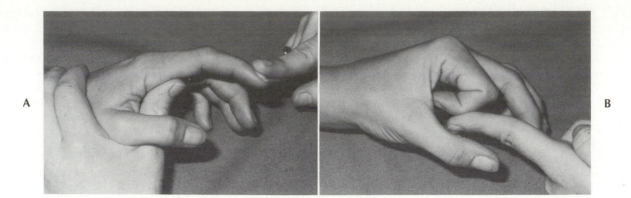

FIG. 29-42. Intrinsic tightness test. **A,** Passive flexion of interphalangeal joints are assessed while metacarpophalangeal joint is supported in extension. One can test radial and ulnar intrinsics separately by deviating finger away from side being tested. **B,** Metacarpophalangeal flexion relaxes intrinsic muscles and lessens tension through extensor tendons, decreasing resistence to passive interphalangeal flexion.

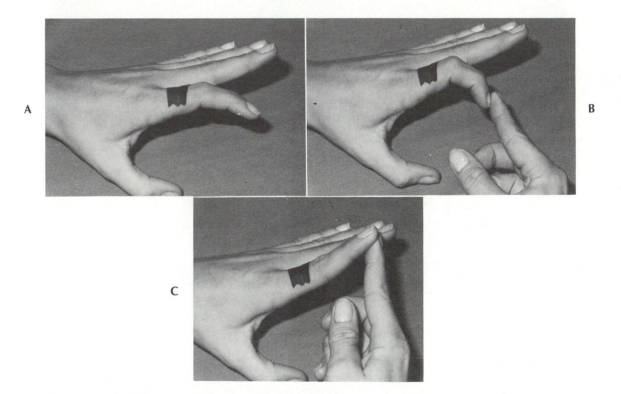

FIG. 29-43. Scar restraint of dorsal apparatus. **A,** Active extension beyond resting position is prevented. **B,** Active and passive flexion is resisted, often feeling "springy." **C,** Passive extension is present if adjacent joints are healthy.

mechanics of finger flexion. Active and passive flexion can be painful with either situation. Scar involving the dorsal apparatus can produce a clinical picture that is indistinguishable from an intrinsic contracture. Intrinsic tightness is tested by passively extending the finger metacarpophalangeal joint while flexing the interphalangeal joints. The individual ulnar and radial intrinsic muscles of each finger may be tested separately by deviating the finger away from the side being evaluated. Intrinsic restraint inferred from testing may reflect scarring of the dorsal apparatus, which can be discerned only at the time of tenolysis (Fig. 29-42).

Proximal phalanx

Scarring of the extensor tendons over the proximal phalanx may involve the central tendon, intrinsic expansions, or the entire dorsal apparatus. The resting position of the proximal interphalangeal joint reflects the positioning of the extensor tendons when motion was arrested at the site of restraint. Active extension of the proximal interphalangeal joint beyond the resting position is lacking. Usually some extensor lag is present, and passive extension to neutral is possible. Active and passive flexion of the proximal interphalangeal joint is blocked, often with an

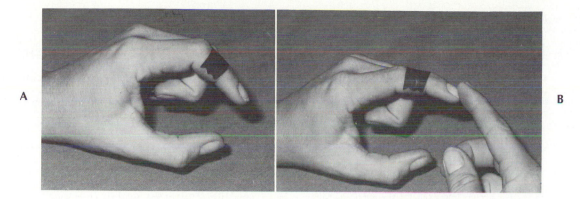

FIG. 29-44. Extensor tendon restraint over middle phalanx. **A,** Active distal interphalangeal joints flexion lacking. Extensor lag may be evident. **B,** Passive distal joint flexion "springy" or blocked. Associated tightness of proximal interphalangeal joint flexion suggests restraint of lateral bands and dorsal fibers of transverse retinacular ligament.

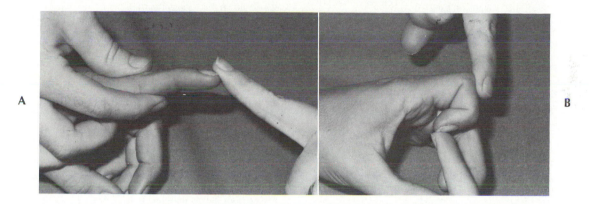

FIG. 29-45. Retinacular tightness or intrinsic intrinsic-plus phenomenon. **A,** Oblique retinacular ligament tightness tested by passive flexing of distal interphalangeal joint while proximal interphalangeal joint is maintained in extension. Relative resistence indicates a positive test. **B,** Combined flexion of both interphalangeal joints is present normally and in mild ligamentous tightness. Test is dependent on position of proximal interphalangeal joint.

elastic or springy quality during testing (Fig. 29-43).

Flexion of the proximal interphalangeal joint can also be prevented by scarring of the triangular ligament and consolidation of the crisscrossed fibers between central tendon and lateral bands. Both conditions block flexion of the proximal interphalangeal joint by preventing the volar shift of the lateral bands.[10] Limitation of flexion of the proximal interphalangeal joint is usually associated with restraints upon the distal interphalangeal joint.

Middle phalanx

Scarring of the extensor tendon over the middle phalanx restrains flexion of the distal interphalangeal joint. Active and passive restraint unrelated to the position of the proximal interphalangeal joint implies scarring of the extensor tendon. Scarring at this level, however, usually involves the retinacular ligaments, too; and isolated tendon scarring is uncommon clinically (Fig. 29-44).

The oblique retinacular ligaments pass volarly to the axis of motion of the proximal interphalangeal joint and exert a dynamic tenodesis when they extend the distal joint as the proximal interphalangeal joint is extended. Normally they probably do not contribute to the final 45 degrees of distal

joint extension. In the imbalanced or scarred finger, however, they can significantly contribute to limiting distal joint motion and fostering deformity. A contracted oblique retinacular ligament produces a positive retinacular tightness test, also called intrinsic intrinsic-plus phenomenon.[4] Passive flexion of the distal interphalangeal joint is present in the normal finger as the proximal interphalangeal joint is passively extended. This distal joint motion is restrained, however, with shortening or scarring of the oblique retinacular ligament. The dependency on the position of the proximal interphalangeal joint differentiates this restraint from extensor tendon fixation (Fig. 29-45).

REFERENCES

1. Agee, J., and Guidera, M.: The functional significance of the juncturae tendinum in dynamic stabilization of the metacarpophalangeal joints of the fingers, personal communication, Sacramento, Calif., 1982.
2. Blacker, G.J.: The abducted little finger in low ulnar palsy, J. Hand Surg. **1:**190, 1976.
3. Boyes, J.H.: Bunnell's surgery of the hand, ed. 5, Philadelphia, 1970, J.B. Lippincott Co.
4. Bunnell, S.: Rupture of tendons. In Bunnell, S.: Surgery of the hand, ed. 4, Philadelphia, 1964, J.B. Lippincott Co.
5. Burkhart, S.S., Wood, M.B., and Linscheid, R.L.: Posttraumatic

recurrent subluxation of the extensor carpi ulnaris tendon, J. Hand Surg. **7:**1, 1982.

6. Eckhardt, W.A., and Palmer, A.K.: Recurrent dislocation of the extensor carpi ulnaris tendon, J. Hand Surg. **6:**629, 1981.

7. Elliott, R.A.: Boutonnière deformity. In Cramer, L.M., and Chase, R.A.: Symposium of the hand, St. Louis, 1971, The C.V. Mosby Co.

8. Engkvist, O., and Lundborg, G.: Rupture of the extensor pollicis longus tendon after fractures of the lower end of the radius: a clinical and microangiographic study, Hand **11:**76, 1979.

9. Haines, R.W.: The extensor apparatus of the finger, J. Anat. **85:**251, 1951.

10. Harris, C.: The functional anatomy of the extensor mechanism of the finger, J. Bone Joint Surg. **54A:**713, 1972.

11. Hollinshead, W.H.: Anatomy for surgeons: the back and limbs, ed. 2, vol. 3, New York, 1969, Harper & Row, Publishers.

12. Johansson, S.H.: Peritendineous fibrosis of the dorsum of the hand, Fifth World Congress of Plastic and Reconstructive Surgery, London, 1971, Butterworth & Co. (Publishers), Ltd.

13. Kaplan, E.B.: Anatomy, injuries and treatment of extensor apparatus of the hand and digits, Clin. Orthop. **13:**24, 1959.

14. Kaplan, E.B.: Functional and surgical anatomy of the hand, ed. 2, Philadelphia, 1965, J.B. Lippincott Co.

15. Ketchum, L.D., Brand, P.W., Thompson, D., and Pacach, G.S.: The determination of movements for extension of the wrist generated by muscles of the forearm, J. Hand Surg. **3:**205, 1978.

16. Kettelkamp, D.B.: Traumatic dislocation of the long finger extensor tendon, J. Bone Joint Surg. **53A:**229, 1971.

17. Landmeer, J.M.F.: The anatomy of the dorsal aponeurosis of the human finger and its functional significance, Anat. Rec. **104:**31, 1949.

18. Light, T.R.: Buttress pinning techniques, Orthop. Rev. **10:**49, 1981.

19. Littler, J.W.: The finger extensor mechanism, Surg. Clin. North Am. **47:**415, 1967.

20. Milford, L.W.: Retaining ligaments of the digits of the hand, Philadelphia, 1968, W.B. Saunders Co.

21. Milford, L.W.: The hand, St. Louis, 1971, The C.V. Mosby Co.

22. Montant, R., and Baumann, A.: Rupture luxation of the extensor appratus of the finger of the first interphalangeal articulation, Rev. d'Orthop. **25:**5, 1938.

23. Reading, G.: Secretan's syndrome: hard edema of he dorsum of the hand, Plast. Reconstr. Surg. **65:**182, 1980.

24. Redfern, A.B., Curtis, R.M., and Shaw Wilgis, E.F.: Experience with peritendinous fibrosis of the dorsum of the hand, J. Hand Surg. **7:**380, 1982.

25. Riordan, D.: Peritendineous fibrosis of the extensor tendons, J. Bone Joint Surg. **47A:**632, 1965.

26. Saferin, E.H.: Secretan's disease, Plast. Reconstr. Surg. **58:**703, 1976.

27. Schenck, R.R.: Variations of extensor tendons of the fingers, J. Bone Joint Surg. **46A:**103, 1964.

28. Schultz, R.J., Furlong, J., II, and Storace, A.: Detailed anatomy of the extensor mechanism at the proximal aspect of the finger, J. Hand Surg. **6:**493, 1981.

29. Secretan, H.: Œdéma dur et hyperplasie traumatique du métacarpe dorsal, Rev. Med. Suisse Romande **21:**409, 1901.

30. Shrewsbury, M.M.: A systematic study of the oblique retinacular ligament of the human finger: its structure and function, J. Hand Surg. **2:**194, 1977.

31. Smith, R.J.: Factitious lymphedema of the hand, J. Bone Joint Surg. **57A:**89, 1975.

32. Smith, R.J.: Balance and kinetics of the fingers under normal and pathological conditions, Clin. Orthop. **92:**104, 1974.

33. Spinner, M., and Kaplan, E.B.: Extensor carpi ulnaris: its relationship to the stability of the distal radioulnar joint, Clin. Orthop. **68:**124, 1970.

34. Stack, H.G.: Mallet finger, Hand **1:**83, 1969.

35. Stark, H.H., Bayer, J.H., and Wilson, J.N.: Mallet finger, J. Bone Joint Surg. **44A:**1061, 1962.

36. Tubiana, R.: The Hand, Philadelphia, 1981, W.B. Saunders Co. vol. 1, pp. 297-325.

37. Tubiana, R., and Valentin, P.: The anatomy of the extensor apparatus of the fingers, Surg. Clin. North Am. **44:**897, 1964.

38. Zancolli, E.A.: Structural and dynamic basis of hand surgery, ed. 2, Philadelphia, 1979, J.B. Lippincott Co.

39. Zbrodowski, A., Gajisin, S., and Grodecki, J.: Vascularization and anatomical model of the mesotendons of the extensor digitorum and extensor indicis muscles, J. Anat. **130:**697, 1980.

30

Rehabilitation of extensor tendon injuries

VALERIE HOLDEMAN LEE

The rehabilitation of extensor tendon injuries demands that the therapist have a complete working knowledge of extensor tendon anatomy, an understanding of the kinetics of the extensor mechanism both in normal and pathological conditions, and thorough understanding of the surgical technique utilized. Verdan has divided the hand into extensor tendon zones (Fig. 30-1). Because the location of injury dictates the timing and goals of rehabilitation, the zones are used as reference areas throughout this chapter.

ZONES 1 AND 2

A disruption of the terminal tendon in zone 1 or 2 produces a mallet or drop-tip deformity. These injuries may be closed or open, and may or may not be associated with a fracture to the distal phalanx. In open injuries associated with a fracture, internal fixation of the distal interphalangeal joint in neutral position or mild hyperextension, by means of a Kirschner wire, may be performed by the surgeon. The wire is removed at 4 to 6 weeks. Closed injuries may be treated with immobilization, again in neutral or mild hyperextension for 4 to 6 weeks. The splint used for closed mallet fingers may be a padded dorsal splint or a volar splint (Fig. 30-2). The dorsal splint, which is padded to prevent undue pressure, has the advantage of allowing for sensory feedback during immobilization. Whether the splint is dorsal or volar, it should not encumber proximal interphalangeal joint flexion, because immobilization of the proximal interphalangeal (PIP) joint for 4 to 6 weeks will result in a stiff joint.

It is not uncommon for nailbed injuries to accompany extensor tendon injuries in zone 1. In this case a nailbed splint fabricated from a well-molded thermoplastic material may be used to encourage a smoother growth of the nailbed.

For open or closed repair, the patient should receive therapy at an early data. Goals of early treatment should be (1) mobilization of the PIP joint and other unaffected joints and (2) a strengthening program.

The mobilization of all unaffected joints is extremely important; however, emphasis is placed on maintaining maximal PIP joint motion, because that joint is considered the most critical joint in hand function.

An injury to even one digit can lead to weakness, primarily from disuse. Therefore a program utilizing wrist weights and resistive exercises should be considered.

When active motion is begun, the exercise and splinting program must be monitored with care. The newly repaired terminal tendon may be easily overstretched by overpowering of the flexor digitorum profundus. This can lead to a secondary deformity, the swan neck. The extensor force is directed proximally to the PIP joint because of the loss of a more distal attachment. The PIP joint is then hyperextended through the transverse retinacular ligament. To prevent this from becoming a fixed deformity, the following steps should be taken: (1) If a lag at the distal interphalangeal (DIP) joints occurs, the splinting program must be adjusted to increase time in extension splinting. (2) If hyperextension of the PIP joint begins to occur, the patient is placed in a splint that maintains the PIP joint in a mild degree of flexion (Fig. 30-3). This prevents extension of the PIP joint and directs the extensor force distally.

Active exercises include blocking and prehension activities. Patients with simple mallet injuries are splinted protectively for an additional 4 weeks after the initiation of active motion. With proper treatment and rehabilitation these patients should achieve a very functional result with minimal if any disability.

ZONES 3 AND 4

Extensor tendon injuries that occur over the PIP joint or proximal phalanx (zones 3 and 4) are critical injuries because of the complex interaction of the extensor mechanism.

The most common injury at this level occurs when the PIP joint is acutely flexed, tearing the central slip and the medial interosseous band. The lateral bands shift volarly at the time of injury, tearing the triangular ligament. The lateral bands are now volar to the axis of motion of the PIP joint and become flexors of that joint and the extensors of the DIP joint. Initially the lag at the PIP joint may not be significant, but with time the unopposed force of the flexor digitorum superficialis and the shortening of the transverse retinacular ligament and of the oblique retinacular ligament will lead to a boutonnière deformity. If left unattended, secondary joint contractures will develop, and this becomes a fixed deformity.

After surgical repair of the extensor mechanism and internal fixation of the PIP joint, the patients are immobilized for a period of 4 weeks with both the PIP and DIP joints in extension. The metacarpophalangeal joint is not encumbered. If surgical repair involved only the central slip and not the lateral bands, at 10 to 14 days the patient is seen in therapy to begin motion of the DIP joint with the PIP joint stabilized in extension to prevent motion of the central slip (Fig. 30-4). The purpose of this exercise is threefold: (1) to stretch the oblique retinacular ligament (which is located volarly to the axis of the PIP joint motion and dorsally to the axis of motion at the PIP joint), (2) to allow gliding of the lateral bands to prevent them from becoming adherent, and (3) to prevent stiffness of the DIP joint.

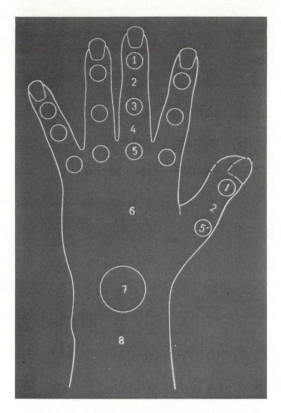

FIG. 30-1. Extensor tendon zones as described by Verdan.

At the end of 4 to 6 weeks, active motion is begun at the PIP joint. Care must be taken that a lag does not develop at the PIP joint because of overstretching of the central slip. Emphasis should be placed on full extension after flexion. If an extensor lag does develop, a small splint supporting the PIP joint in extension is utilized as appropriate. The desired goal is to obtain gradual increases in PIP flexion while maintaining full extension. Velcro loops or buddy taping can be utilized at 5 to 6 weeks to provide active assistive exercises for flexion (Fig. 30-5). At 6 weeks dynamic extension splinting may be used to provide for support in extension and resistance into flexion. A banding metal splint (Fig. 30-6) or other assistive devices may be used at 7 to 8 weeks. Again I must emphasize that the active range of motion be monitored closely, so that if a lag develops the amount of time spent in extension splinting must be increased and the time spent in dynamic flexion splinting decreased.

A pathologic condition such as rheumatoid arthritis may also lead to a boutonnière deformity. Chronic synovitis attenuates the central slip and triangular ligament and allows for volar displacement of the lateral bands. With time, fixed deformities result.

Patients with chronic traumatic boutonnière deformities with fixed flexion contractures need to be seen preoperatively in an attempt to decrease the flexion contracture before surgery. Dynamic extension assist splints are used intermittently during the day. Static splints such as a metal splint or serial plaster cast may be used at night to maintain the degree of extension gains made during the day. The results after surgical repair of a chronic traumatic boutonnière deformity are directly related to the amount of passive extension available preoperatively.

ZONE 5

Laceration to the extensor tendons over the metacarpophalangeal joint (zone 5) results in an inability to extend the proximal phalanx. After surgical repair, the wrist is

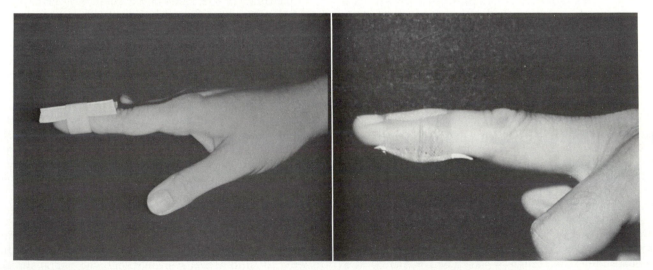

FIG. 30-2. A, Padded dorsal splint for mallet finger. **B,** Volar splint for mallet finger.

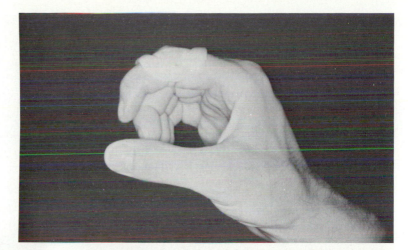

FIG. 30-3. "Swan-neck" splint to prevent proximal interphalangeal hyperextension.

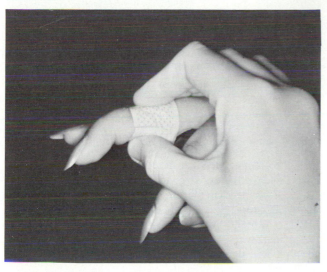

FIG. 30-4. Proximal interphalangeal joint is stabilized and distal interphalangeal joint is actively flexed. This allows motion of the lateral bands while preventing motion of the newly repaired central slip.

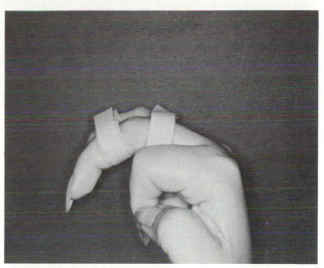

FIG. 30-5. Velcro loops can be used to provide active assistive flexion and extension.

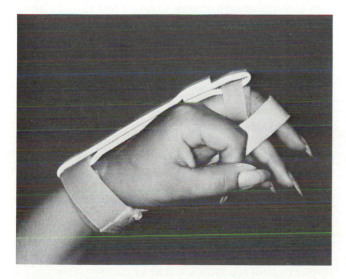

FIG. 30-6. A dorsal banding metal splint with an attached flexion cuff may be used to increase passive flexion.

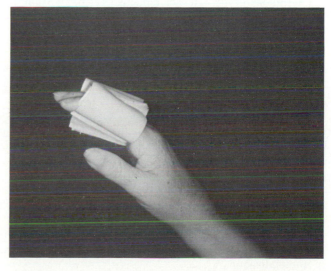

FIG. 30-7. Large velcro loops prevent flexion of interphalangeal joints and encourage flexion at metacarpophalangeal joints.

immobilized in extension with the metacarpophalangeal joints in mild flexion.

At 4 weeks active motion is begun, with protective splinting being carried out for an additional 4 weeks.

Initially an extensor lag may be noticed at the metacarpophalangeal joint because of adherence of skin to the extensor tendon. There may also be an extensor lag at the PIP joint because of adherence of the central slip. Care must be taken that the extensor lag at the PIP joint does not lead to secondary flexion deformities. Prevention of such deformities is aided by intermittent extension splinting of the PIP joint.

The intrinsics may become tight because of the necessary position of immobilization. Intrinsic stretching is done gently, by supporting the proximal joint in extension while simultaneously flexing the interphalangeal joints.

At 4 weeks, when active motion is begun, simultaneous metacarpophalangeal and interphalangeal joint flexion will not be possible, because of tendon adherence. The wrist should be placed in extension when one first asks the patient for metacarpophalangeal and interphalangeal flexion, to reduce stress on the suture line.

To encourage tendon gliding over the metacarpophalangeal joint, large Velcro loops over the interphalangeal joints are used to direct the extensor force proximally (Fig. 30-7). This prevents flexion of the interphalanageal joints.

To maximize metacarpophalangeal joint motion, the wrist is placed in extension. Active exercises to the wrist in flexion and extension are also utilized.

The fingers may be taped in a claw position for muscle reeducation of the extensor digitorum communis. Light resistance to finger flexors may be begun at 5 to 6 weeks. However, resistance to the extensor tendons themselves must be delayed until 7 to 8 weeks.

If the metacarpophalangeal joint is not involved in the injury, full active flexion and extension should be achieved approximately 8 weeks after the injury.

ZONE 6

Lacerations to the extensor tendons over the dorsum of the hand (zone 6) are often associated with crushing trauma, which produces a moderate to severe amount of edema formation. The healing extensor tendons may become adherent in the surrounding infratendinous and supratendinous fasciae. They may also become greatly adherent to the skin. If fractures are involved, they may become adherent volarly to the metacarpals.

After surgical repair, the wrist is splinted in extension with the metacarpophalangeal joints in mild flexion, for a period of 4 weeks. When active motion is begun at 4 weeks, there will be incomplete metacarpophalangeal and interphalangeal flexion because of tendon adherence. Extensor lag at the metacarpophalangeal and interphalangeal joints will increase with increasing wrist extension. Tethering of the tendons in scar will initially result in limited wrist flexion. As with injuries over the metacarpophalangeal joint, intrinsic tightness may be present because of the position of immobilization.

When active flexion of the metacarpophalangeal and interphalangeal joints is initiated, the wrist is placed in ex-

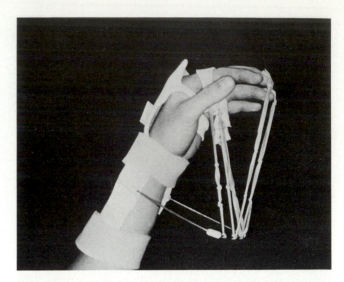

FIG. 30-8. To decrease extensor tendon adherence, proximal phalanx is first flexed until interphalangeal joints extend. Traction is then applied over distal phalanx to place a gentle stretch on extensor tendon.

tension to reduce stress at the site of repair. Over the next 2 to 3 weeks the wrist is held in decreasing degrees of extension to increase the stress on the suture site as further healing occurs.

Extensor tendon tightness is present (provided the joints are normal) when the interphalangeal joints can extend but resist passive flexion when the metacarpophalangeal joints are flexed.

Dynamic splinting may be utilized at 7 to 8 weeks in order to increase joint mobility and to decrease extensor tendon tightness. A dorsal splint (Fig. 30-8) is fabricated. The proximal phalanx is flexed with a moleskin on a leather loop until the interphalangeal joints extend because of the extrinsic tightness. Traction is then applied over the distal phalanx so that a gentle stretch is placed on the extensor tendon. This splint is worn intermittently during the day.

ZONE 7

In zone 7, at the level of the dorsal carpal ligament, there is a potential for injury to 12 tendons. When multiple tendons are injured, the surgeon preserves independent extension of the wrist, fingers, and thumb. Repaired extensors in this zone are generally immobilized for 4 to 6 weeks.

Rehabilitation of the wrist extensors must include exercises in radialulnar deviation and in the flexion-extension plane. For example, maximal excursion of the extensor carpi radialis longus and extensor carpi radialis brevis occurs in flexion and extension. However, maximal excursion of the extensor carpi ulnaris does not occur in flexion-extension but in radioulnar deviation. Because the extensor carpi ulnaris acts more as a stabilizer than as a wrist extensor when the forearm is in pronation, wrist flexion and extension must be performed in both supination and pronation.

ZONE 8

Lacerations in zone 8 must be immobilized with the wrist in extension for a period of up to 8 weeks to prevent rupture of the repair. However, the length of immobilization is conducive to massive adhesion formation. With scarring proximal to the wrist, wrist flexion may result in hyperextension of the metacarpophalangeal joints. But with the wrist in extension, the digits cannot be simultaneously extended. When fingers are fully flexed, the proximal scarring prevents simultaneous wrist flexion. Patients with injuries in zone 8 require aggressive splinting in an attempt to overcome the tendon adherence and may ultimately need to undergo tenolysis.

THUMB

The thumb is divided into four zones. The position of immobilization is with the wrist in extension and the thumb in extension-adduction. At 4 weeks, active motion is begun.

Injuries to the extensor tendons of the thumb may be compared to those of the digits, with some variations. A mallet thumb is almost always associated with a fracture, because the force required to produce this deformity must be significant, whereas a mallet finger is not necessarily associated with a fracture.

Rupture of the extensor pollicis brevis at the metacarpophalangeal joint may result in a boutonnière deformity, the severity of which is in part dependent on the amount of metacarpophalangeal flexion available. The extensor pollicis longus does not always attenuate and will instead stretch the extensor hood ulnarward. This ulnar pull is countered by the radial pull of the thenar lateral extensor tendon. The proximal phalanx flexes with the force of the adductor pollicis augmented by the lateral extensor tendons, which have shifted volarly to the axis of the joint. This produces a deformity that is a cross between the ulnar drift and the typical buttonhole deformity.

Because of the position of immobilization in extension-adduction, a thumb-web contracture may be developed during immobilization. This is corrected with use of a thumb-web spacer.

Because the metacarpophalangeal joint must be immobilized in extension after extensor tendon repair of the thumb, this joint is often stiff after splint removal. To direct all flexor force at the metacarpophalangeal joint, the interphalangeal joint is prevented from flexion by use of a small dorsal splint.

SUMMARY

Although guidelines can be set for timing of extensor tendon rehabilitation, remember that each patient will need to be treated on an individual basis.

The dilemma of extensor tendon rehabilitation is to increase motion after immobilization and repair while preventing overstretching of a newly repaired structure.

The goal of increasing motion while preventing extension lag is best accomplished with a carefully monitored splinting and active range of motion program.

BIBLIOGRAPHY

Bowers, W.H., and Hurst, L.C.: Chronic mallet finger: the use of Fowler's central slip release, J. Hand Surg. **3**:373-376, July 1978.

Dargan, E.L.: Management of extensor tendon injuries of the hand, Surg. Gynecol. Obstet. **128**:1269-1273, June 1969.

Elliott, R.A.: Injuries to the extensor mechanism of the hand, Orthop. Clin. North Am. **1**:335-354, Nov. 1970.

Elliott, R.A.: Boutonnière deformity. In Cramer, L.M., and Chase, R.A.: Symposium of the hand, St. Louis, 1971, The C.V. Mosby Co.

Harris, C., and Rutledge, G.L.: The functional anatomy of extensor mechanism of the finger, J. Bone Joint Surg. **54A**:713-726, June 1972.

Iselin, F., Levane, J., and Godoy, J.: A simplified technique for treating mallet fingers: tenodermodesis, J. Hand Surg. **2**:118-121, March 1977.

Kilgore, E.S., Jr., and Granam, W.P., III: The hand: surgical-nonsurgical management, Philadelphia, 1977, Lea & Febiger, pp. 184-199.

Littler, J.W., and Eaton, R.G.: Redistribution of forces in the correction of the boutonniere deformity, J. Bone Joint Surg. **49A**:1267-1274, Oct. 1967.

Schenck, R.R.: Variations of the extensor tendons of the fingers, J. Bone Joint Surg. **46A**:103-110, Jan. 1964.

Smith, R.J.: Balance and kinetics of the fingers under normal pathological conditions, Clin. Orthop. Rel. Res. **104**:92-111, Oct. 1974.

Smith, R.J.: Intrinsic muscles of the fingers: function, dysfunction, and surgical reconstruction. In American Academy of Orthopaedics Surgeons: Instructional course lectures **24**:200, St. Louis, 1975, The C.V. Mosby Co.

Souter, W.A.: The problem of boutonnière deformity, Clin. Orthop. Rel. Res. **104**:116-133, Oct. 1974.

Tubiana, R., and Valentin, P.: The physiology of the extension of the fingers, Surg. Clin. North Am. **44**:909-918, 1964.

Tubiana, R., and Valentin, P.: The anatomy of the extensor appratus of the fingers, Surg. Clin. North Am. **44**:897-906, 1964.

Tubiana, R.: Injuries to the extensor apparatus on the dorsum of the fingers. In Verdan, C.: Tendon surgery of the hand, New York, Churchill Livingstone, Inc., pp. 119-128.

VII
NERVE INJURIES

31

Nerve response to injury and repair

GEORGE E. OMER, Jr.

The peripheral nerves are extensions of the central nervous sytem and are responsible for integrating the activities of the hand. Interruption of the structural continuity of a peripheral nerve results in derangement of the involved functional units. A functional unit is called a "neuron." The neuron consists of the nerve cell nucleus and cytoplasm (perikaryon) in the anterior column of the spinal cord (motor neurons) or the dorsal root ganglia (sensory neurons), the nerve cell cytoplasm in the peripheral nerve trunk (axon), and the anatomic unit at the synaptic terminal (such as the extrafusal fibers of muscles or Meissner's touch corpuscles) (Fig. 31-1). If the central cell body (perikaryon) were the height of an average man, its axon would be 1 or 2 inches in diameter and would extend more than 2 miles.[17] The number of neurons is constant after birth, and there is no replacement when a nerve cell is destroyed.

The axon may be surrounded by Schwann cells, which form the insulation (myelin) for fast conduction of nerve impulses. External to the Schwann cell layer is a connective tissue sheath termed the "endoneurium" (Fig. 31-2). The endoneurial tube (Schwann tube or Büngner band) may contain only one myelinated axon or several unmyelinated axons. The nerve fiber (axon and sheath) is the smallest structural unit of the peripheral nerve. Nerve fibers are gathered into aggregations called fasciculi, funiculi, or nerve bundles. Each fasciculus is composed usually of a mixture of motor, sensory, and sympathetic fibers. The perineurium is a relatively fine but strong connective tissue sheath that encases each fasciculus. Fasciculi are arranged usually in groups as they proceed peripherally. The groups (bundles) of fasciculi are embedded in epineurium (intraneurial epineurium, intrafascicular epineurium, or epineurial connective tissue). The amount of epineurial tissue within a peripheral nerve trunk may range from 25% to 75% of the cross-sectional area[68] (Fig. 31-3). The epineurium is condensed at the surface of the nerve trunk to form a definite encasing sheath, the epineurial sheath (nerve sheath or circumferential sheath).

INJURY

After injury to the axon there are retrograde reactions involving the central cell body. The more proximal the extremity injury (axonal level) and the greater the violence to the axon (stretch avulsion as opposed to transection), the more severe the reaction of the central cell body. Estimates of neuronal death range from 30% to 75%.[68] Even if the nerve cell survives, the volume (length) of axon that must be regenerated may exceed the metabolic capacity of the central cell body. Retrograde effects will be more serious in sensory than in motor neurons, and sensory recovery will be slower and less satisfactory than motor recovery.[64] A child has a greater regeneration potential than an adult and a shorter axon distance between the spinal cord and functional end organs.

In the distal nerve stump all the neuronal elements undergo secondary degeneration. Morphologic changes occur within 24 hours after injury, and all unmyelinated axons degenerate within 1 week.[50] Muscles respond to nerve stimulation for 4 or 5 days, and ascending (sensory) nerve action potentials can be recorded for 6 to 8 days after axon division.[70] By 3 weeks after injury most of the axon and myelin have been digested by the Schwann cells, and by 8 weeks the débridement is complete.[16] With subsequent collapse of the individual endoneurial tubes, the reentry of regenerating axons may be difficult. This shrinkage of the distal stump is maximal at approximately 3 months after injury.[70] Endoneurial tubes within the distal segment of a disrupted nerve may wither to 10% of their original diameter,[25] and to what extent the endoneurial tube can expand in response to ingrowing axons is unknown. The conduction velocity in sutured human nerves frequently remains slow (20% to 60% of normal) even with clinical return of function.[25] The prognosis for functional recovery is better when nerve suture is performed within 3 months after injury.

For nerve regeneration to occur, myelinated axon sprouts must enter a distal endoneurial tube (Schwann tube or Büngner band) and be invaginated by Schwann cells and then remyelinated. Schwann cells of unmyelinated axons do not form compact columns analogous to the bands of Büngner. In a mixed nerve perhaps 50% of the regenerating motor neurons will grow down sensory pathways and the remainder correctly enter motor pathways.[20] However, many neurons in the motor pathway may be inappropriate in that they previously served antagonists of the muscle being reinnervated.[11] In like manner, sympathetic axons regenerating through endoneurial tubes destined for muscle form no functional end-organ connections and deny the entry of motor axons. Only slight rotation of either end of a severed nerve would produce misdirected axons or appose significant numbers of axons to an impervious epineurium and perineurium. The amount of tension, both circumferential and longitu-

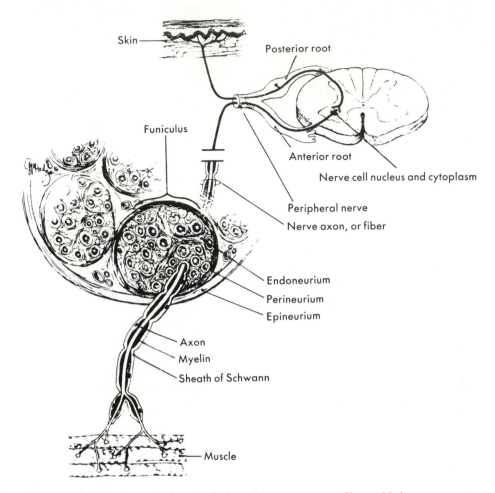

FIG. 31-1. Anatomy of nerve cell, showing cell body and nerve axon, or fiber, with its component parts. (From Grabb, W.C.: Orthop. Clin. North Am. **1**:419, 1970.)

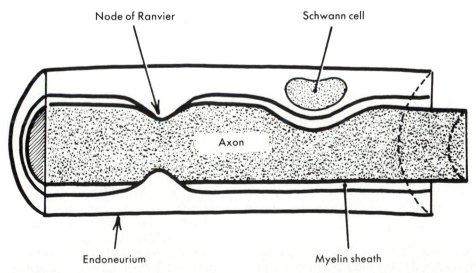

FIG. 31-2. Basic anatomy of a myelinated nerve fiber. (From Urbaniak, J.R., and Warren, F.H.: Application of microsurgical techniques in the care of the injured peripheral nerve. In American Academy of Orthopaedic Surgeons: Symposium on microsurgery, St. Louis, 1979, The C.V. Mosby Co.)

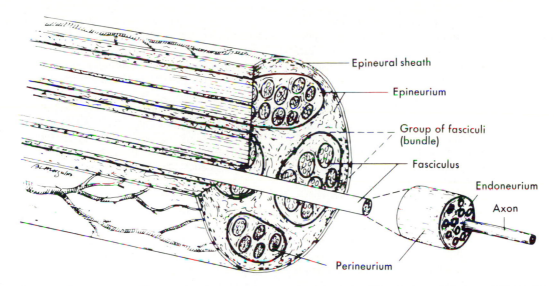

FIG. 31-3. Basic structures of a peripheral nerve. (From Urbaniak, J.R.: Clin. Orthop. Rel. Res. **163**:57, March 1982.)

dinal, within a sutured nuerve is directly related to connective tissue proliferation at the anastomosis.[35] The maturing scar tissue will shrink and constrict the axons. The regenerating axons may fail to achieve myelination, which would then lead to anatomic but not functional innervation of the end organs.

Denervation of skeletal muscle results in progressive shrinkage of muscle fibers and ultimate destruction. After 3 months the motor end plates become increasingly distorted by proliferating connective tissue. Denervated muscle does survive for relatively long periods, as evidenced by biopsy material and the persistence of fibrillations.[65] Muscle fiber viability can be demonstrated up to 3 years after denervation, but atrophy and connective tissue proliferation may preclude functional recovery after reinnervation.[70] The clinical impression that electrical stimulation of denervated muscle delays muscle fiber derangement and motor end-plate destruction has not been supported by human microscopic studies or measured work capacity of the muscle before and after denervation.[47,73] However, experimental long-term stimulation of muscle has demonstrated histochemical evidence of fiber-type transformation[55] and the prevention of decreased oxidative enzymes.[41] Muscle regeneration will occur under the stimulus of a functional nerve to supply both afferent and efferent pathways of the neural reflexes controlling muscle contraction.[4]

The extent to which biologic mechanisms are influenced by electrical forces is unknown.[6,7,9] Direct electrical current has been shown to stimulate growth of neurons in vitro[60] similar to the facilitatory effects of nerve growth factor, which has a predominant role only on embryonal neural tissues. There is current research[42] on the effect of minute direct electrical currents to the area of a nerve repair (suture site) after laceration. Insufficient data are available to determine if nerve regeneration will be enhanced by electrical forces.

Sensory receptor end organs that are denervated undergo progressive degeneration over several months, and it is probable that adult mammals lack the ability to form new sensory receptors after nerve transection.[50] After 4 months the Meissner corpuscle is incapable of full response to a regenerating axon.[15] The Meissner corpuscle appears to be about midway in the rate of degeneration between the rapid Merkel cell–neurite complex and the more stable pacinian corpuscle. It is unknown whether a regenerating axon can innervate a different sensory receptor, such as a quickly adapting axon innervating a Merkel cell–neurite complex, nor is the potential functional result known. It would appear that sensory end organs are even more susceptible to degeneration than skeletal muscle is, and a delay longer than 6 months between injury and suture will handicap the recovery of sensation.

The rate at which the axon regenerates has clinical importance. There are three periods of delay: neuronal survival, crossing the area of nerve disruption, and the end-organ connection. The patient's age and the tissue homeostasis of the involved extremity are important factors. The rate of growth gradually slows as the length of the axon increases. For practical use, after suture of a divided peripheral nerve there is a 3- to 4-week latent period, followed by axon advance of approximately 1 mm per day.[58]

In the clinical situation, there are three basic injury-regeneration patterns to consider, as outlined by Seddon[56]: Minimal nerve injury is termed ''neurapraxia,'' in which the nerve is intact but conduction is impaired. Moderate injury, termed ''axonotmesis,'' is characterized by interruption of the axons and their myelin sheaths; however, the endoneurial tubes remain intact and guide the regenerating axons to their appropriate peripheral connections. Severe injury, termed ''neurotmesis,'' describes a nerve that has either been completely severed or is so seriously disorganized that spontaneous regeneration is impossible. Most traumatic accidents, including fractures, dislocations, and gunshot wounds, can result in any one of these three types of injury. Lacerations usually result in neurotmesis. Total loss of nerve function after this injury demands exploration and suture of the affected nerve.

NOCICEPTIVE COMPLICATIONS OF NERVE INJURY

Current investigation indicates that pain may be a specific sensory event and not merely excessive stimulation of other sensory modalities. Current investigation has resulted in better definition of the specific pain receptors in the skin, viscera, and deep somatic structures. All these receptors respond to innocuous stimulation, whether it is mechanical, thermal, electrical, or chemical. A significant portion of the bare nerve endings are termed "nociceptors" and respond only to strong stimulation that is potentially damaging to tissue. In the periphaeral nervous system, the small myelinated axons are called "A-delta" (class III) and conduct at 12 to 80 meters per second. Approximately 25% of these axons are nociceptors and are stimulated by temperatures above 45° C or below 10 ° C and by intense mechanical stimulation. The even smaller unmyelinated axons are termed "C-delta" (class IV) and conduct at 0.4 to 1.0 meters per second. Approximately 50% of these axons are nociceptors. Iggo has defined the characteristics of the nociceptors as follows: very high thresholds to mechanical or thermal stimuli, relatively small receptive fields, and persistent after discharges for any suprathreshold stimulus.[27] There are three groups of nociceptors: high-threshold mechanoreceptors, heat nociceptors, and "polymodal" nociceptors responsive to both noxious mechanical and noxious thermal stimuli.[8] Polymodal and heat nociceptors can be sensitized after repeated or prolonged stimulation, or during regeneration after section of nerve, so that their thresholds for activation can be lowered to levels of stimulus intensity that are ordinarily innocuous. This could account for the pain states occurring after burns or nerve injury.[61]

The sympathetic nervous system of the upper extremity is concentrated in the thoracic portion of the spinal cord. Myelinated sympathetic axons exist through the anterior nerve root and then separate to form the white rami that enter the thoracic ganglia. A synapse occurs, and the postganglionic unmyelinated axons exit from the thoracic ganglia and enter the peripheral nerve. Since preganglionic axons form plexuses and synapses with many different postganglionic axons, a sympathetic discharge may affect several different target organs represented in more than one dermatome. Activation of a sympathetic discharge may elicit either an excitatory or an inhibitory response in different target organs, based on the relative potencies of the various catecholamines released at the neuroeffector junction. During an abnormal process, such as reflex sympathetic dystrophy, there may be great variations in the extremity, such as vasodilatation or vasoconstriction, increased redness or pallor, sweating or dryness, coolness or heat, depending on the severity or the state of involvement of different organs.

Injured nerve axons are excited by norepinephrine, which is the substance released at the neuroeffector junction by efferent impulses in the sympathetic nervous system. In the normal intact sensory nerve, sympathetic transmitters do not evoke obvious injury signals, although they may modulate sensitivity. Partially damaged nerve membrane and the unmyelinated axons (sprouts) within a neuroma are highly sensitive to norepinephrine. Stimulation of myelinated axons releases local endorphins, which dampen or stop the oversensitive spontaneous activity of these unmyelinated axons at the spinal cord level. When tissue is injured, the nociceptors are influenced by sympathetic efferents, the chemical environment, the vasculature, the temperature, and high-frequency antidromic impulses.

The study of peripheral receptors led to an understanding of the relationship between humoral mediators and pain. Acute inflammation invokes an exudative response that results in hydrolysis of extracellular macromolecules and breakdown of intracellular compounds.[59] The immediate mediators include histamine, released from basophils and mast cells, and serotonin, released from platelets. At the same time, plasma precursors are activated to form materials with a low molecular weight that provoke acute vascular inflammation and pain. All injured cells release prostaglandins and thromboxanes. These mediators are also liberated by mechanical pressure, electrical stimulation, radiation, or thermal injury. They induce pain in two ways: (1) direct irritation or stimulation of the nociceptors and (2) sensitizing the nociceptors to the pain-provoking effect of kinins and similar substances. The humoral mediators lower the threshold to pain transmission and increase the intensity of the stimulus.

We would suffer unrelenting pain if there were no endogenous defense against these humoral mediators. The mechanisms that limit their activity are being identified. For example, histaminase is produced to break down histamine, and peptidases degrade the kinins. Specific drugs can interrupt metabolic reactions such as the injury of cells to form prostaglandins and thromboxanes. The clinical value of nonsteroidal anti-inflammatory agents, such as aspirin or indomethacin, is that they block the metabolic pathway for the formation of prostaglandins and thromboxanes.[71]

The action potential produced by stimulation of the nociceptors passes to the dorsal horn of the spinal cord, which has six laminae of cell networks that both process and transmit the impulses.[53] There appear to be two types of pain-related sensory neurons in the dorsal horn. Class 1 nociceptive neurons are located in the most superficial layer of the dorsal horn (lamina 1). Class 1 neurons are responsive to injurious levels of stimulation.[14] Class 2 nociceptive neurons are located primarily in lamina 5 and respond to low-intensity stimulation, but as the intensity of stimulation is increased these neurons follow with more vigorous and sustained discharge.[72] Class 2 neurons are impinged upon by both somatic and visceral sources and may be involved in visceral referred pain.[24] Melzack and Wall[34] postulated a dynamic interaction (control gate) among large and small afferent neurons, mediated through the small cells of the substantia gelatinosa (lamina 2 and 3). Large afferent neurons excite the cells of the substantia gelatinosa and increase presynaptic inhibition (closing the gate) to noxious impulses incoming on small afferent neurons. Small afferent neurons inhibit the cells of the substantia gelatinosa and thus decrease the presynaptic inhibition (opening the gate). Pain is perceived when a threshold level of nociceptive action potential is attained by the central transmission neurons.

Nociceptive impulses are transmitted from the dorsal horn of the spinal cord to all levels of the central nervous system. The neurons in laminae I, IV, V, and VI of the dorsal horn connect to the spinothalamic system, the neospinothalamic tract, and the paleospinothalamic tract.[13,69] The neospinothalamic tract runs to the thalamus, where it synapses with central neurons that pass to the somatosensory cortex. This tract conveys information for perception of sharp, well-localized pain. The older paleospinothalamic tract projects to the spinal cord and the thalamus, where it synapses with neurons that connect with the limbic forebrain structures. This tract conveys information for the perception of poorly localized, dull, aching, burning pain. Impulses transmitted by this tract provoke suprasegmental reflex responses concerned with circulation, respiration, and endocrine function. In addition, there are multisynaptic afferent systems, including the spinoreticular system, spinocervicothalamic system, dorsal intracornu system, and other complex tracts. In this infinitely duplicated system for the reception, transmission, and perception of pain, there is specificity at the periphery, but in the central nervous system the specificity is lost completely.

Supraspinal descending neural systems modify the nociceptive impulses. The pyramidal tracts, rubrospinal tracts, and retinculospinal tracts influence transmission in the dorsal horn.[22,62] The descending fibers from the cortex of the brain affect transmission in the thalamus, reticular formation, dorsal column of the cord, and other relay stations.

In 1969, Reynolds[54] stimulated cells in the periaqueductal periventricular gray matter and produced profound analgesia at the spinal cord level. This stimulation-produced analgesia can completely inhibit the pain-evoked discharges of class 2 dorsal horn neurons, without affecting their responsiveness to nonpainful stimuli.[43] This appears to be the same descending circuit affected by morphine to produce analgesia.[31] One particular spinal pathway conveying these descending pain-modulatory impulses is the dorsolateral funiculus, which terminates in the dorsal horn of the spinal cord. The neurotransmitter carried by these cells and released in the spinal cord is serotonin.[2,61] Either chemical or dietary depletion of brain serotonin levels increases sensitivity to pain. Tolerance develops to stimulation-produced analgesia, and cross-tolerance is found between morphine and stimulation-induced analgesia.[32] The morphine antagonist naloxone reverses stimulation-produced analgesia[1] when the stimulator is located ventrally within the periaqueductal gray matter, but it does not block analgesia when the stimulator is located dorsally within the periaqueductal gray matter.[3]

There are stereospecific receptors for the alkaloids from the opium poppy in the brain.[19] These receptors are confined to nervous tissue and perhaps the transmission of pain.[51] Hughes and colleagues[26] extracted a peptide of low molecular weight from the brain that acted as an agonist at opiate receptor sites, and its action was prevented by narcotic antagonists. The peptide was named "enkephalin." Others noted that the amino acid sequence of enkephalin was identical to that of beta-lipotropin C-fragment, a pituitary peptide. A higher opiate activity was exhibited by the beta-lipotropin C-fragment peptide than by enkephalin.[10] The C-fragment is now named "beta-endorphin." Beta-endorphin produces analgesic effects 3 to 4 times more potent than those of morphine when injected intravenously.[67] Pretreatment with naloxone eliminates the analgesia. A possible neurotransmitter or neuromodulator role for these neuropeptides is suggested by studies showing that they affect the action or release of dopamine and acetylcholine.[29,30,38] Acupuncture analgesia may be mediated by morphine-like hormones or neuropeptides released by the pituitary.[52] Thus it may be possible that the physiologic role of opiates and endogenous opiate-like neuropeptides involves the transmission of pain. The endogenous opiate-like neuropeptides may act on both presynaptic and postsynaptic opiate receptors in the spinal cord and brain. The same substance may be used as a neurotransmitter in one instance, a neuromodulator in another, and a hormone in still another situation.[21,44]

In addition to the endogenous opioid mechanism for analgesia, there may be a nonopioid mechanism. Mayer and colleagues[31] reported that naloxone blocked acupunctural analgesia, but not hypnotic analgesia in humans. Stimulation-produced analgesia is effective when the stimulator is in one portion of the periaqueductal gray matter but is not effective when the stimulator is moved to nearby sites.[3] Mayer and Price[33] have proposed that the descending pain-inhibitory mechanism may involve both a serotonergic and an enkephalin-like neurotransmitter system. Endorphins (enkephalins) may act as hormone-releasing or -inhibiting factors in peripheral target organs such as the adrenal medulla and the pancreas.[5] Electrical or chemical stimulation of either system produces analgesia, while chemical or surgical blockade of either prevents analgesia.

TIMING OF NERVE REPAIR

No controlled prospective study comparing clinical function after primary and secondary nerve suture has been reported. Clinical studies in the human show considerable variation because the return of useful function depends as much on the total response of the extremity to the injury as on the regeneration of the injured nerve.[45,46]

Our preference is to suture a severed nerve during the first 24 hours when there is a "clean" laceration and to wait 3 to 5 days when there is an injury to an extremity that is managed best with a delayed primary closure.[48] An extensive extremity wound dictates that nerve suture be delayed until after there is homeostasis of the involved tissues and the correct level of demarcation of the nerve injury can be determined.

Advantages of nerve suture at the time of acute injury include the following: (1) nerve stumps require minimal mobilization and débridement because the cut ends have not retracted and become embedded in scar tissue; (2) extensive dissection of the extremity is not required in order to remove scar tissue; (3) the axonal bundles at the nerve ends are more likely to correspond; (4) satisfactory suture can be performed without tension; (5) immediate suture reduces the time for which peripheral tissues are denervated and the patient is impaired; and (6) if a second operation is required, it is technically easier because the nerve ends are not retracted and the amount of nerve to be débrided (and therefore the gap to be closed) is reduced. Primary suture should be reserved for those cases in which the conditions of injury justify immediate closure and in which surgery can be done by an adequate operating room staff.

Advantages of delayed primary closure over acute closure include the following: (1) a contaminated wound will have become either clinically infected or safe for reconstructive surgery; (2) the repair is an elective procedure performed by an experienced surgeon; and (3) wound closure can incorporate additional débridement, stabilization of skeletal elements, and distal flap coverage.[12]

Advantages of delayed nerve suture (after 3 weeks) include the following: (1) the total injury to the extremity can be evaluated; nerves are only as functional as their sensory receptors and the viable muscle-tendon motor units; (2) multiple nerve involvement can be approached with incisions clear of the primary scar; (3) the extent of intraneural fibrosis and axonal damage at the nerve ends can be accurately determined, and débridement will offer the potential for less blocking scar; and (4) the epineurium is then thicker and facilitates epineurial sheath suture technique, and the intraneurial epineurium is also thicker for group fascicular (axonal bundles) suture technique.

Closed fractures of long bones with associated nerve injuries present a problem concerning the time for elective exploration and possible nerve suture. Approximately 85% have spontaneous recovery. A poorer prognosis usually involves a fracture adjacent to a joint, a fracture-dislocation with stretching of the nerve, or a severely comminuted fracture. Complete and precise physical examination of peripheral nerve function at the time of injury offers the best baseline for management. Electrodiagnostic studies should be initiated after 1 month and recorded periodically for evaluation of the course of clinical recovery. It is appropriate to explore at 3 to 4 months nerve lesions that result in total functional loss and that are associated with missile and gunshot wounds above the elbow, stretch injuries from dislocation of joints, or fractures that are severely comminuted or adjacent to joint.[49]

NERVE SUTURE

There are only two principles in the techniques for suture of nerves: (1) align the axons (fascicular groups), and (2) avoid tension in all suture lines. The technique of nerve suture is the only factor affecting the return of function that is fully under the control of the surgeon.[35,46]

The controversy of whether epineurial or some type of fascicular (fiber-bundle) repair gives better results is yet to be resolved[68] (Fig. 31-4). Most cleanly severed peripheral nerves should be repaired by the epineurial technique, especially proximal (high)lesions where there are many groups of fascicles (fiber bundles) that cannot be easily identified or matched. Epineurial repair should be selected when a slight amount of tension is necessary at the suture line.[68] Group fascicular (fiber-bundle) repair is indicated for median and ulnar nerves severed at the wrist (Fig. 31-5). The dorsal cutaneous branch of the ulnar nerve and the thenar branch of the median nerve should be separated from the

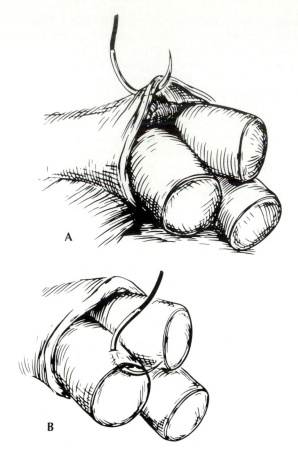

Fig. 31-4. Epineurial and fascicular suturing. **A,** Epineurial repair. Suture is passed through epineurium surrounding three fasciculi. **B,** Fascicular repair. Suture is carefully passed through perineurium of individual fasciculus. Care is taken not to injure intrafascicular contents. (From Urbaniak, J.R.: Clin. Orthop. Rel. Res. **163**:57, March 1982.)

main nerve trunk in these lesions.[37] Group fascicular (fiber-bundle) repair is indicated in nerve-graft anastomoses and is probably responsible for the improved results that can now be expected from that method of repair.[37,65]

Epineurial suture

The wound must be debrided and the nerve inspected for orientation. The most difficult technical step is the operative transection of the nerve. The goal of transection is to achieve a flat stump for the nerve end and to obtain a flush joint for the anastomosis. The nerve may be wrapped with a slip of paper, or fitted into a neurotome, and then cut with a surgical bladder or microsurgical scissors so that the transverse matched surface between the nerve stumps can be fashioned. If a significant amount of scar is present within the nerve, the transection procedure is repeated until easily identified axonal bundles are seen.

Histologic examination of epineurial repairs done without magnification and fine suture material demonstrate funicular malalignment with gaps, overriding buckling, and straddling.[18] The amount of tension in a sutured nerve is directly related to connective tissue proliferation at the anastomo-

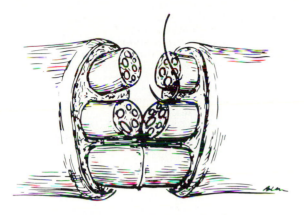

FIG. 31-5. Group fascicular repair. Epineurium has been stripped. Matching groups of fasciculi (bundles) are identified and united by two 10-0 nylon sutures in each bundle of fasciculi. (From Urbaniak, J.R.: Fascicular nerve suture, Clin. Orthop. Rel. Res. **163**:57, March 1982.)

sis.[36] Circumferential tension, with decrease in the cross-sectional area, causes deflection of the funicular alignment with many regenerating axons ending blindly in the endoneurium. Longitudinal tension may result in subepineurial and intrafunicular hemorrhages with fibrosis.

Group fascicular suture

Each fasciculus is usually a mixture of motor, sensory, and sympathetic axons encased by the perineurium. Fasciculi are usually arranged in groups and embedded in epineurium. Epineurium not only is the sheath around the nerve trunk, but also generally comprises 30 to 75 per cent of the cross-sectional area of the nerve.[68] It is important to note that fascicular group repairs have the sutures placed in the deep epineurium and not the perineurium.

Electrophysiologic techniques have been used to aid in fascicular group orientation in acute injuries.[23] It is common to produce motor responses with electrical stimulation of the distal nerve stump for 4 to 5 days after injury. Stimulation of the proximal stump elicits subjective sensations from the patient as long as the cells of origin in the dorsal root ganglia are intact. Studies on the internal structure of nerve trunks are available to indicate the location of motor and sensory fascicular groups.[28,66]

Immobilization periods and methods of mobilization are the same for epineurial and group fascicular suture repairs. The extremity should be splinted 3 to 4 weeks for healing of the surgical procedure. Hyperflexion of joints should be avoided and should not be greater than 30 degrees under any immobilization program. After the healing period is complete, joints are mobilized 10 degrees per week.[57,58]

Nerve graft

A nerve graft is indicated to close a gap in a nerve and provides a scaffold that assists the regenerating axons to find their way into the distal nerve stump and restore the original pattern of innervation. The nerve graft must be acceptable to the body without producing an inflammatory response or constrictive fibrosis: it should be small enough

in diameter to revascularize readily, and it should have a fascicular (funicular) pattern similar to selected fascicular groups in the proximal and distal suture lines.

Seddon popularized the cable graft; his technique involves suturing multiple nerve segments together to equal the diameter of the disrupted nerve, thus forming a multiple-segment cable.[57] The cable graft is superior to grafting of a single large-diameter nerve, because the multiple cables develop an adequate intergraft circulation, while a large-diameter nerve will undergo central necrosis. The multiple cable graft is sutured proximally and distally to bridge the gap in the disrupted nerve.

Millesi and associates have improved the multiple cable graft by developing a technique that emphasizes no tension at suture lines, accurate group fascicular alignment, and excision of the epineurium.[36] The healthy epineurium of the nerve trunk is opened longitudinally, both proximally to the neuroma and distally to the fibroma. Groups of fasciculi that have the approximate cross-sectional area of the donor nerve are cut at different levels in both the proximal and distal stumps. The local epineurium, which has been opened, is excised. A sketch of the group fascicular pattern of the nerve ends is made so that one can plan the connecting multiple cable grafts. Each donor nerve graft is sectioned to fit the gap in the disrupted nerve. Each segment of donor nerve graft should be without tension. An operating microscope is most useful, because 10-0 suture material should be used. One suture connects the epifascicular epineurium of the selected fascicular group to the epineurium of the donor nerve graft. Occasionally, as determined under magnification, an additional 10-0 suture is necessary to establish optimal alignment and contact. Natural fibrin clotting provides sufficient tensile strength to prevent disruption, if the graft is long enough to neutralize any tension in the longitudinal direction. If indicated, a tourniquet should be used in nerve grafting, but the pressure is released and meticulous hemostasis is obtained before wound closure. The involved limb is immobilized in comfortable extension for 3 to 4 weeks, and then activity is begun.

After the nerve graft has been performed, the axons cross the proximal suture site and regenerate toward the distal suture site. In a long nerve graft the distal site may scar and block before the axons reach that level. Clinically, this becomes apparent as the Tinel sign stops advancing. After a 45-day delay at this point, the distal suture site should be exposed for evaluation of the neuroma in continuity by electrodiagnostic techniques (nerve-action potentials). If there is no distal electrical conduction, the distal suture site should be resected and a second neurorrhaphy should be performed.

REGENERATION AFTER REPAIR

It has been a clinical assumption that neurons would become degenerated unless peripheral connections are established during regeneration after repair. Recent laboratory studies suggest that neurons do retain the capacity for function for long periods. Sumner[63] allowed the hypoglossal nerve of rats to regenerate after an 84-day delay. Degenerative appearances of perikaryons and dendrites reversed, numbers of synapses per dendrite increased, and somatic bouton frequencies increased slowly.[50]

Morris and associates[39,40] demonstrated two aspects of regeneration with an electron microscopic study in rats. A certain proportion of Schwann cells and their axons are found in "groups." These groups are of two types: one contains a single myelinated axon associated with a variable number of unmyelinated axons; the other type has all axons initially unmyelinated, but by the tenth day possesses at least one myelinated axon. Axons of both groups are believed to be derived from a single transected myelinated axon and are termed "regenerating units."

The second process in regeneration is termed "compartmentation."[40] During the first 6 weeks after division, the original single or dual fascicular configuration of the rat sciatic nerve is replaced by a series of small fascicles, each surrounded by its own perineurium. The change is stimulated by axonal regeneration and is coordinated by changes in Schwann cells and endoneurial fibroblasts, which begin to resemble perineurial cells.

There is extensive reorganization within the regenerating nerve, as demonstrated by "regenerating units" and their "compartmentation." Present surgical concepts that coapt endoneurial tubes in the proximal and distal stumps of the disrupted nerve offer little possibility that appropriate matching will be accomplished. There should be other techniques to promote control between central and peripheral connections.

REFERENCES

1. Adams, J.E.: Naloxone reversal of analgesia produced by brain stimulation in the human, Pain **2**:161-166, 1976.
2. Akil, H., and Liebeskind, J.C.: Monoaminergic mechanisms of stimulation-produced analgesia, Brain Res. **94**:279-296, 1975.
3. Akil, H., Mayer, D.J., and Leibeskind, J.C.: Antagonism of stimulation-produced analgesia by naloxone, a narcotic antagonist, Science **191**:961-962, 1976.
4. Allbrook, D.: Skeletal muscle regeneration, Muscle and Nerve **4**:234-245, 1981.
5. Amir, S., Brown, Z.W., and Amit, Z.: The role of endorphins in stress: evidence and speculations, Neurosci. Behav. Rev. **4**:77-86, 1980.
6. Becker, R.O., and Spadaro, J.A.: Electrical stimulation of partial limb regeneration in mammals, Bull. N.Y. Acad. Med. **48**:627-641, 1972.
7. Becker, R.O.: The bioelectric factors in amphibian-limb regeneration, J. Bone Joint Surg. **43A**:643-655, 1961.
8. Bessou, P., and Perl, E.R.: Response of cutaneous sensory units with unmyelinated fibers to noxious stimuli, J. Neurophysiol. **32**:1025-1043, 1969.
9. Borgens, R.B., Roederer, E., and Cohen, M.J.: Enhanced spinal cord regeneration in lamprey by applied electric fields, Science **213**:611-617, 1981.
10. Bradbury, A., Smyth, D., Snell, C., Deakin, J., and Wendlant, S.: Comparison of the analgesic properties of lipotropin C-fragment and stabilized enkephalins in the rat, Biochem. Biophys. Res. Commun. **74**:478-754, 1977.
11. Brushart, T.M., and Mesulam, M.M.: Alteration in connections between muscle and anterior horn motorneurons after peripheral nerve repair, Science **208**:603-605, 1980.
12. Burkhalter, W.E., Butler, B., Metz, W., and Omer, G.E.: Experiences with delayed primary closure of war wounds of the hand in Viet Nam, J. Bone Joint Surg. **50A**:945-954, 1968.
13. Casey, K.L.: Pain: a current view of neural mechanisms, Am. Sci. **61**:194-200, 1973.
14. Christensen, B.N., and Perl, E.R.: Spinal neurons specifically excited by noxious or thermal stimuli: marginal zone of the dorsal horn, J. Neurophysiol. **33**:293-307, 1970.
15. Dellon, A.L.: Evaluation of sensibility and re-education of sensation in the hand, Baltimore, 1981, The Williams & Wilkins Co.
16. Ducker, T.B.: Metabolic factors in surgery of peripheral nerves, Surg. Clin. North Am. **52**:1109-1122, 1972.
17. Ducker, T.B.: Metabolic consequences of axotomy and regrowth. In Jewett, D.L., and McCarroll, H.R., Jr., editors: Nerve repair and regeneration: its clincal and experimental basis, St. Louis, 1980, The C.V. Mosby Co.
18. Edshage, S.: Peripheral nerve repair: a technique for improved intraneural topography, evaluation of some suture materials, Acta. Chir. Scand. (Suppl.) 331, 1964.
19. Goldstein, A., Lowney, L.I., and Pal, B.K.: Stereospecific and nonspecific interactions of the morphine congener levorphanol in subcellular fractions of mouse brain, Proc. Natl. Acad. Sci. U.S.A. **68**:1742-1747, 1971.
20. Grabb, W.C.: Management of nerve injuries in the forearm and hand, Orthop. Clin. North Am. **1**:419-431, 1970.
21. Guillemin, R.: Discussion in Reichlin, S., Baldessarini, R.J., and Martin, J.B., editors: The hypothalamus, New York, 1978, Raven Press.
22. Hagbarth, K.E., and Kerr, D.I.B.: Central influences on spinal afferent conduction, J. Neurophysiol. **17**:295-307, 1954.
23. Hakstian, R.W.: Funicular orientation by direct stimulation, J. Bone Joint Surg. **50A**:1178-1186, 1968.
24. Handwerker, H.O., Iggo, A., and Zimmermann, M.: Segmental and supraspinal actions on dorsal horn neurons responding to noxious and non-noxious skin stimuli, Pain **1**:147-165, 1975.
25. Hubbard, J.H.: The quality of nerve regeneration factors independent of the most skillful repair, Surg. Clin. North Am. **52**:1099-1108, 1972.
26. Hughes, J., Smith, T.W., Morgan, B.A., and Fothergill, L.A.: Purification and properties of enkephalin—the possibile endogenous ligand for the morphine receptor, Life Sci. **16**:1753-1758, 1975.
27. Iggo, A.: Pain receptors. In Bonica, J.J., Procacci, P., and Pugni, C.A., editors: Recent advances on pain: pathophysiology and clinical aspects, Springfield, Ill., 1974, Charles C Thomas, Publisher.
28. Jabaley, M.E., Wallace, W.H., and Heckler, R.H.: Internal topography of major nerves of the forearm and hand: a current view, J. Hand Surg. **5**:1-18, 1980.
29. Jhamandos, K., Swaynok, J., and Sutak, M.: Enkephalin effects on release of brain acetylcholine, Nature **269**:433-439, 1977.
30. Loh, H., Brase, D., Sampath-Khanna, S., Mar, J., Way, E., and Li, C.: Beta-endorphin in vitro inhibition of striatal dopamine release, Nature **264**:567-568, 1976.
31. Mayer, D.J., Wolfle, T.E., Akil, H., Carder, B., and Liebeskind, J.C.: Analgesia from electrical stimulation in the brainstem of the rat, Science **174**:1351-1354, 1971.
32. Mayer, D.J., and Hayes, R.: Stimulation-produced analgesia: development of tolerance and cross-tolerance to morphine, Science **188**:941-943, 1975.
33. Mayer, D.J., and Price, D.D.: Central nervous system mechanisms of analgesia, Pain **2**:379-404, 1976.
34. Melzack, R., and Wall, P.D.: Pain mechanisms: a new theory, Science **150**:971-979, 1965.
35. Millesi, H., Meissl, G., and Berger, A.: The interfascicular nerve-grafting of the median and ulnar nerves, J. Bone Joint Surg. **54A**:727-750, 1972.
36. Millesi, H.: Interfascicular nerve grafting, Orthop. Clin. North Am. **12**:287-301, 1981.
37. Moneim, M.S.: Interfascicular nerve grafting, Clin. Orthop. **163**:65-74, 1982.
38. Moroni, F., Cheney, D., and Costa, E.: Beta-endorphin inhibits ACH turnover in nuclei of rat brain, Nature **267**:267-268, 1977.
39. Morris, J.H., Hudson, A.R., and Weddell, G.: A study of degeneration and regeneration in the divided rat sciatic nerve based on electron microscopy. II. The development of the "regenerating" unit, Z. Zellforsch. **124**:103-130, 1972.
40. Morris, J.H., Hudson, A.R., and Weddell, G.: A study of degeneration and regeneration in the divided rat sciatic nerve based on electron microscopy. IV. Chnages in fascicular microtopography, perineurium and endoneurial fibroblasts, Z. Zellforsch. **124**:165-203, 1972.
41. Nemeth, P.M.: Electrical stimulation of denervated muscle prevents decreases in oxidative enzymes, Muscle and Nerve **5**:134-139, 1982.
42. O'Brien, W.J., and Orgel, M.G.: The electrical stimulation of nerve regeneration. Research in progress, July 1979 through May 1982, University of New Mexico, Albuquerque, N. Mex.

43. Oliveras, J.L., Besson, J.M., Guilbaud, G., and Liebeskind, J.C.: Behavioral and electrophysiological evidence of pain inhibition from midbrain stimulation in the cat, Exp. Brain Res. **20:**32-44, 1974.

44. Olson, G.A., Olson, R.D., Kastin, A.J., and Coy, D.H.: The opioid neuropeptides enkephalin and endorphin and their hypothesized relation to pain. In Smith, W.L., Mersky, H., and Gross, S.C., editors: Pain: meaning and management, New York, 1980, SP Medical and Scientific Books.

45. Omer, G.E., Jr.: Injuries to nerves of the upper extermity, J. Bone Joint Surg. **56A:**1615-1624, 1974.

46. Omer, G.E., Jr., and Spinner, M.: Peripheral nerve testing and suture techniques. In American Academy of Orthopaedic Surgeons: Instructional course lectures **24:**122-143, St. Louis, 1975, The C.V. Mosby Co.

47. Omer, G.E., Jr.: Complications of treatment of peripheral nerve injuries. In Epps, C.H., Jr., editor: Complications in orthopaedic surgery, Philadelphia, 1978, J.B. Lippincott Co.

48. Omer, G.E., Jr.: The management of traumatic injuries of peripheral nerves in the extremities, Surg. Rounds **4:**22-32, 1981.

49. Omer, G.E., Jr.: Results of untreated peripheral nerve injuries, Clin. Orthop. **163:**15-19, 1982.

50. Orgel, M.G.: Experimental studies with clinical application to peripheral nerve injury: a review of the past decade, Clin. Orthop. **163:**98-106, 1982.

51. Pert, C., and Snyder, S.: Opiate receptor: demonstration in nervous tissue, Science **179:**1011-1014, 1973.

52. Pomeranz, B., Cheng, R., and Law, P.: Acupuncture reduces electrophysiological and behavioral responses to noxious stimuli: pituitary is implicated, Exp. Neurol. **54:**172-178, 1977.

53. Rexed, B.: The cytoarchitecture organization of the spinal cord of the cat, J. Comp. Neurol. **96:**415-496, 1952.

54. Reynolds, D.V.: Surgery in the rat during electrical analgesia induced by focal brain stimulation, Science **164:**444-445, 1969.

55. Salmons, S., and Henriksson, J.: The adaptive response of skeletal muscle to increased use, Muscle and Nerve **4:**94:105, 1981.

56. Seddon, H.J.: Three types of nerve injury, Brain **66:**237-288, 1943.

57. Seddon, H.J., editor: Peripheral nerve injuries, Medical research Council Spec. Rep. Ser. 282, London, 1954, Her Majesty's Stationery Office.

58. Seddon, H.J.: Surgical disorders of the peripheral nerves, ed. 2, Edinburgh, 1975, Churchill Livingstone.

59. Singer, S.J.: Architecture and topography of biologic membranes. In Weissman, G., and Claiborne, R., editors: Cell membranes: biochemistry, cell biology, and pathology, New York, 1975, Hospital Practice Publishing Co.

60. Sisken, B.F., and Smith, S.D.: The effects of minute direct electrical currents on cultured chick embryo trigeminal ganglia, J. Embryol. Exp. Morphol. **33:**29-41, 1975.

61. Sternback, R.A.: Modern concepts of pain. In Dalessio, D.J., editor: Wolff's headache and other head pain, ed. 4, New York, 1980, Oxford University Press.

62. Stilz, R.J., Carron, H., and Sanders, D.B.: Reflex sympathetic dystrophy in a 6-year-old: successful treatment by transcutaneous nerve stimulation, Anesth. Analg. **56:**38-443, 1977.

63. Sumner, B.E.H.: Responses in the hypoglossal nucleus to delayed regeneration of the transected hypoglossal nerve: a quantitative ultrastructural study, Exp. Brain Res. **29:**219-231, 1977.

64. Sunderland, S.: Nerves and nerve injuries, ed. 2, Edinburgh, 1978, Churchill Livingstone.

65. Sunderland, S.: Clinical and experimental approaches to nerve repair, in perspective. In Jewett, D.L., and McCarroll, H.R., Jr., editors: Nerve repair and regeneration: its clinical and experimental basis, St. Louis, 1980, The C.V. Mosby Co.

66. Sutherland, S.: The anatomic foundation of peripheral nerve repair techniques, Orthop. Clin. North Am. **12:**245-266, 1981.

67. Tseng, L.F., Loh, H., and Li, C.: Beta-endorphin as a potent analgesic by intravenous injection, Nature **263:**239-240, 1976.

68. Urbaniak, J.R.: Fascicular nerve repair, Clin. Orthop. **163:**57-64, 1982.

69. Webster, K.E.: Somaesthetic pathways, Br. Med. Bull. **33:**113-120, 1977.

70. Weeks, P.M., and Wray, R.C.: Management of acute hand injuries: a biological approach, St. Louis, 1978, The C.V. Mosby Co.

71. Weissman, G.: Pain mediators and pain receptors. In Bonica, J.J., editor: Considerations in management of acute pain. New York, 1977, Hospital Practice Publishing Co.

72. Willis, W.D., Trevino, D.L., Coulter, J.D., and Maunz, R.A.: Responses of primate spinothalamic tract neurons to natural stimulation of hindlimb, J. Neurophysiol. **37:**358-372, 1974.

73. Wynn Parry, C.B.: Rehabilitation of the hand, ed. 3, London, 1973, Butterworths & Co. (Publishers), Ltd.

32

Nerve lesions in continuity

MORTON SPINNER

Nerve compression lesions are a major and significant cause of peripheral neuropathy. Lesions of the upper extremity may potentially involve any nerve. The compressed region usually is localized to a discrete portion of a segment of the nerve, which, because of its anatomic position, is particularly susceptible to entrapment. When a nerve is compressed, it is the peripheral axons within the nerve that suffer the greatest injury. At first, the central fibers may be spared, but as the compression continues or worsens, the central fibers may also become involved. Within the central region, the motor, proprioceptive, light touch, and vibratory sensory axons, which are heavily myelinated, are more vulnerable than the thinly myelinated pain and sympathetic fibers. However, when the compression is of sufficient duration and magnitude, all the fibers are paralyzed.

CLASSIFICATION OF NERVE-COMPRESSION LESIONS

There are two methods of classifying neural compression lesions. Sir Herbert Seddon's method utilizes the three terms "neurapraxia," "axonotmesis," and "neurotmesis." Sir Sidney Sunderland's classification has five degrees of nerve injury. Only the first four apply to nerve lesions in continuity, since the fifth degree refers to an injury in which the nerve is severed and the two ends retract.

Neurapraxia

Sunderland's first-degree lesion corresponds to Seddon's neurapraxia. Neurapraxia is a reversible syndrome. The prognosis for recovery is excellent.

There are three types of neurapractic lesions: ionic, vascular, and mechanical. The first, ionic, is related to electrolyte-imbalance potassium, sodium, and ATPase disturbance at the node of Ranvier. The second type, vascular, is believed to be attributable to an anoxia at the capillary level within the funiculi, caused by venous obstruction in the epineurium. The third neurapractic lesion, mechanical, has structural changes in the nerve fibers because of compression-shear forces.

There are two basic ultrastructural mechanical lesions of neurapraxia. The first is bulbous myelin lesions with segmental tapering of internodal segments. The second type is paranodal myelin intussusception at the node of Ranvier; in this condition acute local compression produces the myelin

invagination. Both lesions occur away from the site of the compression. Initially there is segmental demyelinization, and with healing, there is segmental remyelinization. In neurapractic lesions, there is no wallerian degeneration. The basement membrane of the neural fiber is intact.

Most neurapractic lesions respond to conservative treatment within 3 months. If a patient has a persistent neural compression lesion of spontaneous or traumatic origin that lasts more than 3 months, surgery is indicated, at which time the nerve should be explored at the level of the lesion. When neurolysis is performed, the speed of return of function often suggests the type of neurapractic lesion. If the recovery occurs rapidly, within hours of the procedure, the ionic or anoxic type of lesion is suggested. However, some neurapractic lesions require 30 to 60 days for recovery because a process of demyelinization and remyelinization occurs, indicating a possible structural neurapractic lesion. If a neurapractic lesion is left untreated and the mechanical factors—compression, traction, and friction—persist, the severity may increase.

Axonotmesis

The next level of severity is Seddon's axonotmesis and Sunderland's second-degree lesion. Minor third-degree lesions also fall within this category. With a pure axonotmetic lesion, the axon fiber is damaged at the point of compression. The basement membrane of the axon is maintained, but there is complete wallerian degeneration distal to the level of the compression. The healing process consists in new axonal sprouting and growth, from the point of axon disruption distally. Although there is a good prognosis for this degree of injury, the rate of the recovery depends on the distance between the muscle to reinnervate and the site of the lesion. The closer the motor end plates, the earlier the recovery.

Sunderland's third-degree lesion may correspond either to Seddon's classification of axonotmesis or to the next category, neurotmesis, depending on the severity of the injury. In a third-degree lesion, the nerve fibers, including their Schwann tubes, are damaged within intact nerve trunk. The perineurium is basically intact, but there is internal fibrosis and damage within the fascicles. Mild lesions, which are reversible, fall within the axonotmetic category. However, in a more severe injury, when the damage may be irreversible as a result of the number of axons involved and the degree of fibrosis within the funiculi, the lesions are classified as neurotmetic.

Neurotmesis

This category is composed of all fourth-degree lesions and the more severe third-degree lesions. A fourth-degree lesion is characterized by extensive or complete fibrosis of a segment of the nerve. The internal structure of the funiculi is severely altered, and neuroma is present. In a complete neurotmetic lesion, there is a nonfunctioning, nonconductive neuroma in continuity.

In the case of a neurotmetic lesion, excision of the neuroma and repair is indicated. It can best be achieved by epineurial repair. If the gap is too great for direct approximation, interfunicular grafting is necessary.

In general, the prognosis for motor recovery after nerve repair is poor if paralysis has been clinically and electrically complete for 10 to 15 months. In such cases, successful recovery after neurorrhaphy depends on the specific nerve involved, the duration of the paralysis, the age of the patient, and the level of the complete lesion. There is little hope for a high ulnar-nerve complete lesion if more than 10 months have elapsed. However, a low median-nerve complete lesion can recover after repair for well beyond 10 months. If the paralysis has extended beyond the critical time, the treatment of choice would be primary muscle transfer.

The prognosis for sensory recovery is much better than for motor recovery. Useful sensory recovery after repair has been achieved with a 25-year-old neurotmetic lesion.

EVALUATION OF NERVE-COMPRESSION LESIONS

To determine the extent of the neural-compression lesion and to decide upon the appropriate treatment, one must consider the age of the patient, the complete history, the duration of the paralysis, and the clinical and operative findings. Hereditary factors may also play a part in neural-compression lesions. At this time, however, it is purely hypothetical as to whether any chromosomal-enzymatic factors play a role in the incidence of neural-compression lesions. Families and isolated cases in which the patient's nerves were pressure sensitive have been reported. Recurrent episodes and multiple peripheral nerve involvement have also been reported.

It is unusual to have a pure first-, second-, third-, or fourth-degree lesion; most often, they are mixed. Furthermore, when a peripheral nerve can be compressed at more than one level in its passage through the arm, it is known as "double-crush nerve entrapment." Improvement in the symptoms can be achieved with release of one of the site compressions, but it may be necessary to explore additional sites as well.

In order to predict the lesion mix of a compression syndrome and the extent of each of the degrees, serial clinical examinations may be necessary. Prompt recovery can follow release. The fibers most sensitive to compression are the large myelinated fibers—motor, proprioceptive, light touch, and vibratory. Partial neural-entrapment lesions respond well to surgical release even after 2 to 3 years of sensory and motor symptomatology.

In general, if there has not been progressive improvement in a neural-compression lesion within 3 to 4 months, surgery is indicated.

There are a number of well-known neural-compression lesions that present distinct symptoms. These include the carpal tunnel, Guyon's tunnel, pronator, and cubital tunnel syndromes. The lesion can be confirmed with electroneuromyographic testing. It is essential that the level of the lesion be located accurately, so that decompression is performed at the proper level. For example, if the patient has a high median nerve lesion, intervention at the wrist is no help. Occasionally, there are anatomic variations or unusual clinical patterns, such as the presence of Sudeck's atrophy in association with a nerve entrapment, which can make the problem more difficult to diagnose.

MANAGEMENT OF NERVE-COMPRESSION LESIONS

The extent of the exposure at surgery is always much greater than the site of the lesion would initially suggest. For example, a lesion an inch long would have an incision of at least 5 inches. Indeed, only with careful anatomic exposure of both the gross neural structure and the fine internal structure in normal tissue proximal and distal to the lesion can conversion of the lesion to one of the more advanced degree be avoided. Particular care must be taken to avoid injury to the superficial skin nerves, because postoperative neurotoma of them can be a major postoperative complication.

During the surgery, the neural structure is identified grossly in the normal tissue proximal and distal to its entrapment. The dissection proceeds, separating the epineurium from its scarred bed, from both the proximal and distal sides. If there is a fibrotic band at the area of maximum entrapment, release of the binding structure causes the entire nerve to be liberated. It is possible that there may be a small residual area of indentation in the nerve, but with an intraneural injection of saline solution one can observe the flow. If any obstruction is noted, a localized neurolysis is necessary.

Neurolysis usually separates the epineurium from its scarred bed or removes crossing thrombosed vessels or thickened fascia. At times, however, the funiculi may require internal dissection.

When it is utilized, internal neurolysis should be adapted to the individual case. For example, in a carpal tunnel syndrome with advanced thenar atrophy and minimal sensory disturbance, after release of the flexor retinaculum, the motor branch is identified and is traced from its departure point from the median nerve distally into the thenar muscles. In the distal course, it frequently penetrates a separate foramen in the flexor retinaculum, which may be the offending obstructive site. The compression can occur at the proximal or distal level of this retinaculum; so the motor funiculus is traced proximally through the main median nerve trunk, including the area distal and proximal to the edges of the flexor retinaculum.

Often with the carpal tunnel syndrome, pain and numbness are the major complaints, with the long finger most involved. In these cases, after opening the epineurium, one separates the medial two or three funiculi as a group, be-

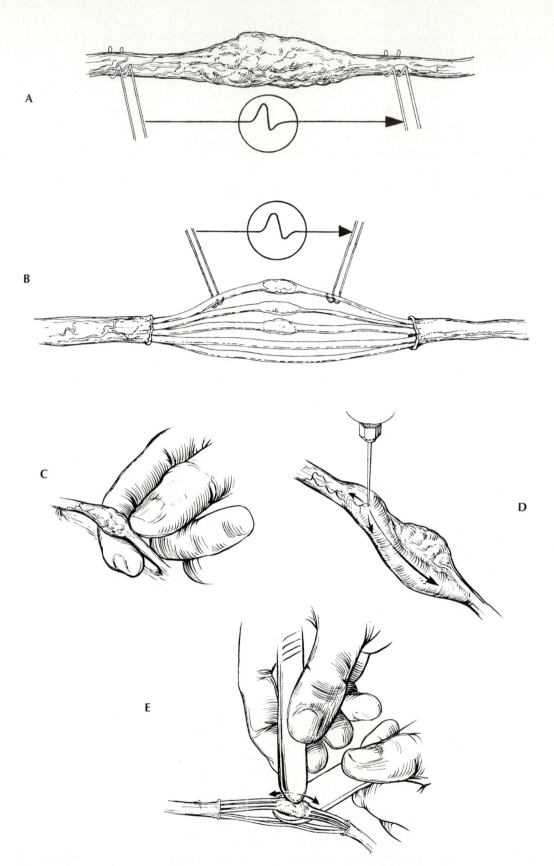

FIG. 32-1. Intraoperative techniques for nerve lesions. **A** and **B,** Intraoperative nerve conduction study across the neuroma may be helpful in evaluation of lesion in continuity. **C,** Palpation of nerve may reveal a rock-hard neuroma with little likelihood of intact fascicles. **D,** Injection of saline deep to the epineurial sheath can help differentiate intact from damaged fascicles. **E,** Intrafascicular dissection separates intact fascicular bundles from those that are involved in a neuroma. Firmness of a funicular neuroma can be evaluated further with the aid of a scalpel handle.

ginning distal or proximal to the transverse carpal ligament in the normal median nerve. The internal neurolysis should include the region of the median nerve compressed by the proximal and distal edges of this ligament. One leaves the adjacent funiculi, which are clinically uninvolved, as they are. In elderly patients, long-finger discomfort and dysesthesias may persist for an extended period after isolated carpal tunnel release. Since selective internal neurolysis has been added to the procedure for patients with this syndrome, in which long-finger pain predominates preoperatively, this morbidity has been improved significantly.

When internal neurolysis is utilized, it should be limited to the fasciculi that are clinically involved. Extensive internal neurolysis can induce fibrosis throughout the neural layers. The integrity of the perineurium is crucial for normal neural function. It acts as a supporting structure for maintenance of normal pressure gradient within the funiculus. It maintains the internal envirnoment within the funiculus, and acts as a barrier for the passage of proteins and other large molecules. Furthermore, the perineurium is a mirror in the peripheral nerve of the central blood-brain barrier. When the perineurium is violated, there is a herniation of axons. The axons that bulge out of the perineurial window undergo pathologic changes. At first, there is segmental demyelinization, followed by localized remyelinization with restoration of the perineurium. In clinical cases for which pain is attributable to a localized lesion, the epineurium is frequently opened, but the perineurium is only opened rarely. However, there are specific indications for violating the perineurium. For example, opening may be necessary when the patient has a third-degree lesion with intraneural fibrosis. The degree of the internal fibrosis and therefore the extent of the third-degree lesion within the nerve may not be clear. Thus, on rare occasion it may be necessary to open the perineurium to improve neural function.

EVALUATION OF NEUROMA IN CONTINUITY

Several methods may be used to evaluate a neuroma in continuity (Fig. 32-1). Once it has been determined that surgery is required, there are intraoperative techniques that can be used to evaluate the lesion. During surgery, electrical stimulation proximal and distal to the neuroma before one frees it completely is useful, with observation of the peripheral muscle and limb response. There are other intraoperative conduction studies that may be made across the neuroma, but they require more refined instrumentation. If the neuroma is stony-hard to palpation, the prognosis is poor for neural recovery by neurolysis. However, a soft enlargement of the nerve is a favorable sign for restoration of neural function. Intraneural saline injection followed by external and internal neurolysis, if necessary, with use of the operating microscope or ocular magnification can be helpful. Magnification is essential in the evaluation of the appearance of the funiculi. The firmness of the funicular neuromas can be evaluated with the aid of the scalpel handle, but the single fascicular electrical recording technique offers the most critical intraoperative evaluation.

When intraoperative evaluation indicates that a complete neuroma in continuity exists, excision of the neural lesion and neurorrhaphy constitute the treatment of choice.

When managing injuries, one must evaluate each on its own merits. After humeral fracture, the radial nerve may have had relatively minor trauma and may recovery spontaneously in 3 to 4 months. On other occasions, it may have been lacerated and require prompt repair, or it may be entrapped in scar tissue and require neurolysis. It may also have sustained a fourth-degree neural lesion, necessitating excision of a neuroma in continuity and neurorrhaphy (Fig. 32-2).

CLINICAL HIGHLIGHTS
Median nerve syndromes

The carpal tunnel syndrome is the result of median nerve compression in a narrowed carpal tunnel. It is a fairly common entrapment syndrome, seen most frequently in women between 40 and 60 years of age. Pain and paresthesia in a distal median nerve distribution are the usual complaints, with nocturnal burning pain in the hand often being reported as well.

There are many significant symptoms and signs of carpal tunnel syndrome, including numbness of the radial $3\frac{1}{2}$ digits, atrophy of the thenar muscles, a Tinel sign at the wrist, a Phalen sign, increased symptoms on application of an arm tourniquet, and motor and sensory nerve electromyographic abnormalities. Often, however, numbness may be restricted to the long finger, and there may be no atrophy of the thenar muscles, and no Tinel and Phalen signs. In approximately 25% of patients with carpal tunnel syndrome, the electromyogram may be normal. Sensitivity to cold may be the major presenting symptom. Sympathetic overflow associated with the carpal tunnel syndrome has been observed by Linscheid.

After fractures and dislocations at the wrist, median and ulnar nerve entrapment can be the cause of reflex dystrophy of the hand. It may be necessary to release one or both of these nerves to relieve the pain and stiffness characteristic of reflex dystrophy. The diagnosis of nerve entrapment can be confirmed by electromyographic studies.

Patients with carpal tunnel syndrome respond to conservative measures of treatment. The combined treatment of splinting the wrist in a neutral position and administering a diuretic is effective in these patients. Vitamin B_6 (100 mg twice a day) has also been helpful in some cases. Any underlying systemic disease should be brought under control. If conservative methods do not provide relief, it may be necessary to release the transverse carpal ligament through surgery. The incision is made on the ulnar side of the carpal tunnel, with step-cutting at the distal flexion crease of the wrist and extention of the incision to the ulnar side of the distal forearm if additional exposure is necessary. Care must be taken to preserve the median palmar cutaneous nerve, because injury to it often causes postoperative pain.

The pronator syndrome is caused by entrapment of the median nerve in the proximal part of the forearm. This syndrome is difficult to diagnose with certainty. Usually the patient has a 9-month to 2-year history of nonlocalized forearm pain. The most consistent finding has been reproduction of pain in the proximal part of the forearm on resistance to pronation of the forearm and resistance to flexion of the superficial flexor muscle of the long and ring fingers. Pa-

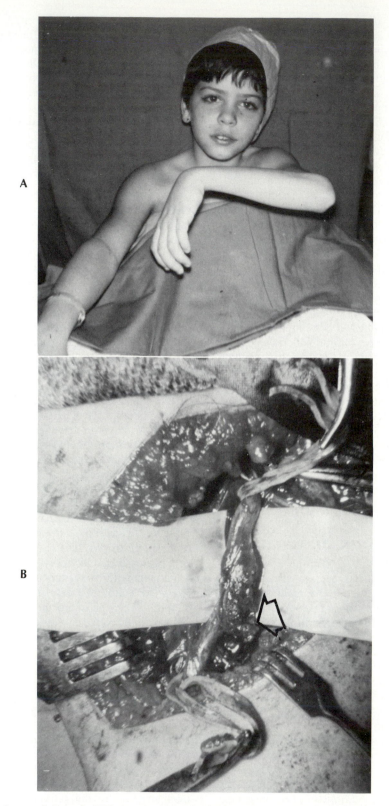

FIG. 32-2. Radial nerve injury. **A,** This boy had a healed humeral fracture but no evidence of radial nerve function 6 months after injury. **B,** Surgical exploration revealed a fourth-degree lesion of the radial nerve.

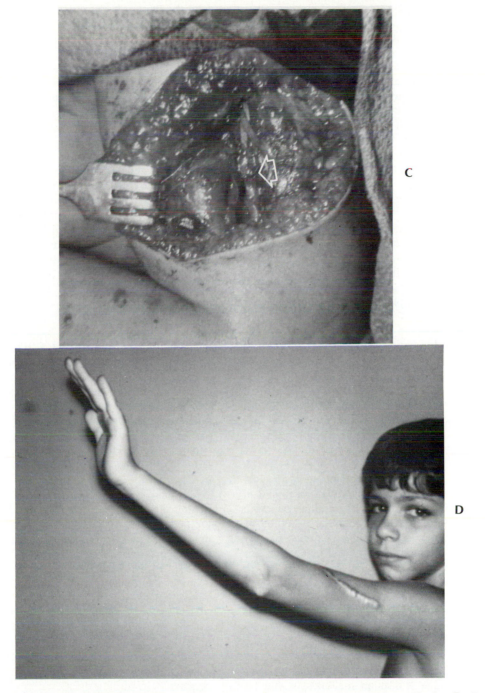

FIG. 32-2, cont'd. C, Neurorrhaphy has been performed after excision of the neuroma in continuity. **D,** Excellent recovery of radial nerve function is demonstrated 1 year later.

tients may report numbness in some digits innervated by the median nerve. Even though the Tinel sign may aid localization, it may not appear for 4 to 5 months after the initial examination. Electromyographic studies may aid in the diagnosis, particularly when the results of several examinations are compared.

Anatomic abnormalities observed in the pronator syndrome are (1) hypertrophy of the pronator teres, (2) fibrous bands within the pronator teres, (3) a thickening of the lacertus fibrosus, (4) passage of the median nerve deep to both heads of the pronator teres, and (5) a thickening of the flexor superficialis arch. Median nerve thickening at the level of the compression has been observed; the degree of thickening seems to be directly related to the duration of symptoms.

The surgical procedure, when necessary, consists in release of the lacertus fibrosus and all compressing fibrous structures crossing the nerve. Translocation of the median nerve anterior to the pronator teres to a subcutaneous position is occasionally necessary. When this is done, the pronator teres is lengthened at its musculotendinous junction and brought posterior to the median nerve. If the flexor superficialis arch is thickened, it is released to allow the median nerve to be superficial in the middle third of the forearm. The skin incision should be S or chevron shaped, through which the lacertus fibrosus is initially visualized. The median nerve is identified proximal to the lacertus and then traced distally. Continuity of the branches of the medial cutaneous nerve of the forearm must be carefully preserved, since severance may result in a postoperative symptomatic neuroma.

The anterior interosseous nerve syndrome results from the compression of the anterior interosseous branch, usually at a site close to its origin from the median nerve. The paralysis of the long flexor of the thumb and the flexor digitorum profundus to the index and long fingers causes the hand to display a typical pinch attitude. Paralysis of the pronator quadratus muscle is also observed. Sometimes paralysis is limited to the distal phalanx of the thumb or index finger. There are usually no sensory abnormalities. If a Martin-Gruber anastomosis, a connection between the anterior interosseous nerve and the ulnar nerve, is present, the entrapment of the anterior interosseous nerve may produce paralysis of some of the intrinsic muscles of the hand. There are anatomic variations in the anastomosis between the ulnar and median nerves within the flexor digitorum profundus, and so the muscle is innervated to variable degrees by both nerves, and flexion of the distal phalanx of the digits may be impaired variably in this neural-entrapment lesion.

Exploration of the anterior interosseous nerve is indicated if the paralysis does not subside spontaneously within 8 to 12 weeks. The median nerve should be identified proximal to the lacertus fibrosus and traced through the region of the pronator teres where the anterior interosseous nerve usually originates. The most common restraining structure is a tendinous origin of the deep head of the pronator teres, which crosses the anterior interosseous nerve at its origin from the median nerve. Other causes of anterior interosseous nerve entrapment are enlarged bicipital bursas, other tendinous structures, thrombosed ulnar collateral vessels, old penetrating local scars, and anomalous passage of the radial artery.

A supracondyloid process is another cause of high median-nerve entrapment. It is an anomalous spur found 3 to 5 cm above the medial epicondyle in 1% of limbs. The connection between the two bony prominences is the ligament of Struthers, which completes the fibro-osseous tunnel. The median nerve passes through the tunnel, usually accompanied by the ulnar artery. This anomaly is usually asymptomatic, but after trauma it may produce median neuritis.

Radial nerve syndromes

Posterior interosseous-nerve syndrome may present in two ways, but there is no sensory deficit in either one. In the first pattern, all the muscles supplied by the posterior interosseous nerve do not function. The patient cannot extend the thumb, long, index, ring, and little fingers at the metacarpophalangeal joints. The wrist can dorsiflex only in a dorsoradial direction, as a result of a muscular imbalance of the wrist extensors because of paralysis of the extensor digitorum communis and the extensor carpi ulnaris.

The second pattern is characterized by a lack of extension of one or more of the digits at the metacarpophalangeal level. Paralysis of the remaining digits often develops when the neural lesion is not recognized or treated. Frequently, posterior interosseous nerve entrapment occurs where the nerve pierces the two heads of the supinator muscle. This area, the arcade of Frohse, is fibrotendinous in 30% of limbs. Other causes for entrapment of the posterior interosseous nerve may be compression by a soft-tissue tumor, synovial proliferation in rheumatoid disease, Volkmann's ischemia, and fractures or dislocations of the head of the radius. The symptom complex known as lateral epicondylitis, or tennis elbow, characterized by pain about the lateral aspect of the elbow, can be attributable to posterior interosseous-nerve compression at the arcade of Frohse. It is confirmed by reproducing the pain at the common extensor origin on resistance to long-finger extension with the elbow extended. Direct pressure along the course of the radial nerve anteriorly is also painful. Electrical conduction studies of the radial nerve across the elbow may reveal motor-latency prolongation. Some patients who have not responded to conservative treatment, to release of the lateral epicondylar soft tissues, or to excision of a portion of the orbicular ligament, have been helped by release of the posterior interosseous nerve as it enters the supinator. If pain persists after the customary surgery for tennis elbow, posterior interosseous nerve compression should be considered as a possibility.

There are two surgical approaches to use in exposing and tracing the entrapped posterior interosseous nerve. Either the radial nerve is identified above the elbow, proximal to its site of division, or the superficial radial nerve is identified under the fascia of the brachioradialis in the forearm and traced proximally to the main radial nerve trunk. Then the posterior interosseous nerve is identified and traced through the two heads of the supinator.

Superficial radial nerve entrapment is a syndrome characterized by pain in the proximal part of the forearm and hypesthesia on the dorsum of the thumb. There is no associated muscle weakness or paralysis, and no motor-conduction abnormalities can be observed by electromyography.

Ulnar nerve syndromes

In the wrist, the ulnar nerve can be involved in Guyon's tunnel. There may be a purely motor or a purely sensory deficit, or a combination of the two. Either the main ulnar nerve or one of its terminal branches may be entrapped, depending on the localization of the compression. In the cubital tunnel syndrome the ulnar nerve can be compressed just distally to the medial epicondyle as it passes through the two heads of the flexor carpi ulnaris.

When one is translocating the ulnar nerve anteriorly, subcutaneous or deep to the flexor-pronator group of muscles, it is important to trace the ulnar nerve 8 cm proximally to the medial epicondyle to the region of the arcade of Struthers, where the ulnar nerve passes from the anterior compartment of the arm to the posterior in the distal third of the arm. Release of this arcade and excision of the adjacent medial intermuscular septum prevent a secondary entrapment of the ulnar nerve at the level of the arcade of Struthers.

In the thoracic outlet syndrome, which occurs at the base of the neck, the ulnar nerve is most frequently compressed at the level of the first rib or at the costoclavicular area. It presents with radicular pain along the medial aspect of the arm to the hand. There are motor and sensory disturbances in the distribution of the ulnar nerve. If appropriate confirmatory tests are positive and conservative treatment is unsuccessful, surgery is indicated.

Cervical arthritis can cause symptoms of numbness in the ring and little fingers with weakness of the digits. On rotation, extension and lateral bending of the neck with reduplication of the radicular complaints are produced. Such clinical findings can help localize the cause of the symptoms. Pain on direct pressure or percussion along the course of the nerve can also help to locate the level of the pathologic condition.

Bowler's thumb

Bowler's thumb is characterized by pain in the thumb, numbness most noticeable on its ulnar aspect, a palpable mass at the base of the thumb, a Tinel sign on percussion of this mass, and a history of bowling. The use of a protective thumb guard and redrilling of the bowling ball so that it is "scythed" at the top are helpful conservative measures for a short period. Surgery is indicated when conservative measures do not relieve the symptoms. Neurolysis, excision of the markedly thickened epineurium, and rerouting of the involved digital nerve into a new soft-tissue bed are indicated.

Similar localized digital compression neuropathy has been seen with baseball batters, and its management is identical in principle.

Multiple entrapment lesions

A nerve can be entrapped simultaneously at two levels; similarly, more than one nerve can be entrapped in a limb. Electromyographic studies are not always sensitive enough to localize a double lesion. It may be necessary to explore a peripheral nerve at two sites. It is also possible that a patient may have two completely separate neurologic conditions, such as syringomyelia of the neck and a compressed peripheral nerve. Furthermore, it is important to avoid a mistaken diagnosis of a localized process that causes a conduction delay, if the problem is instead actually a diffuse peripheral neuropathy. Examination of other peripheral nerves will serve to prevent this error.

33

Thoracic outlet syndrome: diagnosis and treatment

SCOTT H. JAEGER, RICHARD READ, STANTON N. SMULLENS, and PAULA BREME

"Thoracic outlet syndrome" is a general term referring to compression neuropathies and vasculopathies of the brachial plexus and the subclavian vessels. The syndrome has had many names, reflecting its various specific causes and presentations: scalenus anticus syndrome, scalenus medius band syndrome, scalenus minimus syndrome, costoclavicular compression syndrome, hyperabduction syndrome, acroparesthesia, cervical rib syndrome, and Paget-Schroeder syndrome.

The vascular expression of the syndrome is well known, but uncommon. The neurologic expression of the syndrome is much more common, but not well appreciated. The purpose of this chapter is to acquaint those who deal with disorders of the upper extremity with this complicated and at times perplexing malady.

The key to the diagnosis of the syndrome is awareness of its occurrence and the ability to support the clinical impression with objective testing. The presentation of the syndrome may be quite bizarre, but it should be considered in any case of pain and paresthesias of the upper extremity.

HISTORICAL BACKGROUND

Understanding of the pathophysiology of thoracic outlet syndrome has come about through a process of historical evolution. The first recognized and treated cases were related to congenital cervical ribs. The recognition of cervical ribs dates back to the early origins of medicine; they were described by Galen and Vesalius. In 1740, Hunauld[14] described the anomaly with his observations. In 1818, A. Cooper[5] was treating symptoms of cervical ribs medically with some success. Willshire,[47] in 1860, and Gruber,[12] in 1869, were among the first to report the condition and its diagnosis. In 1861, Coote[6] performed the first operation for removal of a cervical rib and relieved the patient's symptoms. By 1895, eight operations had been performed for this condition. In 1907, W.W. Kean[17] reviewed the matter extensively and described 42 cases in which patients had been operated on to that year. In 1916, Halsted[13] reviewed a series of 716 patients with cervical ribs. Thirty-five percent had vascular symptoms. His interest in the observed poststenotic dilatation seen in these patients led to his later research on the subject.

It became apparent, however, to many observers that cases simulating the symptoms of cervical rib were present in patients who did not have this anomaly. In 1903, Bramwell[2] had noted a relationship between pressure of a first rib and the first dorsal nerve root. In 1910, Thomas Murphy[25] of Australia was the first to resect a normal first rib with relief of the patient's symptoms. English pathology literature then recorded cases of patients with cervical rib symptoms who were relieved by removal of normal or abnormal first ribs. These included cases by Morley[24] in 1913 and Stopford and Telford in 1919.[39] In 1927, Brickner[3] in the United States reported his own cases and supported their findings that symptoms were relieved with removal of the first rib.

In that same year of 1927, a monumental paper by Adson and Coffey[1] significantly changed the thinking regarding the pathophysiology of this condition. It was their belief that the symptoms were related to the scalenus anticus muscle in relationship to the cervical rib rather than the cervical rib itself. They based this view on their operative findings and clinical results as well as on the observation that most cases of cervical ribs were asymptomatic. The well-known Adson test was introduced at this time. Support for the scalenus anticus muscle as the etiologic factor was emphasized by Ochsner, Gage, and DeBakey in 1935,[29] who credited the concept to Naffziger. Further articles were published by Craig and Knepper in 1937[7] and Naffziger and Grant in 1938,[26] and the "scalenus anticus syndrome," or "Naffziger syndrome," became firmly entrenched in medical literature and in medical thinking.

Although the acceptance of the scalenus anticus muscle as the major etiologic factor was quick, others still sought to explain the symptoms as being attributed to other mechanisms. Lewis and Pickering in 1934[19] and Eden[9] in 1939 suggested that compression of the neurovascular bundle between the clavicle in front and the cervical and first rib behind was the cause of the symptoms. This concept of compression was characterized by Falconer and Weddell[11] in 1943 as the "costoclavicular compression syndrome." Anomalies of the first rib were also described in this regard.

Another concept was introduced into the etiologic factors of these cases by Wright[48] in 1945 when he described symptoms caused by hyperabduction of the arms. He believed that there were two zones of pressure. One was posterior to the pectoralis minor muscle and its attachments to the coracoid process, and the second was between the clavicle and the first rib. However, the scalenus anticus remained the most popular etiologic factor, and scalenotomy was the usual operation carried out at this time.

Lord[20], in 1953, gave support to the concept of compression as the cause of the hyperabduction, costoclavicular, cervical rib, and scalenus anticus syndromes by suggesting that removal of the clavicle would relieve the patient's symptoms. Scalenotomy at this time was the preferred treatment. However, Raaf[31] and others maintained that fewer than 50% of their patients were improved by this procedure.

In 1956, Peet and his associates[30] made an important contribution to the understanding and treatment of this disorder by emphasizing that all the patients with neurovascular compression in this area, although it was attibutable to different causes, shared the characteristics of stretching and compression as their etiology. They suggested, therefore, that all patients in this category be grouped together under the name "thoracic outlet syndrome." At that same time they emphasized the importance of a nonoperative approach to relief of symptoms in many of these patients. They stressed the idea of the "sagging shoulders" type of habitus seen in many of the middle-aged women who presented with these complaints and believed that this was an important etiologic factor in these conditions. In 1958, Rob and Standeven[33] amplified the term to "thoracic outlet compression syndrome" and presented their experience.

Disenchantment with scalenotomy and the necessity of operating on a certain number of patients not relieved by nonoperative means revived interest in removal of the first rib. In 1962, Falconer and Li[10] supported the idea of resection of the first rib for relief of costoclavicular compression of the brachial plexus. However, it was the presidential address before the American Association of Thoracic Surgery by O. Theron Clagett in 1962[4] that firmly focused attention on the first rib as a common denominator in the pathophysiology of the many forms of thoracic outlet compression syndrome. He stressed the concept of a unified nomenclature and suggested that resection of the first rib was the best approach for these patients. He advocated a posterior thoracotomy approach, much like the thoracoplasty incisions used in the past.

In 1966, Roos[34] introduced the transaxillary approach to first rib resection. Using this technique, he found a 93% improvement in the patients operated on by this approach. Others, including Urschel[43-45] and Rainer[32], reported similar excellent results using the transaxillary approach.

Other techniques for first-rib removal were also advocated. The superior approach was the technique used by Dr. Murphy in 1910[25], which has been supported by Thomas[41], Tyson[42], and others. Articles by Nelson and associates[27,28] reported good results when an anterior infraclavicular incision was used.

Further important work was reported by Roos in 1976[35] when he described the high incidence of associated congenital anomalies found in patients with thoracic outlet syndrome. In 1920, Law[18] had called attention to the fact that patients with symptoms suggestive of cervical rib involvement, but in which none were found, had adventitial ligaments that should be divided in addition to the scalenous

anticus muscle. Roos reported seven distinct types of congenital fibrous or muscular bands that he had found in the work-up of patients with this disease. It was his belief that these anomalies were the major factor, since 98% of his patients who underwent operation had an anomalous band whereas only 67% of cadaver dissections displayed abnormalities. It was his belief that these anomalies explain the presence of symptoms in patients who do not have cervical ribs.

In 1982, Roos[36] made a further contribution to the pathophysiology of the syndrome by suggesting there was a group of patients whose major symptoms were in the upper brachial plexus rather than in the lower.

Our present understanding of this syndrome is based on this historical foundation. To some extent the plethora of causes has confused clinicians, and the diagnosis has been frequently overlooked. This situation has been to the detriment of a significant number of patients who have this problem.

FUNCTIONAL ANATOMY

In consideration of the regional functional anatomy of the brachial plexus, the C8 and T1 nerve roots form the lower trunk of the brachial plexus. The C8 component of the lower trunk then makes a contribution to the posterior cord, which ultimately becomes the peripheral radial nerve. The remainder of the lower trunk then becomes the medial cord and eventually becomes the ulnar nerve and along with components of the lateral cord becomes the median nerve (Fig. 33-1). Considering this pattern of distribution, it is unusual but not unlikely to have symptomatic presentation in median, ulnar, or radial distribution, either isolated or in combined fashion.

In the neurologic component of the thoracic outlet syndrome, this distribution is subject to irritation or compression at multiple sites along its pathway.

The lower trunk of the plexus may be affected (1) if it passes out of the intervertebral foramen as the nerve root passes behind Sibson's fascia, (2) if it rubs across the bony surface of the first rib or of a cervical rib or elongated transverse process of C7 or (3) if it is compressed between the clavicle and first rib with such maneuvers as shoulder-girdle retraction or either horizontal or vertical hyperabduction.

The medial cord of the plexus may be affected (1) where it rubs across the posterior border of the scalenus anterior muscle, (2) if it is compressed between the intramuscular cleft of the scalenus medius and minimus muscles or between the scalenus anterior and medius muscles, (3) if it is compressed by an aneurysm from the subclavian artery, (4) if it is compressed as a result of a space-occupying lesion such as a hypertrophied subclavian muscle, or (5) if it is compressed by a Pancoast's tumor of the lung, or secondary to irregular or accentuated S-shape of the clavicle, or an abnormal exostosis of the clavicle from a previous fracture.

The peripheral components of the distal plexus can be affected (1) in extreme positions of the arm, in which they are stretched under the insertion of the pectoralis minor to the coracoid process, or (2) in vertical or horizontal hyperabduction of the shoulder girdle and arm or in shoulder-

FIG. 33-1. Diagram of brachial plexus.

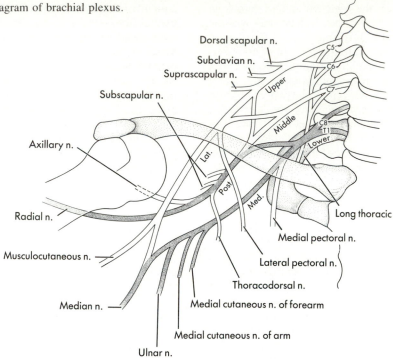

girdle retraction, in both of which they are pressed against or stretched over the humeral head.

One must also consider that as the long thoracic nerve descends, it lies immediately posterior to the lower trunk because they both cross over the proximal portion of the first rib. Pressure at this point can produce, in addition to the traditional ulnar or median nerve symptoms, an isolated weakness or paresis of the serratus anterior. This weakness or paresis is seen occasionally as an additional finding.

CLINICAL PRESENTATION

It becomes extremely important for a clinician to understand the varied clinical manifestations of thoracic outlet syndrome as a proximal entity with symptoms referable distally into the forearm and hand. Failure to consider this in the differential assessment can lead to an erroneous diagnostic conclusion. Sometimes unnecessary distal surgery is performed, and the label of malingerer or neurotic is applied to the patient if the symptoms fail to disappear after the surgery or within an appropriate conservative course of therapy.

ETIOLOGY

Thoracic outlet syndrome results from the compression of the brachial plexus or the subclavian vessels. A variety of mechanisms can result in this compression. The mechanisms can be divided into two categories: primary and secondary.

Primary thoracic outlet syndrome

The primary form of the syndrome is caused by anatomic abnormalities of the thoracic outlet. These abnormalities can involve bone or fibrous tissue, or both. The thoracic outlet is bounded by the first rib inferiorly, the costoclavicular ligament and the scalenus muscle posteriorly, and the clavicle superiorly. The most common bony mechanisms involve cervical ribs and malunited clavicular fractures. Congenital or acquired fibrous bands of the scalenus anterior and medius muscles are the most common fibrous tissue mechanisms of compression. In addition, tumors occurring in this area, such as those arising from the apex of the lung, may cause compression.

Secondary thoracic outlet syndrome

In the absence of any anatomic abnormalities, the muscles surrounding the thoracic outlet are quite supple and do not compress the neurovascular structures that pass through the aperture. However, chronic pain secondary to trauma to the arm, shoulder, or cervical spine can alter the posture of the shoulder. This alteration in posture can result in an acute, intermittent compression of the neurovascular bundle at the thoracic outlet. If the altered posture is maintained, nerve irritation can cause inappropriate and continuous stimulation of nerves, perpetuating muscle spasm and actual development of fibrous cords, which create a vicious cycle of chronic, intermittent, and continuous compression of the neurovascular bundle. Occasionally, the compression is aggravated by improper activities of the arm and can be alleviated occasionally by behavioral modifications. If the compression is aggravated by a distal painful stimulus such as a painful neuroma, the distal disorder must be treated. In addition, secondary thoracic outlet syndrome is often accompanied to some degree by an element of reflex sympathetic dystrophy or a shoulder-hand syndrome.

Symptoms

The symptoms associated with thoracic outlet syndrome result from compression of the brachial plexus or the subclavian vessels.

Neurologic symptoms. The neurologic expression of the syndrome is much more common than the vascular expression. The most common symptoms are pain and paresthe-

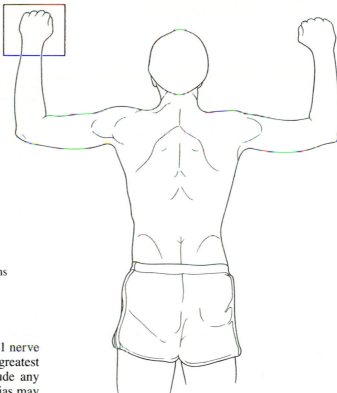

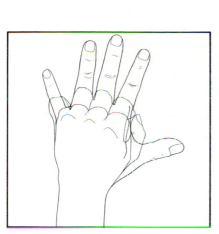

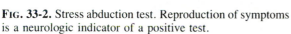

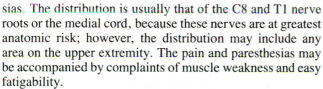

FIG. 33-2. Stress abduction test. Reproduction of symptoms is a neurologic indicator of a positive test.

sias. The distribution is usually that of the C8 and T1 nerve roots or the medial cord, because these nerves are at greatest anatomic risk; however, the distribution may include any area on the upper extremity. The pain and paresthesias may be accompanied by complaints of muscle weakness and easy fatigability.

It is important to be aware that since the compression is occurring at the level of the brachial plexus, the distribution of the symptoms may be quite bizarre.

Vascular symptoms. The vascular expression of the syndrome is uncommon, but it may accompany the neurologic aspects to some degree. The most common vascular symptoms are related to arterial insufficiency and venous congestion and are expressed as claudication, cold intolerance, and swelling. Occasionally the vascular aspects of the syndrome are seen as Raynaud's phenomenon. In severe cases of vascular compression poststenotic aneurysms can be produced, and they lead to the symptoms associated with thrombosis and embolism seen as actual ischemia and even necrosis of fingertips.

HISTORY

The history can give significant clues to the diagnosis of thoracic outlet syndrome. Posture and certain types of upper extremity activity can aggravate the compression of the neurovascular bundle in both the primary and the secondary forms of the syndrome. The most common aggravating factor is activity with the arms held above shoulder level. Here the symptoms are initiated or increased by activities, especially repetitive ones. Combing one's hair is an especially common aggravating activity. Sleeping on the affected side may lead to increased symptoms upon awakening. The manner in which a patient can temporarily relieve the symptoms may also give a clue to the diagnosis.

EXAMINATION

The physical examination for thoracic outlet syndrome involves the discovery of the results of chronic compression

of the neurovascular bundle, as well as maneuvers to elicit neurologic and vascular indicators of intermittent compression related to posture.

Neurologic signs

An extensive sensory examination is essential because the distribution of the paresthesias may be in peculiar patterns of no one particular nerve root or peripheral nerve. The most common distribution is that of the usual ulnar nerve pattern, since the C8 and T1 nerve roots are at greatest risk of compression. However, if the compression is more distal, the medial cord is involved and the pattern may extend to include the median nerve. No nerve root or cord is free of possible involvement.

Evidence of motor loss is another valuable clue to the diagnosis. Palsy of the ulnar nerve–innervated intrinsic muscle is the most common motor finding, but the additional involvement of the median nerve–innervated muscles is a very strong indicator of thoracic outlet syndrome versus an ulnar neuropathy.

In the thoracic outlet syndrome, especially in its purely neurologic expression, the most consistent clinical tests are maneuvers that have a neurologic indicator. The two tests are the 3-minute abduction stress test and supraclavicular Tinel's sign. In our experience these tests were positive in 80% of the cases of the syndrome. The 3-minute abduction stress test is performed by directing the patient to abduct his arms and repetitively flex and extend his fingers (Fig. 33-2). The test is considered positive if the symptoms are increased before a 3-minute period expires. Supraclavicular Tinel's sign can be elicited by direct palpation or percussion of the brachial plexus in the supraclavicular area.

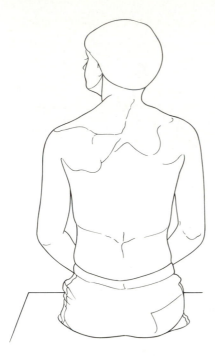

FIG. 33-3. Adson's test. Loss of radial pulse is a vascular indicator.

Vascular signs

In severe cases of vascular expression of the syndrome, evidence of vascular disturbance can be detected with the limb at rest. Here the signs include a thrill or bruit in the supraclavicular area and differences in blood presssure between the limbs in unilateral involvement. In addition, there can be color and temperature differences, and if venous occlusion is present, the involved limb can be edematous.

In cases of the syndrome in which the vascular element is less severe, it is necessary to perform certain maneuvers to elicit the vascular disturbance. Note that these maneuvers may produce a disturbance in many normal subjects if the vascular indicator alone is considered. However, if the maneuvers result in the reproduction of the patient's symptoms, whether they are vascular or neurologic in nature, a positive result can be considered a true sign of the syndrome with more certainty. The maneuvers reproduce postures that can exaggerate the compression of the neurovascular bundle. Adson's sign is performed by directing the patient to brace the shoulder posteriorly, rotate his head to the affected side, elevate the chin, and hold his breath in full inspiration (Fig. 33-3). The vascular indicator is a diminution of the radial pulse. The hyperabduction, or Wright's, test is performed with the same posture as Adson's test. In addition the arm is abducted to 90 degrees in full external rotation of the shoulder. Diminution of the radial pulse is again the indicator. Costoclavicular compression is another maneuver. Here the patient allows his shoulders to slump, and the arms are pulled inferiorly by application of traction. The positive indicator may be either vascular or neurologic.

OBJECTIVE STUDIES

Once the surgeon suspects thoracic outlet syndrome from the history and physical examination, a number of objective studies are necessary to confirm the diagnosis and rule out other entities.

Chest roentgenography

Roentgenograms of the chest in the posteroanterior and lateral projections are very important. They can give information with regard to the presence of cervical cysts and thoracic masses.

Cervical spine roentgenography

Roentgenograms of the cervical spine are an essential part of the evaluation of thoracic outlet syndrome. Cervical spondylosis can simulate the syndrome and can be ruled out; however, the presence of degenerate changes need not exclude the possibility of the presence of thoracic outlet syndrome. Cervical ribs, malunited fractures of the clavicle, and roentgenologic evidence of compressing masses can be objectively noted by this study (Fig. 33-4).

Angiography

Transfemoral subclavian angiography can be helpful when the vascular expression is severe, but it is rarely indicated when the neurologic expresssion of the syndrome is dominant. The possible morbidity associated with the study does not usually justify the study in these cases.

Electroneuromyographic evaluation

Electromyography and nerve conduction velocity studies have been one of the traditional methods of evaluating a thoracic outlet syndrome. A classic measurement is to calculate the motor conduction velocity of the ulnar nerve across the supraclavicular transaxillary segment of the ulnar nerve component of the medial cord of the brachial plexus. Normal values for conduction velocity for this segment have been calculated at 72 meters per second, with a normal and acceptable range being between 60 and 72 meters per second. When conduction velocities of less than 60 meters per second were seen, a thoracic outlet syndrome was a suspected diagnosis, and surgical resection of the first rib was carried out in the presence of failed conservative therapy.

The validity of this technique of assessment has come under challenge. Some patients who exhibit many signs and symptoms of thoracic outlet syndrome would have normal supraclavicular transaxillary ulnar conduction velocities. This seeming paradox may be explained in part because the site of supraclavicular stimulation, which is Erb's point, may be distal to the site of irritation or compression. In this situation, the small area of segmental injury would be proximal to the site of stimulation, and with normal conduction velocity values, a diagnosis of thoracic outlet syndrome might be erroneously ruled out.

In an attempt to evaluate more accurately the probability of injury to the proximal region of the lower trunk of the brachial plexus, a technique of C8 root level stimulation has been described by MacLean and Taylor[21] and later by Johnson[15]. This involves the use of stimulation with intramuscular needle electrodes placed at the C8 root level. When this technique is used in conjunction with traditional methods of supraclavicular ulnar nerve stimulation and distal recording over the ulnar abductor digiti quinti, they present a way of objectively evaluating the entire peripheral and

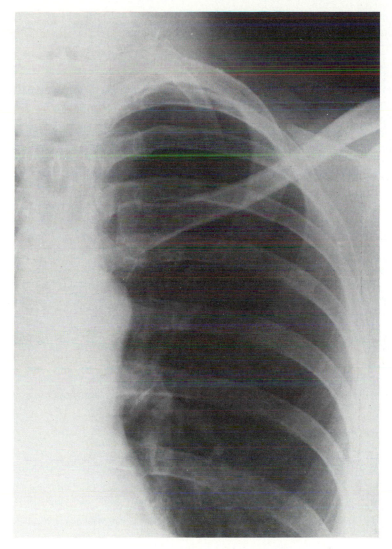

FIG. 33-4. Chest radiograph showing a cervical rib.

plexus components of the ulnar nerve, including the proximal portion of the lower trunk where it may be irritated or compressed as it transverses the proximal region of the first rib.

A protocol for performing electrophysiologic testing for thoracic outlet syndrome was developed at the Hand Rehabilitation Center in Philadelphia using both traditional ulnar nerve conduction parameters and the C8 root level stimulation techniques. The C8 root level stimulation technique was further developed to include testing the patient not only in traditional resting positions but also in positions of provocation that would impart intermittent stress on the lower trunk of the brachial plexus. These positions included both long-axis traction postures and shoulder-girdle depression that would stretch the lower trunk and the medial cord over the first rib. Additionally, overhead positions of hyperabduction and vertical flexion that would press the lower trunk and the medial cord between the clavicle and first rib and/or stretch the distal plexus nerves under the coracoid process and pectoralis minor or over the humeral head were employed.

During conduction-velocity studies, one evaluates the parameters of latency, amplitude, and conduction velocity and looks for abnormal changes in any of these parameters,

which may indicate a neuropathy. Spinner[38] writes: "It is the peripheral axons within a compressed nerve that suffer the greatest injury. Central fibers may be spared completely. As the compression continues or increases, the central fibers become involved as well. In this central region the more heavily myelinated fibers (the motor, proprioceptive, light touch, and vibratory sensory axons) are more vulnerable than the thinly myelinated pain and sympathetic fibers. If the compression lasts long enough and is of sufficient degree, all the fibers both sensory and motor within the nerve are paralyzed." Sunderland[40] further writes: "In some patients the appearance of symptoms indicative of a plexus lesion was preceded by a bout of unaccustomed work involving carrying heavy objects on the shoulder or vigorous movements of the limb. Once weakness develops, the constant friction of the lower trunk on the first rib or around the scalenus anterior leads to intraneural changes which disturb conduction in some nerves and block conduction in others." Since evoked motor amplitude is a function of the number of viable motor axons conducting, it is reasonable to consider amplitudinal changes as a sensitive indicator of segmental neuropathy. Accordingly, we at the Philadelphia Hand Rehabilitation Center hypothesized that changes in evoked amplitude would be the most sensitive indicator of conduction anomaly and could be evaluated relative to fiber population or drop out while one is evaluating the changes in peak-to-peak amplitude at rest and under stress-testing positions of provocation.

Testing protocol. The thoracic outlet test protocol developed at the Hand Rehabilitation Center using both electromyography and nerve conduction studies has the following objectives: (1) to rule out any concomitant distal peripheral nerve entrapment, (2) to allow evaluation of the conduction velocity of the supraclavicular segment of the ulnar nerve, and (3) to allow evaluation of the conduction parameters of the proximal portion of the lower trunk of the brachial plexus and the effects intermittent stress positioning would have on the evoked motor amplitude as an indicator of segmental neuropathy.

The step-by-step testing protocol is as follows:

A. Nerve-conduction studies
   1. Where possible the median and ulnar nerves should be evaluted bilaterally for comparative purposes.
   2. When bilateral evaluation is not possible, unilateral evaluation should be carried out on a symptomatic extremity as follows:
      a. The median-nerve distal sensory and motor latencies and motor conduction velocity in the forearm and across the carpal tunnel are performed and evaluated to rule out a carpal tunnel neuropathy.
      b. The ulnar-nerve distal sensory and motor latencies are performed across the wrist and through the canal of Guyon. The ulnar nerve is then segmentally tested in the proximal direction to rule out local entrapment neuropathies at the elbow cubital tunnel, supracondylar region, axilla, and brachial plexus distal to Erb's point.

c. The cervical root stimulation technique is then administered as follows:
   (1) The spinous process of C6 is located by manual palpation techniques.
   (2) Paired monopolar needle electrodes of either 50 or 75 mm in length are then inserted 2 cm laterally and 1 cm inferiorly to the tip of the C7 spinous process. This should place the stimulating electrode adjacent to the C8 nerve root proximal to its articulation over the first rib (Fig. 33-5).

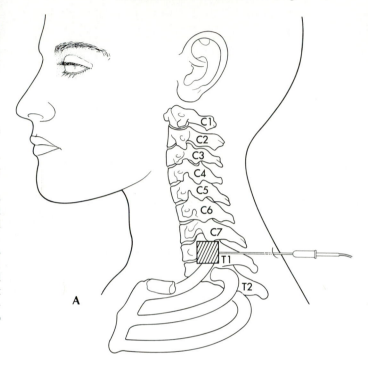

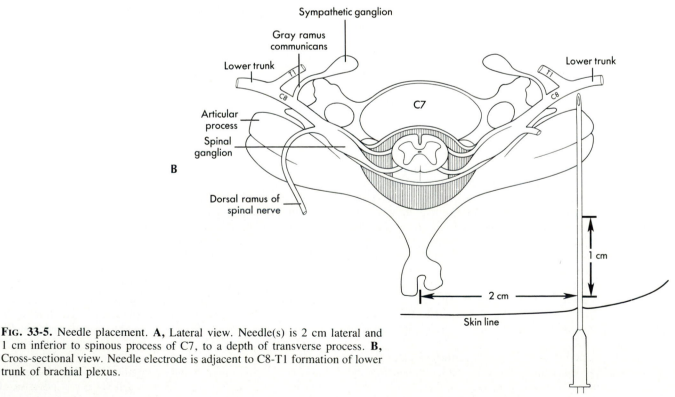

FIG. 33-5. Needle placement. **A,** Lateral view. Needle(s) is 2 cm lateral and 1 cm inferior to spinous process of C7, to a depth of transverse process. **B,** Cross-sectional view. Needle electrode is adjacent to C8-T1 formation of lower trunk of brachial plexus.

(3) Recording is performed with surface electrodes over the motor point of the abductor digiti quinti in the hand.
(4) The patient is tested while sitting, and the test is carried out in the following five positions:
  (a) The arm is held at the patient's side in extension and internal rotation, and the shoulder girdle is depressed (Fig. 33-6, *A*).
  (b) The same position is maintained, and a 5- or 10-pound weight is then placed in the hand to provide long-axis hanging traction causing the lower trunk to be stretched over the first rib (Fig. 33-6, *B*).

  (c) The weight is withdrawn, and the patient now raises the arm into hyperabduction with the shoulder joint in 90 degrees of abduction in the frontal plane, 10 degrees or greater of abduction in the sagittal plane, and 90 degrees of elbow flexion, with the forearm in full supination. There is neutral cervical rotation and side bend in this position (Fig. 33-6, *C*).
  (d) The same position is maintained, and the cervical spine is now taken into the end range of contralateral side bend and rotation (Fig. 33-6, *D*).
  (e) The cervical spine is returned to neutral rotation and side bend, and the arm is now vertically flexed to 165 degrees (Fig. 33-6, *E*).

B. Electromyography. The median and ulnar distal muscles are now sampled to establish the presence of any denervation activity, increased polyphasia, or loss of voluntary motor unit recruitment ability. These abnormal observations in the presence of normal plexus and peripheral conduction parameters would suggest a proximal root level pathologic condition. Accordingly, paraspinal muscles should then be tested. Normal or abnormal paraspinal electromyogram ac-

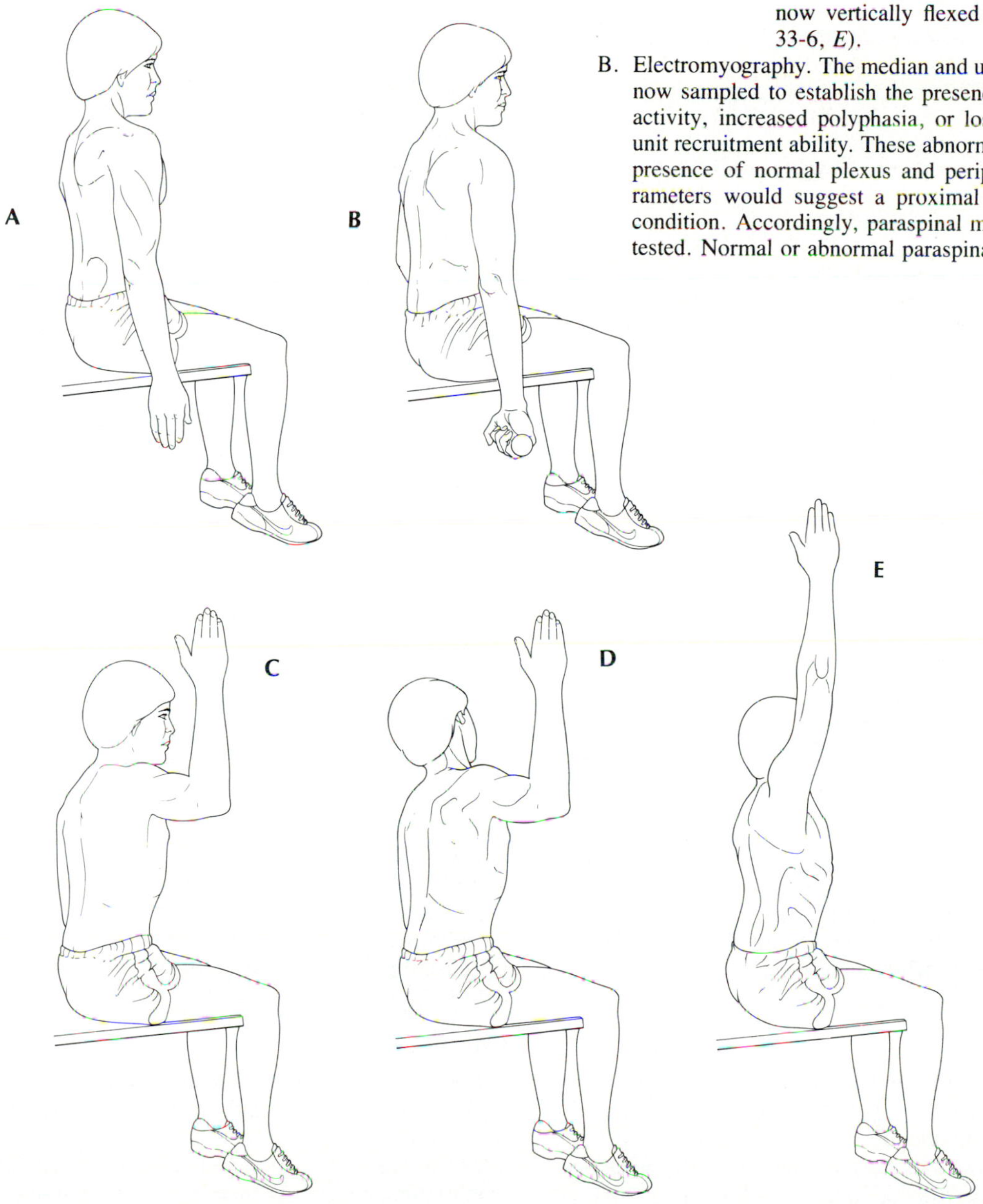

FIG. 33-6. Stress positions. **A,** Resting test position. Baseline amplitudinal comparison may be established between this level and that obtained from supraclavicular stimulation. **B,** Long-axis traction stress position. **C,** Hyperabduction stress position—minimal tension on ipsilateral neck flexor muscles. **D,** Hyperabduction stress position—maximum tension on ipsilateral neck flexor muscles. **E,** Vertical overhead stress position.

tivity would assist in further differential localization of root versus plexus or peripheral involvement.

  C. Summary

    1. Where possible, bilateral median and ulnar nerves are tested to rule out peripheral entrapment syndrome.

    2. The involved ulnar nerve should show normal conduction parameters for all segments between the axilla and the wrist.

    3. The supraclavicular segment of the ulnar nerve may show a slowing of the conduction velocity of less than 60 meters per second, or 10 meters per second slower than the humeral segment. This would suggest a lesion at the distal brachial plexus level.

    4. The C8 root stimulation technique may show a drop in the evoked motor amplitude measured peak to peak, and may be seen in any one or all of the previously described stress positions. Amplitudinal drops in excess of 25% from the supraclavicular level are considered to be significant so long as the correct stimulating electrode placement has been maintained. Abnormalities seen at this level suggest a proximal lower trunk level lesion.

    5. The electromyogram may show denervation activity, increased polyphasia, or loss of motor unit recruitment power. These findings could also suggest a C8 root level lesion proximal to the lower trunk level of the brachial plexus, and accordingly the cervical paraspinals would then need to be evaluated to assist in differentiation between a root level of a plexus level lesion.

DIFFERENTIAL DIAGNOSIS

The thoracic outlet syndrome can have an extremely varied presentation, and it is important to consider and rule out other disorders that may mimic or occur along with the syndrome. Such disorders are the following:

1. Ulnar nerve compression
2. Median nerve compression
3. Cervical spondylosis
4. Syringomyelia
5. Progressive muscular atrophy

NONOPERATIVE TREATMENT

Once the diagnosis of thoracic outlet syndrome is confirmed, the initial treatment is nonoperative. The treatment plan includes evaluation, patient education, behavior modification, and, if indicated, exercise and joint mobilization. The patient must be aware that symptoms can be relieved if one adheres to a specific plan. Thoracic outlet syndrome should not be treated on a one-time basis but instead must be followed closely by the patient and the therapist so that alterations can be made when appropriate.

Evaluation

Along with information obtained by the physician, electromyogram, and nerve-conduction velocity testing, the therapist must evaluate the patient to establish a baseline of condition. These data are used to determine appropriate behavior modifications, exercises, and joint mobilization techniques. A comparison of initial to subsequent assessments will determine if treatment is effective. A comprehensive evaluation includes a history and assessments of posture, upper extremity range of motion, strength, mobility, pain, and sensory changes.

An accurate history will give indications of the cause and propagation of thoracic outlet syndrome. For example, a patient may report symptoms occurring after a new job involving overhead activities, in which case behavior modification eliminating that motion is indicated. Another patient may claim a gradual onset, in which case a postural assessment could indicate an imbalance of upper quarter musculature. Treatment would then focus on exercises and postural correction. Documentation of pain and paresthesia patterns indicate the structures within the brachial plexus that are most involved, along with secondary developments such as muscle atrophy or poor tissue nutrition.

Postural inadequacies must be recognized and corrected. Common deficits are rounded or retracted shoulders, increased thoracic kyphosis, and an increased compensatory cervical lordosis resulting in a foward head posture. Muscular imbalances and soft-tissue elongation or shortening in the cervical region will alter the position of the posterior triangle. For the same reason, hypertrophy of the upper trapezius muscles and pendulous breasts can be a contributing factor. Subtle soft-tissue contractures of the craniovertebral, cervical, and scapulothoracic joints are often secondary manifestations of the thoracic outlet syndrome.

Test maneuvers to cause compression of the neurovascular bundle and recreation of the symptoms will clue the therapist to one of the specific structures at fault. In the Adson maneuver the examiner looks for a decrease in radial pulse, or an increase in symptoms, as a positive test. The mechanism involves decreasing the space between the anterior and middle scalene, through which the brachial plexus and the subclavian artery lie. The hyperabduction test provides two points of compression to the neurovascular bundle. The first is in the decreased costoclavicular space, and the second is at the pulley formed by the insertion of the pectoralis minor muscle into the coracoid process of the scapula, beneath which the bundle passes. In the costoclavicular maneuver the neurovascular bundle is compromised by the approximation of the clavical and the first rib, thus reproducing symptoms. Passive hyperextension of the glenohumeral joint will also increase symptoms by trapping structures beneath the coracoid insertion of the pectoralis minor. Manual compression superior and posterior to the medial one third of the clavical will also produce symptoms.

Once the pattern for symptom production is identified— that is, scalene hypertonicity or decrease of costoclavicular space—the goals of therapy are easily established. Constant reassessment of the test maneuvers and subjective reports of sensation will allow the effectiveness of the protocol to be monitored.

Patient education

Education of the patient to the mechanics of the thoracic outlet syndrome is essential to treatment. The physician or the therapist should explain how the syndrome began, and what structures are involved. Discussion in easily understood language and by means of clear diagrams will make the condition tangible. Once he has visualized the condition, the patient will understand why certain positions aggravate the symptoms. Individual problem solving will be simpler when the patient is properly informed.

Behavior modification

Once the patient is educated about thoracic outlet syndrome, he is asked to apply this knowledge to everyday activities to control the symptoms. With a therapist's assistance, behavior can be consciously modified. The following suggestions are made to the patient.

Sleeping. The positions that aggravate the thoracic outlet syndrome during sleep are the following: bringing the arms up overhead, lying on the affected side, and lying on the stomach with the head turned to one side. A position that reduces symptoms is side-lying on the unaffected side with one pillow under the head and another pillow in the line of the trunk to support the upper arm. Another position of comfort is lying on the back with one pillow under the head and shoulders and one pillow under each arm.

Working. Whether one is working at home or in the office, there are certain activities to avoid. Guard against working above shoulder level, because this compresses the neurovascular bundle in the costoclavicular space and beneath the coracoid insertion of the pectoralis minor muscle. Using a step stool to reach high objects is an easy solution. One must prevent traction of the plexus over the glenohumeral joint, which is produced when one is carrying items with the affected arms. Briefcases and grocery bags are the biggest offenders in this regard, and alternative solutions must be developed. When sitting at a desk or armchair, make sure there is a forearm-supporting surface that will not cause excessive elevation or depression of the shoulders.

Driving. A hint to minimize symptoms during driving is to keep the hands low and relaxed on the steering wheel. A small pillow should support the arm if the armrest is not present on the affected side, or it is at an improper height.

General precautions. There are some situations occurring in all activities that should be modified. Stressful situations will lead to tension of the cervical musculature. Alternative methods of relieving stress, either in sharing a burden with others or avoidance altogether, must be arranged. Large breasts contribute to poor posture by pulling the chest down and protracting the shoulders. Thin bra straps add to discomfort by applying a great force to a small area. Thick bra straps, strapless bras, or bralessness will assist in decreasing the direct pressure on the thoracic outlet. Strenuous breathing requires the action of secondary respiratory masculature whose function is elevation of the ribs. With the first rib placed in this manner symptoms are provoked. Cold weather creates shivering and hypertonicity of the body's muscles, including those of the upper cervical region. Wearing several layers of light clothing will reduce shivering.

• • •

In patients with a minimally progressed thoracic outlet syndrome, the mere application of behavior modification is enough to control the symptoms. Adherence to these principles will decrease the chance of recurrence.

Exercises

All exercises must be tailored to a patient's needs as determined through evaluation. Results of compression testing, range-of-motion measurements, and postural assessment will direct treatment goals. Exercises should be clearly written and demonstrated so that the patient can perform them three or four times daily.

Hypertonicity of the scalene muscles is one mechanism that can give rise to a positive Adson's maneuver. To reduce the tightness, begin in the supine position and actively or passively sidebend to the uninvolved side. Initially, rotation is avoided until the muscle's flexibility improves, at which time rotation toward the opposite side of the sidebend is incorporated. The stretch should be held and then relaxed and repeated bilaterally. Contraction-relaxation patterns of inhibitory proprioceptive neuromuscular facilitation can be employed to gain mobility. Sometimes evident from a positive hyperabduction and hyperextension test, increased tone of the pectoralis minor muscle should be reduced. Initial performance should be in a supine position with the arms abducted to 90 degrees, in neutral, and with the elbows flexed to 90 degrees. The arms are slowly externally rotated until a pulling sensation across the anterior glenohumeral joint is felt. Again, contraction-relaxation patterns are used to gain mobility. Once the patient achieves good external rotation, the exercise is performed while the patient stands. The patient will face the corner with shoulders 90 degrees abducted, full external rotation, elbow flexed 90 degrees, and forearms resting against the wall. The patient leans toward the corner to achieve the same stretching sensation. As with all exercises to increase muscular mobility, a sustained stretch will facilitate the inhibitory activity of the muscle spindle.

Faulty posture, especially for a prolonged time, will result in adaptive soft-tissue shortening. Shoulder contraction will eventually limit the scapulothoracic joint in its medial glide across the rib cage. Instructing the patient in shoulder circles with emphasis on gradual scapular retraction will increase joint motion. This is easily performed when one is sitting relaxed, with forearms supported to avoid elevation or depression. A forward head posture involves increased lordosis of the middle cervical spine along with forward glide of the occiput on the atlas and a forward bend of the lower cervical and thoracic spine. Axial extension exercises performed actively by the patient will reverse forward head posture and increase mobility of the craniovertebral and cervical articulations. The patient begins by sitting comfortably and then is asked to push his head back (chin tuck), being careful not to tilt anteriorly or posteriorly. A finger on the chin will assist in avoiding movement up or down. This exercise is a glide of the occiput on the atlas posteriorly and straightening of the cervical spine. Many times the scapula will fall into a desired relaxed position naturally when one is performing axial extension. Diaphragmatic breathing exercises are often indicated when the majority of respiratory action evolves from the accessory muscles. The elevation of the rib cage by the pectoralis minor and scalenes should be eliminated because this action decreases the thoracic outlet space.

The position assumed when one is performing these exercises may recreate symptoms; however, once the exercise is completed, the symptoms will stop. As mobility improves, symptoms should not reappear as easily.

If indicated through bilateral testing, weak musculature

should be strengthened. Since upper extremity weakness in the appropriate myotomal distribution can be a result of the thoracic outlet syndrome, strength will improve as the neuropraxia is relieved. Upper trunk muscles commonly weak because of disuse rather than the compression are the serratus anterior, middle and lower trapezius, latissimus dorsi, and the rhomboids. Although the long thoracodorsal nerve may be involved by stretching over an increased thoracic kyphosis, producing secondary weakness of the latissimus dorsi, this too will increase strength with postural correction.

Very rarely are the upper trapezius and deltoid weak secondary to the thoracic outlet syndrome. Attempting to strengthen by adding a weight to the gravity-dependent arm increases the traction force on the brachial plexus over the humeral head, ultimately aggravating the symptoms.

Joint mobilization

Joint-mobilization techniques of the sternoclavicular, acromioclavicular, and scapulothoracic joints and the first and second rib articulations provide a reliable method of increasing the costoclavicular space. Mobilization of the occiput on the atlas will also facilitate axial extension movement. However, the patient must be willing to make daily therapy visits initially and follow the exercise program faithfully. The additional joint mobility produced by mobilization techniques is maintained with exercises by the patient at home. Reduction of pain and paresthesias is often successful with this method. The rationale for joint mobilization is described by Cyriax,[8] Kaltenborn,[16] Maitland,[22] and Smith.[37] Techniques of joint mobilization should be performed only by persons with appropriate training in manual therapy.

• • •

A successful nonoperative treatment program should produce a decrease in symptoms within 1 month. If this is noted, nonsurgical treatment should be continued in the effort to eliminate the symptoms. However, if the patient has not progressed or has in fact regressed through the natural course of the syndrome, the physician must select an alternative method of intervention.

SURGICAL TREATMENT

It has been reported that 50% to 70% of people with thoracic outlet syndrome can be relieved by the nonoperative treatment discussed earlier. However, there is a group of patients with severe neurologic symptoms who are not improved by the physical therapy and may, indeed, be worsened by such treatment. Patients with severe intractable pain and disability, particularly if physical therapy has not been effective, are candidates for surgical treatment. In addition, those patients with arterial or venous components to their symptoms are best treated surgically. Although one or several different causes may be present to produce the thoracic outlet symptoms, the first rib appears to be a common denominator in most, if not all, of these. Surgical removal of the first rib, therefore, with any congenital bands associated with it, including a cervical rib, gives the most consistent results in the treatment of this syndrome. Scalenotomy has been virtually abandoned because of the poor overall results. Removal of the clavicle has also been abandoned because

of the discomfort and poor cosmetic appearance after its removal.

First rib resection through the axillary approach as described by Roos in 1966[34] is the simplest and most acceptable way of removing the first rib. Other techniques that have been described include the limited posterior thoracotomy incision popularized by Clagett in 1962[4] and recently by Martinez.[23] However, the operation is more extensive and cosmetically inferior to the transaxillary procedure. Supraclavicular and infraclavicular approaches have also been reported and have their advocates.

With the use of careful technique, postoperative complications have been few. It is particularly important to avoid undue traction on the nerves to prevent postoperative brachial plexus dysfunction.

Excellent results of therapy have been reported in 85% to 90% of patients treated through the transaxillary approach. Ten percent have had a mild improvement, and 5% to 10% have had no improvement.

Occasionally one sees patients in whom symptoms of reflex sympathetic dystrophy are severe. Although many patients with the thoracic outlet syndrome have such symptoms and need only the first rib removed, some with more severe findings are benefited by the addition of a thoracic sympathectomy performed through the same transaxillary approach after the first rib has been excised. It is usually necessary to remove only the lower part of T1, T2, and T3 ganglia.

Some patients may initially have an excellent response and then have a recurrence of some or all of their symptoms. This is believed to be attributable to scar formation about the plexus. Urschel[46] suggests using the posterior approach in these patients with excision of the distal portion of the first rib as well as a neurolysis of the brachial plexus if necessary.

The place of scalenectomy, as recently described by Roos,[36] in those with predominantly upper plexus symptoms has yet to be established.

SUMMARY

Thoracic outlet syndrome is a general term for compression neuropathies and vasculopathies of the brachial plexus and the subclavian vessels. The vascular expression of the syndrome is uncommon, while the neurologic expression is common and often not appreciated. The key to the diagnosis of the syndrome is awareness of its occurrence and the ability to support the clinical impression with objective testing. The presentation of the syndrome may be bizarre, but it should be considered in any case of pain and paresthesias of the upper extremity.

REFERENCES

1. Adson, A.W., and Coffey, J.R.: Cervical rib: a method of anterior approach for relief of symptoms by division of the scalenus anticus, Ann. Surg. **85:**839-857, 1927.
2. Bramwell, E.: Lesion of the first dorsal nerve root, Rev. Neurol. Psychiat. **1:**299, 1903.
3. Brickner, W.M.: Brachial plexus pressure by the normal first rib, Ann. Surg. **85:**858-872, June 1927.
4. Clagett, O.T.: Presidential address, American Association of Thoracic Surgery, Research and Prosearch, April 16-18, 1962, J. Thorac. Cardiovasc. Surg. **44**(2):153-166, Aug. 1962.

5. Cooper, A.: Cited by Adson, A.W., and Coffee, J.R.: Cervical rib: method of anterior approach for relief of symptoms by division of scalenus anticus, Ann. Surg. **85:**839-857, 1927.

6. Coote, H.: Pressure on the axillary vessels and nerve by an exostosis from a cervical rib: interference with the circulation of the arm, removal of the rib and exostosis: recovery, Medical Times and Gazette. **II:**108, 1861.

7. Craig, W.M. and Knepper, P.A.: Cervical rib and scalenus anticus syndrome, Ann. Surg. **105:**556-563, 1937.

8. Cyriax, J.: Textbook of orthopedic medicine, ed. 6, London, 1976, HK Lewis & Co., ed. 6, vol. 1, pp. 61-98, 169-179.

9. Eden, K.C.: The vascular complications of cervical ribs and first thoracic rib abnormalities, Brit. J. Surg. **27:**111-139, 1939-1940.

10. Falconer, M.A., and Li, F.W.P.: Resection of the first rib in costoclavicular compression of the brachial plexus, Lancet, **1:**59-63, Jan. 13, 1962.

11. Falconer, M.A., and Weddell, G.: Costoclavicular compression of the subclavian artery and vein: relation to the scalenus anticus syndrome, Lancet **2:**539-544, Oct. 30, 1943.

12. Gruber, W.: Über die Halsrippen des Menschen mit vergleichend-anatomischen Bemerkung, St. Petersburg, 1869.

13. Halsted, W.S.: An experimental study of circumscribed dilation of an artery immediately distal to a partially occluding band, and its bearing on the dilation of the subclavian artery observed in certain cases of cervical rib, J. Exp. Med. **24:**271, 1916.

14. Hunauld: Sur le nombre des côtes, moindre ou plus grand a l'ordinaire, Hist. Acad. Roy. des Sci. de Paris, 1740.

15. Johnson, E.W.: Practical electromyography, Baltimore, 1980, The Williams & Wilkins Co.

16. Kaltenborn, F.M.: Manual therapy for the extremity joints, Oslo, 1974, Olaf Norlis Bokhandel, pp. 86 and 87.

17. Kean, W.W.: The symptomatology, diagnosis, and surgical treatment of cervical ribs, Am. J. Med. Sci. **133:**173-218, 1907.

18. Law, A.A.: Adventitious ligaments simulating cervical ribs, Ann. Surg. **28:**109, 1954.

19. Lewis, T., and Pickering, G.: Observations upon maladies in which the blood supply to the digits ceases intermittently or permanently, Clin. Sci. **9:**327, 1934.

20. Lord, J.W., Jr.: Surgical management of shoulder girdle syndromes, A.M.A. Arch. Surg. **66:**69, 1953.

21. MacLean, I., and Taylor, R.: Nerve root stimulation to evaluate brachial plexus conduction, abstracts of communications of the Fifth International Congress of Electromyography, Rochester, Minn., 1975, p. 47.

22. Maitland, G.D.: Peripheral manipulation, London, 1974, Butterworth & Co., pp. 148 and 149.

23. Martinez, N.S.: Posterior first rib resection for total thoracic outlet syndrome decompression, Contemp. Surg. **15:**13-21, July 1979.

24. Morley, J.: Brachial pressure neuritis due to a normal first thoracic rib: its diagnosis and treatment by excision of rib, Clin. J. **42:**461, Oct. 23, 1913.

25. Murphy, T.: Brachial neuritis caused by pressure of first rib, Aust. Med. J. **15:**582, Oct. 20, 1910.

26. Naffziger, H.C., and Grant, W.T.: Neuritis of the brachial plexus mechanical in origin: the scalenus syndrome, Surg. Gynecol. Obstet. **67:**722-730, Dec. 1938.

27. Nelson, R.M., and Davis, R.W.: Thoracic outlet compression syndrome: collective review, Ann. Thorac. Surg. **8**(5):437-451, Nov. 1969.

28. Nelson, R.M., and Jensen, C.B.: Anterior approach for excision of the first rib: surgical technique, Ann. Thorac. Surg. **9**(1):30-35, 1970.

29. Ochsner, A., Gage, M., and DeBakey, M.: Scalenus anticus (Naffziger) syndrome, New Orleans, 1935, Departments of Surgery, Tulane University School of Medicine, Charity Hospital, and Touro Infirmary.

30. Peet, R.M., Henriksen, J.D., Anderson, T.P., Martin, G.M.: Thoracic outlet syndrome: evaluation of a therapeutic exercise program, Staff Meetings Mayo Clin., pp. 281-287, May 2, 1956.

31. Raaf, J.: Surgery for cervical rib and scalenus anticus syndrome, J.A.M.A. **157:**219-223, Jan. 15, 1955.

32. Rainer, W.G., Vigor, W., and Newby, J.P.: Surgical treatment of thoracic outlet compression, Am. J. Surg. **116:**704-707, Nov. 1968.

33. Rob, C.G., and Standeven, A.: Arterial occlusion complicating thoracic outlet compression syndrome, Brit. Med. J., pp. 709-712, Sept. 20, 1958.

34. Roos, D.B.: Transaxillary approach for first rib resection to relieve thoracic outlet syndrome, Ann. Surg. **163**(3):354-358, 1966.

35. Roos, D.B.: Congenital anomalies associated with thoracic outlet syndrome, Am. J. Surg. **132:**771-778, Dec. 1976.

36. Roos, D.B.: The place for scalenectomy and first rib resection in thoracic outlet syndrome, Boston, June 18, 1982, Society for Vascular Surgery, p. 50.

37. Smith, K.F.: The thoracic outlet syndrome: a protocol of treatment, J. Orthop. Sports, Am. Phys. Thera. Assoc. **1**(2):89-99, Fall 1979.

38. Spinner, M.: Injuries to major branches of the peripheral nerves of the forearm, ed. 2, Philadelphia, 1978, W.B. Saunders Co.

39. Stopford, J.S.B., and Telford E.D.: Compression of the lower trunk of the brachial plexus by a first dorsal rib, with note on surgical treatment, Brit. J. Surg. **8:**168, 1919.

40. Sunderland, S.: Nerves and nerve injuries, ed. 2, New York, 1978, Churchill Livingstone.

41. Thomas, G.L., Jones, T.W., Stavney, L.S., and Manhas Dev, R.: Thoracic outlet syndrome, Am. Surg. **16:**483-495, Aug. 1978.

42. Tyson, R.R., and Kaplan, G.F.: Modern concepts of d diagnosis and the treatment of the thoracic outlet syndrome, Orthop. Clin. North Am. **6**(2):507-549, April 1975.

43. Urschel, H., Razzuk, M., Wood, R., Parekh, M., and Paulson, B.: Objective diagnosis (ulnar nerve conduction velocity) and current therapy of the thoracic outlet syndrome, Ann. Thorac. Surg. **12**(6):608-620, Dec. 1979.

44. Urschel, H., Paulson, B., and McNamara, J.: Thoracic outlet syndrome, Ann. Surg. **6**(1): July 1968.

45. Urschel, H.C., Jr.: Management of the thoracic-outlet syndrome, N. Engl. J. Med. **286:**1140-1143, May 1972.

46. Urschel, H.C., Jr., Razzuk, M.A., Albers, J.E., Wood, R.E., and Paulson, D.L.: Reoperation for recurrent thoracic outlet syndrome, Ann. Thorac. Surg. **21**(1):19-25, 1979.

47. Willshire, W.H.: Supernumerary first rib: clinical records, Lancet **2:**633, 1860.

48. Wright, I.S.: The neurovascular syndrome produced by hyperabduction of the arm, original communication, Am. Heart J. **29**(1):1-19, 1945.

BIBLIOGRAPHY

Adson, A.W.: Surgical treatment for symptoms produced by cervical ribs and scalenus anticus muscle, Surg. Gynecol. Obstet. **85:**687, 1927.

Brain, W.R.: Spontaneous compression of both median nerves in the carpal tunnel, Lancet, pp. 277-282, 1927.

Caldwell, J.W., Crain, C.R., and Cruzen, E.M.: Nerve conduction studies: an aid in diagnosis of thoracic outlet syndrome, South. Med. J. **6**(2):210-212, 1971.

Gelberman, R., Hergenroeder, D., Hargens, A., Lundberg, G., and Akeson, W.: The carpal tunnel syndrome: a study of carpal canal pressures, J. Bone Joint Surg. **63**(3):380-383, 1981.

Gol, A., Patrick, D.W., and McNeel, D.P.: Relief of costoclavicular syndrome by infraclavicular removal of first rib: technical note, J. Neurosurg. **28:**81-84, 1968.

Hughes, E.S.R.: Venous obstruction in the upper extremity (Paget-Schroetter's syndrome): collective review, Int. Abstr. Surg. **88**(2):89-127, 1949.

Liveson, J., and Speilholz, N.: Peripheral neurology: case studies and electrodiagnosis, Philadelphia, 1979, F.A. Davis Co.

Lord, J.W., and Stone, P.W.: Pectoralis minor tenotomy and anterior scalenotomy with special reference to the hyperabduction syndrome and "effort thrombosis" of the subclavian vein, Circulation **13:**537, 1956.

Roos, D.B.: Experience with first rib resection for thoracic outlet syndrome, Ann. Surg. **173**(3):429-442, 1971.

Rydevik, B., Lundborg, G., and Bagge, U.: Effects of graded compression on intraneural blood flow, original communication, J. Hand Surg. **6**(1):3-11, 1981.

Sanders, R.J., Monsour, J.W., and Baer, S.B.: Transaxillary first rib resection for the thoracic outlet syndrome, Arch Surg. **97:**1014-1023, Dec. 1968.

Spinner, M., and Omer, G.: Management of peripheral nerve problems, Philadelphia, 1980, W.B. Saunders Co.

Telford, E.D., and Stopford, J.S.B.: The vascular complications of the cervical rib, Brit. J. Surg. **18:**559, 1937.

Upton, A., and McComas, A.: The double crush and nerve entrapment syndromes, Lancet, pp. 359-361, 1973.

34

Sensibility testing: state of the art

JUDITH A. BELL

The true design and function of cutaneous sensibility have defied simple description. Compared with available knowledge of vision, hearing, and other sensory processes, there is much to be learned of this important sensory function.

Many tests have been popularized for measurement of cutaneous sensibility. These, in fact, represent a multitude of thought processes and perspectives. They are of value in attesting to the complexities involved in measuring a system that is as yet incompletely defined.

One finds in the literature conflicting opinions that are often perpetuated by repetition. There exists an inability to directly compare one testing method with another[14,27] and an apparent limited communication of one discipline with another. If these are confusing to the novice, they are confusing as well to the initiated.

The differing opinions and problems in testing would be simplified if objective tests were available. Some tests are more objective than others, but a reliable, repeatable, consistent test has yet to be developed. *What tests have been believed to be objective in the past can be demonstrated to be subjective in application[3,7,13] and are further dependent on the technique of the examiner or the individual response of the patient.*

The examiner of cutaneous sensory function is cautioned against placing too much weight on a particular measurement or test. An examiner would be better counseled to remain open to developments in testing, taking all tests and measurements only as samples of the function he or she is trying to measure. As with all samples, they can be misleading when viewed out of context with the whole and are likely to represent only a part of the whole picture. *It is always possible that additional samples will describe a totally different picture.*

What has to be weighed and balanced in sensibility testing is the need for a simple test versus the need for detailed testing (Fig. 34-1). In clinical testing one begins early to feel that to do justice to the patient needing sensory evaluation one would have to devote a professional lifetime to the sorting of information, justification of testing procedure, and documentation of testing results. Most examiners do not have the time for such detailed investigation. There has long been a search for a simple, objective, easy-to-perform sensory test of neural status and hand function. It is recognized that there is a need for a simple test that would be readily available and of little cost for use in a wide variety of clinical settings. It may be that in time there will be such a test. Within the confines of one's own practice, one has to do the best that can be done with what is available. But when possible, it may be wise for the cautious examiner to trade the idea of a simple test for that of thorough testing. *The patient is our real concern. Do we do him justice if we tell him that he does not have a problem on the basis of a simple test?* Can it be determined how one patient functions much better than another with what appears to be an identical injury? How do we really know if one type of surgical repair is better than another in restoring sensory function, or if sensory reeducation is worth the time and effort? These and other questions are as yet unanswered and may not be able to be answered by a simple test.

WHERE DO THE ANSWERS COME FROM?
Literature

There is much to be learned from the literature if one accepts as fact only those things that can be demonstrated as fact, and as theory all else. Many fascinating studies of cutaneous sensibility have been executed since the age of Aristotle. Each study offers insight into the concepts of sensory function and into what has and has not been attempted in measurement. One need not review every paper that has ever been written on the subject, but it is important that the serious examiner search for original sources of information that might otherwise be taken for granted.

All papers list a bibliography of their information sources referenced. By reading these references, and the studies they in turn reference, one comes into contact directly with the original sources of information. It is often a surprise to find that one's own interpretation of the original study is quite different from the interpretation of the study by another author. For instance, it was in this way that I discovered that von Frey,[32,33] credited as one of the earliest experimental investigators of cutaneous sensation, actually had a better test in the 1890s than presently available renditions of his test. Through the translation of von Frey's original German articles, one discovers that von Frey has a lot to say to us one century later.[34,35] He had anticipated many problems we are now describing with our modern instruments, and modern technology with which to measure them. Much of his original work has been lost through various translations and interpretations. The same is true of other authors.

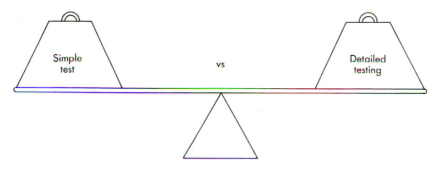

FIG. 34-1. Examiner of cutaneous sensibility must weigh and balance need for simple test versus need for thorough testing. Examiner needs a simple test for use in office and in field situations. He or she also needs information that is not forthcoming from a simple test.

A standardized test

Beyond consideration of a simple versus detailed test, the question remains, What test could be utilized to provide information internally in a clinic and externally from clinic to clinic? So many tests are available, each with its own respected advocate, that it is difficult for the clinician to decide which to use. The danger herein is that many clinicians are likely to use the most popular method advocated by the strongest examiner. The "most popular method" is not necessarily the most objective or reliable test. Other examiners choose to determine for themselves which test they believe to be optimum. Still others abstain from judgment completely, seeking alternative ways of solving their patient's problems.

One solution to the many varied tests and testing techniques presently utilized in clinical testing might be for examiners to adopt one test in common for reporting results and so on. This sounds reasonable enough, but still another problem remains: one cannot standardize a test until there is one to standardize. So long as our clinical tests can be demonstrated to be subjective, the clinician is left "at risk" in making decisions as to neural status based on any test.

There seems to be no escaping the homework required for either finding an objective test or finding ways in which present tests can be made more objective. *It is not enough to identify a single test or to say subjectivity does matter when one cannot know the effect of subjective variables on the interpretation of test results.* The subjective nature of our tests in a day of modern technology where better tests are possible dictates that we first seek an objective test and then seek to standardize it.

One might argue that it is impossible to control all variables in a test situation. Psychologists face this problem in their work even more than examiners of sensibility. In their test design, they first make the test as objective as possible, dealing with variables that can be eliminated. Then when faced with variables that cannot be eliminated such as a test requiring the subjective response of a patient, they minimize the error by finding ways to deal statistically with the subjective element. In sensibility testing, a forced-choice test that would deal with guessing statistically has been suggested by Dyck and LaMotte.[15,19] In a forced-choice procedure of testing a patient is given a series of stimulations, and the patient must decide on which number of the series he felt the stimulation. According to LaMotte, in a forced-choice procedure of testing, the response bias plays a relatively minor role because a subject can get no better than 50% correct by guessing.

Test battery

There are other considerations that make it disadvantageous at this time to decide only upon one clinical test, even an objective test. Were every clinic to choose only one method of obtaining information, the result might be that of inhibiting the development of other needed information. Suppose the technique chosen contained an unknown variable that eventually rendered all clinical testing invalid? Depending so heavily on one test is comparable to investing all of one's money on one horse in a race. There are ways of predicting which methods might be more advantageous than another in sensibility testing, but the final champion is only proved once it has made its way to the finish. Efforts to utilize a single test in the past have had to be abandoned by changes in thought and evidence leading in another direction.[8] There does have to be some common base of communication. If every clinic could use perhaps one or two tests in common, along with their own particular test they believe provides them with the most reliable information, there would be at least some common ground for communication. In addition, clinicians then would be more likely to use at least one clinical test that would later prove reliable and could serve as a basis for comparison with other tests.[6]

Another consideration is that a test battery may in fact be required to provide clinicians with a complete picture of the patient's problem. Many test designs are directed only at one aspect of sensory function. It has become almost universal in thinking recently for examiners to seek a test that not only provides information as to neural status, but includes as well an indication of the patient's actual ability to function with his present or absent sensibility. Although such a test would be convenient, it may be impossible for only one test to supply this much information. In testing we are asking many questions. As with any investigation, to be assured of clear answers, we may need to break down our questions into their simplest components.

Take, for example, testing of the vision of the eye. In testing the eye, we surely want to known how the eye preceives its environment with whatever vision is present or absent. In our testing we might wish to include the ability to distinguish colors and the ability to visualize objects without perceptual distortion, as well as the visual acuity with which the eyes focus. We would not, however, attempt to test all of the above together by only one test. To do so would complicate our efforts to obtain clear and useful n-formation. We would test first for acuity and then for these other functions (Fig. 34-2).

In cutaneous sensibility testing there exists at least a two-fold objective: that of determining sensory acuity and that of determining the patient's function with his acuity. The first is the patient's potential to function; the second depends on the patient's actual ability to function. Most of our tests for peripheral nerve function can be said to fall in a spectrum between these two ends (Fig. 34-3).

In sensibility testing it may be very important to make a difference in the patient's potential and actual ability. An optimum test for peripheral nerve acuity might be independent of the patient's ability to retrain or compensate for his injury. If our question about a nerve after it was repaired is whether it has improved to an acceptable level or will require corrective intervention, we wish to known the specific status of the nerve repair, not if the patient has been able to compensate for the injury by clues and intelligence. Tests such as nerve-conduction velocity, pinprick, and Tinel's sign[30] would fall on the acuity end of the spectrum.

An optimum test for patient function might depend heavily on the patient's ability to compensate for his injury. The blind can be taught to see with their hands. The ''blind hand'' may also be taught to see through reeducation and compensation.[9,10,23] Tests for stereognosis, graphesthesia, ridge/edge perception,[27,28] and Moberg's timed object pickup[24] would fall on the adaptation-compensation end of the spectrum.

It is possible that there will be a test designed that will meet these two ends: both the patient's potential and his ability to function through adaptation and compensation. It is probable that more than one test will be needed to provide a clear picture.

Neurophysiology

Contrary to what might be conceived by a literature review, neurophysiologists are still trying to isolate the components of ''normal'' sensibility. Quite naturally, the neurophysiologist is interested in ''normal'' sensory function, and his test requirements are adjusted accordingly for normal thresholds.[21,25,26] The clinician is interested in abnormal thresholds, and his tests are focused accordingly. Measurements of both normal thresholds and abnormality contribute to the understanding of sensory neurophysiology. Collaboration of the neurophysiologist and the clinical examiner could prove productive. Such collaboration may in fact be required for resolution of problems inherent in clinical testing, and an accurate description of normal physiology versus abnormality. *If our understanding of neurophysiology is as yet incomplete and an objective test is as yet unknown, the clinician finds himself in the situation of trying to use an unknown test to define an unknown system.* Either an ob-

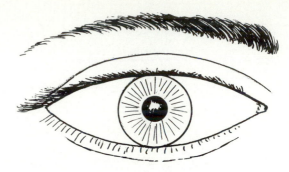

FIG. 34-2. In testing vision of eye, one tests first for visual acuity and then for astigmatism and color blindness. Attempts to measure these three functions together would complicate efforts toward obtaining clear and useful information.

jective test will have to be identified to shed light on the neurophysiology, or the neurophysiology will have to be identified to shed light on an objective test (Fig. 34-4).

Future objective tests

Because there can be no agreement on the optimum test or tests for sensibility until more is learned about the actual physical properties of the tests and the exact nature and function of cutaneous end organs, there is much to be said both about cooperative studies in general among testing clinics and for the idea of test batteries. There will be no one person who will find the solution to our problems in cutaneous sensibility testing. The answers will come from a composite of information from many investigators representing many disciplines. If ways could be found to compare information, it is believed that so doing could advance testing by several years.

LABORATORY FINDINGS VERSUS CLINICAL TESTING

In the cutaneous layers of the skin are found billions of end organs, which represent the receptive end of the human nervous system. Many advances have been made in laboratory measurements of end-organ function in controlled settings.[17,21,26,39] However, what is found to be true in test conditions in a laboratory cannot alwayͺ be applied directly to a clinical situation. As with trying to study the internal structure of the atom, were we able to introduce something into the atom with which to measure its physical characteristics, we would have created an artificial situation. Likewise, with end organs, once we have introduced something into an end organ with which to measure it, we have created an artificial situation.

Even when end-organ response can be isolated individually, the response of an end organ to a stimulus individually tells us very little about how that end organ works in concert with the others to produce what we know as cutaneous sensibility. For example, in some instances it is conceivable that some end organ or organs may have to be stimulated to a certain threshold before another can react. It is also conceivable that the response of quickly adapting end organs in some instances give to slowly adapting end organs or vice versa clues or signals that are not measurable by changes in electrical conduction as is commonly done in the lab.[12,14,20,21]

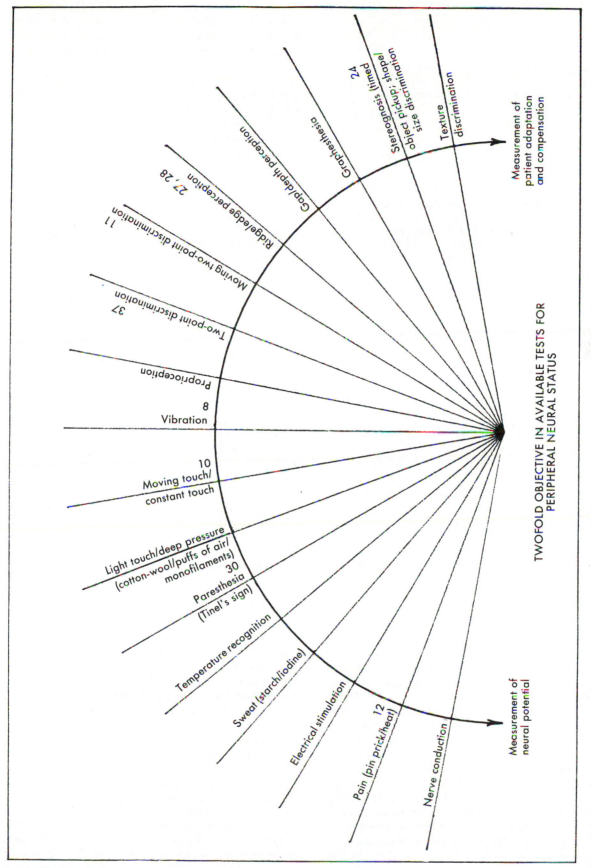

TWOFOLD OBJECTIVE IN AVAILABLE TESTS FOR PERIPHERAL NEURAL STATUS

FIG. 34-3. In testing for peripheral nerve status, there exists a twofold objective: determining a patient's neural potential and determining adaptation or compensation for neural diminution. Most tests of neural status can be said to fall in a range between these two ends.

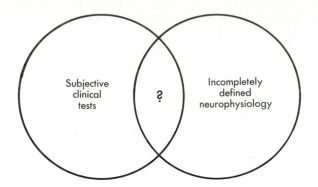

FIG. 34-4. If our understanding of neurophysiology is as yet incomplete and an objective test is as yet unknown, we are left with an unknown test trying to define an unknown system. Either an objective test will have to identified to shed light on neurophysiology, or the neurophysiology will have to be identified to shed light on an objective test.

Organ-specific tests

Attempts have been made by some examiners to divide clinical testing instruments into those that test the slowly adapting end organs and those that test the quickly adapting end organs. Although this at first appears to be a sophisticated approach to testing, it is believed that such efforts are premature at this time. In any given skin area 10 mm² there are close to 3000 end organs.[24] Any stimulation of the skin is quite likely to bombard these end organs with stimuli. It would be surprising if any stimulation of an area so densely populated with end organs (both slowly and rapidly adapting) (Fig. 34-5) could select out only quickly adapting fibers, or only slowly adapting fibers at the total exclusion of the others.

Although there are some end organs that can be shown in a laboratory situation to be rapidly adapting in response to a stimulus, and other end organs to be slowly adapting; there are still others that respond in between and are possibly moderators of the other two types. What would be their roll in response to a stimulus? And still further, how is all this interpreted at the central cortex level?

Even if our clinical instruments did not stimulate a broad area of end organs in comparison with isolation of a single end organ in the lab, there are other reasons to believe that our current instruments cannot yet be divided into specific organs for which they test. Our testing instruments provide signals to the end organs in the form of energy produced when the instrument is applied to the skin. This energy can be measured as to its frequency content on a spectrum ranging from low to high frequency. We are more familiar with the frequency spectrum of audible sound waves and of visual light waves. The sound waves in particular are a good analogy because they not only range from low to high frequency, but also stimulate delicate end organs in the ear at specific frequencies to provide one with the sense of hearing. Measurements of cutaneous end organs in the lab have shown slowly adapting fibers to be responsive to low-frequency signals, and rapidly adapting fibers to be responsive to high-frequency signals. *This does not mean, of course, that they*

do not respond to other frequencies! It might seem plausible to test differentially the slowly adapting end organs against the rapidly adapting end organs if our testing instruments provide a pure low-frequency or high-frequency signal. However, this is not the case. In a test analysis of the signal produced by the application of test instruments to a strain gauge, currently available clinical test instruments were found to produce signals throughout a broad frequency spectrum.[7] Although providing strong signals at their reported measured frequency, they also produce signals at both low and high frequencies, which would, in fact, stimulate both slowly and rapidly adapting end organs.[4]

Much has been made of the roll of the response of end organs to different frequencies in the lab. Such analysis may eventually decode the response of the end organs to stimuli. But even in the lab, the end organs have been measured mostly in a frequency range from 0 to 300 Hz because of instrumentation limited in the measurement of stimuli at these frequencies. It is possible that end organs are even more sensitive at higher frequencies. Just because the stimulus signal on instrumentation can be measured only for a certain portion of an energy spectrum, it does not mean that other portions of the spectrum do not exist or that end organs are not more sensitive at frequencies higher than 300 Hz. Thus information that has been gathered about end organs in the lab is reflective of only part of the spectrum. Newer instrumentation is being designed to measure end-organ function in greater detail at higher frequencies.

Neurophysiology incompletely defined

One of the most interesting studies of end-organ function up to now is a study by Arrington on the sensation of the cornea of the eye.[1] To the cornea of the eye can be attributed the sensations of pain, touch and pressure, heat, and cold. Yet the cornea of the eye is reported to contain mostly unmyelinated c fibers, which are believed to be pain receptors. If an area populated mostly by c fibers can respond to all these stimuli, what then is the roll of the other receptors? A touch-pressure test of the sensibility of the eye patterned after the touch-pressure testing of von Frey has been developed.

Both von Frey and Weber attempted, as later Head did, to establish a direct relationship between a specific sensory perception and a specific cutaneous end organ.[5] After exhaustive attempts to do so, they began to believe that there was little evidence for organ-specific function and that the receptors must work in some concert with each other to provide what we identify as distinct sensory perceptions.

Von Frey established the doctrine of four energies in the form of pressure, warmth, cold, and pain. The other senses he believed to be perceptual interactions of pressure and sensations of pain. Von Frey succeeded in demonstrating that there are end organs and that these end organs play a definite but specifically undetermined roll in the recognition of pressure, warmth, cold, and pain.

Weber[36,37] described his two-point discrimination test in his paper "De Tactu," in 1834. He intended in his test to show only that a touch on the skin can be distinguished as to the pressure, temperature, and position. Weber was reportedly at great pains not to separate these function but to

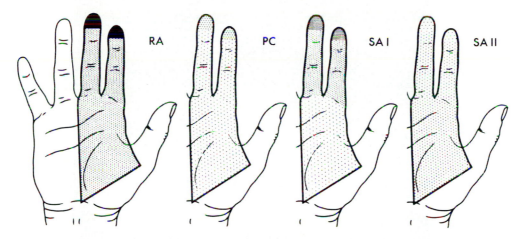

FIG. 34-5. Estimated absolute densities of four types of tactile sensory units in glabrous skin. Each dot represents a single sensory unit innervating skin area. It should be emphasized that this figure illustrates only average unit density within region whereas dot size and exact location of individual dot in relation to neighbours has no relevance with regard to receptive field size and spatial distribution of fields. (From Vallbo, A.B., and Johansen, R.S.: The tactile sensory innervation of the glabrous skin of the human hand. In Gordon, G., editor: Active touch, Oxford, 1978, Pergamon Press Ltd.)

show that they do go together and are interdependent.

Consider Weber's example of a recumbent man who has two coins placed on his forehead, for example, a nickel and a quarter. If the nickel and the quarter were of the same temperature, the quarter would be perceived as heavier in weight. If the nickel were cold, however, and the quarter warm, the nickel would be perceived as the same weight or even heavier than the quarter. Weber concluded that if temperature affects perceived pressure the cutaneous "senses" cannot be separate.

In the years since these early studies, many investigators have continued attempts to identify specific functions of the end organs and to assign them a name. The end organs have been identified as to their size, shape, location, depth from the skin surface, myelination or lack of it, and response in the laboratory to a specific controlled stimulus, but they have not been identified as to their specific function. They have been classified as encapsulated, expanded, and free; as nociceptors (pain), thermoreceptors (heat), and mechanoreceptors (mechanical deformation); and most recently as quickly adapting fibers, slowly adapting fibers type I and type II, and pacinian corpuscles.[31] That the receptors can be measured in some way in response to a given stimulus and can be given a name is somewhat misleading. Even with the best of studies, much of what is believed to be the function of the end organs is theoretical at this time and is subject to change with new information, as it has been in the past. The pacinian corpuscle, a rapid adapter, has been the most studied because it is more easily tested and is the largest in size. Much of what has been found in its response in testing has sometimes been assumed to apply to other tactile receptors. Such assumption may be incorrect, or may be only partially correct.

TWO-POINT DISCRIMINATION TEST: A CLOSER LOOK

The Weber two-point discrimination test[36] was in most common use when I first began testing patients in 1969. This test undoubtably supplies useful information to examiners of sensibility. However, it is believed significant that many authors became interested in other sensibility tests solely because the two-point discrimination test did not supply answers to many of the problems of patients presenting themselves for evaluation. I sadly watched as many patients were told they had normal "feeling" by earnest physicians who believed two-point discrimination testing to make a definitive diagnosis. History and an examination of probing the affected area belied a normal tactile cutaneous sensibility in these patients who would often repeatedly return for evaluation because their problems had not been resolved. It was found that blindfolding these patients and having them identify an area that changed in feeling as a probe was drawn across their hand would result in a repeatable mapping (the examiner would have to recognize a delay in response in an affected area in order to obtain a clear line between areas easily felt by the probe and areas of diminution). When this type of testing was repeated on successive visits of the patient and the test results proved identical to those previously mapped, it was deemed that these patients must have discernible areas of diminution or loss of sensibility that were not measured by two-point discrimination testing.

This was found again in later tests with other patients in cases with nerve compressions.[2] Werner and Omer[40] noted in a review of 4000 tests with the filaments that the presence of light touch does not necessarily indicate that two-point discrimination is present. Specific examples cited were in

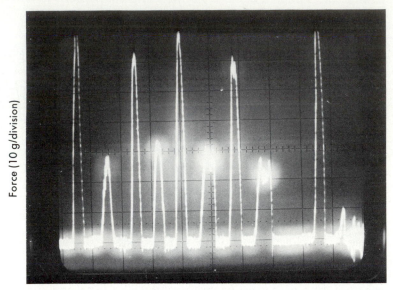

Force (10 g/division)

Time (1 sec/division)

FIG. 34-6. Oscilliscope screen showing application force of one and two points of a hand-held paper clip. Variation in force is over 30 gm.

such conditions as radiculitis, causalgia, and entrapment syndromes. It has recently been reported that patients with experimentally induced nerve compressions have been shown to have a normal two-point discrimination test when there was a considerable decrease in nerve-conduction sensory fiber amplitude.[16,22] In one subject two-point discrimination was still normal at a point when sensory fiber amplitude approached zero. In rephrasing of the discussion of testing with any one test, I wonder how one would have discovered that some patients with a nerve compression may have a normal two-point discrimination examination if only the two-point discrimination test had been used as a measure? Patients with nerve lacerations may also have injuries with nerve-compression components attributable to post-injury swelling. How can we determine to what extent patients with nerve lacerations and other injuries have nerve compression as opposed to swelling internal or external to the nerve that may render the two-point discrimination test less accurate? The common use of the two-point discrimination test as a primary measure in the past has most likely delayed recognition of exceptions in testing. The same may be true of other tests. There is no way of knowing until objective testing is available, and the tests can be directly compared.

In the past the two-point discrimination test has frequently been assumed to be objective because it can be reported on in numerical terms. In clinical practice, there is considerable variation in the force and velocity of application among clinicians, a situation that renders the test subjective (Fig. 34-6). For instance, it would be expected to be easier for a patient to distinguish the difference between one and two points applied at 37 gm of force than to distinguish between one and two points applied at only 19 gm of force (Table 34-1). The reproducibility of a consistent application force

by an examiner applying two points to the same spot on the same patient has been found to vary widely, even when blanching of the skin is used as a control.[4] In the same study it was found that blanching of the fingers occurs at different forces on separate fingers; thus this difference brought into question the common use of blanching as a valid control of application force.

The lack of control on application force is even more pronounced when the stimulus is moved, such as in the recently popularized test of moving two-point discrimination.[11] Here the force applied by the examiner is made to vary even greater by the "hills" and "valleys" of the skin topography as the examiner draws the testing instrument against the finger. This does not, of course, mean that the two-point discrimination tests are meaningless, but only that the effect of variations in application force on the accuracy of the tests needs to be further studied. Otherwise, how can the examiner determine if a patient is responding to a difference in recognition of one or two points, or of a heavier and lighter application force?

The problems with control of application force and velocity are not limited to the two-point discrimination tests, but apply to any of our tests that are hand applied. Only the monofilament design of testing[18,29,35] attempts to control the force of application. This test is not without its problems, which are discussed in Chapter 35,[29,38] but it does approach an objective test of cutaneous sensibility.

It is possible that the two-point discrimination tests and the monofilaments and other frequently utilized tests of cutaneous sensibility as well could be made objective by instrument design that would control the force of application and the velocity of application. The force and velocity of application are foremost in the minds of neurophysiologists and others who are developing controlled laboratory testing

TABLE 34-1. Stimulus force of a paper clip applied to blanching*

Tester	Two points in contact		One point in contact	
	Mean (gm)	Standard deviation (gm)	Mean (gm)	Standard deviation (gm)
1	**19.16**	7.27	**13.49**	2.83
2	28.32	5.55	16.08	3.95
3	20.53	5.87	14.83	4.79
4	19.39	6.01	17.01	4.81
5	32.15	8.61	17.24	4.04
6	**36.49**	4.94	**17.09**	5.47
Overall	26.01	6.38	17.09	4.32

*Six testers, 20 applications each, alternating between two points in contact and one point in contact.

of end-organ function. A few prototype instruments are available, some expensive and complicated, and others not quite so complicated. When these instruments are available to the clinician, it may then be possible for direct comparison of our clinical tests.

SUMMARY

Cutaneous tactile sensation is no simple perception. It may be that in the end there will be some simple tests to measure it, but one must always appreciate the intricacies and sensitivity of the system. There will be no one person who will find the solution to our problems in sensory testing. The answers will come from a composite of information obtained by many investigators over time. It is important for the examiner to realize that although much useful information can be derived from current clinical tests and instruments, there are no "cookbooks." He or she must keep a critical eye toward factors that render tests subjective and carefully integrate test results with the needs and problems of the patient.

REFERENCES

1. Arrington, J.: Corneal sensation measurement, Presented at the fourteenth annual meeting of the United States Public Health Service Professional Association, Phoenix, Ariz., April 1977.
2. Bell, J.A.: Sensibility evaluation: In Hunter, J., Schneider, L., Mackin, E., and Bell, J., editors: Rehabilitation of the hand, St. Louis, 1978, The C.V. Mosby Co.
3. Bell, J.A., and Buford, W.L., Jr.: Assessment of levels of cutaneous sensibility, Presented at the sixteenth annual meeting of the United States Public Health Professional Association, Houston, Tex., 1979.
4. Bell, J.A., and Buford, W.L., Jr.: The force time relationship of clinically used sensory testing instruments, Presented at the thirty-seventh annual meeting of the American Society for Surgery of the Hand, Aurora, Colo., 1982.
5. Boring, E.G.: Sensation and perception in the history of experimental psychology, New York, 1942, Appleton-Century-Crofts.
6. Brand, P.W.: Symposium, Assessment of cutaneous sensibility, Comments of chairman, National Hansen's Disease Center, Carville, La., 1980.
7. Buford, W.L., and Bell, J.A.: Dynamic properties of hand held tactile assessment stimuli, Proceedings of the thirty-fourth annual conference of Engineering in Medicine and Biology, 23:307, 1981.
8. Caine, D.B., and Pallis, C.A.: Vibratory sense: a critical review, Brain 89:723, 1966.
9. Curtis, R.M.: Sensory reeducation after peripheral nerve injury. In Fredricks, S. and Brody, G.S., editors: Symposium on the neurologic aspects of plastic surgery, St. Louis, 1978, The C.V. Mosby Co., vol. 17.
10. Dellon, A.L., Curtis, R.M., and Edgerton, M.T.: Reeducation of sensation of the hand after nerve injury and repair, Plast. Reconst. Surg. 53:297, 1974.
11. Dellon, A.L.: The moving two-point discrimination test: clinical evaluation of the quickly adapting fiber/receptor system, J. Hand Surg. 3(5):474, 1978.
12. Demichelis, F., Giaretti, W.A., Barberis, M.L., and Teich-Alesia, S.: Biomedical instrumentation for the measurements of skin sensitivity, Trans. Biomed. Eng. BMR-26(6):326-330, June 1979.
13. Dyck, P.J.: Quantitation of cutaneous sensations in man, In Dyck, P.J., and Thomas, P.K., editors: Peripheral neuropathy, Philadelphia, 1975, W.B. Saunders Co.
14. Dyck, P.J., O'Brien, P.C., Bushek, W., and others: Clinical vs quantitative evaluation of cutaneous sensation, Arch. Neurol. 33(9):651-656, 1976.
15. Dyck, P.J.: Symposium, Assessment of cutaneous sensibility, National Hansen's Disease Center, Carville, La., 1980.
16. Gelberman, R.H., Szabo, R.M., Williamson, R.V., and Dimick, M.P.: Sensibility testing in peripheral nerve compression syndromes: a human experiment study, San Diego, 1982. (Unpublished paper.)
17. Gray, J.A.B., and Malcom, J.L.: The initiation of nerve impulses by mesenteric pacinian corpuscles, Proc. R. Soc. Lond. (Biol.) 137:96, 1950.
18. Jamison, D.G.: Sensitivity testing as a means of differentiating the various forms of leprosy found in Nigeria, Int. J. Lepr. 39(2):504-507, 1972.
19. LaMotte, R.H.: Symposium, assessment of cutaneous sensibility, sensory discrimination and neural correlation, National Hansen's Disease Center, Carville, La., 1980.
20. LaMotte, R.H., and Mountcastle, V.B.: Capacities of humans and monkeys to discriminate between vibratory stimuli of different frequency and amplitude: a correlation between neural events and psychophysical measurements, J. Neurophysiol. 38:539-559, 1979.
21. Looft, F.J., and Williams, W.J.: One-line receptive field mapping of cutaneous receptors, Trans. Biomed. Eng. BME-26(6):350-356, June 1979.
22. Lundborg, G., Gelberman, R.H., Minteer-Convery, M., Lee, Y.F., Hargens, A.R.: Median nerve compression in the carpal tunnel: functional response to experimentally induced controlled pressure, J. Hand Surg. 7(3):252-259, May 1982.
23. Millesi, H., and Renderer, D.: A method of training and testing sensibility of the fingertips, from the Department of Plastic and Reconstructive Surgery, Surgical University Clinic of Vienna and Ludwig-Boltzmann Institute for Experimental Plastic Surgery, Vienna, Austria, 1978.
24. Moberg, E.: Objective methods of determining the functional value of sensibility of the hand, J. Bone Joint Surg. 40B:454-476, 1958.
25. Mountcastle, V.B.: Medical physiology, ed. 12, St. Louis, 1968, The C.V. Mosby Co., vol. 2, pp. 1345-1371.
26. Paul, R.L., Merzesich, M., and Goodman, H.: Representations of slowly and rapidly adpating mechanoreceptors of the hand in Broadmann's areas 3 and 1 of *Macaca mulatta*, Brain Res. 36:229, 1972.

27. Poppen, N.K.: Sensibility evaluation following peripheral nerve suture: critical assessment of the von Frey, two-point discrimination, and ridge tests. In Jewett, D.L., and McCarroll, H.K., Jr., editors: Symposium on nerve repair: its clinical and experimental basis, St. Louis, 1979, The C.V. Mosby Co.
28. Renfrew, S.: Fingertip sensation: a routine neurological test, Lancet, **1:**396-397, Feb. 22, 1969.
29. Semmes, J., Weinstein, S., Ghent, L., and Teuber, H.-L.: Somatosensory changes after penetrating brain wounds in man, Cambridge, Mass., 1960, Harvard University Press.
30. Tinel, J.: The "tingling" sign in peripheral nerve lesions (Translated by B. Kaplan), Presse Med. **47:**388-389, 1915.
31. Vallbo, A.B., and Johansson, R.S.: The tactile sensory innervation of the glabrous skin of the human hand: In Gordon, G., editor: Active touch, Oxford, Eng. 1978, Pergamon Press Ltd.
32. von Frey, M.: Berichte der Sachlichen Gesellschaft der Wissenschaften, Leipzig, **46:**185-283, 1894.
33. von Frey, M.: Gibt es tiefe Druckempfindungen (?) Dtsch. Med. Wochenschr. **51:**113-124, 1925.
34. von Frey, M.: Physiologie des Sinnesorgane der menschlichen Haut, Ergebn. Physiol. **9:**351-368, 1910.
35. von Frey, M.: Zur Physiologie der Juckempfindung, Arch. Neurol. Physiol. **7:**142-145, 1922.
36. Weber, E.H.: Data cited by Sherrington, C.S., in Shafer's Textbook of physiology, Edinburgh, 1900, Young, J. Pentland.
37. Weber, E.H.: Ueber den Tastsinn, Müller Archiv, pp. 152-159, 1935.
38. Weinstein, S.: Tactile sensitivity of the phalanges, Percept. Motor Skills **14:**351-354, 1962.
39. Werner, G., and Mountcastle, V.B.: Neural activity in mechanoreceptive cutaneous afferents: stimulus-response relations, Weber functions and information transmission, J. Neurophysiol. **28:**359, 1965.
40. Werner, J.L., and Omer, G.E.: Evaluating cutaneous pressure sensation of the hand, Am. J. Occup. Ther. **24:**5, 1970.

BIBLIOGRAPHY

Chochinov, R.H., Ullyot, L.E., and Moorehouse, J.A.: Sensory perception thresholds in patients' juvenile diabetes and their close relatives, N. Engl. J. Med. **286**(23):1233, 1969.
Conomy, J.P., Barnes, K.L., and Cruse, R.P.: Quantitative cutaneous sensory testing in children and adolescents: Cleve. Clin. Q. **45**(2):197-206, 1978.
Gelberman, R., Urbaniak, J., Bright, D., and Levin, L.: Digital sensibility following replantation, J. Hand Surg. **3:**313-319, 1978.
Jabaley, M.E.: Recovery of sensation following peripheral nerve repair. In Fredricks, S., and Brody, G.S., editors: Symposium on the neurologic aspects of plastic surgery, St. Louis, 1978, The C.V. Mosby Co., vol. 17.
Jabaley, M.E., and Bryant, M.W.: The effect of denervation and reinnervation of encapsulated receptors in digital skin. In Marchac, C., and Hueston, J.T., editors: Transactions of the Sixth International Congress of Plastic and Reconstructive Surgery, Paris, 1976, Masson, pp. 103-106.
Moberg, E.: Criticism and study of methods for examining sensibility of the hand, Neurology **12:**8-9, 1962.
Naafs, B., and Dagne, T.: Sensory testing: a sensitive method in the follow-up of nerve involvement, Int. J. Lepr. **45**(4):364-368, 1978.
Omer, G.E., Jr.: Evaluation and reconstruction of the forearm and hand after acute traumatic peripheral nerve injuries. In American Academy of Orthopaedic Surgeons: Instructional course lectures **18:**1454-1478, St. Louis, 1973, The C.V. Mosby Co.
Omer, G.E., and Spinner, M.: Management of peripheral nerve problems, Philadelphia, 1980, W.B. Saunders Co.
Terzis, J.: Metabolism of peripheral nerve injuries. In Fredricks, S., and Brody, G.S., editors: Symposium on the neurologic aspects of plastic surgery, St. Louis, 1978, The C.V. Mosby Co., vol. 17.

35

Light touch–deep pressure testing using Semmes-Weinstein monofilaments

JUDITH A. BELL

ADVANTAGES OF MONOFILAMENT TESTING

Light touch–deep pressure testing with monofilaments of increasing forces has been described as one of the most objective tests for measuring cutaneous sensibility.[2-4,7,13] The filaments bend when the peak-force threshold has been achieved. A relatively consistent force is continued by the filaments until they are either removed from the skin contact or are severely curved. When they are severely curved, the force on the skin is less than the desired threshold. In addition to controlling the force of application, the filament design attempts to control the velocity of application. If applied too quickly, the filament force will exceed the desired threshold. Otherwise, the bending of the filament minimizes the vibration of the examiner's hand.

The currently available testing instrument is the Semmes-Weinstein[7] Aesthesiometer monofilament testing set. (Fig. 35-1). This testing set contains 20 filaments. Smaller sets containing fewer filaments are available on request from the manufacturer. Although not a perfect testing instrument because of variations in the tip geometry of the filaments, the Semmes-Weinstein monofilament set produces results that are repeatable within a certain force range, usually in milligrams. The instrument set succeeds in demonstrating gradients of sensibility diminution.

Color coding of the filament force produces a mapping that provides the examiner with differential thresholds of touch in areas of normal or relatively normal sensibility and areas of diminution (Fig. 35-2). If the application technique is consistent, the mappings produced can be serially compared for changes in neural status (Fig. 35-3). The mappings can be predictors of the rate of neural return or diminution. They can be predictors as well of the quality of neural return, or severity of diminution (Fig. 35-4). Attempts to correlate increasing or decreasing touch thresholds with levels of patient function at this time appear promising, and correlation is perhaps superior to that associated with many other forms of testing.

The filament testing is not recommended as an ''only'' test at this time, for reasons explained in Chapter 34. Used in combination with other clinical tests of sensory function, particularly a test of sensory nerve conduction, the test can lead to the resolution of patient problems that are not resolved by other forms of testing and can clarify other test results. The filaments are often used by neurophysiologists in studies to determine end-organ response. Like the other tests of sensibility, they could be made more objective through careful consideration of their physical properties.

HISTORY OF THE INSTRUMENT

Although von Frey[8] was the inventor of the monofilaments, the currently available testing sets are not identical to the test instrument he described. Von Frey was at pains to put a consistent tip on the ends of each of his filaments. The consistent tip allows that portion of the tip of the filament coming into contact with the skin while the filament is bent, to be held constant in size, and only the force to vary from one filament to another. This simplifies and makes more accurate calculations of pressures produced when the filaments are applied to the skin. A consistent tip in addition makes the effect of increasing diameters of the filaments inconsequential.

The current testing instrument was developed by Semmes and Weinstein and is described in their book *Somatosensory Changes After Penetrating Brain Wounds in Man.*[7] Semmes and Weinstein desired a measure that would be applicable over a wider range of intensities than von Frey's and one that would provide an interval scale. The investigators attempted to show with their filaments, which increase in diameter to exert increased forces, that the common logarithm of the force increases in an approximately linear fashion with the ordinal rank of the filaments. The intervals between filaments are not equal. This unequal increment in the forces has presented problems in testing scales that have been adjusted for believed differences in sensitivities of the thumb, fingers, and palm. A close examination of the interpretation scales in common use reveals that the filaments have been adjusted by a change to the next heaviest filament. The next heaviest filament in some instances represents an increment of 18.5 mg and in other instances an increment of 165.5 gm of force (Table 35-1). Thus, such adjustments in the scale are rendered disproportionate and confusing.

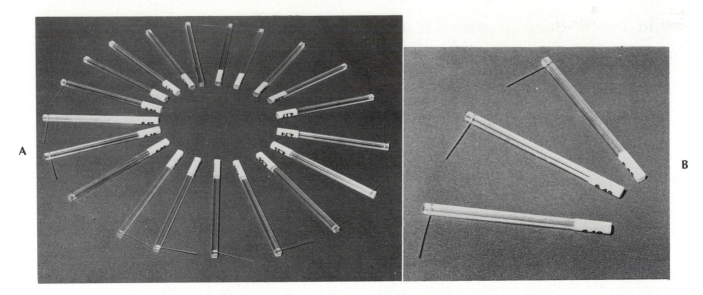

FIG. 35-1. **A,** Semmes-Weinstein Anesthesiometer monofilament testing set. **B,** Close-up view of filaments.

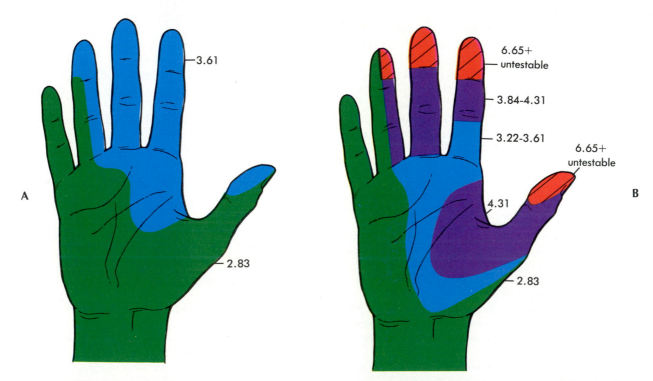

FIG. 35-2. **A,** Monofilament mapping showing a median nerve compression as measured in woman with history of numbness for 2 years and no corrective intervention. **B,** Same patient as measured 4 months later. Touch pressure recognition has become downgraded from diminished light touch to untestable with monofilaments.

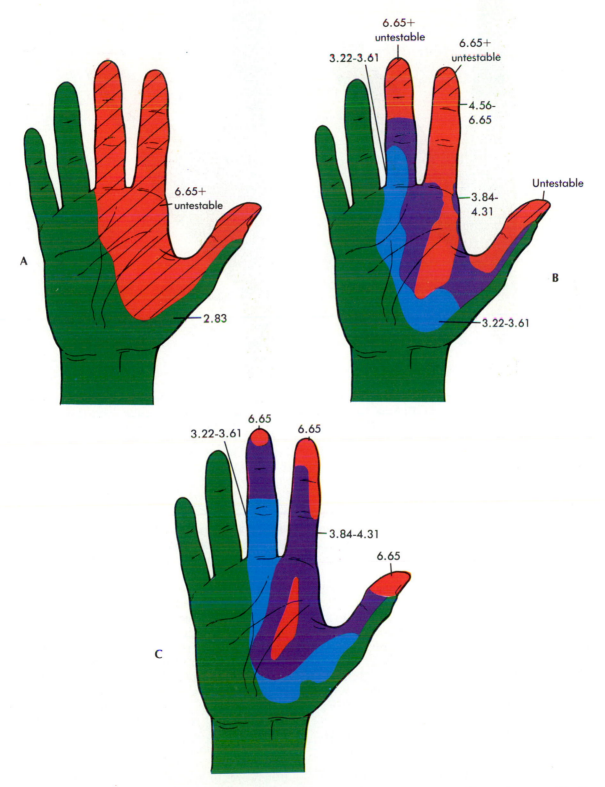

FIG. 35-3. A, Monofilament mapping showing a median nerve laceration before surgery. Two-point untestable. **B,** Same patient 3 months after surgery. Two-point untestable. **C,** Same patient 7 months after surgery. Two-point untestable. Fingertips now testable with monofilaments.

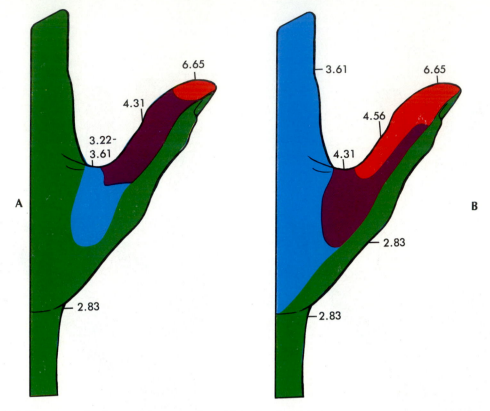

Fig. 35-4. A, Two years after incomplete amputation of right thumb. Digital nerves were not resutured. Small centimeter pedicle of dorsal skin was intact. **B,** Same patient after injection of lidocaine around median nerve to determine if innervation was radial nerve or median. Notice that although the volar thumb sensation was downgraded, it and the palmar area of the median nerve did not become asensory. This finding brings into question the blocking of the contralateral nerve in testing. Such blocks may be incomplete and lead to false conclusions.

Semmes and Weinstein,[7,12] using the currently available monofilaments, established a threshold below which stimuli are never (or rarely) perceived and above which they are always (or nearly always) perceived. In their studies of 20 normal subjects each with two hands, they found the left hand only slightly more sensitive than the right, with only the left thumb reaching a significant level of difference. The left hand exhibited a more pronounced gradient of sensitivity between parts (thumb and palm) than the right hand, in which there was *no* significant difference in parts (thumb and palm). Thus, even if the monofilaments were ordered with equal force increments between filaments, there are few clear lines if any in threshold differences between fingers, thumbs, and palms for adjustments in the testing scales. Testing scales then cannot be arbitrarily altered for fingers, thumb, and palm areas, as examiners frequently do, without invalidation of data from areas altered. Such adjustment in a testing scale produces an unrealistic mapping.

I recommend that the examiner use one consistent scale and allow for slight diminutions in sensibility in areas of the skin believed to be slightly less sensitive in touch pressure thresholds. An example would as with testing of the plantar surface of the foot. One would not be concerned if this surface reflects a diminished light touch, because one knows the keratin layer of the plantar cutaneous skin to be relatively thick. One would, however, be quite concerned if the plantar surface reflected a diminished protective sensation. It is emphasized that variations in cutaneous sensitivity thresholds, if any, can be measured in milligrams. The force range of the monofilaments is from 4.5 mg to 447 gm.

Although the early investigators utilizing the filaments did succeed in standardizing the filaments with normal subjects, and referenced the filaments of increasing or decreasing forces to "normal" thresholds as has been stated, the filaments were not standardized to functional levels of diminution in the manner they are most typically utilized today. Their greatest value at present is their sensitivity, which allows testing of normal thresholds of sensibility. Once an area of normal sensibility has been established, the other filaments of increasing forces can be referenced to this area of normal sensibility to establish a light touch–deep pressure differential in sensory areas, as between the ulnar and median nerves or between the median nerves of the right and left hands.

The credit for equating increasing levels of forces required by the monofilaments to levels of diminution in sensory function goes to Kilulu von Prince.[9,10] Von Prince began grouping the filaments into levels that could be equated with expected levels of function on the part of the patient. Von

TABLE 35-1. Rod markings versus calculated force in gram increments from filament to filament

Rod markings (Log 10 force, 0.1 mg)	Calculated force (gm)*		
	Force between filaments	Force between filaments	
Loss of protective sensation			
6.65		447.0	
6.45	165.5 {	281.5	
6.10		127.0	154.5
5.88	52 {	75.00	
5.46		29.00	46
5.18	14 {	15.00	
5.07		11.70	3.3
4.94	3.05 {	8.650	
4.74		5.500	3.15
4.56	1.868 {	3.632	
Diminished protective sensation			1.57
4.31		2.052	
4.17	0.568 {	1.494	
4.08		1.194	0.3746
3.84	0.4972 {	0.6958	
Diminished light touch			0.2886
3.61		0.4082	
3.22	0.2422 {	0.1660	
Normal			0.0983
2.83		0.0677	
2.44	0.0402 {	0.0275	
2.36		0.0230	0.0045
1.65	0.0185 {	0.0045	

*Scale is linear but not at regular increments.

Prince was greatly influenced by the work of Napier[6] and of Moberg.[5] Concurrently with studies being done by Semmes in sensory losses arising from central origin, von Prince began to investigate the residual function of patients who had received a multiple variety of peripheral nerve injuries from war wounds. Von Prince realized that although some patients would have injuries similar to those of other patients, there was a considerable difference in the level of function of the patients. For example, of two patients who could not tell a difference in testing between one and two points, one could feel a match that would burn his finger and the other could not. Thus she perceived that there must be a protective level of sensation that was not measured by the other test. Of two patients who would have a response to a pinprick, one would have the ability to discriminate textures and one would not. Thus she perceived that there must be a light touch level of sensation that would be equated with the patient's ability to discriminate textures.

Von Prince may have been one of the earliest hand therapists. She was considered rather radical in ideas at the time she developed her concepts of sensory testing. She broke with what was then tradition for therapists in the armed services to develop a common base of training. Considering the development of testing to measure the level of function of peripheral nerve injuries so important, she requested 6 months in which to investigate this area and develop testing scales.

In her early scales, von Prince attempted to equate levels of diminished sensory function with levels of two-point discimination testing. This was a logical assumption, since the Weber[11] two-point discrimination test was frequently used in practice. This would be changed in later scales when it would be found that although there appears to be a relationship between diminishing levels of two-point discrimination and increasing levels of force required by the monofilaments, the two tests cannot be directly equated.

Omer in particular realized the value of von Prince's work and was instrumental in assuring that her work would continue by other investigators when von Prince was sent to other assignments. He published a paper with Werner in 1970[13] that would add to the "classic" publications in sensibility testing. The testing scale of von Prince was changed in the article by Werner and Omer to omit two-point discrimination as a consideration in the filament testing and treat it as a separate test.

The scales of von Prince and of Werner and Omer have been frequently utilized and additional variations developed for sensory testing in the ensuing years. In 1976, the Bicentennial year, so many scales were available with limited history as to their origin that one utilizing the filaments was unsure of their accuracy and unable to justify this form of testing as a sensitive monitor of peripheral nerve function for presurgical and postsurgical hand cases. An attempt was launched to identify the scale most commonly used for testing.

After much comparison it was discovered that the scale chosen for interpretation of the filaments (Table 35-2) (since other scales were eliminated through clinical use) was identical to that of the "area-localization" scale described by Werner and Omer. If their level of diminished light touch is further divided and the full range of filaments included, this comparison can be seen.[1,13] (Werner and Omer chose to leave out a few filaments.) The chances that two independent investigators would settle upon the same interpretation scale for clinical use are quite small unless there are indeed differences in the patient's level of sensory function—that is, light touch and protective sensation—that are measurable at specific forces in a spectrum from light touch to deep pressure.

James M. Hunter, at the Hand Rehabilitation Center in Philadelphia, realized the value of the filament mapping in producing information on the patient's neural status that was not forthcoming from other sensory examinations. He has encouraged this form of testing with his surgical patients, many of whom came to him with long-standing unresolved peripheral nerve problems.

The filaments have recently been used to map sensibility diminutions and losses of patients with Hansen's disease. These patients can have diminution or loss of feeling in one of three ways—through end organ invasion by bacilli, through nerve trunk invasion by bacilli, or through nerve compression secondary to swelling. The involvement of peripheral nerves can mimic a peripheral nerve lesion or compression from other causes. Much can be learned of neural function in these patients, and they are a challenge to any of our present tests. The filaments are being used as a sensitive monitor of early changes in sensory status in these patients, who can have reversal or improvement of their neural damage through timely use of steroids and other medications.

PRESENT TECHNIQUE

Testing with the monofilaments begins with filaments in the normal threshold level and progresses to filaments of increasing pressure until touch is identified by the patient (Table 35-2). The filaments 1.65 to 4.08 are applied three times to the same spot. This was found necessary in measurements of the filament forces. One touch may not reach the required threshold of these light filaments. All the filaments are applied in a perpendicular fashion in 1 to 1.5 seconds, continued in pressure in 1 to 1.5 seconds, and lifted in 1 to 1.5 seconds. The filaments 1.65 to 6.45 should bend to exert the specific pressure. Filaments 4.17 to 6.65 are applied only one time. All sensibility testing is performed with careful attention to the normal distribution of the sensory nerves and common variations. A detailed history is taken from the patient and charted as an aid in close examination of the nerve distribution of suspected involvement and the screening of other areas. Unless a higher lesion is suspected from the history, it is often necessary to examine only the hands with the filaments, though *it is possible to test the entire extremity with the filaments.* As nerve return progresses proximally to distally, except for cases such as syringomyelia and localized partial lesions, the fingertip in the median and ulnar nerve distributions will be the first area to lose sensibility and the last area for return of sensibility.

It is considered more accurate for the same examiners to repeat successive evaluation, but because this is not always possible, the testing can be repeated by other examiners using the same technique. Testing by other examiners is possible when a double-blind situation is desired for studies.

What is mandatory is a quiet testing area; unfortunately this makes the use of the filaments questionable in an open clinic. It is sometimes very difficult for the patient to attend the filaments in a diminished sensory area. As one patient described the problem, it is like asking him to read a technical journal when he does not recognize all the words. Any sound is distracting, and sounds such as people walking by or typing can make it impossible for some patients to feel filaments they may feel in a quiet area. To assure an accurate examination it is most critical for the examiner to be quite certain the patient can and is attending the filaments.

The testing technique described is in contrast to that of

TABLE 35-2. Scale of interpretation of monofilaments

		Filament markings	Calculated force (gm)*
Green	Normal	1.65-2.83	0.0045-0.068
Blue	Diminished light touch	3.22-3.61	0.166-0.408
Purple	Diminished protective sensation	3.84-4.31	0.697-2.06
Red	Loss of protective sensation	4.56-6.65	3.63-447
Red-lined	Untestable	Greater than 6.65	Greater than 447

*Data from Semmes, J., and Weinstein, S.: Somatosensory changes after penetrating brain wounds in man, Cambridge, Mass., 1980, Harvard University Press.

other authors who have required area and point localization when testing with the monofilaments. In area localization, after being touched, the patient responds by indicating the *area* that was touched. In point localization, the patient responds by covering the *point* touched with a wooden dowel within a centimeter. Testing the latter method is more time consuming and is sometimes confusing to patients who have referred touch. It is believed that point localization may reflect the cognitive ability of a patient to adapt to new sensory pathways more than the actual level of return of the nerve and its response to touch. If what we are actually attempting to test is threshold of touch, it is believed that it can be more simply and aptly measured by having the patient respond to stimulation by the monofilament by saying the word "touch." An argument to this effect is that under nerve retraining we can effect an improvement in a patient's point localization and discrimination of sensory input, but few examiners would believe we are actually effecting a change in the physiologic status of the nerve. Point localization is tested in the sensory evaluation but is treated as a tactile discrimination requiring cortical participation. It can be quickly tested, and a note made of the direction and distance in centimeters into another point, area, or finger where the touch is referred.

Consistent colors from cool to warm are used to correspond with the diminishing sensibility levels. These allow a quickly read, consistent, easily comparable mapping of sensibility.

Procedure

1. Draw a probe (a Boley gauge) across the area to be tested in a radial-to-ulnar and proximal-to-distal manner. Ask the patient to describe where and if his feeling changes. *Do not ask for numbness, because the patient's interpretation of numbness varies.*

Dot the area described as "different" with an ink pen. The examination is easier if the patient can identify the gross area of involvement as a reference; if he cannot, proceed the same way on testing but allow more testing time.

2. Establish an area of *normal sensibility* as a reference. Familiarize the patient with the filament to be used, and demonstrate it in the proximal area believed to be normal. Then, with the patient's eyes occluded, demonstrate the filament until the patient can easily identify the filament on the low side of normal (2.83). (The filaments lighter than 2.83 are not necessary unless the examiner is attempting to obtain a differential in a normal range of touch.)

If possible, test the volar surface of the uninvolved hand first, applying the monofilaments to the fingertips and proceeding proximally. If testing is within normal limits, proceed to the dorsum of the hand and then to the involved hand.

Test the involved hand (volar surface) by applying the same filament (2.83) to the fingertips first and working proximally. Dot the spots correctly identified with a *green* felt-tip pen. (Explain to the patient that the second touch he feels is a marking of the pen.) In general, the patient is tested distally to proximally, but a consistent pattern is not used to avoid patient anticipation of the area to be touched. When all the area on the volar surface of the hand that can

be identified as within normal limits is marked in green, proceed to the dorsum of the hand and test in the same fashion. Since the sensibility on the dorsum of the hand is not always so well defined as the volar surface, it is easier to establish areas of decreased sensibility on the volar surface first. *Now the gross areas of normal and decreased sensibility have been defined* (Fig. 35-2, *B*).

3. Return to the volar surface of the hand. Proceed to the filaments within the level of *diminished light touch* (Table 35-2), but change the color of the marking pen for this level to *blue*. Test as above in the unidentified areas remaining, working again first on the volar surface and then on the dorsum (Fig. 35-2, *B*).

4. If areas remain unidentified, proceed to the filaments in the *diminished protective sensation* level *(purple)* and then *loss of protective sensation level* (red) and continue testing until all the areas have been identified (Fig. 35-2, *B*).

5. Record the colors and filament numbers on the report form to produce a sensory mapping. (Color and mark hands on form.) Note any variations and unusual responses, especially delayed responses. Delayed responses (more than 3 seconds) are considered abnormal. Note the presence and direction of referred touch with arrows. Note and draw on the form any unusual appearances on the hands, including sweat patterns, blisters, dry or shiny skin, calluses, cuts, blanching of the skin, and so on.

INTERPRETATION

Turning the data from testing into levels of sensibility and levels of expected patient function, as when one initially tests sensibility, can appear an impossible task at first. With a little experience, however, and some sensitivity to the needs of the patients, it not only can be done, but it becomes easier as well.

Normal touch is a recognition of light touch, and therefore deep pressure, that is within normal limits. This level is the most significant of all levels because it allows the examiner to distinguish between areas of normal and areas of sensory diminution.

Diminished light touch is diminished recognition of light touch. If a patient has diminished light touch, provided that his motor status and cognitive abilities are in play, he has fair use of his hand, his graphesthesia and stereognosis are both close to normal and adaptable, he has good temperature appreciation, he definitely has good protective sensation, he most often will have fair to good two-point discrimination, and he may not even realize he has had a sensory loss.

Diminished protective sensation is just that. If a patient has diminished protective sensation, he will have diminished use of his hands, he will have difficulty manipulating some objects, he will have a tendency to drop some objects, and he may complain of weakness of his hand, but he will have an appreciation of the pain and temperature that should help keep him from injury, and he will have some manipulative skill. Sensory reeducation can be begun at this level. It is possible for a patient to have a gross appreciation of two-point discrimination at this level (7 to 10 mm).

Loss of protective sensation is again what it says. If a patient has loss of protective sensation he will have little use of his hand, he will have a diminished, if not absent, temperature appreciation, he will not be able to manipulate objects outside his line of vision, he will have a tendency to injure himself easily, and it may even be dangerous for him to be around machinery. He will, however, be able to feel a pinprick and have deep pressure sensation, which does not make him totally asensory. Instructions on protective care are helpful to prevent injury.

If a patient is *untestable*, he may or may not feel a pinprick but will have no other discrimination of levels of feeling. If a patient feels a pinprick in an area otherwise untestable, it is important to note this during the mapping. Instructions on protective care of the hand are mandatory at this level to prevent the normally occurring problems associated with the asensory hand.

Further interpretation of the effect the decrease or loss of sensibility has on patient function depends on the area and extent of loss and whether musculature is diminished.

FUTURE CONSIDERATIONS

A few cases of suspected nerve compression have been found in which all the testing of neural status described is within normal limits, and a patient history is the only indicative finding. A review of the literature quickly shows similar cases. It is suspected that in these cases the patient is not always being tested at the time of his symptoms. He comes in for testing after he has slept late, had a good breakfast, and had a more quietly paced and lighter duty morning than his normal routine, while in reality he complains of problems only after heavy-duty work of a few hours' duration. Hunter has termed this condition "transient stress neuropathy." It is a challenge to our future testing.

The recognition of threshold levels of light touch–deep pressure is invaluable in peripheral nerve evaluation. Mappings of such thresholds enable the examiner to "see" what is otherwise invisible. I believe this testing method will clearly be validated by improved testing technique and instruments.

ACKNOWLEDGMENT

The author gratefully acknowledges Bill Buford, Bioengineer at the U.S. Public Health Service Hospital, Carville, Louisiana, for his help in reviewing the monofilament calculations in developing instrument measurements, and collaborating on sensibility test design.

REFERENCES

1. Bell, J.A., and Buford, W.: Comparison of forces and interpretation scales as used with the von Frey Aesthesiometer, Presented at Hand Surgery Correlated with Hand Therapy meeting, Philadelphia, 1978.
2. Bell, J.A., and Buford, W.L.: The force time relationship of clinically used sensory testing instruments, Presented at the thirty-seventh annual meeting of The American Society for Surgery of the Hand, Aurora, Colorado, 1982.
3. Buford, W.L., Jr., and Bell, J.A.: Dynamic properties of hand held tactile assessment stimuli, Proceedings of the thirty-fourth annual conference of Engineering in Medicine and Biology **23**:307, 1981.
4. Gelberman, R.H., Szabo, R.M., Williamson, R.V., and Dimick, M.P.: Sensibility testing in peripheral nerve compression syndromes: a human experimental study, San Diego, 1982. (Unpublished paper.)
5. Moberg, E.: Objective methods of determining the functional value of sensibility of the hand, J. Bone Joint Surg. **40B**:454-476, 1958.
6. Napier, J.R.: Hands, New York, 1980, Pantheon Press.
7. Semmes, J., Weinstein, S., Ghent, L., Teuber, H.-L.: Somatosensory changes after penetrating brain wounds in man, Cambridge, Mass., 1960, Harvard University Press.
8. von Frey, M.: Zur Physiologie der Juckempfindung, Arch. Neurol. Physiol. **7**:142-145, 1922.
9. von Prince, K.: Occupational therapy's interest in sensory function following peripheral nerve injury, Med. Bull., U.S. Army, Europe **23**:143-147, 1966.
10. von Prince, K., and Butler, B.: Measuring sensory function of the hand in peripheral nerve injuries, Am. J. Occup. Ther. **21**:385-396, 1967.
11. Weber, E.H.: Data cited by Sherrington, C.S., in Shafer's textbook of physiology, Edinburgh, 1900, Young, J. Pentland.
12. Weinstein, S.: Tactile sensitivity of the phalanges, Percept. Motor Skills **14**:351-354, 1962.
13. Werner, J.L., and Omer, G.E.: Evaluating cutaneous pressure sensation of the hand, Am. J. Occup. Ther. **24**:5, 1970.

BIBLIOGRAPHY

Arrington, J.: Corneal sensation measurement, Presented to the fourteenth annual meeting of the United States Public Health Service Professional Association, Phoenix, Ariz., April, 1977.
Chochinov, R.H., Ullyot, L.E., and Moorehouse, J.A.: Sensory perception thresholds in patients' with juvenile diabetes and their close relatives, N. Engl. J. Med. **286**(23):1233, 1969.
Demichelis, F., Giaretti, W.A., Barberis, M.L., and Teich-Alexia, S.: Biomedical instrumentation for the measurements of skin sensitivity, Trans. Biomed. Eng. **BMR-26**(6):326-330, June 1979.
Jamison, D.G.: Sensitivity testing as a means of differentiating the various forms of leprosy found in Nigeria, Int. J. Lepr. **39**(2):504-507, 1972.
Naafs, B., and Dagne, T.: Sensory testing: a sensitive method in the follow-up of nerve involvement, Int. J. Lepro. **45**(4):364-368, 1978.

36

Sensibility testing: clinical methods

ANNE D. CALLAHAN

The surgeon and the therapist are faced daily with the challenge of evaluating the hand with diminished sensibility after peripheral nerve injury. The challenge arises because sensibility is so complex. It affords the skin protection and provides a means of exploring and interacting with the environment. How then can the busy clinician accurately assess the scope of sensibility? Cottonwool and the safety pin, traditional tools of the neurologist, are recognized as inadequate for the task. Many additional tests[7,11,34,37,38,47] have been devised in an effort to find a quick, reliable means of gaining useful information about the nature of a sensibility deficit. The challenge to the clinician has therefore expanded to include deciding which tests of the many available should be used to assess sensibility. The purpose of this chapter is to discuss general considerations in sensibility testing in the clinic, describe the most commonly used tests, and offer guidelines for selection of tests based upon the history presented when the examiner's goal is to obtain a comprehensive assessment of the level of sensibility present in a nerve-damaged hand.

GENERAL CONSIDERATIONS IN SENSIBILITY TESTING
Relevant definitions

Sensation versus sensibility. Confusion sometimes exists regarding these two terms, such that seemingly opposite definitions can be found in current literature.[12,29] For the purpose of this chapter, sensation is defined as "an impression conveyed by an afferent nerve to the sensorium," whereas sensibility is "susceptibility of feeling; ability to feel or perceive."[14] It is these concepts that seem to have the widest use in the medical literature today.

Academic versus functional sensibility. A distinction is made between return of sensibility as evidenced by the ability to perceive pinprick, touch, and temperature ("academic") and the return of sensibility sufficient to enable the hand to engage in full activities of daily living, including those activities in which vision is essentially occluded while the hand manipulates an object ("functional"). Seddon[40] and Bowden[5] were among the first to make this distinction in assessing recovery of sensibility. Functional sensibility enables one to identify objects in a pocket, manipulate garment fasteners on the back, and perform many work-related activities. Moberg[25,27] has probably been the most influential

in emphasizing the importance of testing functional sensibility.

Tactile gnosis. Tactile gnosis (*gnōsis,* Greek "knowledge") is a term popularized by Moberg[7] to denote the capacity of the hand to "see" while gripping or manipulating an object even when the eyes are closed, that is, functional sensibility. A distinction is made between tactile gnosis and the central nervous system function described as stereognosis.

Candidates for evaluation

Patients may be referred for sensibility evaluation for any of the following reasons: (1) to aid in diagnosis (partial versus complete nerve injury, assessment of sensory changes in carpal tunnel syndrome, and so on); (2) to aid in serial follow-up after nerve repair; (3) to aid in disability assessment in compensation cases; and (4) to determine the need or readiness for sensory reeducation.

Essentials of a sensibility evaluation

A thorough assessment of sensibility includes the following: a careful history; examination of sympathetic function in the hand; appropriate selection of tests, based upon the specific information desired; administration of the tests in a standard manner so that as many testing variables as possible can be minimized and so that follow-up evaluation can be reliably compared; and knowledgeable interpretation of information gathered. These components of evaluation will be discussed in this chapter.

OBTAINING THE HISTORY

A careful history, based upon medical chart information and skillful interviewing of the patient, will provide the examiner with information that cannot be gained by any specific clinical test. Such information will aid in shortening the time required for testing and will help determine the prognosis for recovery.

A history should include name, age, sex, dominance, and occupation. Age will influence prognosis for recovery. Occupation and whether the dominant or nondominant extremity was injured will help in estimating degree of sensibility recovery required for functional use of the extremity in work and leisure activities.

The date, nature, and level of injury should also be re-

407

corded. The time elapsed since the date of injury or repair helps in proper assessment of Tinel's sign and in better interpretation of the presence or absence of sympathetic function. The nature of the injury (such as laceration, crush, traction, compression, or infection) will influence the amount of scarring that occurs, in turn influencing the quality of regeneration. Prognosis for recovery of distal sensory function is partially dependent on the level of the injury; injuries at or proximal to the wrist level rarely result in good functional sensation in the adult.[10,27,29]

The medical chart will frequently document a patient's involvement in litigation. This is important information for the examiner because litigation will tend to influence the level of cooperation of the patient. The best candidate for sensibility evaluation is one who has nothing to gain by negative results from the tests.

Skillful interviewing will result in useful information on the current status of sensibility. Questions should be phrased in such a way as to avoid leading or suggesting to the patient. Thus an appropriately worded initial question would be, "Please tell me what problems you have in this hand." The patient will then tend to give precedence to his nerve-related complaints without artificial emphasis on sensory disturbances. For example, a patient with carpal tunnel syndrome may not describe any sensory-related problems, limiting his complaint to a weakness in grip strength. In this case one could expect that he would probably test with normal or only slightly diminished sensibility. On the other hand, if he states, "It feels like there is a veil on my fingertips when I try to pick up something," he could be expected to test with slight to moderate loss of sensibility. Terms such as "numbness," "dead," "asleep," and "pins and needles" may refer to hypesthesia, anesthesia, or parasthesia depending on that particular patient's meaning of the term.

Once the patient has described his dysfunction in his own words, the examiner can ask more leading questions to elicit greater detail about the current status of sensibility. Such questioning will help the nonsophisticated or nonobservant patient to articulate his problems. The examiner will want to know if sensibility is improving, getting worse, or staying the same. Are symptoms aggravated by certain positions or activities, and are they relieved by certain positions or motions (such as "shaking of the arm")? Does the sensibility deficit affect performance of activities of daily living?

At this time in the examination it is convenient to assess briefly motor function, including grip and pinch strength, and in selected cases individual muscle strength because motor function will affect performance on certain sensibility tests that may be used. The patient's performance during these motor tests can suggest to the examiner his general level of cooperation, as evidence by the shape of his strength curve on the Jamar Dynamometer (refer to Chapter 4) and exertion of maximal effort during muscle testing.

EXAMINATION OF SYMPATHETIC FUNCTION IN THE HAND

Sympathetic fibers subserve vasomotor (*vas*, Latin "vessel"), sudomotor (*sudor*, Latin "sweat"), and pilomotor (*pilus*, Latin "hair") functions in the extremity. After nerve injury the area of loss of sympathetic function closely corresponds to the area of loss of sensory function because the cutaneous sympathetic fibers follow essentially the same pathway to the periphery as the cutaneous sensory fibers.[44] The actual autonomous area of sympathetic function may be smaller than the corresponding autonomous area of cutaneous sensory function because there is more overlap between sympathetic fibers than between sensory fibers.[19] The combination of sympathetic and sensory dysfunction results in characteristic trophic (*trophē*, Greek "nourishment") changes in all tissues of the involved area.[44] Examination of the sympathetic function and trophic changes in the hand (Table 36-1) will provide definitie information on the nutritional state of the part and suggestive information on sensory function in the part.

The correlation between presence of sympathetic function and sensibility is greatest immediately after nerve laceration and in long-term cases where little or no regeneration occurs. However, if the original injury were partial or the nerve undergoes incomplete regeneration, there may be return of sympathetic function without significant return of sensation.[30,32,43,44]

TABLE 36-1. Sympathetic changes after nerve injury

	Sympathetic function	Early changes	Late changes
Vasomotor	Skin color	Rosy	Mottled or cyanotic
	Skin temperature	Warm	Cool
Sudomotor	Sweat	Dry skin	Dry or overly moist
Pilomotor	Gooseflesh response	Absent	Absent
Trophic	Skin texture	Soft; smooth	Smooth; nonelastic
	Soft-tissue atrophy	Slight	More pronounced, especially in finger pulps
	Nail changes	Blemishes	Curved in longitudinal and horizontal planes; "talonlike"
	Hair growth	May fall out or become longer and finer	May fall out or become longer and finer
	Rate of healing	Slowed	Slowed

Vasomotor changes

Vasomotor function is reflected in temperature, color, and edema. For 2 to 3 weeks after complete denervation, or longer in some incomplete lesions, the skin feels warm to the touch because of vasodilatation secondary to paralysis of the vasoconstrictors.[41] This warm phase is gradually superseded, for reasons not completely understood, by a phase in which the skin feels cool to the touch. During the cold phase the patient may complain of cold intolerance. The skin temperature is abnormally influenced by environmental temperature, particularly cold, and when exposed to cold, the part becomes cold and rewarms slowly.[44] Cold intolerance may extend beyond the denervated part to include the entire hand and will recovery only as reinnervation restores normal circulation.[41,44] According to Richards,[39] normal warmth of the skin, perceived subjectively by the patient and objectively by the examiner, does not occur until there is a high degree of sensory recovery.

Skin temperature is quickly assessed by use of the dorsum of the examiner's hand to compare the involved cutaneous area with the contralateral normal area. The dorsum is used because it is rich in temperature receptors and is less likely than the warm, moist volar skin to result in a false reading.

During the warm phase, the skin is flushed or rosy. During the cold phase it is usually mottled (a combination of pallor and cyanosis) or, in severe cases, reddish blue from stasis.[8] Color is assessed by comparison with the uninvolved hand.

Edema may occur as a result of decreased circulatory function and is more likely after brachial plexus injuries than distal injuries.[41]

Sudomotor changes

Lack of sweating occurs in the autonomous area of the sympathetic fibers immediately after denervation. Abnormally increased sweating, such that beads of sweat are clearly visible, may occur after partial nerve injury, especially when the nerve is irritated and pain is present, or during regeneration of a lacerated nerve.[19]

The presence of sweating does not imply the return of sensory function.[24,30,32] However, the absence of sweating in a recent nerve laceration or in a long-term injury does strongly correlate with a lack of discrimination sensation.[15,25]

Pilomotor changes

Absence of the ''gooseflesh'' response occurs when there is complete interruption of sympathetic supply to an area.[19] Since this phenomenon can be observed only at opportune moments, it is not regularly included in a sensibility evaluation.

Trophic changes

Interruption of normal nerve supply results in interruption of the normal nutritive process of the tissues, thereby causing some atrophy of all tissues from skin to bone.[8] Decreased nutrition will be evident in skin texture, the soft tissue of the finger pulps, nail changes, hair growth, increased susceptibility to injury, and slowed healing.

Trophic changes are reversible as regeneration occurs. Persistent changes are associated with failure of regeneration

or persistent irritation of a partial nerve lesion. Some nerves carry more sympathetic fibers than others; thus median nerve lesions result in more trophic changes (particularly noticeable in the index finger) than ulnar nerve lesions, which result in more changes than the radial nerve. Trophic changes will be more pronounced in causalgic states and in brachial plexus lesions than in simple nerve lacerations.[8,44]

Skin texture. Early on, the skin is thin and smooth, almost ''velvety,'' as the papillary ridges and finger creases become less distinct because of atrophy of the epidermis. In long-term cases, the skin becomes shiny, smooth, and inelastic.[44] Examination is by visual observation and by palpation with the dorsum of the examining hand.

Atrophy of finger pulps. The generalized atrophy that follows denervation is most obvious in the pulps of the fingers, which may take on a tapered appearance. In fact, the entire digit may appear noticeably smaller than its corresponding digit on the other hand. This change occurs with long-term denervation because of irreparable injury or failure of regeneration; therefore it is not generally observed to reverse itself.[44]

Nail changes. Changes within the first few months include striations, ridges and similar blemishes, slowed growth, and increased hardness.[44] Later, in response to atrophy of the soft tissue of the digits, the nails conform to the shape of the atrophied pulp. They become smaller than the corresponding nail on the opposite hand and curve in the longitudinal and horizontal planes. They may become talonlike in appearance. The lunula is diminished or absent (Fig. 36-1). Severe nail changes are signs of long-term denervation and therefore are not likely to improve with time.[44]

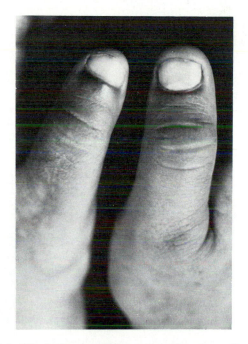

FIG. 36-1. Thumbnail changes in a case of chronic median nerve denervation. Notice that nail on left is smaller than one on right and has no visible lunula. Thumb has atrophied, and nail has curved to conform to tapered tip.

Hair growth. Hair may fall out in the region of denervation or may become longer and finer.[8] Occasionally it may demonstrate increased growth, termed "hypertrichosis," which state is most frequently noted on the forearm in radial nerve and median nerve injuries and occasionally in injures of the brachial plexus.[19] Seddon[41] states that the apparent increase in growth of hair on the forearm is often attributable to atrophy of the denervated part. In causalgia, there is loss of hair where the skin is atrophic and shiny.[44]

Susceptibility to injury and slowed healing. Atrophy of the epidermis and underlying tissue causes the skin to become more delicate and therefore more susceptible to injury from noxious stimuli, including pressure, temperature, and sharp objects. This is clearly exemplified when atrophic skin is penetrated by a sharp pin and responds with a minute spot of blood whereas normal skin on the same extremity does not. Healing takes longer than in normal skin because of decreased nutrition and vascularity, a condition that reverses itself as reinnervation occurs.[44] The patient who does not compensate for increased susceptibility to injury will frequently present with blisters and ulcers on the denervated skin (Fig. 36-2), whereas the presence of "wear" marks,[25] such as dirt stains and calluses, indicates functional use of the hand and is a sign of useful sensibility. Absence of "wear" marks on skin that has undergone reinnervation and has adequate motor function while other parts of the same hand demonstrate them indicates lack of use and useful sensibility of the unmarked parts (Fig. 36-3).

• • •

A thorough history and examination of the hand will clue the experienced examiner to the status of sensibility in the hand. However, the details of sensory dysfunction and the progress of regeneration can only be determined through the administration of specific clinical tests designed to assess sensibility.

CHARACTERISTIC PATTERNS OF LOSS AND RECOVERY OF SENSIBILITY AFTER DENERVATION

Certain characteristics of sensibility loss and recovery have been observed by clinicians after denervation. These are described below.

Immediately after denervation the autonomous area of nerve supply is anesthetic. Overlapping areas of supply with neighboring cutaneous nerves are hypesthetic. Therefore careful testing should elicit a borderline transition area between the zones of normal and absent sensibility. The transition area is smaller for touch sensibility than for pain sensibility.[41]

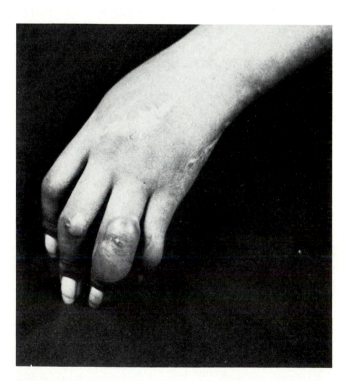

FIG. 36-2. This hand with median and ulnar nerve injury was allowed to rest against a hot radiator, resulting in second-degree burns to ulnar three digits.

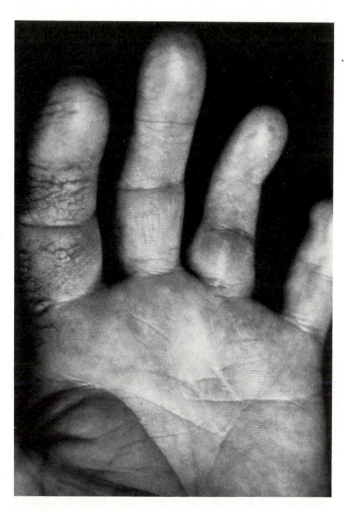

FIG. 36-3. "Wear marks" on this hand of a mechanic indicate that index finger is used for functional activities, but ulnar three digits, which had sustained digital nerve injury 1 year previously, are not. Testing revealed presence of light touch but poor discriminative sensation in involved digits.

Some ingrowth of nerve supply along the borders of the anesthetic area occurs during the early weeks after denervation, thereby causing apparent shrinkage of the anesthetic zone. The exact mechanism for initiation of this phenomenon is not known.[41,44]

The rate of regeneration of sensory fibers in humans generally falls within an average range of 1 to 2 mm per day, with wider ranges reported by some investigators.[40,44] An initial recovery rate of 3 mm per day is not unusual, with slowing of the rate over time.[40] Factors affecting the rate of regeneration within an individual include the nature and level of the lesion and the age of the patient.[48]

Pain elicited by pinch is a very early sign of sensory recovery and may precede a positive Tinel's sign.[44] Tenderness to pressure and to pinprick precede sensitivity to moving touch, which precedes light touch and discriminative touch.[8,41,44] At first, perceptions are poorly localized and may radiate proximally or distally. Accurate localization is among the last sensory functions to recover.[46]

Determination and interpretation of Tinel's sign

Tinel's sign[45] is assessed by gentle percussion from distal to proximal along the nerve trunk. The most distal point at which the patient experiences a tingling sensation that radiates peripherally in the cutaneous distribution of the nerve is the point of positive Tinel's sign. This sign is said to represent the advancing terminations of the regenerating sensory axons. Progress in regeneration can be documented by recording the level of Tinel's sign in successive examinations, using an anatomic landmark as a point of reference.

Seddon[41] states that this sign has come to be regarded as unreliable because a positive sign can occur in the presence of a partial, unrepaired nerve lesion, thereby falsely indicating regeneration. He credits Henderson[20] with making the sign more informative by his repeated observations on 400 cases of nerve injury in prisoner-of-war hospitals in World War II. Seddon states, "Henderson found that Tinel's sign became important about 4 months after the time of injury. If it was strongly positive at the level of the lesion but persistently absent below, spontaneous regeneration could not be expected. If the sign was strongly positive at the site of damage and also appeared weakly distal to it, the quality of regeneration would be poor. But a strongly positive sign at the level of the lesion that gradually faded as the response moved peripherally and became stronger in the distal part of the nerve indicated that satisfactory regeneration was in progress."

One must always assess the meaning of Tinel's sign in the context of other information gathered about sensory function. The sign may be absent where too much muscle lies over the nerve to allow adequate percussion of it.[41]

In cases of nerve compression, such as carpal tunnel syndrome, Tinel's sign may be present at the level of compression, but its absence does not indicate an absence of compression.

Mapping the area of dysfunction

Assessment of sensibility after nerve injury is made faster and more precise when one maps out the area of sensibility dysfunction before the administration fo specific tests. This can be done in two ways.

Mapping by examiner. The examiner draws a probe, such as the blunt end of a pen, lightly over the skin, starting from an area of normal sensibility and proceeding to the area of suspected abnormal sensibility. The patient, whose vision is occluded, is asked to immediately say "now" when the sensation produced by the probe is suddenly "different." Using a felt-tip pen, the examiner marks the skin at the spot where the patient said "now," and then proceeds to approach the area of dysfunction from another starting point. The area is thus approached from all directions—proximal, distal, radial, and ulnar—until all boundaries are marked (Fig. 36-4). (Note that in later stages of regeneration the patient may not experience a "suddenly different" sensation during application of the probe and so a map of sensory dysfunction is not obtained. This sign is interpreted as excellent progression in recovery of light touch.)

Mapping by patient. Some examiners prefer to have the patient map the area of dysfunction. With vision unoccluded, the patient draws the probe across his skin as described above and marks on the skin where the sensation produced

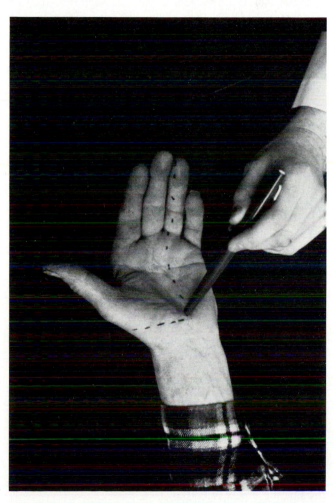

FIG. 36-4. Mapping area of dysfunction helps make subsequent testing faster and more accurate.

by the probe suddenly feels different. This method may allow for a more precise mapping.

With either method of mapping, the probe should be drawn fairly slowly across the skin with a light touch so that no drag is produced. In a reliable patient the path from normal to abnormal, the patient will say "now" at the same location. The results can be made even more specific if the patient is required to state each time he feels a sudden change as the probe continues across the area of dysfunction, thereby demarcating the boundaries between the normal and hypesthetic and anesthetic areas. Progress in reinnervation will be reflected in a progressively diminishing "map" size over time. The results of mapping should be transferred to an outline of the hand or photographed, to provide a permanent record.

CATEGORIES OF SENSIBILITY TESTS

Generally speaking, the sensibility tests most commonly used today can be divided into three main categories: modality tests, functional tests, and objective tests.

Modality tests

Modality tests include tests for the four classic cutaneous functions: pain, heat, cold, and touch-pressure. They are sometimes called "academic" tests because they seek to assess the presence or absence of a specific modality of sensation without being able to relate directly the information gained to function. The modality tests can, however, answer the following questions:

1. Is protective sensation present as measured by the ability to perceive a sharp object, deep pressure, or hot and cold?

2. Is light touch present? Light touch perception is a necessary component of functional sensibility, but its presence is not sufficient to confirm the presence of functional sensibilty. The modality tests are most useful in the early stages of regeneration.

Functional tests

Functional tests allow one to assess the quality of sensibility. For example, is sensibility present on a gross level only, or on a fine discriminative level? Is it useful for fine-prehension tasks? Is it sufficient for daily activities and work tasks where vision is occluded during manipulation of objects? It is these qualitites that Moberg has termed "tactile gnosis." These tests might also be considered as integrative tests because they require a higher level of sensory processing than the modality tests do.

Functional tests include two-point discrimination, moving two-point discrimination, ridge sensitometer, Seddon coin test, Moberg pickup test, and others.[7,37] Some of these require active manipulation of an object rather than simply passive recognition of a stimulus. The requirement for active manipulation is based upon recognition that touch is an active, exploratory process of the hand, not merely a passive receptive sense, and therefore touch can be more accurately assessed if the hand is permitted to actively explore and "scan" the object presented.[16]

Objective tests

This category includes the Ninhydrin sweat test and other tests of sudomotor function, nerve-conduction studies, and the wrinkle test.[31] These are termed "objective" because they require only passive cooperation of the patient and not his subjective interpretation of a stimulus. They do not directly correlate with functional sensation after nerve repair.[1,30,32,43] However, the sudomotor and wrinkle tests can be useful in obtaining information about the function of a nerve in children and malingerers and nerve-conduction tests do provide useful information about conduction parameters in a nerve (see Chapter 44).

CONTROL OF VARIABLES IN TESTING

Regardless of which tests are used, one must keep in mind that many variables contribute to the subjective nature of sensibility testing. Some variables can be controlled by the careful tester; others are not yet under our control but are being studied (see Chapter 34). The examiner's knowledge of the nature of these variables and attempt to control them will help make testing more accurate and reliable.

Environment-related variables

Background noise is distracting to the patient and tester. A test administered in a noisy environment is not the same as one administered in a quiet environment. To minimize the effect of noise, all testing should be done in a quiet room. The examiner must be alert for sound made by a testing instrument before or during the application of a stimulus, which will cue the patient as to a change in stimulus. Similarly, the sound of a starched coat sleeve as the examiner moves about will cue the patient to the arrival of a stimulus. These extraneous noises, and other sources of noise, must be eliminated from the sensibility examination.

Patient-related variables

Patient-related variables have to do with patient attitude, level of concentration, and possibly anxiety level. Each patient will bring his own agenda to a sensibility test. Some will want to test well; others will not. Some are suggestible and may imagine a stimulus when there is none; others admit a sensation only if they are absolutely positive it was felt. Methods are being sought to control for some of these patient-related psychological variables.[9]

Normal callused skin has a higher sensory threshold than normal uncallused skin in the hand because a given stimulus will deform callused skin less than soft, supple skin. Therefore areas of callosity should be noted so that test results can be more validly assessed. Because there is variation of sensitivity within the normal population, the uninvolved hand is always the best control in the determination of sensibility dysfunction.

Instrument-related variables

Instrument-related variables include quality control in the manufacturing of instruments and variations in the same instrument over time.[24] Instruments that are designed to exert a specific pressure should be calibrated regularly. The examiner should be aware of the idiosyncrasies of each instrument that he uses. For example, certain two-point discrimination instruments are heavier than others; so the examiner must be careful not to exert a heavier pressure when testing with the heavier instrument.

Method-related variables

The same test instrument, even a cotton ball, in two different examiner's hands can produce different results because of differences in the methods of administration. For example, one examiner may use more pressure than the other or may stimulate with a moving instead of a constant touch. Control of method-related variables can be assisted by the following:

1. Standardized instructions to the patient before each test.
2. Use of a standard method of supporting the hand during testing for modalities and certain functional tests.

Brand[6] has recommended that the hand be fully supported in the examiner's hand so that inadvertent stretch of tissues and movement of joints can be avoided (Fig. 36-5, *A*). He has further suggested that a better method of support would be to rest the hand in putty or similar medium that would provide full support (Fig. 36-5, *B*). Use of such a medium would have the advantage of eliminating transmission of vibration inherent in the supporting hand to the hand being tested.[4,6]

3. Criteria for application of the stimulus must remain the same within a test and between tests. Important criteria include speed of stimulus application, which is known to affect perception,[17] the amount of pressure exerted on the skin, and whether the stimulus is moving or constant.

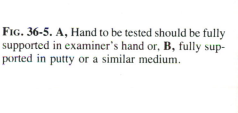

FIG. 36-5. **A,** Hand to be tested should be fully supported in examiner's hand or, **B,** fully supported in putty or a similar medium.

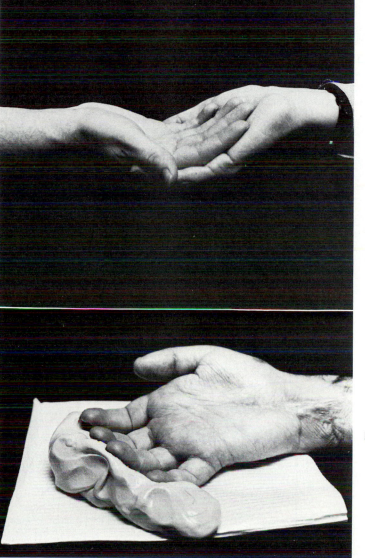

4. The time interval between applications of the stimulus and the spacing of stimuli must be varied so that the patient cannot anticipate the timing or location of the next stimulus.
5. Results should be carefully documented for better comparison between successive tests.

Examiner-related variables

Experience, attention to detail, and concern for adherence to methods of administration will affect test results, as will the examiner's level of concentration and fatigue. To minimize the former variables, the same examiner should perform successive tests on a given patient.

ADMINISTRATION OF SPECIFIC TESTS
Modality tests

Modality tests are particularly useful in cases of nerve laceration to monitor return of protective sensibility and touch and pressure sensibility. In cases of nontraumatic nerve compression, modality testing, particularly light touch and pressure, is useful to assess early changes in sensibility function.

A goal in modality testing is to record information in a way that allows for valid comparison with follow-up reports. When testing for any of the modalities—pain, temperature, or touch-pressure—one can make testing more systematic and documentation more accurate by use of a worksheet that has a grid superimposed on an outline of the hand (Fig. 36-6). The grid is divided into zones, whose longitudinal lines parallel the rays of the hand and whose horizontal lines correspond to the flexion creases of the digits and palm. This grid was devised by von Prince[46] for use in her studies of light-touch dysfunction in nerve-injured patients in the 1960s. I have found this grid useful for all modality tests. During testing, the examiner visualizes the grid on the patient's hand and applies the test stimulus to a particular zone. Correct and incorrect responses are recorded in the corresponding zone on the work sheet. A different work sheet can be used for each modality test, and the work sheets can be filed for permanent records or the information on the work sheet can be transferred to a more formal report. The use of this grid will be elaborated on below in the description of methodology for each modality test.

During all modality tests the hand is fully supported in the examiner's hand or in putty (Fig. 36-5). Vision is occluded by use of a blindfold, by the patient simply closing his eyes, or by a screen (Fig. 36-7). The last method is ideal because it allows test instruments and recording sheets to be hidden from view even between tests when vision might not otherwise be occluded.

Pinprick perception. Protective sensation is defined as the ability to perceive painful or potentially harmful stimuli on the skin and in the subcutaneous tissue. Heat, cold, deep pressure, low-grade repetitive pressure, and superficial pain are examples of such stimuli. Of these, the most commonly tested and the one regarded as the best test of protective sensation is superficial pain tested with a safety pin. It is not sufficient simply to require the patient to say "now" when touched with the sharp end of the pin because he may respond simply to pressure of the stimulus and not sharpness

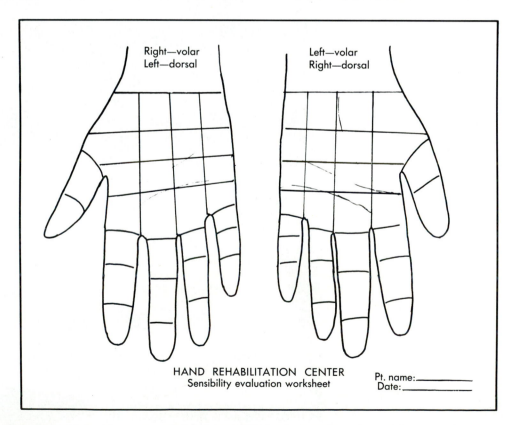

FIG. 36-6. Grid worksheet is recommended during modality testing to make testing and documentation more systematic.

of the stimulus. A more accurate assessment of protective sensation requires that he discriminate between the sharp and dull sides of the pin.

When testing with a pin, the examiner should keep in mind that during nerve regeneration there will occur a period of hypersensitivity to pinprick. In the area of hyperanalgesia, the response to pinprick will be hyperacute, that is, abnormally unpleasant. Therefore testing should proceed in such a way that the number of applications of the stimulus in one "zone" of the hand are minimized.

The amount of pressure necessary to elicit correct responses on the uninvolved hand is used as a guide for pressure to be used on the involved hand. It is not unusual to observe minute spots of blood where the pin has penetrated the fragile outer layer of skin in a denervated hand, even though only light pressure has been used.

The grid is used as a work sheet during testing. The examiner alternates randomly between the sharp and dull sides of the pin, being sure that each zone has been stimulated at least once by each end of the pin so that true discrimination within an area has been ascertained. A code is used to mark each zone tested on the work sheet, as follows: $+S$ (correct response to sharp), $-S$ (no response to sharp), $+D$ (correct response to dull), $-D$ (no response to dull), "S" (reported dull stimulus as "sharp"), and "D" reported sharp stimulus as "dull"). The entire area of dysfunction, as determined previously by mapping, is tested.

Results within a zone are interpreted as follows: correct response to both sharp and dull, intact protective sensation; incorrect response to both sharp and dull, absent protective sensation; "S," hyperanalgesic; "D," pressure awareness.

Sunderland notes that the perception of pinprick ranges along a hierarchy that includes absence of awareness, pressure sensation without distinguishing between sharp and dull, hyperanalgesia with radiation, sharp sensation with some radiation and gross localization, sensation of sharpness with or without slight stinging or radiation and fair localization, and, finally, normal perception.[44] Seddon likewise grades the response to pinprick along several parameters.[41]

It should be noted that Kirk and Denny-Brown[22] found pin scratch to be a more reliable stimulus than pinprick in their studies of dorsal-root lesions in monkeys; however, pin scratch has not been generally adopted clinically.

Moberg[27] and Dellon,[13] among others, have stated that they do not test for pinprick because of the discomfort involved to the patient and because the information gained does not correlate directly with functional sensation. However, one can argue for testing pinprick in cases where functional tests and other modality tests have proved negative or can be predicted to be negative by the history of the patient. Certainly, protective sensation is "functional" sensation of a sort, and therefore its presence when other indications of sensibility are absent is important to ascertain.

Temperature perception. Test tubes or metal cylinders filled with hot and cold fluids are the usual instruments used for clinical testing of temperature perception. The limitation of these instruments is that the information obtained is gross if the temperatures are not carefully controlled. The clinician can determine if the patient can distinguish between hot and cold, but not if he can distinguish between temperatures 1° to 5° C apart, as in the normal hand, or if he can distinguish between temperatures along the entire range of very cold to very hot. Therefore the tester must be cautious about reporting that the patient has normal temperature sensation, which implies good discriminative ability, if he has simply tested hot and cold at one interval in the range.

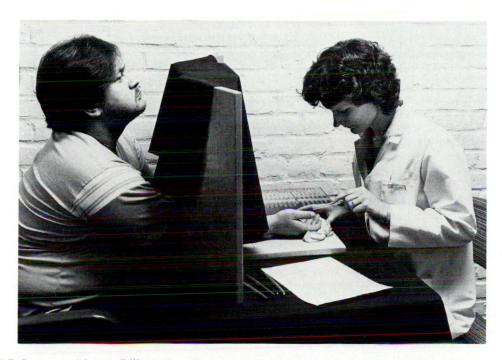

FIG. 36-7. Screen used for sensibility testing allows test instruments and worksheets to be hidden from patient's view.

Because of the difficulties in controlling test conditions within a test and between tests and the lack of correlation with functional sensation, many clinicians do not test for temperature discrimination.[13,26,41,44] Some clinicians satisfy themselves with testing simply for the perception of hot and cold on a gross level; others do not test for temperature at all, preferring to allow the presence of pinprick perception to be sufficient evidence of protective sensation.

If one chooses to test for temperature, one should keep in mind that in the early stages of regeneration cold will be perceived more intensely than normal and hot may not be perceived. Therefore, in responding "cold" and "hot" the patient may merely be responding to a "cold" and a "not-cold" stimulus. To ascertain that the patient can perceive both cold and hot, one should use three identical material containers to administer the stimulus: one cold, one hot, and one neutral in temperature. When testing, one should hold the stimulus in place in the selected zone for identical periods of time per stimulus (1 second is suggested), and the patient must be able to correctly identify within the zone tested the cold and hot stimuli and be able to differentiate each from the neutral temperature stimulus. Stimuli are not applied successively to the same zone but at random to the zones of suspected dysfunction. As when testing for pinprick perception, a code is used on the work sheet to identify correct and incorrect responses, for example, $+C$ (correct identification of cold), $-C$ (incorrect response to cold), $+H$, $-H$, $+N$, and $-N$. In this way one will ascertain if cold only is present, or if perception of both hot and cold is present.

Light touch–deep pressure (using nongraded instruments). Light touch sensibility and deep pressure sensibility are considered to represent two ends of a continuum of cutaneous sensibility, with light touch being perceived by receptors in the superficial skin layers and pressure being perceived by receptors in the subcutaneous and deeper tissue.[44] Pressure sensibility is a form of protective sensation, since it warns of deep pressure or of low-grade repetitive pressure, which might result in injury to the skin. Light touch sensibility is a necessary component of fine discrimination.

Light touch sensibility has been tested in clinical settings by use of cotton, the eraser end of a pencil, and the examiner's fingertip. These instruments all have one thing in common: they cannot reliably be graded to provide different amounts of pressure along the light touch–deep pressure continuum. If one assumes that the instrument is applied to the skin with the same amount of pressure on each trial, the patient will have been tested at only one interval on the continuum. Either he will feel the stimulus or he will not. One does not know if the stimulus is felt more distinctly in one location or another, or if a slightly higher or lower pressure would have resulted in a positive response. As long as one recognizes the limitations of these instruments and the information they provide, they can be used properly in the hands of a skilled and experienced examiner.

Skilled use includes care in the application of the stimulus. If only a limited interval on the light touch–deep pressure continuum is to be tested, that interval should be at the light end of the range. Certainly, a light touch stimulus

should never produce blanching. The examiner should be guided by the knowledge of the normal hand's ability to perceive the touch of a feather, and he should apply a similar pressure to the patient's skin.

The stimulus can be applied with a constant or moving touch, but the same type of stimulus should be applied throughout the test. Since there are more receptors for moving touch than constant touch in the hand and since moving touch returns before constant touch,[10] it is more valid to test with a constant touch if the patient is to be declared as having normal light touch.

As with the other modality tests, the use of the grid is recommended for better documentation during this test. The stimulus is applied to the center of a zone in the case of constant touch, or to the entire zone in the case of moving touch. Duration of the stimulus in either case is 1 second. The patient is asked to "touch" each time he feels the stimulus. Localization is not a requirement for a positive response, since it is the presence only of light touch, not the ability to localize it, that is being tested. A simple "$+$" (positive response) or "$-$" (negative response) is sufficient as a code on the worksheet. There should be variable time intervals between trials, and trials should be spaced so that the patient does not anticipate the timing or location of the stimulus. Two nonsuccessive stimuli are applied to each zone. All zones in the area of dysfunction, as previously determined by mapping, are tested.

The interpretation of responses is as follows: two correct responses out of two trials = light touch intact; one correct out of two trials = diminished light touch; neither of two trials correct = absent light touch in the zone tested.

Light touch–deep pressure (using a graded instrument). Many have sought to improve the testing of light touch by using an instrument that could grade the amount of pressure applied to the skin from light to deep.[21,41,46] Such instruments have been developed to enable more precise monitoring and documentation of progress in return of light touch and the quality of that touch. These test instruments are all variations upon the graded stimulus developed by von Frey in 1895 in his classic studies of touch threshold.

In 1960, Semmes and Weinstein[42] developed a graded light touch testing instrument for use in a study of somatosensory changes in brain-injured adults. The instrument is now known as the Semmes-Weinstein Pressure Aesthesiometer* and includes a kit of 20 probes (Fig. 36-8, *A*), each probe consisting of a nylon monofilament attached to a polymethylmethacrylate (Lucite) rod (Fig. 36-8, *B*). Each probe is marked with a number ranging from 1.65 to 6.65 that represents the logarithm of 10 times the force in milligrams required to bow the monofilament (log 10 F_{mg}).[24] Thus the finest filament, labeled 1.65, will "bow" when it is applied at a perpendicular angle to the skin with a force of 0.0045 gm, and the thickest filament, labeled 6.65, will bow at 448 gm (Fig. 36-8, *C* and *D*).

In 1967, von Prince[47] introduced this instrument into the clinic for use in testing light touch–deep pressure sensibility in the nerve-injured hand. Her pioneering efforts were taken

*Research Designs, Inc., 7320 Ashcroft, Suite 103, Houston, Tex. 77081.

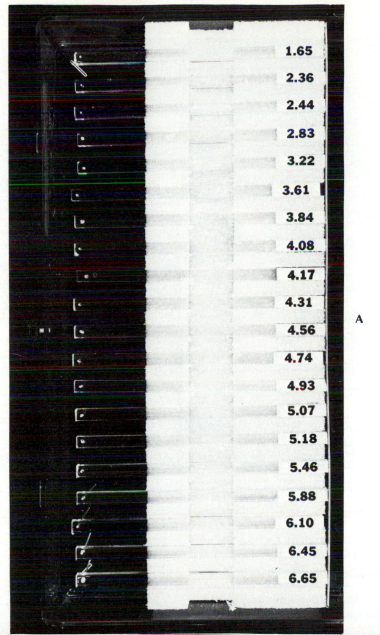

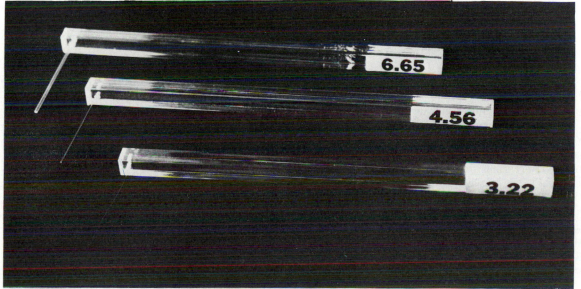

FIG. 36-8. A, Semmes-Weinstein Pressure Aesthesiometer. **B,** Each probe consists of a nylon monofilament attached to a Lucite rod.

Continued.

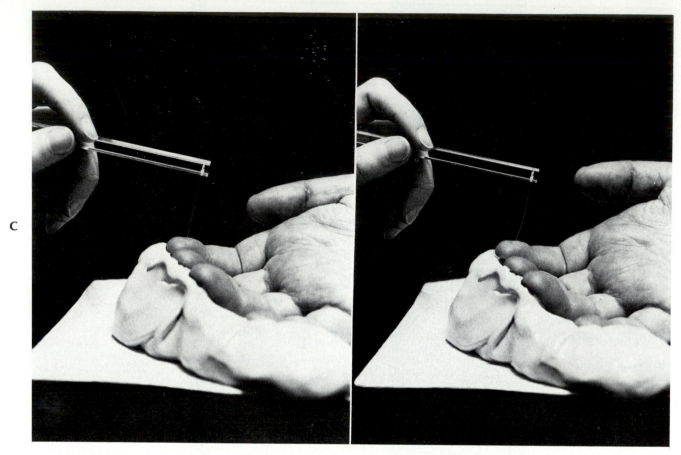

C   D

Fig. 36-8, cont'd. C, Proper application requires that the filaments be applied perpendicularly to skin. D, Until they become bowed.

up by Werner and Omer[49] and Bell.[3] The methods of administration and interpretation of this test are described in detail in Chapter 35. In keeping with the emphasis of this chapter on standardization of method and documentation, the methods presented below demonstrate how the grid work sheet can be used to facilitate administration and documentation of this test. These methods draw heavily upon those described by the clinicians mentioned above.

The corresponding skin area on the uninvolved hand serves as a control. Initially, both surfaces of the involved hand are tested, with special emphasis on the area of dysfunction as determined by mapping (Fig. 36-4). In follow-up tests only the area of dysfunction determined by the initial test need be reevaluated.

When testing, the examiner visualizes the grid on the patient's hand and chooses the center of any zone for the application of the stimulus. Should a more detailed test be desired, as after digital nerve repair, the zones can be subdivided one or more times in the area of special concern. Testing is usually begun with the filament marked 2.83, which is considered to test for normal light touch.[3,47,48] If the history suggests moderate-to-severe dysfunction, however, testing is begun with a higher marked filament, chosen at the examiner's discretion. The filament is applied perpendicularly to the skin until it bows (Fig. 36-8, C and D). In a given zone, one trial with any filament marked 1.65

through 4.08 consists in three applications of the stimulus as described by Bell[3]: the filament is applied to the skin in 1 to 1.5 seconds, held in place for 1 to 1.5 seconds, lifted for 1 to 1.5 seconds, and applied twice more in the same manner. Filaments marked 4.17 through 6.65 are applied only once per trial in a given zone. Control of the speed of application is necessary because a quickly applied stimulus will be more easily perceived than an equal amount of pressure slowly introduced.[17] The monofilament must not slip or slide on the skin during application because this will result in a more easily perceived stimulus than that applied by a stationary monofilament on the skin.

The hand is fully supported, and the patient is familiarized with the test by observing several applications of the stimulus on the uninvolved hand. Then vision is occluded, and he is instructed to say "touch" each time he feels a touch. He must respond accurately to a particular filament on two nonsuccessive trials before testing in a zone is considered complete. If the first response is accurate and the second inaccurate, a third trial is made to reach a final assessment in that zone. When responses are inaccurate for two trials with a given filament in a zone, the examiner returns to that zone at random intervals with successively thicker filaments until a correct response is obtained. If no response is obtained with the filament marked 6.65 in a given zone, the pinprick test is used as a final test of sensibility in that zone.

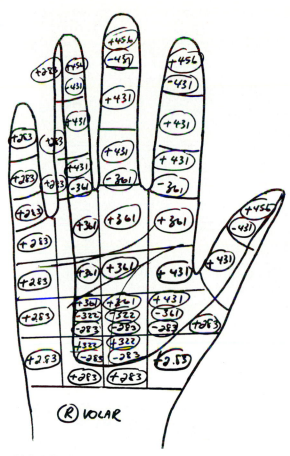

FIG. 36-9. Life-sized outline of hand, subdivided into zones allows detailed recording of responses to the Semmes-Weinstein Pressure Aesthesiometer.

TABLE 36-2. Scale of interpretation for Semmes-Weinstein Pressure Aesthesiometer: light touch–deep pressure

Code	Level	Filaments
Green	Normal light touch	2.36-2.83
Blue	Diminished light touch	3.22-3.61
Purple	Diminished protective sensation	3.84-4.31
Red	Loss of protective sensation	4.56-6.65
Red lined	Unresponsive to 6.65	

Modified from Levin, S., Pearsall, G., and Ruderman, R.: J. Hand Surg. **3**(3):211, 1978.

The zones are tested in a random sequence.

It is essential in this test to carefully record accurate and inaccurate responses, because it is easy to forget where a stimulus has been previously applied and how the patient responded. Careful recording makes the test shorter, more accurate, and more validly compared to follow-up tests. Careful recording has the further advantage of documenting inconsistencies in the responses of a suspected malingerer. An example of a useful code for the work sheet is the following: +2.83 (first positive response to 2.83 monofil-

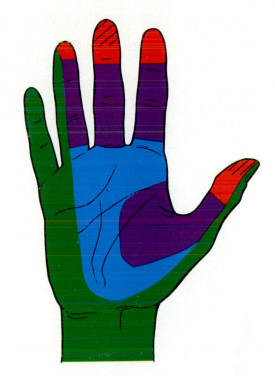

FIG. 36-10. Color-coded mapping of hand is used to report results of the Semmes-Weinstein light touch–deep pressure test. (From Bell, J.A.: Sensibility Evaluation. In Hunter, J.M., Schneider, L.H., Mackin, E.J., and Bell, J.A., editors: Rehabilitation of the hand, St. Louis, 1978, The C.V. Mosby Co.)

ament); +2.83 (second positive response; testing complete in that zone); −2.83 (first negative response to 2.83); −2.83 (second negative response to 2.83; test at random intervals with thicker filaments until accurate responses are obtained); +3.22 (first positive response to 3.22); and so on. Detailed documentation of this nature requires a work sheet with a life-sized outline of the hand to provide space for notations (Fig. 36-9). Each examiner can devise his own code, so long as it facilitates accuracy in recording.

A scale of interpretation[3] (Table 36-2) is used to assess the results of this test. The norms in this scale have not been standardized but are based upon clinical observation of light-touch function in hundreds of nerve-injured hands (see Chapter 35). The information on the grid work sheet is transferred to a color-coded outline of the hand for a formal report (Fig. 36-10). The following colors, for example, correspond to the four levels of sensibility in the scale of interpretation: Green on the outline indicates an area in which 2.83, the filament representing normal light touch, was perceived. Blue indicates areas where filaments marked 3.22 or 3.61, corresponding to diminished light touch, were perceived. Purple represents area where filaments marked 3.84 to 4.31, corresponding to diminished protective sensation, were perceived. Red represents areas of loss of protective sensation, where only filaments marked 4.56 to 6.65 were perceived, and a red-lined area would indicate that no filament was perceived. Clinical interpretation of the levels of sensibility is described more fully in Chapter 35.

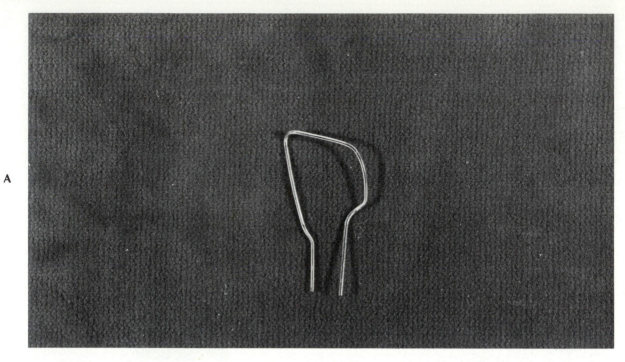

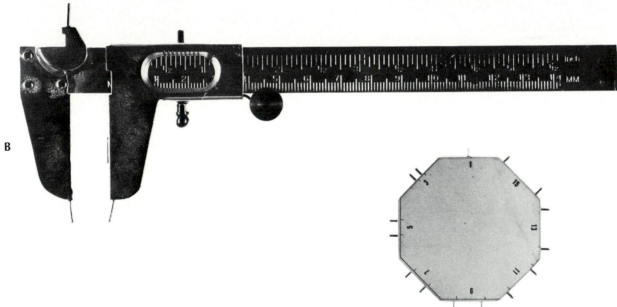

FIG. 36-11. A, Paper clip is not recommended for testing two-point discrimination because manufacturing process results in a barb on one end; therefore testing ends are not uniform. **B,** Caliper with blunt ends, such as Boley gauge, *top left,* or DeMayo 2-Point Discrimination Device, *bottom right,* is recommended.

The time required for this test varies with the severity of the dysfunction and the experience of the tester. The experienced tester may require as little as 10 minutes or as much as 30 minutes or longer to carefully perform the test.

For greater reliability of the instrument, Levin has recommended that the kit be stored at "reasonably constant temperatures and moderate humidity" in order to preserve the correct mechanical properties of the filaments.[24] Serial

tests should be carried out by the same examiner. If a filament is not perpendicular within its Lucite handle and cannot be manually realigned by the examiner, it should not be used. Storage for several days or weeks will frequently result in perpendicular realignment of filament; if not realigned, it should be replaced. Ideally, the filaments should be recalibrated periodically.[24] If this is not feasible, the finer filaments, which lose their mechanical properties more easily, should be replaced periodically.

Functional tests

The presence of fine discriminative sensation determines the usefulness of the sensibility in daily activities. Therefore selection of tests and interpretation of results must be done carefully before one declares that a patient has normal discriminative sensibility.

Two-point discrimination. Two-point discrimination (2PD) is the classic test of functional sensibility because it is generally acknowledged to relate to the ability to use the hand for fine tasks.[25,30] (However, Dellon[13] has summarized several studies that refute this correlation.) Moberg has stated that 6 mm of two-point discrimination is required for winding a watch, 6 to 8 mm for sewing, and 12 mm for handling precision tools, and that above 15 mm gross tool handling may be possible, but only with decreased speed and skill.

The test instrument should be light and have blunt testing ends. A paper clip (Fig. 36-11, *A*), though light, is not recommended because the manufacturing process results in a sharp barb on one end, which the examiner must be careful to apply away from the skin to avoid stimulation of pain receptors. A Boley Gauge* or other caliper with blunt ends such as the DeMayo 2-Point Discrimination Device† (Fig. 36-11, *B*) is recommended. The measuring scales incorporated into these instruments make them convenient to use. The Boley Gauge has the further advantage of being adjustable in 1-mm increments; however, one must be careful to avoid applying too much pressure with the relatively heavy Boley Gauge.

Regardless of the instrument used, the patient's hand should be fully supported. During the test vision is occluded. Only the fingertips need be tested because it is the fingertips that are the most important in active exploration and tactile scanning of an object. Testing is begun with the instrument set at a 5-mm distance between the two points. One or two ends are applied lightly to the fingertip in a random sequence in a longitudinal orientation to avoid crossover from overlapping digital nerves (Fig. 36-12). A common error is to apply too much pressure. Since it is light touch discrimination that is being tested and the patient is to be compared to the normal population, the pressure applied should be very light and stop just at the point of blanching.[6] Seven out of 10 responses must be accurate for scoring. If the responses are inaccurate, the distance between the ends is increased by increments of 1, 2, or 5 mm, depending on the suspected severity of the dysfunction, until the required accurate responses are elicited. Testing is stopped at 15 mm (or less, if the pulp is not of sufficient length) if responses are inaccurate at that level.

Interpretation of scores is based on the guidelines set by the American Society for Surgery of the Hand[2] (Table 36-3).

Localization of touch. None of the tests described thus far have required localization of a stimulus. Localization represents a more integrated level of perception than simple

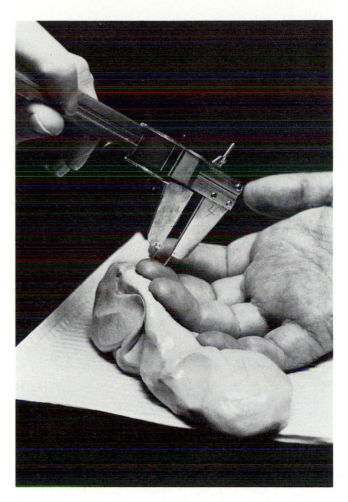

FIG. 36-12. The two-point discrimination instrument is applied lightly to fingertip in a longitudinal orientation.

TABLE 36-3. Two-point discrimination norms

Normal:	Less than 6 mm
Fair:	6 to 10 mm
Poor:	11 to 15 mm
Protective:	One point perceived
Anesthetic:	No points perceived

recognition of a stimulus; therefore it should be tested as a separate function. The ability to localize was found by Weinstein[48] in a study of 48 normal adults to have a high correlation with two-point discrimination (.92), while neither two-point discrimination nor localization was found to have a high correlation with light touch threshold (.17 and .28 respectively). Because of its high correlation with two-point discrimination, localization is considered to be a test of functional sensation.

Localization is most appropriate for testing after nerve repair because the poor localization that typically occurs after repair can seriously limit function. The stimulus used is the same as that used for light touch, that is, cotton ball,

---

*Boley Gauge, Research Designs, Inc., 7320 Ashcroft, Suite 103, Houston, Tex. 77081.
†DeMayo 2-Point Discrimination Device, Padgett Instruments, 2838 Warwick Trafficway, Kansas City, Mo. 64108.

fingertip, and so on, or the finest Semmes-Weinstein mono-filament that resulted in a positive response during light touch testing. Unlike two-point discrimination, which is tested only on the fingertips, localization is tested over the entire area of dysfunction.

The grid is most useful for recording the results of this test.[49] With the patient's vision occluded and the hand fully supported, a stimulus is applied to the center of a given zone. The patient is instructed to open his eyes each time he feels a touch and point to the exact spot touched. His responses will be more accurate if he uses his vision to help localize than if he attempts to localize with his eyes closed.[18] If the stimulus is correctly localized, a dot is marked in the corresponding zone on the work sheet. If the stimulus is incorrectly localized, an arrow is drawn on the work sheet from the site of stimulation to the site of referral (Fig. 36-13). Each zone is stimulated only once. The resulting data on the work sheet are used as the permanent record. The work sheet gives the examiner and the patient a graphic representation of the quality of localization and points out patterns of referral that might be amenable to sensory reeducation. With improvement in localization over time, the localization worksheets should demonstrate fewer and shorter arrows.

Moving two-point discrimination. The rationale for this test, devised by Dellon,[11,12] is that since fingertip sensibility is highly dependent on motion the stimulus for discrimination testing should be moving. Dellon recommends a reshaped paper clip for testing, with the barb pointing away from the surface to be tested. However, for the reasons stated above, one might choose instead to use a Boley Gauge* or similar caliper. Testing is begun with the instrument set at an 8 mm distance between the two points. The instrument is moved proximally to distally on the fingertip parallel to the long axis of the finger, with the testing ends side by side (Fig. 36-14). The pressure used is just light enough so that the subject can appreciate the stimulus. Once the patient is inaccurate or hesistant in responding, he is required to respond accurately to seven out of 10 stimuli before the distance is narrowed. Testing is stopped at 2 mm, which represents normal moving two-point discrimination (m2PD).[11]

Dellon has reported that moving two-point discrimination always returns earlier than two-point discrimination after nerve laceration and approaches normal 2 to 6 months before two-point discrimination reaches normal. Therefore he advocates this test as a more valid assessment of discrimination and as an earlier means of assessing return of discrimination than the classic 2-point test.

Ridge sensitometer. The Ridge Sensitometer,† or plastic ridge device, was designed by Poppen[34,35] as a modification of a depth-sensitivity device described by Renfrew.[38] The instrument is a clear plastic rectangular block (Fig. 36-15, A). Along the center of the testing surface is a smooth ridge that progresses from a height of zero at one end to 1.5 mm at the opposite end. The opposite surface is marked at centimeter intervals for scoring. Values of 0.5, 1.5, and 2.5 cm on that scale correspond to ridge heights of 0.15, 0.30, and 0.45 mm respectively.[34]

This device was first reported for use in assessment of

---

*Boley Gauge, Research Designs Inc., 7320 Ashcroft, Suite 103, Houston, Tex. 77081.
†Ridge Sensitometer, Howmedica, Inc., Orthopedics Division, 359 Veterans Blvd, Rutherford, N.J. 07070.

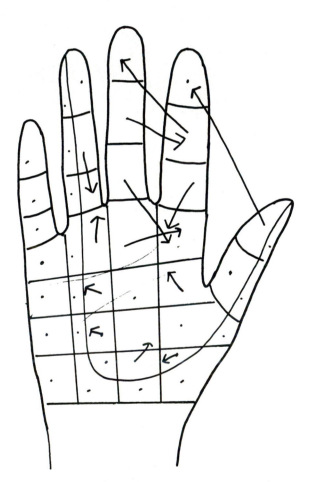

Fig. 36-13. Mapping of localization. *Dot,* Stimulus that was accurately perceived; *arrow,* referred stimulus; *arrowhead,* point to which stimulus was referred.

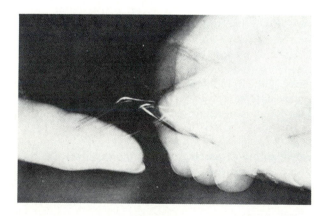

Fig. 36-14. The m2PD instrument is applied to fingertip with testing ends side by side. Instrument is moved lightly across fingertip from proximal to distal position. (From Dellon, A.L.: J. Hand Surg. **3**:474-481, 1978.)

sensibility after suture of digital nerves.[34] After the area of dysfunction has been mapped, the digit to be tested is supported in the examiner's hand and the patient's vision is occluded. The ridge device is lightly moved over the area of maximal deficit in a proximal-to-distal direction, with care being taken to avoid touching areas of normal sensibility (Fig. 36-15, *B*). The ridge should be moved at a rate of 1 cm/sec, over the area being tested. A pause of 7 to 10 seconds is necessary between repeat trials to obtain maximum threshold sensibility. The patient is instructed to say ''now'' when the surface is not smooth when the device is applied.[34,35]

The ridge device measures the depth-sense limen.[36] On the normal finger the ridge will be perceived at or before the first centimeter marking, corresponding to a ridge height of approximately 0.23 mm. Poppen states that testing results can be interpreted functionally and are most useful for de-

termining the presence or absence of tactile gnosis in patients whose two-point discrimination results fall between 8 and 12 mm, a range that, according to Poppen, may or may not indicate tactile gnosis. If the ridge can be felt at or before the 2-cm mark, tactile gnosis is present and the two-point discrimination is ≤10 mm. If the ridge device cannot be felt, tactile gnosis is absent and the two-point discrimination is ≥8 mm.[34,35]

According to Poppen, then, the advantage of this test is that it yields a more accurate assessment of tactile gnosis in less than one tenth the time required for two-point discrimination testing.

Seddon coin test. The Seddon coin test is a functional test that requires both motor and sensory participation; it is indicated for median or combined medioulnar lesions. Although Seddon popularized the test, he states that he did not originate it.[41] He also states that it is often described

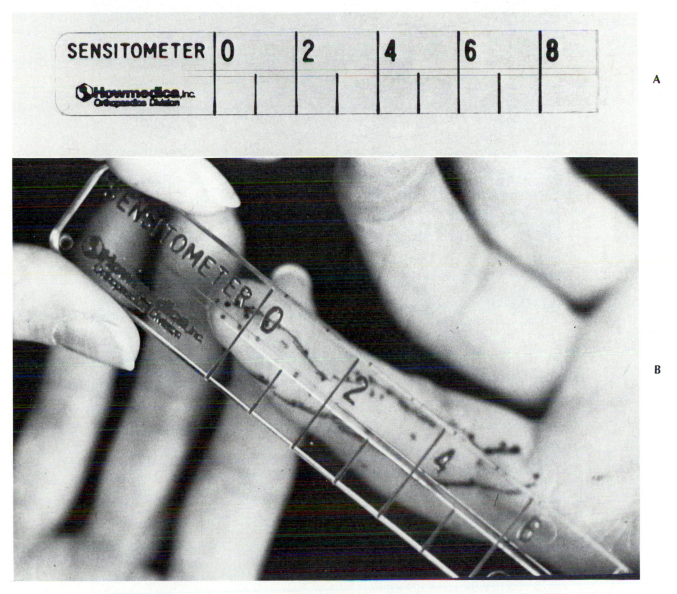

A

B

FIG. 36-15. **A,** Ridge Sensitometer. **B,** Device is lightly moved over area of maximal deficit in a proximal-to-distal direction.

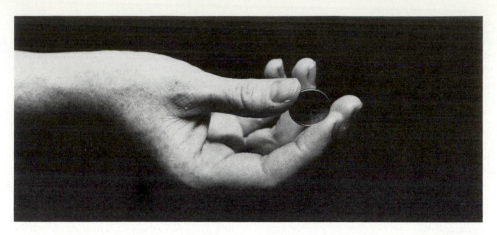

FIG. 36-16. Correct administration of Seddon coin test requires that coin be actively manipulated by patient.

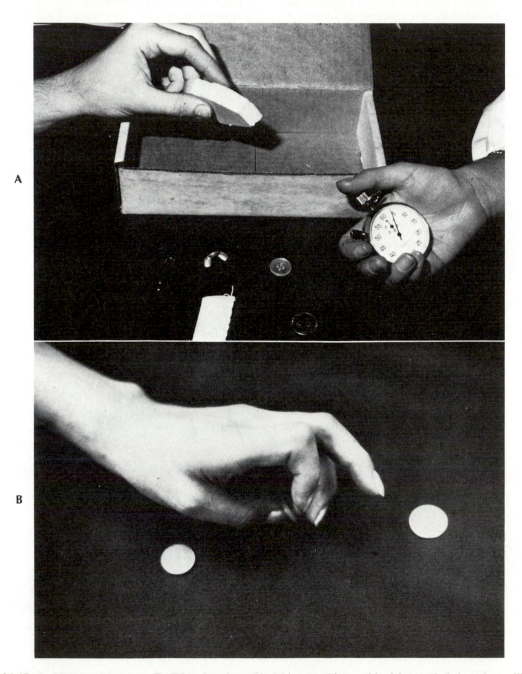

FIG. 36-17. A, Moberg pickup test. B, When locating and picking up objects with vision occluded, patient will tend not to use sensory surfaces that have poor sensibility.

inaccurately as one in which the skin involved is stroked with a smooth-edged coin and then with a milled-edged coin and the patient is asked to discriminate between the two. The correct method entails placing the coin in the patient's hand and asking him to manipulate it to determine whether it is smooth or milled (Fig. 36-16). As such, this test was a precursor to the Moberg pickup test.[41]

There are no norms associated with this test, but as an observational test it can provide information regarding gross discrimination ability in the fingertips.

Moberg pickup test. The Moberg pickup test,[25,26] a functional test like the coin test, requires motor participation and is most appropriate for median or combined medioulnar lesions. An assortment of everyday objects, the number and nature of which are selected by the examiner, is placed on a table in front of the patient. He is instructed to pick them up one at a time, as fast as he can, and place them into a box using his involved hand (Fig. 36-17, *A*). The examiner times him and notes which digits are used for prehension. The patient repeats the task with his uninvolved hand. Finally, he is asked to pick up objects again, but this time with eyes closed. Again, time required and manner of prehension are noted. When locating and picking up objects with vision occluded, the patient will tend not to use sensory surfaces that have poor sensibility (Fig. 36-17, *B*).

Norms have not been established for this test. Its value lies in the observations that can be made during the brief time it requires to administer. Taking into account motor deficits, the best comparison for the involved hand is the performance by the uninvolved hand. The test can be made more difficult by requiring the patient to identify the objects as he picks them up.

Dellon modification of Moberg pickup test. Dellon has modified the pickup test by standardizing the items used and requiring identification of them. He chose objects of similar material to avoid giving cues by texture or temperature and objects graded to require increasing ability to discriminate (Fig. 36-18).[12]

In cases in which the ulnar nerve is not involved, the ulnar digits are taped to the palm. The patient is timed as he picks up the objects and places them into a box. If the motor deficit is judged too severe during this sighted part of the test, the test is discontinued. If the deficit is not too severe, vision is occluded and the examiner places one item at a time into the median three digits for patient identification. The time required for identification is recorded; no more than 30 seconds is permitted per object. Each object is presented twice. Normal values, based upon the performance of 10 adults, for the pickup and recognition parts of this test are presented in Tables 36-4 and 36-5.

Objective tests

Two objective tests, the Ninhydrin sweat test and the wrinkle test, are described below because of their occasional usefulness in testing, especially for children and suspected malingerers. As stated previously, they can give suggestive evidence of sensory function early after nerve laceration and in long-term cases where regeneration has failed, but they do not correlate directly with the presence or absence of sensibility during regeneration.[24,32,33,44]

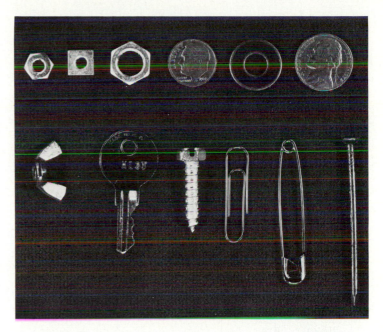

FIG. 36-18. Items used in Dellon modification of Moberg pickup test.

TABLE 36-4. Modified picking-up test—normal values for object pick-up*

Trial I		Trial II	
Mean (sec)	**Range (sec)**	**Mean (sec)**	**Range (sec)**
13	10-19	11	9-16

From Dellon, A.L.: Evaluation of sensibility and re-education of sensation in the hand, Baltimore, 1981, The Williams & Wilkins Co. © 1981, The Williams & Wilkins Co., Baltimore.
*n = 8.

TABLE 36-5. Modified picking-up test—normal values for object recognition*

Object	Trial I		Trial II	
	Mean (sec)	**Range (sec)**	**Mean (sec)**	**Range (sec)**
1. Wing nut	1.7	1-3	2.0	1-3
2. Screw	1.4	1-2	1.5	1-2
3. Key	1.5	1-3	1.6	1-2
4. Nail	1.7	1-4	1.5	1-2
5. Large nut	1.8	1-3	1.4	1-2
6. Nickel	1.8	1-3	2.0	2
7. Dime	1.7	1-5	1.3	1-2
8. Washer	1.8	1-3	1.7	1-3
9. Safety pin	1.6	1-2	1.6	1-2
10. Paper clip	2.3	1-5	2.1	1-3
11. Small nut (hex)	2.1	1-3	1.6	1-3
12. Small nut (square)	1.6	1-3	1.6	1-3

From Dellon, A.L.: Evaluation of sensibility and re-education of sensation in the hand, Baltimore, 1981, The Williams & Wilkins Co. © 1981, The Williams & Wilkins Co., Baltimore.
*n = 8.

Ninhydrin sweat test. The method of administration has been described by several authors,[15,25,32,33,43] but those described by Perry[32] and Phelps[33] are the easiest to follow since they make use of commercially available Ninhydrin developer and fixer (Fig. 36-19). The essentials of their techniques are presented below.

The patient's hand is cleansed thoroughly with soap and warm water, rinsed thoroughly, and then wiped with ether, alcohol, or acetone. Perry recommends a 5-minute waiting period to allow the normal sweating process to ensue, while Phelps requires a 20- to 30-minute period to elapse before proceeding with the test. During the waiting period, the patient's fingertips must not come into contact with any surface.

At the end of the waiting period, the fingertips are pressed with a moderate amount of pressure against a good quality bond paper (no. 20) that has previously been untouched. The fingertips are traced with a pencil and held in place for 15 seconds. During this time the examiner must be careful not to touch any part of the paper and the patient's fingertips must not slide on the paper to avoid contamination of the results.

The paper is then sprayed with Ninhydrin spray reagent (N-0507)* and allowed to dry for 24 hours or heated in an

oven for 5 to 10 minutes at 200° F (93° C). During the development period the Ninhydrin stains purple the amino acids and lower peptide components of sweat that have penetrated the paper. After development, the prints are sprayed with Ninhydrin fixer reagent (N-0757)* for a permanent record of the results.

According to Perry, a good normal print is one in which dots can be clearly visualized representing discrete sweat gland orifices. A blank print indicates that no sweating has occurred. A smudged print may represent a finger that moved during testing, or hyperhidrosis that has stained beyond its boundaries and may be masking an area of anhidrosis.[32]

Moberg has scored Ninhydrin test results on a 0 to 3 scale, with 0 representing absent sweating and 3 representing normal sweating.[25]

Wrinkle test. The wrinkle test was described by O-Riain[31] in 1973. He observed that a denervated hand placed in warm water (40° C; 104° F) for 30 minutes does not wrinkle in the denervated area as normal skin does. He associated this phenomenon with an absence of sensory function, and the return of wrinkling with a return of sensory function.

In a study of 41 nerve-injured patients, using the same finger-wrinkling method, Phelps[33] found that only after recent complete laceration did an absence of finger wrinkling always correlate with an absence of sensibility. In patients

---

*Sigma Chemical Company, P.O. Box 14508, St. Louis, Mo. 63178.

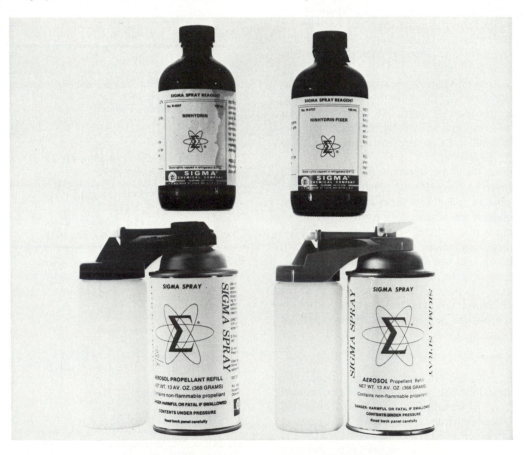

FIG. 36-19. Materials required for ninhydrin sweat test.

with nerve compression, the presence of wrinkling does not indicate intact sensibility. Therefore the wrinkle test appears to be of most use after recent nerve laceration, particularly in children and others unable or unwilling to cooperate with a sensibility examination.

Phelps noted that the results of finger wrinkling are difficult to document, even photographically. She used the same 0 to 3 scoring system to rate the amount of wrinkling that Moberg used for scoring the Ninhydrin test.

SENSIBILITY EVALUATION BATTERY

This chapter has considered the essentials of a sensibility evaluation, the variety of tests in current use, and methods of controlling variables during testing; the question now arises as to which tests are appropriate for different types of nerve dysfunction. Certainly, no single test can adequately assess the complexity of sensibility. Evaluation is best approached by a battery of tests selected to answer specific questions depending on the history presented and the information desired. Other pertinent factors in selection include time available for testing, examiner familiarity with a particular test, and age and concentration level of the patient. Presented below are guidelines for selection of tests. In all cases, the selected battery of tests must be supplemented by the other essentials of a sensibility evaluation: history, examination of the hand, and knowledgeable interpretation of results.

Guidelines for test selection after laceration, severe crush, or traction injury

In assessing a patient after severe nerve injury, inspection of the hand for evidence of sympathetic dysfunction is always indicated, as well as determination of the area of sensory dysfunction by mapping. Further selection of tests is based upon the specific information desired, as presented below:

1. Is regeneration of sensory fibers progressing? Here, Tinel's sign and serial mapping to determine shrinkage or lack of shrinkage of the area of sensory dysfunction are indicated.
2. Is protective sensation present? Pinprick perception is the most accepted measure of protective sensation. Suggestive evidence is provided by inspection of the hand for blisters, ulcers, and other trophic changes associated with long-term denervation, as well as by the patient's subjective statements regarding function.
3. Is light touch present? This can be answered grossly by the use of a cotton ball, fingertip, pencil eraser, or cottonwool, applied lightly with either a constant touch (preferred) or moving touch. If information regarding the relative differences in the touch threshold between adjacent skin areas is desired, testing with a graded touch stimulus such as the Semmes-Weinstein Pressure Aesthesiometer is indicated.
4. Is functional sensibility (tactile gnosis) present? Two-point discrimination testing on the fingertips provides information that is easily interpreted by other professionals. Localization of touch tested on the entire area of dysfunction provides information on the amount

and patterns of referral and is a good evaluation tool to indicate a need for sensory reeducation. Moving two-point discrimination and the ridge sensitometer are quickly applied tests of fingertip function. Both are reported to correlate with tactile gnosis, but neither is currently used as widely as classic two-point discrimination. The Seddon coin test, Moberg pickup test, and Dellon modification of the pickup test integrate motor and sensory function and are all quickly administered. They are most appropriate for median or combined medioulnar nerve dysfunction. (Only one of these need be administered.) Inspection of the hand for "wear marks" and the patient's report of functional use of the hand in activities of daily living will provide further evidence of functional sensibility.

The above questions are listed in a hierarchy progressing from a state of minimal sensibility to normal sensibility (Table 36-6). If a patient presents early after nerve injury or presents with severe trophic changes, it is most appropriate to ask questions and select tests from the bottom of the hierarchy (for example, Is regeneration progressing?). If the patient presents late after nerve repair, if sympathetic function looks good, and if he reports functional use of the hand, it is most appropriate to start with the question, Is functional sensation present? and proceed to the other questions if the answer is no.

For those suspected of malingering, the Semmes-Weinstein Pressure Aesthesiometer can be especially useful in documenting inconsistencies in responses. For the child, the wrinkle test, possibly the ninhydrin sweat test, and the Moberg pickup test may provide the information desired regarding function.

TABLE 36-6. Guidelines for test selection after laceration, severe crush, or traction injury

Information desired	Indicators
1. Is regeneration progressing?	Tinel's sign Serial mapping
2. Is protective sensation present?	Pin prick Skin inspection
3. Is light touch present?	Nongraded tests (cotton ball, fingertip, and so on) Graded tests (Semmes-Weinstein Pressure Aesthesiometer)
4. Is functional sensibility present?	Two-point discrimination Localization Moving two-point discrimination Ridge Sensitometer Pickup test Dellon modification of pickup test "Wear marks" on skin

HAND REHABILITATION CENTER   P.1
901 Walnut Street
Philadelphia, Pa. 19107

SENSIBILITY EVALUATION SUMMARY

Name_____   Eval. #_____

Chart #_____   Date:_____

Dominance_____   Ex: _____

Age _____

HISTORY:

_____

PATIENT SUBJECTIVE DESCRIPTION

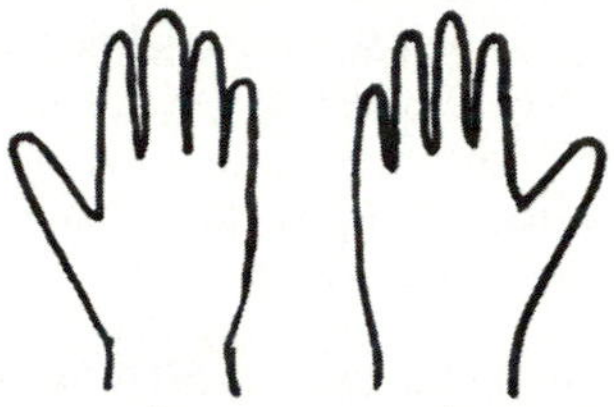

                                         L/R   L/R
                                   Sensation Decreased
                                   Sensation Absent
                                   Paraesthesia

ROM | SYMPATHETIC FUNCTION

MUSCLE FUNCTION

_____

Grip (lbs.)   (Jamar #_____)   Pinch (lbs.)

R) 1_____   L) 1_____   Lateral R)____   L)_____

   2_____   2_____   Pulp   R)____   L)_____

   3_____   3_____

   4_____   4_____

   5_____   5_____   6/82

FIG. 36-20. Sensibility evaluation forms used at Hand Rehabilitation Center in Philadelphia, Pa.

SENSIBILITY EVALUATION SUMMARY   P.2

Chart#: _____

Eval. #: _____

Tactile Gnosis   (Moberg Pick-Up Test: _____objects)

Date: _____

	R	sec.	L	sec.
Eyes Open		sec.		sec.
Eyes Closed		sec.		sec.

Comments:

TWO POINT DISCRIMINATION (mm.)

LIGHT TOUCH - DEEP PRESSURE (VON FREY)

Two Point Discrimination (mm.)

	I	II	III	IV	V
R				/	
L				/	

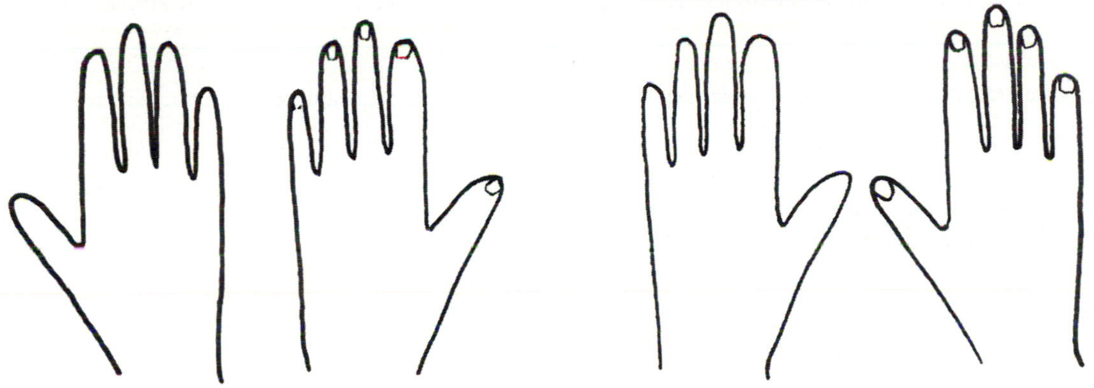

(L) VOLAR   (L) DORSAL   (R) VOLAR   (R) DORSAL

ASSH 2 P.D. SCALE

0mm - 6mm	Normal
6mm - 10mm	Fair
11mm - 15mm	Poor

1 Point Perceived:
            Protective

No Point Perceived:
            Anesthetic

LIGHT TOUCH - DEEP PRESSURE: SCALE OF INTERPRETATION

Green	Normal	2.36 - 2.83
Blue	Diminished light touch	3.22 - 3.61
Purple	Diminished protective sensation	3.84 - 4.31
Red	Loss of protective sensation	4.56 - 6.65
Red Lined	Unresponsive to 6.65	

6/82

FIG. 36-20, cont'd. For legend see opposite page.

Guidelines for test selection for nontraumatic nerve compression

Early changes in sensibility because of nontraumatic compression of the median and ulnar nerves will generally be reflected in the fingertips, particularly the index fingertip for the median nerve and the little fingertip for the ulnar nerve. Since early changes are subtle, it is most appropriate to begin with the more subtle tests such as two-point discrimination and possibly moving two-point discrimination. Even if these are normal, testing for light touch using a graded stimulus is indicated, because the only early change may be a slight decrease in light touch sensibility on a fingertip.[28] The other functional tests and modality tests will not pick up these early changes though they will pick up advanced changes.

Hand rehabilitation center sensibility battery

The sensibility battery used at the Hand Rehabilitation Center in Philadelphia includes patient history, patient's description of his nerve-related problems, examination of the sympathetic function in the hand, mapping, grip and pinch tests, manual muscle testing in selected cases, and a core group of tests: light touch–deep pressure using the Semmes Weinstein Pressure Aesthesiometer, two-point discrimination, and the Moberg pickup test (Fig. 36-20). We have found that this particular battery provides the desired information in most patients referred for sensibility evaluation. In selected cases the battery has been supplemented by each of the other tests described above. In different settings, different batteries will be appropriate.

SUMMARY

A thorough and accurate sensibility evaluation requires a careful history, knowledgeable examination of sympathetic function in the hand, skillful interviewing of the patient, and knowledge of the tests available and their correct administration. Additionally, the examiner must strive to control the variables associated with testing and select a battery of tests designed to answer specific questions based upon the patient's history. The careful examiner who criticizes his methods and who listens to his patients will learn from each patient and will become a skilled examiner. The skilled examiner will accept the challenge of sensibility as an always interesting and at times fascinating task.

REFERENCES

1. Almquist, E., and Eeg-Olofsson, O.: Sensory nerve conduction velocity and two-point discrimination in sutured nerves, J. Bone Joint Surg. **52A:**791, 1970.
2. American Society for Surgery of the Hand: The hand: examination and diagnosis, Aurora, Colo., 1978, The Society.
3. Bell, J.A.: Sensibility evaluation. In Hunter, J.M., Schneider, L.H., Mackin, E.J., and Bell, J.A., editors: Rehabilitation of the hand, St. Louis, 1978, The C.V. Mosby Co.
4. Bell, J.A., and Buford, W.L.: The force/time relationship of clinically used sensory testing instruments. Presented at the thirty-seventh annual meeting of the American Society for Surgery of the Hand, New Orleans, 1982.
5. Bowden, R.E.M.: Factors influencing functional recovery. In Seddon, H.J., editor: Peripheral nerve injuries, London, 1954, Her Majesty's Stationery Office.
6. Brand, P.W.: Functional manifestations of sensory loss. Presented at symposium, Assessment of levels of cutaneous sensibility, U.S. Public Health Service Hospital, Carville, La., Sept. 1980.
7. Brunelli, S.G.: Gnostic rings for assessment of tactile gnosis, American Society for Surgery of the Hand Newsletter, no. 53, 1981.
8. Bunnell, S.: Surgery of the hand, ed. 5, revised by Boyes, J.H., Philadelphia, 1970, J.B. Lippincott Co.
9. Clark, W.C.: Pain sensitivity and the report of pain: an introduction to sensory decision theory, Anesthesiology **40:**272, 1974.
10. Dellon, A.L., Curtis, R.M., and Edgerton, M.T.: Reeducation of sensation in the hand after nerve injury and repair, Plast. Reconstr. Surg. **53:**297, 1974.
11. Dellon, A.L.: The moving two-point discrimination test: clinical evaluation of the quickly-adapting fiber/receptor system, J. Hand Surg. **3:**474, 1978.
12. Dellon, A.L.: The paper clip: light hardware to evaluate sensibility in the hand, Contemp. Orthop. **1**(3):39-42, 1979.
13. Dellon, A.L.: Evaluation of sensibility and reeducation of sensation in the hand, Baltimore, 1981, The Williams & Wilkins Co.
14. Dorland's illustrated medical dictionary, ed. 26, Philadelphia, 1981, W.B. Saunders Co.
15. Flynn, J.E., and Flynn, W.F.: Median and ulnar nerve injuries: a long range study with evaluation of the Ninhydrin test, sensory and motor return, Ann. Surg. **156:**1002, 1962.
16. Gibson, J.: Observations on active touch, Psychol. Rev. **69:**477, 1962.
17. Grindley, G.C.: The variation of sensory thresholds with the rate of application of the stimulus, Br. J. Psychol. **27:**86, 1936.
18. Halnan, C.R.E., and Wright, G.H.: Tactile localization, Brain **83:**677, 1960.
19. Haymaker, W., and Woodhall, B.: Peripheral nerve injuries: principles of diagnosis, ed. 2, Philadelphia, 1953, W.B. Saunders Co.
20. Henderson, W.R.: Clinical assessment of peripheral nerve injuries: Tinel's test, Lancet **2:**801, 1948.
21. Kanatani, F.N.: A steel wire aesthesiometer. Presented at symposium, Assessment of levels of cutaneous sensibility, U.S. Public Health Service Hospital, Carville, La., Sept. 1980.
22. Kirk, E.J., and Denny-Brown, D.: Functional variation in dermatomes in the macaque monkey following dorsal root lesions, J. Comp. Neurol. **139:**307, 1970.
23. LaMotte, R.H.: Sensory discrimination and neural correlation. Presented at symposium, Assessment of levels of cutaneous sensibility, U.S. Public Health Service Hospital, Carville, La., Sept. 1980.
24. Levin, S., Pearsall, G., and Ruderman, R.J.: Von Frey's method of measuring pressure sensibility in the hand: an engineering analysis of the Weinstein-Semmes Pressure Aesthesiometer, J. Hand Surg. **3:**211, 1978.
25. Moberg, E.: Objective methods for determining the functional value of sensibility in the hand, J. Bone Joint Surg. **40B:**454, 1958.
26. Moberg, E.: Criticism and study of methods for examining sensibility in the hand, Neurology **12:**8, 1962.
27. Moberg, E.: Nerve repair in hand surgery: an analysis, Surg. Clin. North Am. **48:**985, 1968.
28. Moran, C.A.: Comparison of sensory testing methods using carpal tunnel syndrome patients, Unpublished master's thesis, Medical College of Virginia/Virginia Commonwealth University, Richmond, Va., 1981.
29. Omer, G.E.: Sensation and sensibility in the upper extremity, Clin. Orthop. Rel. Res. **104:**30, 1974.
30. Onne, L.: Recovery of sensibility and sudomotor activity in the hand after nerve suture, Acta Chir. Scand. (Suppl.) **300:**1, 1962.
31. O'Riain, S.: New and simple test of nerve function in the hand, Br. Med. J. **22:**615, 1973.
32. Perry, J.F., Hamilton, G.F., Lachenbruch, P.A., and others: Protective sensation in the hand and its correlation to the Ninhydrin sweat test following nerve laceration, Am. J. Phys. Med. **53:**113, 1974.
33. Phelps, P., and Walker, E.: Comparison of the finger wrinkling test results to established sensory tests in peripheral nerve injury, Am. J. Occup. Ther. **31:**9, 1977.
34. Poppen, N.K., McCarroll, H.R., Doyle, J.R., and others: Recovery of sensibility after suture of digital nerves, J. Hand Surg. **4:**212, 1979.
35. Poppen, N.K.: Clinical evaluation of the von Frey and two-point discrimination tests and correlation with a dynamic test of sensibility.

In Jewett, D.L., and McCarroll, H.K., editors: Symposium on nerve repair: its clinical and experimental basis, St. Louis, 1979, The C.V. Mosby Co.

36. Poppen, N.K., and McCarroll, H.R.: The plastic ridge device and moving 2-point discrimination (Letter to the editor), J. Hand Surg. **5:**92, 1980.

37. Porter, R.W.: New test for fingertip sensation, Br. Med. J. **2:**927, 1966.

38. Renfrew, S.: Fingertip sensation: a routine neurological test, Lancet **1:**396, 1969.

39. Richards, R.L.: Vasomotor and nutritional disturbances following injuries to peripheral nerves. In Seddon, H.J., editor: Peripheral nerve injuries, London, 1954, Her Majesty's Stationery Office.

40. Seddon, H.J., editor: Peripheral nerve injuries, London, 1954, Her Majesty's Printing Office.

41. Seddon, H.J.: Surgical disorders of the peripheral nerves, ed. 2, New York, 1975, Churchill Livingstone.

42. Semmes, J., Weinstein, S., Ghent, L., Teuber, H.-L.: Somatosensory changes after penetrating brain wounds in man, Cambridge, Mass., 1960, Harvard University Press.

43. Stromberg, W.B., McFarlane, R.M., Bell, J.L., and others: Injury of the median and ulnar nerves: one hundred and fifty cases with an evaluation of Moberg's Ninhydrin test, J. Bone Joint Surg. **43A:**717, 1961.

44. Sunderland, S.: Nerves and nerve injuries, ed. 2, New York, 1978, Churchill Livingstone.

45. Tinel, J.: The "tingling" sign in peripheral nerve lesions (Translated by Emanuel B. Kaplan). In Spinner, M.: Injuries to the major branches of peripheral nerves of the forearm, ed. 2, Philadelphia, 1978, W.B. Saunders Co.

46. Trotter, W., and Davies, H.M.: Experimental studies in the innervation of the skin, J. Physiol. **38:**134, 1909.

47. von Prince, K., and Butler, B.: Measuring sensory function of the hand in peripheral nerve injuries, Am. J. Occup. Ther. **21:**385, 1967.

48. Weinstein, S.: Intensive and extensive aspects of tactile sensitivity as a function of body part, sex and laterality. In Kenshalo, D.R., editor: The skin senses, Springfield, Ill., 1968, Charles C Thomas, Publisher.

49. Werner, J.L., and Omer, G.E.: Evaluating cutaneous pressure sensation of the hand, Am. J. Occup. Ther. **24:**347, 1970.

37

Methods of compensation and reeducation for sensory dysfunction

ANNE D. CALLAHAN

The quality of sensibility that returns to the hand after nerve repair in the adult is well documented in the literature: results are poor, as measured by localization, two-point discrimination, tactile gnosis, and other tests of functional sensation. Numerous investigators* have noted the poor localization that occurs after nerve repair even when there has been good return of pain, temperature, and touch perception. Regarding two-point discrimination Stromberg[23] found that in 150 cases of nerve repair, of which half were at least 2 years after repair, normal or near-normal two-point discrimination was recovered in all children less than 10 years old—but in only three adults. In Onne's[19] classic study of results after "ideal" nerve suture, two-point discrimination was found to correspond with the patient's age up to 20 years. Between the ages of 20 and 30, results varied but were mainly poor. After 30 to 35 years, two-point discrimination was poor in all cases of median or ulnar nerve repair. Similarly, Almquist and Eeg-Olofsson[1] found a linear relationship between two-point discrimination and age until the time of puberty, with adults demonstrating poor clinical results. The universal conclusion is that the prognosis for return of normal sensibility after nerve repair is good in the child but poor in the adult.

WHY THE RETURN OF FUNCTIONAL SENSATION IS POOR

Functional sensation is poor after nerve repair because regeneration of sensory fibers is imperfect. Sunderland[26] has clearly described several of the factors that contribute to imperfect regeneration, as follows.

1. Injury to nerve axons causes injury to the parent neurons. The higher the level of the initial injury, the greater the retrograde damage to the parent cells. The health of the parent cell, in turn, influences the quantity and diameter of the regenerating axons.

2. Regenerating axons must successfully cross the suture site and enter a funiculus (bundle of axons protectively ensheathed by perineurium) in the distal nerve stump. However, the amount and nature of the scar tissue at the suture site will affect the ability of the axons to cross the site. Clean lacerations result in less scarring and better regeneration than either missile or stretch injuries. The denser the scar tissue, the more likely that a regenerating axon will "dead-end" and turn back in its path, thereby contributing to formation of a neuroma at the suture site.

Those axons that successfully bridge the suture site will come upon a distal stump that has atrophied and has a cross-sectional pattern of funiculi that does not exactly match that found in the proximal stump. The result is that axons may fail to enter the distal stump at all or, if they do, may fail to enter a funiculus, terminating instead either in connective tissue outside the nerve or in connective tissue between the funiculi (Fig. 37-1).

3. Successful entry of a regenerating axon into a funiculus still does not ensure successful reinnervation of an end organ. Each funiculus is usually comprised of motor, sensory, and sympathetic fibers in varying proportions, and each fiber is housed in an endoneurial sheath. The regenerating sensory axon must therefore find its way into an endoneurial sheath that formerly housed a sensory axon. Even if an axon does enter a functionally similar sheath, chances are that it will not enter the same sheath as previously, and therefore the spatial (somatotopic) organization of the nerve will be altered. This explains why functional results are better after a crush injury to a nerve than after a laceration. In a crush injury where the endoneurial tubes have not been interrupted the regenerating axons will be able to follow their original endoneurial sheath all the way to the same end organ as before the injury.

4. The final challenge to the regenerating axon is that of successfully reinnervating a sensory end organ. The state of atrophy of the end organ and the degree of myelinization of the regenerated axon are additional factors that will influence quality of regeneration.

It is clear from Sunderland's explanation of factors contributing to imperfect regeneration that the result of regeneration is fewer and smaller nerve fibers and receptors and a pattern of reinnervation that differs from the preinjury pattern. The effect on function of fewer and smaller fibers and receptors is not clear. According to Horch,[15] that particular deficit after nerve repair in a cleanly transected nerve may be less than what naturally occurs in man in the normal process of aging and so may be of less significance than has previously been believed. On the other hand, the effect of the disturbed somatotopic pattern of organization is undisputed. Such a disturbance will result in functional deficits

---

*See references 2, 14, 17, 23, 24, 26, and 27.

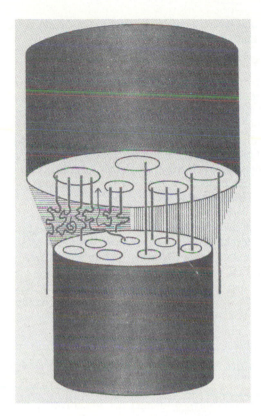

FIG. 37-1. Factors influencing nerve regeneration at suture site include amount and nature of scar tissue, atrophy of distal stump, and a cross-sectional pattern of funiculi that differs from that in proximal stump. (From Sunderland, S.: Nerves and nerve injuries, ed. 2, New York, 1978, Churchill Livingstone.)

in localization, two-point discrimination, and tactile gnosis, even when there is normal or near-normal perception of pain, temperature, and touch.

IS IT POSSIBLE TO IMPROVE THE LEVEL OF FUNCTIONAL SENSATION AFTER NERVE REPAIR?

At this time it is not clear to what degree it is possible to improve the level of functional sensation that typically occurs after nerve repair. Clinicians have observed for many years that two people with the same level of "academic" sensory recovery after nerve repair may have considerably different levels of function in their nerve-injured hands. Stopford attributed this higher functioning level in some people to "educability" of a "capable patient."[24] Davis[6] reviewed 82 patients after peripheral nerve injury and found that functional recovery was significantly better in those who were motivated to incorporate their injured hand into their occupational and leisure activities, especially if the involved hand was their dominant hand. Bowden[2] was in agreement with Davis's findings and stated that constant use of an involved extremity can lead to greater function in that extremity. Onne[19] also observed the capacity to adapt to sensibility deficits in the hand, depending on the extent to which the hand was consciously used in daily activities and the motivation of the patient. What these investigators and

others[15,26] have in common is the notion that a sensibility deficit can be compensated for, and therefore sensibility function improved, by such factors as attitude, persistence, and trainability (that is, motivation)[15] and attention, storage, and recall[26] (that is, learning). Thus, given a certain motivation and opportunity for learning, one person may overcome a sensibility deficit while another of lesser motivation and trainability will not.

Given that it is possible to improve overall function in a hand with a sensibility deficit, is it possible to relearn specific sensory skills, such as two-point discrimination, localization, and tactile gnosis? Opinions and findings vary on this question. Ford,[12] Sperry,[23] Hawkins,[14] Bowden,[2] and Horch[15] all opposed the concept of actual relearning of sensory skills after nerve injury, with special emphasis on repeated observation of patients' inability to accurately localize touch several years after nerve repair. Omer[18] noted that patients with poor sensibility could learn to recognize objects used in a daily test over several months, but this skill could not be generalized to other objects. He also pointed out that patients with neurovascular-cutaneous island pedicle transfer could learn to localize correctly at the site of the transfer but that under stress this ability was lost.[17]

In contrast, Parry[20,21] and Dellon[7-10] hold that sensory reeducation as measured by long-term improvements in localization, tactile gnosis, and two-point discrimination is possible in the adult after nerve repair. Parry has incorporated formal sensory reeducation into his rehabilitation program since 1966.[20] In 1976, he reported on the results of his program for the previous 9 years.[21] Patients who had undergone median or medioulnar nerve repair and who had some return of sensation in the fingers were candidates for sensory reeducation. Training divided into localization exercises and stereognosis tasks. All patients underwent four 10-minute training sessions daily on an in-patient basis. Assessment of results was based on improvements in localization, time and accuracy in recognition of textures, and time and accuracy in recognition of objects. Parry did not use improvement in two-point discrimination as a criterion for success because he believes that it cannot provide a measure of dynamic function after nerve repair. Individual results were not given in his report, but he states that 22 out of 23 patients achieved normal ability to localize within 3 months of training and that in his experience localization almost invariably returns to normal with training.[21] On the whole, the patients also improved in their ability to recognize textures and objects different from the training objects, and the time required for such identification lessened. The length of follow-up is not clear, but Parry states that improvements were exceeded in those who conscientiously incorporated their involved hand into daily activities and were decreased, but still significantly better than previously, in those who did not require use of their hands in daily activities.

In 1974, Dellon, Curtis, and Edgerton[10] reported the results of their sensory reeducation program. Nine patients participated in the program on an out-patient basis, including five who underwent median or ulnar nerve repair, one who underwent ulnar neurolysis, and three who had sustained a compression or crush to the median and ulnar nerves. The program was divided into early-phase and late-phase reeducation. Patients entered the program when their sensory return appeared to have plateaued for at least three weeks. Early-phase reeducation was focused on training in the perception of moving and light touch and localization of those perceptions. Training was initiated when the patient could perceive a 30-cps vibration administered through a tuning fork but not moving touch to the same distal point, or could perceive a 256-cps vibration but not constant touch to the same distal point. Use of vibratory perception as a guideline for initiating early reeducation was based on a sequence of sensory recovery observed by Dellon and co-workers in an earlier study.[9] Late-phase reeducation was initiated when moving and constant touch could be perceived at the fingertips with good localization. Late-phase exercises focused on size and shape discrimination and object recognition with use of familiar household objects.[7] Late-phase reeducation continued until two-point discrimination reached normal or had plateaued. Using two-point discrimination as the measure of success, Dellon determined that all six adults who entered the late-phase program recovered normal or nearly normal functional sensation within 2 to 6 weeks of training.[10]

Why were Parry and Dellon successful when others have been so pessimistic? Each made use of higher cortical functions—that is, attention, learning, and memory—to maximize sensory function. Typically, the patient was given a sensory stimulus or task while his vision was occluded, then allowed to open his eyes to integrate the tactile experience with his vision, and finally instructed to repeat the task with his eyes closed for reinforcement of what he had just learned. Attention was maximized by training in a quiet room for short intervals. Daily practice sessions over several weeks reinforced the learning. Thus all the factors noted by earlier observers as important in maximizing function were incorporated into their formal training programs. Their training techniques are similar to those used with success earlier by Forster and Shields[13] and Vinograd[28] in their studies of sensory retraining after insult to the central nervous system.

Thus, although the full potential for sensory reeducation is not known at this time, it appears that the motivated patient can learn to compensate for sensory deficits and, in a structured program that makes use of learning principles, can improve specific sensory skills that contribute to functional sensation.

CANDIDATES FOR SENSORY REEDUCATION

Two groups of patients are considered to be candidates for sensory reeducation after peripheral nerve injury:
1. Those in whom protective sensation is lacking or severely decreased as evidenced by inability to perceive stimuli that are potentially or overtly damaging to the tissues, including pinprick, deep pressure, hot and cold, and repetitive low-grade friction that can result in bruises or blisters. These patients are candidates for protective sensory reeducation.
2. Those who have the ability to perceive pinprick, temperature, and touch, but who lack discriminative sensation (that is, localization, two-point discrimination,

and tactile gnosis). These are candidates for discriminative sensory reeducation.

PROTECTIVE SENSORY REEDUCATION

The purpose of protective sensory reeducation is to teach the patient to compensate for the lack of protective sensory input. Because the hand that lacks protective sensation does not always experience pain under the same conditions that normally innervated skin does, it is more likely to be subjected to forces and stimuli that a normally innervated hand would withdraw from. The danger from inadvertently subjecting the hand to excessively hot or cold objects or sharp objects is obvious; however, other dangers are more subtle. In his work with patients with Hansen's disease and other neuropathies, Dr. Paul Brand[3] has observed other ways in which the hand without protective sensation is vulnerable to tissue damage because of "uninhibited" use.

The first of these dangers occurs from using excessive force when gripping or manipulating objects. A hand that has decreased proprioceptive and pressure feedback will have a tendency to be used with too much force even in simple familiar activities such as turning a key in a door. The unaware person will unconsciously exert too much force in an effort to achieve some sensory feedback from the hand. The result of such activity will be lacerations, abrasions, and other forms of damage to underlying tissues.[5]

A second source of danger lies in subjecting the hand to low-grade repetitive pressure when the hand is engaged in a grip or pinch activity. The hand with normal motor and sensory innervation will accommodate itself to tissue stress by subtle changes in grip or pinch when holding an object for a period of time. These accommodations will occur because the person will experience discomfort or pain from prolonged pressure or shear forces applied by an object upon the skin. The hand with decreased sensibility will not experience the discomfort or pain and so will not make the necessary accommodations or will lack the motor ability to change the grip or pinch position to ward off tissue damage. The result is the formation of blisters and bruises. Adapted grips are especially prone to result in damage to tissue from local stress because areas normally not involved in grip or pinch may be subject to prolonged or repetitive pressure[3] (Fig. 37-2).

A third source of danger in the hand that lacks protective sensation is a result of the lack of sweating that frequently characterizes such a hand. The skin is dry and smooth and prone to become inelastic and crack from lack of moisture. Dry, cracked skin is more likely to be damaged from daily use than soft, pliant skin and has the further disadvantage of making pinch and grip more difficult because of the lack of friction that moisture adds to the skin.

Methods of compensation for lack of protective sensation

A patient who lacks protective sensation should be instructed in the guidelines listed below[3-5] and observed in follow-through during functional activities in occupational therapy.
1. Avoid exposure of the involved area to heat, cold, and sharp objects.

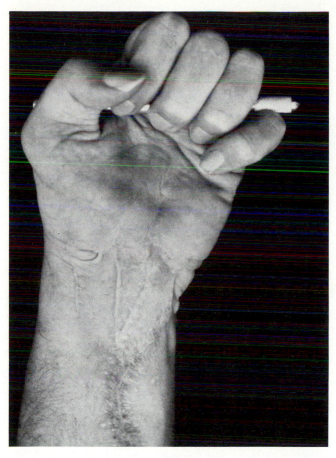

FIG. 37-2. Adapted grips, such as that demonstrated in this replanted hand with reduced sensibility and motor function, are especially prone to result in tissue damage from stress to areas that do not normally contact an object during grip or pinch.

2. When gripping a tool or object, be conscious of not applying more force than necessary.
3. Beware that the smaller the handle, the less distribution of pressure over the gripping surfaces. Avoid small handles by building up the handle or by using a different tool whenever possible.
4. Avoid tasks that require use of one tool for long periods of time, especially if the hand is unable to adapt by changing the manner of grip.
5. Change tools frequently at work to rest tissue areas.
6. Observe the skin for signs of stress, that is, redness, edema, and warmth, from excessive force or repetitive pressure, and rest the hand if these signs occur.
7. If blisters, lacerations, or other wounds occur, treat them with the utmost care to avoid further injury to the skin and possible infection.
8. To keep skin soft and pliant, follow a daily routine of skin care, including soaking and oil massage to lock in moisture.

At the Hand Rehabilitation Center in Philadelphia, patients who lack protective sensation are monitored by visual observation and volumetric readings for signs of stress in the hand after active use that requires gripping or tool han-

dling. Tool handles are built up to accommodate grips and distribute pressure. Patients are instructed in proper skin care and taught to inspect their skin frequently for signs of damage. By following the steps outlined above, one can compensate for a lack of protective sensation and the hand can be successfully reincorporated into gainful activity.

DISCRIMINATIVE SENSORY REEDUCATION

The purpose of discriminative sensory reeducation is to teach the patient to better attend to residual sensory cues so that the brain can better interpret sensory messages transmitted by an altered somatotopic organization at the periphery.

Prerequisites for training

For optimum results for discrimination training certain requirements must be met regarding level of return, selection of patients, selection of exercises or tasks that challenge the sensory system, and time allotted for training.

The level of return must be such that protective sensation is present and there is a return of touch to the fingertips as measured by the patient's ability to perceive the touch of the examiner's fingertip or by ability to perceive the touch of the Semmes-Weinstein Pressure Aesthesiometer* at a level of 4.31 or better (see Chapter 36). The presence of touch at the fingertips indicates that sufficient regeneration has occurred to initiate retraining. Retraining will occur throughout the hand but with special emphasis on the fingertips, since these are the most important discriminative sensory surfaces.

The patient must be motivated, intelligent, and able to concentrate. He must be willing to devote time daily to achieve a goal that is not so tangible as motor reeducation. He must be willing to incorporate the hand consciously into daily activities that may at first seem easier to perform without use of the involved area.

The patient and therapist must be patient and work to achieve successive short-term goals. Neither should hope for or expect normal sensibility but should work for noticeably increased function from training.

Appropriate choice of activities presents the greatest challenge to the therapist because those that are too easy do not result in learning and those are too hard will frustrate. Sensory discrimination demands active exploration by the digits, but often the hand with sensory impairment also has motor impairment. Therefore early tasks may involve movement of a stimulus over the digits rather than active exploration by the digits. Tactile cues to uninvolved sensory surfaces on either hand must be avoided at certain times in the training to maximize learning.

At the Hand Rehabilitation Center in Philadelphia, the discriminative reeducation program is divided into tasks that require localization and those that require graded discrimination. These two avenues of training are traveled simultaneously with an ultimate goal of successful incorporating of the hand into work-related tasks.

---

*Research Designs, Inc., 7320 Ashcroft, Suite 103, Houston, Tex. 77081.

Training in localization

Ability to localize is tested and mapped (see Chapter 36) to establish a base line for training. The stimulus used initially for training is the therapist's fingertip or the eraser end of a pencil applied with a moving or constant touch over a specific area.[10] The therapist or trainer can use the grid work sheet described in Chapter 36 during training. The grid is visualized on the patient's hand, and the touch stimulus, whether moving or constant, is applied to only one arbitrary zone at a time. Training in this way will help to better identify local areas of poor localization.

With his eyes closed, the patient concentrates on the stimulus as it is applied to a selected zone. He is asked to open his eyes and point to the area stimulated. If he is incorrect, the stimulus is reapplied while he watches so that he can integrate the visual image with the tactile perception. The stimulus is then repeated with the eyes closed, so that he can integrate the tactile experience with his memory of what he just observed when his eyes were open. The entire process is then repeated with a touch stimulus to a different area. Through this process of concentration, immediate feedback, integration of visual and sensory information and memory, and reinforcement by repetition, the higher centers of the cortex can begin to compensate for impaired localization. Through further practice and reinforcement, learning, that is, reeducation, is achieved. The learning principles involved in this training are common to other formal programs.[7,10,13,20,21,28]

Twice a month, localization is formally reevaluated for monitoring improvements. As the patient improves in his ability to localize the relatively widespread and heavy pressure applied by a fingertip or pencil eraser, the training stimulus becomes smaller and lighter. Our ideal goal is that the patient be able to localize the constant touch of a stimulus (as from a Semmes-Weinstein monofilament) that is close to the level of his touch threshold. Therefore our program training in localization tends to continue throughout the reeducation program. This differs from the programs described by Parry[20,21] and Dellon[7,10] in which "normal localization" is reached early in training but appears to be measured by the ability to localize a blunt and fairly widespread stimulus.

Training in discrimination

Activities used at the Hand Rehabilitation Center to encourage discrimination are designed as much as possible to be carried out by the patient without assistance from the therapist or another party at home, thereby reducing therapist time and patient dependence on another person to assist in frequent training sessions. The activities are graded to require gross to fine discrimination. Within each activity there are three levels of difficulty:

1. Are these (stimuli) the same or different?
2. In what way are they the same or different?
3. Identify the texture, object, and so on.

Choice of difficulty level within an activity depends on assessment of the patient's present skills. Some tasks require motor function; others do not because sensory dysfunction is usually accompanied by motor dysfunction. When a stimulus is to be applied to different areas of the skin for training, the examiner or trainer uses the grid work sheet (p. 414)

for selection of a zone for stimulating and recording of results. The patient is also familiarized with the grid work sheet and, when working by himself, is instructed to apply a selected stimulus to only a small area at a time. In this way, training is somewhat standardized between patient and therapist.

Texture and shape discrimination tasks. The following activities do not require advanced motor skills. Each task uses the eyes-closed, eyes-open, eyes-closed sequence with appropriate feedback as described above.

Texture discrimination with sandpaper or other textures on dowels. A coarse grade of sandpaper is attached to one end of several dowels. At the opposite end is attached either the same grade or a different grade, varying from coarse to extra fine (Fig. 37-3, *A*). Both ends of a selected dowel are lightly moved over a selected arbitrary zone of dysfunction while the patient's eyes are closed. He is asked to state whether the two ends are the same or different. If he is incorrect, he watches while the same stimuli are reapplied to the same area and then closes his eyes for further reinforcement while they are applied once again. He will require further practice in this area of involved skin. If he is correct, he is given the appropriate feedback, and training proceeds to other areas of the hand. As discrimination improves, the grades of sandpaper chosen for practice become more similar.

The sandpaper is attached to dowels so that the patient can engage in this task without assistance from another person and without inadvertently receiving tactile cues on uninvolved sensory surfaces (Fig. 37-3, *B*). After appropriate evaluation, the therapist selects certain dowels for practice. The patient can then apply the reeducation technique to himself at home or in the therapy department. That is, with eyes closed he can pick up any dowel at the center, apply first one end and then the other to an involved sensory area to test himself, and then open his eyes and check the accuracy of his response without having received any cues to uninvolved skin areas. Because the dowel is moved over the involved surface, motor function can be impaired and still allow for reeducation, but the fingers can also be moved over the dowel, if preferred.

Similarly, other textures or substances can be applied to dowel ends (or pencils) (Fig. 37-4) and applied in the same way. The patient can make his own reeducation kit for home use.

Texture discrimination using fabrics. At first, a sample fabric is placed in front of the patient whose eyes are closed, and he is asked to match that fabric with one of three fabric choices (Fig. 37-5, *A*). When matching from a small group is no longer challenging, matching from a larger group is required, and the patient may be asked to describe the qualities of the fabrics.

One can also carry out this activity independently at home by attaching the sample fabrics to cards in a book that has a circular binding so that the patient can flip the book open to any page, with eyes closed, and match the fabric on that page with one from a group of possibilities (Fig. 37-5, *B*).

Differentiation of roughness and smoothness. Differentiation of the rough and smooth edges of coins, nuts, bolts, and washers is another discrimination task. Dellon[10] has

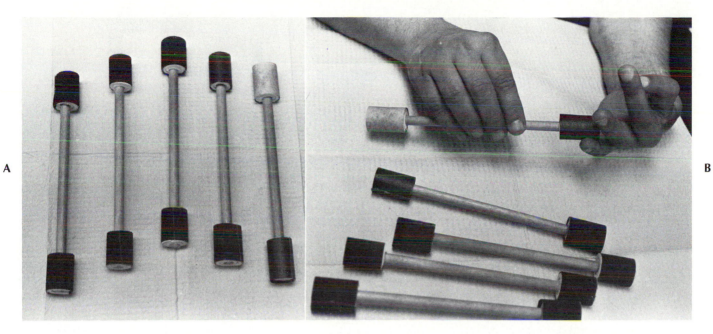

FIG. 37-3. A, Early reeducation task requires identification of two identical or different grades of sandpaper attached to either end of a dowel. **B,** Dowels are used to allow patient to self-administer the task without receiving cues on uninvolved sensory surfaces.

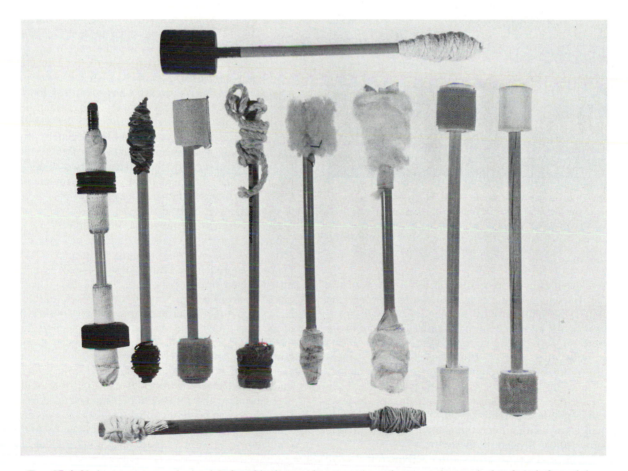

FIG. 37-4. Various textures and materials found in therapy department or at home can be attached to dowels for training in discrimination.

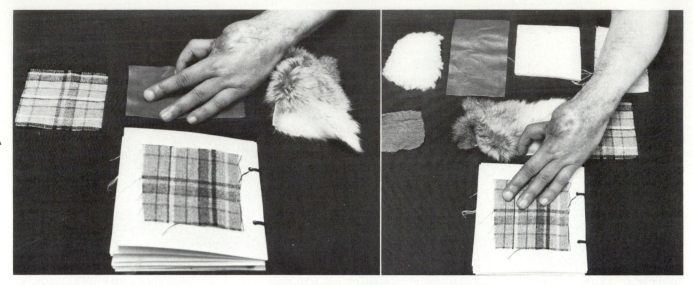

FIG. 37-5. Texture discrimination using fabrics. **A,** Early task requires matching test fabric with one of three choices. **B,** Later task requires matching test fabric with one from a group of possibilities. If properly set up, this task can be carried out independently by patient.

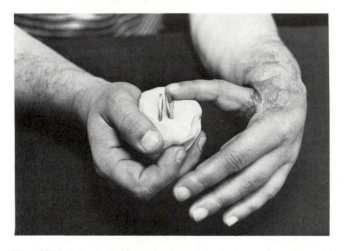

FIG. 37-6. Discrimination of coins, nuts, bolts, and washers. If patient lacks motor ability to manipulate these small objects, or tactile cues to a normally innervated thumb are not desired, task can be carried out independently by seating the objects in putty.

recommended that these objects be carried in the patient's pocket for frequent home training sessions. However, if the patient lacks the motor ability to manipulate such small items, or if tactile cues to a normally innervated thumb are not desired, the activity can be carried out with the objects seated in putty (Fig. 37-6). With eyes closed, the patient rotates the putty before attempting to locate and identify objects in it using involved sensory surfaces.

Graphesthesia. The therapist or a third person traces a number or a geometric figure on an involved fingertip or other small area, using a fingertip or blunt instrument, and requires the patient to identify the figure.

Games and puzzles. Discrimination activities that have a game or puzzle quality are generally more enjoyable and challenging to the patient. The more he is mentally involved in the activity, the more he will be able to benefit from it. Three types of activities have been useful in training.

Identification of letters. Block letters formed from adhesive-backed Velcro are superimposed on square blocks of wood (Fig. 37-7, *A*). The blocks are laid facedown. Each one is notched at the top so that the patient can pick it up with his eyes closed and orient it correctly in his uninvolved hand while he tries to identify the letter using his involved fingers. When he believes he has identified the letter, he opens his eyes to check his accuracy. If incorrect, he retraces the letter with his eyes closed to try to determine why he was incorrect. If he is correct, he immediately proceeds to another block. A time limit makes this activity more challenging. As described, the letters are two dimensional. If the patient has sufficient motor function for manipulation, three-dimensional letters cut out of wood are recommended to make the task more difficult.

Braille designs. Millesi[16] has described the use of braille geometric figures for sensory training, and Walsh[29] has described the use of braille designs for training. With use of Walsh's approach, a braille design, such as a house, is imprinted on braille paper (Fig. 37-7, *B*). The design is placed in front of the patient, whose eyes are closed, and he is given a particular task, for example, outline the frame of the house, determine the number of windows, and locate the door. One can grade this task in difficulty depending on how closely spaced the different components of the design are. Patients with a severe problem in localization generally find his task easier to do with one digit than with several digits because the information from several cross-reinnervated digits can be very confusing when the eyes are closed.

Finger mazes. Finger mazes are devised by use of a colored epoxy* to form a raised design on cardboard (Fig. 37-

---

*Hi-Marks, Mark-Tex Corp., Englewood, N.J. 07631.

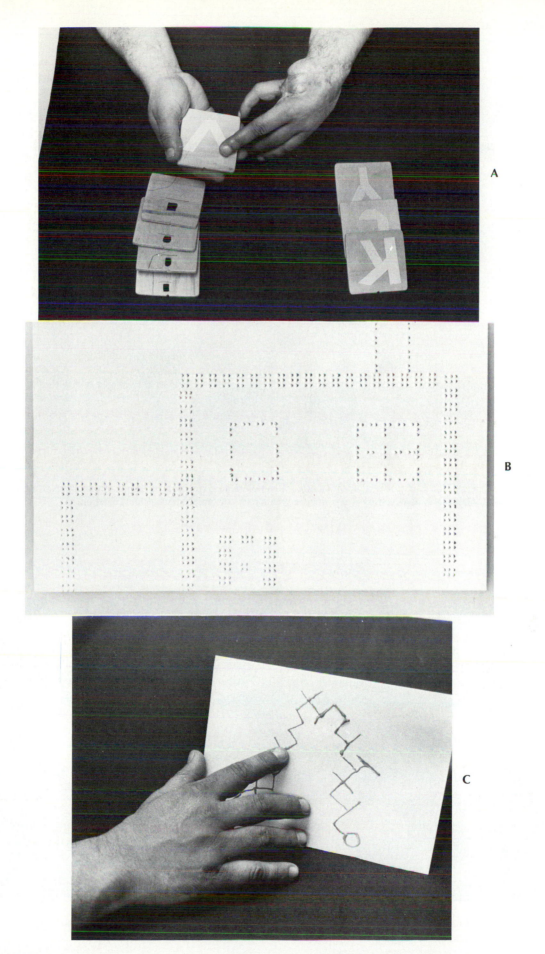

FIG. 37-7. Games and puzzles used to train sensory discrimination. **A,** Velcro letters superimposed on blocks of wood. **B,** Braille designs. **C,** Finger maze.

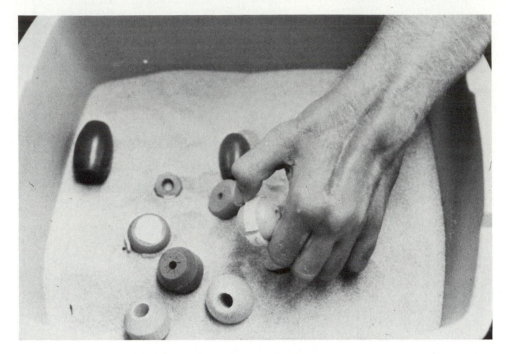

Fig. 37-8. Early reeducation task dependent on motor function requires picking out objects from a background medium, such as sand. Grading is achieved by using smaller, similar objects and requiring identification.

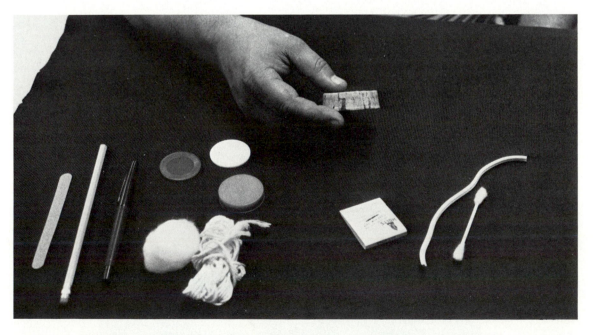

Fig. 37-9. Identification of everyday objects requires manipulation and discrimination.

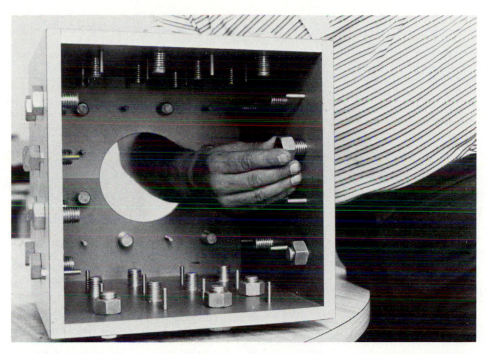

FIG. 37-10. As motor skills improve, appropriate sensory-training activities include work-simulated tasks that require use of involved sensory surfaces.

7, *C*). The patient's fingertip is then placed at the starting point, and he is asked to find his way through the maze to the ending point (indicated by a circle or other sign). Variations of this activity are limited only by the ingenuity of the therapist and patient. The latter will frequently suggest ways to make training easier or more difficult.

Tasks that require motor function. The following tasks are considered to be more difficult because they require greater integration of motor or sensory function and require object recognition. However, these too can be graded from gross to fine and, as long as sufficient motor function is present, can be prescribed concurrently with the above tasks.

Picking out objects from a bowl of sand, wool, styrofoam, rice, etc. (Fig. 37-8). This activity requires differentiation of an object from its background medium. At first, large geometric shapes can be used; later, smaller objects can be used.

Identification of common objects. The patient is asked to select and identify an object from a box of objects. The objects in the box have been chosen either because they are dissimilar to make the task easier or similar to make the task more difficult (Fig. 37-9).

Activities of daily living with vision occluded. Many of our daily grooming and work tasks require manipulation of objects without the assistance of vision. As motor skills improve, activities in occupational therapy should include activities of daily living and work tasks that require use of the involved part (Fig. 37-10).

Selection of activities

The exact choice of activity for each patient is based upon evaluation of his baseline discrimination skills by use of tests of functional sensation including two-point discrimination, localization, and tests of tactile gnosis. Each treatment session should be brief, approximately 10 to 15 minutes, because concentration must remain high for maximum learning. A minimum of one session per day is recommended, though two or three sessions are ideal. Each session should include practice and training from each category of tasks: localization, texture and shape discrimination, puzzles or games, and incorporation of the involved part into a motor activity. The relationship between the therapist and the patient is dynamic in that the therapist designs the content of the program and gives feedback to the patient, while the patient gives feedback to the therapist regarding relative difficulty of specific tasks and the cues used to discriminate and identify objects.

ASSESSMENT OF RESULTS

The results of training for the patient who requires protective sensory reeducation are measured by a lack of inflammation, blisters, ulcers, and other signs of tissue breakdown over time. The person who has truly learned to protect his hyposensitive hand will not develop these signs of abuse of his hand.

Results in the patient who requires training in discriminative sensation are more difficult to assess and cannot be precisely measured. The following are some of the parameters that are clinically useful for periodic assessment:

1. Mapping. An example of mapping is the use of an outline of the hand to record progress in the ability to localize a stimulus (see Chapter 36, Fig. 36-13).
2. Number of accurate responses. How many objects or

textures are identified or matched in a given time period?

3. Time required to complete a task. How long does it take to locate and remove 15 objects from a bowl of rice? How long does it take to complete a finger maze?

4. Improvement in two-point discrimination. Two-point discrimination is a commonly used measure of improvement in sensory reeducation[10,22]; however, some clinicians state that this test is not a valid measurement of functional sensation after nerve repair.[11,20]

5. Patient's report of increased function in activities of daily living. This, after all, is the most important measure of success. If sensory reeducation results in a person's increased ability to perform activities of daily living, or to handle his tools better on the job, or to better enjoy the tactile sensations of everyday living, then reeducation has been meaningful and successful.

LONG-TERM EFFECTS OF SENSORY REEDUCATION

Patients who have been followed for several years after sensory reeducation have been observed to maintain and increase their functional gains if they continued to use the hand actively for fine activities after discharge from therapy. Some function was lost in those whose work did not require a high degree of sensory function.[21] The finding that maintenance depends on continued use of the hand has been supported by other clinicians.[6,18,19]

SUMMARY

Patients who lack protective sensory function are candidates for training in compensation for lack of protective sensation. Patients who lack discriminative sensation are candidates for training in discriminative sensation. The rationale for reeducation programs is that the higher cortical levels of the brain can compensate through attention, integration, and recall for sensory dysfunction. Reeducation requires a patient who is intelligent, motivated, and willing to make a conscious effort to incorporate the involved hand into daily activities and to carry out a structured program on a daily basis. The success of sensory reeducation can be measured along several parameters, the most important of which is improvement in function in activities of daily living, including work activities. Long-term maintenance of gains will depend on the patient's persistence in using the hand in work and other daily activities that challenge its sensory function. Important gains have been made in reeducation, but studies are still needed to determine the best approach in reeducation and to better define its capabilities.

REFERENCES

1. Almquist, E., and Eeg-Olofsson, O.: Sensory nerve conduction velocity and two-point discrimination in sutured nerves, J. Bone Joint Surg. **52A:**791, 1970.
2. Bowden, R.E.M.: Factors influencing functional recovery. In Seddon, H.J., editor: Peripheral nerve injuries, London, 1954, Her Majesty's Stationery Office.
3. Brand, P.W.: Rehabilitation of the hand with motor and sensory impairment, Orthop. Clin. North Am. **4:**1135, 1973.
4. Brand, P.W.: Management of sensory loss in the extremities. In Omer, G.E., and Spinner, M., editors: Management of peripheral nerve problems, Philadelphia, 1980, W.B. Saunders Co.
5. Brand, P.W., and Ebner, J.D.: A pain substitute: pressure assessment in the insensitive limb, Am. J. Occup. Ther. **23:**479, 1969.
6. Davis, D.R.: Some factors affecting the results of treatment of peripheral nerve injuries, Lancet **1:**877, 1949.
7. Dellon, A.L.: Evaluation of sensibility and reeducation of sensation in the hand, Baltimore, 1981, The Williams & Wilkins Co.
8. Dellon, A.L., and Jabaley, M.E.: Reeducation of sensation in the hand following nerve suture, Clin. Orthop. **163:**75, 1982.
9. Dellon, A.L., Curtis, R.M., and Edgerton, M.T.: Evaluating recovery of sensation in the hand following nerve injury, Hopkins Med. J. **130:**235, 1972.
10. Dellon, A.L., Curtis, R.M., and Edgerton, M.T.: Reeducation of sensation in the hand after nerve injury and repair, Plast. Reconstr. Surg. **53:**297, 1974.
11. Edshage, S.: Experience with clinical methods of testing sensation after peripheral nerve surgery. In Jewett, D.L., McCarroll, H.K., Jr., and Relton, H., editors: Nerve repair and regeneration: its clinical and experimental basis, St. Louis, 1979, The C.V. Mosby Co.
12. Ford, F.R., and Woodhall, B.: Phenomena due to misdirection of regenerating fibers of cranial, spinal and autonomic nerves, Arch. Surg. **36:**480, 1938.
13. Foster, F.M., and Shields, C.D.: Cortical sensory deficits causing disability, Arch. Phys. Med. Rehabil. **40:**56, 1959.
14. Hawkins, G.E.: Faulty sensory localization in nerve regeneration, J. Neurosurg. **5:**11, 1948.
15. Horch, K.W., and Burgess, P.R.: Functional specificity and somatotopic organization during peripheral nerve regeneration. In Jewett, D.L., McCarroll, H.K., Jr., and Relton, H., editors: Nerve repair and regeneration: its clinical and experimental basis, St. Louis, 1979, The C.V. Mosby Co.
16. Millesi, H., and Rinderer, D.: A method for training and testing sensibility of the fingertips, Department of Plastic and Reconstructive Surgery, Surgical University Clinic of Vienna and Ludwig-Boltzmann Institute for Experimental Plastic Surgery, Vienna, Austria, 1978.
17. Omer, G.E.: Sensation and sensibility in the upper extremity, Clin. Orthop. Rel. Res. **104:**30, 1974.
18. Omer, G.E.: Sensory evaluation by the pickup test. In Jewett, D.L., McCarroll, H.K., Jr., and Relton, H., editors: Nerve repair and regeneration: its clinical and experimental basis, St. Louis, 1979, The C.V. Mosby Co.
19. Önne, L.: Recovery of sensibility and sudomotor activity in the hand after nerve suture, Axta. Chir. Scand. (Suppl.) **300:**1, 1962.
20. Parry, C.B.W.: Rehabilitation of the hand, ed. 4, London, 1981, Butterworth & Co. (Publishers), Ltd.
21. Parry, C.B.W., and Salter, M.: Sensory reeducation after median nerve lesion, Hand **8:**250, 1976.
22. Reid, R.L.: Preliminary results of sensibility reeducation following repair of median nerve, American Society for Surgery of the Hand, Newsletter 15, 1977.
23. Sperry, R.W.: The problem of central nervous reorganization after nerve regeneration and muscle transposition, Q. Rev. Biol. **20:**311, 1945.
24. Stopford, J.S.B.: An explanation of the two-stage recovery of sensation during regeneration of a peripheral nerve, Brain **49:**372, 1926.
25. Stromberg, W.B., McFarlane, R.M., Bell, J.L., and others: Injury of the median and ulnar nerves: one hundred and fifty cases with an evaluation of Moberg's Ninhydrin test, J. Bone Joint Surg. **43A:**717, 1961.
26. Sunderland, S.: Nerves and nerve injuries, ed. 2, New York, 1978, Churchill Livingstone.
27. Trotter, W., and Davies, H.M.: Experimental studies in the innervation of the skin, J. Physiol. **38:**134, 1909.
28. Vinograd A., Taylor, E., and Grossman, S.: Sensory retraining of the hemiplegic hand, Am. J. Occup. Ther. **5:**246, 1962.
29. Walsh, W.W.: Sensory modalities vs. functional use approach to reeducation, Symposium, Assessment of levels of cutaneous sensibility, United States Public Health Service Hospital, Carville, La., Sept. 1980.

38

Rehabilitation of the patient with an injury to the brachial plexus

ROBERT D. LEFFERT

The problem of rehabilitation of a patient with an injury to the brachial plexus is difficult, not only for the patient, to whom it may assume enormous proportions,[7] but in a different way to those who participate in his care. The anatomy of the nerves is complex and difficult to remember, and the infrequency of such cases in most individual practitioners' experience makes the lack of familiarity a significant handicap. The time intervals required for spontaneous resolution of those lesions that heal, as well as the results of central or peripheral reconstruction, involve long-term commitment to patients.

Since patients and their problems present as a series of questions, this chapter will be similarly arranged.

Who are the patients, and what are the mechanisms of injury?

The majority of brachial plexus injuries are due to traction, which generally results from high-velocity motorcycle accidents or occasionally bicycle or automobile trauma. Far fewer result from falls or industrial injuries in which the weight falls on the shoulder or traction on the arm. The common mechanism is a forceful separation of the head and shoulder during a fall. This stretching of the nerves causes a variety of distributions and degrees of injury, which are the clinically observed deficits. Patients are usually young males in their late teens or early twenties, often unskilled or beginning manual occupations. A considerably smaller number of patients sustain open injuries to the brachial plexus, and these as well as postanaesthetic palsies will be briefly discussed.

What are the pertinent clinico-anatomic correlations?

The anatomy is fascinating, complex, and frustrating because although one could memorize a textbook diagram of how the plexus is arranged, it would not be adequate for application to a significant percentage of clinical situations. A detailed discussion of the anatomy is beyond the scope of this chapter, but fortunately a number of excellent references are available.* Suffice it to say that the classic brachial plexus is formed by the anterior primary rami of

---

*See references 6, 15, 18, 21, 22, 23, 27, and 51.

C5, C6, C7, C8, and T1 and their terminal outflow (Fig. 38-1). If C4 contributes a significant branch to C5, and it does so in a high percentage of patients, then the term "prefixed" is used. If T2 contributes significantly to T1, then the plexus is said to be "postfixed." This occurs in a significantly smaller group of patients. The importance of these particular variations is that in our dealings with the brachial plexus we will rely heavily on indirect methods of neurologic diagnosis. Therefore, one must be prepared to anticipate variations by at least one spinal level in determining the location of the lesion. Furthermore, in traction lesions, actual avulsion of the nerve roots from the spinal cord may occur. Hence, knowledge of the location of branches known to be given off immediately after the spinal nerve exits from the intervertebral foramen allows for identification of such supraganglionic lesions, which have no potential for useful spontaneous recovery or successful surgical manipulation. For example, if a patient has a traction lesion involving C5, C6, or C7 and the scapula is clinically winged, this indicates denervation of the serratus anterior muscle, the nerves for which are root collaterals arising at the spinal canal. On the other hand, an intact serratus in a patient who has paralysis of the lateral rotators of the humerus would indicate a lesion located farther distally. All grades of nerve injury are possible distally, from nondegenerative neurapraxias to frank rupture of the nerves within the substance of the plexus itself. Finally, the presence of an ipsilateral Horner's syndrome in a patient with a traction lesion of the brachial plexus indicates a supraganglionic lesion involving the T1 nerve root and a poor prognosis for that particular root, although in a few cases, some recovery may occur.[46]

What are the clinically observed patterns of injury?

Among patients who have sustained traction injury to the brachial plexus by means of the mechanism described above, there are four commonly observed patterns: (1) the C5-6 lesion, (2) the C5, C6, C7 lesion, (3) the (C7), C8, T1 lesion, and (4) the whole-plexus lesion.

The C5-6 lesion is a common type of injury, it results in paralysis of the deltoid, the lateral rotators of the humerus, and the elbow flexors. The wrist extensors may or may not be paralyzed as well, and if they are, the patient still may

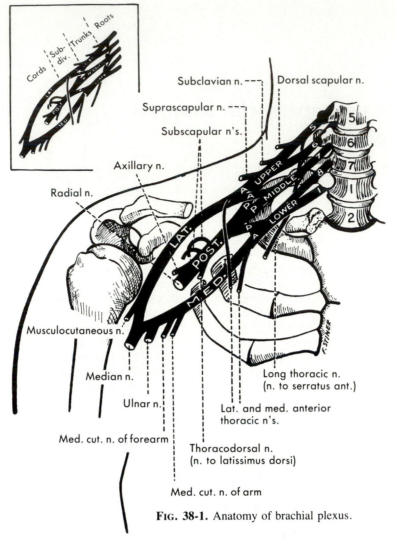

FIG. 38-1. Anatomy of brachial plexus.

be able to dorsiflex the wrist if the finger extensors are intact. The functional deficit is the inability to control the shoulder, which can be neither abducted nor forward flexed, and although the elbow can be extended, it cannot be actively flexed. The sensory loss involves the thumb and the index finger. The incidence of nondegenerative lesions that recover spontaneously is highest in this group, and avulsion of the roots from the cord does not occur frequently. Isolated injuries to the upper trunk have the best prognosis.[4,46]

The C5, C6, C7 lesion includes all of the deficits in the previous group, with the addition of a loss of active wrist and elbow extension as well as finger extension. It is as if a radial nerve palsy were superimposed upon the C5-6 lesion. There is slightly more sensory loss, which involves the middle finger. The prognosis for spontaneous recovery is less favorable.[4]

The (C7), C8, and T1 lesion represents only a small portion of the adult traction lesions, being considerably more common in obstetrical palsies, in which the term "Klumpke's palsy" identifies it. While the shoulder and elbow control as well as wrist extension are preserved, there is loss of active finger flexion and extension as well as all intrinsic function of the hand. The sensory loss is usually confined to the little and ring fingers, although if C7 is involved, the middle finger will lose sesnsation as well.

The whole-plexus lesion is the most disastrous of the traction lesions of the brachial plexus, not only in terms of the extent of the lesion, but also in terms of severity and prognosis.[5] While the three former categories can be significantly benefited by peripheral reconstructive surgery, the whole-plexus lesion must be thought of and treated differently, because not only is there profound motor weakness, but total loss of sensibility in the limb as well. This is the "flail-anesthetic limb," which has an extremely poor prognosis for spontaneous recovery.

Before I proceed, note should be taken of three other types of injury to the brachial plexus. These are (1) closed infraclavicular injury, (2) postanesthetic palsy, and (3) open injury to the brachial plexus.

Closed infraclavicular injury to the brachial plexus occurs as a result of skeletal injury in the region of the shoulder, usually fractures or fracture-dislocations of the glenohumeral joint or the scapula.[30,32] The nerves are injured by the stretch or compression of the humeral head or the fracture fragments, and usually the prognosis for recovery is considerably better than for the closed supraclavicular injuries.

It should be noted, however, that nerves may actually be cut by sharp fracture fragments, which can also produce significant vascular injury. It is important to make sure that a supraclavicular injury does not exist in a patient who has had a shoulder girdle injury, since it will be the supraclavicular injury that determines the prognosis in that case.

Postanesthetic palsy may occur in patients who are under general anesthesia in the operating room.[25,29] This is a preventable type of nerve injury resulting from malposition of the head, neck, or arm at surgery. In almost all cases, even though the paralysis may be widespread, it is usually not permanent and it is of lesser severity than would be seen with a high-velocity injury. The prognosis for full recovery is excellent.

Open injuries to the brachial plexus[8,45] fortunately occur infrequently in civilian practice. If they are the result of gunshot wounds without either vascular or pulmonary complications, they should be treated expectantly, since many of them will recovery spontaneously. For patients who have sharp wounds of the plexus involving the upper or intermediate trunk, microsurgical techniques have improved the possibility of functional recovery following direct surgery. Nevertheless, such a case should not be considered an emergency unless, of course, there is a concomitant vascular lesion. In the past 6 months I have explored two patients who had had their brachial plexuses severed by chain saws that they had been operating. The damage was extensive in both patients, although in one we were able to do limited neurologic reconstruction.

What methods of documentation and evaluation are available?

The clinical history is of extreme importance, although sometimes the patient will have sustained a head injury at the time he injures the brachial plexus, and so will be amnesic in regard to the event. Nevertheless, it is important to know the date and the circumstances of the injury, whether there was a head injury, and what the initial neurologic deficit in the limb was. The presence of concomitant fractures should be ascertained. Obviously one should know such things as the hand dominance of the patient, his occupation, and whether he has a history of neurologic deficit or injury to the limb. Only then will it be possible to ascertain whether there has been a change since the injury, if the patient is not seen immediately thereafter. Patients who are seen late should be encouraged to obtain all medical records, including their prior workups. Finally, since many patients with brachial plexus injuries have pain, a history regarding its presence, its course, factors influencing it, and so on will be important.

The physical examination must be conducted in a systematic fashion and recorded so that nothing is omitted. For this purpose, a number of schemes and charts have been devised. I use one that is adapted from Professor Merle d'Aubigne (Fig. 38-2). It includes space not only for the historical data but also for range of motion of all joints in the shoulder girdle and upper limb, manual muscle testing, and sensation. Each muscle in the limb must be tested and its strength recorded. Sensation is evaluated by pin and touch. The face should be examined for the presence of Horner's syndrome, and the supraclavicular fossa should be palpated and percussed. If Tinel's sign can be elicited in the supraclavicular fossa of a patient with a flail-anesthetic arm following a traction injury, then it is extremely likely that at least one root is ruptured distally in the neck rather than avulsed centrally at the spinal cord.

For all patients, it is important to perform a general neurologic examination that inclues the lower extremities. The presence of "long tract signs" would indicate spinal cord injury.

Plain radiographs of the cervical spine, ipsilateral shoulder girdle, and any fractures that might be reported or found to be present are taken at the original evaluation.

Myelography is a useful adjunct to clinical evaluation[39,40] but should be delayed in most cases until 1 month after injury to avoid injecting the contrast material into a possibly bloody spinal fluid, since not only may the pertinent details be obscured by blood clot, but there is a possibility of producing arachnoiditis. Although in the past Pantopaque has been the contrast material that has been used, we have recently used water-soluble materials such as Metrizamide, combined with polytomography so that greater detail of the spinal nerve roots at the level the cord may be seen. When a myelogram in a patient with a root avulsion is done several months after the injury, the retracted and scarred meninges will form a traumatic pseudomeningocele, which will appear as a pouch at the level of the root avulsion. It should be emphasized that although myelography offers good presumptive evidence of root avulsion, it is by no means completely reliable,[20,26] and some surgeons have disgarded its use altogether. I continue to use myelography, with knowledge of its limitations.

Both electromyography and nerve conduction velocity determinations can be used to provide important additional information in the evaluation of a patient with a traction injury to the brachial plexus. Bufalini and Pescatori[9] have shown that since the deep layers of the posterior cervical musculature are serially innervated by the posterior primary rami of the same spinal nerves that provide the anterior primary rami that form the brachial plexus, needle electromyography of these muscles will identify and differentiate root avulsions from distal ruptures. If, for example, the limb musculature is denervated and the erector spinae muscles are not, then the posterior primary rami are intact, and since they are given off immediately after the spinal nerves exist the intervertebral foramina, the lesion must be further distally in the plexus, and therefore be a rupture rather than an avulsion. If, on the other hand, both sets of musculature are denervated, an avulsion is present. The electromyogram may be used on serial examination to identify evidences of reinnervation in appendicular musculature that appears to be clinically paralyzed. The test can be done anytime after 3 weeks in a patient who is clinically paralyzed, since that interval is necessary for the development of wallerian degeneration and the appearance of fibrillations on the electromyogram.

Nerve conduction velocity determinations can also be used to distinguish avulsions from distal ruptures. In patients who have root avulsions with paralysis and sensory loss, although motor nerve conduction velocity determination

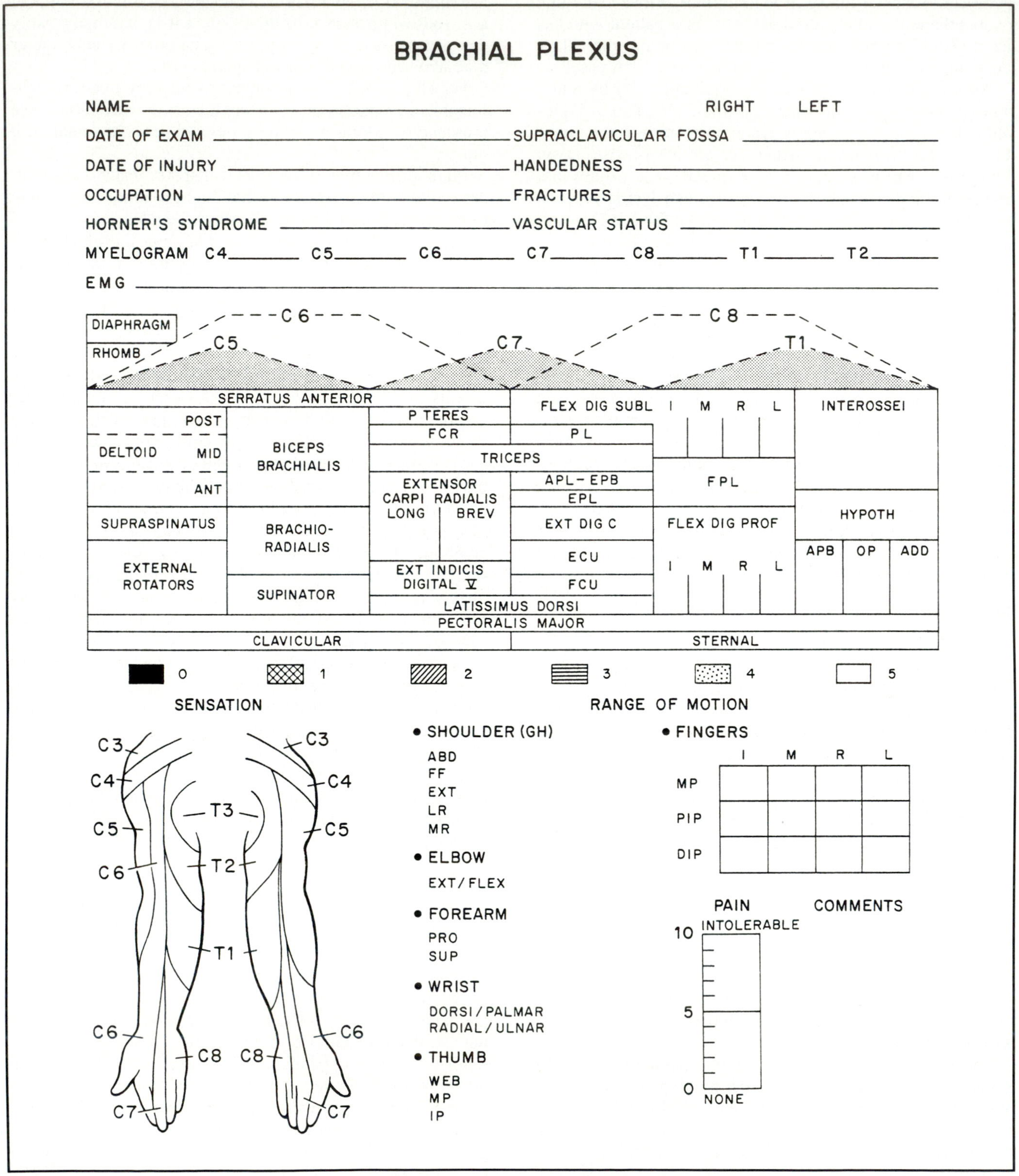

BRACHIAL PLEXUS

NAME _____   RIGHT   LEFT

DATE OF EXAM _____ SUPRACLAVICULAR FOSSA _____

DATE OF INJURY _____ HANDEDNESS _____

OCCUPATION _____ FRACTURES _____

HORNER'S SYNDROME _____ VASCULAR STATUS _____

MYELOGRAM C4_____ C5_____ C6_____ C7_____ C8_____ T1_____ T2_____

EMG _____

	C6		C8	
DIAPHRAGM	C5	C7	T1	
RHOMB				

SERRATUS ANTERIOR		P TERES	FLEX DIG SUBL I M R L		INTEROSSEI
POST	BICEPS BRACHIALIS	FCR	PL		
DELTOID MID		TRICEPS		FPL	
ANT		EXTENSOR CARPI RADIALIS LONG BREV	APL–EPB		
			EPL		HYPOTH
SUPRASPINATUS	BRACHIO-RADIALIS		EXT DIG C	FLEX DIG PROF	APB OP ADD
EXTERNAL ROTATORS		EXT INDICIS DIGITAL V	ECU	I M R L	
	SUPINATOR		FCU		
		LATISSIMUS DORSI			
		PECTORALIS MAJOR			
CLAVICULAR			STERNAL		

■ 0   ▨ 1   ▧ 2   ▤ 3   ▨ 4   □ 5

SENSATION

C3 C3
C4 C4
T3
C5 C5
C6 T2
T1
C6 C6
C8 C8
C7 C7

RANGE OF MOTION

- SHOULDER (GH)
  - ABD
  - FF
  - EXT
  - LR
  - MR
- ELBOW
  - EXT/FLEX
- FOREARM
  - PRO
  - SUP
- WRIST
  - DORSI/PALMAR
  - RADIAL/ULNAR
- THUMB
  - WEB
  - MP
  - IP

- FINGERS

	I	M	R	L
MP				
PIP				
DIP				

PAIN   COMMENTS

10 INTOLERABLE

5

0 NONE

FIG. 38-2. Chart for recording results of physical examination for brachial plexus injury.

will be impossible since the axon would have been separated from the anterior horn cell in the spinal cord, sensory conduction will be preserved because the dorsal root ganglion is in continuity with the axon or dendrite. Hence, intact sensory conduction in the anesthetic limb is a poor prognostic sign.

The sequence of steps in the evaluation of a brachial plexus injury can be recapitulated as follows: One would perform a detailed history and physical examination initially, whether the patient has just been injured or is being seen after time has elapsed. If electrodiagnostic studies have not been done, they should be and duly recorded. If, for example, electromyograms are done on a patient with a fresh brachial plexus injury and there is evidence of degeneration, there must have been prior injury, since it normally takes 3 weeks for this phenomenon to develop. Plain radiographs are taken initially, and if there are any fractures, updated films are obtained. As stated, myelography is usually delayed for 1 month after injury. With the clinical and ancillary studies having been completed, one is ready to formulate the plan for therapy.

How is the treatment plan formulated?[30,31]

In addition to the physician's evaluation, patients should be seen by the occupational therapist and the physical therapist for evaluation and input. Arrangements should be made for detailed and thorough follow-up, which provides increased observation and the possibility of further explanations or ventilating of the patient's concerns. All information that is compiled from these evaluations is explained to the patients in detail, by means of diagrams and models. Several explanatory sessions may be required because of the technical nature of what is being discussed or anxiety on the part of the patients. It is most important that this information be shared with the patients as soon as it is solidly established, so that as little time as possible is lost in planning the therapy and whatever modifications will be necessary in life-style or ultimate goals.

What operative techniques are available for central neurological reconstruction of the traumatized brachial plexus?

Although the early years of the twentieth century witnessed brave and imaginative attempts to reconstruct the traumatized brachial plexus, enthusiasm gradually waned with the passage of time and more rigorous scrutiny of end results. Notwithstanding some spectacular results, by the time of the Second World War and for the next two decades, brachial plexus exploration was done largely for the establishment of the extent of the lesions and for formulation of a prognosis.[49] The advent of microsurgery stimulated a new group of surgeons in various parts of the world to reexamine the possibility of reconstructing the injured nerves. The work of Millesi,[36,37,38] Narakas,[41,42,43] Allieu,[1] Alnot,[2,3] Lusskin, Campbell and Thompson,[34] and Sedel[48] should be consulted for their specific results. However, it is difficult, and sometimes impossible to compare the various reported series in terms of their ultimate functional results. Furthermore, in those patients in whom partial lesions exist, and who have the possibliity of peripheral reconstruction by means

of conventional techniques of arthrodesis and tendon transfer, the lack of a standardized approach to evaluation has thus far made comparison difficult. For those patients with flail anestheic arms and no possibility of peripheral reconstruction, central neurologic reconstruction remains the only possibility for enhancing neurologic and, ultimately, functional improvement. The general consensus seems to be that the adult traction injuries are best explored within the first 6 months following injury[38] (optimally after 3 months, to allow for whatever diagnostic workup is to be done and the possibility of spontaneous recovery). Although useful results have been reported after the 6-month period and as long as 18 months after injury, the low probability of significant benefit from surgery done after the 6-month period makes it often not worthwhile. Although in our present state of technology, it is impossible to replant a spinal nerve that has been avulsed from the cord, if there is sufficient length of nerve available distal to the intervertebral foramen to serve as a source of axons, then surgical manipulation may be attempted. Since most traction injuries involve extensive longitudinal damage to the nerves, it is highly unlikely that direct suture will be successful in these situations, and some type of nerve graft will be necessary. The sural nerves are often used as donors, and occasionally the medial cutaneous nerve of the forearm taken in the arm or even the ipsilateral ulnar nerve if it is defunctionalized by reason of a supraganglionic lesion of C8 and T1. The prognosis for recovery after grafts of the lower trunk, even in situations in which avulsion has not taken place, is so poor that grafting is hardly worthwhile. The best prognosis is for grafts of the upper and intermediate trunks with the possibility of some shoulder control as well as recovery of elbow flexion and some wrist motors.[38,43] Occasionally finger flexion can be restored. The restoration of sensibility is, of course, of primary importance, and there have been some successes, particularly with reference to the radial side of the hand. Needless to say, the results obtained from direct neurologic reconstruction are far from normal, but compared to the absolutely hopeless prognosis for the patient with a flail-anesthetic arm that is not operated on, they are sufficiently worthwhile to be recommended, as long as the patient realizes that the objectives are quite limited.

For the patient with partial function in the limb, there is considerably more controversy as to what should be done—either central neurologic reconstruction or peripheral reconstructive surgery. My preference in this group is for peripheral reconstruction, which will be described below.[31] Suffice it to say that further documentation of results of these techniques is needed, and I hope it will be forthcoming in the near future.

What are the important nonoperative considerations in patient management during the periods spent waiting either for spontaneous recovery or the results of surgery?

As has been previously noted, patients with brachial plexus injuries have multiple problems resulting not only from the often extensive motor and sensory deficits in the limb, but from contractures, edema. subluxations, and the possibility of further injury of insensate parts. These patients require careful monitoring by all concerned with their management and continued education so that they can contribute to their care. The control of anxiety and the provision of psychological support during this difficult time are necessary and ongoing areas of concern. The management of pain will be discussed in a later section.

The shoulder, normally the most mobile joint in the body, not only can become very stiff in a relatively short period of time because of failure to move it passively when active control has been lost, but also is subject to painful subluxation because of the weight of the arm unsupported by the paralyzed muscles. Sometimes the patient will take to unrelenting use of slings to prevent or correct subluxation, with the result that the shoulder loses passive range, particularly in abduction and lateral rotation. Many varieties of orthosis have been designed to offset this problem. Unfortunately there is no universally applicable orthosis, and each case must be dealt with individually.

The elbow, which may have been injured at the same time the brachial plexus palsy occurred, may become stiff because of continual use of a sling or failure to put it through a full range of motion every day. The hand tends to conform to the contour of the abdomen, against which it rests, with the result that very quickly the metacarpophalangeal joints are ankylosed in full extension and a thumb is in the plane of the palm and therefore useless even if motor control were reestablished. The judicious use of physiologic orthoses and passive range of motion exercise, as well as scrupulous attention to the integrity of the skin, is mandatory if the hand is to be returned to a functional status. The patient must be educated to protect his insensitive skin from trauma and to avoid persistent edema, since it too will sometimes prove devastatingly permanent once it is established.

Whether to attempt to supply a patient with a functional orthosis to accommodate his flail-anesthetic limb has been a subject of some controversy. Wynn-Parry in England has been particularly successful in providing his patients with functional splints.[53]

What can be obtained from peripheral reconstruction of the shoulder?

The complexity of the motions of the shoulder and the number of muscle couples that are required for normal function make the criteria for results of neurologic reconstruction of the plexus for the paretic or paralyzed shoulder particularly demanding. Even if the deltoid can be reinnervated, it is also necessary to have a functioning rotator cuff. Sometimes the cuff can be substituted for my means of tendon transfer.[17] However, with extensive paralysis, even that option is not available, and usually the flail shoulder must either be accepted as such or be fused. It is important to understand the concept of arthrodesis of the shoulder and to realize that it does not mean that a shoulder that is completely stiff. The operation makes use of the fact that in normal shoulder motion, the scapula accounts for significant elevation and forward flexion of the arm. If the trapezius and serratus anterior muscles are intact, even in the presence of significant plexus injury, it may well be possible by means of an arthodesis of the glenohumeral joint in a functional position to significantly aid the control of the limb.[47] Specifically, with the glenohumeral joint fused, the patient may forward flex to the horizontal and may be able to reach the other shoulder, the front trousers pocket, and the rear. A number of techniques are available, but the one that I have used for the last 10 years involves internal fixation with compression screws and a postoperative period of immobilization in a shoulder spica for 12 weeks. The result is usually significant enhancement of the limb in its role as an assistive member.

Tendon transfer about the shoulder has been practiced in the past, particularly in the treatment of patients with poliomyelitis.[17] Unfortunately, the techniques are not directly applicable to the brachial plexus population, because the number of available muscles in the latter group is usually considerably less than in the former. Nevertheless, for patients with partial lesions, multiple tendon transfers may be quite useful. One of the most successful is that described by L'Episcopo[33] for the restoration of shoulder control in patients who have some deltoid function but lack active lateral rotation control. In these patients, the latissimus dorsi and teres major may be transferred posterolaterally with significant benefit. The important concept in regard to the patient who is considered for tendon transfer about the shoulder is that no single muscle transfer will restore function, and multiple transfers must always be done. It is obvious that a shoulder that has important contractures cannot be expected to benefit from tendon transfer unless those contractures are overcome by means of either physical therapy or direct surgical release.

What techniques are available for the restoration of control to the paralyzed elbow?

Although few would argue about the importance of elbow extension power in normal activities of daily living, the focus of reconstruction in the paralyzed elbow has been flexion. Numerous techniques have, again, been adapted from the experience in poliomyelitis, and the same cautions exist as for the shoulder. Although one can restore active elbow flexion by means of a transfer of the sternocleidomastoid,[10] few use that technique today. The major thrust of surgical reconstruction has been toward the use of closer muscles, such as the pectoralis and the flexor-pronator muscles at the elbow.

The flexor-pronator muscles of the forearm and wrist are auxiliary elbow flexors. In 1918, Arthur Steindler reported their use in the "flexorplasty," which was the standard treatment of the elbow paralyzed by poliomyelitis.[50] The operation involves transposition of the muscle origins from the medial epicondyle proximally to either the medial intermuscular septum or directly to the bone anteriorly a distance of about 7 cm.[35] This imparts a greater flexion moment to the elbow and may allow the hand to be brought to the mouth or to assist the normal other side. The power attained is usually not more than the ability to lift a few pounds.[28] The elbow is immobilized postoperatively for 4 to 6 weeks, and then a long period of postoperative muscle reeducation is required. If the shoulder is either under good control or fused, the ability to forward flex it and thereby eliminate gravity will enhance the power of elbow flexion by eliminating the weight of the limb. The pectoral transfer, originally described by Clark[13] in 1946, and its modifications,[12] can provide excellent and powerful elbow flexion to the paralyzed elbow if the shoulder is either strong or fused. Failure to recognize this requirement results in loss of power because of the uncontrolled joint and subsequent medial rotation and arm adduction rather than elbow flexion. Although the operative exposure is an extensive one, the postoperative morbidity is not great, and the therapy program is similar to that of the Steindler flexor plasty. In both of these procedures, it is desirable to maintain a permanent flexion contracture of approximately 30 degrees because it adds to the mechanical advantage of the transfer. It is for this reason that I encourage the use of a sling for 2 to 3 months after either operation.

Transfer of the latissimus dorsi for elbow flexion may be employed in the brachial plexus patient if the muscle is of good quality and power preoperatively.[24,56] Unfortunately, in extensive paralysis, as is often the case, it is not available.

Triceps transfer, again adapted from the polio literature, is available for use to restore active elbow flexion.[10,11] The advantages may be outweighed, however, by the functional loss that forfeiture of active extension implies. Obviously, one would not want to do the operation in a patient who walks on crutches, and certainly not bilaterally. Fortunately, bilateral brachial plexus injuries are rare. Furthermore, the loss of the stabilization and positioning of the forearm and hand that are conveyed by an intact triceps is a significant consideration in use of this transfer. Postoperative phase conversion has not been a significant problem in my experience. However, either preceding or as a substitute for a surgical reconstruction, one might consider the use of a static or dynamic orthosis, with the power for the latter being provided by cable or external power sources.

The timing of these reconstructive procedures must obviously depend on the needs of the patient. In general, when a chronic state has been reached and no further spontaneous recovery has occurred or is deemed likely to occur, then surgical reconstruction may begin. Because of technical considerations, it is wise to begin distally in the limb and work proximally, although the Clark pectoral transfer will have to be preceded by the arthrodesis of the shoulder. If shoulder fusion is done before a Steindler flexor plasty, it becomes very awkward to perform the surgery. Ordinarily I do not advocate arthrodesis of the shoulder before 9 months after injury, but surgery around the elbow distally may be done at 6 months or so, as long as the neurologic status of the limb has been clarified.

What are the problems with the wrist of the brachial plexus–injured patient?

As has already been described, there is a very real danger of development of flexion contracture in the wrist of a patient with major paralysis who is allowed to remain unsplinted and uses a sling. Obviously, the kinesiologic benefits of a mobile wrist need not be justified. However, it should be emphasized that the ability to utilize the tenodesis mechanism of either flexors or extensors by maintenance of wrist mobility is of significant benefit. For the patient who is expected to regain function, the judicious use of long wrist supports, with due regard being given to the possiblity of skin breakdown, will maximize the ultimate functional result. For patients with lesions of the lower and intermediate trunk, if active voluntary control of the fingers and thumb is to be even partially restored, it will be necessary to arthrodese the wrist to allow for liberation of the wrist motors and their subsequent use to power the fingers and thumb. The technique of Haddad and Riordan,[16] in which an iliac crest bone graft is inserted from the radial side, is of advantage because it does not produce scarring on the dorsum of the wrist, which might interfere with the gliding of the extensor tendons at a later date. The normal postoperative healing time after that procedure is 8 weeks, during which time it is necessary to maintain the mobility of the joints of the fingers and thumb. Certainly, special situations will sometimes dictate the use of other techniques.

How does the management of the hand of a patient with a brachial plexus injury differ from the management of the hands of patients with other nerve injuries?

The answer to this question is a highly individualized one, depending on the degree of loss in a particular limb. Sometimes, all of the considerations in regard to tendon transfer and arthrodesis that are applicable to patients with more simple, peripheral nerve injuries are entirely transferable to the patient with a brachial plexus injury. It is really a matter of degree, in that the plexus injury patient usually has a more complicated problem that will impose additional restrictions because of involvement of adjacent joints. For these patients, as has been previously stated, the reconstruction of the hand, if it is to be salvaged, should precede consideration of the other joints, for several reasons. The first is that the remainder of the limb has as its purpose the placement of the hand, or terminal device, and if that fails, there is less pressure to reconstruct the other joints. Nevertheless, sometimes the more proximal joints may be all that is potentially salvageable in a limb. If the patient is demonstrated to be uncooperative in the conduct of the reconstruction of the hand, the situation may merit serious reconsideration before the physician proceeds proximally. Then, since the ease of the surgical technique may depend on the placement of the hand on a "hand table," it is certainly easier to do that if the remainder of the limb is mobile.

All of the techniques that are available to maintain mobility, prevent or treat edema, and protect the hand from further injury must be systematically applied to the hand of a patient with a brachial plexus injury. Since these are discussed in great detail in the other chapters of this book, they will not be repeated here.

How is pain managed in the brachial plexus injury patient?

A high percentage of patients with traction injuries to the brachial plexus have pain that may initially be very severe. Fortunately, the discomfort usually diminishes with time, and although it may persist, the patient's reaction to it may improve. It is particularly important to identify and deal with anxiety and depression; they may have been present in the premorbid state, but if they are present as a result of injury they may seriously worsen the reaction of the patient to his pain. The treatment of the pain with narcotics on a long-term basis is contraindicated, since this is chronic, "benign" pain. Unfortunately, many patients are started by well-meaning physicians on narcotic medications, and some patients are drug abusers before they are injured. Both classes of patient may be very difficult to wean from their narcotics, and in some cases, which fortunately are rare, it may be impossible. The use of phenytoin (Dilantin) or carbamazepine (Tegretol) is usually suggested but in my experience is rarely predictively successful. In addition, since Tegretol has potentially serious side effects, its use must be monitored closely. Some patients will respond positively to the transcutaneous nerve stimulator, and some maintain that acupuncture has been helpful. I have seen very few patients whose pain has been significantly benefited by hypnosis or psychotherapy, although the latter may be helpful in the management of anxiety or depression.

The surgery for pain of brachial plexus injury has had a long and difficult history. Although at one time it was thought that resection of the traumatic pseudomeningoceles might favorably influence the pain, this procedure does not enjoy popular support today, nor is there great enthusiasm for cordotomy, rhizotomy, or sympathectomy. The question of whether neurolysis is of value in the treatment of pain in brachial plexus injury is still unresolved. Several workers have the impression that reconstructing the plexus itself and augmenting input in a sensory-deprived situation may improve pain. The dorsal column stimulator[52] and implanted electrodes are of interest and have been used in some carefully selected patients. Further work needs to be done in this area. There are some favorable preliminary reports on the use of selective surgical lesions of the substantia gelantinosa of the spinal cord, by Dr. Nashold at Duke University.[44] Suffice it to say that the problem of the pain of brachial plexus injury continues to be a difficult one for which no clearly dependable solution exists.

How are the permanently flail-anesthetic arm and hand managed?

Until the recent resurgence of interest in microsurgical reconstruction of the brachial plexus, the standard option for treatment of the flail-anesthetic limb was ablation. Actually, there were three choices, the first of which was to do nothing and to have the patient keep the arm in a sling or his hand in a pocket. For some patients whose life-styles or occupations were not significantly prejudiced by this approach, it could suffice. As long as the limb was not injured, it would be possible for many patients to live relatively unencumbered. Some, however, found that the limb was heavy, annoying, and in the way, and so opted to have it amputated. Often there was no consideration of functional restoration by means of prosthetic fitting, and so the standard treatment was a high humeral amputation. If the patient was not to be fitted with a prosthesis, there really was no time constraint. However, if prosthetic fitting was to be done and the patient was to use the prosthesis, it was best done before 2 years had elapsed since the time of injury.[55] This particular approach, combined with an arthrodesis of the shoulder, did

result in some minimal use of the limb, and in some patients, use of the limb in the course of gainful employment. The experience was well documented by Yeoman and Seddon.[54]

Although a flail-anesthetic arm could technically be reconstructed by a series of tenodeses and arthodeses, as documented by Hendry,[19] this particular approach has not been appealing because of the vulnerability of the limb to injury of the insensate skin in the course of normal use.

For patients who may by some combination of central and peripheral reconstruction regain the proximal control of the limb but not have a useful hand, there may be significant benefit from the performance of a forearm amputation and fitting of a prosthesis. Even in those patients who do not have active control of the elbow, or sensation over the proposed forearm stump, if there is proprioception in the elbow a forearm amputation may be done with the beneficial fitting of a prosthesis. We have used this approach for 10 years and have been gratified both by the use of the prosthesis and by the lack of stump complications.

Finally, the question arises as to whether a patient with a painful flail-anesthetic limb can be relieved of his pain by amputation of the limb. Fletcher[14] has objected to amputation in such a situation, as has Seddon,[49] and our experiences has been similar.

REFERENCES

1. Allieu, Y.: Exploration et traitement direct des lesions nerveuses dans les paralysies traumatiques par élongation du plexus brachial chez l'adulte, Rev. Chir. Orthop. **63:**107, 1977.
2. Alnot, J.Y.: Technique chirgicale dans les paralysies du plexus brachial, Rev. Chir. Orthop. **63:**75, 1977.
3. Alnot, J.Y., Augereau, B., and Frot, B.: Traitement direct des lesions nerveuses dans les paralysies traumatiques par élongation du plexus brachial chez l'adulte, Chirurgie **103:**935, 1977.
4. Barnes, R.: Traction injuries of the brachial plexus in adults, J. Bone Joint Surg. **31B:**10, 1949.
5. Bonney, G.: Prognosis in traction lesions of the brachial plexus, J. Bone Joint Surg. **41B:**4, 1959.
6. Bowden, R.E.M.: The applied anatomy of the cervical spine and brachial plexus, Proc. R. Soc. Med. **59:**1141, 1966.
7. Brewerton, D.A., and Daniel, J.W.: Factors influencing return to work, Br. Med. J. **4:**277, 1971.
8. Brooks, D.M.: Open wounds of the brachial plexus, J. Bone Joint Surg. **31B:**17, 1949.
9. Bufalini, C., and Pescatori, G.: Posterior cervical electromyography in the diagnosis and prognosis of brachial plexus injuries, J. Bone Joint Surg. **51B:**627, 1969.
10. Bunnell, S.: Restoring flexion to the paralytic elbow, J. Bone Joint Surg. **33A:**566, 1951.
11. Carroll, R.E.: Restoration of flexor power to the flail elbow by transplantation of the triceps tendon, Surg. Gynecol. Obstet. **95:**685, 1952.
12. Carroll, R.E., and Kleinman, W.B.: Pectoralis major transplantation to restore elbow flexion to the paralytic limb, J. Hand Surg. **4:**501, 1979.
13. Clark, J.M.P.: Reconstruction of biceps brachii by pectoral muscle transplantation, Br. J. Surg. **34:**180, 1946.
14. Fletcher, I.: Management of severe traction lesions of the brachial plexus, J. Bone Joint Surg. **48B:**178, 1966.
15. Goss, C.H.: Gray's anatomy, ed. 28, Philadelphia, 1966, Lea & Febiger.
16. Haddad, R.J., Jr., and Riordan, D.C.: Arthrodesis of the wrist: a surgical technique, J. Bone Joint Surg. **49A:**950, 1967.
17. Harmon, P.H.: Surgical reconstruction of the paralytic shoulder by multiple muscle transplantations, J. Bone Joint Surg. **32A:**583, 1950.
18. Harris, W.: The true form of the brachial plexus and its motor distribution, J. Anat. Physiol. **38:**399, 1904.
19. Hendry, A.M.: The treatment of residual paralysis after brachial plexus injuries, J. Bone Joint Surg. **31B:**42, 1949.

20. Heon, M.: Myelogram: a questionable aid in diagnosis and prognosis in avulsion of brachial plexus components by traction injuries, Conn. Med. **29:**260, 1965.
21. Herringham, W.P.: The minute anatomy of the brachial plexus, Proc. R. Soc. Lond. **41:**423, 1886.
22. Hollinshead, W.H.: Anatomy for surgeons, vol. 3, The back and limbs, New York, 1969, Harper & Row, Publishers, Inc., Ch. 4.
23. Hovelacque, A.: Anatomie des nerfs craniens et rachidiens et du système grand sympathique, Paris, 1927, Gaston, Dion, p. 385.
24. Hovnanian, A.P.: Latissimus dorsi transplantation for loss of flexion or extension at the elbow: a preliminary report on technique, Ann. Surg. **143:**493, 1956.
25. Jackson, L., and Keats, A.S.: Mechanism of brachial plexus palsy following anesthesia, Anaesthesia **26:**190, 1965.
26. Jelasic, F., and Piepgres, U.: Functional restitution after cervical avulsion injury with "typical" myelographic findings, Eur. Neurol. **11:**158, 1974.
27. Kerr, A.T.: The brachial plexus of nerves in man, the variations in its formation and branches, Am. J. Anat. **23:**285, 1918.
28. Kettlekemp, D.B., and Larson, C.B.: Evaluation of the Steindler flexorplasty, J. Bone Joint Surg. **45A:**513, 1963.
29. Kwaan, J.H.M., and Rappaport, I.: Postoperative brachial plexus palsy—a study on the mechanism, Arch. Surg. **101:**612, 1970.
30. Leffert, R.D.: Brachial plexus injuries, N. Engl. J. Med. **291:**1059, 1974.
31. Leffert, R.D.: Lesions of the brachial plexus, including thoracic outlet syndrome. In American Academy of Orthopaedic Surgeons: Instructional course lectures, vol. XXVI, St Louis, 1977, The C.V. Mosby Co.
32. Leffert, R.D., and Seddon, H.: Infraclavicular brachial plexus injuries, J. Bone Joint Surg. **47B:**9, 1965.
33. L'Episcopo, J.B.: Restoration of muscle balance in the treatment of obstetrical paralysis, N.Y. State J. Med. **39:**357, 1939.
34. Lusskin, R., Campbell, J.B., and Thompson, W.A.L.: Post-traumatic lesions of the brachial plexus: treatment by transclavicular exploration and neurolysis or autograft reconstruction, J. Bone Joint Surg. **55A:**1159, 1973.
35. Mayer, L., and Green, W.: Experiences with the Steindler flexorplasty at the elbow, J. Bone Joint Surg. **36A:**775, 1954.
36. Millesi, H.: Microsurgery of peripheral nerves, Hand **5:**157,1973.
37. Millesi, H.: Indications et resultats des interventions direct, Rev. Chir. Orthop. **63:**82, 1977.
38. Millesi, H.: Surgical management of brachial plexus injuries. J. Hand Surg. **2:**367, 1977.
39. Murphy, F., Hartung, W., and Kirklin, J.W.: Myelographic demonstration of avulsing injury of the brachial plexus, Am. J. Roentgenol. Radium Ther. Nucl. Med. **58:**102, 1947.
40. Murphy, F., and Kirklin, J.: Myelographic demonstration of avulsing injuries of the nerve roots of the brachial plexus—a method of determining the point of injury and the possibility of repair, Clin. Neurosurg. **20:**18, 1972.
41. Narakas, A.: Indications et resultats du traitement chirurgical direct dans les lesions par élongation du plexus brachial, Rev. Chir. Orthop. **63:**88, 1977.
42. Narakas, A.: The surgical management of brachial plexus injuries. In Daniel, R.K., and Terzis, J.K., Editors: Reconstructive micro-surgery, Boston, 1977, Little, Brown & Co., vol. 1, Ch. 9.
43. Narakas, A.: Surgical treatment of traction injuries of the brachial plexus, Clin. Orthop. **133:**71, 1978.
44. Nashold, B.S., Jr., and Ostdahl, R.H.: Dorsal root entry zone lesions for pain relief, J. Neurosurg. **51:**59, 1979.
45. Nelson, K.G., Jolly, P.C., and Thomas, P.A.: Brachial plexus injuries associated with missile wounds of the chest: a report of 9 cases from Vietnam, J. Trauma **8:**268, 1968.
46. Rorabeck, C.H., and Harris, W.R.: Factors affecting the prognosis of brachial plexus injuries, J. Bone Joint Surg. **63B:**404-407, 1981.
47. Rowe, C.R.: Reevaluation of the position of the arm in arthrodesis of the shoulder in the adult, J. Bone Joint Surg. **56A:**913, 1974.
48. Sedel, L.: The results of surgical repair of brachial plexus injuries, J. Bone Joint Surg. **64B:**54, 1982.
49. Seddon, H.J.: Surgical disorders of the peripheral nerves, Edinburgh, 1972, Churchill Livingstone.
50. Steindler, A.: Reconstruction work on hand and forearm. N.Y. State Med. J. **108:**117, 1918.
51. Stevens, J.H.: Brachial plexus paralysis. In Codman, E.A.: The shoulder, Brooklyn, N.Y., 1934, G. Miller & Co.
52. Sweet, W., and Wepsic, J.: Stimulation of the posterior columns of the spinal cord for pain control: indications, techniques and results, Clin. Neurosurg. **21:**378, 1974.
53. Wynn-Parry, C.B.: Rehabilitation of the hand, ed. 4, London, 1981, Butterworth & Co. (Publishers), Ltd.
54. Yeoman, P.M.: Cervical myelopathy in traction injuries of the brachial plexus, J. Bone Joint Surg. **50B:**253, 1968.
55. Yeoman, P.M., and Seddon, H.J.: Brachial plexus injuries: treatment of the flail arm, J. Bone Joint Surg. **43B:**493, 1961.
56. Zancolli, E., and Mitre, H.: Latissimus dorsi transfer to restore elbow flexion: an appraisal of eight cases, J. Bone Joint Surg. **55A:**1265, 1973.

39

Splinting the nerve-injured hand

SHIRLEY OLLOS PEARSON

All three nerves supplying the hand are liable to damage that may result in very severe loss of function. The severity of the injury depends not only on the amount of damage to the nerve but also on the degree of soft-tissue damage and the type of injury. While many times tendons are injured and the nerve remains intact, generally if a nerve is lacerated or compressed, tendon and vascular injury also occur. Even though the repair of a nerve is successful and the regeneration of that nerve is complete, the damage to the tendons and the soft tissue with subsequent fibrosis and stiffening of the joints can produce a crippled hand for life. Splinting in conjunction with a good program of therapy and physician follow-up is a valuable tool in preventing this and in correcting deformity if it has already occurred. While injury to a nerve can result in neurapraxia, axonotmesis, or neurotmesis, the splinting principles would be the same and only the duration of splintage and the durability of the materials used might vary.

PURPOSES OF SPLINTING

Splinting for the nerve-injured hand can be divided into the following three purposes: (1) to restore the hand to suppleness with full passive range of motion of the entire extremity and to assist in restoring active range of motion and strength in the muscles not affected by the nerve injury, (2) to prevent deformities from occurring because of the lack of balance of muscle power in the extremity, and (3) to position the hand or to add mechanical assistance so that hand can be used functionally.

Restoration of suppleness

The first stage in the treatment of most nerve injuries would be to correct the deformity caused by the acute injury and emergency treatment. Before functional splints can be easily used, it is necessary to first mobilize the hand as much as possible and to regain control of the wrist. Especially in cases involving lacerated nerves at the wrist level that also involve tendon and vascualr injuries, a cast will have been applied to the wrist to eliminate stress on the approximated nerve ends and the repaired structures. In median and ulnar nerve repairs the wrist will have been held in palmar flexion for 3 to 4 weeks; consequently, the patient often begins treatment with a tight flexion contracture of the wrist, a tough scar, and a variable amount of edema.

At this time a program of gentle active and passive exercise, elevation of the extremity, and splinting should begin. A static splint may be needed to hold the patient's wrist in as close to functional position as is comfortable. Unless it is necessary to immobilize the fingers, they should be left free so the patient is able to exercise them easily. Usually a wrist-control splint is sufficient, but it will need to be adjusted serially at the wrist every few days until the desired position is reached. This splint can be constructed on either the volar or the dorsal portion of the hand and forearm, depending on which is comfortable for the patient. Sometimes it is advisable not to apply the splint over a severe wound. Splinting the wrist will make it easier for the patient to maintain his arm in elevation, thus reducing the edema. When the patient is able to maintain his wrist in slight dorsiflexion, the static splint can be used only as a night splint and a functional splint can be applied.

When patients have severe contractures that do not respond to treatment, it may be necessary to use dynamic traction splinting to assist in restoring the hand to suppleness. Contractures that were present for several years have been reduced with a strenuous program of dynamic splinting. Consequently, the patient can proceed to functional splints and finally to tendon transfers that will restore good hand function.

Prevention of deformities resulting from lack of balance of the muscles in the hand

When a muscle is paralyzed, its antagonist, now unopposed, draws the limb into deformity so that the paralyzed muscles become too long. When the nerve finally regenerates, the elongated muscle is at such a disadvantage in trying to work against the resistance of the healthy muscle that recovery will be limited or greatly delayed until the muscle regains its ability to contract. Structures such as collateral ligaments shorten, adherences occur, and after long periods bony changes may be seen. Therefore splinting is necessary to prevent these occurrences. The splint need not hold the limb overcorrected to the opposite deformity; it should merely hold it in the position of balance.

Positional or mechanical assistance for hand function

The need for corrective splintage in peripheral nerve injuries is easy to recognize, but it is just as essential that a good splint should do more than merely correct deformity;

452

it should also encourage function. Some correctional splints are not designed to encourage movement and, in fact, often hinder it. Many movements are available in the nerve-injured hand, and if a splint is designed both to correct deformity and to make use of these movements for function, the patient will make more use of his hand. Movement patterns will not be lost in the brain during the long period of paralysis; circulation is retained with the consequent reduction of edema, and the patient is able to return to a more normal life-style.

NERVE INJURIES AND SPLINTS

There are many different designs for splints for each nerve injury. It is important to carefully analyze each hand, assess the lack of function, and design the splint for the individual patient and his needs. These splints may need to be altered, since the fit will change with the wasting or recovery of muscle bulk. In order for the patient to wear a splint for a long period of time, the splint should be light, easy to clean, and as esthetically pleasing as possible, and it should not immobilize any more of the hand than is necessary.

Median nerve palsy

Lesions or compressions of the median nerve at any level will produce deformity in the hand. Deformities caused by lower forearm or wrist injuries are commonly known as the "ape" hand, because of the flat appearance of the hand resulting from wasting of the thenar eminence and lack of opposition. The thumb is held beside the index finger because the abductor brevis and opponens muscles are paralyzed and, therefore, their antagonists, the extensor pollicis longus and the adductor pollicis, act unopposed. There is paralysis of the first and second lumbricals, so there may be a hyperextension deformity at the metacarpophalangeal joints of the index and middle fingers.

The purpose of the splint in median nerve palsy is to position the thumb in abduction to counteract the deforming action of the long extensor and to encourage opposition by the long flexor. While it is possible to dynamically

achieve this position with an elastic band and sling attached to a wrist band, stability of the thumb is needed for most hand function. An abducted position with stability can be achieved with a C-bar opponens splint (Fig. 39-1, *A*), which allows full wrist movement; interphalangeal flexion of the thumb, while holding the thumb in opposition to the index and middle fingers; and full flexion of the fingers. A thumb post splint (Fig. 39-1, *B*) will also hold this thumb position, and it has the advantage of maintaining a palmar arch.

Ulnar nerve palsy

The classic deformity caused by an ulnar nerve palsy is the "clawhand," which will occur if the lesion is present in the wrist, elbow, or even the neck. The metacarpophalangeal joints are held in varying degrees of hyperextension owing to the overaction of the extensor digitorum communis and the extensor digiti minimi, which are acting against the paralyzed third and fourth lumbricals. The interphalangeal joints are held in flexion owing to the overpull of the flexors sublimus and profundus, which are unopposed by the paralyzed interossei.

If the lesion is at the elbow, the flexor profundus of the ring and little fingers will also be paralyzed, thus minimizing the deformity of the fingers. However, when the nerve regenerates and innervates the flexor profundus, the deformity will increase.

The principle of the ulnar nerve splint is to prevent hyperextension of the metacarpophalangeal joints. If the hand is supple and the splint effectively stops metacarpophalangeal hyperextension, the support at the metacarpophalangeal joints allows the extensor digitorum to act on the interphalangeal joints.

There are many ways to splint a hand with ulnar nerve palsy. A simple wrist band with rubber bands and slings (Fig. 39-2, *A*) may be effective if the hand is very supple and the patient has no difficulty in maintaining his wrist in slight extension. However, many patients have already developed a wrist flexion pattern when they flex their fingers; hence, it is necessary to attach the finger loops and rubber

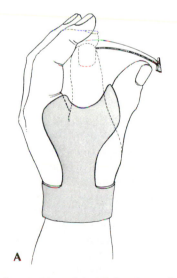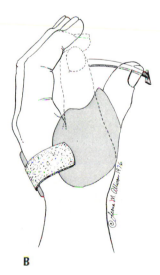

A   **B**

FIG. 39-1. Lack of opposition of thumb is primary functional loss in median nerve palsy; thus splint such as, **A,** C-bar opponens splint or, **B,** thumb post splint may be used to position thumb and provide function to hand.

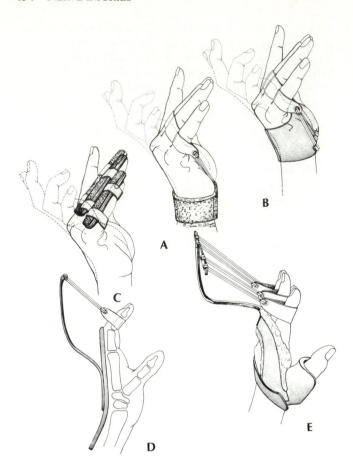

FIG. 39-2. Hand with ulnar nerve loss can be splinted in many ways depending on status of deformity. **A,** Wrist band with finger loops and rubber bands will control hyperextension of metacarpophalangeal joints in supple hand with good wrist control. **B,** If patient does not have good control of his wrist, finger loops will need to be attached to hand cuff. **C,** Finger splints will allow all flexion power to be exerted at metacarpophalangeal joints. **D,** Dynamic traction may be needed to reduce flexion contractures at proximal interphalangeal joints. **E,** Thumb opposition post can be added for hand with combined median and ulnar nerve palsy.

bands to a pliable cuff that is fitted to the hand (Fig. 39-2, *B*). Both these splints will allow the patient to use his hand functionally and are easy to apply. Finger splints (Fig. 39-2, *C*) can be an effective way to eliminate finger flexion and allow the entire pull of the flexor profundus and flexor sublimus to increase metacarpophalangeal flexion. Spring-wire splints or a molded plastic metacarpalphalangeal block may also effectively control metacarpalphalangeal joint hyperextension and allow functional use of the hand.

When contractures are already present, it may be necessary to use dynamic-traction splinting (Fig. 39-2, *D*) to reduce the deformities and then proceed with less cumbersome splinting. When both ulnar and median nerves are paralyzed, an effective splint would be a thumb post splint with a metacarpophalangeal bar to prevent hyperextension. If deformities need correcting, an outrigger to dynamically extend the interphalangeal joints (Fig. 39-2, *E*) can be used, and then the outrigger can be eliminated when the contracture is eliminated.

Radial nerve palsy

The most obvious deformity in radial nerve palsy is a wristdrop. The wrist is held in 45 degrees of palmar flexion owing to the overaction of the wrist flexors unopposed by their antagonists, the paralyzed wrist extensors. The thumb is held in palmar abduction and slight flexion, owing to the unopposed action of the short flexor and short abductor

working against their paralyzed antagonists, the long abductor and the short and long extensors of the thumb. The paralyzed extensor digitorum allows the lumbricals to pull the metacarpophalangeal joints into flexion. Extension in the interphalangeal joints is preserved, since they are extended by the interossei, which are not innervated by the radial nerve.

It is not necessary in all cases to splint the hand with a radial nerve palsy. Because extension of the interphalangeal joints is preserved, the patient may be able to use his hand quite functionally in the wristdrop position (Fig. 39-3, *A*), thus preventing stiffness from occurring. The patient can sometimes be taught to grasp objects in a wristdrop position and then supinate, thus allowing gravity to assist him in holding objects.

If the wristdrop position is painful or uncomfortable, the patient may prefer to wear a wrist control splint even though it will decrease the function of his hand. Some patients prefer a splint to dynamically extend the fingers, even though it is cumbersome.

When the wrist must be immobilized for radial nerve repair or to heal an accompanying fracture, it is advisable to attach outriggers (Fig. 39-3, *B*) to the cast to extend the fingers and thumb. The most effective way to splint a radial nerve palsy would be to construct the splint with a hinged wrist and a dynamic extension force (Fig. 39-3, *C*). This would allow the patient to flex his wrist, thus setting up a tenodesis action that would give good hand function.

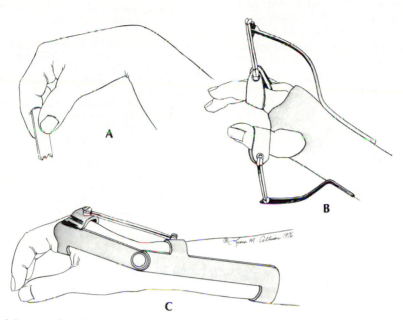

FIG. 39-3. Loss of finger and wrist extension is primary functional loss in radial nerve palsy. **A,** Unless wristdrop position is painful, patient can maintain use of his hand in this position. **B,** If it is necessary to immobilize patient's wrist in cast, outriggers need to be added to provide any finger function. **C,** Splint with hinged wrist and dynamic wrist extension will provide patient with functional hand if he finds wristdrop position comfortable.

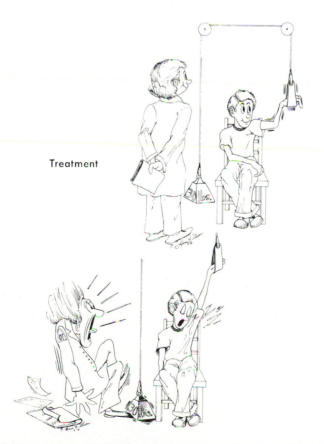

FIG. 39-4. Outcome of treatment depends on combination of exercise, splinting, and activity in which patient is an *active participant*.

• • •

With splinting, as with any other part of the patient's treatment, the patient must be an *active* participant (Fig. 39-4). To be successful with a program involving splinting, the patient must understand the purposes of the splint, the precautions that need to be observed, and how to apply the splint correctly, and he must want to *participate* in a program that will restore hand function to him.

ACKNOWLEDGMENT

The illustrations in this chapter were done by Leona Allison.

BIBLIOGRAPHY

Boyes, J.H.: Bunnell's surgery of the hand, ed. 5, Philadelphia, 1970, J.B. Lippincott Co.

Chase, R.A.: Surgery of the hand, N. Engl. J. Med. **287:**1174-1181; 1227-1234, 1972.

Fess, E.E., Gettle, K.S., and Strickland, J.W.: Hand splinting principles and methods, vol. 1, St. Louis, 1981, The C.V. Mosby Co.

Littler, J.W.: Dynamic splinting and immobilization. In Converse, J.M.: Reconstructive plastic surgery, vol. 4, Philadelphia, 1964, W.B. Saunders Co.

Malick, M.H.: Manual on static hand splinting, Pittsburgh, 1973, Harmarville Rehabilitation Center.

Malick, M.H.: Manual on dynamic hand splinting with thermoplastic materials, ed. 2, Pittsburgh, 1978, Harmarville Rehabilitation Center.

Parry, C.B.W: Rehabilitation of the Hand, ed. 4, London, 1981, Butterworth & Co. (Publishers), Ltd.

Rockwood, C.A., Jr., and Green, D.P.: Fractures, vol. 1, Philadelphia, J.B. Lippincott Co. 1975.

Seddon, H.: Surgical disorders of the peripheral nerves, ed. 2, Edinburgh, 1975, Churchill-Livingstone.

Swan, D.: Hand disability. Paper presented at a South Australian Association of Occupational Therapists Members Meeting, Commonwealth Rehabilitation Center, Felixstow, South Africa.

40

Mechanics of tendon transfers

PAUL W. BRAND

The whole object of tendon transfer operations is to restore balance to a hand, after one or more of its muscles have been paralyzed or destroyed. In so doing the surgeon must compare the usefulness of the action of the lost muscle with that of the muscle that will have to be transferred, leaving a defect in the place where it was before.

It is not enough to consider the function and usefulness of these muscles in a qualitative sense. One has also to make an attempt to quantify the gains and losses at each joint, so that one does not *overbalance* a hand in an attempt to restore balance.

In this process of planning tendon transfers it is useful to think about those mechanical qualities that are transferred with a tendon and those that remain in the distal part of the limb as passive structures that have to be moved and that sometimes resist movement.

FACTORS TRANSFERRED WITH A MUSCLE

When a muscle-tendon unit is transferred, it carries with it some but not all of the qualities it had in its original situation.

Strength

In this context, by strength I mean ability to generate tension in the tendon. The tension capability of a muscle depends on the number of muscle fibers that it has and on the total cross-sectional area of all its fibers. Its ability to sustain its tension over a period of time, and over a number of repeated contractions, depends also on the adequacy of its blood supply, but the act of transferring a tendon should not change the vascular supply or the nerve supply of its muscle. There used to be a widely quoted rule that said when a muscle-tendon unit was transferred, its strength dropped one level in the scale of 0 to 5 by which muscles were graded.[4,7,9,10,13] This rule was worked out in the days when polio was the most common cause of paralysis demanding tendon transfers, and surgeons had to grade muscles carefully, not just as "paralyzed" and "unparalyzed" but in various grades of paralysis. We were warned not to use a grade 3 muscle without realizing that after transfer it would only work as grade 2. Any truth in this generalization must have been due to factors other than muscle strength, such as "drag," which we shall discuss later. The actual strength of a muscle is unchanged by transfer.

Just within the last few years surgeons have started to transplant muscles by microvascular and nerve anastomosis. This is quite a different thing from simple transfer; it involves removing a muscle from another limb, with its major artery, vein, and nerve, and placing it in a new situation, using locally available vessels and the motor nerve of the muscle that it is to replace. This is a new challenge, and one for which the rules have not yet been worked out. The fascicular patterns of the grafted nerve and the recipient stump may be very different, and even with the highest skill there is no chance that every nerve fiber will get through to a muscle unit. The published reports[3,8] have so far indicated that the successful cases are those in which the transplanted muscles are bigger and bulkier than the muscles they are to replace, presumably to allow for considerable loss of muscle units and yet allow for adequate survival. How much discrepancy to allow between the strength of the donor and the required strength after transplant has not yet been estimated. I would suspect that a ratio of two to one would be a conservative estimate.

For transfer, however, the task is simpler. Here the muscle remains in situ. Only the tendon is redirected, or "transferred." We choose a muscle that is about the right size to restore the balance of the hand that has been disturbed by paralysis. This is not the same as choosing a muscle of the same size as the one it is to replace. In most cases of paralysis the sum of the strengths of all the muscles that remain will be substantially less than the original total. Therefore, to obtain a new balance for the hand, the surgeon should be content to replace only part of the strength of the muscles that have been paralyzed.

Fortunately, there is a good deal of flexibility in this choice because muscles fairly quickly adapt their tension output to the demand. A strong muscle will become weaker if it is not used, and a weak muscle will become stronger, up to a point, so long as it is used to its maximum tension capability. However, it will become stronger only if it is used, and used in phase. A muscle will not become stronger just by being placed in a situation that demands strength. It must be daily and hourly used to its maximum by active contraction. Passive lengthening may occur from the activity of other muscles, but active contraction results from the recognition by the patient of the new function of the muscle. Here the therapist may be a great help. As an aid in the selection of a muscle of the right strength the tables published by Brand, Beach and Thompson may be used. At operation the relative diameters of exposed tendons serve as a good approximation. If one muscle is twice as strong as another, then the cross-sectional area of all its muscle fibers will be double that of the other, and the cross-sectional area of its tendon will also be about double that of the other tendon.[2] This is true only of the preparalysis strength. The extent to which tendon diameters change after periods of paralysis or of hypertrophy of the muscle is not known.

Excursion

Another feature of a muscle that is transferred with it is its potential range of excursion. However, this statement needs to be qualified by defining terms. We may recognize three kinds of excursion: *potential, required,* and *available.* If a muscle is freed from all its connective tissue attachments, and the naked muscle is stimulated from its fully stretched position, it should contract through a distance that is about equal to the resting length of its individual muscle fibers. This is a basic quality of muscle fibers, depending on the number of sarcomeres they contain. We have called this the *potential* excursion of the muscle. However, in the intact limb, very few muscles are able to achieve their full potential range of excursion, either because of restrictions imposed by surrounding connective tissue or because the joints they control do not have the range of motion that requires that much excursion. *Required* excursion is determined more by joints than by muscles. It is the excursion that is needed to put the joints through their whole range of motion. The extensor carpi radialis brevis, for example, has fibers that are about 6 cm long and, therefore, could potentially contract through 6 cm. However, the full range of motion of the average wrist can be accomplished with about 3.5 cm. Thus in the average hand this muscle never uses more than 3.5 cm of excursion. Previously published lists of tendon excursions have been mostly estimates of what we now call required excursion.[2] Perhaps the most significant information needed by the surgeon is the *available* excursion, as Freehafer[5] calls it, which he measures at operation after cutting the tendon distally, and which we think is that excursion permitted by the investing connective tissue. This available excursion varies from case to case and probably is largely dependent on the extent to which the patient has actually used the joints and muscles during the previous months. Connective tissue is responsive to the pattern of use. For example, people who have not previously done jogging or ballet dancing find that they cannot stretch their calf muscles far enough to run or dance effectively. By persistent stretching exercises they finally obtain a larger range. Probably they have not actually lengthened their muscle fibers; they have merely lengthened the connective tissue of the paratenon and perimysium. After such activity their available excursion would have increased.

Available excursion may be measured at operation after the tendon to be transferred has been divided. It may be held at its end by a hemostat or stitch and pulled out to its full stretch. At this point the muscle is stimulated by a tetanizing current while the movement of the tendon is measured. If the patient is awake he may make the contraction voluntarily. The figure should be recorded for reference after

surgery. Available excursion is transferred to the new site at operation only if the transfer involves minimal change of position and minimal dissection. Sometimes a long-fibered (long potential excursion) muscle is transferred from a site where it had a short required excursion to a site where it has a long required excursion. In such a case it will take time and active use to lengthen the connective tissue in and around the muscle and tendon so that the available excursion increases to match the new required excursion. If a tendon is to be widely rerouted and if the transfer is done through open wounds, then the normally compliant connective tissue and paratenon are divided and will be replaced by scar. In many operations for tendon transfer the final success or failure is determined more by the mechanical qualities of the paratendinous scar than by any other single factor. It is difficult enough for the patient to have to learn to use a muscle for a new action in an unfamiliar situation, but if that action cannot be accomplished until scar has been mobilized and lengthened, it may never be accomplished at all.

There is wide variation in the mechanical qualities of various types of connective tissue. Paratenon typically is easily stretchable. It has a long, low length-tension curve. This means that a great deal of lengthening results from a very little tension. This situation permits nearly free tendon movement over a wide range of excursion. The common fatty areolar connective tissue that serves to fill spaces between structures in the body is not quite so compliant, but it also will lengthen with moderate tension and then, with repeated movement, will become modified into a kind of paratenon.

Fascia and retinaculum, fibrous septa, and scar all tend to have steep length-tension curves, lengthening only about 10% even under considerable tension. Thus if a tendon comes to lie on a ligament that has been cut or scarified at surgery, the tendon may become united to the ligament through a collagen scar whose short fibers become parallel oriented by the pull of the tendon. Such fibers, only 1 or 2 mm long, would allow almost no tendon movement. If, instead, the transferred tendon is passed through a tunnel in loose fat and connective tissue, then the scar that forms around the tendon will attach it only to the soft and complaint tissues through which the tendon tunneler has found its way. When traction is applied to that tendon, the new scar may not stretch, but the surrounding fat and areolar tissue will stretch and move with the tendon through several millimeters. This early movement will allow the patient to sense the new action and use it. Thus, he will continue to stimulate further muscle contraction and movement and further stretch and then lengthening and remodeling of the new paratendinous tissue.

Thus the concept of excursion of a tendon is complex and involves many factors. The true potential excursion, dependent only on the number of sarcomeres in each fiber, is not responsive to movement or active use; it is responsive to the tension in the resting fiber. Tarbary and others[11,12] have shown in experimental animals that if a muscle fiber is immobilized in a slack position it becomes shorter by loss of sarcomeres, and if it is immobilized in a stretched position it becomes longer by adding of sarcomeres, until neutral tension is achieved.

MECHANICAL FACTORS AT DISTAL END OF TRANSFER

Leverage

All that a muscle can give to a joint is tension and excursion of the tendon. At the joint this is turned into action according to the leverage. The actual movement of a joint around an axis is accomplished by "torque," or "moment." These two terms mean the same thing, and are the product of force times leverage, or tension times moment arm. We all know that a lever enables a small force to move heavy objects (Fig. 40-1). We also know that a heavy weight can be moved most easily by a small force if the force is applied far up the lever, away from the axis, or if the load is close to the axis. This increases the *mechanical advantage*. (Mechanical advantage is equal to the moment arm of the force divided by the moment arm of the load.) What we often forget is that the force has to move farther if its lever arm is long and that the load will move very little if its lever arm is short.

Now this concept must be translated into the terminology of tendons and joints. The leverage that a tendon has at a joint is the perpendicular distance between the joint axis and the tendon as it crosses the joint. The lever arm beyond that is the length of the bone or digit distal to the joint axis. Thus it must be obvious at once that in the body almost all levers work with the force at the short end of the lever and the load at the long end. We are using a system of muscles that can produce enormous forces over rather short distances. The lever and pulley systems around joints are designed to take big forces with short ranges and make them effective over bigger ranges, with reduced force. There is no way to beat this system. The price of increased power is reduced range. I often hear surgeons say that they have found a way to increase the "strength" of a transfer at a joint. I rarely hear them mention the amount of excursion that has been used up, leaving less "strength" for other joints in the same sequence, or the fact that the transfer will now be effective over a smaller range.

One reason that surgeons usually do not try to work out the moments or leverages of the tendons they transfer is that they know it is so difficult to identify exactly where the axis of a joint is located. Therefore, it is not possible at surgery to measure the perpendicular distance between the axis and the tendon.

There is, however, a simple and practical method of estimating the moment arms of tendons at joints that will enable surgeons to know exactly how effective each tendon will be at each joint it crosses. The method is based on two rules of geometry (Fig. 40-2). The first is that when a lever (bone) moves around an axis (joint), every point on the lever moves through a distance proportional to its own distance from the axis. The second rule grows out of the first, and is an example of it (Fig. 40-3). If a lever moves around an axis through an angle of 57.29 degrees, then every point on the lever moves a distance *equal* to its own distance from the axis. If a length of a radius is marked on the circumference of a circle, and the two ends of that radius are joined to the center, the angle between them is called a radian and measures about 57.29 degrees (Fig. 40-4). As a lever moves around an axis a number of points on its length may be thought of as marking out a number of arcs of concentric circles. When the lever has moved a radian, every arc that has been described is the same length as the distance (radius) of that point on the lever from the axis. This becomes a way to relate angles to distances; angles of joint movement can be related to excursions of the tendons that cause the movement or are affected by it.

In the stressful, time-dominated atmosphere of the operating room, nobody is going to measure tenths of a degree, or even single degrees. I find it useful to have in the operating room a metal triangle with angles of 30, 60, and 90 degrees (Fig. 40-5). I also have a metal millimeter scale. Keeping a little tension on a tendon, I move a joint through 60 degrees, while my assistant measures exactly how far the tendon has moved. *The excursion of the tendon that matches 60 degrees of joint movement is the same as the*

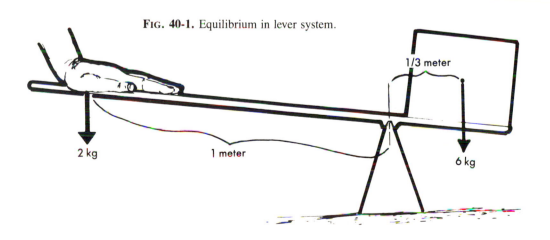

FIG. 40-1. Equilibrium in lever system.

Mechanical advantage of arm = 3:1
Moment of hand = 2 kg-m
Moment of weight = 2 kg-m

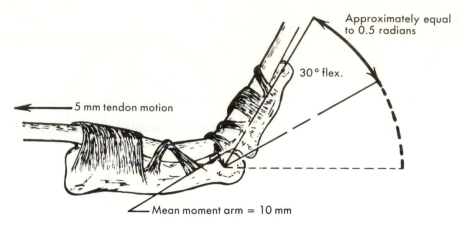

FIG. 40-7. Tendon excursion that matches 30 degrees of joint motion is approximately equal to half the moment arm of that tendon at that joint.

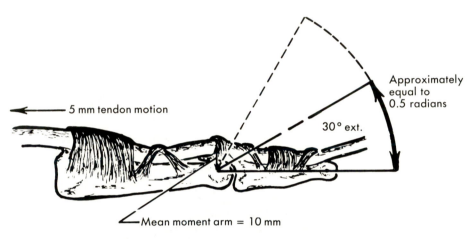

FIG. 40-8. When joint is nearly straight, tendon hugs skeletal plane. Moment arm measured through 30 degrees of flexion is 5 mm.

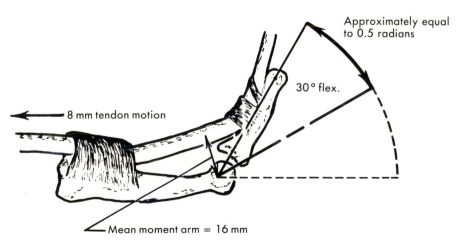

FIG. 40-9. As joint flexes, with excised flexor sheath, tendon bowstrings. Next 30 degrees of flexion takes 8 mm of tendon excursion. Demonstration of increasing moment arm.

useful to take two readings (Figs. 40-7 and 40-8), one of the first 30 degrees of motion and the other of the last 30 degrees of motion. In the case of a flexor tendon graft that has no sheath at the metacarpophalangeal joint and that has had a new pulley reconstruction, the surgeon may measure the tendon excursion that matches 0 to 30 degrees, and then 60 to 90 degrees, of metacarpophalangeal joint motion (Fig. 40-9). A normal finger might give readings of 5 mm and 6 mm, indicating a moment arm of 10 mm (near extension) and 12 mm (near flexion). The measured excursion has been doubled to obtain the moment arm, because the joint has been moved only 30 degrees at a time rather than 60 degrees. With a well reconstructed pulley a surgeon might find readings of 5 mm and 7 mm, showing just a little increase in bowstringing. However, if the surgeon gets readings of 5 mm and 10 mm, he or she will know that there is severe bowstringing. The new pulley is either too loose or too far up the finger away from the axis. If the surgeon accepts that result, some poor patient will struggle vainly to obtain flexion of the proximal interphalangeal joint while the metacarpophalangeal joint flexes too strongly, using up the best of the available excursion.

Two axes

In placing a tendon transfer the surgeon must consider all the possible directions in which the joint may move in response to the transferred tendon. In many cases there will be an axis for flexion and extension, and another axis for abduction and adduction. The tendon may cross the joint in an oblique direction so that the surgeon may be uncertain exactly how the joint will respond. Here I suggest a quick test. Keep tension on the tendon by a stitch marker while the joint is moved first through 60 degrees of flexion-extension and then through 30 degrees of abduction-adduction. I suggest 30 degrees because few joints can do a full 60 degrees of lateral movement. Do not forget to double the 30-degree reading to obtain the abduction-adduction moment arm. Now the two vector moment arms can be plotted on a graph to give the real or resultant moment arm as the diagonal of the rectangle so formed (Fig. 40-10).

The third axis—rotation

The third movement is rotation and the axis is longitudinal, at right angles to both the other axes. Many joints, such as metacarpophalangeal joints, do not have much active rotation in normal strong hands but may develop significant rotation if the finger either is hypermobile or has damaged stabilizing ligaments as in rheumatoid arthritis. This becomes a more severe problem if a tendon transfer is added that is unopposed in a rotational sense.

Joints in series

In severe paralysis a single tendon is sometimes placed across a series of joints, without the support of other muscles at the proximal joints. This might be satisfactory if each segment of a digit were always supported by external opposing forces as it is when one grasps a cylinder. However, if the distal segment alone is opposed by a force, as in pinch, the proximal segments may buckle. The surgeon must remember the following: (1) A tendon crossing several joints exerts equal force at each. There is no way a person can instruct his muscle to apply more force at one joint than at another. The actual moment or torque that is exerted at each joint varies only according to the moment arms of that tendon at each joint. (2) The distal external force or load at the tip of the digit exerts an opposing moment or torque at each joint, and this also varies according to the moment arm of the external force, at that joint. The moment arms of tendons in the hand are usually small, because tendons are held close to the skeleton and are only a little larger at proximal joints as the skeleton becomes thicker. However, the moment arms of the external force or load are based on the length of the bones and the length of the digit, and thus become enormously greater at proximal joints. Thus an unopposed digit may be flexed by a single muscle-tendon unit acting on all of the joints. The flexor profundus, unaided by other muscles, produces a full sweep from extended finger to clenched fist. As soon as the finger tip is opposed by a load or external force, it becomes necessary to recruit the flexor superficialis for the proximal interphalangeal and metacarpophalangeal joints plus the intrinsic muscles for the metacarpophalangeal joints, or the fingers will flex distally and hyperextend proximally.[1]

Consider the mechanism of the well-known Froment sign in the thumb. When the short flexors and adductor muscles are paralyzed, the long flexor will have equal tension along its length and will exert flexion moment at the metacarpophalangeal and interphalangeal joints in proportion to the moment arms at each joint, which are only marginally different from each other. When a firm pinch is used, the index

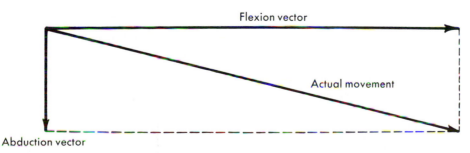

FIG. 40-10. Vector diagram of motion at joint in two planes. There is also a rotational vector, with axis at right angles to the plane of this page.

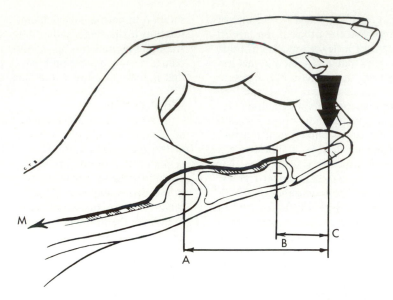

FIG. 40-11. Diagram of a tendon that crosses more than one joint. External force of pinch, *arrow at C*, has a tendency to force joints *A* and *B* into extension. Turning moment at *A* is proportional to *A-C*, while that at *B* is proportional to *B-C*. (From Brand, P.W.: Tendon transfers in the forearm. In Flynn, J.E.: Hand surgery, ed. 3, Baltimore, 1982, The Williams & Wilkins Co.)

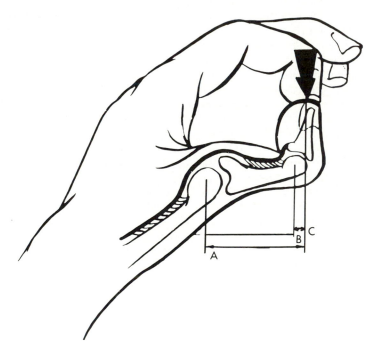

FIG. 40-12. Deformity that results from having only one flexor tendon crossing two joints. (From Brand, P.W.: Tendon transfers in the forearm. In Flynn, J.E.: Hand surgery, ed. 3, Baltimore, 1982, The Williams & Wilkins Co.)

finger (Fig. 40-11) may push the thumb toward extension. The long flexor, though, immediately increases its tension to oppose the index finger and stabilize the pinch. However, the *extension* moment resulting from the index finger is far greater at the metacarpophalangeal joint of the thumb, where it has more than double the moment arm that it has at the interphalangeal joint.

The long flexor increases its tension to prevent hyper-

extension at the metacarpophalangeal joint, and, thereby unavoidably flexes the interphalangeal joint, at which less moment is needed. In flexing the interphalangeal joint, the terminal phalanx is brought to a position end-on to the index finger, so that the force from the index is applied still closer to the axis, or even at the axis (Fig. 40-12). Thus the Z-shaped buckling of the thumb becomes irreversible. Many surgeons, noting the flexed tip of the thumb, have assumed that it can be corrected by adding extra power to the extensor. *Not so*. The problem can be corrected only by adding an extra *flexor* to the metacarpophalangeal joint so that the long flexor can relax at this joint and avoid overflexing the interphalangeal joint. Because it is so difficult to balance a series of joints against a distal load, it is often wise to arthrodese one or more joints in the chain so that the few remaining muscles may effectively control the joints that remain. In the example above, arthrodesis of the metacarpophalangeal joint of the thumb will allow a strong pinch without the ''Froment'' flexion of the tip.

Drag

In any operation for tendon transfer, we consider first the capability of the motor, the muscle-tendon unit that we transfer. Then we consider the geometry and mechanics by which the tension of the motor is transformed into the torque at each joint, and thus into effective movement of segments of limbs. Finally we have to realize that at each stage of this process we shall encounter internal resistance in the form of friction and the need to stretch passive soft tissues. This we may collectively call ''drag,'' which we must recognize as an obstacle that may frustrate all of our endeavors, unless we plan a way to minimize its effect, and work to overcome its unavoidable residue.

Friction. Friction occurs whenever two objects move against each other. It is minimized when their surfaces are congruous and smooth, and when the materials have a low coefficient of friction. I am not going to discuss this very much because true independent movement of surfaces over each other occurs only in joints and in synovial tendon sheaths. All the features of the architecture, the selection of low-friction materials for joint surfaces, and the lubrication systems involved, are so amazingly well designed, and work so efficiently, that it is hard to imitate or match them. There is little we can do to restore them if they are lost. In the case of transferred tendons, true gliding may occur in a sheath if it was there before we interfered, and if the transferred tendon has a blood supply. If true gliding is needed after transfer in a place where it was not present before, the only thing we can do is to restore movement of the tendon, which is accomplished by stretching and relaxing the investing connective tissue, and wait for the synovial space to open up in its own good time. Such synovial spaces usually develop on the concave side of a curving tendon, but it takes months to happen.

Lengthening of soft tissue. Except in the limited areas where synovial spaces occur, all movement within limbs is permitted by the lengthening and shortening of connective tissue. We often use the word ''gliding'' in referring to tendon movement, but it is not real gliding in most cases. A tendon does not move over the tissue next to it. It is attached to the paratenon that surrounds it. That tissue is usually relaxed when the tendon is at its midpoint of motion. It stretches and lengthens when the tendon needs to move. Peritendinous tissues are made of collagen and elastin, and of some interesting structureless ground substance that is semifluid and that has gel-like qualities. When this composite soft tissue is subjected to tension, it becomes longer. When relaxed, it shortens back to where it was before. When

the tissue is pulled, it takes energy to make it longer. When it is allowed to shorten, it gives up energy.

The application of this simple concept is very straightforward. Every time a tendon is placed in a new situation, it becomes attached there by soft tissue. Therefore, every time it moves it takes energy to lengthen that soft tissue, and it tends to get pulled back to its original position of attachment when it is no longer under tension. The amount of force that it takes to lengthen that soft tissue and the distance through which it has to be lengthened are absolutely critical to the success of any tendon transfer. Yet they are the least studied aspect of tendon transfer. I have made it sound very simple in order that you may be willing to follow me into a step or two of complexity so that we may be in a position to understand and control this most important aspect of tendon transfer operations and postoperative rehabilitation.

Most studies on the mechanical qualities of soft tissues have been done on excised tissue.[6,14] A piece of skin, ligament, tendon, or connective tissue is removed, placed in a machine, and tested under various levels of stress and varying rates of stretch. From these studies we are able to identify the elasticity of a tissue, and its viscosity. We may note that there is a hysteresis, in that when a tissue is stretched it lengthens, but when it is relaxed it comes back to its resting state by a different curve and takes longer in the process. We also may note a ''creep,'' which means that when it is overstretched it does not come back to its first length, but remains a little longer (Figs. 40-13, 40-14). This type of study gives a good background for understanding soft-tissue mechanics, but it may give a false impression of what happens in living tissue. For example, if living soft tissue is overstretched, it also will exhibit creep, but this may be accompanied by an inflammatory reaction that occurs in response to the violence that has been done to some elements of the tissue fabric. That inflammation may result in the exudation of some tissue fluid containing fibrinogen, and there may be an incursion of inflammatory cells. The final result may be the laying down of some new interstitial collagen scar that will make the tissue more contracted and less compliant in the future.

We have to study the qualities of *living* soft tissue in response to mechanical force. This must include its ability to *remodel* or to be remodeled. It is this remodeling that is the basis for the gradual increase in range of motion at a joint that is limited by a soft-tissue contracture. It does not improve simply by passive stretching or by creep but by *growing* in length, or remodeling of the shortened tissue. This is the basis by which a transferred tendon gradually becomes free to move. The adhesions have not just been stretched; they have been remodeled, or have grown to accommodate to new requirements. Now some of this remodeling may be just a change in the bonding of collagen, but it is accomplished by living cells, by fibroblasts that act in response to mechanical and biomechanical orders that they understand. Our duty is to learn the type of mechanical stimulus to which these cells respond, and to use these stimuli as our instruments to change the pattern of adhesions and scar.

It is very difficult to study the behavior of collagen and

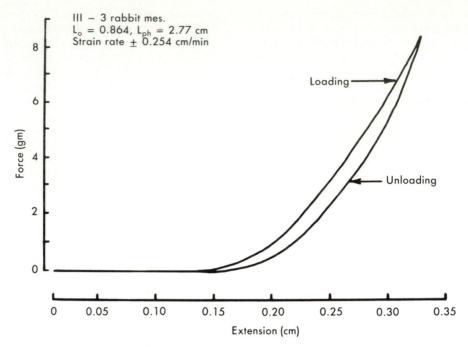

FIG. 40-13. Hysteresis curve. Rabbit mesentery. Load and unloading curves after Y.C.B. Fung. Note that the stretched length of this tissue is more than three times the relaxed length. This curve shows only the end part of the length-tension curve of a piece of mesentery. The full curve is five times as long and is all flat; that is, the tension needed to lengthen or stretch the mesentery is so small that it is not measurable until the mesentery is nearly fully stretched. This is very much like the behavior of paratenon tissue, for which we do not yet have a precise curve. (From Fung, Y.C.B.: Am. J. Physiol. **213**(6):1532-1544, Dec. 1967.)

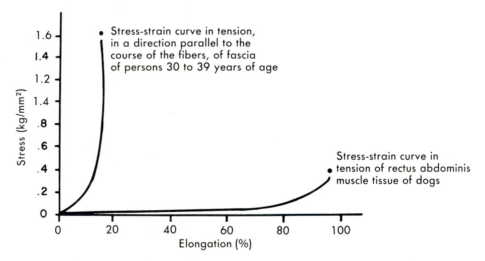

FIG. 40-14. Length-tension curves for fascia *(left)* and muscle (passive stretch only). Note that even fascia and tendon are lengthened 10% to 20% under tension and that muscle fiber is lengthened nearly 60% to 80% before it offers increasing resistance. This is from the fully relaxed length, not the physiological resting length in situ. (Composite of curves after Yamada, H.: Strength of biological materials, edited by F.G. Evans, Baltimore, 1970, The Williams & Wilkins Co.)

elastin and connective tissue complexes in the intact hand because, as we open the tissues to look, it ceases to be an intact hand. However, even without knowing exactly how these tissues respond, at a molecular level, we may study total tissue response to a known input of mechanical stress.

This involves the discipline of the measurement of stress input, recorded against range-of-motion output. Our present methods of prescribing the forces that are intended to lengthen adhesions are usually completely nonquantitative (''use *gentle* passive movement''), and even our measurements of range of motion are partly subjective in that we tend to pull or press a little harder when we measure the range of

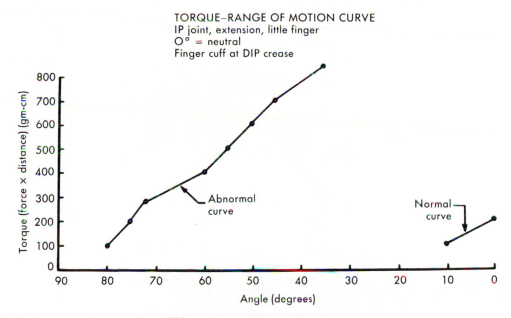

TORQUE–RANGE OF MOTION CURVE
IP joint, extension, little finger
O° = neutral
Finger cuff at DIP crease

FIG. 40-15. Torque-angle curve of a stiff interphalangeal joint moving into extension. The segment of curve on the right shows that a normal proximal interphalangeal joint would need only a small torque to achieve 0 degrees (full extension). The curve of a stiff finger shows a gradually increasing angle with gradually increasing torque. This says that the stiffness is "soft"; that is, the resistance is due to tissues that can be progressively stretched and that therefore may be expected to grow longer with sustained therapy.

passive motion if we are expecting or hoping that it has improved.

I suggest, therefore, that all serious hand surgeons and therapists adopt a "torque–range of motion" (T-ROM) principle in monitoring the progress of tendon movement or joint stiffness preoperatively and postoperatively.

The principle of T-ROM is based on the recognition that although we can rarely measure the actual lengthening of any tissue or any adhesion without cutting the skin, their lengthening can be monitored by measuring the angular movement of the joint against the torque applied to it, because all the tissues that concern us have an effect on a joint. Thus we need to have a repeatable way to apply known force at a known distance from the axis while we measure the range of joint motion in response to it.

The key word, for most of us, is *repeatable*. For research workers the actual moment arms and exact forces are very important, but for understanding a given case and for following the progress of scar lengthening it is enough if we use repeatable criteria.

For the measurement of torque I suggest that we apply a known force—say 1 kg—at a standard position, such as at a skin crease, at right angles to a segment of the digit. We measure the joint angle while the torque is being applied. A day later, or a week later, the same force is applied at the same skin crease so that the torque is the same, and then we know for sure that any change in angle represents a change in the tissue restraints at the joint (or around the tendon).

There are three ways to increase the usefulness (and the complexity) of this measurement, each of which will teach us something different.

1. Use a series of forces, to vary the torque. This results in a T-ROM curve (Fig. 40-15). We often use 200, 400, 600, 800, and 1000 gm, applied by a spring scale at the same distance from the joint axis. We measure the joint angle at each level of torque. In general, we find that the *shape* of the curve gives some idea of the quality of the restricting adhesions. A shallow curve shows a complaint tissue. A steep curve means a more rigid tissue, or a tissue with shorter fibers and therefore poor prognosis for great increase in length.

2. Repeat the T-ROM measurement on the finger joint with different positions of the proximal joints (wrist). This gives a good idea of the relative role played by proximal tendon and muscle restrictions as compared to distal joint stiffness.

3. Repeat the T-ROM measurement in a time sequence, such as early morning, before exercise, after exercise, or, if the hand is swollen, before and after hand elevation.

Although a T-ROM curve is based on a sequence of angles, it may be interpreted in terms of the length of the soft-tissue restraints that cross the joint, and those that limit the excursion of the tendon that crosses the joint.

I recognize that surgeons and therapists will find, at first, that these measurements are time consuming, and that it requires manual dexterity to manipulate a joint, a protractor, and a spring at the same time with only one pair of hands. This will become easier with practice, and there are a couple of tricks that make it simple. One is to have a "sunburst" protractor drawn on a card that lies flat on a table (Fig. 40-16). Above it is a single light source that projects a beam downward. Now the therapist positions the digit over the card and pulls on the finger segment with a spring while he or she reads off the angles from the shadows on the card.

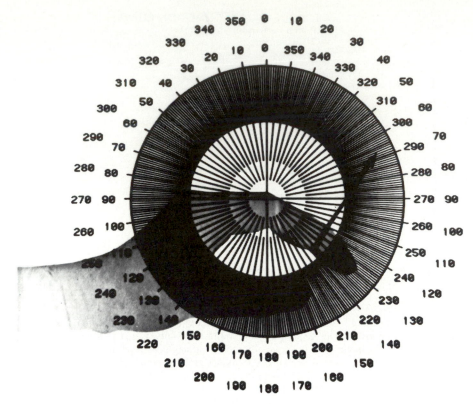

FIG. 40-16. Sunburst protractor. One way to measure torque angles is to have an overhead lamp with a parallel beam (an old slide projector will do). The operator holds the patient's finger level, over the sunburst protractor, and applies tension to a segment of the digit. By moving the hand so that the back of each segment is parallel to rays of the sunburst, the angle can be read without the need to hold a protractor.

This may be done more easily if a pointer is fixed on the back of a segment of a digit with adhesive tape.

With such a monitoring system, it will be possible to be quite precise about relating the therapy program to the changes that result from it. For example, it will be possible to compare the results of intermittent high-torque exercises with the results of continuous immobilization in low-torque extension (or flexion).

In general it will be found that where restraints to joint movement have a viscous element to them, it is best to prescribe a great deal of movement and exercise. Where the restraint is mainly elastic, there may be more benefit from continuous low-torque stretching (for a digit this torque may be as low as 250 gm-cm). To distinguish viscous from elastic resistance, one needs only to measure range of motion before and after a short period of active movement. Since viscous damping of range of motion is mostly due to movement of fluids in tissues, there would be marked changes in range of motion at the same torque after just minutes of exercise.

• • •

In this chapter on mechanics of tendon transfers I have written mostly about methods of measurement and methods of monitoring change rather than giving instructions about methods of treatment. This is because there is very little available quantitative information on the relative merits of different types of transfer, and of different methods of mobilizing stiff joints or adherent tendons. Rather than giving my opinions to rival opinions of others, I want to stress the fact that we need to develop disciplines of measurement so that we can each find out for ourselves whether procedure A is more effective than procedure B. It is numbers that we need, not more theories.

Finally, we have to keep in mind that whenever we direct therapy with the object of changing just one tissue, we will always have some effect on the whole hand, and often on the whole person. If we want to lengthen a contracture on the flexor side of a hand, and if we use long-term low-torque extension, by splinting, we may achieve that goal. At the same time we may produce loss of length in dorsal structures, and limit flexion. Other fingers in the same hand may lose range of motion just by disuse. Any form of immobilization will tend to cause loss of compliance in capsular tissues and loss of fluid components of hyaline cartilage. Thus, whenever possible, we should avoid single-minded mechanical approaches to any deformity. If long-term tension is called for, at least 1 hour per day should be reserved for free, active exercise and purposeful movement to keep tissue fluids moving, to move collagen fiber on collagen fiber, and to encourage the restoration of normal balance between the fluids and gels in cartilage and in paratenon tissues. Then with restored homeostasis, relaxed fibroblasts, and contented fat cells, we may return to the discipline of tension and torque to accomplish a specific objective.

REFERENCES

1. Brand, P.W.: Tendon transfers in the forearm. In Flynn, J.E., editor: Hand surgery, ed. 2, Baltimore, 1975, The Williams & Wilkins Co.
2. Brand, P.W., Beach, R.B., and Thompson, D.E.: Relative tension and potential excursion of muscles in the forearm and hand, J. Hand Surg. **6:**209-219, May 1981.
3. Buncke, H.J.: The role of microsurgery in hand surgery (presidential address, American Society for Surgery of the Hand), J. Hand Surg. **6:**533-536, Nov. 1981.
4. Daniels, L., Williams, M., and Worthingham, C.: Muscle testing: techniques of manual examination, ed. 2, Philadelphia, 1956, W.B. Saunders Co.
5. Freehafer, A.A., Peckham, H., and Keith, M.W.: Determination of muscle-tendon unit properties during tendon transfer, J. Hand Surg. **4:**331-339, July 1979.
6. Fung, Y.C.B.: Elasticity of soft tissues in simple elongation, Am. J. Physiol. **213:**1532-1544, Dec. 1967.
7. Legg, A.T., and Merrill, J.B.: Physical therapy in infantile paralysis. Reprinted from Mock, Pemberton, and Coulter, editors: Principles and practices of physical therapy, Hagerstown, Md., 1932, W.F. Prior Co., Inc., pp. 45-71.
8. Manktelow, R.T., Zuker, R.M., and McKee, N.H.: Functioning free muscle transplantation. Presented at the Thirty-Seventh Annual Meeting of the American Society for Surgery of the Hand, January 18-20, 1982, New Orleans, La. (In press.)
9. Nelson, N.: Factors to be considered in evaluating effect of treatment in anterior poliomyelitis, Arch. Phys. Med. **28:**358-363, 1947.
10. Sharrard, W.J.W.: Muscle recovery in poliomyelitis, J. Bone Joint Surg. [Br.] **37B:**63-79, 1955.
11. Tabary, J.C., Tabary, C., Tardieu, C., and others: Physiological and structural changes in the cat's soleus muscle due to immobilization at different lengths by plaster casts, J. Physiol. **224:**231-244, 1972.
12. Tabary, J.C., Tardieu, C., Tardieu, G., and others: Functional adaptation of sarcomere number of normal cat muscle, J. Physiol. (Paris) **72:**277-291, 1976.
13. Wright, W.G.: Muscle training in the treatment of infantile paralysis, Boston Med. Surg. **167:**567-574, 1912.
14. Yamada, H.: Strength of biological materials edited by Evans, F.G., Baltimore, 1970, The Williams and Wilkins Co., pp. 96-97.

41

Tendon transfers in the upper extremity

LAWRENCE H. SCHNEIDER

The application of the motor power of one muscle to another weaker or paralyzed muscle by the transfer of its tendinous insertion is now well established. This technique, "tendon transfer," was originally referred to as "tendon transplanation," a differentiation that is subtle. "Transplant" implies complete removal of the muscle and "replanting" it in a new location, while the term "transfer" seems to describe better the act of redirecting the insertion. "Tendon grafting," quite a different procedure, was a term used interchangeably in the early literature to describe this technique, further adding to the confusion of terminology.

HISTORY

Study of the evolution of the techniques that are now widely accepted takes one through an exciting period in the history of reconstructive extremity surgery. Excellent reviews have been written by Waterman[21] and Adamson and Wilson.[1]

Carl Nicoladoni is given credit by most historians for the first tendon transfer performed in 1880. He took the peroneal tendons and sutured them into the tendo Achillis for talipes calcaneus deformity secondary to infantile paralysis. Soon after the operation, which was carried out in Vienna, he moved to Innsbruck leaving the aftercare to an associate who reported, according to Waterman,[21] that the "anastomosis separated and the procedure was a failure." Interestingly, although be became a great contributor to surgical knowledge, Nicoladoni never performed his procedure again.

What is not commonly acknowledged is that authors for about 100 years had been advocating the repair of severed tendons by "grafting" the distal segment onto adjacent intact tendons. Missa in 1770 sutured the lacerated extensor tendon of the long finger into that of the intact ring finger. Nicoladoni's case probably rates then only as the first reported use of the technique in infantile paralysis but certainly an ingenious contribution nonetheless.[21]

After 1880 there were scattered reports of tendon transfers, but because of technical failures interest generally waned. Then in 1896 Drobnik published 16 cases with follow-up and overall had a successful experience. Included in his list was case number 5, the first tendon transfer for paralysis in the upper extremity. In a patient with partial finger extensor paralysis, Drobnik transferred the extensor carpi radialis longus into the extensor digitorum communis. He also took one half of the extensor carpi radialis brevis and put it into the extensor pollicis longus.[21]

Franke was the first to transfer the wrist flexors for paralysis of the finger extensors, a technique widely used today after radial nerve injury (Fig. 41-1). He also first performed tendon transfers for infantile spastic paralysis of cerebral origin.[21]

In the 1890s Parrish and Milliken in New York and Goldthwait in Boston established the technique in the United States. Apparently they were not familiar with each other's work or that of Nicoladoni.[21] In 1897 Bradford of Boston published 27 personal examples of what he called "tenoplastic operations."[3] This further popularized the procedure in the United States.

Meanwhile in Germany, Vulpius in Heidelberg, Lange in Munich, and Biesalski in Berlin developed the procedures further. There were disagreements, usually on technical points, among the world leaders. For example, Vulpius believed that the transfer should be fixed to the tendon of the recipient muscle, while Codovilla[9] of Bologna and Jones in England believed that periosteal fixation was superior. Codovilla, an innovator, introduced the concept of transfer through the sheath of the paralyzed tendon. He also lengthened tendons too short to reach the periosteal insertion by fascial strips. Lange approached the length problem with silk thread prolongation of the motor tendon. The problem of fixation of the transferred tendons by adhesions was a serious one, and Mayer of New York worked on this aspect in Lange's clinic, later continuing his work in Berlin under Biesalski. It was Mayer who published, with his mentor, the monograph *The Physiology of Tendon Transplantation*. This work, subsequently published in English in three articles in *The Journal of Surgery, Gynecology, and Obstetrics*[14] in 1916, renewed interest in tendon surgery in the United States. In this work the need for gentle tissue handling was stressed along with the importance of clean-gliding tissue planes for successful tendon transfer. Mayer returned to the United States and established himself as a leading orthopedic surgeon.[15] Working in Iowa City, Steindler[20] contributed and perfected many surgical techniques in tendon transfer. Bunnell,[8] the father of American

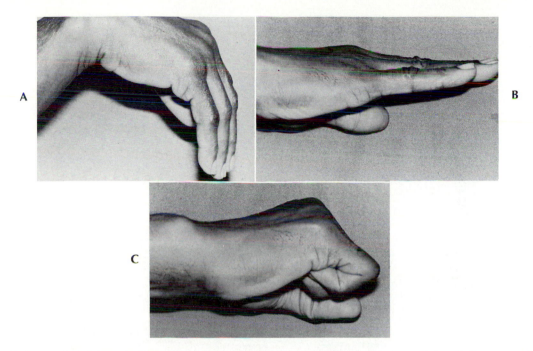

FIG. 41-1. Transfer of the wrist flexor (flexor carpi ulnaris) to extensor digitorum communis in radial nerve paralysis. **A,** Wristdrop and loss of metacarpophalangeal joint extension seen after high radial nerve injury. **B** and **C,** Range of extension and flexion seen 6 months after transfer.

hand surgery, refined much of the work and added a large clinical experience in the upper extremity. He was influenced by his long friendship with Mayer.

Based on the work of these men are the pinciples of tendon transfer in the upper extremity. Although many of the original procedures were developed in patients with poliomyelitis, in present day surgery most tendon transfers are carried out on patients afflicted with peripheral nerve damage or traumatic muscle loss. Patients with central nervous system disorders are probably the third most frequent group aided by tendon transfer.

The more recent refiners of the work of the masters are many. Leading these would be Brand,[7] Boyes,[4-6] Curtis,[10] Fowler, Littler[12,13] Omer,[16,17] Riordan,[18] White,[22] and Zancolli.[23]

INDICATIONS FOR TENDON TRANSFER

The absence of a particular needed function after irreparable nerve injury, nerve disease, or muscle loss should bring up a consideration for tendon transfer. Time should be allowed for wound healing to occur and for recovery of function, either spontaneously in the case of neuropraxia or axonotmesis or for reinnervation after a nerve repair. This usually requires a delay of 4 to 6 months. During this period it is the obligation of the treating physician and therapist to maintain passive mobility in the involved joints. This would be achieved through passive motion exercises and by the use of dynamic splints where indicated. Nerve loss in itself is not always an indication for tendon surgery, since patients can at times perform unexpectedly through substitutive or adaptive methods or can function because of dual innervated musculature and/or variations in innervation. For example, median nerve injury at the wrist may not result in loss of

true thumb opposition in many patients, because this action may be performed by use of thenar eminence muscles partially or completely ulnar nerve innervated.[19] However, when it does occur, loss of opposition is a functional loss worthy of tendon transfer (Fig. 41-2). The point here is that each problem must be individualized in terms of the loss of function, its severity, the reconstructive possibilities, and the patient's needs and desires. Also to be stressed is the fact that tendon transfer is a palliative procedure that usually does not restore full and normal function. It is a redistribution of available power in an attempt to improve functional impairment.[2]

Once it is decided that tendon transfer has a place in the solution of a particular patient's problem, certain basic conditions must be satisfied.

Joint mobility. The participating joints in the function in question must be capable of passive motion if the transfer is to succeed. Hand therapy using physical modalities, including dynamic splinting, is needed to keep the joints mobile. This therapy can be carried out by the patient himself or through the supervision and guidance of trained therapists. At times, if joints have stiffened and do not respond to therapy, one must do preliminary surgical releases to restore passive mobility.

Adequate soft-tissue coverage. Well-healed and pliable soft tissues must be present to provide gliding planes through which the transfer can function. This may require the preliminary shifting of skin and the use of local or distant pedicle skin flaps.

Available motor tendons. A donor muscle must be available in the extremity. In single motor nerve injury in the upper extremity several motor tendons may be available. If two of the three major nerves in the extremity are irreparably

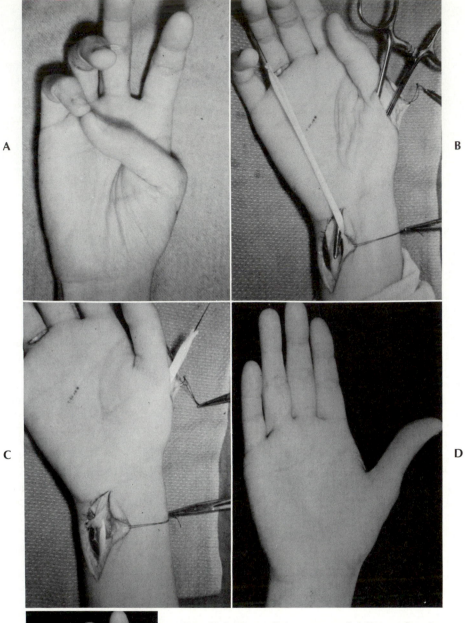

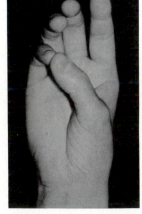

FIG. 41-2. Flexor digitorum superficialis transferred to thumb to restore opposition. **A,** True opposition has been lost because of irreparable injury to median motor nerve branch in thenar eminence. **B** and **C,** Flexor superficialis of ring finger has been removed to wrist level and passed around flexor carpi ulnaris at wrist and then subcutaneously to metacarpophalangeal joint region of thumb. **D** and **E,** Extension of thumb and opposition performed, photographs taken 2 years later.

damaged, choices are limited and prognosis in terms of function will be greatly reduced. Tendons available in the upper extremity vary with the injury and include wrist flexors, wrist extensors, flexor digitorum superficialis, proprius extensors, and brachioradialis.

SELECTION OF A MOTOR TENDON FOR TRANSFER

Boyes in 1962[5] discussed the factors involved in selection of a motor tendon. Amplitude of the donor tendon and power are the prime factors in tendon selection.

Amplitude. The distance that a muscle can shorten from its maximum length is the excursion or amplitude. Average amplitude of the wrist flexors and extensors is about 3.5 cm. Full finger extension at the metacarpophalageneal joints requires 5 cm and the flexor digitorum profundus group an amplitude of 7 cm for full function. As motor tendons, the flexor digitorum superficialis group, which provide an amplitude of about 6 cm, are the only availble tendons that can approach the necessary amplitude to replace the profundus. (Obviously when the extensor carpi radialis longus is used to power the flexor digitorum profundus, some sacrifice in range of motion must be accepted [Fig. 41-3]). This deficit is partially overcome by the additional amplitude provided the system by the tenodesis effect of the mobile wrist joint. Restoration of the long extensor system by transfer of a wrist flexor is a better matched situation as far as their respective amplitudes of motion are concerned.

Power. The ability of a muscle to perform work, power, is directly proportional to its cross-sectional diameter. Examples of the relative power of muscles in the forearm are as follows:

Pronator teres, 1.2 meters/kilogram
Brachioradialis, 1.9
Flexor carpi ulnaris, 2.0
Flexor carpi radialis, 0.8
Extensor carpi radialis longus, 1.1
Extensor carpi ulnaris, 1.1

In the preoperative period accurate muscle testing is essential in the evaluation of a potential motor tendon. Each available muscle must be graded to assure adequate strength for transfer. The rating system 0 to 5 is used:

0—Total paralysis
1—Flicker of muscle action
2—Muscle contracts and moves joint with gravity eliminated
3—Muscle moves joint through a full range of motion against gravity
4—Muscle moves joint through a full range of motion against resistance
5—Normal muscle

Because the procedure of tendon transfer weakens the donor muscle by at least one grade, a four-power muscle may be inadequate for transfer.

Direction (Fig. 41-4). The pathway of the transferred muscle should be as straight as possible to its new insertion. This may require extensive proximal mobilization of the muscle. Care must be taken to avoid injury to the nerve and vascular supply of the muscle.

Phase. Wrist extensors and digital flexors perform synergistically and are said to function in phase. The same applies for the activities of wrist flexors and digital extensors. Although it may be true that transfers within the phasic groupings are easier to train, the phasic action of a transfer is no longer regarded as a major factor in the selection of a motor tendon for transfer. In fact, muscles 180 degrees out of phase are not uncommonly used, an example being the use of the flexor superficialis as a motor for the extensor digitorum communis in radial nerve paralysis.

TECHNICAL ASPECTS OF TENDON TRANSFERS

When one is setting up a transfer procedure, it is helpful to have a plan of action in which available assets are listed against functional needs. Then an attempt is made to rebalance the situation providing power for lost functions while only minimally affecting present function. The importance of a stable functioning wrist is important for success in many transfers, and wrist fusion is contraindicated except in extreme situations. For the same reason, it is necessary to preserve at least one wrist extensor and one wrist flexor when these tendons are used as transfers.

The general rules of tendon surgery have to be observed. Gentle handling of the tendon to avoid damage to its surface is recommended. Wherever possible the tendon is passed through soft gliding planes. Appropriate incisions are planned that cross transversely to the planned direction of

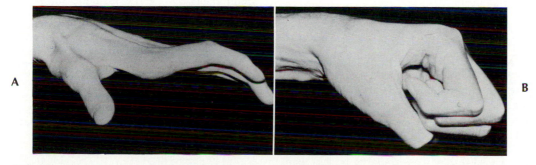

FIG. 41-3. Postoperative photos of patient with severe injury to median and ulnar nerves in proximal forearm, who had undergone transfer of extensor carpi radialis longus into flexor profundi in attempt to restore finger flexion. **A,** Extension of fingers. **B,** Flexion through transfer is surprisingly good.

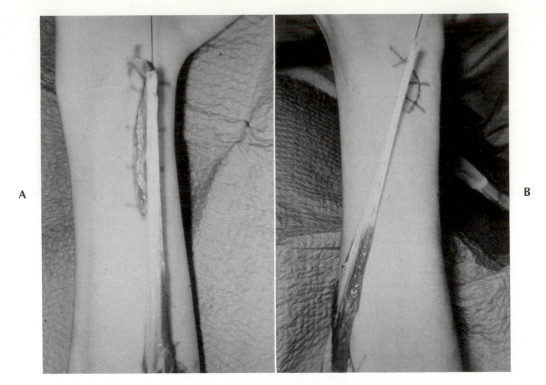

FIG. 41-4. Direction of tendon transfer should be as straight as possible to its new insertion. **A,** Flexor carpi ulnaris is freed from its insertion and taken back into proximal forearm. **B,** Tendon is as straight as possible in its route to its new insertion at the radial wrist extensors in this patient with spastic paralysis.

the transfer, thereby reducing the area of potential adhesion formation.

Tendon junctures can be carried out end to end, side to side, or by interweaving techniques. The junctures should be strong when nonabsorbable low-reactive 2-0 or 3-0 suture material is used. As a general rule, the transfers are put in so as to err on the tight side. This especially applies when tranfers are done into the extensor system, where failures are likely to occur if the transfer is too loose.

Plaster immobilization is used for 3 to 4 weeks before removal for exercises. Splint protection is usually added for an additional 3 weeks while the muscle is educated in its new role. If the rules are obeyed, this usually is a rapid relearning process but may at times tax the ingenuity of both surgeon and therapist.

CAUSES FOR DISAPPOINTMENT IN TENDON TRANSFERS

Suboptimal results do occur in tendon transfer, and this is a more likely event where an overly ambitious program is attempted in severe functional loss. This can be avoided if realistic attainable goals are established. Although the reinstitution of active motion is desirable, the treating surgeon should not lose sight of the place for tenodeses and arthrodeses in the reconstructive program.

When patients whose results were found to be less than expected were analyzed, the following pitfalls were seen to be prominent:

1. Acceptance of less than full passive range of motion before transfer
2. Overestimation of the strength of the donor muscle—careful here especially when transferring a reinnervated muscle
3. Adhesions along the course of transfer
4. Technical failures
   a. Breakdown of the juncture
   b. Transfer put in too loose

The solutions to the above problems are obvious—careful attention to the details of evaluation and surgery.

SUMMARY

The dynamic procedure of the transfer of the action of a muscle from its usual function to a widely different one is still an exciting and challenging area of reconstructive extremity surgery. Careful planning and preoperative patient evaluation, along with strict attention to the rules and details of the procedure, can reward patient, therapist, and surgeon.

REFERENCES

1. Adamson, J.E., and Wilson, J.N.: The history of flexor tendon grafting, J. Bone Joint Surg. **43A:**709-716, 1961.
2. Beasley, R.W.: Basic considerations for tendon transfer operations in the upper extremity. In American Academy of Othopaedic Surgeons: Symposium on tendon surgery in the hand, St. Louis, 1975, The C.V. Mosby Co., pp. 163-170.
3. Bick, E.M.: Source book of orthopaedics, ed. 2, New York, 1968, Hafner Publishing Co.
4. Boyes, J.H.: Tendon transfers for radial palsy, Bull. Hosp. Joint Dis. **21:**97-105, 1961.
5. Boyes, J.H.: Selection of a donor motor for tendon transfer, Bull. Hosp. Joint Dis. **23:**1-4, 1962.

6. Boyes, J.H.: Bunnell's surgery of the hand, ed. 4, Philadelphia, 1964, J.B. Lippincott Co.

7. Brand, P.W.: Biomechanics of tendon transfer, Orthop. Clin. North Am. **5:**205-230, 1974.

8. Bunnell, S.: Tendon transfers in the hand and forearm. In American Academy of Orthopaedic Surgeons: Instructional course lectures **6:**106-112, Ann Arbor, Mich., 1949, J.W. Edwards Co.

9. Codovilla, A.: Tendon transplants in orthopaedic practice, 1899, translated in Clin. Orthop. **118:**2-6, 1976.

10. Curtis, R.M.: Fundamental principles of tendon transfer, Orthop. Clin. North Am. **5:**231-242, 1974.

11. Erlacher, P.J.: The development of tendon surgery in Germany, In American Academy of Orthopaedic Surgeons: Instructional course lectures **13:**110-115, Ann Arbor, Mich., 1956, J.W. Edwards Co.

12. Littler, J.W.: Tendon transfers and arthrodeses in combined median and ulnar palsies, J. Bone Joint Surg. **31A:**225-234, 1949.

13. Littler, J.W.: Restoration of power and stability in the partially paralyzed hand. In Converse, J.M.: Reconstructive plastic surgery, Philadelphia, 1964, W.B. Saunders Co., vol. 4, pp. 1674-1695.

14. Mayer, L.: The physiological method of tendon transplantation, Surg. Gynecol. Obstet. **22:**182-197; 298-306; 472-481, 1916.

15. Mayer, L.: The physiological method of tendon transplants renewed after forty years. In American Academy of Orthopaedic Surgeons: Instructional course lectures **12:**116-120, Ann Arbor, Mich., 1955, J.W. Edwards Co.

16. Omer, G.E.: Evaluation and reconstruction of the forearm and hand after acute traumatic peripheral nerve injuries, J. Bone Surg. **50A:**1454-1478, 1968.

17. Omer, G.E.: The technique and timing of tendon transfers, Orthop. Clin. North Am. **5:**243-252, 1974.

18. Riordan, D.C.: Surgery of the paralytic hand. In American Academy of Orthopaedic Surgeons: Instructional course lectures **16:**79-90, St. Louis, 1959, The C.V. Mosby Co.

19. Rowntree, T.: Anomalous innervations of the hand muscles, J. Bone Joint Surg. **31B:**505-510, 1949.

20. Steindler, A.: Tendon transplantation in the upper extremity, Am. J. Surg. **44:**260-271, 1939.

21. Waterman, J.H.: Tendon transplantation: its history, indications and technique, Med. News **12:**54-61, 1902.

22. White, W.L.: Restoration of function and balance of the wrist and hand by tendon transfers, Surg. Clin. North Am. **40:**427-459, 1960.

23. Zancolli, E.: Structural and dynamic bases of hand surgery, Philadelphia, 1968, J.B. Lippincott Co.

42

Preoperative and postoperative management of tendon transfers

S.L. KOLUMBAN

The decision to transfer a tendon should never be made until a full assessment of the entire upper extremity is completed. It is this assessment that will provide the facts that will determine the feasibility of a transfer and the selection of the tendon and its reattachment site. Therefore the initial step in the tendon-transfer procedure is to establish a baseline assessment of the upper extremity, for which there is no substitute and no shortcut.

BASELINE ASSESSMENT

The purpose of the baseline assessment is to provide accurate and objective data about the upper extremity. It is not my intention here to give an elaborate description of the various assessment techniques, since they will be dealt with elsewhere in this book, but any such assessment should provide information about the following:

1. The history
2. All nerves—normal or involved
3. All muscles—normal, weak (what grade?), or paralyzed
4. All joints—active and passive range of motion, contractures, deformities
5. The skin—sensory loss, contractures, scar tissue, edema, open wounds, signs of inflammation, and quality
6. Hand-function capability—precision and power pinch and grasp, general dexterity, and activities of daily living

SELECTION OF TRANSFER TENDON

Perhaps the assessment reveals that no transfer is really necessary or advisable or possible and that a conservative, nonsurgical program of therapy will suffice or is even preferable. However, if there is a definite indication for surgery, the surgeon will select a suitable tendon for transfer only *after* taking into consideration several factors: (1) the strength of the transfer muscle must be strong enough to do the job intended; (2) the preoperative excursion of the transferred tendon must be adequate at the postoperative attachment site; (3) the removal of a tendon must not result in unbalancing a key joint; (4) a tendon whose muscle is synergistic with the desired postoperative movement generally will be easier to reeducate than one that is not synergistic; however, it has been shown that nonsynergistic muscles also do well in transfers[6] (refer to Chapter 41 for further details).

After all the above considerations the surgical plan may be formulated or perhaps delayed pending results of treatment. In any case the plan is shared with the hand therapist. The therapist's understanding of the total plan for the patient is vital to the planning of the preoperative and postoperative treatment program and in helping the patient to understand what is to be done and what is expected.

PREOPERATIVE MANAGEMENT

A patient may or may not need a preoperative treatment program; whether he needs one depends on the condition of the extremity. Many patients in our unit do undergo the following preoperative program:

1. Heat (when indicated)
2. Massage
3. Exercise
4. Splinting
5. Home program

The typical daily treatment program begins with some form of heat (paraffin dips or whirlpool bath) followed by massage (Fig. 42-1). Both of these help to increase circulation, nutrition, and quality of the skin. If there are joint contractures, massage can be applied in a distal direction to help passively stretch the tight tissues. This is followed by active or passive exercises, or both, to help strengthen muscles and increase joint range of motion. Then the reeducation movement pattern is taught in preparation for tendon transfer (see the discussion on reeducation, on p. 477).

Finally, some type of static or dynamic splint is usually indicated to help increase, maintain, prevent, or control joint range of motion and provide for better hand function. Home instructions are given.

This routine is generally followed each time the patient attends therapy.

The main concerns and problems for the therapist in preoperative management of tendon transfers are the following:

1. Extent of nerve damage, if any, as determined by the preoperative assessment
2. Strength of muscles, especially transfer muscle
3. Range of motion of the joints of the upper extremity, especially those directly affected by the transfer
4. Condition of the skin and tissues
5. Reeducation exercise, which is to be taught before surgery and continued postoperatively

476

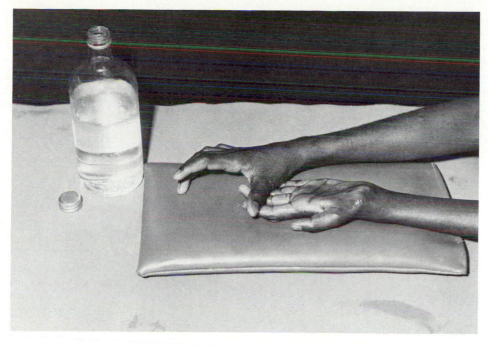

FIG. 42-1. Oil massage for stretching finger flexion contractures.

The strength problem of the transfer muscle

The standard muscle test,[3] perhaps augmented by electrical tests, will give a concise picture of the state of individual muscle power. It is important in the preoperative stage to strengthen maximally the transfer muscle so that it can be more effective postoperatively. Any weakened muscles of the upper extremity, regardless of whether they are selected for transfer, should be strengthened as a matter of routine to increase the chances of a better postoperative result.

Progressive resistive exercises are used to increase strength. If a less than normal muscle selected for transfer does not respond to exercise and fails to become stronger, this fact should be reported to the surgeon, who may then alter the plan.

The joint problem

It is essential to ensure as much range of motion as possible to joints before surgery so as not to handicap the transfer. If there is limitation, the cause must be determined, since it may be a factor in the treatment plan. If the limitation is attributable to a bony block, no further improvement is expected; however, if the limitation is attributable to soft-tissue contractures, a splint is fabricated.[5]

Although heat, massage, and exercises will increase joint range of motion, the effect is usually temporary and the joint will revert to the original (or nearly so) contracted range if nothing else is done. A joint cannot be expected to gain in range if it is stretched for only 1 hour a day and allowed to rest in the contracted state for the remaining 23 hours. The value of the splint is that it maintains the temporary gain in range of motion (after heat, exercises, and so on) and helps prevent the joint from reverting to the

original contracture angle. The preferred way of correcting contractures is by a steady stretch with minimal force applied to a maximum skin area for relatively long periods of time. The temptation to use strong passive forces must be resisted, since "short-term gain mobility is followed by long-term stiffness."[2]

The therapist can estimate the response to treatment by the "end feel." If the movement ends with a springy feeling, the prognosis is encouraging. The more springy the "end feel," the better the chances for improvement.

The skin problem

The use of some form of heat followed by oil massage helps to increase the circulation and nutrition of the skin and softens it so that it becomes more supple and easier to stretch. The actual stretching of the skin is done by active and passive exercises and splints.

Reeducation

The general principle in preoperative muscle reeducation is to try to have the patient isolate the action of the muscle whose tendon is to be transferred. The movement should be as specific as possible so that it activates the best quality contraction of the muscle while at the same time minimizing or completely eliminating the action of other muscles; for example, the movement that extracts the best contraction of the extensor carpi radialis longus and minimizes the other wrist extensors is wrist extension with radial deviation.

During the reeducation exercise there should be no active movements of any other joints, because this would activate other muscles, an effect that would defeat the purpose of isolated contraction.

The time it takes to perform the reeducation exercise

correctly and consistently varies from patient to patient, but usually it can be learned in a very short time. It should be reinforced at each treatment session until the day of surgery.

Readiness for surgery

The hand should now be ready for surgery if all the joint, skin, muscle, and reeducation problems have been eliminated or minimized to the least possible and acceptable degree. The length of preoperative treatment depends on the degree and number of complications to be corrected. Some hands may have no complications at all and can be operated upon immediately. Moderate joint contractures could take a month or more to resolve and severe ones much longer. If the hand is being splinted for joint contractures, these splints must be applied until the day of surgery; otherwise, if there is a gap between splint removal and surgery, the contracture could rapidly return.

SURGERY

Sometimes, during the surgery, technical difficulties may be encountered or anomalous structures and adhesions discovered that will cause the surgeon to alter the original plan. The planned insertion site or tendon route may be changed, or a different tendon may be transferred. Whatever these changes may be, it is essential that the hand therapist be made aware of them and understand their implications so that adjustment in the postoperative therapy can be planned accordingly.

The best and most detailed information is obtained if the therapist actually observes the surgery, but this, of course, is not always feasible or possible. In addition, the therapist should read the operative report as soon as possible after surgery. Any questions should be clarified with the surgeon.

POSTOPERATIVE MANAGEMENT
Immediate postoperative stage

Immediately after surgery edema is a main concern of the hand therapist. If edema is encountered, its presence can lead to soft-tissue joint contractures, which may prove to be unyielding. The treatment at this time consists in keeping the hand elevated.

The patient's hand is immobilized postoperatively; however, uninvolved parts of the hand should be maintained in an active motion program.

In most cases the surgeon will begin mobilization of the transfer at 3 to 4 weeks postoperatively; however, some transfers may be immobilized up to 6 weeks.

One to 3 weeks after cast removal

The first 3 weeks after the cast is removed constitute the tissue-stretching period, which is the optimum when "tendon junctures are just strong enough to take strain and adhesions weak enough to be stretched."[1] If treatment is delayed beyond this period, stretching becomes more difficult, since the adhesions will be thicker and stronger.

For the first postimmobilization week treatment consists of whirlpool bath, massage, gentle active exercises, and protective splinting.

Soaks. For the first week whirlpool bath treatments can help cleanse the hand, remove dead skin, and soften the tissues. If there are open wounds, sterile techniques must be followed.

Massage. Massage is used after the whirlpool bath treatment, except around open wounds. Retrograde massage will be useful in reducing any edema that may be present.

Exercises. Initially, active range-of-motion exercise is used to increase joint motion and muscle strength and reeducate the transferred muscle. Active motion should be gentle so that the transfer muscle is not overstretched.

Increasing range of motion and strength. During the first week after the cast is removed all the joints immobilized in the cast for the 3 to 4 weeks will be stiff, even the ones with normal range preoperatively. The muscles will also be generally weak from disuse. On the first day after cast removal there may be only two or three exercise sessions of 5 minutes' duration, to lessen the danger of overstretch to the transfer. The patient is asked to move the joints gently through a small arc of all possible movements and to increase this range gradually at each session.

For some operations there may be particular joint movements that need to be restricted for longer periods.

Reeducation. The general principle of muscle reeducation after a tendon transfer is to get the patient to attempt the same movement that the muscle did before transfer. This is by no means an automatic process, although it is perhaps easier if the transferred muscle was preoperatively synergistic with the desired postoperative movement. It is not reasonable to expect a muscle that has been performing a specific movement for many years to suddenly start performing another, altogether different movement. Reeducation exercises therefore are needed so that the transferred muscle can learn the new motion.

If the patient has learned the correct reeducation exercise preoperatively, it should be easier postoperatively. On the first day the patient should do the exercise only a few times, using minimal contraction force, and then gradually increase the number of repetitions and the strength of muscle contractions.

Faradic stimulation of the transferred muscle may be of some help when the patient finds it difficult to activate the transfer. Of course, the difficulty may be attributable to complications, which should be checked. The fault may lie in a malfunctioning transfer. Faradic stimulation can usually verify this quickly.

The following are some reasons for transfer failure or partial failure that a therapist should keep in mind:

1. Tendon adhesions
2. Limitation of joint range of motion
3. Low tension of transferred tendon
4. Preoperative tendon excursion inadequate
5. Excessive tension of the transfer
6. Detached tendon
7. Muscle weakness

Tendon adhesions are probably the most common cause of failure and should be suspected first when there is a partial failure. The presence of skin puckering, especially at incision sites, confirms the suspicion. Adhesions of the transfer tendon can occur anywhere along the tendon route. They are more common at incision sites or areas of tissue trauma, where the tendon can become bound to the surrounding healing tissues.[7,8] They may become partially (more common) or wholly bound down. If the latter, none of the muscle contraction force will be conveyed to the insertion site and so there will be no transfer movement.

Adhesions are commonly identified by observation of puckering skin, especially at incision areas. If the tendon has a superficial route, one may be able to locate the site or sites of adhesions by palpating the gliding tendon, starting proximally and moving distally.

One may determine the extent of the adhesion by placing the pulp of one finger over the adhesion site and rolling the skin in all directions to see and feel if it is stuck fast to unyielding underlying tissue.

If adhesions are suspected, they should be treated immediately, since it is easier to stretch or break them before they get thickened and organized. Ultrasound and friction massage can be given at the adhesion site.

Limitation of joint range of motion is an obvious cause that can be seen and measured.

Low tension is suspected when there is partial function and absence of any adhesions or puckering.

Excess tension in the transfer is suspected when faradic stimulation shows partial movement and there is bowstringing of the transfer tendon. There is also considerable resistance to passive movement of the joint in the direction opposite to the transfer action.

A detached tendon may be suspected when no transfer movement is elicited from the reeducation exercise or faradic stimulation.

Testing the transfer. Sometime during the first week after cast removal it should be established whether the transfer is acting well, partially, or not at all. This is accomplished in several ways. The first method is by observation of the effects on joint movement when the patient actively attempts the reeducation exercise. Thus, if the extensor carpi radialis longus is transferred anteriorly to replace paralyzed intrinsics, the expected movements to watch for would be metacarpophalangeal flexion and interphalangeal extension. However, in certain operations it is possible that these transfer movements may be caused by a passive tenodesis force. In this case the extensor carpi radialis longus, because of its anterior route, would be stretched passively during wrist extension and the transfer movement would result. In the first week after cast removal, because all the joints are still stiff, it is not easy to distinguish between active and passive transfer movements.

The second method of transfer testing is by electrical stimulation (Fig. 42-2). If the transfer muscle is superficial, it is stimulated with the strong faradic current, and if the expected joint movement takes place, the transfer is capable of active functioning. However, this does not rule out a tenodesis effect, but most likely, if the faradic test elicits the transfer movement, the transfer is functioning. If there is no movement or only partial movement, the explanation will be one of the causes of failure mentioned above.

A third but less exact way of transfer testing is to palpate, if possible, the gliding movement of the superficial transfer tendon during the reeducation exercise (Fig. 42-3).

Other complications

Edema. Postoperative edema has several causes. If it is present immediately at cast removal, it may be attributable to the effects of operative trauma. This will take several days to subside. If the edema appears only on the second or third day after cast removal it could be caused by the effects of loss of skin support after the cast is removed. This is seen after extended periods of cast application. This edema should subside in a few days. Edema may occur after overexercising or overstretching of tissues. This may require

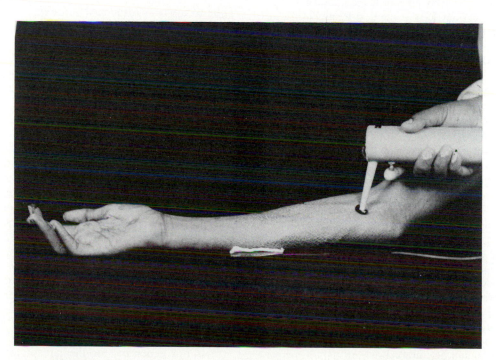

FIG. 42-2. Faradic stimulation testing of pronator teres transfer to wrist extensors.

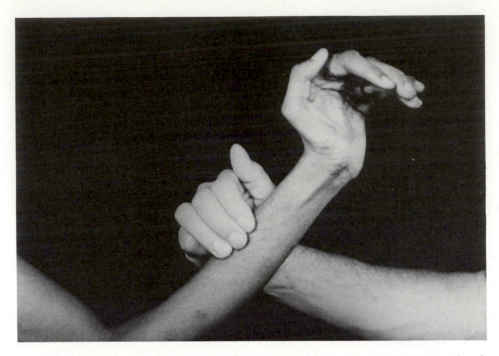

FIG. 42-3. Palpating gliding tendon of extensor carpi radialis longus as it courses anteriorly during reeducation exercise

reduction of the treatment program and allowance of more time for rest and healing.

In all cases the edema must be reduced. At all times, even during the treatment if possible, the hand should be elevated. Other physical methods include massage, active exercise, ice, string wrapping,[4] pneumatic cuffs, and elastic gloves. Edema should be monitored daily.

Open wounds. If incisions are not healed, care must be taken to prevent infection. Rest is the best treatment for an open wound; however, total rest may be impossible because of the necessity to mobilize the tendon transfer.

Usual contraindications for open wounds must be observed. Gentle active exercises several times a day for a few minutes can be done during this time to prevent adhesions and contractures.

Splinting. There are three main reasons for splinting postoperatively:

1. To protect a joint from excessive early movement
2. To prevent the possible formation of new deformities or the recurrence of preoperative ones
3. To provide needed rest for proper tissue healing

Movement of a joint acted upon by a tendon transfer must take place gradually. Excessive early movement in the opposite direction to the movement intended by the tendon transfer could be harmful. For example, if the purpose of the transfer is to extend the proximal and distal interphalangeal joints, flexion of them too soon should be avoided. Such movement is best prevented for the first week or two by a splint, which will not permit it.

If it is suspected that the joints are becoming stiff in the operative position, earlier removal of the splint and range-of-motion exercises can be initiated.

The splint is taken off during the treatment period and reapplied for the intervening times. It is usually the static type, because dynamic splints permit movement.

There is a strong tendency for corrected contractures and deformities, such as a contracted thumb web or proximal interphalangeal flexion contracture, to recur postoperatively. The postoperative splint helps to prevent such recurrence by opposing the deforming forces.

Four to 6 weeks after cast removal

The range of motion is evaluated. The program is similar to that of the first 3 weeks, with some changes. One increases the exercise time and intensity by adding more repetitions and requiring stronger muscle contractions, but always keeping in mind the limitations and watching for the signs of inflammation or overstretching.

Active use during activities of daily living is initiated.

About the fifth postcast week, if there have been no complications, daytime splinting can be discontinued but nighttime splinting may continue. Removal of the daytime splint will encourage the patient to begin to move the joints more freely and help restore full range more quickly. However, if the preoperative deformities or contractures begin to recur after the splint is removed, it should be reapplied on a schedule appropriate to the severity of the contractures.

By the end of the fifth postcast week, there should be about 50% to 75% of the expected range of motion of the joints of most transfers and the transfer should be activated easily. The patient should be using the hand in activities of daily living (Fig. 42-4).

Home instructions and discharge

It is not necessary for the patient to obtain 100% of possible function before discharge from formal treatment,

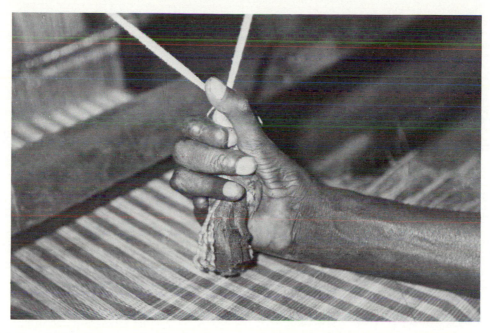

FIG. 42-4. Functional activity exercise for thumb opponens replacement using ring flexor digitorum superficialis. Notice active participation of transfer tendon.

which may occur at 8 to 12 weeks postoperatively. The patient may be given a home program to further increase the strength of the transfer. Night splints may be continued and reviewed at follow-up visits.

SUMMARY

A comprehensive preoperative and postoperative therapy program for management of tendon transfers has been described. Not every patient will require such an intensive program. However, knowledge of the principles and techniques described will aid in the management of the more difficult cases.

REFERENCES

1. Brand, P.W.: Tendon transfers in the forearm. In Flynn, J.E., editor: Hand surgery, ed. 2, Baltimore, 1975, The Williams & Wilkins Co.
2. Brand, P.W.: The forces of dynamic splinting: ten questions before applying a dynamic splint. In Hunter, J.M., Scheider, L.H., Mackin, E.J., and Bell, J.A., editors: Rehabilitation of the hand, St. Louis, 1978, The C.V. Mosby Co.
3. Daniels, L., and Worthingham, C.: Muscle testing: techniques of manual examination, Philadelphia, 1980, W.B. Saunders Co.
4. Hunter, J.M., and Mackin, E.J.: Edema and bandaging. In Hunter, J.M., Schneider, L.H., Mackin, E.J., and Bell, J.A., editors: Rehabilitation of the hand, St. Louis, 1978, The C.V. Mosby Co.
5. Kolumban, S.L.: The role of static and dynamic splints: physiotherapy techniques and time in straightening contracted interphalangeal joints, Leprosy in India, pp. 323-328, Oct. 1969.
6. Leffert, R.D., and Meister, M.: Patterns of neuromuscular activity following tendon transfer in the upper limb: a preliminary study, J. Hand Surg. **1:**181, 1976.
7. Madden, J.W.: Current concepts of wound healing as applied to hand surgery, Orthop. Clin. North Am. **1:**325, 1970.
8. Peacock, E.E., Jr.: Fundamental aspects of wound healing relating to the restoration of gliding function after tendon repairs, Surg. Gynecol. Obstet. **119:**241, 1964.

43

Electromyography and electrical testing in hand rehabilitation

WILLIAM J. ERDMAN II

Before performing electrical testing, one should make a determination, by a careful history and clinical evaluation of the patient, of which tests to use and how extensive they need to be. Electromyography and other electrodiagnostic studies are dynamic evaluations of living tissue, and it is imperative that the areas tested and the procedures used be thoughtfully studied and that adjustments be made in response to findings. Usually there is a specific question about diagnosis or prognosis that is being pursued, but in the process the electrical findings may indicate that additional muscles, nerves, or extremities require testing. In this chapter I examine some common problems, not the esoteric ones. It is neither a text on performing electrical testing nor a compendium of equipment available, but an effort to correlate the value of electrical testing in clinical hand impairment.

Both the upper extremities and the head and neck should be carefully inspected for limitation in range of motion, atrophy, and weakness on manual muscle testing. Reflexes should be evaluated. A reflected light may reveal sweating alterations. New or long-standing scars may have deeper tissue implications. Limitation in range of motion of the head on the neck or on the trunk may suggest that the pathologic condition is more proximal than an obvious injury. Careful sensory mapping, including touch with Frey hairs, pain with an algesimeter, two-point discrimination, perception and discrimination of heat and cold, deep pressure, Tinel's sign, and evidence of correct localization versus mislocalization, will indicate where one may most likely expect abnormalities to appear in electrical testing.

There is a fascination with electromyography, which has superseded some of the simpler noninvasive tests, which still are very useful. Skin that is normally innervated has a low resistance to electrical current. Resistance is increased substantially by pressure or damage to the sympathetic nerve supply at any place along the course of the fiber. The amount of current flow, measured by a dermometer, can show injury to sympathetic fibers and may substantiate sensory changes. Hysterical sensory alterations may be suggested by an inconsistency between sensory and sweating loss. This inconsistency may be an indication of posterior ramus pressure before the junction of the posterior ramus with the sympathetic root.

The responses to stimulation by a faradic or galvanic current in a grossly denervated muscle may be more tolerable to the patient than puncturing the skin with even a monopolar needle. Those responses actually show two of the points of the strength-duration curve for the muscle. One is a point on the curve where it is asymptotic to the y-axis, and the other is a point where it is asymptotic to the x-axis. Similarly, a chronaxie test uses two points from the curve. In chronaxic determinations the rheobase, or least amount of current required to stimulate biologic tissue when applied over a long interval (up to 0.3 seconds), is first determined, and then the strength is doubled. The rheobase is the voltage of the strength-duration curve at the point it is asymptotic to the x-axis. The doubled voltage, or twice the rheobase, is the second point on the curve, and its distance from the y-axis is the chronaxie. The curve shifts dramatically to the right when denervation has occurred at any point along the peripheral nerve from the anterior horn cell to the neuromyal junction. Slight changes in chronaxic values need not be overinterpreted any more than irregular or incomplete strength-duration curves if the examiner sets a standard sufficiently above normal to rule out all experimental errors. One millisecond is such a safe standard. Chronaxic determinations are noninvasive and relatively comfortable for a patient. It is worth noting that partial prior neuropathy from disease or injury may significantly decrease the patient's tolerance to electrical current and may cause heightened discomfort in a variety of testing procedures requiring the application of transcutaneous or intraneural stimulation. The twitch-tetanus ratio of current strengths occasionally has usefulness as a confirming test, but it is less comfortable.

The results obtained in the above tests should corroborate findings in electromyography and help avoid the pitfall of overreading or overinterpreting the findings in any one testing technique. Normal muscle may show fibrillations, and it is helpful to have parallel testing procedures to give appropriate weight to the findings. False-positive conclusions should not arise from appropriate and careful testing, and the incidence of false-negative findings is decreased by more extensive and overlapping procedures.

ELECTROMYOGRAPHY

The motor unit consists of a lower motor neuron and the muscle fibers that are supplied by it. Similarly, a sensory unit consists of sensory perceptors and the sensory neuron, which carries impulses toward the cental nervous system. A peripheral nerve is made up of either or both motor and sensory pathways, the connective tissue, and the nerve covering. Electromyography is a means of studying the motor unit or the sensory unit in part or in whole. Disease or injury may affect the anterior horn cell, the ramus, the plexus, the peripheral nerve, the neuromyal junction, or the muscle itself. If the nerve interruption is complete, as when a nerve is cut, the patient's problems are usually so obvious that electrical testing is employed to corroborate only. An advancing Tinel sign is usually the best indication of recovery after death of the Schwann cell and total interruption of nerve transmission. Electromyography plays an important role in determining neuropraxia with nerve recovery and the degree or presence of neuropraxia as well. Neuropraxia is an abnormality in conduction with preservation of the axon, which temporarily is not transmitting impulses. In upper extremity pathologic conditions it is helpful to know whether early exploration of injury, removal of pressure in the carpal tunnel, transposition in ulnar nerve neuropraxia, differentiation between posterior interosseous entrapment and tennis elbow, localization of brachial plexus injury, or root disease is indicated. Patients are referred for electrical testing because specific localized information is sought, and the reports should be inclusive enough to allow conclusions to be reached, with data to confirm the conclusions. Reporting too many minor and inconsequential variations is more confusing than helpful.

Electromyographic equipment includes electrodes, which are placed on the surface of the skin, or needles, which are inserted into the muscles or nerves. The needles may be monopolar, bipolar, or tripolar. For patient comfort those inserted should be of the smallest caliber consistent with the desired results. Currents picked up are evoked potentials secondary to stimulation, to voluntary activity, or to involuntary discharge. They are passed through an amplifier and displayed on an oscilloscope with or without sound. Auditory amplification is frequently helpful to the examiner and sometimes to the patient in learning by biofeedback. Information may be stored, averaged, or manipulated by computer to give the examiner better interpretation of the findings. The integrity of the peripheral nerve may be checked also by spinally or cortically evoked potentials, a subject that is beyond the scope of this presentation.

Electromyographic examination of the muscles is performed by insertion of the electrodes while one observes and listens for insertional potentials. Resting fibrillation potentials, the involuntary discharge of muscle electrical activity, have been reported in some part of normal muscles in up to 5% of normal muscles but they generally are pathognomonic of denervation, polymyositis, or hyperkalemic periodic paralysis. Localized injury to a muscle, as from a tight-fitting shoe or tourniquet or from pounding of the fist, may lead to fibrillations without denervation. The frequency and area of occurrence have diagnostic and, in serial studies, prognostic value. Polyphasic potentials, particularly the large ones, are valuable also in differentiating denervation from reinnervation. However, as fibrous tissue replaces dying denervated muscle fibers, the frequency of fibrillations decreases also, and so a decrease frequency is not always a favorable sign and must be correlated with the entire clinical and electrical picture.

MEASUREMENT OF CONDUCTION VELOCITIES

In hand rehabilitation cases the electrodiagnostician most frequently is asked to demonstrate evidence of neuropraxic injuries occurring with other injuries or of peripheral nerve entrapment. Localization of the site of injury or disease may be possible by careful study of the muscles alone. Usually, measurement of motor and sensory nerve conduction velocities, with localization of the area of slowing, is the best technique. Velocities change with age and temperature, and they vary according to the particular laboratory performing the test.

Median nerve

Motor. Motor conduction is measured between a cathodal stimulation approximately 8 cm proximal to the point of a recording electrode and a surface electrode on the thenar eminence at the motor point of the abductor pollicis brevis, which is over the proximal end of the first phalanx. If the recording electrode is over the motor point of the muscle, the initial deflection is negative. If not negative, it may not be the motor point and should be moved, or it may be an indication of aberrant innervation. The velocity of nerve conduction is determined by dividing the distance between the stimulator and the recorder by the time elapsed; the result is usually expressed in meters per second (derived by dividing milliseconds into millimeters). It may be necessary or preferable to use a needle electrode to pick up the evoked potential. The stimulus must be supramaximal.

The median nerve may also be stimulated in the antecubital fossa medial to the biceps tendon, on the medial aspect of the humerus, in the supraclavicular fossa, or at the C8 root. In each instance conduction times and velocities are calculated as above. Inferences may then be drawn as to the point of injury along the efferent pathway of the nerve, and correlations can be made with the clinical history.

Because of the frequency of crossover innervation between the ulnar and median nerves, it is important to stimulate the ulnar nerve at the wrist and elbow while one is recording from median nerve muscles, and vice versa. This information may explain apparent clinical inconsistencies and aid in surgical decisions. Unfortunately, failure to make this differentation may also explain the failure of surgical release to give clinical relief.

Sensory. Sensory conduction may be measured orthodromically by stimulating surface electrodes placed on the index or middle fingers and recording at various, progressively more proximal points along the median nerve—at the wrist, the elbow, and all the way to the roots. If only a digital sensory nerve is being tested, the area of the digit that is denervated must receive the stimulus and the recording must be made before the nerve's junction with other digital nerves.

It is also possible to determine sensory conduction velocities antidromically, by placing recording circumferential electrodes on the fingers and stimulating proximally at any convenient point. The current required is less and the response greater, but the test may be more painful.

Compression of the median nerve at the wrist, which has been known clinically for over a century, is one of the most frequent hand complications. If it is suspected and found, testing should be done bilaterally, since compression occurs frequently on both sides. Bilateral testing is usually important for determination of the significance, if any, of unilateral findings, and discovery of the presence of abnormalities on both sides may avoid erroneous conclusions. Serial testing may show changes that indicate that medical treatment without release is sufficient, as in neuropraxia, or that indicate the importance of decompression or explain the reaction to surgery.

There may be injuries to branches of the median nerve forearm muscles with significant evidence of motor denervation to the involved muscles and no sensory changes. The differential susceptibility to compression may give rise to more severe sensory and pain changes than to motor loss, as after extravasation and edema in antecubital fossa injections, or under tight casts or tourniquets.

Normal values for upper extremity nerve conduction. Normal values for median nerve conduction are as follows: motor, 53 to 61 meters per second; sensory, 54 to 62 meters per second; distal latency or conduction time from wrist to thenar eminence, motor, 3.4 to 4.0 milliseconds, and sensory, 2.8 to 3.2 milliseconds. If arbitrary values higher than these, such as 4.6 msec motor and 3.8 msec sensory, are adopted, unnecessary decompressions of nerves that might have responded to conservative treatment or to time alone will be prevented. These ranges for normal values in conduction velocity also are normal for other upper extremity nerves.

Ulnar nerve

Motor. The recording electrode is placed over the motor point of the abductor digiti quinti or first dorsal interosseous (less painful unless ulnar sensory loss exists), and the reference electrode is placed over the proximal phalanx. Cathodal stimulation is applied at the wrist, medial condyle of the elbow, and up to the C8 root, as with the median nerve. Stimulation of the ulnar nerve 1 cm distally and 1 cm proximally to the edges of the medial condyle will permit a determination of the time required for an impulse to cross this area. If is the location where the ulnar nerve is most susceptible to injury after fracture and healing or to compression during surgery, prolonged pressure from reading in bed or falling asleep with elbows on armrests, or single or repeated blows to the "crazy bone." Careful avoidance of pressure may allow spontaneous improvement. Anterior transposition may be required.

Sensory. Sensory conduction measurement may be performed orthodromically or antidromically with ring electrodes on the fifth digit and the recording or stimulating electrode over the ulnar nerve at the wrist approximately 14 cm proximally. It may also be placed more proximally at any available point. Measurements greater than 1 milli-

second across the medial condylar space are abnormally slow.

Radial nerve

Motor. The recording electrode is placed over or in the motor point of the extensor indicis proprius muscle because this muscle receives the most distal branch of the radial nerve. The motor point is approximately one third of the distance from the wrist to the elbow, on the dorsal surface. Stimulation with the cathode is applied just medially to the brachial radialis or just posteriorly to the deltoid, over the muscular spiral groove of the humerus.

Because the radial nerve is subject to compression in the axilla, as it wraps around the humerus, or the deep motor branch of the radial nerve can become entrapped by the supinator muscle, this nerve should be stimulated at several points. It may be affected in anesthesia, sleep, or "Saturday night palsy." Differentiating "tennis elbow" from posterior interosseus nerve compression is easy electrically, and there are obvious differences in treatment.

Sensory. Accurate measurements of the radial nerve conduction velocity must be done antidromically. Ring recording electrodes are placed around the thumb, and the cathode-stimulating electrode is placed over the dorsolateral radius, about one third of the distance from the wrist to the elbow.

Musculocutaneous nerve

Motor. The nerve conduction velocity is easiest to record in the biceps brachii, with surface or needle electrode recording from the medial head and the stimulating cathode in the axilla or in the supraclavicular fossa of the anterior triangle of the neck. The musculocutaneous nerve may be injured when the lateral cord of the superior trunk of the brachial plexus is injured or when that nerve is directly injured.

Sensory. Measurement is antidromic. The recording electrode is placed on the volar aspect of the forearm in the distal radial area, with the reference electrode 4 cm away. The cathode-stimulating electrode is placed just laterally to the biceps tendon in the antecubital fossa. This determination is necessary only in edema or direct injury, and then only rarely.

Brachial plexus. The variety of injuries to the brachial plexus makes an interesting challenge when one is isolating the involved area. Partial root injuries give rise to electrical changes in many of the muscles supplied by the injured root, but in complete root injuries all of the muscles show electrical changes. Testing the contralateral side is imperative, to rule out pressure in the canal or a cervical disk. Herniated disks usually give rise to bilateral electrical changes even though the symptoms and clinical changes are unilateral. A useful technique in suspected root irritation at the foramina is to move the head actively and passively on the neck and trunk, looking and listening for electrical discharge produced by the mechanical root irritation in the recording electrode. If it occurs, slight manual traction with the same movement may eliminate the mechanical irritation and confirm the location.

Stimulation of the brachial plexus trunk is best accomplished at Erb's point. Recording electrodes are inserted into the infraspinatus, supraspinatus, deltoid, biceps, and triceps. Surface electrodes may be used in some of these muscles. Erb's point lies just laterally to the insertion of the sternocleidomastoid into the clavicle above and as far posteriorly as possible. The cathode stimulator should be at Erb's point.

Lesions in the roots may be difficult to differentiate from trunk lesions, because both affect motor nerve conduction velocity. However, plexus lesions may and usually do have sensory conduction slowing, which roots do not.

CONCLUSION

Electrical testing is well established as a useful clinical tool and may be the most important test available. The field and its literature are expanding as new tests and equipment become available. This discussion gives some of the common and hopefully useful findings and conclusions. It is not exhaustive.

44

Implications of electromyographic examinations for hand therapy

ARTHUR J. NELSON

For clarification of the electrophysiologic report it is helpful to review the neuropathology of the peripheral nerve. The clinical problems that may be encountered in hand care can be subdivided into disorders of the nerve trunk, the axon, its myelin sheath, the motor neuron, the myoneural junction, and the skeletal muscle.

MOTOR UNIT

The anterior horn cell, its axon, and all the muscle fibers supplied by that one neuron are called the "motor unit." The number of muscle fibers supplied may vary from five or six to 1000 or more. Because the all-or-none law ensures complete firing of the whole motor unit, the smaller the ratio of axon to muscle fibers, the more refined the motor control possible. The smaller motor units are recruited first in progressively more intense contractions, followed by the larger ones in an orderly progression according to the size-order principle of Henneman.

The electromyographic (EMG) appearance of a motor unit has a biphasic or triphasic pattern with a duration of 6 to 12 msec and an amplitude of 300 μV to 5 mV or more. The duration of the motor unit is dependent on the spread of the endplate zone as it relates to the total length of the muscle fibers. For example, the abductor pollicis brevis muscle has an end plate zone that represents 50% of the total length of the muscle fibers, resulting in a longer duration, while the biceps brachii muscle has an endplate zone of approximately 10% of the total length of the muscle, which results in a shorter duration.

The amplitude of the motor unit potential is the result of the relative size of the muscle fiber membranes that are active within the same period of time. The electromyographic potential visualized on the screen is a compound one resulting from an amalgamation of all the individualized muscle fiber discharges. The size of the muscle fibers (membranes) coupled with the total conductive area available within the muscle contributes toward the amplitude of the motor unit action potential (MAP). Amplitude comparisons are difficult to utilize for assessment of strength, but large differences from one side to the other can have value in making clinical judgments.

Skeletal muscle is structured in such a way that the motor units are in a somewhat checkerboard configuration. According to Buchthal[1] a motor unit occupies approximately 5 to 11 mm^2 of a given muscle. If the electrical discharges are to be effectively displayed on the electromyogram, the needle electrode must be within the vicinity of the motor unit that is active. Movement of the electrode even a few millimeters away from the active motor unit will decrease the amplitude of the response by 90%. This factor explains why surface electrodes are not employed for the accurate delineation of the motor unit potentials and can only determine gross electrical discharge.

The nerve trunk contains thousands of axons with varying diameters organized in bundles with connective tissue sheaths. These bundles are then enveloped in an overall sheath called the "epineurium." The speed of conduction along the nerve trunk is a reflection on the collective diameters plus the amount of myelin coating of the axons contained therein. Because the fibers are in a braided configuration, it is necessary to provide a more than maximum (supramaximal) stimulation to ensure that all the fibers are stimulated.

NEUROPATHOLOGIC CORRELATES OF ELECTROMYOGRAPHIC FINDINGS

Disorders of the motor neuron, its axon, the nerve trunk or any of its components, the myoneural junction, or the muscle itself may be involved in hand problems. To rank neural disorders affecting the hand from the most frequently encountered to the least frequently encountered, one would start with entrapment of the peripheral nerve, which is quite commonly encountered. Then come peripheral nerve injuries, followed by axonal or motor neuron disease, which is not a commonly encountered problem, and, finally, myoneural junction and myopathic disorders, which are rarely encountered.

Entrapment syndromes

There are many sites of entrapment or compromise of peripheral nerves, but a common site is the *median nerve at the wrist*. It is believed that the median nerve is compromised by either lack of space in the carpal tunnel or inflammation of the tendons, blood vessels, or other contents of the tunnel.[2] The compression affects the fibers that are more metabolically dependent, the thickest fibers. Many

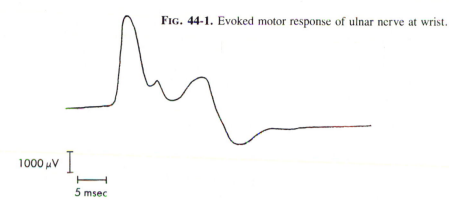

FIG. 44-1. Evoked motor response of ulnar nerve at wrist.

1000 µV

5 msec

sensory fibers are in the thicker category, except for those involved with pain and temperature, which thereby results in a loss of light touch sensibility but a retention of pinprick and crude touch sensibility. The thicker motor axons may also be affected early in the course of this disorder. Because the evoked electrical stimulation of the nerve trunk will activate all the fibers capable of conduction, the ones that conduct the fastest will be observed as the first component of the response wave (Fig. 44-1). In some patients the sensory component will reveal a prolonged latency while the motor component may be within normal limits (that is, 3.7 ± 0.3 msec for the median nerve at 8 cm from stimulating to pickup electrode). When the distal latencies are near the borders of normal, it usually proves helpful to compare the two limbs and to compare the findings with the distal latency of the ulnar nerve because there should be no more than a 1 msec difference with distance held constant.

Another feature of the evoked response to note is the amplitude of the evoked response. If there is a loss of more than 50% of the amplitude when compared to the opposite side and the recording technique has been completed with care on both sides, it is to be noted and may be of clinical significance if other electrical findings correlate with this change.

The electromyogram may reveal motor action potential (MAP) changes such as increased amounts of polyphasic MAP in muscles innervated by the median nerve distal to the wrist where the nerve has been compromised for several months (Fig. 44-2). It is essential to survey muscles from each of the major peripheral nerves and the cervical nerve roots to assure that the complaints are not from other neuronal disorders.

Many patients with carpal tunnel syndrome reveal bilateral changes in their median nerves. When this occurs, it is important to determine if the other peripheral nerves, such as the ulnar nerve, have any distal delays or evidence of neuronal disorder that might suggest a peripheral neuropathy multiplex. Persons suffering from generalized peripheral nerve disease are typically more vulnerable to compression. The therapist should know if the compressed lesion is superimposed on a generalized peripheral neuropathy because he or she must exercise care when providing splinting that will avoid compression of other peripheral nerves while keeping the median nerve from being com-

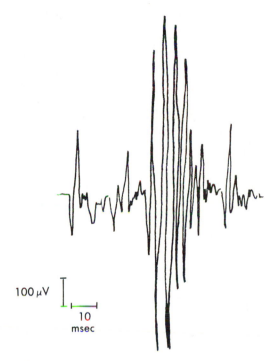

100 µV

10 msec

FIG. 44-2. Chronic neuropathic motor unit potential and normal motor units.

pressed against the carpal tunnel's superior surface when in extension. A neutral wrist position provides the least compromise.

The case that presents a mild distal delay of the motor or sensory component of the median nerve is typically treated with neutral wrist support coupled with steroid infiltration of the carpal tunnel. There are no exact boundaries of the test results that determine surgical intervention or conservative care. Operative intervention is considered most effective in those suffering from more prolonged latencies that are the result of mechanical disruption of the nerve without other neuropathy present.

Tardy ulnar palsy

Another compressive disorder of somewhat frequent occurrence is compromise of the ulnar nerve at the region of the elbow. One should flex the elbow while recording to avoid a false-positive determination of slowing of conduction across the elbow. A significant slowing of conduction of the ulnar nerve across the elbow may or may not result in any motor impairment of the intrinsic hand muscles innervated by the ulnar nerve, because slowing does not stop function.

In addition to a local change in the conduction velocity across the elbow, as the compression of the ulnar nerve continues there will be a reduction in the amplitude of the sensory nerve action potential (SNAP). At this stage the motor action potential (MAP) may be of normal amplitude. There may be concomitant electomyographic changes consisting of complex, polyphasic MAPs that result from collateral sprouting from the noncompressed intact axons to the denervated muscle fibers. The muscles affected will extend from the elbow distally to the forearm muscles and to the intrinsic hand muscles innervated by the ulnar nerve. When there is motor affectation, it is helpful to determine by means of the electrophysiologic data if there is axonal degeneration. The use of electrical stimulation would be influenced by its presence. In a recent study by Pachter and others[6] they noted that electrical stimulation performed when fibillation had decreased resulted in greater muscle bulk and strength than a nontreated sample of rats with peripheral nerve lesions. Vrbová indicates that stimulation of a fibrilating muscle tends to decrease the fibrillation, and she suggests that too early stimulation may retard reinnervation.

What type of stimulation is best? The duration of the pulse of direct current applied by the negative pole should be as close to the optimal chronaxie value (minimal duration) as possible. Also it appears that the more the pattern of stimulation simulates functional motion or is actually involved in performance of some activity, the more effective the reinnervation. This would mean placing the electrical stimulation on muscles during the time they are needed to carry out an activity.

As soon as the muscle is fully reinnervated, conventional strengthening through active and resistive exercise should begin. The relative intensity of muscle contraction may be monitored with a surface electrode electromyograph. Training with an electromyograph should utilize the information to predict the muscle's needed output. This is best done if the activity is performed rhythmically and with a regular, predictable pattern to it. To simply confirm muscle action with electromyographic feedback is of some help, but more gains can be obtained by using this information for prediction of outcome.

Patients should be instructed to keep their forearm in supination if they have to rest on the affected elbow, because this will draw the ulnar nerve away from the site of pressure.

Deep branch of the ulnar nerve

The deep branch of the ulnar nerve, which sweeps into the palm of the hand, is subject to entrapment in the canal de Guyon. This involvement is tested by stimulation of the ulnar nerve at the wrist and placement of pickup electrodes over the abductor digiti minimi muscle and over the first dorsal interosseous muscle. One might expect that a latency difference between the two pickup points will be less than 0.7 msec. Additionally, one might expect to find normal electromyographic findings in the hypothenar musculature,

but the other intrinsic musculature innervated by the ulnar nerve may reveal neuropathic electomyographic changes, such as polyphasic MAPs, or spontaneous activity at rest, such as positive sharp waves or fibrillation potentials, as well as reduction in the recruitment of motor action potentials.[3]

Stimulation would be instituted when fibrillation had subsided. After a 6- or 8-week interval the evoked response should be repeated for comparison with the previous study to determine changes in latency or amplitude.

Deep interosseous branch of the radial nerve

Protracted compression is most frequently a part of the history of patients' suffering from radial nerve palsy, but lead poisoning may also affect the radial nerve selectively. The deep interosseous branch departs from the main radial trunk in the region of the spiral groove of the humerus, and stimulation applied there is directed distally to pickup electrodes placed over an outcropping muscle on the dorsum of the forearm (such as the extensor pollicis longus). Another point of stimulation of this branch would be the anterolateral cubital fossa. If the nerve has a simple blockade of conduction (neuropraxia), typically there will be no response proximal to the area of the block but a normal response distal to it. The electromyographic findings in distal muscles will not reveal any evidence of denervation (such as fibrillation or positive sharp waves) in a neuropraxia lesion. It is important to recall that if the distal portion of the nerve degenerates (as occurs in the wallerian type) it takes 14 to 18 days; therefore the electromyogram taken during that interval will probably reveal an absence of motor action potentials but not a specific indication of denervation. If no electromyographic evidence of axonal degeneration occurs after 14 days, it is quite probable that the defect is one of blockade. Recovery may be expected spontaneously within the next 2 weeks if the lesion is a local block (neuropraxia).

Median nerve entrapped in pronator teres

The median nerve may be compromised in the region of the elbow, possibly where it pierces the pronator teres or where it passes beneath the ligament of Struthers. When this is the area of encroachment, it may be recognized by a loss of conduction of evoked responses from above the elbow through the forearm area. This is usually coupled with good conduction below the elbow (antecubital fossa) before axonal degenerative changes are manifested. If the electromyograph detects evidence of axonal degeneration such as fibrillation, positive sharp waves at rest, or increased polyphasicity with moderate contraction in the long flexor of the thumb and other muscles below the pronator teres, such evidence would implicate this area. As the thenar muscles innervated by the median nerve will also reveal neuropathic electromyographic findings, a complete study must include muscles proximal to the wrist so that this identification of the lesion is ensured.

Deep interosseous branch of median nerve

The deep interosseous branch of the median nerve splits from the main trunk soon after it leaves the pronator teres and innervates the flexor pollicis longus and the pronator quadratus.[5] The electrodiagnostic findings will be confined to prolonged conduction time over this branch to the flexor pollicis longus or to the pronator quadratus, and if axonal degeneration has taken place only to these muscles, the electromyographic findings associated with denervation (such as fibrillation and positive sharp waves) will be evident. The most obvious deficit functionally will be loss of flexion strength of the distal phalanx of the thumb. This lesion may easily be confused with the carpal tunnel syndrome. To distinguish between them, sampling from the flexor pollicis longus and the musculature distal to the wrist as well must be made.

Peripheral nerve injuries of median and ulnar nerves

Traumatic lesions of the median and ulnar nerves induced by lacerations at the wrist are frequently encountered by the hand therapist. The electromyographer provides clarification as to the extent of neural impairment. When tendons have been severed, it is sometimes difficult to determine if lack of motion is the result of pain and restriction or of denervation.[3]

During the denervation phase, fibrillation potentials of short duration (1 to 3 msec) and of relatively low amplitude (100 to 300 μV) and positive sharp waves (Fig. 44-3) may be seen 7 to 14 days from the time of the injury. When several months have passed, the fibrillation and positive sharp waves found at rest usually decrease. For monitoring of the amount of spontaneous activity (fibrillation and positive sharp waves) the following four categories have been established:

1. Few scattered fibrillation potentials
2. Consistently found fibrillation potentials for brief periods
3. Relatively prolonged periods of fibrillation and trains of positive sharp waves

FIBRILLATION POTENTIALS

50 μV

10 msec

POSITIVE SHARP WAVES

100 μV

10 msec

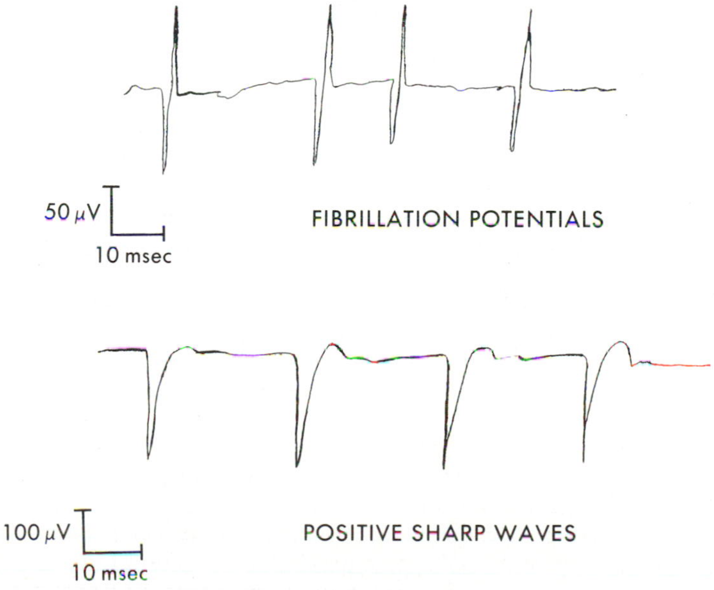

FIG. 44-3. Denervation potentials at rest.

4. Prolonged periods of fibrillation potentials and sustained trains of positive sharp waves (Fig. 44-3)

The appearance of brief-duration, low-amplitude, polyphasic motor unit potentials (BLAP) (sometimes called "nascent" potentials) are indicative of reinnervation and typically precede the onset of clinical return of movement. At this stage, electrical stimulation and exercise are indicated, because the muscle has lost some of its denervation sensitivity and is physiologically capable of receiving electrical stimulation without detracting from reinnervation. As the muscle responds to activity and resistance may be added, the fibers hypertrophy and subsequently an increased amplitude of the electromyographic potential results. Possibly because of collateral sprouting (spreading of an endplate zone), the motor action potential increases its duration (to 20 msec or more). The combination of these two factors results in higher amplitude potentials and longer duration (15 to 20 msec) (HALD) (Fig. 44-2).

The intensity of exercise should be increased with graduated stress on the effected musculature so that the muscle will become capable of sustaining activity for the period of time required for accomplishing specified activities of daily living. For example, one should consider the duration of palmar prehension needed for bringing the utensil to the mouth and also for the repetition needed for feeding oneself a meal. What is the duration of total activity? How may rest be obtained and at what intervals? If the exercise program may be enhanced by use of electromyographic (integrated) information, not only will the patient get augmented sensory feedback but will also be provided with information about the efficiency of the muscle. When the electomyograph tracing line falls off, it can be the result of fatigue or it could also be caused by lack of effort. Sometimes a very highly motivated person may synchronize motor units in such a manner that the integrated electromyogram line becomes slightly increased over a previously maximum effort.[4]

FUNCTIONAL ELECTRICAL STIMULATION

The electromyographic findings also provide the therapist with information that is useful for initiation of functional electrical stimulation (FES). In stimulating weakened, denervated muscles, it can be more effective if included within a functional pattern of motion. The pattern of stimulation must take into consideration the rate of tension development, the amplitude or intensity of the contraction, and its duration. The number of repetitions is determined by the needs of the activity under usual circumstances. Most intrinsic hand muscle activity appears to involve rapid, mild-intensity contractions that are alternately sustained for several seconds, giving way to a low-grade activity that might be sustained for several minutes. This sequence should then be repeated for the usual duration of the activity (for example, from 6 to 10 minutes for feeding).

Radial nerve injury in spiral groove of humerus

Injury to the deep interosseous branch of the radial nerve results in loss of wrist and finger extension along with the extension and abduction movements of the thumb.

The evoked responses of this branch of the radial nerve

result in amplitudes of approximately 4 to 7 μV. If there is a loss of axons, that loss will be reflected in a proportional reduction of amplitude of the evoked response. The preinjury amplitude may be estimated by reference to the evoked response of the opposite nonaffected side.

The functional implication of reduced amplitude in the response wave would be a corresponding loss of strength in the early stages of the problem. As the intact axons sprout to the affected ones, the number of active muscle fibers increases proportionately. As they are exercised, the strength will be expected to increase progressively even if there is no further reinnervation by the original axons that were damaged. If the percentage of damaged axons is considerable, the compensatory hypertrophy of the remaining intact fibers may not be adequate to bring the muscle tension to a functional level.

The electromyographic findings can be of further assistance by showing the relative number of motor units available, which is evidenced by the recruitment pattern during maximum effort. The smoother the progression of the recruitment of motor units from smaller to the larger ones, the more refined the control will be. Where the larger motor units are available, the movements become tremendous and have an all-or-nothing quality.

Proximal peripheral nervous disorders

The hand may be affected by any number of problems affecting the peripheral nervous system. Electromyography can be helpful in delineating where the lesion may be located. In addition to the distal sites noted previously, there are some proximal lesions to consider, such as the brachial plexus or the cervical nerve roots or spinal cord.

Brachial plexus

Some typical electrophysiologic findings from a relatively acute brachial plexus affectation would typically include electromyographic findings consisting of fibrillation and positive sharp waves at rest, with diminished recruitment of motor units proportional to the severity of the disorder. The anatomic pattern is of greatest importance for identification of the site of involvement. For example, if the hypothenar muscles and the extensors of the thumb are involved, it is evident that the problem is not confined to the ulnar nerve. It is possible that the disorder could result from involvement of two peripheral nerves, but as a general rule one should seek out a single source such as the lower trunk of the brachial plexus or the eighth cervical and first thoracic nerve roots.[7]

To further distinguish involvement between the lower trunk (brachial plexus) and the cervical nerve root, the evoked responses (conduction studies) can be instructive. The motor conduction studies will be normal because conduction does not change in axonal degeneration unless more than 80% of the fibers are degenerated. If a significant number of axons are lost, the amplitude of the evoked response will be reduced (especially when compared to the opposite side). If the problem is distal to the dorsal root ganglion, the sensory evoked response will be reduced proportional to the degree of affectation.

In compromise of the lower trunk, the sensory action

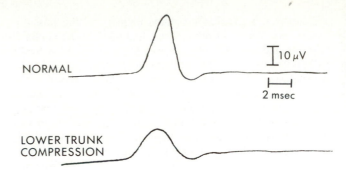

FIG. 44-4. Sensory action potential. Normal versus brachial plexus compression.

potential (SAP) can frequently be reduced to 50% of the nonaffected side, while in cervical radiculopathies there is no reduction in the SAP (Fig. 44-4).

There are also some conduction studies that may be used to investigate the proximal portions of the involved nerves, such as the F wave or somatosensory cortically evoked responses. The F wave involves the delivery of an electrical stimulus to the median or ulnar nerve, and with a sufficient sweep (duration) available on the oscilloscope, two distinct responses usually are obtained (Fig. 44-5). The first, or larger, amplitude is the M response (the response obtained during conventional conduction studies), and the second, or smaller, amplitude (100 to 200 μV) will appear somewhere between 24 and 29 msec delay (latency). The longer the arm, the longer the latency will be; therefore the involved arm should be compared to that of the opposite side.

With pickup electrodes affixed to the hand area of the somatosensory cortex opposite to the stimulated median nerve, one may study the evoked responses elicited by a train of 500 stimuli to identify if there is any delay between Erb's point to the spinal cord. This type of study requires special instrumentation but can be an added valuable resource in differentiation between radiculopathies and distal peripheral nerve disorders.

The differentiation between a cervical radiculopathy and a brachial plexus lesion is furthered by electromyographic examination of the paraspinal muscles in the cervical area. If there are neuropathic electromyographic findings in the erector spinae muscles corresponding to the same segmental distribution through the anterior ramus, the lesion would be proximal to the division of anterior and posterior rami (Fig. 44-6).

A further distinction between ventral root and dorsal root involvement in cervical radiculopathies may be made on the basis of electromyographic studies and clinical symptomatology. In ventral root affectation, there will be more electromyographic findings associated with axonal degeneration (such as fibrillation, positive sharp waves, and complex motor unit action potentials). Deep throbbing or aching pain within the myotome is more typical of ventral root compression. The dorsal root symptoms is characterized by lancinating or shocklike pain that follows the dermatome or sclerotome, reaching a maximum in the fingers or palm of the hand. These symptoms may also be correlated with

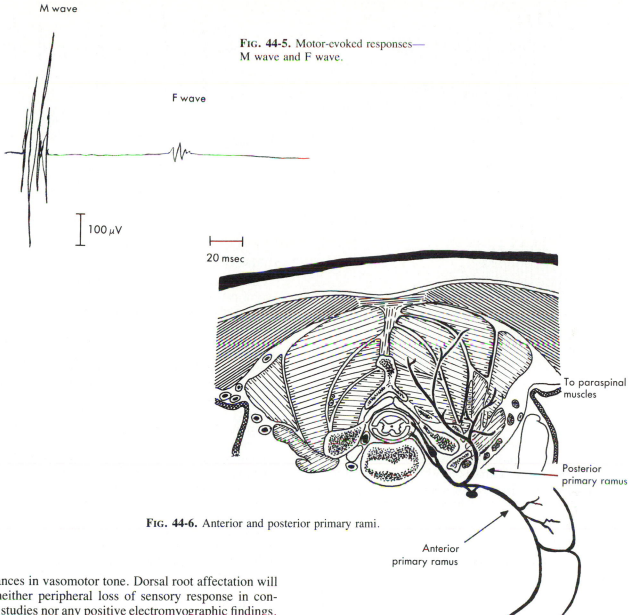

M wave

FIG. 44-5. Motor-evoked responses— M wave and F wave.

F wave

100 μV

20 msec

To paraspinal muscles

Posterior primary ramus

Anterior primary ramus

To limbs and abdomen

FIG. 44-6. Anterior and posterior primary rami.

disturbances in vasomotor tone. Dorsal root affectation will reveal neither peripheral loss of sensory response in conduction studies nor any positive electromyographic findings. Extensive disk protrusions may compromise both ventral and dorsal components resulting in both sets of symptoms.

NEURONOPATHIES

Electromyography is essential to the delineation of anterior horn cell disease in patients who demonstrate atrophy and wasting of intrinsic hand musculature plus difficulty chewing and swallowing or spasticity. In disorders such as amyotrophic lateral sclerosis, the intrinsic hand muscles frequently demonstrate electromyographic signs of denervation, such as fibrillation potentials at rest and diminution of motor unit recruitment. The conduction studies are usually within normal limits except for some loss of amplitude in the response wave. Because the reduced amplitude can also result from the more benign disuse atrophy, it must be correlated with electromyographic evidence of denervation, such as fibrillation at rest, to be indicative of anterior horn cell disease.

MYELOPATHIES

Myelopathies (spinal cord disorders) do not manifest specific electromyographic or conduction changes. Somatosensory evoked responses will be helpful in delineating spinal cord disturbances by monitoring conduction along the spinal cord. However, the detection of minor or early myelopathy may not be readily made with any certainty using current technology.

MYONEURAL JUNCTIONAL DISORDERS

The myasthenic syndrome and myasthenia gravis generally do not produce changes specific to the hand. When a patient manifests a generalized lack of endurance or weakness, one should conduct repetitive stimulation (Jolly test)

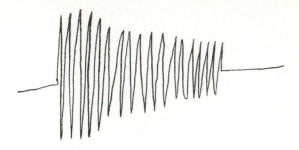

MYASTHENIA GRAVIS

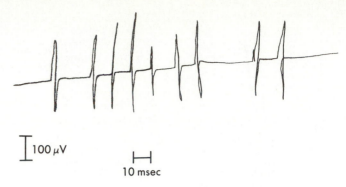

$\bar{I}$ 100 μV

$\vdash\dashv$
10 msec

Fig. 44-8. Myopathic motor unit potentials.

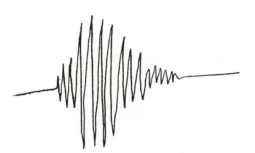

MYASTHENIC SYNDROME

Fig. 44-7. Response to repetitive stimulation in myasthenia gravis and in myasthenic syndrome.

studies to look for a decrement in the motor-response wave. Generally in myasthenia gravis there is a decrement in the response to repetitive stimulation, while in the myasthenic syndrome there is a potentiated response after a brief exercise bout, followed by a decrement of the response (Fig. 44-7).

MYOPATHIES

Many myopathic disorders are made manifest through weakness of the proximal muscles, and only relatively few myopathies manifest themselves with distal weakness. The majority of myopathies reveal electromyographic motor unit potentials that are of brief duration and relatively low amplitude (BLAP potentials) with voluntary contractions. Another characteristic finding would be good recruitment (complete interference pattern) of motor units with relatively minor exertions (Fig. 44-8).

Some myopathies may manifest electromyographic changes that are more typically associated with neuropathic disorders. It is sometimes difficult to discern with electrophysiologic methods alone which type of disorder is involved. From the view point of developing therapeutic strategies, the type of electromyographic findings are not specific, but fatigue is to be avoided for optimal care of persons with primary muscle disease. Exercise of myopathic muscle is indicated but not to the point of exhaustion.

SUMMARY

Conduction studies and electromyographic studies for the care of patients with hand disorders are mainly concerned with the identification of the site and nature of the lesion and its magnitude. Slowing of the conduction will not result in any significant loss of strength but rather a loss of motor control. Presence of conduction of evoked stimuli and a decrease in fibrillation after a peripheral nerve injury would signal the time to start electrical stimulation and eventually exercise. When weakness if present, the recruitment of motor units visualized on the electromyogram can assist in determining the optimal exercise or other treatment recommended.

Hand symptoms associated with neuropathies may be traced to lesions of the brachial plexus or cervical nerve roots as well as to local lesions of peripheral nerves. The electromyogram can assist in localizing the lesion and therefore directing treatment at the correct area.

Differentiation between motor neuron disorder, muscle disease, myoneural junctional disorders, and neurologic problems is of importance to direct treatment of the source of the disorder.

REFERENCES

1. Buchthal, F., and Rosenfalck, P.: Action potential parameters in different human muscles, Acta Psychiatr. Neurol. Scand. **30**:125, 1955.
2. Eliasson, S.G., Prensky, A.L., and Hardin, W.B.: Neurological pathophysiology, London, 1975, Oxford University Press.
3. Liveson, J., and Spielholz, N.I.: Peripheral neurology, Philadelphia, 1979, F.A. Davis Co.
4. Nelson, A.J., Moffroid, M., and Whipple, R.: Relationship of integrated EMG to isokinetic contractions of ankle dorsi and plantar flexors. In Desmedt, J.E., editor: Recent advances in EMG and clinical neurology, vol. 3, Basel, 1973, S. Karger, A.G.
5. Nelson, R.M., and Currier, D.P.: Anterior interosseous syndrome, Phys. Ther. **60**:194, 1980.
6. Pachter, B.R., Eberstein, A., and Goodgold, J.G.: Electrical stimulation effect on denervated skeletal myofibers in rats, Arch. Phys. Med. Rehabil. **63**(9):427-433, 1982.
7. Waylonis, G.W.: Electromyographic findings in chronic cervical radicular syndromes, Arch. Phys. Med. Rehabil. **49**:407, 1968.

45

Desensitization of the traumatized hand

LOIS M. BARBER

The patient with hypersensitivity occurring after hand trauma presents the physician and the therapist with a unique challenge, both in evaluation and in treatment of the problem. The lack of an objective assessment of both the complaint and the improvement, as well as the deficiency of published formalized treatment procedures, has made hand hypersensitivity particularly thought provoking.

The purposes of this chapter are to discuss the development of and indications for a method of desensitization treatment, to describe the Downey Hand Center Hand Sensitivity Test (DHCHST), an instrument for measuring the status and improvement of hypersensitivity, and to outline the progress of 124 patients who completed the desensitization test and treatment at the Downey Hand Center (DHC).*

LITERATURE REVIEW

Methods for decreasing hypersensitivity of the injured hand are just now appearing in the literature.[1,3,7,18] Several earlier approaches to the desensitization of painful scars and amputation stumps have been documented.[2,6,9,10,12-15] Rubin recorded complete relief of pain and tenderness caused by phantom limb, neuroma, and scar origin, in 23 of 37 areas of hypersensitivity, with the use of ultrasound treatment.[12] Vibration has historically been used in the treatment of hypersensitive scars. Russell and Wall theorized that the nerve fibers concerned with firing hyperpathic sensations are very easily traumatized into inactivity by a vibrator.[14,17] Hochreiter, in her study of the effect of vibration of 80 Hz on tactile sensitivity, stated that vibration results in an elevated tactile threshold and that the increase lasts for at least 10 minutes but not as long as 15 minutes, a duration indicating that vibration actually reduces tactile sensitivity.[8] Brown hypothesized that in dropping particles from a height over the involved area one can elicit a response similar to vibration.[3] Melzak relates that vibration is also able to modify the amount of pain produced by noxious stimulation of the skin in normal subjects.[10]

Russell theorized about the use of percussion to treat painful amputation stumps and phantom limbs. He posited that conduction in a mixed nerve is easily interrupted by repeated pressure without causing pain and that the regenerating nerve fibers, which form neuromas in an amputation stump, might well be even more vulnerable to minor trauma than normal nerves and nerve endings are. It was considered likely, therefore, that if painful neuromas are repeatedly percussed, their nerve fibers would gradually degenerate and be replaced by fibrous tissue.[15] A survey of phantom limb treatment lists a number of approaches to the problem of painful stumps in phantom limb, only one of which is stump conditioning or desensitization.[16]

Hardy described a sequential method of desensitizing the traumatized hand. Five levels of desensitization included use of paraffin, vibration, massage, constant touch-pressure, textures, object identification, and specific tools to simulate common job activities. Work simulation was included as a final level of the desensitization program.[7] Brown stated that desensitization techniques aided in the physiologic and psychological change toward normalcy and advocated the use of textural stimulation and the judicious use of vibration as well as the performance of functional activities as means of desensitization.[3]

A survey of 32 surgeons and therapists by me in 1982 indicated that desensitization is included as part of the treatment regimen of a number of therapists and physicians and that the majority of them would like to see a proved method of desensitization developed.

DEFINITIONS

Hypersensitivity, as used in this chapter, is defined as a condition of extreme discomfort or irritability in response to normally nonnoxious tactile stimulation.[20] It is important to point out that the hypersensitivity referred to throughout this chapter occurs at or near the injury site and is not to be confused with the general manifestations of pain, as seen in causalgia or the shoulder-hand syndrome.

Two relevant dictionary definitions of "desensitize" are as follows: "to lessen the sensitiveness of, to eliminate the native or acquired reactivity or sensitivity of an animal, organ, tissue, etc., to an external stimulus such as an allergen" (*Random House Dictionary*) and "to render less sensitive or insensitive as to light or pain" (*American Heritage Dictionary*).

Treatment in this chapter is defined as the use of modalities and procedures designed to diminish or reduce symptoms. Desensitization treatment as described here is spe-

*Downey Community Hospital Hand Center, 11500 Brookshire Ave., Downey, Calif. 90241.

cifically designed to reduce the symptom of hypersensitivity in the injured hand. Although a connection may be theorized, it is not to be confused with that used for sensibility reeducation.

DEVELOPMENT OF TREATMENT

After working with a significant number of patients at the Downey Hand Center, it became evident to the staff that the natural tendency for many patients was to protect the sensitive areas after injury or surgery. Use of parts of the hand commonly involved in pinch and grasp was avoided, a situation that resulted in awkward pinch patterns, such as extensor habitus. Patients found use of the hand with areas of hypersensitivity dangerous in that when they were touched inadvertently they might withdraw and drop whatever they were working on, possibly hurting themselves or others. This condition was a definite deterrent to returning to work. Part of the therapist's role became to inform the patient that it was not only all right but actually beneficial to touch the hypersensitive areas.

In 1976, as a first step in organizing our program, a hierarchical method of treatment of the hypersensitive hand injury was begun at the Downy Hand Center. Our staff arbitrarily picked 10 different textures and 10 different particles and lined them up in what was considered a logical hierarchy of least irritating to most irritating. I published a general description of this method in 1978.[1] Three types of modalities were used: dowel textures, with use of materials glued onto ½-inch dowel sticks; contact, with use of particles such as rice and beans; and vibration, with use of battery-operated and electric plug-in vibrators (Fig. 45-1). These first two modalities were then divided into 10 sub-categories each, four in the case of vibration, and organized in what was considered a logical hierarchy of least irritating to most irritating.

These textures and particles were chosen on the basis of how tactilely stimulating they seemed to be, from giving very little tactile sensation to giving a significant amount. We can only speculate as to whether subjects are sensitive to the textures or to the pressure exerted by the modalities employed.[20] Another consideration was availability of the materials so that the treatment could be standardized if desired.

After this method was used over a period of several months, it was determined that the predetermined hierarchy was not a sound basis for treatment. Many patients found some particles and textures irritating that were not irritating to the normal, and vice versa. It was therefore decided to have the patient determine his own hierarchy of hypersensitivity for the contact and immersion textures and base his treatment on this. This method of treatment proved effective, in that most patients improved and progressed in their treatment hierarchy. In many cases, for comparison, we also recorded the patient's hierarchy on the normal side, the results of which will be the subject of a future article.

In the process of researching the subject, it was noted that a type of hierarchical desensitization was also used with phobias and in the art of karate. Anxiety hierarchies consisting of sequentially more threatening situations were introduced in the late 1950s to treat phobias. The therapy was terminated when the final item on the hierarchy could be tolerated by the patient.[19] The rationale of having a patient touch progressively irritating textures, in theory, is not unlike any progressive exercises that we do from gross to fine

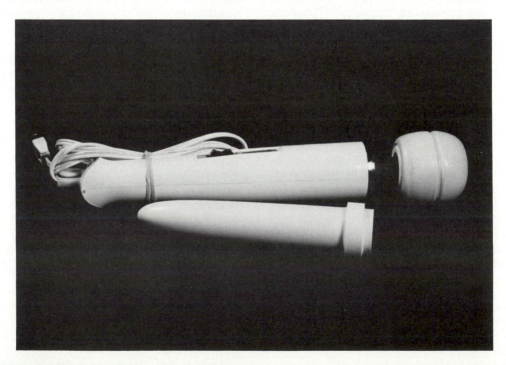

Fig. 45-1. Vibrators. Electric vibrator with speeds of 83 cycles and 100 cycles used for clinic treatment *(top)*. Battery-operated vibrator with speeds of 23 cycles and 53 cycles used for home treatment *(bottom)*. (Vibrators available from Fred Sammons, Inc., 145 Tower Drive, Burr Ridge, Ill. 60521, BK 5207 and BK 5203.)

and from light to heavy. Progressing from nonirritating to irritating seemed the logical way to proceed. This process is also based on a fundamental tenet of occupational therapy, in that it is "given in increasing doses as the patient's condition improves."[11]

DOWNEY HAND CENTER HAND SENSITIVITY TEST

The staff was gratified by the patients' improvement with this method and felt a need to validate the procedure so that it could be more confidently used and shared with others. Therefore, in 1980, a new instrument, the Downey Hand Center Hand Sensitivity Test (DHCHST), was developed to measure the effects of desensitization treatment.[20] First, detailed instructions were written for administration of the test so that use of the tool could be consistent. In the case of the dowel textures, the tester randomly selected one of the 10, instructing the patient to rub, roll, or tap the texture over the hypersensitive area. Then a random dowel was selected and the patient was asked, "Which of these is the most irritating?" Dowel textures ranged from moleskin to Velcro hooks, as follows:

1. Moleskin
2. Felt
3. Quickstick
4. Velvet
5. Semirough cloth
6. Velcro loops*
7. Hard T-Foam
8. Burlap
9. Rug back
10. Velcro hooks

The contact or immersion particles were contained in 3-pound coffee cans into which the patient was instructed to immerse the hand. The 10 particles ranged from cotton to plastic squares and were numbered for recording purposes as follows:

1. Cotton
2. Terry cloth pieces
3. Dry rice
4. Popcorn
5. Pinto beans
6. Macaroni (salad)
7. Plastic wire insulation pieces
8. Small beebees or buckshot
9. Large beebees or buckshot
10. Plastic squares

The tester randomly selected one of the 10, instructing the patient to repeatedly immerse his hand in it. Then another random texture was selected and the patient was asked, "Which of these is the most irritating?" This procedure was repeated until a sequence was established of all 10, ranging from the least irritating to the most.

To keep a consistent number of 10 with all three modalities, a hierarchy of 10 was also established for vibration, based both on speed of vibration and on amount of contact. The 83- and 100-cycle vibrator was used only in the clinic, and the 23- and 53-cycle vibrator was used at home. The

*Velcro USA, Inc., 681 Fifth Ave., New York, N.Y. 10022.

patient continued the vibration step for 10 minutes a session. The hierarchy is as follows:

1. 83 cycles, near but no actual contact on the area
2. 83 cycles, near but no actual contact; 23 cycles, near but no actual contact
3. 83 cycles, no contact; 23 cycles, intermittent contact
4. 83 cycles, intermittent contact; 23 cycles, intermittent contact
5. 83 cycles, intermittent contact; 23 cycles, continuous contact
6. 83 cycles, continuous contact; 23 cycles, intermittent contact
7. 100 cycles, intermittent contact; 53 cycles, intermittent contact
8. 100 cycles, intermittent contact; 53 cycles, continuous contact
9. 100 cycles, continuous contact; 53 cycles, continuous contact
10. No problem with vibration.

The method was the same as that used for the dowel and contact modalities.

To determine how reliable the tool was for normal persons and whether differences in reliability existed because of ethnicity, sex, or the hand being tested, a standardization sample of 40 volunteers with normal hands, 20 to 40 years of age, consisting of 10 male and 10 female Anglo-Americans and 10 male and 10 female Mexican-Americans were selected. A normal hand was defined as a hand presenting without pain, neurologic deficit, or skin abnormality. Each subject's hierarchy of sensitivity of both hands was determined as described above. The subjects were retested in 2 weeks. The test-retest reliability figures were as follows: dowel textures—right hand .77, left hand, .79; contact particles—right hand .74, left hand, .80; vibration—right hand .82, left hand .82. There were no statistically significant differences in reliability because of sex, ethnicity, or which hand was being tested. Therefore it was concluded that the Downey Hand Center Hand Sensitivity Test could be used as both a research and a clinical tool.[20]

Because the same modalities were used in both testing and clinical practice, which might be confusing, it was important to differentiate the use of the DHCHST, the actual testing tool, from the desensitization treatment, which is described next. Because its function is to measure change, the DHCHST could be used to test the effectiveness of other forms of treatment in addition to the regimen described in this paper. Despite the fact that the DHCHST was validated on normal hands, the experience gained using the instrument in the study described in this paper demonstrated its value as a tool in assessing change in the injured hand.

DESENSITIZATION TREATMENT AND DOCUMENTATION

Any patient referred to the Downey Hand Center who had an area of hypersensitivity on the hand that exhibited extreme irritability to the touch was a candidate for desensitization treatment. How disabling the hypersensitivity was to him was determined by administration of the DHCHST and observation of the patient's use of the hand. Before initiation of treatment, the results of the DHCHST and other

THE DOWNEY HAND CENTER HAND SENSITIVITY TEST (DHCHST)
DOWNEY COMMUNITY HOSPITAL - HAND REHABILITATION CENTER

1. Name________ Age____ Sex____ Language Barrier Yes___ No___ Hispanic Yes___ No___
2. Diagnosis________
3. Source of pain: Amputation___ Scar___ Crush___ Neuroma___ Burn___ Other________
4. Description of painful area: Initial:________
5. Dominance: Right___ Left___ Discharge________
6. How injury occurred________
7. Date(s) of injury________ Date(s) of Surgery________ Date of 1st Rx after surgery________
8. No. of weeks from DOI to 1st Des. Rx:____ No. of weeks from surgery to 1st Des. Rx:________
9. No. of weeks between 1st and last Rx:____ No. of treatments____ Referring M.D.________
10. Occupation________ Return to Work: Yes___ No___ Previous job? Yes___ No___

		Dowel Textures - Date				Contact Textures - Date				Vibration - Date
11.										
12.	1				1				1	
13.	2				2				2	
14.	3				3				3	
15.	4				4				4	
16.	5				5				5	
17.	6				6				6	
18.	7				7				7	
19.	8				8				8	
20.	9				9				9	
21.	10				10				10	
22.	Init		N	DC	Init		N	DC		

23. Int. Did the Desensitization Treatment affect your sensitivity today? Yes___ No___
24. How? Increased it? Yes___ No___ Decreased it? Yes___ No___
25. How much? A Lot___ Some___ Very Little___ How much? A Lot___ Some___ Very Little___
26. 2 Wks Has the Desensitization Treatment affected your sensitivity? Yes___ No___
27. How? Increased it? Yes___ No___ Decreased it? Yes___ No___
28. How much? A Lot___ Some___ Very Little___ How much? A Lot___ Some___ Very Little___
29. DC Did the Desensitization Treatment affect your sensitivity? Yes___ No___
30. How? Increased it? Yes___ No___ Decreased it? Yes___ No___
31. How much? A Lot___ Some___ Very Little___ How much? A Lot___ Some___ Very Little___
32. DC Which Treatment affected your sensitivity the most?________ Comments________

INSTRUMENT USED: DOWNEY HAND CENTER HAND SENSITIVITY TEST

FIG. 45-2. Desensitization form.

information were recorded on the desensitization treatment form (Fig. 45-2).

After documentation and testing, treatment was begun with the texture, particle, and vibration level the patient could use; the treatment was done for 10 minutes, three or four times a day. In the case of the dowel textures (Fig. 45-3), he was instructed to use one that was slightly irritating but that he could tolerate rubbing, rolling, or tapping on the sensitive area for a 10-mintue period (Fig. 45-4). Dowel textures were convenient in that they could be carried with the patient and used during the day.

Contact particles (Fig. 45-5) were generally used in the clinic; however, when indicated, the patient was given a home program as well. The patient was instructed to put his hand in the particles and either move the hand about in the particles or drop them onto the area, such as the back of the hand or other parts not involved in grasp. Again, the patient was asked to choose the particle that was slightly irritating but tolerable for 10 minutes (Fig. 45-6). This was indicated by writing the date next to the number of the particle on the record form.

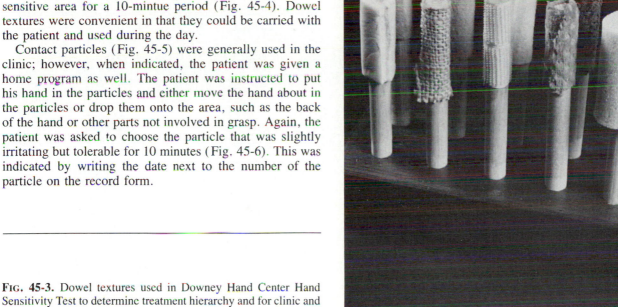

FIG. 45-3. Dowel textures used in Downey Hand Center Hand Sensitivity Test to determine treatment hierarchy and for clinic and home treatment. Range from smooth fabric to Velcro Hook.

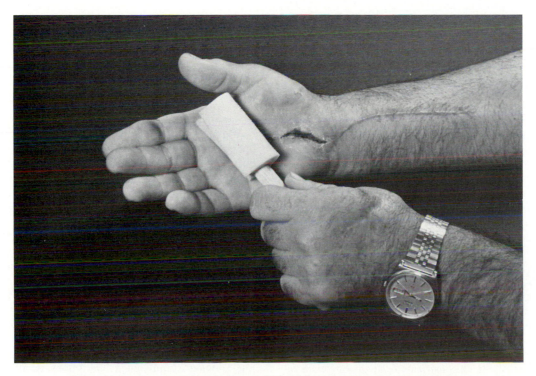

FIG. 45-4. Patient using dowel texture near healing wound and over healed area.

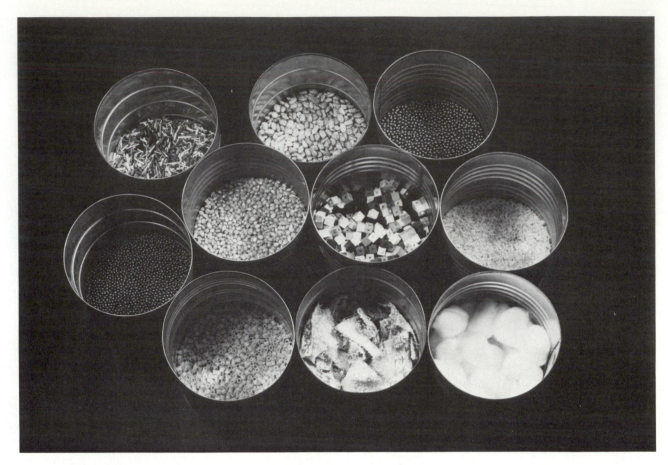

Fig. 45-5. Contact particles in 3-pound cans used to determine treatment hierarchy and for treatment. Range from soft cotton to Velcro Hook.

In the case of vibration, the patient chose where he was on the predetermined vibration hierarchy by going through as much of the sequence as possible with the therapist. He was then started on the level of the hierarchy that he could tolerate for 10 minutes, two or three times a day. The vibration hierarchy was based on the cycles per second of the two vibrators plus the amount of contact on or near the area. In the beginning stages the vibrator might not touch the scar or wound site at all but touched as close to the periphery as possible. The predetermined vibration hierarchy has not been foolproof in that more cycles per second were not necessarily more irritating to the injured hand than less. For instance, in a few cases the home-vibrator speed of 23 cycles per second was more irritating than when set at 53 cycles. Since few patients reached 9 or 10 on the hierarchy, it appeared that the highest levels were the most irritating.

The patient's treatment regimen included other therapeutic activities such as exercises and therapeutic handicrafts. Use of the hypersensitive part was encouraged (Fig. 45-7). The actual desensitization treatment was done by the patient, took approximately 20 minutes of the 2- to 3-hour treatment session, and was done any time during the treatment session, depending on the availability of equipment and the patient's preference. Part of the desensitization treatment, such as use of the battery-operated vibrator and the dowel textures, was done by the patients at home. These modalities were also kept by the patient after discharge.

PSYCHOLOGICAL IMPLICATIONS

The major effect of the motivation and the psychological status of the patient must be acknowledged. In the case of neuromas occurring after amputation, Grant[6] stated that in the majority of patients these symptoms gradually faded and use of shortened members resumed with little or no disability. Of the two major reasons for persistence of pain after amputation, one was infection, with resulting excessive scar, and the other was a greater or lesser instability of the psyche of the patient. Of course, the psychological implications are great when one is dealing with the subject of hypersensitivity. Russell in 1957[14] stated that the physician should at all times be prepared to embark on what might be termed "a game of bluff with the patient's higher cerebral mechanisms." Clark[4] reported that suggestion directed toward increasing the tolerance of thermal pain decreased the probability of withdrawal response.

The power of suggestion, no doubt, has some influence. The therapists supervising the desensitization treatment at the Downey Hand Center had a positive attitude regarding

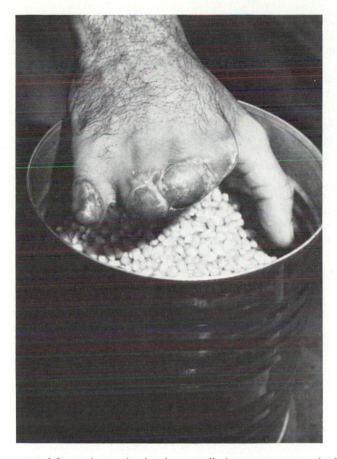

FIG. 45-6. Patient with amputated fingers immersing hand repeatedly in popcorn as step in desensitization treatment.

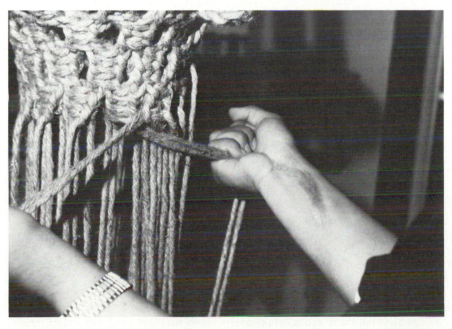

FIG. 45-7. Patient using therapeutic craft (macramé knotting) to repeatedly stimulate sensitive palmar scar and provide stretch to scar over distal part of forearm.

the potential benefits to the patient, based primarily on positive experience with its use. They estimated that 75% to 80% of the patients were significantly helped by the desensitization treatment.

In responding to the aforementioned survey, one physician who works with farmers who sustained hand injuries stated, "I treat mostly well-motivated, self-employed farmers and ranchers who don't complain about neuromas, etc., except under dire circumstances. Because of the mechanized nature of farms these days, we get quite a few crush amputations, yet the percentage that get problems is quite small. Perhaps it has something to do with the motivation aspect. The patients just don't seem worried."[5]

Looking at groups and generalizing conclusions does not necessarily demonstrate the impact that reduction in hypersensitivity may have on a person. The clinician needs to be alert to each person's needs.

J.E. was a 25-year old Mexican-American male machine operator who suffered a degloving injury to the ulnar aspect of his right, dominant hand 2 years before referral to the Downey Hand Center. He had been unemployed since injury. He had had a number of surgical procedures in attempts to gain function in the small finger and reduce hypersensitivity in the ulnar aspect of his hand. On first interview at the DHC, he was unable to hold anything in the hand that might touch this hypersensitive area and was unable to touch this part to any surface, as would be required for writing. He was referred specifically for transfer of dominance. Because of the generally healthy status of his right hand, which demonstrated good range of motion except in the little and ring fingers and exhibited a 25-pound palmar pinch and a 30-pound lateral pinch, the patient was begun on a treatment program with emphasis on desensitization. Hypersensitivity was unquestionably the patient's most limiting problem. He was extremely apprehensive about even lightly touching the sensitive area and incredulous when he was told it was beneficial for him to do so. After a couple of days of therapy he began to feel a change and participated maximally in his program.

At discharge, after participating in 32 therapy sessions over a period of 6 weeks, each including desensitization treatment, he complained of only a small area of hypersensitivity about the size of a dime on the ulnar aspect of his palm. He was able to use the hand for all functional activities, including writing, and could handle such things as macramé cord and a hammer without difficulty. He reached 10 on both the dowel and contact textures and 9 on the vibration hierarchy, having started on level 6 dowels, 4 contact, and 3 vibration. He felt that vibration was the most beneficial modality. At discharge he was scheduled to begin training as a mechanical draftsman. The rehabilitation counselor and the therapist were optimistic about his future vocational potential. The patient expressed sincere gratitude and had an optimistic outlook on his future.

This is a dramatic example of someone who, prior to the initiation of a desensitization program, believed "If it hurts, you should not touch it," and had not been instructed otherwise. It is an example of how beneficial desensitization treatment can be.

Description of group studied (n = 124)		
Hypersensitive scars 67	Amputations 44	Crush injuries 13
Male 90		Female 34
Mexican-Americans 74		Anglo-Americans 50

DESCRIPTION OF GROUP STUDIED

The patient group described in this chapter participated in treatment as described above at the Downey Hand Center between March 1980 and March 1982. During this time approximately 400 patients participated in desensitization treatment, approximately 40% of the total population of patients seen at the DHC. Of the 400 who participated to some extent in desensitization treatment, 124 patients had complete records of their DHCHST and the treatment and were used in the following conclusions. The majority of the patients were manual laborers; 67 had hypersensitive scars, 44 amputations, and 13 crush injuries. Other diagnoses such as grafts, burns, and neuromas were also treated, but the numbers were too small for comparisons and the records were incomplete. Seventy-four (60%) of the total were Mexican and 50 (40%) Anglo-Americans; only 34 (28%) were females (see boxed material).

The term "hypersensitive scars" referred to scars caused by surgical procedures, lacerations, or other injuries and included digital nerve lacerations and neuromas. These pateints were started with the desensitization program as soon as healing had occurred or as soon as the patient could touch the vibrator or the dowel texture near the scar.

Amputations were divided into tip amputations, phalangeal amputations, and a mixture of these. The total group of 44 amputations included 23 with tip amputations of one or two fingers, 16 who had amputations of one phalanx and tip or two of each of these, and five who had amputations of more than two sites.

The term "crush injuries" referred to those patients who had a hand injury primarily involving a crush. The injury might also have involved fractures and minor lacerations as well.

SUMMARY OF FINDINGS

The patient's hypersensitivity was considered improved each time he progressed a step in his hierarchy. Maximum improvement was assumed when the patient had reached step 10 in all three modalities.

I will not speculate regarding the physiologic reasons for the improvement made. Since all patients participated in a variety of treatment tasks, many including touching the hypersensitive area, along with desensitization treatment, caution must be exercised when one concludes that the improvement demonstrated was attributable to desensitization treatment by itself.

TABLE 45-1. Number of weeks between first treatment and first change (rounded to nearest 0.5 week)

	Scar (*n* = 67)		Amputation (*n* = 44)		Crush (*n* = 13)	
	Range	Average	Range	Average	Range	Average
Dowel textures	0.5 to 10	2	0.5 to 14	3	0.5 to 3	1.5
Contact particles	0.5 to 10	2	0.5 to 8	2	0.5 to 20	3.5
Vibration	0.5 to 24	3	0.5 to 9	2.5	0.5 to 4	2

TABLE 45-2. Patients reaching level 10 and patients' responses

	Dowel textures	Contact particles	Vibration	Unknown
Patients reaching level 10 on modality				
Scar	76%	63%	21%	
Amputation	61%	23%	7%	
Crush	62%	54%	22%	
Patients' responses: which treatment affected sensitivity the most				
Scar	11%	21%	60%	8%
Amputation	9%	49%	35%	7%
Crush	16½%	37½%	46%	0

TABLE 45-3. Time to first treatment and length of treatment (average, nearest 0.5 week)

	Time between onset and first treatment	Length of treatment
Scar (n = 67)	11	6.5
Amputation (n = 44)	13	7
Crush (n = 13)	8.5	7.5

The end of treatment came when the patient had made improvement in hand function and was no longer vocationally limited by his hypersensitivity. In many patients other factors, such as loss of strength, limited range of motion, or loss of digits, were the most disabling factors. Maximum improvement (level 10 on the three modalities) in hypersensitivity was not imperative to return to work. How disabling hypersensitivity was depended on many factors, such as hand affected, severity of injury, and location and extent of hypersensitivity. All patients were given the option to continue desensitization after discharge and were provided with dowel sticks and a home vibrator.

In our analysis of the number of weeks between the first treatment and the first change within the three major categories of patients and the categories of treatment modalities (Table 45-1), we found that within 2 to 3 weeks almost all patients had made one change in their hierarchy in at least one modality.

In looking at how many subjects reached the highest level (10) on any of the hierarchies, we found that anywhere from 60% to 75% in all three groups reached that level on the dowel hierarchy. The patients with amputations seemed significantly more sensitive to the vibration hierarchy. Al-

though only 7% of amputation patients whose vibration responses were recorded reached 10 on the vibration hierarchy, 35% believed that vibration was the modality that helped the most. It is also interesting to note that when we look at the patients' responses regarding which modality they believed affected sensitivity the most, the smallest percentage of people in each of the three categories believed that the dowel textures were the most effective. However, the greatest percentage in each category reached 10 on the dowel hierarchies (Table 45-2).

The length of treatment averaged about 7 weeks and was initiated an average of 8½ to 13 weeks after injury. Amputations, on the average, required a longer healing period before treatment could be begun (Table 45-3).

The logical next question when one looks at results is, "How many of those patients returned to gainful employment?" Olivia Diaz, M.S., C.R.C., consultant to the Downey Hand Center between April 1981 and May 1982, interviewed a randomly selected group of 24 patients at least 6 weeks after discharge. Diaz found that 18 of them were working, all at their previous jobs. Two, not currently working, had returned to their previous jobs after discharge but were later laid off because of lack of work. The other four of those not working had physical problems other than hypersensitivity that prevented their return to work. The jobs they returned to were machine operator, machinist, warehouseman, butcher, hand assembler, general steel worker, wood assembler, welding technician, and press-brake operator in a sheet-metal shop, all of which require heavy and constant use of the hands. Twenty-two of the 24 said that they continue to experience sensitivity but not to a degree that prevents their return to work.

CONCLUSION

A method of desensitizing the traumatized hand that presents with hypersensitivity attributable to scar, crush, or amputation was presented. The 124 patients included in the Downey Hand Center study improved to the extent that they were discharged from treatment without hypersensitivity severe enough to prevent them from returning to work. Objectively, they all showed improvement in some aspect of the Downey Hand Center Hand Sensitivity Test. In retrospect, a major value of this study may have been in the questions it raised. Would it be just as effective to have a hierarchy of five steps in each modality? Are there some contact particles and textures that could be eliminated? Which would be the best to maintain? Is the value mainly in the fact that the patient is in a somewhat elaborate manner guided in merely touching the sensitive area? It is also interesting to speculate if the patient might progress in his hierarchies in the DHCHST by doing other activities, such as crafts alone or exercises not necessarily so finely graded as those presented. The subject, indeed, remains mysterious. Although many patients, one can legitimately argue, can do very well without direction, there are those who definitely need it, as the case study illustrated. A case study such as this also invalidates the philosophy "Leave him alone and he will get better on his own," which is claimed by some. In the case of the motivated farmers, this may often be true. However, it is also hard to quantify the importance of a casual bit of encouragement, like "Touch it a lot; it will make it better," by a trusted physician.

Future analyses of these procedures could perhaps deal with such interesting factors as location of hypersensitivity, effect of handedness, occupation, and time after onset in relation to level of improvement, all questions that were not thoroughly dealt with in this analysis.

Although the subject is complex and the questions are endless, there was significant evidence presented to suggest strongly that stimulating hypersensitive areas helped reduce hypersensitivity. The systematic approach described gave and therapist and the patient a guide and focused attention on the problem. This method gave the patient the necessary guidelines to do his own desensitization treatment. It also had the element of gratification in that progress could be periodically assessed and documented.

Although the subject is complex and many questions remain unanswered, I hope this information is both stimulating and helpful, and even more so do I hope that the clinician will continue to pursue the unanswered questions.

ACKNOWLEDGMENTS

I wish to acknowledge Dr. Elizabeth J. Yerxa for her assistance in compiling and editing the manuscript; Andres Rosales, C.O.T.A., and Wendy Black, C.O.T.A., for compiling data; Dr. Garry Brody, Laurie Meadows, O.T.R., and the Downey Hand Center staff and patients for their support of the desensitization project; and Frances Robertson for invaluable assistance in typing, editing, and data organization. All photographs were taken by Susie Lee.

Desensitization testing and treatment materials are available from LMB Hand Rehab Products, Inc., P.O. Box 1181, San Luis Obispo, Calif. 93406, and Mart I Manufacturing, P.O. Box 4814, Whittier, Calif. 90607.

REFERENCES

1. Barber, L.M.: Occupational therapy for the treatment of reflex sympathetic dystrophy and post-traumatic hypersensitivity of the injured hand. In Fredericks, S., and Brody, G.S., editors: Symposium on the neurologic aspects of plastic surgery, St. Louis, 1978, The C.V. Mosby Co., pp. 108-117.
2. Blitz, B., Dinnerstein, A.J., and Lowenthal, M.: Attenuation of experimental pain by tactile stimulation: effect of vibration at different levels of noxious stimulus intensity, Percept. Mot. Skills **19:**311-316, 1964.
3. Brown, D.M., and Ellis, R.A.: A physiological basis for desensitization of the hypersensitive upper extremity, Atlanta, 1982. (Unpublished manuscript.)
4. Clark, W.C.: Pain sensitivity and the report of pain: an introduction to sensory decision theory, Anesthesiology **40:**272, March 1974.
5. Collins, P.: Personal communication, Caldwell, Idaho, 1982.
6. Grant, G.H.: Methods of treatment of neuromata of the hand, J. Bone Joint Surg. **33A:**841-848, Oct. 1951.
7. Hardy, M.A., Moran, C.A., and Merritt, W.H.: Desensitization of the traumatized hand, VA. Med. **109:**134-137, Feb. 1982.
8. Hochreiter, N.W.: Effect of vibration on tactile sensitivity, Phys. Ther. 1983.
9. Mathews, G.J., and Osterholm, J.L.: Painful traumatic neuromas, Surg. Clin. North Am. **51:**1313-1324, Oct. 1972.
10. Melzack, R.: The puzzle of pain, New York, 1973, Basic Books, Inc.
11. Mock, H.E., and Abbey, M.L.: Occupational therapy, J.A.M.A. **91:**797-801, Sept. 15, 1928.
12. Rubin, D., and Kuitert, J.H.: Use of ultrasonic vibration in the treatment of pain arising from phantom limbs, scars and neuromas: a preliminary report, Arch. Phys. Med. Rehabil. **36:**445-451, July 1955.
13. Russell, W.R.: Painful amputation stumps and phantom limbs, Br. Med. J. **1:**1024-1026, June 11, 1949; Treat. Serv. Bull. **4:**48-54, Oct. 1949.
14. Russell, W.R., Espir, M.L.E., and Morgenstern, F.: Treatment of post-herpetic neuralgia, Lancet **1:**242-245, Feb. 2, 1957.
15. Russell, W.R., and Spalding, J.M.K.: Treatment of painful amputation stumps, Br. Med. J. **2:**68-73, July 8, 1950.
16. Sherman, R.A., Sherman, C.J., and Gall, N.G.: A survey of current phantom limb pain treatment in the United States, Pain **8:**85-99, 1980.
17. Wall, P.D., and Cronly-Dillon, J.R.: Pain, itch and vibration, Arch. Neurol. **2:**365-375, April 1960.
18. Wilson, R.L.: Management of pain following peripheral nerve injuries, Orthop. Clin. North Am. **12:**343-359, April 1981.
19. Wolpe, J.: Systematic desensitization, J. Nerv. Ment. Dis. **132:**189, 1961.
20. Yerxa, E.J., Barber, L.M., Diaz, O., Black, W., and Azen, S.P.: Development of a hand sensitivity test for use in desensitization of the hypersensitive hand, Am. J. Occup. Ther. **37**(3):176-181, 1983.

46

Management of pain syndromes in the upper extremity

GEORGE E. OMER, Jr.

The most common reason for patients seeing a physician is pain.[10] Pain is an unpleasant sensory and emotional experience associated with actual or potential tissue damage or described in terms of such damage.[39] Approximately 75 million Americans are afflicted with pain each year.[6] Over 40 million Americans are either partially or totally disabled by chronic pain. As a result nearly 700 million work days are lost, which, together with health care costs and compensation, total approximately 50 billion dollars each year.[6]

Chronic pain is defined as pain that persists or recurs at intervals for months or years.[6] Chronic pain is caused not only by pathologic processes in the nervous system, but also by psychopathology and environmental influences. Chronic pain is a wicked force that imposes excessive psychologic, social, and economic stresses on the patient. The treatment of chronic pain problems is most difficult, since pain is such an intensely personal reaction; Aristotle and Plato considered pain to be a "passion of the soul."[14]

PERCEPTUAL PARAMETERS AND PERSONALITY

The pain threshold is the least stimulus at which a patient perceives pain.[39] The pain-tolerance level is the greatest stimulus intensity causing pain that a patient is prepared to tolerate.[39] In the experimental setting, pain threshold and tolerance can be determined by several techniques that show high reliability.[9,63,68,69,77] Age, sex, race, ethnic group, religion, and other factors influence pain tolerance.[55] Personality is the unique blend of intellectual and emotional qualities reflected in individual behavior.[4,71] A number of traits are characteristic facets of personality, such as anxiety, expressiveness, depression, or hypochondriasis.[29] Clinicians may believe that the patient who complains about pain more than the average person does has a low pain threshold, but this is an error. The readiness to communicate the pain is a function of expressiveness, and this in turn is associated with the degree of extraversion.[63] In experimental studies, Lynn and Eysenck[37] found that pain tolerance in college students was negatively correlated with neuroticism and positively correlated with extraversion. Social learning influences expressiveness as well, including that related to pain communication.

Basic personality attributes may be measured by two tests, the Eysenck Personality Inventory (EPI) and the Minnesota Multiphasic Personality Inventory (MMPI). The EPI test measures two dimensions of personality regarded as fundamental because they are related directly to physiologic activity of the central nervous system. These dimensions are stability-neuroticism (N) and introversion-extraversion (E). The higher the patient's N score, the greater the emotional vulnerability shown. The higher the E score, the more the person will be found to be gregarious and cheerful and to have high levels of energy. In general, thresholds for pain are lower for introverts than for extraverts. The EPI can be completed in 10 to 15 minutes.[4] The MMPI is a checklist of physical and emotional symptoms, including both those from the past and those present at the time of examination. High scores indicate the presence of an emotional disturbance. For patients with chronic pain, significantly higher scores are found on those items measuring hypochondriasis, depression, and hysteria. Patients with acute pain show high scores for hypochondriasis and hysteria, but not for depression. One of the attractions of the MMPI is that the personality profiles permit the identification of groups of characteristics, and on this basis patients with pain problems may be categorized.[4] Sternbach and associates[62] found that patients with low back pain of a duration of less than 6 months obtained MMPI profiles within normal limits, while patients with low back pain of longer duration had greatly elevated scores for depression, hypochondriasis, and hysteria. There is a reported clinical correlation of 86.3% between the topographic pain drawing[11] and the MMPI score.

In a practical sense, the attending surgeon or therapist must learn to identify the unstable emotional personality. In such patients the "pain state" becomes a permanent "memory bank," and the total personality may become focused on the pain. These patients will require much more time and explanation to cope with their pain.

TREATMENT

There are only two principles in the treatment of an established pain syndrome involving the upper extremity: (1) relieve the patient's symptoms, and (2) institute active use of the involved extremity.[45,47-49]

Relief of symptoms

One initiates the relief of pain by attempting to divide the source of the patient's symptoms into categories: (1) increased peripheral nociceptive stimulus, which is often a "trigger point" with an associated local disorder, such as a neuroma; (2) reflex sympathetic summation, usually described as "diffuse, burning, sustained" (when symptoms are overwhelming, this should be termed "causalgia"); (3) inflammatory pain of systemic origin, such as peripheral neuritis of diabetes; (4) personality dysfunction pain, which will overlap with all other categories; and (5) cancer pain.[49]

Pain should be evaluated promptly; one should never wait for the full development of an established pain syndrome before initiating aggressive treatment. For example, the osteoporosis of Sudek's atrophy is not evident by roentgenography for 5 to 8 weeks after injury,[52] but the patient has pain from the time of injury.

Peripheral nociceptive stimulus. Pain may develop after local trauma for many reasons. The damaged portion of the nerve may develop intraneural fibrosis, or external adhesions may transfix the nerve to its bed. Friction upon a nerve will result in inflammatory changes and further fibrosis. The compressed nerve will have venous stasis, capillary leakage, and perineurial edema.[54] Decreased blood flow can be associated with pain, as in any compression syndrome.[15] Any procedure producing vasodilatation may relieve this pain.

A peripheral nerve responds to injury, whether partial or complete, with proliferation of connective tissue and regeneration of damaged axons to form a neuroma. The neuroma becomes symptomatic depending on the quality of regeneration and is influenced by the extent of fibrosis, vascularity, infection, foreign material, and other local factors. Neuromas with inadequate numbers of large myelinated axons or outer fibrous layers develop hyperpathia. Hyperpathia is a painful syndrome characterized by an overreaction or an aftersensation to stimuli.[39] The patient characteristically has extreme sensitivity directly over the neuroma; altered sensibility in at least part of the area supplied by the nerve; and sustained, widely distributed, poorly localized pain.[76]

Percutaneous injection about the painful neuroma should provide local anesthesia. Bupivacaine hydrochloride has a longer duration of anesthesia than lidocaine hydrochloride.[40] Percutaneous injection of triamcinolone acetonide about the neuroma after a cutaneous block with 2% lidocaine hydrochloride has been reported to relieve the pain symptoms in 50% of patients after one injection and in 80% of patients with multiple injections.[59]

Percussion or massage of painful neuromas has been a clinical procedure in amputees since the World War I. Controlled clinical studies have indicated that the technique is useful in selected cases.[21] Rubber mallets, mechanical vibrators, or ultrasonic treatments will provide the repetitious percussion. Anesthesia may be necessary over the trigger area at the onset of treatment, but later the percussion or massage should be done without local anesthesia.

Acupuncture is an ancient technique involving point pressure to relieve pain. Traditional teaching identifies 365 to 400 acupuncture points along the 12 meridian channels that contain the yin and yang forces, that control the energy of life.[72] Modern laboratory studies possibly indicate that acupuncture analgesia is transmitted by the nervous system and requires an intact functional nervous system to be successful.[38,58,70] If an intact dynamic interaction (control gate)

among large and small afferent neurons is required, acupuncture should be ineffective in the disrupted nerve, such as a terminal bulb neuroma. An additional neurophysiologic explanation is that some humeral agent may be responsible, and this may explain the generalized alterations in the pain threshold that have been reported in humans.[64] Acupuncture should be more effective in reflex sympathetic summation than in peripheral nociceptive stimulus.

A peripheral chemical sympathetic block may be performed on the ward.[44,45] A 16-gauge needle is inserted near the nerve just proximal to the "trigger point," and a flexible 18-gauge polyethylene intravenous catheter is inserted through the needle. The needle is removed, leaving the catheter in place. A solution of 0.5 ml of 0.5% lidocaine hydrochloride is injected. If the pain is relieved, the catheter is capped and taped in place, allowing exercise activity. Additional periodic injections of lidocaine solution are based on the length of time of pain-free activity. The periodic perineurial infusion has been continued for a few days up to 2 weeks. If there is more than one trigger point, separate catheters should be used. This method has been less effective in those patients in whom the pain has been untreated for 3 or more months.

A neuroma can be classified as a terminal bulb or a neuroma in continuity. A painful partial nerve disruption may benefit from internal neurolysis and graft repair of some fascicular groups.[46,61] If there is no useful distal sensory or motor function, an end-to-end anastomosis should be performed after removal of the neuroma in continuity. Terminal bulb neuromas typically occur in amputation stumps. Although many procedures have been reported, present methods include simple resection of the neuroma, capping of the terminal portion with silicone, or transposition of the entire neuroma to a new site.[24,65,67] The most reliable procedure is transfer of the neuroma, attached to the proximal nerve stump, to a new site where compression is unlikely and traction is minimal. The neuroma should be placed in an area of good circulation with a thick subcutaneous layer that is free of scar.[13,28] Success has been reported in 82% of patients treated by this technique.

Traction injuries to the brachial plexus are often painful initially, but pain should progressively subside.[76] An increase in pain may represent fibrous tissue involvement. The pain from nerve root avulsion is severe, having the characteristics of causalgia, or maximum reflex sympathetic summation.[78]

Reflex sympathetic summation. Many clinical syndromes, including burning pain, abnormal vasomotor response, and trophic dystrophy, have been described. Classic causalgia may have variants that are termed "Leriche's posttraumatic pain syndrome" (minor causalgia), "Sudek's atrophy," or "shoulder-arm-hand syndrome."[29] Phantom pain is identical to reflex sympathetic dystrophy but adds postural cramping or squeezing. Reflex sympathetic dystrophy may not develop immediately but gradually increase to dominate the clinical picture.

The loss of vascular, sudomotor, pilomotor, and muscle tone controls will result in profound nutritional (trophic) changes. There is atrophy of subcutaneous tissue, skin, muscle, and bone. In the early stages the residual limb is greatly swollen and warm. There is hyperesthesia to light touch and sensitivity to cold. After 2 to 3 months, there is fibrotic brawny edema. Contractures become fixed because of a lack of active motion. Roentgenograms of the distal bones show patchy osteopenia. A bone scan (technetium 99m–labeled diphosphonate) will be positive before the bone resorption is visible on plane roentgenograms. Six to 9 months after the onset of pain, the extremity becomes pale and cool with either hyperhidrosis or dryness. Pain may dominate or the extremity may be absolutely rejected by the patient.

This syndrome is believed to be a prolongation of the normal sympathetic response to injury.[5] The pain impulses to the cortex are greatly amplified, causing intense discomfort. The hypothesis that a partial injury to a major nerve can result in abnormal cross-stimulation between sympathetic and sensory fibers has clinical support.[12] Others have postulated the liberation of a vasodilator substance (neurokinin) at the periphery as the basis for the pain.[2,7]

In those patients with Raynaud's symptoms associated with pain, it is important to measure digital blood flow.[1] We follow Porter's[53] method: the patient sits quietly for 30 minutes in a warm room with the temperature about 24° C (76° F). The digital pulp temperature is determined with an electronic telethermometer. The patient's hands are then immersed in an ice water mixture for 20 seconds, and the digital pulp temperature measured until the temperature returns to the baseline value for 45 minutes. Normal temperature-recovery time is 10 minutes, with a range from 5 to 20 minutes. The digital temperature test can be supplemented with arteriography to differentiate arterial spasm from organic obstructive disease. Medication to decrease peripheral sympathetic activity should be beneficial for the patient with painful Raynaud's symptoms. A variety of drugs have been proposed for intra-arterial injection, including the alpha-receptor blocking drugs tolazoline hydrochloride (Priscoline) and phenoxybenzamine hydrochloride, the beta-adrenergic receptor blocking drug propranolol hydrochloride, and the neuronal norepinephrine depletors reserpine, methyldopa, or guanethidine. Griseofulvin has also been used because it has a direct vasodilator action exclusive of sympathetic innervation. Porter obtained excellent responses in patients with Raynaud's symptoms with repeated brachial artery injections of reserpine (0.25 mg) at approximately 2- to 3-week intervals.[53] Porter also treated 23 patients with oral guanethidine, 10 mg daily, and then increased the level 10 mg each week until there was hypotension or symptomatic improvement. Two patients could not tolerate guanethidine even at the minimal dose of 10 mg daily because of hypotension and were changed to phenoxybenzamine, 10 mg daily. After an average follow-up of 12 months, 19 of the 23 patients had significant reduction in the frequency and severity of the Raynaud's attacks.[53] Similar results have been reported for propranolol hydrochloride in oral dosages of 40 mg every 4 hours.[57]

Chuinard and associates[8] have reported the use of reserpine administered intravenously to relieve pain. The technique is the same as that used for intravenous regional anesthesia. One milligram of reserpine diluted in 50 ml of normal saline solution is injected, and the tourniquet is released after 15 minutes. The authors reported that 21 of 25 patients obtained pain relief.

Hannington-Kiff introduced the regional intravenous sympathetic block technique with guanethidine.[22,23] Wynn Parry[78] records that guanethidine blocks are most valuable and provide instantaneous pain relief. Under tourniquet control, 20 mg of guanethidine in 20 ml of normal saline is injected slowly into a dorsal wrist vein. The tourniquet is deflated in 20 minutes.

Early treatment includes chemical central interruption of the abnormal sympathetic reflex, and a sympathetic block should be performed as a diagnostic test and as a therapeutic procedure. We use solutions of either 1% lidocaine hydrochloride or 1% mepivacaine hydrochloride to produce peripheral warming and loss of sweating, as well as relief of pain. The anterior approach is preferred for the isolated stellate block, with the technique described by Kleinert[27] being used. A series of four or five blocks should be given on consecutive days; one placebo of normal saline solution given during the series will confirm the value of the sympathetic block. Leffert and colleagues at the Massachusetts General Hospital have developed a technique for continuous sympathetic blockade that utilizes an indwelling catheter for injection about the stellate ganglion.[31] The initial technique for periodic chemical sympathetic blocks involved the lumbar area.[66]

Transcutaneous electric nerve stimulation should be considered for those patients whose pain persists after chemical central sympathetic block. Three sites of electrode placement are utilized: (1) over a large nerve trunk proximal to the pain site, (2) at the periphery of a painful area if the lesion appears to be primarily cutaneous, or (3) directly over a pain site if proximal nerve trunks are not readily stimulated.[20] The intensity should be varied by the patient because stimuli that are too intense overcome the inhibition mechanism and produce additional pain. Pain relief is complete in less than one third of patients,[19,20,33,34] and the best results are obtained when the transcutaneous electrical stimulation is initiated within 3 months of the onset of pain.

In 1967, Sweet and Wall[74] implanted electrodes directly on the median and ulnar nerves of a patient with traumatic hyperpathia. Goldner and associates[42] reported 38 peripheral nerves in 35 patients stimulated with electrodes over periods from 4 to 9 years. There was successful relief of pain in 53% of patients with upper extremity pain. Direct stimulation to the peripheral nerve is more effective in the upper extremity than in the lower extremity. Current researchers are implanting electrodes to stimulate cells in the periaqueductal periventricular gray matter to release beta-endorphin and obtain analgesia.[25,36]

Surgery should be performed when the burning pain completely responds to central chemical sympathectomy but requires repeated blocks for the long-term relief of pain. The effectiveness of sympathectomy is not related to interruption of a sensory pathway from the extremity, but to elimination of the sympathetic efferent discharge to the peripheral arteries and sweat glands. Surgical sympathectomy will relieve only burning pain; associated painful neuromas or arthritic pain will not be altered. Horner's syndrome often is not present after the transaxillary approach, which permits removal of only the lower half of the stellate ganglion, but it is more often present after the supraclavicular approach and can be most annoying to the patient. Postoperative precise sudomotor function tests should demonstrate complete sympathetic denervation of the involved extremity.

Inflammatory pain. Corticosteroids are useful for the patient with rheumatoid arthritis, diabetes, Reiter's syndrome, or other conditions that are trapped in a massive episode of painful inflammatory stiffness.[17,18] We have utilized a tourniquet and intravenous regional block with 50 ml of 1% lidocaine hydrochloride and 40 mg of methylprednisolone sodium succinate.[75] During the 20 to 30 minutes of analgesia, one can manipulate stiff joints and stretch contracted web spaces. A different program involves utilization of 250 mg of hydrocortisone sodium succinate intravenously each day for 5 days and then a decrease in the dosage to 100 mg each day for 5 days. These drugs must be monitored and the patients evaluated for adverse reactions. As the pain subsides, the patient is encouraged to employ a gentle lanolin massage and warm water baths. Salicylates should be given to abort ongoing inflammatory metabolic pathways.

Osteoarthritis is managed with aspirin, splinting, physical therapy, and intra-articular steroids as clinically indicated. Compression and massage therapy may be helpful adjuncts, and tissue vibrators at frequencies of 100 to 140 Hz can activate joint mechanoreceptors, which have inhibitory influences in the dorsal horn of the spinal cord. Transcutaneous electric nerve stimulations can activate afferent circuits and induce inhibitory influences. Septic complications require appropriate antibiotics.

Personality dysfunction. Optimal management requires a multifaceted and highly individualized program. The patient's general physical condition may have deteriorated because of inadequate sleep, improper diet and exercise, medication abuse, or other complications. Depression may progress to the point that the patient develops an attitude of hopelessness. An occasional tranquilizer for a particular clinical situation may be effective. Narcotics are not indicated.

Medications for emotional instability include phenytoin (Dilantin Sodium), fluphenazine dihydrochloride (Prolixin), carbamazepine (Tegretal), and amitriptyline hydrochloride (Elavil).[75] Phenytoin may be given up to 300 to 500 mg daily in divided or single doses taken with food. This is the safest phenothiazine. Amitriptyline may be given 25 mg at bedtime and at intervals during the day up to 150 mg maximum daily dosage. Phenytoin and amitriptyline may be used together. Benson also advises a phenothiazine such as fluphenazine hydrochloride (Prolixin), which potentiates any narcotic, possesses an analgesic property of its own, and depresses the response to peripheral stimuli.[3] Recommended dosage is 1 mg three times daily; this may be increased to a total of 10 mg per day.[3,76] Carbamazepine (Tegretal) is the most effective drug but is prone to develop toxic symptoms such as nausea, vomiting, or unsteady gait. Because of hematopoietic suppression, it is appropriate to follow patients on carbamazepine with monthly hemoglobin and white cell count studies.

Electromyographic biofeedback may be utilized to relieve tension. Pain declined significantly in 12 of 18 patients with tension headaches studied at the University of Washington in Seattle,[51] but significant pain relief was obtained in only one of eight patients with back pain. To be effective, this modality must be given with maximal therapist support.

In the latter part of the eighteenth century, the German physician Franz Anton Mesmer developed modern techniques for hypnosis. Experiments in hypnosis have shown that subjects can distort both perception and motor movements, and through hypnosis one can produce partial to total anesthesia. Successful acupuncture and hypnosis both require the cerebral cortex to activate complex conditioned reflexes that raise pain thresholds, remove anxiety and tension, and relieve depression.[41]

Personality dysfunction may result in the physical presentation of a psychological problem with painful symptoms or clinical state. Examples include the clenched fist syndrome,[56,60] Secretan's disease (or peritendinous fibrosis of the dorsum of the hand[43]) and the S-H-A-F-T syndrome.[73] These patients are far more complex than the malingerer, and require supportive psychotherapy. Attempts to manage the pain symptoms without a multidisciplinary approach are doomed to failure.

Cancer pain. Patients should be considered for an invasive operation when their pain is proved to be intractable to nonsurgical techniques.

Spinal dorsal sensory root rhizotomy through a laminectomy is indicated in patients who have unilateral pain involving the brachial plexus and the involved extremity is functionally useless. Leavens[30] has reported long-standing anesthesia in 50 of 71 patients undergoing this procedure. Other reports of rhizotomy have indicated limited success and disappointing long-term results.[26,32,50] Cordotomy is indicated when the pain is diffuse and involving areas innervated by many roots in a functioning upper extremity. Leavens[30] reported unilateral cervical cordotomy in 37 patients; 15 patients experienced some pain relief until death from their disease, an average of 3 months after surgery. Twelve of the 37 patients developed pain in the previously nonpainful side, an average of 1½ months after surgery.

Destructive lesions in the thalamus, brainstem, and frontal lobes have been employed for many years. Cingulotomy is the one technique that is still used for patients in whom anxiety and depression are major factors.[35] None of these procedures provides long-lasting pain relief[16]; they are most useful in patients who are expected to live no more than 1 year. The return of pain after surgery is related to increased activity of polysynaptic systems (paleospinothalamic or spinoreticulothalamic) that are widespread in the brainstem and thalamus. These polysynaptic systems are infinitely complex and diffuse and eventually frustrate any surgical ablation procedure.

Institution of functional activity

The second principle in the treatment program of an established pain syndrome is the institution of functional activity. Passive modalities decrease pain and maintain mobility. Passive modalities will improve circulation, decrease edema, and prepare the patient for voluntary participation in active modalities such as athletics. Active modalities build strength and develop dexterity. Active modalities result in an independent patient.

Passive modalities include massage, vibrators, stump wrapping, faradic muscle stimulation, ice packs, hot packs, paraffin packs, microwaves, ultrasound, and inflatable splints with positive and negative pressure. In the apprehensive patient, use of these modalities may have to be preceded by very delicate techniques, such as stroking the skin with a feather. Some passive modalities may be contraindicated, such as the whirlpool bath, because it is dependent on heat and may increase edema. The passive program should maintain joint motion, prevent contracture, and desensitize hyperesthetic areas.[76]

The more important phase is voluntary functional activity. Special care should be directed to warming up key areas of circulation, such as the rotator cuff muscles in the shoulder-arm-hand syndrome. Total body conditioning is important, and the patient should be ambulatory if possible. Function can be developed with diversional games, athletics, assigned work, and activities of daily living. It is important that the health care team be compassionate, yet obtain maximal effort from the patient. The best functional activity occurs when the patient returns to his usually work. With the continued use of functional activity, patients ultimately "cure" themselves.

REFERENCES

1. Balas, P., Tripolitis, A.J., Kaklamanis, P., Mandalaki, T., and Paracharalampous, N.: Raynaud's phenomenon: primary and secondary causes. Arch. Surg. **114**:1174-1177, 1979.
2. Barnes, R.: The role of sympathectomy in the treatment of causalgia, J. Bone Joint Surg. **35B**:172-180, 1953.
3. Benson, W.F.: Treatment of the painful extremity, American Society for Surgery of the Hand Newsletter 50, 1977.
4. Bond, M.R.: Pain: its nature, analysis, and treatment, Edinburgh, 1979, Churchill Livingstone, pages 35-40.
5. Bonica, J.J.: Causalgia and other reflex sympathetic dystrophies, Postgrad. Med. J. **53**:143-148, 1976.
6. Bonica, J.J.: Current status of pain therapy. In Perry, S., Chairman: The Interagency Committee on New Therapies for Pain and Discomfort, report to the White House: 111-114, May 1979, U.S. Dept. of Health, Education, and Welfare, Public Health Service, National Institutes of Health.
7. Chapman, L.F., Ramos, A.O., Goodell, H., and Wolff, H.G.: Neurohumoral features of afferent fibers in man, Arch. Neurol. **4**:49-82, 1961.
8. Chuinard, R.G., Dabezies, E.J., Gould, J.S., Murphy, G.A., and Mathews, R.E.: Intravenous reserpine for treatment of reflex sympathetic dystrophy, J. Hand Surg. **5**:289, 1980.
9. Craig, K.D., Best, H., and Ward, L.M.: Social modelling influences on psychophysical judgments of electrical stimulation, J. Abnorm. Psychol. **84**:366-373, 1975.
10. de Jong, R.H.: Commentary: Defining pain terms, J.A.M.A. **244**:143,
11. Dennis, M.D., Rocchio, P.O., and Wiltse, L.L.: The topographical pain representation and its correlation with MMPI scores, Orthopedics **5**:432-434, 1981.
12. Doupe, J., Cullen, C.H., and Chance, G.Q.: Post-traumatic pain and causalgic syndrome, J. Neurol. Neurosurg. Psychiatr. **7**:33-48, 1944.
13. Eaton, R.G.: Painful neuromas. In Omer, G.E., Jr., and Spinner, M., editors: Management of peripheral nerve problems, Philadelphia, 1980, W.B. Saunders Co.
14. Gelard, F.A.: The human senses, ed. 2, New York, 1972, John Wiley & Sons, Inc.

15. Gelberman, R.H., Hergenroeder, P.T., Hargens, A.R., Lundborg, G.H., and Akeson, W.H.: The carpal tunnel syndrome: a study of carpal tunnel pressures, J. Bone Joint Surg. **63A**:380-383, 1981.
16. Gildenberg, P.L.: Central surgical procedures for pain of peripheral nerve origin. In Omer, G.E., Jr., and Spinner, M., editors: Management of peripheral nerve problems, Philadelphia, 1980, W.B. Saunders Co.
17. Glick, E.N.: Reflex dystrophy (algoneurodystrophy): results of treatment by corticosteroids, Rheumatol. Rehabil. **12**:84-88, 1973.
18. Glick, E.N., and Helal, B.: Post-traumatic neurodystrophy: treatment by corticosteroids, Hand **8**:45-47, 1976.
19. Goldner, J.L.: Pain: extremities and spine—evaluation and differential diagnosis. In Omer, G.E., Jr., and Spinner, M., editors: Management of peripheral nerve problems, Philadelphia, 1980, W.B. Saunders Co.
20. Goldner, J.L., Nashold, B.S., and Hendrix, P.C.: Peripheral nerve electrical stimulation, Clin. Orthop. **163**:33-41, 1982.
21. Grant, G.H.: Methods of treatment of neuromata of the hand, J. Bone Joint Surg. **33A**:841-848, 1951.
22. Hannington-Kiff, J.G.: Intravenous regional sympathetic block with guanethidine, Lancet **1**:1019-1020, 1974.
23. Hannington-Kiff, J.G.: Relief of Sudek's atrophy by regional intravenous guanethidine, Lancet **1**:1132-1133, 1977.
24. Herndon, J.H., Eaton, R.G., and Littler, J.W.: Management of painful neuromas in the hand, J. Bone Joint Surg. **58A**:369-373, 1976.
25. Hosobuchi, Y., Possier, J., Bloom, F.E., and Guillemin, R.: Stimulation of human periaqueductal grey matter for pain relief increases immuno-reactive beta-endorphin in ventricular fluid, Science **203**:279-281, 1979.
26. Hosobuchi, Y.: The majority of unmyelinated afferent axons in human ventral roots probably conduct pain, Pain **8**:167-180, 1980.
27. Kleinert, H.E., Cole, N.M., and Wayne, L.: Post-traumatic sympathetic dystrophy, Orthop. Clin. North Am. **4**:917-927, 1973.
28. Laborde, K.J., Kalisman, M., and Tsi, T.-M.: Results of surgical treatment of painful neuromas of the hand, J. Hand Surg. **7**:190-193, 1982.
29. Lankford, L.L.: Reflex sympathetic dystrophy. In Omer, G.E., Jr., and Spinner, M., editors: Management of peripheral nerve problems, Philadelphia, 1980, W.B. Saunders Co.
30. Leavens, M.E.: Neurosurgical relief of pain in cancer patients, The Cancer Bulletin **33**:98-100, 1981.
31. Leffert, R.D., Lenson, M.A., and Todd, D.P.: The use of continuous sympathetic blockade in the treatment of reflex dystrophy, Personal communication, Boston, June 19, 1978.
32. Loeser, J.D.: Dorsal rhizotomy for the relief of chronic pain, J. Neurosurg. **36**:745-750, 1972.
33. Loeser, J.D., Black, R.G., and Christman, A.: Relief of pain by transcutaneous stimulation, J. Neurosurg. **43**:308-314, 1975.
34. Long, D.M.: Electrical stimulation for the control of pain, Arch. Surg. **112**:884-888, 1977.
35. Long, D.M.: Relief of cancer pain by surgical and nerve blocking procedures, J.A.M.A. **244**:2759-2761, 1980.
36. Long, D.M.: Neuromodulation for the control of chronic pain, Surg. Rounds **5**:25-34, 1982.
37. Lynn, R., and Eysenck, H.J.: Tolerance for pain, extraversion and neuroticism, Percept. Mot. Skills **12**:161-162, 1961.
38. Matsumoto, T., and Levy, B.A.: Acupuncture for patients, Springfield, Ill., 1975, Charles C Thomas, Publisher.
39. Mersky, H.: Pain terms: a list with definitions and notes on usage (International Association for the Study of Pain (IASP) Subcommittee on Taxonomy), Pain **6**:249-252, 1979.
40. Moore, D.C., Bridenbaugh, L.D., Bridenbaugh, P.O., and Tucker, G.T.: Bupivacaine: a review of 2,077 cases, J.A.M.A. **214**:713-718, 1970.
41. Murphy, T.M., and Bonica, J.J.: Acupuncture analgesia and anesthesia, Arch. Surg. **112**:896-902, 1977.
42. Nashold, B.S., Goldner, J.L., Mullen, J.B., and Bright, D.S.: Long-term pain control by direct peripheral-nerve stimulation, J. Bone Joint Surg. **64A**:1-10, 1982.
43. Omer, G.E., Jr., Riordan, D.C., Conran, P.B., and Winter, R.: Peritendinous fibrosis of the dorsum of the hand in monkeys, Clin. Orthop. **62**:251-259, 1969.

44. Omer, G.E., Jr., and Thomas, S.R.: Treatment of causalgia: review of cases at Brooke General Hospital, Tex. Med. **67:**93-96, 1971.

45. Omer, G.E., Jr., and Thomas, S.R.: The management of chronic pain syndromes in the upper extremity, Clin. Orthop. **104:**37-43, 1974.

46. Omer, G.E., Jr., and Spinner, M.: Peripheral nerve testing and suture techniques. In American Academy of Orthopaedic Surgeons: Instructional Course Lectures **24:**122-143, St. Louis, 1975, The C.V. Mosby Co.

47. Omer, G.E., Jr.: Management of pain syndromes in the upper extremity. In Hunter, J.M., Schneider, L.H., Mackin, E.J., and Bell, J.A., editors: Rehabilitation of the hand, St. Louis, 1978, The C.V. Mosby Co.

48. Omer, G.E., Jr.: Management of the painful extremity. In Ahstrom, J.P., Jr., editor: Current practice in orthopaedic surgery, vol. 8, St. Louis, 1979, The C.V. Mosby Co.

49. Omer, G.E., Jr.: Nerve, neuroma, and pain problems related to upper limb amputations, Orthop. Clin. North Am. **12:**751-762, 1981.

50. Onofrio, B.M., and Campa, H.K.: Evaluation of rhizotomy: review of 12 years' experience, J. Neurosurg. **36:**751-755, 1972.

51. Peck, C.L., and Kraft, G.H.: Electromyographic biofeedback for pain related to muscle tension, Arch. Surg. **112:**889-895, 1977.

52. Plewes, L.W.: Sudek's atrophy in the hand, J. Bone Joint Surg. **38B:**195-203, 1956.

53. Porter, J.M., Snider, R.L., Bardana, E.J., Rosch, J., and Eidemiller, L.R.: The diagnosis and treatment of Raynaud's phenomenon, Surgery **77:**11-23, 1975.

54. Rydevik, B., Lundborg, G., and Bagge, U.: Effects of graded compression on intraneural blood flow, J. Hand Surg. **6:**3-12, 1981.

55. Schachtel, H.J.: Pain and religion, The Cancer Bulletin **33:**84-85, 1981.

56. Simmons, B.P., and Vasile, R.G.: The clenched fist syndrome, J. Hand Surg. **5:**420-427, 1980.

57. Simson, G.: Letters Section: Propranol for causalgia and Sudek atrophy, J.A.M.A. **227:**327, Jan. 21, 1974.

58. Sjölund, B., Terenius, L., and Eriksson, M.: Increased cerebrospinal fluid levels of endorphins after electro-acupuncture, Acta Physiol. Scand. **100:**382-384, 1977.

59. Smith, J.R., and Gomez, N.H.: Local injection therapy of neuromata of the hand with triamcinolone acetonide: a preliminary study of twenty-two patients, J. Bone Joint Surg. **52A:**71-83, 1970.

60. Spiegel, D., and Chase, R.A.: The treatment of contractures of the hand using self-hypnosis, J. Hand Surg. **5**(5):428-432, 1980.

61. Spinner, M.: Injuries to the major branches of peripheral nerves of the forearm, ed. 2, Philadelphia, 1978, W.B. Saunders Co.

62. Sternbach, R.A., Wolf, S.R., Murphy, R.W., and Akeson, W.H.: Traits of pain patients: the low-back "loser," Psychosomatics **14:**226-229, 1973.

63. Sternbach, R.A.: Modern concepts of pain. In Delessio, D.J., editor: Wolff's headache and other head pain, ed. 4, New York, 1980, Oxford University Press.

64. Sufian, S., Pavlides, C., Fischer, C.R., III, Matulewski, T., and Matsumoto, T.: Acupuncture for chronic pain and anesthesia, Surg. Rounds **5:**38-49, Jan. 1982.

65. Swanson, A.B., Boeve, N.R., and Lumsden, R.M.: The prevention and treatment of amputation neuromata by silicone capping, J. Hand Surg. **2:**70-78, 1977.

66. Thomason, J.R., and Moritz, W.H.: Continuous lumbar paravertebral sympathetic block maintained by fractional installation of procaine, Surg. Gynecol. Obstet. **89:**447-453, 1949.

67. Tupper, J.W., and Booth, D.M.: Treatment of painful neuromas of sensory nerves in the hand: a comparison of traditional and newer methods, J. Hand Surg. **1:**144-151, 1976.

68. Tursky, B., and O'Connell, D.: Reliability and interjudgment predictability of subjective judgments of electrocutaneous stimulation, Psychophysiology **9:**290-295, 1972.

69. Tursky, B.: Physical, physiological, and psychological factors that affect pain reaction to electric shock, Psychophysiology **11:**95-112, 1974.

70. Ulett, G.H.: Acupuncture treatments for pain relief, J.A.M.A. **245:**768-769, 1981.

71. Vaux, K.L.: Pain: the moral dimensions, The Cancer Bulletin **33:**86-87, 1981.

72. Veith, I.: Acupuncture in traditional Chinese medicine, Calif. Med. **118:**70-79, 1973.

73. Wallace, P.F., and Fitzmorris, C.S., Jr.: The S-H-A-F-T syndrome in the upper extremity. J. Hand Surg. **3**(5):492, 1978.

74. White, J.C., and Sweet, W.H.: Pain and the neurosurgeon: a forty year experience, Springfield, Ill., 1969, Charles C Thomas, Publisher.

75. Wiley, A.M., Poplawski, Z.B., and Murray, J.: Post-traumatic dystrophy of the hand, Orthop. Rev. **6:**59-61, 1977.

76. Wilson, R.L.: Management of pain following peripheral nerve injuries, Orthop. Clin. North Am. **12:**343-359, 1981.

77. Wolff, B.B., and Jarvik, M.E.: Variations in cutaneous and deep somatic pain sensitivity, Can. J. Psychol. **17:**37-44, 1963.

78. Wynn Parry, C.B.: Brachial plexus lesions, causalgia, and Sudek's atrophy, American Society for Surgery of The Hand Newsletter 2, 1981.

47

Reflex sympathetic dystrophy

L. LEE LANKFORD

Homeostasis is defined as a tendency to stability in the normal body states (internal body condition) of the organism and is achieved by a system of control mechanisms activated by negative feedback in order to return to normalcy any deranged body condition produced by an abnormal stimulus. The body, therefore, has a mechanism designed for the purpose of returning to normalcy (homeostasis) any abnormal state produced by injury or disease. This usually takes place in an orderly fashion, and within the limits of the injury or disease the body will be reinstated in its previous condition. On occasion, however, this orderly mechanism does not function properly and a deranged state persists in the body. Reflex sympathetic dystrophy is an example of such a dysfunction on the part of the body. Instead of an injury or a disease of an extremity healing in the expected fashion, the limb is beset by a condition of increasing pain and dysfunction. Fortunately, however, this happens infrequently, but because of the devastating effect this has on the extremity and the person as a whole, it behooves us to acquaint ourselves with this condition and its diagnosis and treatment.

WHAT IT IS

Reflex sympathetic dystrophy (RSD) is a diseased state of an extremity that is characterized by very severe pain, swelling, stiffness, and discoloration (Fig. 47-1). It usually occurs after a trauma or disease of an extremity, is generated by an abnormal sympathetic reflex, and is characteristically treated by the abolition of this increased sympathetic nerve stimulation. Reflex sympathetic dystrophy is generally considered to be synonymous with "vasomotor and trophic disorders." There are several clinical types of RSD, ranging from a minor involvement of one or more fingers to the severest form, which is major causalgia; therefore RSD presents many different aspects and varying degrees of pain and dysfunction.

WHAT IT IS NOT

It is important to realize that reflex sympathetic dystrophy is not the only condition that causes more stiffness, swelling, pain, discoloration, and dysfunction than is normal for a given severity of trauma or disease in the normal individual. Injury (including surgery) or disease in a hand that has a tendency toward excessive fibrosis ("high up on the fibrosis scale") most likely will produce a greater amount of pain, swelling, stiffness, and dysfunction than the same severity of injury or disease in an otherwise normal person. Although one may well think of this as being a "dystrophic" condition, these findings alone do not make it a case of reflex sympathetic dystrophy. Conditions that fall in this category are as follows: Dupuytren's palmar fasciitis, hypertrophic arthritis, psoriatic arthritis, the primary type of carpal tunnel syndrome (produced by increased fibrosis of the transverse carpal ligament causing thickening and longitudinal contracture of the ligament, thus narrowing the diameter of the carpal tunnel), stenosing tenosynovitis, "knuckle pads" with thickened and inelastic skin over the dorsum of the finger, and long-standing diabetes. One must not be deluded into thinking that all bad results and stiff hands are due to reflex sympathetic dystrophy. It is very important to make this distinction early in the course of the disease so that the appropriate treatment may be given these distinctly different types of dystrophy.

NOMENCLATURE

A Civil War neurologist by the name of Silas Weir Mitchell, working in the Turner's Lane Hospital in Philadelphia,

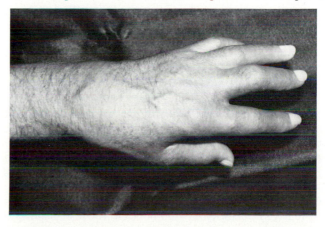

FIG. 47-1. Hand in reflex sympathetic dystrophy is usually swollen and red and has tight shiny skin. (From Lankford, L.L., and Thompson, J.E.: Reflex sympathetic dystrophy, upper and lower extremity: diagnosis and management. In American Academy of Orthopaedic Surgeons: Instructional course lectures, vol. 26., St. Louis, 1977, The C.V. Mosby Co.)

509

is generally credited with the first accurate description of the condition that we now call "reflex sympathetic dystrophy." Although Mitchell's description[42] remains as the classic, many authors previously had written case reports of patients who may well have had one of the clinical forms of reflex sympathetic dystrophy; they are Paré[52] in 1598, Potts[57] in 1736, Denmark[10] in 1813, and Hamilton[22] in 1838. Mitchell, Moorehouse, and Keen[42] published their epochal description in 1864, entitled *Gunshot Wounds and Other Injuries of Nerves*. In the same year, Paget[49] described trophic changes and a glossy appearance of the hand and fingers with severe pain and dysfunction after a nerve injury. Sudeck[64] in 1900 described a condition, which he later called "inflammatory bone atrophy," that produced a reflex sympathetic dystrophy appearance but without specific nerve injury. In 1937 de Takáts[12] described a similar condition, which he called "reflex dystrophy," but in another article,[13] in 1945, he used the name "causalgic state." Homans[23] in 1940 coined the term "minor causalgia." In the years after this, many authors who felt the need to recognize the role of trauma and vasomotor dysfunction suggested terms such as "posttraumatic dystrophy," "painful vasodilatation," "posttraumatic osteoporosis," "posttraumatic causalgia," "sympathetic neurovascular dystrophy," "posttraumatic vasomotor disorders," and "reflex nervous dystrophy."

It was not until 1867 that Mitchell[40] in another publication created the term "causalgia" after the Greek words for 'burning pain'—*kausos* plus *algos* plus *-ia* ("condition").

I[30] believe that all of the above-mentioned vasomotor-trophic conditions are linked together, because all of them owe their existence to an abnormal sympathetic nerve reflex, and therefore all should be classified as reflex sympathetic dystrophy. One should also understand, however, that there are several clinical types of reflex sympathetic dystrophy. Since Mitchell[40-42] described his condition as a partial injury to a major mixed nerve in the proximal part of the extremity and believed that this condition arose only from a nerve injury, I believe that the term "causalgia" should be reserved for those forms of RSD that involve nerves. The designation of a major causalgia will be given to Mitchell's condition, since not only does it describe the fact that a major nerve is involved but also the symptoms are of the greatest severity. There is, however, a clinical type of RSD that involves the trauma of a peripheral digital nerve and produces, in comparison, minor symptoms and dysfunction, and so in our classification it is called "minor causalgia." More frequently, however, reflex sympathetic dystrophy does not involve specific nerve injury but instead involves damage to the soft-tissue, joint, or bone. These non–nerve injury types of RSD therefore are called "minor traumatic dystrophy" or "major traumatic dystrophy," depending on the severity of the inciting trauma or disease and the magnitude of noxious signs and symptoms. The remaining clinical type of reflex sympathetic dystrophy is the shoulder-hand syndrome, which is also precipitated by an abnormal sympathetic nerve reflex but is caused either by a trauma of the proximal part of the body or by damage or disease of a viscus.

SYMPTOMS AND SIGNS

Pain

Certainly the paramount symptom of reflex sympathetic dystrophy is pain, and it is characteristically described as a burning pain. Most traumas and disease states produce pain, but the distinguishing feature in RSD is that the severity of the pain is all out of proportion to the inciting injury or disease state. In most cases, the first complaint is that of a burning pain, but as time goes on, patients often describe the pain as a pressure, crushing, binding, searing, aching, cutting, or cramping pain. Even though the pain in the patient with well-developed RSD is constant, it certainly is aggravated by either active or passive attempts at motion. Another distinguishing feature is the dysesthesia and paresthesia that is produced by even a light touch of the affected skin. It is difficult to do an examination at times because of the patient's withdrawal of the hand from the examiner. At first, the pain is more apt to be the expected degree of pain for the involved injury or disease. Later, however, the pain gets worse, and in many cases it does not start until after the cast has been removed. The initial pain, also, is in the expected nerve distribution area of the injury, but it soon spreads to the whole hand, wrist, forearm, and the entire upper extremity. The severity of the tenderness is also quite pronounced, and it is usually worse around the interphalangeal joints of the fingers.

Swelling

Swelling is usually the first physical sign, occurs initially in the involved area, and then slowly spreads to other areas so that eventually it may encompass the hand, wrist, and distal part of the forearm. The swelling in the fingers, which at first produces a fusiform appearance, gradually changes to periarticular thickening at the joints. At first the swelling is that of a soft edema, but in time it becomes a hard, brawny edema and certainly is one of the factors that produces loss of motion.

Stiffness

As in the case of pain, the stiffness in reflex sympathetic dystrophy is distinctive because it is profoundly worse than one would expect from the antecedent trauma or disease. A trauma without the presence of RSD would be expected to produce some stiffness, but as time goes on and as the wound heals, the stiffness would normally improve. In the case of reflex sympathetic dystrophy, however, one usually finds that the stiffness increases with time. Since any attempt at either active or passive motion is exquisitely painful, it is not hard to understand that the initial lack of motion is attributable to the enforced immobility to escape further aggravation of the pain. Subsequently, the stiffness is attributable to increased fibrosis in the ligamentous structures and adhesion formation around the tendon, which sticks all gliding structures together. All fibrous structures about the joints are thickened and quite hard and inelastic. It is not uncommon to see palmar fasciitis accompanying RSD, and this too, of course, will add to the severity of flexion contractures in the digits.

Discoloration

An ever-present sign is some type of discoloration of the hand. Usually, the discoloration takes the form of redness and initially is most commonly located over the dorsum of the metacarpophalangeal joints and the interphalangeal joints of the fingers, but it may at times involve the whole hand rather diffusely. At some period of the disease the hand may be pale and at other times grayish to cyanotic. A purplish discoloration may often be seen in the flexor creases of the fingers in the palm and this is particularly true if a palmar fasciitis has developed. The omnipresence of increased coloration of the hand has caused me[29] to call RSD the "red hand disease." Pallor is present, of course, where there is vasoconstriction of both arterial and venous systems, and redness is present when there is dilation of both sides of the vascular tree, but blueness or cyanosis is usually present when there is vasoconstriction of the venous system.

Osteoporosis

The next most common and reliable sign of reflex sympathetic dystrophy is osteoporosis, and here again the degree of osteoporosis is distinguished by the fact that it is a great deal more severe than would be expected by the preceding trauma or disease (Fig. 47-2). The initial demineralization in the more severe forms of RSD usually takes place in the carpal bones and produces punched-out areas, which prompted Sudeck[64] to call this condition "inflammatory bone atrophy." There are, however, no distinguishing features of this spotty osteoporosis because with the passage of time the untreated case will progress from the punched-out areas eventually to a diffuse osteoporosis with no particular clinical significance. Also, very early in the disease the demineralization takes place in the polar regions of the long bones of the metacarpals and the phalanges. Although some demineralization would, of course, be present from immobilization alone, the bulk of the washing out of the calcium undoubtedly comes from increased blood flow in the joints. This has recently been shown by Genant.[18]

Sudomotor changes

Sudomotor changes are usually present but may be variable according to several factors. More often than not the early stages of reflex sympathetic dystrophy display hyperhidrosis though in some severe clinical types dryness may be present initially. In the last stages of the disease, dryness is the rule. At times the diaphoresis is great enough to observe beads of sweat dropping from the hand.

Temperature

The temperature of the extremity involved with reflex sympathetic dystrophy also is quite variable. If it is possible to observe the disease at its very earliest onset, one most commonly finds a decrease in the temperature, and this is also usually the case when there is hyperhidrosis. In the early stages when there is drying of the hand or when there is redness, the temperature is more commonly elevated. When there is pallor or cyanosis, the temperature is nearly always diminished. In some instances, one may find concurrently increased temperature over the reddened joints and

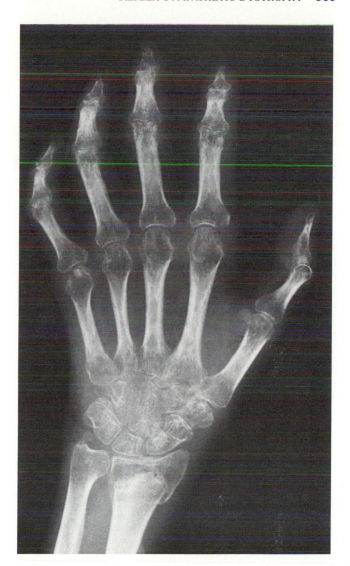

FIG. 47-2. Degree of osteoporosis is distinguished by the fact that it is much greater than would be expected in usual case of trauma with immobilization. (From Lankford, L.L., and Thompson, J.E.: Reflex sympathetic dystrophy, upper and lower extremity: diagnosis and management. In American Academy of Orthopaedic Surgeons: Instructional course lectures, vol. 26, St. Louis, 1977, The C.V. Mosby Co.)

diminished temperature in between the joints where there is pallor. Carron and Weller[6] have used thermograms to demonstrate that most patients have increased heat, but they do not state during which stage the thermograms were taken.

Palmar fasciitis

A palmar fasciitis with acute nodules and thickening of the longitudinal bands of palmar fascia in the fingers or in the hand may be seen in several clinical types of reflex sympathetic dystrophy. The condition may progress as long as the RSD is not successfully treated. This does, of course, tend to produce flexion contractures of the fingers.

Vasomotor instability

Prolonged capillary refill time is commonly found in reflex sympathetic dystrophy, and one may easily demonstrate this by blanching the finger nail with pressure or by pressing on the fat pad areas in the finger. This is generally found with pallor, cyanosis, or excess sweating. A rapid capillary refill may be seen when there is redness in the hand, and this is indicative of vasodilation. In the very early stages of RSD, vasoconstriction is the rule.

Trophic changes

One almost always associates a glossy shiny appearance of the skin with reflex sympathetic dystrophy. In the early stages this appearance is attributable to the swelling and ironing out of the skin wrinkles and is secondary to lack of motion in the joints. Later on, the nutritional changes that produce the glossy, shiny surface of the skin are caused by skin and subcutaneous tissue atrophy. This was prominently mentioned by Mitchell[42] and by Paget[49] and many others subsequently. The skin feels quite tight, and one can readily observe a definite decrease in the mobility of the skin over the dorsum of the fingers and particularly the interphalangeal joints. The ends of the fingers may take on a "pencil-pointing" appearance because of the atrophy of the tip of the fat pad and the concomitant downward curving of the fingernail.

STAGES

The difficulty of diagnosis of reflex sympathetic dystrophy is attributable in part to the variable signs and symptoms depending on when in the course of the disease the examiner first sees the patient. A particular sign or symptom may be present temporarily but not at a subsequent stage. It is therefore important to be cognizant of the great variations according to the duration of the condition. It is possible to divide the course of reflex sympathetic dystrophy into three stages.

Stage I

In the early part of stage I, pain is the most pronounced feature. The pain is usually of a burning nature, and throughout stage I the pain generally increases in severity. Painful paresthesia to light touch may be seen quite early, but aggravation of the constant pain with attempts at motion is seen with greater regularity near the end of stage I. Swelling begins quite early and may cause pitting over the dorsum of the hand if quite prominent (Fig. 47-3). Lack of motion of the fingers or the wrist is seen early and is progressive throughout this stage. The coloration of the hand is variable but most commonly in the early part of the stage is either pale or cyanotic and near the end of the stage becomes red, especially over the dorsum of the metacarpophalangeal joints and the interphalangeal joints. Increased sweating and coolness in the first stage is more frequent than drying or heat, particularly in the early part of stage I. Vasoconstriction or peripheral vasospasm is most commonly noted. Osteoporosis is not present before 3 weeks and often is not seen until the fifth week. The average duration of stage I is 3 months.

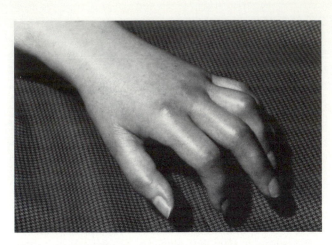

FIG. 47-3. In first stage of reflex sympathetic dystrophy, swelling is usually soft and puffy with redness over joints. (From Lankford, L.L., and Thompson, J.E.: Reflex sympathetic dystrophy, upper and lower extremity: diagnosis and management. In American Academy of Orthopaedic Surgeons: Instructional course lectures, vol. 26, St. Louis, 1977, The C.V. Mosby Co.)

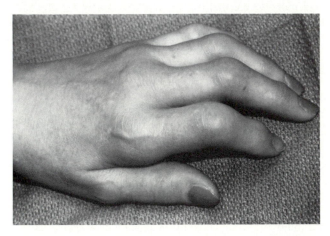

FIG. 47-4. Stage II is characterized by brawny edema with stiffness, as evidenced by flattening out of extensor and flexor wrinkles. (From Lankford, L.L., and Thompson, J.E.: Reflex sympathetic dystrophy, upper and lower extremity: diagnosis and management. In American Academy of Orthopaedic Surgeons: Instructional course lectures, vol. 26, St. Louis, 1977, The C.V. Mosby Co.)

Stage II

Pain continues to be one of the most prominent features of stage II, and it continues to get worse during most of this stage unless treated. The swelling changes from a soft nature to a brawny, hard edema (Fig. 47-4). It is difficult to reduce the swelling by elevation or other standard means during this stage. Stiffness continues to increase throughout most of this stage and again pain is aggravated by attempts at active and passive motion. During stage II redness, increased heat, and decreased sweating are most commonly found. Vasomotor instability is still observed. The demineralization also increases and changes from the spotty demineralization in the carpal bones and the polar deminer-

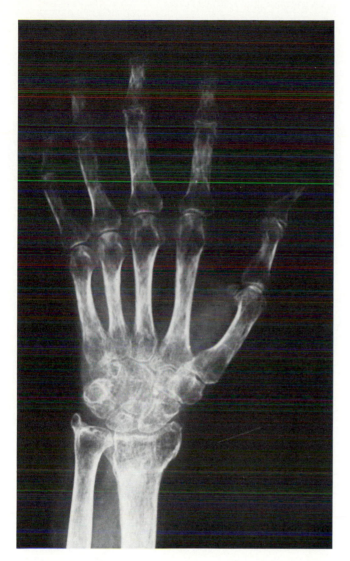

FIG. 47-5. Near end of stage II and early part of stage III, osteoporosis has become uniform and very intense throughout all bones of hand and wrist. (From Lankford, L.L., and Thompson, J.E.: Reflex sympathetic dystrophy, upper and lower extremity: diagnosis and management. In American Academy of Orthopaedic Surgeons: Instructional course lectures, vol. 26, St. Louis, 1977, The C.V. Mosby Co.)

alization in the long bones of the fingers to a more widespread homogeneous appearance (Fig. 47-5). The glossy or shiny appearance of the skin continues to increase. The duration of stage II is most commonly through the ninth month.

Stage III

The severity of the pain in most instances has peaked in stage III and either remains constant for several months or slowly improves. In many cases, however, the pain continues on for at least 2 years and in some cases, indefinitely. John Mitchell, the physician son of Silas Weir Mitchell, continued to follow some of his father's cases and reported in 1895[39] that severe pain and dysfunction lasted for more

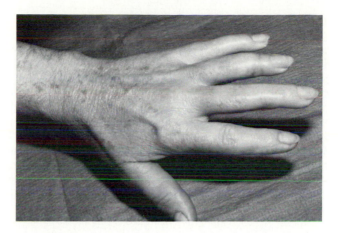

FIG. 47-6. Stage III is characterized by atrophy of skin and subcutaneous tissue, which produces a glossy appearance of skin. (From Lankford, L.L., and Thompson, J.E.: Reflex sympathetic dystrophy, upper and lower extremity: diagnosis and management. In American Academy of Orthopaedic Surgeons: Instructional course lectures, vol. 26, St. Louis, 1977, The C.V. Mosby Co.)

than 20 years. Pain on motion remains fairly severe for several months in stage III even though the constant pain may have subsided somewhat. The fingers and the wrist are usually quite stiff in the untreated case and show very little improvement. The swelling changes from the brawny edema to periarticular thickening of the joints, and such structures as the collateral ligaments are quite obviously thickened. The hand usually becomes pale, dry, and cool. The glossy appearance is usually at its peak in stage III (Fig. 47-6). The skin and subcutaneous tissue atrophy continues with "pencil pointing" of the fingertips at its greatest. Osteoporosis is profound. In most cases the hand is quite dysfunctional. Stage III usually lasts for at least 2 years but in many cases will extend through many years.

CLINICAL TYPES

Evans[16] first suggested that all the many descriptive terms previously used for the various vasomotor conditions be changed to reflex sympathetic dystrophy, since it is apparent that all these conditions are produced by an abnormal sympathetic reflex. I wholeheartedly concur with this name, but at the same time I recognize that there are distinct clinical types and have devised the following classifications[30] of reflex sympathetic dystrophy:
1. Minor causalgia
2. Minor traumatic dystrophy
3. Shoulder-hand syndrome
4. Major traumatic dystrophy
5. Major causalgia

Minor causalgia

Since this clinical type of RSD involves a nerve, it is therefore called a "causalgia," and since the nerve involved is a peripheral nerve with the least severe pain and dysfunction, the term "minor causalgia" is used for this condition. A nerve injury in the upper extremity is seen much more commonly in the hand and wrist than in the elbow and upper arm. The symptoms produced are less noxious and involve a smaller part of the hand and may well be limited to only one or two fingers. The degree of pain, swelling, stiffness, discoloration, and osteoporosis is concomitantly less severe. The antecedent trauma is more frequently to the dorsal superficial sensory branch of the radial nerve overlying the radial styloid area of the wrist, and this site is the most vulnerable to injury. If the injury has produced scarring of the nerve or a nerve was severed and repaired, the nerve very commonly binds itself down to the surrounding fixed structures with adhesions and thus produces a "neurodesis" with the fixation of the nerve distal to the wrist. Any flexion of the wrist will produce a stretching of the nerve, and this stretching excites greater fibrous tissue proliferation with the ultimate production of a painful neuroma. In the past I have recommended that severely traumatized radial sensory nerves not be sutured but instead be cut cleanly proximally as far as possible to avoid the formation of the painful neuroma. It was my hope that with the advent of microsurgery the sacrifice of the dorsal superficial branch of the radial sensory nerve might not be necessary, but so far these hopes have not come to fruition.

The palmar branch of the median nerve just proximal to the wrist is quite often injured with lacerations or because of a surgical procedure in this area, and this branch is our next most common nerve injury site in the minor causalgia type of RSD. This nerve is quite often injured inadvertently with the use of a transverse incision in the volar wrist, and for this reason I have avoided the use of this incision.

The next most common site of nerve injury is the dorsal superficial sensory branch of the ulnar nerve and particularly over the dorsal ulnar aspect of the wrist and hand. The common digital and the proper digital branches of the median and ulnar nerves, though less commonly involved in minor causalgia, quite definitely can represent the inciting trauma producing this type of RSD.

Not every painful neuroma, of course, represents minor causalgia. A neuroma of some degree is always produced at the point of an injury of a nerve, and, of course, not all neuromas are painful. If a neuroma is painful only when pressure is applied and not between those times, it should not be considered a minor causalgia. The pain of minor causalgia is constant, and the other features of RSD such as pain on motion, swelling, stiffness, and osteoporosis are much greater than would be expected from a simple painful neuroma. Only when these findings are present can the diagnosis of reflex sympathetic dystrophy be properly made.

Minor traumatic dystrophy

Minor traumatic dystrophy is the most common clinical type of reflex sympathetic dystrophy because traumas not involving a specific nerve are much more common than nerve injuries and also because minor traumas are more common than major traumas, thereby producing the most frequent painful stimuli. Minor traumatic dystrophy, however, is also the most frequently overlooked type of RSD, since it is not as well known that reflex sympathetic dystrophy can involve only a small segment of a hand. The precipitating painful lesion is usually a trauma of minor proportions such as a mashed finger, fracture, dislocation, a sprain, or even a penetrating wound that does not specifically involve a nerve injury. The degree of involvement may encompass only one or a few fingers rather than the whole hand, but the same type of signs and symptoms such as pain, swelling, stiffness, discoloration, and dysfunction are present. The redness is characteristically found over the dorsum of the metacarpophalangeal and interphalangeal joints as well as over the collateral ligaments. A mild degree of palmar fasciitis may also be present. The digits are usually stiffened in flexion.

Shoulder-hand syndrome

The shoulder-hand syndrome usually starts with considerable pain and progresses to stiffness in the shoulder with spreading of the pain into the whole extremity, producing moderate-to-marked swelling of at least the wrist and the hand and sometimes the entire upper arm as well. The causative painful lesion is either a proximal trauma such as a shoulder, neck, or rib-cage injury, or it may well be from visceral sources such as heart attacks, strokes, stomach ulcers, or a Pancoast tumor of the apex of the lung. In most instances in shoulder-hand syndrome, there is a fusiform type of swelling and the fingers are stiffened in extension rather than in flexion (Fig. 47-7). Redness, when present, is more diffuse rather than being solely over the metacarpophalangeal and interphalangeal joints, and the hand is usually warmer and dryer than normal. Palmar fasciitis with acute nodules is more likely to be present in this form of RSD than in any other clinical form. The sex distribution of all forms of RSD is heavily weighted toward the female, but the differential is greatest of all in shoulder-hand syndrome. The highest incidence of age distribution is between 45 and 55.

Otto Steinbrocker[62,63] first described this condition in 1947. At that time, apparently he did not fully appreciate

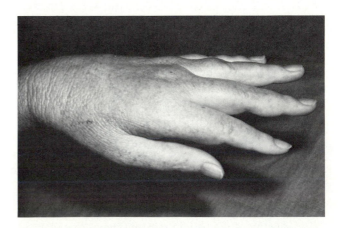

FIG. 47-7. Extension contractures of fingers are usually noted in shoulder-hand clinical type of reflex sympathetic dystrophy, as contrasted to flexion contractures, which are usually noted in other clinical types. (From Lankford, L.L., and Thompson, J.E.: Reflex sympathetic dystrophy, upper and lower extremity: diagnosis and management. In American Academy of Orthopaedic Surgeons: Instructional course lectures, vol. 26, St. Louis, 1977, The C.V. Mosby Co.)

the role of the abnormal sympathetic reflex and very likely included in his series several cases of shoulder stiffness that probably should have been diagnosed as adhesive capsulitis or arthritis. It should be emphasized that not all stiff, painful shoulders with swelling in the upper extremities that follow heart attacks or strokes fit into the category of reflex sympathetic dystrophy. Statistically, of course, the majority of painful stiff shoulders have their origin in disuse from trauma, rotator cuff tendinitis, or adhesive capsulitis, and if these conditions are properly diagnosed early, they can usually be successfully treated with physical means. If, however, the degree of pain, swelling, stiffness, dysfunction, and especially osteoporosis is much greater than otherwise expected and the vasomotor component is recognized, they should be considered as possible reflex sympathetic dystrophy of the shoulder-hand clinical type and be so treated.

Major traumatic dystrophy

Major traumatic dystrophy is the clinical type that has given reflex sympathetic dystrophy such a bad name. The persistent painful lesion that triggers major traumatic dystrophy is usually a major trauma such as a crushed hand, Colles' fracture, or a severe fracture dislocation of the wrist. In a high percentage of cases, this type of trauma produces an acute traumatic carpal tunnel syndrome, which is most likely responsible for the painful lesion that activates RSD.[29] The acute carpal tunnel syndrome, however, need not be from trauma but may well be from an acute flare-up of arthritis. A high percentage of patients with Colles' fracture who have subsequently developed RSD were found to also have carpal tunnel syndromes in our series of cases. Major

traumatic dystrophy is the clinical type of RSD that produces the greatest pain, stiffness, swelling, and dysfunction in the non–nerve injury cases. As in all cases of RSD, the degree of pain, swelling, stiffness, dysfunction, and osteoporosis is very much greater than one would expect to find with the same type of antecedent trauma or disease in an otherwise normal person. Flexion contractures of the digits in this type are more frequent than extension contractures. Wrist motion is usually extremely limited, and flexion deformities are present along with a definite limitation of rotary motion of the forearm.

Major causalgia

Major causalgia is the clinical type of reflex sympathetic dystrophy that produces the greatest degree of pain and devastation to the patient (Fig. 47-8). This is the clinical type of RSD that was noted by Mitchell,[42] who described the inciting painful lesion as being a partial nerve injury in a mixed major nerve in the proximal part of the extremity. In the case of the upper extremity, the median nerve is usually involved, while in the lower extremity the sciatic nerve is involved more frequently. Sunderland[65] has shown that these two nerves have a much greater sympathetic nerve fiber population than other nerves do, and this is believed to be significant in the production of this clinical type of reflex sympathetic dystrophy. Without a doubt, pain is the most prominent symptom of a major causalgia and may, on occasion, begin at the time of injury, but most commonly it makes its appearance within the first week after injury. Characteristically the pain is described as burning. The pain usually progresses through all three stages and becomes

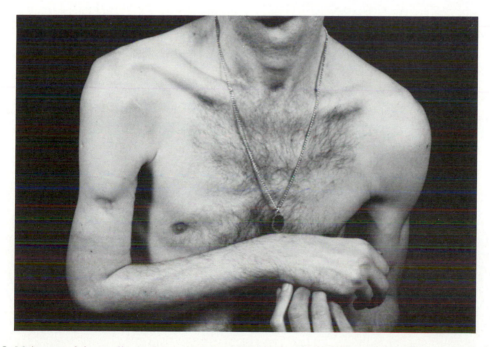

FIG. 47-8. Major causalgia usually produces greatest degree of pain and dysfunction of all types of reflex sympathetic dystrophy. It is usually caused by an injury to a major mixed nerve in proximal portion of extremity. In this case, initiating trauma was a partial injury to median nerve from gunshot wound. (From Lankford, L.L., and Thompson, J.E.: Reflex sympathetic dystrophy, upper and lower extremity: diagnosis and management. In American Academy of Orthopaedic Surgeons: Instructional course lectures, vol. 26, St. Louis, 1977, The C.V. Mosby Co.)

extreme. The patient may seek relief by wrapping his hand and upper extremity in wet towels. An exacerbation of the pain may be brought on by light touch of the skin or even by auditory stimuli such as hearing a squeaky noise or by becoming emotionally upset. The vibration of riding in an automobile or even of another person walking across the floor may cause an aggravation of the pain. The pain may, at times, become so severe that the patient will beg for an amputation of the part. There is generally less red coloration in this type of reflex sympathetic dystrophy than in other types, and the early stages are almost always pale or cyanotic in color. Sweating and coolness are usually a prominent feature. At first the pain is confined to the distribution of the nerve that was injured but soon begins to spread over the entire hand and eventually the upper extremity. Flexion contractures of the fingers occur, but although the stiffness is extreme, the degree of flexion contracture is often not so

great as in major traumatic dystrophy. The pain, stiffness, and dysfunction if untreated may be expected to continue indefinitely.

According to Mitchell[42] his malady developed after the partial injury to a major mixed nerve, but this has subsequently been disproved by Nathan,[45] Kirklin,[25] and Shumacker,[58] who found that it was also caused by complete nerve lacerations. Doupe[14] in 1944 advanced the hypothesis that major causalgia was caused by the loss of the myelin sheath in the afferent sensory fibers in the partially injured nerve and this produced an "artificial synapse" that allowed a "short circuiting" of the afferent pain impulses and the efferent sympathetic nerve stimulation. Doupe described a physiologic breakdown of the normal insulating material around the afferent fibers as a "fiber interaction" between the normally nonmyelinated sympathetic efferent fibers and the recently demyelinated pain fibers (Fig. 47-9). With this

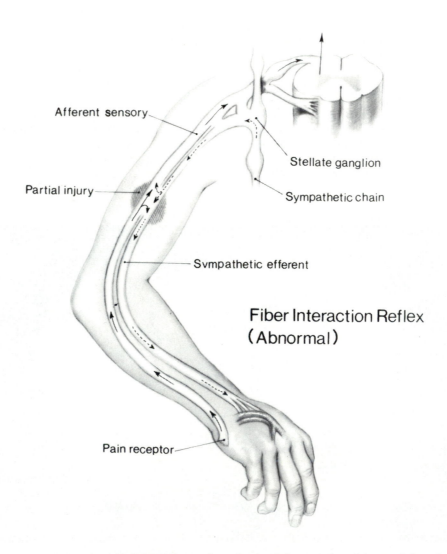

Afferent sensory

Partial injury

Stellate ganglion

Sympathetic chain

Sympathetic efferent

Fiber Interaction Reflex (Abnormal)

Pain receptor

FIG. 47-9. Doupe described a physiologic breakdown of myelin sheath in area of partial nerve injury that produced a "fiber interaction" of efferent and afferent impulses, which results in increased sympathetic nerve activity and increased pain. (From Lankford, L.L., and Thompson, J.E.: Reflex sympathetic dystrophy, upper and lower extremity: diagnosis and management. In American Academy of Orthopaedic Surgeons: Instructional course lectures, vol. 26, St. Louis, 1977, The C.V. Mosby Co.)

being the case, the efferent sympathetic fibers could be "short-circuited" in an antidromic direction and would be interpreted by the cerebral cortex as pain. Also, the afferent pain fibers with the loss of their myelin sheath could be "short-circuited" across the "artificial synapse" so that the pain impulses would then be turned distally (antidromic) as sympathetic fiber impulses and cause a greater sympathetic activity. Granit[21] in 1944 has shown in an experimental model that it is possible to produce this cross-stimulation effect from an "artificial synapse."

DIAGNOSTIC CRITERIA

It is of utmost importance to make an early diagnosis in cases of reflex sympathetic dystrophy because early treatment is much more effective than treatment at a later stage. This, at times, becomes somewhat difficult because of the varied symptoms in each of the three clinical stages and the variation of the symptoms in the five clinical types of RSD. It is also of utmost importance to rule out other conditions that are characteristically known to produce pain, swelling, stiffness, and dysfunction but do not come under the classification of reflex sympathetic dystrophy. As pointed out earlier, traumas or diseases occurring in patients who have a tendency toward increased fibrosis (such as patients with Dupuytren's contracture, arthritis, long-standing diabetes, the primary type of carpal tunnel syndrome, and other collagen disorders) will often produce a stiff-hand syndrome. Although it is not uncommon to see a "flare reaction" in these types of patients after injury or disease, it is very important not to confuse them with reflex sympathetic dystrophy.

The dominant characteristic of RSD is that the symptoms and signs are much more profound than ordinarily would be expected from a trauma or disease occurring in an otherwise normal individual. In a normal individual the signs and symptoms will improve with time, but in the patient with RSD they get progressively worse. The four cardinal symptoms and signs are as follows:

1. Pain
2. Swelling
3. Stiffness
4. Discoloration

The secondary symptoms and signs, which are most often present but not necessarily inevitable, are as follows:

1. Osseous demineralization
2. Sudomotor changes
3. Temperature changes
4. Trophic changes
5. Vasomotor instability
6. Palmar fibromatosis

If all four of the cardinal symptoms and signs are present and at least several of the secondary symptoms and signs are found and they exist to a degree much greater than normally expected, a *presumptive* diagnosis of reflex sympathetic dystrophy can be made. Actual *confirmation* of this diagnosis, however, comes after interruption of the sympathetic nerve reflex has produced some amelioration of the patient's condition. One cannot, however, rule out RSD upon a single attempt to interrupt the sympathetic reflex arc. At least three or more blocks with completely negative ef-

fects should be used so that RSD may be conclusively ruled out. It is also important to make sure that the attempted interruption in the sympathetic reflex arc has been technically successful as evidenced by Horner's sign and by warmth and dryness of the extremity.

ETIOLOGY

Because of the lack of confirmatory laboratory experimentation, the many theories of the etiology and genesis of reflex sympathetic dystrophy have yet to be proved. My clinical impression[29] is that the following three factors must occur concurrently before a patient can develop RSD:

1. Persistent painful lesion (trauma or disease)
2. Diathesis (predisposition, susceptibility, or inherent trait)
3. Abnormal sympathetic reflex

If all three of these conditions are present at the same time in the same patient, it is expected that reflex sympathetic dystrophy will occur. This explains why RSD develops in only a few persons even though their traumas and treatment may have been identical to those of patients who did not develop RSD.

Persistent painful lesion

A significant characteristic of RSD is that the magnitude of the inciting trauma or disease is not necessarily equivalent to the severity of the patient's symptoms and signs. In general, minor traumas will produce the minor-traumatic-dystrophy clinical type of RSD and the more severe traumas will produce the major traumatic dystrophy, but almost invariably one is struck by the fact that it is not reasonable to expect the very severe symptoms and signs that are sometimes produced from a very minor trauma. One usually finds himself asking the question, "How could this severe condition result from such a minor injury?"

Most persistent painful lesions that initiate RSD are of traumatic origin, but in some cases pain from a disease will also be sufficient to initiate the process, such as a severe flare-up of arthritis, an acute carpal tunnel syndrome, Pancoast's tumor, tissue ischemia, nerve entrapment, a heart attack, or stroke. Acute traumatic carpal tunnel syndrome has been the initiating persistent painful lesion in a high percentage of my patients with Colles' fracture who developed major traumatic dystrophy. The trauma, however, need not be very severe and may be as inconsequential as a mashed fingertip, a bruised nerve over the radial styloid, or an interphalangeal joint sprain.

Diathesis

I[29] have long believed that certain patients are susceptible to the development of reflex sympathetic dystrophy while others are not. There appears to be a predisposition, inherent characteristic, natural tendency, a bodily constitutional trait, or diathesis that allows some patients to develop reflex sympathetic dystrophy while others receiving the same degree of trauma are not so afflicted. The diathesis in all probability is an inherited trait, which cannot be changed. I have had as patients a mother and daughter who had Colles' fractures (many years apart), both of whom developed reflex sym-

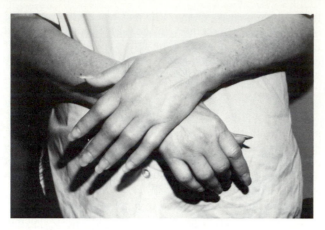

FIG. 47-10. This patient developed bilateral major traumatic type of reflex sympathetic dystrophy from bilateral traumatic carpal tunnel syndromes, which resulted from minimally displaced bilateral Colles' fractures. (From Lankford, L.L., and Thompson, J.E.: Reflex sympathetic dystrophy, upper and lower extremity: diagnosis and management. In American Academy of Orthopaedic Surgeons: Instructional course lectures, vol. 26, St. Louis, 1977, The C.V. Mosby Co.)

pathetic dystrophy after their fractures. Another patient in whom RSD developed in the lower extremity and again several years later in a traumatized upper extremity has been observed. I have also seen bilateral RSD occurring simultaneously from a bilateral Colles' fracture (Fig. 47-10). Coffman[9] reported in 1975 the occurrence of RSD in the same person on several occasions after different traumas.

Two different types of diathesis are recognized. The first diathesis is the tendency of the patient to be a "hypersympathetic reactor." These patients have increased sympathetic nerve activity.[48] When a history is being taken, the patient is always asked if he has sweaty palms (hyperhidrosis) or other evidence of increased sympathetic nerve activity, such as a history of pallor or excessive coolness of fingers and toes when they are exposed to colder temperatures. On physical examination one often finds evidence of peripheral vasoconstriction and poor capillary refill on the uninvolved extremity. Also, other historical evidence of vasomotor dysfunctions such as fainting, excessive blushing, or even migraine headaches is often obtained in patients with RSD.

The second diathesis has to do with the psychological makeup of the patient. This type of diathesis is more difficult to determine than the hypersympathetic reactor. However, in most patients with reflex sympathetic dystrophy it is possible to recognize that they have certain psychological traits that are often described by psychiatrists as "fearful, suspicious, emotionally labile, inadequate personality, chronic complainer, dependent personality, insecure and unstable personality." I almost never discover a psychological trait in a patient with RSD who is described as being stoic or a "Spartan." Patients who develop reflex sympathetic dystrophy also have the tendency to have a very low pain threshold. This type of patient will usually not be very cooperative in carrying out the doctor's orders, will think up many excuses for not doing what he is told, and will try

to control his own treatment and seek to place the blame for his condition on others.

One therefore would have to be suspicious that a patient has the diathesis for RSD if he has a very low pain threshold and cold, sweaty hands, asks a multitude of irrelevant questions, and tries to manipulate the doctor. This should not be construed to imply that patients with reflex sympathetic dystrophy are malingerers. The patient cannot control this diathesis and therefore cannot willfully cause this to happen to himself. However, patient gain or the emotional element can never be fully ruled out of any condition producing pain, stiffness, and dysfunction.

Abnormal sympathetic reflex

Even if a person had a normal tendency toward having increased sympathetic nerve activity, reflex sympathetic dystrophy could not take place unless a grossly abnormal situation arose in the sympathetic nerve reflex to perpetuate the extreme increase in sympathetic nerve activity for a prolonged period of time. It would therefore have to be an abnormal sympathetic reflex to cause this to happen.

There is a normal sympathetic reflex arc that comes into play with trauma. When afferent nerves transmit a message of pain from the extremity, these nerve fibers synapse in the posterior root ganglion and then again in the posterior horn and finally in the lateral horn, where the message of pain is transferred to the sympathetic nerve cell bodies. The sympathetic reflex is activated when efferent sympathetic impulses are sent out the anterior horn through the anterior root to the sympathetic chain and then through the white ramus into the sympathetic ganglion, where a synapse occurs; the postganglionic sympathetic fiber then leaves the ganglia through the gray ramus, where it enters the peripheral nerve and goes distally into the extremity to produce vasoconstriction of the small vessels (Fig. 47-11). This is a normal reflex, and it is the body's attempt to begin a process to return the injured tissue to normalcy.

The vasoconstrictive reflex is necessary to prevent excessive bleeding in the injured tissue, but after a few hours it gives way to vasodilation, which is a part of the reparative process in an orderly stepwise progression to healing. If for some reason, however, this normal sympathetic reflex arc does not shut down at the appropriate time but in fact continues on in an accelerated fashion, it will produce ultimately an intense degree of sympathetic nerve activity. The increased vasoconstriction produces ischemia in the tissue, which is painful and causes increased afferent pain impulses to be sent centrally, thus activating the sympathetic reflex arc, and increased sympathetic nerve activity results.[65] This "sympathetic-pain reflex" sets into motion the abnormal sympathetic reflex, which is necessary for the production of reflex sympathetic dystrophy. There are many theories as to the exact cause of this abnormal sympathetic reflex, but up to now none seems to present a satisfactory explanation.

PATHOGENESIS

The lack of a satisfactory laboratory experimental animal model has hampered the basic research necessary to help

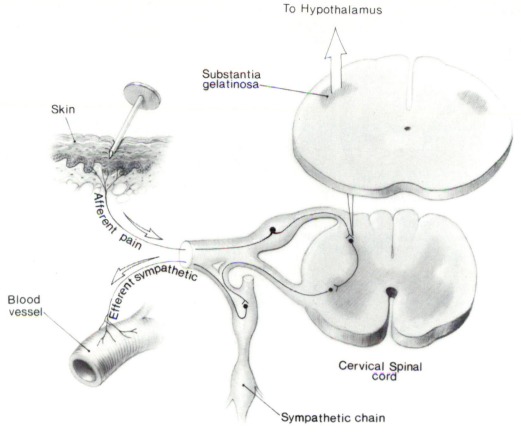

To Hypothalamus

Substantia gelatinosa

Skin

Afferent pain

Efferent sympathetic

Blood vessel

Cervical Spinal cord

Sympathetic chain

FIG. 47-11. A normal sympathetic nerve reflex arc is set into motion with any painful stimuli; it results in a temporary vasoconstrictive action of the small vessels. However, if this normal sympathetic reflex arc fails to shut down at the appropriate time, an abnormal sympathetic reflex may develop, thus producing one of the etiologic factors of reflex sympathetic dystrophy. (From Lankford, L.L., and Thompson, J.E.: Reflex sympathetic dystrophy, upper and lower extremity: diagnosis and management. In American Academy of Orthopaedic Surgeons: Instructional course lectures, vol. 26, St. Louis, 1977, The C.V. Mosby Co.)

answer some of the many questions concerning the pathogenicity of this enigmatic problem.

Livingston,[32] Gerard,[19] and Kennard[24] have further developed a concept first proposed by Lorente de Nó[34] that an abnormal sympathetic reflex was put into play because of an abnormal "feedback mechanism" that occurred in the "internuncial pool" of the posterior and lateral horns of the spinal cord. This increased sympathetic nerve activity producing tissue ischemia, which in turn generates more pain, turns into a "vicious cycle," which can certainly account for the severe pain and the increased sympathetic nerve activity seen in reflex sympathetic dystrophy (Fig. 47-12).

Pool[53] stimulated the proximal end of the distal segment of a severed sensory nerve and produced pain in the sensory distribution of this nerve and found that by blocking adjacent nerves with a local anesthesia he could eliminate the pain produced by stimulation of the cut nerve. This suggests that intensive sympathetic nerve fiber stimulation might well produce a pain-evoking substance. Chapman[8] produced a substance he called "neurokinin" by electrically stimulating the distal end of a divided nerve. He found that this substance was the mediator of neurogenic vasodilation of skin. This certainly could explain why in reflex sympathetic dystrophy we have some areas of vasoconstriction and at the same time in adjacent areas we have vasodilation. When neurokinin was injected subcutaneously, it produced a "flare" reaction, which lowered the pain threshold in the injected area. This might well help to explain the intense dysesthesia noted in patients with reflex sympathetic dystrophy when stimulated with light touch. Further evidence of the presence of the abnormal sympathetic reflex is given by Walker[66] and Procacci.[55]

It is generally agreed that afferent pain impulse projection centrally is produced through the small-diameter, slow-conducting, nonmyelinated C fibers and the thinly myelinated A-delta fibers, whereas the heavily myelinated large-diameter A-alpha fibers are responsible for conducting light pressure and proprioceptive sense. Melzack and Wall[37] in 1965 helped to give us some understanding of how some people can perceive a great deal of pain with a minimal stimulus and others feel little or no pain. Their "gate-control" theory of pain proposed that the large-diameter (light

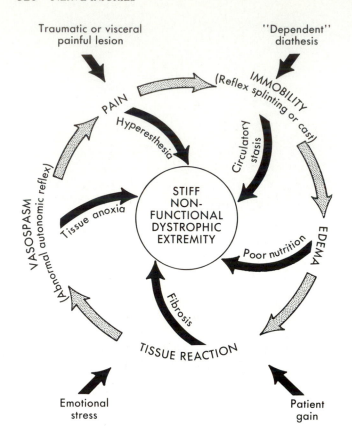

Fig. 47-12. Vicious cycle is produced when tissue ischemia produces greater tissue reaction and pain secondary to vasoconstrictive action of increased sympathetic nerve activity, resulting in a painful, stiff, swollen, and dystrophic extremity, as seen in reflex sympathetic dystrophy. (From Lankford, L.L., and Thompson, J.E.: Reflex sympathetic dystrophy, upper and lower extremity: diagnosis and management. In American Academy of Orthopaedic Surgeons: Instructional course lectures, vol. 26, St. Louis, 1977, The C.V. Mosby Co.)

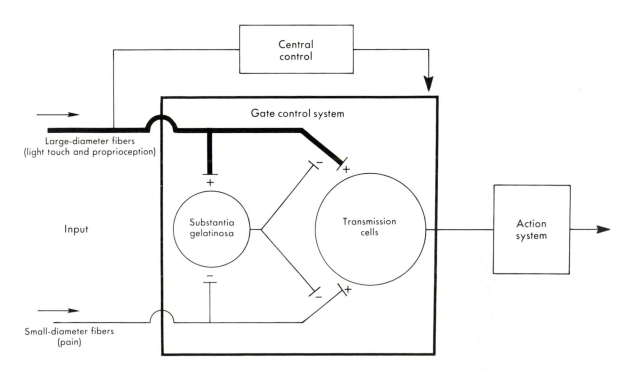

Fig. 47-13. Melzack and Wall's gate-control theory of pain. Melzack and Wall have theorized that large-diameter fibers of light touch and proprioceptive sense impulses can "close the gate" to slower-acting, small-diameter, non-myelinated nerve fibers of pain. On the other hand, absence of large-diameter fiber stimulation will "open the gate" for pain impulses to be projected centrally so that a minimal pain impulse is interpreted as severe pain by cerebral cortex. (From Melzack, R., and Wall, P.D.: Science **150:**971-979, Nov. 1965.)

touch pressure and proprioceptive sense) afferent fibers have the ability to "close the gate" on the slower conducting nonmyelinated C fibers, which conduct pain. This "modulation" of pain impulses takes place in the substantia gelatinosa of the dorsal horn in the spinal cord. They further propose that there is a central control of the gating mechanism that is activated in the higher centers of the central nervous system that can influence the forward projection of pain (Fig. 47-13). Although not all of the theories of this gating mechanism have been proved in the laboratory, it goes a long way to help with our understanding of this complex problem. The central control mechanism that alters the forward projection of pain helps to explain how psychological and emotional factors can greatly influence the amount and quality of pain perceived by some patients. It also helps to explain how light touch and gentle exercise tends to eliminate pain in reflex sympathetic dystrophy and why painful stimuli will cause a self-sustaining aggravation of pain. Casey[7] in 1973 defined pain as "the private experience of unpleasantness and the interpretation of the stimulation in terms of present and past experience. Moreover, pain is profoundly modified by attention, emotions, and suggestion and by pathologic conditions of a central or peripheral nervous system that can increase or decrease the intensity."

TREATMENT

The old axiom that early diagnosis and early treatment produce the best result has never been more correct than in the case of reflex sympathetic dystrophy. Delay in starting the treatment because of the difficulty of diagnosis is certain to produce a greater residual in the form of pain, stiffness, and dysfunction. It is therefore important to rule out other forms of dystrophies that produce similar but not so severe symptoms so that the appropriate treatment for RSD may be given without delay.

It has already been stated that there are three etiologic factors (persistent painful lesion, diathesis, and abnormal sympathetic reflex) that must be present at the same time before reflex sympathetic dystrophy can occur. The treatment is therefore to remove one or more of these factors, and one would hope the vicious cycle can be broken. Although this may stop the forward progress of the disease, it cannot return the patient to normalcy. It would follow therefore that treatment should include attempts to eliminate the initiating painful state, modify the patient's diathesis if possible, and interrupt the abnormal sympathetic reflex.

Of these three approaches to the treatment, the elimination of the abnormal sympathetic reflex is usually the easiest to perform and by all odds the most direct and successful approach. Depending on the severity and the duration of RSD, this may be accomplished with the use of one or more of the following regimens: use of sympatholytic drugs, local anesthetic blocks on somatic nerves or "trigger points," pharmacologic or chemical blocks of the stellate ganglion and the upper thoracic chain, or use of an upper thoracic sympathectomy.*

---

*See references 3, 5, 25, 36, 58, 59, and 68.

Sympatholytic drugs

Sympatholytic medications are alpha-adrenergic blocking agents, which effectively reduce the sympathetic vasoconstrictive action of the peripheral vessels in the involved extremity. This may, at the same time, produce orthostatic hypotension and should therefore be used with caution. Phenoxybenzamine (Dibenzyline)[11,15,17] seems to be the most effective alpha-adrenergic blocking agent, with the only really significant complication being orthostatic hypotension with excessive dosing. A 10-mg capsule is given orally twice a day as a starting dose. If there has been no adverse effect after 5 days, this can be increased to three times a day; and after another 5 days if RSD symptoms are not distinctly improved and no orthostatic hypotension has occurred, the patient may be tried on four times a day. However, with the occurrence of any undesirable side effect, the medication should be either reduced or stopped. As with any medication one should not operate a machine or drive a car until he has had time to determine whether the medication would disturb him in this activity. When a patient is believed either to have the diathesis for reflex sympathetic dystrophy or if he has an obvious vasospastic tendency, phenoxybenzamine may be used prophylactically to help reduce the sympathetic nerve activity and possibly prevent the occurrence of RSD.

Phentolamine (Regitine) and tolazoline (Priscoline) are also alpha-adrenergic blocking agents, but they have definite disadvantages over Dibenzyline. Propranolol (Inderal) has not been found effective in my experience, and it also has some undesirable side effects.

Reserpine is also used for sympathetic blockage because of the catecholamine (norepinephrine)–depleting action at the neurotransmitter junction on the vessel wall. Reserpine may be given by intra-arterial injection[54] and regionally by intravenous injection[60] but requires considerable expertise for its use. Oral reserpine (Serpasil) has also been used for the treatment of RSD, but it certainly has limited application because the effective dosage may also bring on undesirable side effects.

Guanethidine, which prevents the storage of catecholamines in the sympathetic nerve terminals at the neuroeffector junction, has been used experimentally as a sympatholytic drug with mixed success. Although it has been used clinically in Europe for several years, it has not been released for general use in this country.

Somatic nerve blocks

A pharmacologic somatic nerve block with a local anesthetic agent does produce an interruption of the abnormal sympathetic reflex inasmuch as the somatic nerves do carry the sympathetic nerve fibers and a blockade at this point would, of course, prevent the increased sympathetic stimulation from reaching the involved area. It is also of benefit because it does, in addition, knock out any afferent nerve impulses of pain that would otherwise help fuel the vicious cycle. Somatic nerve blocks are more commonly used for the minor types of RSD such as minor causalgia and minor traumatic dystrophy. One may accomplish this by giving a median, ulnar, or radial nerve block at the wrist, or even in some cases a metacarpal block in the hand will suffice.

Ordinarily lidocaine (Xylocaine) or mepivacaine (Carbocaine) is the pharmacologic agent used for the first somatic nerve blocks so that its benefits can be definitely established, and then any future blocks are usually given with bupivacaine (Marcaine). All ordinary precautions are observed, of course, with the use of any local anesthetic, and the patients should be made aware that since their digits are anesthetic they must take precautions to avoid injury. Axillary blocks may also be given as well as median, ulnar, and radial nerve blocks at the wrist. These are less desirable, however, because they leave a greater area anesthetic and temporarily paralyzed. The effective length of time of the sympathetic blockade increases, however, the more proximally the block is performed. The more distal blocks are accepted better by patients than are the more proximal blocks, and they can be given two and three times a week without causing local irritation.

Periodic perineural infusion

Omer and Thomas[46,47] described a method of implanting a small flexible catheter into the site of a "trigger point" by insertion of a large-bore hypodermic needle under local anesthesia into the involved area and periodically infusing it with a small amount of local anesthesia. This method can be quite effective if the trigger point is easily delineated. The same technique can also be used to infuse larger nerves in the forearm, such as the median, ulnar, and radial ones. The exact details of this technique can be found in an anesthesia textbook.

Stellate ganglion blocks

Certainly the most effective treatment for reflex sympathetic dystrophy is the interruption of the abnormal sympathetic reflex, and the most effective way to accomplish this is through blockade of all the sympathetic efferent impulses into the extremity by a stellate ganglion block. Although this prevents any sympathetic nerve activity in the extremity, it does not block out any somatic nerve and will therefore not produce a temporary anesthesia or paralysis (unless there is unusual spreading of the anesthetic agent). If a technically satisfactory block has been accomplished, there will be a generalized warming, drying, and return to a more normal coloration of the skin of the entire upper extremity. When the upper two thirds of the stellate ganglion has been adequately perfused with the local anesthetic agent, Horner's sign with drooping of the eyelid, enophthalmos, hyperemia of the conjunctival vessels, constriction of the pupil, and drying and warming of the ipsilateral side of the face will occur. If only the upper thoracic sympathetic ganglia have been blocked, it is possible for the extremity to have been effectively sympathectomized without the presence of Horner's sign, which is usually the hallmark of a successful stellate ganglion block. With the accomplishment of a successful blockade of the sympathetic impulses, the patients are generally amazed at the immediate change in the condition of their hands. There is usually a very prompt and distinct improvement of pain and a generalized feeling of well-being. In our Hand Rehabilitation Unit, for the last several years we have obtained measurements of joint motion, volume, and grip strength of the extremities before

and after stellate ganglion blocks, and it has been demonstrated that improvement in all three categories is generally evidenced. Even though there may still be some pain on strenuous joint motion, almost always the burning or constant pain has been relieved after the block. It is only after satisfactory sympathetic blockade that an effective exercise program is beneficial to the patient. Before the block, the pain is usually so great that the patient cannot participate in a vigorous exercise program. It is not wise to subject the patient to strenuous passive exercise before the sympathetic blockade because it is usually very painful and this increased pain simply accelerates the "pain–sympathetic reflex" cycle, and the condition is actually made worse rather than better. The sympathetic block is not only therapeutic but also acts to confirm the diagnosis of reflex sympathetic dystrophy. If, on the other hand, the block has been technically unsatisfactory (as evidenced by the absence of drying and warming of the extremity and Horner's sign), or has failed to produce subjective or objective improvement, it cannot on the basis of one block rule out the diagnosis of reflex sympathetic dystrophy. In my experience, there has been one patient who had four technically successful blocks without any subjective improvement but on the fifth and subsequent blocks showed dramatic improvement.

Generally, not more than one or two blocks are given each week unless the patient is in very severe distress. Only rarely can this condition be completely reversed after only one block. The average number of blocks necessary for the reversal of this abnormal sympathetic reflex is between four and five stellate ganglion blocks. On one occasion it was necessary to use 16 blocks before the forward progress of the disease was reversed. The number of blocks necessary for benefit certainly depends on the duration and the severity of the condition. When blocks alone are used, there is usually a fairly good chance of producing the desired benefit to the patient if sympathetic blockade is started within the first 3 to 4 months. Much later on, however, it is less likely that the sole use of stellate ganglion blocks will be sufficient, and a surgical sympathectomy would need to be considered.

Stellate ganglion block technique. The stellate ganglion block should not be performed by anyone who is not thoroughly familiar with the anatomy and the possible complications of the block. The stellate ganglion lies anterior to the seventh cervical lateral mass and may be located when one first palpates Chassaignac's tubercle, which lies at the level of the sixth cervical vertebral lateral mass. In essence, this is approximately 4 cm lateral to the midcervical line and 4 cm superior to the sternal notch. Before doing the stellate ganglion block, one must be prepared to treat any complication such as an intravascular injection of the anesthetic agent, a "time overdose" (a rapid absorption of an otherwise normal amount of the anesthetic agent), a drug idiosyncrasy reaction, or an anaphylactic shock reaction. Oxygen also should be available in case a pneumothorax has been inadvertently produced. Details of the treatment of a complication of a stellate ganglion block will not be given at this point, but one must understand that a means of giving oxygen and intravenous medication to stabilize the blood pressure should be available.

Moore[43] fully describes the anterior paratracheal ap-

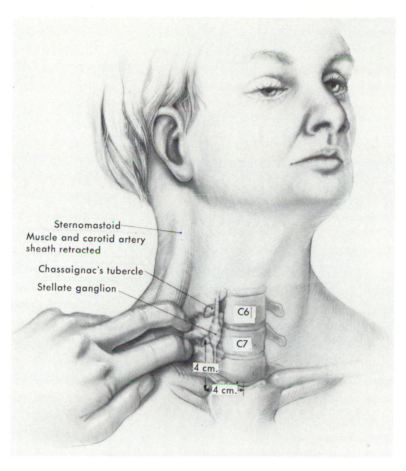

FIG. 47-14. Stellate ganglion of sympathetic chain is located opposite seventh cervical vertebra, which is palpated less than 2 cm inferior to Chassaignac's tubercle and can be found when sternocleidomastoid muscle and great vessels are retracted laterally. (From Lankford, L.L., and Thompson, J.E.: Reflex sympathetic dystrophy, upper and lower extremity: diagnosis and management. In American Academy of Orthopaedic Surgeons: Instructional course lectures, vol. 26, St. Louis, 1977, The C.V. Mosby Co.)

proach, which I favor, and for a detailed discussion of this approach I recommend that one use this reference. It is preferred that the first block be done with a short-acting local anesthetic agent with 1:200,000 epinephrine concentration. The short-acting anesthetic agent may be either 1% lidocaine (Xylocaine) or 1% mepivacaine (Carbocaine) for the initial block, and subsequent blocks may be accomplished with 0.5% bupivacaine (Marcaine). The patient should be positioned in a 45-degree semi-Fowler's position with the head not using a pillow and turned 45 degrees to the contralateral side. Chassaignac's tubercle is located by deep palpation while the nondominant index and long fingers are retracting the sternocleidomastoid muscle and the great vessels in the carotid sheath laterally (Fig. 47-14). After sterile preparation and with sterile technique being used throughout, a small wheel of local anesthesia is given with a short 25-gauge needle on a 10 ml Luer-Lok syringe. The point of injection is about 1½ cm inferior to Chassaignac's tubercle, which would make it immediately over the seventh cervical lateral mass. The 25-gauge ¾-inch (2 cm) needle is directed straight posteriorly without angulation and should

touch the seventh cervical lateral mass. After this bony landmark has been touched with the needle, one should then withdraw the needle 0.5 to 0.8 cm to clear the prevertebral fascia and muscles and after adequate aspiration (to check for intravascular penetration) inject a test dose of 2 ml (Fig. 47-15). An observation period of 1 minute should be allowed, and if no adverse effects such as ringing in the ear, dizziness, nausea, or cardiac palpitations are detected, 3 ml of the local anesthetic is slowly injected without displacement of the needle. Another period of observation of 1 minute should be allowed, and if no uncomfortable sensations have occurred, the remaining 5 ml of the local anesthetic agent should be injected slowly. A similar technique is employed when bupivacaine is used. In most cases, 10 ml of the anesthetic agent is adequate to get a technically satisfactory block. The first signs of improvement may be apparent within 5 minutes of removal of the needle, but it is not unusual for benefit not to occur for 30 to 45 minutes. Bilateral blocks should not be attempted at the same time for fear of pneumothorax or a bilateral paralysis of the recurrent laryngeal nerve. The patient should remain in the

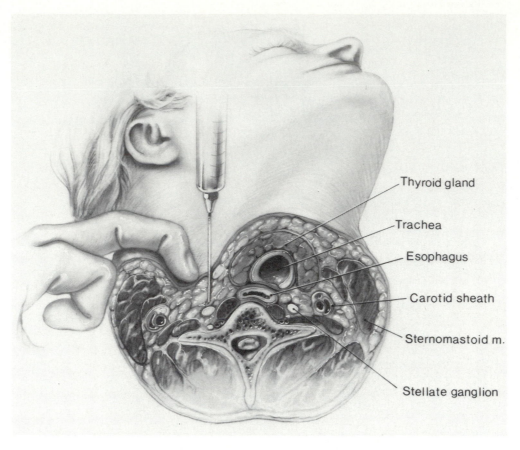

Thyroid gland

Trachea

Esophagus

Carotid sheath

Sternomastoid m.

Stellate ganglion

FIG. 47-15. Anterior paratracheal approach to stellate ganglion is made by inserting needle straight down to seventh cervical lateral mass and then withdrawing it about 0.5 to 0.8 cm to clear prevertebral fascia and muscles. (From Lankford, L.L.: Reflex sympathetic dystrophy. In Evarts, C.McC., editor: Surgery of the musculoskeletal system, New York, 1983, Churchill Livingstone, Inc.)

semi-Fowler's position for at least 30 minutes after completion of the block. Although the normal physiologic interruption of the function of nerve fibers using lidocaine (Xylocaine) and mepivacaine (Carbocaine) is approximately 1½ to 2½ hours and the length of action of bupivacaine (Marcaine) may last from 9 to 18 hours, the benefit as far as the interruption of the abnormal sympathetic reflex is concerned may well last from 1 to 3 days before the sympathetic nerve hyperactivity has regenerated itself to the point that the abnormal sympathetic reflex has again been produced. Because of irritation of the tissues surrounding the stellate ganglion, it is seldom advisable to give more than two blocks per week. If a successful block has been produced, the patient should then be sent to the hand therapy department for physical treatment.

Continuous stellate blockade

Betcher, Bean, and Casten[4] in 1953 described a technique for continuous blocking of the stellate ganglion when it is necessary to produce a longer period of blockade of the sympathetic efferent impulses. Although continuous stellate blockade is not ordinarily advised, it may well be necessary if the patient is having a great deal of pain or is too appre-

hensive to tolerate interrupted stellate ganglion blocks. A 16-gauge needle is inserted down to the stellate ganglion under local anesthesia and with image intensification roentgenographic control. After the needle has been introduced down to the seventh cervical lateral mass, it is again withdrawn a little over 0.5 cm and a flexible polyvinyl venicatheter is inserted into the 16-gauge needle and the large-bore needle is then withdrawn. The catheter is taped into place and the exact position of the tip of the catheter can be determined by a very small injection of absorbable radiopaque solution. A female Luer-Lok adapter is then attached to the catheter and periodic injections of any of the above-mentioned anesthetic agents are given. In between injections a sterile adapter is used to maintain the sterility. With the catheter taped securely into place the patient may become ambulatory but is requested to minimize motions of the neck and shoulder to prevent dislodgment of the catheter. If bupivacaine (Marcaine) is used, injections need not be more frequent than 18- to 24-hour intervals. The shorter acting anesthetic agents would need to be injected more often. While the patient is experiencing the benefit of the blockade of the abnormal sympathetic reflex, he should take full advantage of it to perform his exercises and functional activities. If the patient should develop distressing hoarseness or difficulty in swallowing, the catheter should be removed and the patient not allowed to take anything orally until the swallowing function has been regained. The catheter may be left in place for 2 weeks or until there is any evidence of infection around the catheter.

Sympathectomy

If stellate ganglion blocks have not been started early enough in the course of reflex sympathetic dystrophy, it may not be possible to break up adequately the abnormal sympathetic reflex with blocks alone. This is especially true in the very severe cases of major traumatic dystrophy and causalgia. If definite benefit has accrued from at least one to three blocks and yet the duration of benefit is not long enough or the relief of pain is less than complete, and especially if the duration of this disease has been at least 4 to 5 months, in all likelihood a surgical sympathectomy will be required in order to give the patient the desired relief. In many cases, one can reach a decision to do surgery after the second block, but at other times one may need to use four to six blocks before determining whether the intermittent blockade will be sufficient or a surgical sympathectomy will be necessary. If one believes that surgical relief of a carpal tunnel syndrome or some type of reconstructive surgery will be required, I regard that as an indication for sympathectomy. The first four thoracic sympathetic ganglia should be removed for complete ablation of the abnormal sympathetic reflex. If only the upper thoracic ganglia are removed, Horner's syndrome is seldom seen. Some techniques include removal of the lower third of the stellate ganglion with relatively little risk of producing permanent Horner's syndrome. One should expect, however, that the patient with reflex sympathetic dystrophy has a diathesis that may make him more likely to complain of pain around the sympathectomy operative site. Fortunately, this postsurgical neuritis seldom lasts more than a few weeks.

After a successful sympathectomy, the greatest benefit to the patient has been the reversal of the process that has given him so much torment. There is usually a dramatic relief of pain, especially of burning or constant pain, though some pain on joint motion may continue, at least for a while. Concomitantly there is a decrease in swelling, improvement in the coloration, and some slow improvement in motion and function. At least after the elimination of the abnormal sympathetic reflex, it is then possible for the patient to do the exercises necessary to improve motion and function (which he was unable to do satisfactorily while he was in the grips of this consuming pain). McGrath[35] in 1974 reported that blood flow in the hands of a sympathectomized patient was increased from sixfold to tenfold over the preoperative state.

On rare occasions when a sympathectomy is needed but the patient for some reason is unable to undergo a surgical operation, a chemical sympathectomy may be indicated wherein the stellate ganglion block is performed with either 50% alcohol or 6% phenol to produce a semipermanent sympathectomy.[5] This, of course, is a somewhat dangerous procedure and should be done only by a person with great expertise in the use of alcohol and phenol for nerve blocks.

Leriche[31] first alluded to the possible connection of an abnormal sympathetic nervous system and Mitchell's causalgia. In 1916, he did a postganglionic sympathectomy of the brachial artery by stripping the adventitia away from the artery. This did provide some relief but only temporarily. Spurling,[61] however, in 1928 did the first successful upper thoracic sympathectomy by removing a portion of the upper thoracic chain. Kwan[28] in 1931 also successfully treated reflex sympathetic dystrophy with an upper thoracic chain sympathectomy. The surgical technique for upper thoracic sympathectomy should, of course, be done by someone with special training and will not be discussed in detail in this volume. There are, however, three general types of upper thoracic sympathectomy that are being currently used: (1) the posterior approach, which was first described by Adson[1] and was later modified by Smithwick[59] in 1940; (2) the transthoracic approaches through the axilla suggested by Adkins[2] and Palumbo;[51] and (3) more recently the thoracic endoscopic sympathectomy as described by Kux[27] in 1978. The supraclavicular anterior cervical approach is seldom used at this time unless the posterior or transthoracic approaches are contraindicated by a scar.

ADJUNCTIVE TREATMENT

Certainly, the most important treatment for reflex sympathetic dystrophy is the interruption of the abnormal sympathetic reflex arc,[68] and this should be done as soon as possible by one of the above-mentioned methods, whether it be a sympathetic nerve block or a surgical sympathectomy. There are, however, other forms of treatment that are helpful and are based on the three etiologic factors. I should emphasize that these methods of treatment should not be used to the exclusion of the blockade of the sympathetic reflex arc.

Treatment of a painful lesion

Since the persistently painful lesion that initiated the reflex sympathetic dystrophy continues to fuel this "vicious cycle," it may well be of some help to try to eliminate the pain. This is expected to decelerate the vicious cycle. One should do no surgery, however, without making sure that the capability of eliminating the abnormal reflex arc exists. It goes without saying that tight casts or casts with pressure points on bony prominences should be promptly rectified. If there has been painful pressure over a nerve, the cast can be windowed and local injections of an anesthetic agent used on this trigger point. A painful amputation stump may require revision so that there is provision of a loose flap coverage or dissection of a neuroma. I would not, however, advise significant shortening of a ray with the mistaken impression that the neuroma can be eliminated by further amputation. It is especially recommended that a ray amputation not be done for treatment of a painful neuroma. The neuroma should be treated with repeated local blocks of an anesthetic agent. If a "neurodesis" (binding down of a nerve distal to a joint) appears to be causing considerable pain, this may be completely resected proximally in the case of a dorsal superficial sensory branch of the radial or ulnar nerve or of the palmar branch of the median nerve. If the nerve in question is a digital nerve, a nerve graft can be

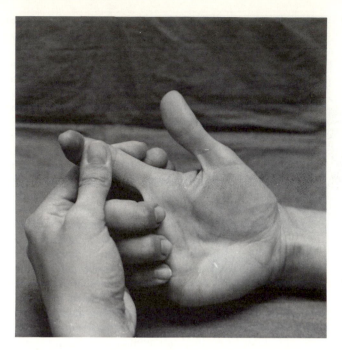

FIG. 47-17. Flexion exercises should be done gently but with 10-second sustained effort and maximum power just short of pain. Note that proximal two joints are being held in extension so that all of tendon excursion will be used to flex the distal interphalangeal joint.

all planes of motion (extension, flexion, radial and ulnar deviation, and supination and pronation). If shoulder and elbow joints have also stiffened, they too are exercised.

At first the patient should have a volume measurement of the hand taken before and after the exercise periods, to make sure the exercises are not done too vigorously. Later on, the need for frequent volume measurement is not so great. With each visit to the therapy department, accurate measurements of active flexion and extension movements of the joints are made and recorded so that the hand therapist can closely monitor the patient's progress or lack of progress. If necessary the exercise program may then be modified. When the patient is able to show some improvement without any flare-ups in the part involved, his exercise period is then increased to 5 minutes out of each 30 minutes while he is awake.

Heat

In many cases, gentle heat can be used effectively to reduce muscle spasm and to allow the patient to do his exercises with less pain and a greater gain of motion. Heat is helpful, however, only if it is used with elevation. Heat with the extremity in dependence should not be used because this will cause stagnation in the lymphatic and venous system, which will result in greater swelling. This would then eliminate the use of the whirlpool bath in the treatment of RSD for fear of causing increased swelling and reaction. Hot, wet towels, the paraffin bath, and a heating pad all can be used with elevation, however, and can easily be applied at home by the patient after sufficient instructions have been given by the therapist. Swelling can also be

reduced with the use of the thermoelastic glove, which will provide warmth and a gentle compression to help control swelling and reduce pain. Patients should be warned that they should avoid cold temperatures because this will increase vasoconstriction; they should therefore always wear warm gloves when going outside in cold weather. Since it has also been shown that smoking of tobacco produces tissue ischemia by increasing vasoconstriction,[9] they should be advised to stop smoking so that at least this factor can be removed from the many causes of tissue ischemia in the patient with RSD.

Transcutaneous nerve stimulation

As already pointed out above, some benefit may well occur from the use of transcutaneous nerve stimulation over the trigger points, and instructions for this are given to the patient by the hand therapist. The patient should wear the stimulation unit while he is doing his exercises and functional activities. It is frequently necessary for the therapist to change the position of the electrodes so that the patient can obtain maximum benefit.

Splinting

The purpose of splinting at first is to rest the hand, to relieve pain on motion, and to relieve muscle spasm. The splints should be light and should be made of a thermoplastic material so that they can be frequently reheated and changed in position. The ultimate goal is to return the position of the hand to the "resting-hand" or "balanced-hand" position, which is approximately 45 degrees of wrist extension, slight ulnar deviation of the wrist, 70 degrees of flexion in the metacarpophalangeal joint and 30 degrees of flexion in the proximal interphalangeal joint. The reason we call this the resting-hand or balanced-hand position is that it is the result of all the forces exerted by the extrinsic muscle pull, the intrinsic muscle forces, and the static forces. This position would then be in a balanced state or a resting state. This is the position where there are fewer deforming forces being exerted on the joints. There are also fewer pathologic forces present when the hand is in this position.

The wrist is the "keystone" of the positioning of the hand, and one cannot expect to reduce the extension contractures of the metacarpophalangeal joints or the flexion contractures of the proximal interphalangeal joints without first getting the wrist into extension. To accomplish this, a volar thermoplastic splint with Velcro straps is customized for the patient with as much extension of the wrist as the patient can comfortably tolerate (Fig. 47-18).

As time goes on, the splint is periodically reheated and the wrist extension is increased. After reducing the wrist flexion contracture and getting the wrist up into at least mild extension, one can then become more vigorous in reducing extension contractures of the metacarpophalangeal joints and flexion contractures of the proximal interphalangeal joints. This reduction is accomplished with a dorsal thermoplastic splint with an outrigger and rubber-band slings to produce a gentle extension force on the interphalangeal joints. It can be achieved, however, only if an equal or greater force is exerted on flexing of the metacarpophalangeal joints. This exertion is done by use of a lumbrical bar

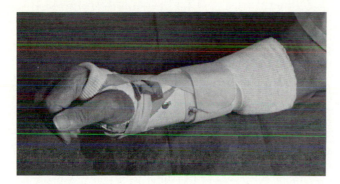

FIG. 47-18. Every effort should be made to obtain wrist extension, since this is keystone of mobilization of hand. Thermoplastic volar wrist splint should be used so that it can be reheated periodically to obtain increased extension of wrist.

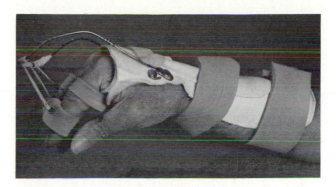

FIG. 47-19. Claw-hand deformities are splinted with a dorsal wrist splint and a dorsal outrigger and slings to produce extension in the proximal interphalangeal joints, but flexion slings must be used on the metacarpophalangeal joints to prevent hyperextension of these joints.

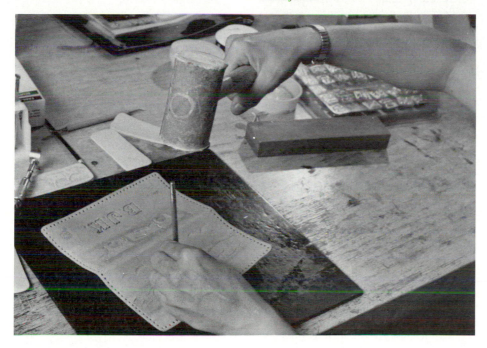

FIG. 47-20. After some motion and power are regained with exercises and splinting, functional activities should be begun in order to teach the patient how to use his hand again. Initially, functional activities are very simple, but they gradually become more sophisticated, requiring greater motion, power, and dexterity.

that presses down on the dorsum of the proximal segments of the fingers (to produce metacarpophalangeal joint flexion) with the same or greater force than is used to extend the interphalangeal joints. This can also be accomplished by use of flexion rubber bands and slings affixed to a wristlet band so that a very respectable flexion force can be applied to the metacarpophalangeal joints (Fig. 47-19).

These dynamic splints, of course, exert passive motion on the joint, and our rule about never allowing a passive force to become painful certainly applies to splinting. Pain produced by an ill-fitting splint or splint adjusted too tightly can be just as detrimental to the patient's stiff hand as a painful passive manipulation. The splints should be worn most of the time but should be removed every 30 minutes for the prescribed exercise program.

Functional activities

In many cases, the patient with RSD has a very poor self-image and is quite despondent over his wretched condition. Many patients have given up any hope of using their hands again and have, in fact, produced a psychological amputation of the part. It is therefore extremely important to teach the patient how to use his hand again and how to achieve useful function for himself. When the hand is very stiff, certainly there will be only a few types of functional activities in which the patient may participate.

In the beginning, activity may be as simple as placing wooden rings over round pegs or stacking blocks, but as better motion is accomplished and the patient has more confidence, the therapist will be able to teach him to do more sophisticated functional activities (Fig. 47-20). The therapist needs to be very observant so that he can pick up any new degree of motion or power developed by the patient, which can then be put to work in doing a different and more advanced type of functional activity. The therapist should be one step ahead of the patient in setting goals for physical accomplishments. Each new accomplishment by the patient is acclaimed with pride and elation, and this spurs him on to even greater heights. The realization by the patient that he has actually made something and performed some useful function provides him with a great psychological boost. Eventually the hand therapist should have the patient doing functional activities that simulate the type of work he will be doing when he returns to his employment.

REHABILITATIVE SURGERY

It should be the goal of the hand surgeon and the hand therapist to return motion, strength, and function of the hand to as nearly normal a state as possible. In most instances, it is not realistic to expect that this can be completely accomplished with physical methods of exercise, massage, and splinting.

At some point in the recovery of the patient, evaluation must be made according to the needs of the patient as to what degree of motion is required and to what extent a contracture can be acceptable for the required degree of function necessary for the patient's well-being. One should have a very limited expectation of regaining a considerable degree of motion after rehabilitative surgery, but at times it may be deemed necessary to gain even a few degrees of motion so that the patient is provided with his required extent of function. There are therefore some very restricted indications for rehabilitative surgery to regain motion in the patient with reflex sympathetic dystrophy though this in general should be discouraged.

One should do surgery of any kind only under the protection of either an upper thoracic sympathectomy or stellate ganglion block to eliminate the abnormal sympathetic reflex. Also the surgery should be delayed until the patient's pain has disappeared or until the reactivity and the excessive fibrosis in the joints have diminished as much as possible and the tissues around the joints have returned to a state of homeostasis to the greatest degree possible. Rehabilitative surgery also should not be done so long as the patient shows progressive improvement with the exercise and splinting and functional activity regimens.

The types of surgical procedures most likely to provide the patient with improved motion are as follows:
1. Capsulotomies of metacarpophalangeal joints
2. Capsulotomies of the proximal interphalangeal joint (with or without resection of the volar plate)
3. Capsulotomy of the volar wrist joint to relieve flexion contracture; tenolysis of the flexor tendon with release of the transverse carpal ligament
4. Resection of the tenodesed flexor digitorum superficialis tendon at the level of the proximal interphalangeal joint

If the wrist cannot be passively moved into extension, the transverse carpal ligament should not be simply incised or excised but should be lengthened by the step-cut method so that it will not be binding on the tendons or the nerve

but will still function to prevent the tendons from "falling out" of the carpal tunnel. Better results with proximal interphalangeal joint capsulotomies are obtained when the contracture is in extension rather than in flexion.

The exact details of these surgical procedures are found in Chapter 15 and are not repeated here. When the operator starts out to do any of the above-mentioned surgical procedures, he must be prepared to do all of them if necessary. In other words, if he does only a capsulotomy but a tenolysis of the flexor tendons is also indicated, he will not obtain benefit by doing *only* the capsulotomy; instead, he must do everything necessary at that time to regain motion. Postoperatively, very early motion should be started. If the patient's reflex sympathetic dystrophy was eliminated with stellate ganglion blocks only, it is advisable for the patient to have another two to three blocks to help prevent the regeneration of RSD.

SUMMARY

1. "Reflex sympathetic dystrophy" should be the name used for all of the vasomotor-trophic disturbances, which have been given various names in the past.
2. These three etiological conditions must be present at the same time for reflex sympathetic dystrophy to develop:
   a. Persistent painful lesion
   b. Diathesis (patient's susceptibility)
   c. Abnormal sympathetic reflex
3. These are the five clinical types of reflex sympathetic dystrophy (listed in ascending order of severity):
   a. Minor causalgia
   b. Minor traumatic dystrophy
   c. Shoulder-hand syndrome
   d. Major traumatic dystrophy
   e. Major causalgia
4. In order for one to make a presumptive diagnosis of reflex sympathetic dystrophy, these four cardinal symptoms and signs should be present:
   a. Pain
   b. Swelling
   c. Stiffness
   d. Discoloration
5. At least several of the following secondary symptoms and signs must also be present before a presumptive diagnosis of reflex sympathetic dystrophy can be made:
   a. Osteoporosis
   b. Sudomotor changes
   c. Temperature changes
   d. Trophic changes
   e. Vasomotor instability
   f. Palmar fasciitis
6. The dominant distinguishing feature of reflex sympathetic dystrophy is the fact that all the symptoms and signs are very much more severe than would ordinarily be expected for a similar type of inciting painful trauma or disease in an otherwise normal individual.
7. The most important treatment of reflex sympathetic dystrophy is some type of interruption of the sympathetic reflex arc so that the abnormal sympathetic reflex is eliminated.

8. The earlier the sympathetic reflex arc is eliminated, the better the result.

9. A confirmed diagnosis of reflex sympathetic dystrophy can only be made when the interruption of the sympathetic reflex arc has been shown to produce at least a definite measure of improvement.

10. There is a high incidence of traumatic carpal tunnel syndrome occurring in the major traumatic dystrophy type of reflex sympathetic dystrophy; when this condition is found to be present, the compression of the nerve should be relieved surgically.

11. No surgery should be performed without having the "protective umbrella" of either a sympathectomy or a stellate ganglion block.

12. The hand therapist should use great care to avoid any painful active or passive exercise on the part of the patient and should be equally as cautious to make sure that no pain is created by the splinting program. The therapist should be only a teacher and not a manipulator.

13. Indications for reconstructive surgery to regain motion should be very restrictive, and the expectations should be limited.

REFERENCES

1. Adson, A.W., and Brown, G.E.: Raynaud's disease of upper extremities: successful treatment by resection of sympathetic cervicothoracic and second thoracic ganglions and intervening trunk, J.A.M.A. **92**:444-449, 1929.
2. Atkins, H.J.B.: Sympathectomy by axillary approach, Lancet **1**:538-539, 1954.
3. Barnes, R.: The role of sympathectomy in the treatment of causalgia, J. Bone Joint Surg. **35B**:172-180, 1953.
4. Betcher, A.M., Bean, G., and Casten, D.F.: Continuous procaine block of paravertebral sympathetic ganglions, J.A.M.A. **151**:288-292, 1953.
5. Bonica, J.J.: Causalgia and other reflex sympathetic dystrophies, Postgrad. Med. **53**:143-148, May 1973.
6. Carron, H., and Weller, R.M.: Treatment of post-traumatic sympathetic dystrophy, Adv. Neurol. **4**:485-490, 1974.
7. Casey, K.L.: The neurophysiologic basis of pain, Postgrad. Med. **53**:58-75, May 1973.
8. Chapman, L.F., Ramos, A.O., Goodell, H., and Wolff, H.G.: Neurohumeral features of afferent fibers in man, Arch. Neurol. **4**:617-650, 1961.
9. Coffman, J.D., and Davies, W.T.: Vasospastic disease: a review, Progr. Cardiovasc. Dis. **18**:123-146, 1975.
10. Denmark, A.: An example of symptoms resembling tic douleureux produced by a wound in the radial nerve, Royal Med. Chir. Trans. **4**:48-52, 1813.
11. DeSaussure, R.L.: Causalgia, Clin. Neurosurg. **25**:626-636, 1978.
12. de Takáts, G.: Reflex dystrophy of extremities, Arch. Surg. **34**:939-956, 1937.
13. de Takáts, G.: Causalgic states in peace and war, J.A.M.A. **128**:699-704, 1945.
14. Doupe, J., Cullen, C.H., and Chance, G.Q.: Post-traumatic pain and causalgia syndrome, J. Neurol. Neurosurg. Psychiatry **7**:33-48, 1944.
15. Edmundson, A.S., and Calandruccio, R.A.: Drug therapy for causalgia, Mississippi Doctor **34**:239-241, 1957.
16. Evans, J.A.: Reflex sympathetic dystrophy: report on 57 cases, Ann. Intern. Med. **26**:417-426, 1947.
17. Fowler, F.D., and Moser, M.: Use of hexamethonium and Dibenzyline in diagnosis and treatment of causalgia, J.A.M.A. **161**:1051-1053, 1956.
18. Genant, H.K., Kozin, F., Bakerman, C., McCarty, D.J., and Sims, J.: The reflex sympathetic dystrophy syndrome, Radiology **117**:21-32, 1975.
19. Gerard, R.W.: The physiology of pain: Abnormal neuron states in causalgia and related phenomena, Anesthesiology **12**:1-13, 1951.
20. Glick, E.M.: Reflex dystrophy (algoneurodystrophy): results of treatment by corticosteroids, Rheumatol. Rehabil. **12**:84-88, 1973.
21. Granit, R., Leskell, L., and Skoglund, C.R.: Fiber interaction in injured or compressed region of nerve, Brain **67**:125-140, 1944.
22. Hamilton, J.: On some effects resulting from wounds of nerves, Dublin J. Med. Sci. **13**:38-55, 1838.
23. Homans, J.: Minor causalgia: a hyperesthetic neurovascular syndrome, N. Engl. J. Med. **222**:870-874, 1940.
24. Kennard, M.A.: Sensitization of spinal cord of cat to pain-inducing stimuli, J. Neurosurg. **10**:169-177, 1953.
25. Kirklin, J.W., Chenoweth, A.I., and Murphey, F.: Causalgia: a review of its characteristics, diagnosis, and treatment, Surgery **21**:321-342, 1947.
26. Kleinert, H.E., Cole, N.M., Wayne, L., and others: Post-traumatic sympathetic dystrophy, Orthop. Clin. North Am. **4**:917-927, 1973.
27. Kux, M.: Thoracic endoscopic sympathectomy in palmar and axillary hyperhidrosis, Arch. Surg. **113**:264-266, 1978.
28. Kwan, S.T.: The treatment of causalgia by thoracic sympathetic ganglionectomy, Ann. Surg. **101**:222-227, 1935.
29. Lankford, L.L.: Reflex sympathetic dystrophy. In Omer, G.E., Jr., and Spinner, M., editors: Management of peripheral nerve problems, Philadelphia, 1980, W.B. Saunders Co.
30. Lankford, L.L., and Thompson, J.E.: Reflex sympathetic dystrophy, upper and lower extremity: diagnosis and management. In American Academy of Orthopaedic Surgeons: Instructional course lectures, vol. 26, St. Louis, 1977, The C.V. Mosby Co.
31. Leriche, R.: The surgery of pain (translated and edited by A. Young), London, 1939, Baillière, Tindall & Cox.
32. Livingston, W.K.: Pain mechanisms: a physiological interpretation of causalgia and its related states, New York, 1943, The MacMillan Co.
33. Long, D.M.: Electrical stimulation for relief of pain from chronic nerve injury, J. Neurosurg. **39**:718-722, 1973.
34. Lorente de Nó, R.: Analysis of the activity of the chains of internuncial neurons, J. Neurophysiol. **1**:207-244, 1938.
35. McGrath, M.A., and Penny, R.: The mechanisms of Raynaud's phenomenon, Part 1, Med. J. Aust. **2**:328-333, 1974.
36. Mayfield, F.H., and Devine, J.W.: Causalgia, Surg. Gynecol. Obstet. **80**:631-635, 1945.
37. Melzack, R., and Wall, P.D.: Pain mechanisms: a new theory, Science **150**:971-979, 1965.
38. Meyer, G.A., and Fields, H.L.: Causalgia treated by selective large fibre stimulation of peripheral nerve, Brain **95**:163-168, 1972.
39. Mitchell, J.K.: Remote consequences of injuries of nerves and their treatment, Philadelphia, 1895, Lea Brothers.
40. Mitchell, S.W.: On the diseases of nerves resulting from injuries in contributions relating to the causation and prevention of disease, and to camp disease. In Flint, A., editor: United States Sanitary Commission Memoirs, New York, 1867.
41. Mitchell, S.W.: Injuries of nerves and their consequences, Philadelphia, 1872, J.B. Lippincott Co.
42. Mitchell, S.W., Morehouse, G.R., and Keen, W.W.: Gunshot wounds and other injuries of nerves, Philadelphia, 1864, J.B. Lippincott Co.
43. Moore, D.C.: Regional block, Springfield, Ill., 1967, Charles C Thomas, Publisher.
44. Nashold, B.S., Jr., and Friedman, H.: Dorsal column stimulation for control of pain, J. Neurosurg. **36**:590-597, 1972.
45. Nathan, P.W.: On the pathogenesis of causalgia and peripheral nerve injuries, Brain **70**:145-170, 1947.
46. Omer, G.E., Jr., and Thomas, S.R.: Treatment of causalgia: review of cases at Brooke General Hospital, Tex. Med. **67**:93-96, Jan. 1971.
47. Omer, G.E., Jr., and Thomas, S.R.: The management of chronic pain syndromes in the upper extremity, Clin. Orthop. Rel. Res. **104**:37-45, 1974.
48. Owens, J.C.: Causalgia, Am. Surg. **23**:636-643, 1957.
49. Paget, J.: Clinical lecture on some cases of local paralysis, Med. Times **1**:331-332, 1864.
50. Pak, T.J., Martin, G.M., Magness, J.L., and Kavanaugh, G.J.: Reflex sympathetic dystrophy, review of 140 cases, Minn. Med. **53**:507-512, 1970.

51. Palumbo, L.T.: Upper dorsal sympathectomy without Horner's syndrome, Arch. Surg. **27**:743-751, 1955.

52. Paré, A.: Les œuvres d'Ambroise Paré (histoire de defunct), Roy Charles IX, Tenth Book. **41**:401, Paris, 1598, Gabriel Buon.

53. Pool, J.L., and Brabson, J.A.: Pain on stimulating the distal segment of divided peripheral nerves, J. Neurosurg. **3**:468-473, 1946.

54. Porter, J.M., Lindell, T.D., Leung, B.S., and Reiney, C.G.: Effect of intra-arterial injection of reserpine on vascular wall catecholamine content, Surg. Forum **22**:183-185, 1972.

55. Procacci, P., Francini, F., Maresca, M., and Zoppi, M.: Skin potentials and EMG changes induced by cutaneous electrical stimulation. II. Subjects with reflex sympathetic dystrophies, Appl. Neurophysiol. **42**:125-134, 1979.

56. Rosen, P.S., and Graham, W.: The shoulder-hand syndrome: historical review with observations on 73 patients, Can. Med. Assoc. J. **77**:86-91, 1957.

56. Rosen, P.S., and Graham, W.: The shoulder-hand syndrome: historical review with observations on 73 patients, Can. Med. Assoc. J. **77**:86-91, 1957.

57. Ross, J.P.: Causalgia, St. Barthol. Hosp. Rep. **65**:103-188, 1932.

58. Shumacker, H.B., Speigel, I.J., and Upjohn, R.H.: Causalgia: the role of sympathetic interruption in treatment, Surg. Gynecol. Obstet. **86**:76-86, 1948.

59. Smithwick, R.H.: The rationale and technique of sympathectomy for the relief of vascular spasm of the extremity, N. Engl. J. Med. **222**:699, 1940.

60. Snider, R.L., and Porter, J.M.: Treatment of experimental frostbite with intra-arterial sympathetic blocking drugs, Surgery **77**:557-561, 1975.

61. Spurling, R.G.: Causalgia of the upper extremity: treatment by dorsal sympathetic ganglionectomy, Arch. Neurol. Psychiatry **23**:784-788, 1930.

62. Steinbrocker, O.: The shoulder-hand syndrome: associated painful homolateral disability of the shoulder and hand with swelling and atrophy of the hand, Am. J. Med. **3**:402-407, 1947.

63. Steinbrocker, O.: The shoulder-hand syndrome: present perspective, Arch. Phys. Med. Rehabil. **49**:388-395, 1968.

64. Sudeck, P.H.M.: Ueber die acute entzündliche Knockenatrophie, Arch. Klin. Chir. **62**:147-156, 1900.

65. Sunderland, S.: Pain mechanisms in causalgia, J. Neurol. Neurosurg. Psychiatry **39**:471-480, 1976.

66. Walker, A.E., and Nulson, F.: Electrical stimulation of the upper thoracic portion of the sympathetic chain in man, Arch. Neurol. Psychiatry **59**:559-560, 1948.

67. Wall, P.D., and Sweet, W.H.: Temporary abolition of pain in man, Science **155**:108-109, 1967.

68. White, J.C.: Sympathectomy for relief of pain. In Bonica, J.J., editor: Advances in neurology, International Symposium on Pain, vol. 4, New York, 1974, Raven Press.

48

Therapist's management of reflex sympathetic dystrophy

JANET WAYLETT

BEHAVIORAL PATTERNS IN REFLEX SYMPATHETIC DYSTROPHY

More than 30 terms have been used to describe the symptom complex of reflex sympathetic dystrophy (RSD). Whatever the term chosen, references in the medical literature describe the RSD patient as follows: emotionally labile with low pain threshold, dependent or inadequate personality, introspective, worrying, apprehensive, hysterical, defensive, and hostile.[1,6-11]

Lankford[10] has discussed a predisposition or diathesis to develop RSD that involves (1) abnormal sympathetic reflex, (2) vasoconstrictive reactions resulting in abnormally cold extremities and possible migraine headaches, and (3) predisposing psychological make-up. The belief that individuals with certain personality traits are most likely to develop RSD is further supported by Ehlers and Zachariae.[7] In their report of a study completed in 1964, 33 male patients with Dupuytren's contracture were seen preoperatively by a psychiatrist, who assessed each one's character and gave a statement containing a prediction regarding the postoperative course. The surgeon was unaware of the contents of the statement. A few months later the real course was compared with the predicted postoperative course. "In 30 out of 33 patients there was conformity between pre-operative psychiatric statement and the real post-operative course, and the conclusion is that an interested psychiatrist can foretell in a great deal of cases whether a hand operation will be complicated by post-operative dystrophic symptoms or not".[7] These 30 men had reflex sympathetic dystrophy.

Because of the frequent frustrations and difficulty encountered in treating this type of individual, Loma Linda University Medical Center and Downey Community Hospital Hand Center became interested in trying to identify some of the more subtle behavioral traits of RSD that might affect such a patient's progress in hand therapy. We noticed that as a group such patients failed to progress as rapidly as other patients and that a few, when seen by the physician after discharge from therapy, had not progressed further on their own.

In 1975 we initiated a survey between our two facilities that involved the standardized Buhler-Coleman Life Goals Inventory[2] and written observations by staff members and students.

BUHLER-COLEMAN LIFE GOALS INVENTORY

The standardized Buhler-Coleman Life Goals Inventory is a self-administered instrument designed to assess personality in terms of an individual's life expectations—what that person wants most and least from life. The four basic tendencies measured by this instrument are as follows:

1. Need satisfaction—need for survival, love, and pleasure
2. Creative expansion—drive toward accomplishment
3. Self-limiting adaptation—limits own needs and satisfaction
4. Upholding the internal order—moral or social values integrated into personality

We studied three groups of patients: In the *control group* were 17 hand patients—seven women and 10 men—of which eight had suffered industrial injuries. The *suspected RSD group* consisted of five women, two of whom had experienced industrial injuries. In the *diagnosed RSD group* were 12 patients who were known to have the disorder.

In the control group all of the 17 patients evaluated had normal profiles except 1 male. Two out of five suspected RSD patients had abnormal profiles. Of the 12 diagnosed RSD patients, five refused to fill out the inventory and one found it too difficult to complete; of the six scored inventories none was in the normal range. In the normally scoring individual there is a well organized hierarchy of needs. In the diagnosed RSD group there was a trend toward self-limiting behavior, with conflicting goals. As a group such patients do not show creative or enterprising tendencies. Because half of this group refused to complete the inventory, one would suspect that these individuals are resistant to the implication that their physical problem is in any way related to their psychological state.

CLINICAL OBSERVATIONS

It was decided that thorough, written observations, recorded on an observation sheet or an outline, could be the means of identifying the more subtle behavioral traits in RSD patients. Four separate observation sheets were completed for each patient. The observers were a physician, a therapist, a psychologist, a rehabilitation nurse, a secretary, and a student. Three of the observers had formed strong opinions on reflex dystrophy prior to the observation; the remaining three for the most part had not heard of the disorder.

The most obvious observation, of course, is the complaint of the constant, often burning pain that seems to totally preoccupy the patient. Interestingly enough, our patients did not have very acute or severe physiologic problems, such as partial amputations or range loss. Another observation made by the staff members was an inability to problem solve, which was seemingly universal among this patient group. This was noted not just in regard to exercises and treatment modalities, which would be unfamiliar to most lay persons, but these patients had difficulty solving very simple tasks. For example, a patient attempted to help out in the center by filling a 30-cup coffee maker with water. She proceeded to do it one cup at a time instead of filling the urn from the faucet. In addition, these patients tended to ignore the most traumatized patients, not displaying any open concern for them.

Behavioral traits based on observations

Control group. The control group demonstrated consistent behavior in at least three out of four observations for each question. In addition they displayed the following positive traits:

1. Did not present the same picture to each observer, suggesting inconsistent behavior
2. Conversation dominated by either pain or disability
3. Typical initial behavior was to be in a roomful of people but withdrawn (this gradually changed but persisted much longer than in control group)
4. Inability to retain instructions from session to session
5. Inability to perform exercises and use modalities without supervision (for example, did not increase weights when on strengthening program)
6. Inability to make decisions about changes needed in splinting (for example, whether rubber band traction is comfortable, whether straps are becoming worn)

Suspected RSD group. The suspected group was so varied that the results were inconclusive.

Diagnosed RSD group. The traits of the diagnosed group, found in over 50% of its members, were as follows:

1. Did not present the same picture to each observer, suggesting inconsistent behavior
2. Conversation dominated by either pain or disability
3. Typical initial behavior was to be in a roomful of people but withdrawn (this gradually changed but persisted much longer than in control group)
4. Inability to retain instructions from session to session
5. Inability to perform exercises and use modalities without supervision (for example, did not increase weights when on strengthening program)
6. Inability to make decisions about changes needed in splinting (for example, whether rubber band traction is comfortable, whether straps are becoming worn)

Conclusions based on observations

The reflex sympathetic dystrophy patient requires:
1. Constant supervision initially, which should be reduced only as the patient demonstrates understanding of his condition, which usually takes a longer period of time than is necessary for the control group.
2. A very highly structured and simplified program, which should include step-by-step teaching by demonstration and written instructions. The use of splints must be explained in a way that is easy to understand, and splints must be easy to apply and wear.
3. Motivation to be an active agent in his own treatment. The idea that he has the *power* to improve must be instilled in him.

A psychologist who reviewed our survey suggested that reflex dystrophy may represent a form of communication disorder, both receptive and expressive, in which emotional distress is expressed physically. He later tested 12 additional RSD patients with the Minnesota Multiphasic Personality Inventory and found they showed the "conversion hysteria profile." He also expressed the opinion that these patients would probably not benefit greatly from psychological counseling, since they would resist the implication that anything might be wrong with them emotionally.

HAND TREATMENT PHILOSOPHY AND PROGRAM

On the basis of the results of our survey, we believe that treatment should be started very early after injury or operation in individuals whom the physician suspects may develop reflex dystrophy. For example, wrist fractures should be seen 1 or 2 days following cast application, to provide early motion of joints proximal and distal to the cast. Early treatment can help to prevent the typical severe edema and trophic changes seen in Fig. 48-1.

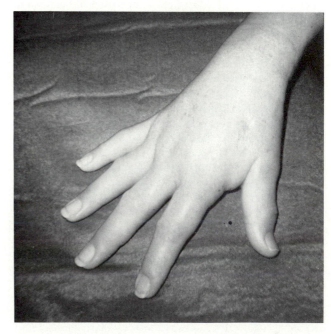

FIG. 48-1. Severe edema as seen in reflex dystrophy.

MODALITIES
Jobst treatment

Edema is usually a serious problem in the RSD hand (because of minimal active movement by the patient), and treatment of this problem is begun on initial contact. The Jobst intermittent compression unit (refer to Chapter 11) is utilized to decrease edema, in combination with elevation and the use of pressure wraps and compression gloves or splints. The Jobst treatment is most effective with patients demonstrating "pitting edema." It is 45 minutes to 1 hour long, with compression being set between 60 and 90 mm Hg. If the Jobst unit is used to increase passive interphalangeal flexion, the compression must be reduced to 30 to 60 mm Hg and the fingers should be alternately positioned in flexion and extension.

Ice treatment

A 20-minute ice treatment can also be used to decrease edema; however, it is not tolerated by RSD patients as well as the other edema-reducing modalities.

Retrograde massage

Retrograde massage is very helpful with this patient group, to decrease edema and at the same time desensitize the fingers and hand and soften any scar tissue present. Retrograde massage is performed for 10 to 15 minutes, with a lanolin-base cream used as a lubricant.

Heat treatment

Once the swelling has decreased, the patient can proceed to heat modalities such as hot packs or a paraffin bath to relax muscles and soften scar tissue. The paraffin bath is used to obtain finger flexion; the patient's fingers are taped into flexion with paper tape to ensure that maximum passive flexion is maintained throughout the bath. The hand is dipped six times into the bath; the patient then soaks the hand for 10 minutes in paraffin if he can tolerate the heat. After removal of the hand from the bath, the paraffin glove is left in place and covered with a plastic bag. With the uninvolved hand the patient passively flexes the involved fingers. Hot packs are used to gain extension range of motion, since their flat, square configuration lends itself well to holding the fingers in extension. Both the paraffin bath and the hot packs are followed by passive or active range-of-motion exercises and strengthening exercises, as indicated by the patient's clinical picture.

Exercise

Active exercise is excellent for decreasing edema, because the pumping action of the muscles assists in venous return.

The exercise program must be painstakingly simple, with a set number of repetitions and predetermined weights. Weight increases must be supervised by either the clinic aide or the therapist.

Skateboard exercises, as shown in Fig. 48-2, are performed on an adjustable-height table and are used to provide gravity-eliminated active exercises to shoulder and elbow in the horizontal plane. These exercises can be made resistive by attaching a weight to the skate through a pulley mechanism. Skateboard exercises are designed to improve shoulder and elbow range of motion, which are often involved in RSD when the patient has a "shoulder-hand syndrome."

Reciprocal pulleys are used to provide assistive range-of-motion exercise to shoulder and elbow musculature and are excellent for home use when applied to a doorway.

Dowel or wand exercises, an example of which is shown in Fig. 48-3, are given for home as well as clinic programs to increase shoulder, elbow, and forearm strength and range

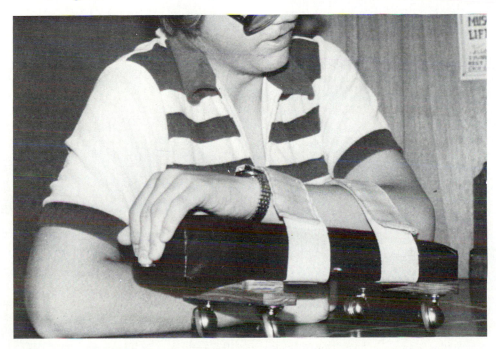

FIG. 48-2. Skateboard exercise for shoulder and elbow.

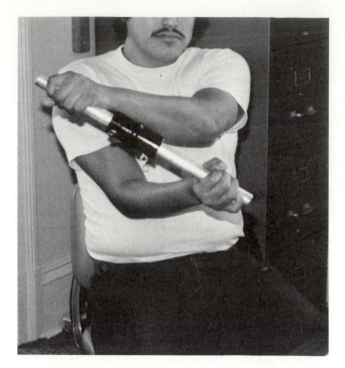

FIG. 48-3. Dowel exercise to increase shoulder, elbow, and forearm strength and range of motions.

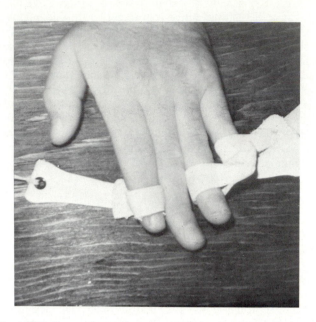

FIG. 48-4. Progressive resistance exercise to finger abductors and adductors.

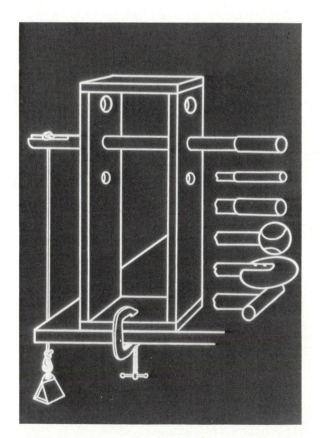

FIG. 48-5. Weight well exercise device with interchangeable handles for wrist and hand exercises.

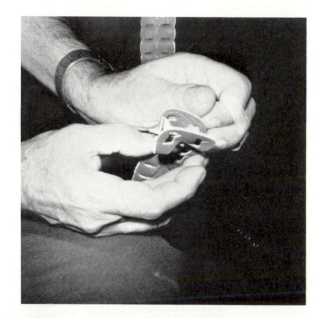

FIG. 48-6. The link belt is a simple rote craft used to rehabilitate the patient with reflex sympathetic dystrophy.

of motion. A Velcro cuff weight can be added to the dowel to provide resistance.

Progressive resistive exercises (PRE) are the method of choice to increase the strength of the upper extremity musculature. PRE to finger abductors and adductors is shown in Fig. 48-4. The treppe, or "staircase," method is utilized to gradually "warm up" the muscle for maximum exertion without the risk of overstretching the muscle. Treppe (the German word for staircase) is the term used to describe the phenomenon of increasing muscle contractions against gradually increasing resistance. The system employs a series of 10 contractions against 50% of maximum weight, 10 contractions against 75% of maximum weight, and finally 10 contractions against 100% of maximum weight.[4,5] Isotonic exercises are preferred to isometric exercises, since isotonic exercises produce joint movement and thereby increase range of motion as well as strength. Patients are seen preferably three times weekly for this strengthening program.

Weight well exercises, as shown in Fig. 48-5, consist of a wide variety of wrist and hand exercises, as demonstrated with the different handles. These exercises also elevate the hand to decrease edema, and they assist venous flow through the pumping action of the forearm and hand musculature. Weight wells can be checked out for home use.

Splinting

Splinting follows the basic principles used with any hand-injured patient. However, splints must be very comfortable, accommodate for swelling, and be very easy to apply, with minimal adjustments.

Activities of daily living and craft activities

Activities of daily living and concurrent craft activities are most important with RSD patients, since these patients characteristically avoid using the involved extremity. They require a highly structured, purposeful activity to reincorporate the spontaneous use of the injured hand into their lives. Simple rote crafts, such as the link belt shown in Fig. 48-6, are excellent because they are bilateral and repetitious and require very little problem solving. Through the initial use of crafts, it is possible to motivate the patient to use the injured hand in everyday activities, since the rigid RSD patient is often unwilling to accept substandard performances in self-feeding and so on, but has no set expectations about a craft activity that was never before attempted. Through simple accomplishments in craft projects, the patient is made aware that the hand is functional and will begin using it once again. Inquiries should be made frequently about how and when the patient is using the hand at home, so that functional use can be upgraded.

SUMMARY

Knowledge of the RSD personality, with its dependency, worry, and apprehensive and hysterical behavior, can assist the therapist in direction of the patient's treatment program. To alleviate apprehension and worry, the therapist should try to tell the patient, in simple terms, exactly what is being done. The patient should be told what is expected of him and when. The therapist should not assume that the patient understands either how to apply a splint or how to perform an exercise until the therapist has observed the patient accomplishing the task, properly, since this type of patient does not seem to attend to directions very well (possibly because he is worrying when he should be listening). This type of patient may not solicit help when he needs it. It is best initially to direct every aspect of the patient's treatment, gradually allowing the patient to assume more responsibility as he demonstrates the ability to do so. This patient group presents a supreme challenge to the therapist's interpersonal skills, since the therapist must relate to the patient socially as an adult peer and in treatment as a dependent or child, and at the same time not offend or alienate him.

REFERENCES

1. Boyes, J.H.: Bunnell's surgery of the hand, ed. 5, Philadelphia, 1970, J.B. Lippincott Co., pp. 643-651.
2. Buhler, C., and Coleman, W.E.: Life goals inventory manual, Los Angeles, 1965, University of Southern California School of Medicine.
3. Caillet, R.: Hand pain and impairment, Philadelphia, 1971, F.A. Davis Co., pp. 72-75.
4. DeLorme, T.L.: Restoration of muscle power by heavy-resistance exercises, J. Bone Joint Surg. 27:645-667, 1945.
5. DeLorme, T.L., and Watkins, A.L.: Technics of progressive resistive exercise, Arch. Phys. Med. 29:263-273, 1948.
6. de Takáts, G.: Causalgic states in peace and war, J. A.M.A. **128**:699-704, 1945.
7. Ehlers, H., and Zachariae, L.: Mentality and dystrophy, Acta Orthop. Scand. **1**:109-113, 1964.
8. Erickson, J.C., III: Evaluation and management of autonomic dystrophies of the upper extremity. In Hunter, J.M., Schneider, L., Mackin, E., and Bell, J., editors: Rehabilitation of the hand, St. Louis, 1978, The C.V. Mosby Co.
9. Kleinert, H.E., Cole, N.M., Wagne, L., and others: Post traumatic sympathetic dystrophy, Orthop. Clin. North Am. **4**(4):917-926, 1973.
10. Lankford, L.L.: Reflex sympathetic dystrophy. In Omer, G., and Spinner, M., editors: Management of peripheral nerve problems, Philadelphia, 1980, W.B. Saunders Co.
11. Parry, C.B.W.: Rehabilitation of the Hand, ed. 3, London, 1973, Butterworth & Co. (Publishers), Ltd., pp. 217-219.

49

Clinical application of the transcutaneous electrical nerve stimulator in patients with upper extremity pain

VALERIE HOLDEMAN LEE and C. CHRISTOPHER REYNOLDS

Transcutaneous electrical nerve stimulation (TENS) has gained universal recognition as a method of producing analgesia in a number of patients with acute or chronic pain. The efficacy of this treatment modality is dependent upon a clear understanding of the neuromechanisms for pain modulation. Choosing the proper electrical stimulator and a thorough knowledge of its clinical applicability are equally imperative. The objective of this chapter is to discuss this technique whereby pain management in the upper extremity might be enhanced.

COMPONENTS OF TENS UNITS

The transcutaneous electrical nerve stimulator is an electrical device that emits a pulsed current in the form of a biphasic asymmetric wave form. Pulsed current is neither alternating nor direct but has components of each (Fig. 49-1).

TENS units generally have three controls: (1) output or amplitude, which is expressed in milliamps; (2) pulse rate or frequency, which is expressed in pulses per second, or Hertz; and (3) pulse width, which is expressed in microseconds.

On some TENS units pulse width is not an option and is set internally. On one commercially available stimulator, the Empi, the pulse width is tied to the amplitude control. As the amplitude increases, the pulse width also increases.

TENS units commonly have either one channel (two electrodes), or two channels (four electrodes). Each channel has the capacity for application of two electrodes. Several models permit additional electrode incorporation on a single channel. This is referred to as a "piggyback arrangement." For patients with upper extremity pain, the two-channel unit is more practical.

Generally, it is not possible to adjust rate and width controls for each channel independently. Characteristically, however, amplitude adjustments maintain their independence on each channel.

Several varieties of electrodes are available. The standard carbon electrode must be covered evenly with conducting gel before it is applied to the patient, to prevent skin irritation or burning. Increasingly popular are the caraya and self-adhesive electrodes. Gel is not necessary and skin reaction is rare. Electrodes are available in various sizes and can be

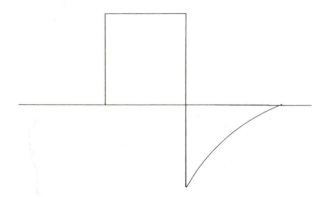

FIG. 49-1. Biphasic asymmetric wave form.

trimmed to meet specific needs. When one is reducing the size of one electrode in a channel, it is important to remember that a 2:1 ratio should not be exceeded, in order to prevent burning under the small electrode. To assure adequate contact for good electrical conduction, one may need to shave the skin. Commercial skin preparations are also available to enhance conduction.

Precut adhesive patches or hypoallergenic paper tape can be used to secure the electrodes to the patient.

Energy sources for TENS units vary. In most instances rechargeable pencil or transistor batteries with rechargers can be obtained. Other units offer separate rechargeable battery packs.

MODES OF TREATMENT

There are several different treatment modes to choose from when TENS is being used for pain relief. These different forms of stimulation are achieved by adjustment of the characteristics (amplitude, pulse rate, pulse width) of the pulsed wave form and are termed "conventional," "brief intense," and "low-frequency (low-rate) TENS" (Fig. 49-2).

Conventional TENS

The success of conventional TENS is based on the gate-control theory proposed by Melzack and Wall[8] in 1965 and further clarified by more recent studies. Receptors that detect pain (nociceptors) transmit information to the central ner-

	RATE	PULSE WIDTH	AMPLITUDE
HIGH RATE (conventional)	60 to 120 pps	50 to 100 microseconds	Comfortable No muscle contraction
LOW RATE	1 to 5 pps	150 to 200 microseconds	Slightly uncomfortable Strong muscle contraction
BRIEF INTENSE	60 to 120 pps	200 microseconds	Tolerable Tetanic or sustained muscle contraction

FIG. 49-2. Modes of TENS treatment.

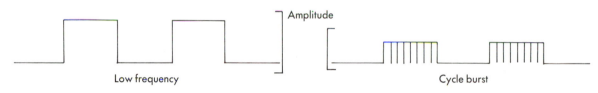

FIG. 49-3

vous system via A-delta and unmyelinated (C) fibers. When these nociceptive impulses reach the posterior horn of the spinal cord, a gating or control mechanism determines which signals ascend in the spinothalamic tract to the brain, where pain is perceived. The gate is facilitated or inhibited by peripheral afferents other than those carrying messages and by impulses descending from the brain. The mechanism of this control and its location are unknown, as is the exact function of substantia gelatinosa. The balance between the activity in the A-delta and C fibers may be critical. Increased C-fiber action inhibits the gate, allowing passage of impulses, while a relative increase in large myelinated A-fiber activity closes the gate, blocking pain.

The parameters for conventional TENS are as follows: rate, which is high (60 to 120 pulses per second [PPS]); width, which is low (50 to 100 microseconds); and amplitude, which is increased until the patient perceives a pleasant, tingling sensation in the area that was previously painful. The onset of pain relief is sudden, and carry-over varies from a few minutes to several hours.

Low-frequency TENS

Pain relief after low-frequency TENS is at present attributed to the release of naturally occurring morphine-like substances called "opioid peptides (endorphins)."[1,5] Elevated endorphin levels have been reported in patients after low-frequency TENS, while patients with chronic pain have been reported to have depleted levels of endorphins.[12,13] Naloxone, a specific opiate antagonist, counteracts the pain relief achieved with low-frequency stimulation.[2,4,5] To achieve low-frequency stimulation, the pulse rate must be low (1 to 5 pps), the pulse width high (150 to 200 μsec), and the amplitude increased until a visible muscle contraction occurs. TENS units with a preset width cannot be adjusted adequately for low-rate stimulation. One should keep these factors in mind when acquiring TENS units for clinical purposes. Low-frequency TENS is perceived by most patients with upper extremity pain to be more comfortable when delivered in a pulsed train or bursting mode. The same low-frequency settings are used, whereas trains of high-frequency bursts are incorporated in each pulse. Less current intensity is necessary to elicit muscle contraction and stimulation may be more tolerable (Fig. 49-3).[12] Pain relief occurs approximately 15 to 30 minutes after initiation of low-rate TENS or cycle-bursting TENS. Carry-over relief can vary anywhere from 30 minutes to several hours. Because a muscle contraction occurs with this mode of treatment, the patient must be cleared for active exercise before its use.

Brief intense TENS

Brief intense TENS has also been labeled "hyperstimulation analgesia."[10] It is in effect a form of counterstimulation. Melzack suggests that areas in the brainstem act as a "central biasing mechanism" and inhibit formation transmission. He states that intense stimulation would produce a predominantly small fiber input, which would give rise to pain, but would also activate the "central biasing mechanism," which would inhibit pain signals from other areas such as sources of pathologic pain.[9,10] To deliver brief intense TENS, the rate is set high (60 to 120 pps), the pulse width is also set high (200 μsec), and the amplitude is adjusted until a strong muscle contraction occurs. Onset of relief should be sudden, treatment time is short, and carryover is extremely variable. Brief intense TENS has several useful clinical applications. Procedures such as wound débridement and suture removal may be simplified. In addition to a sustained muscle contraction, sensation is almost completely inhibited within the electrode field. Muscle fatigue occurs rather rapidly, however, and stimulation time must be brief.

Modulation

Accommodation and sensory adaptation may occur during stimulation.[3] To prevent these phenomena from occurring, a number of TENS units provide modulation controls for rate or amplitude, or both. These controls may increase effectiveness of treatment and aid in patient comfort.

POSTOPERATIVE TENS

Transcutaneous electrical nerve stimulation may be used to reduce pain postoperatively. Sterile electrodes are available and may be placed intraoperatively or in the recovery room. Best results with pain relief have been reported when the patient awakes from anesthesia with the TENS functioning. The patient should be seen by the therapist before surgery to experience the stimulation and allay any apprehension. Conventional TENS is usually the method of choice. It delivers a pleasant sensation to the patient and provides immediate pain relief, and a muscle contraction is unnecessary.

Postoperative TENS may be extremely beneficial in facilitating early motion in patients with fractures or after such surgical procedures as capsulectomies, neurolysis, and tenolysis and is of particular value with patients who have a history of reflex sympathetic dystrophy or a chronic pain problem.

One must, however, remember that pain can be an important feedback mechanism to prevent damage to newly repaired structures. Therefore the therapist must closely monitor the exercise program to prevent the patient from overexercising while experiencing pain relief from the TENS.

USE OF TENS FOR PAIN OTHER THAN POSTOPERATIVE

The use of TENS has been beneficial in a number of upper extremity problems. Particularly, neurostimulators have proved beneficial in reducing pain for persons with a diagnosis of peripheral nerve injury, reflex sympathetic dystrophy, or crush injuries. Sensitive scars resulting from fingertip injuries and surgeries about cutaneous branches of peripheral nerves have been desensitized with TENS.

Selection of mode of treatment

Although no set rules have been established, it appears that conventional TENS is best used for initial trial treatment. Onset of pain relief is immediate, and many patients achieve good results with conventional TENS alone. If satisfactory pain relief does not occur after 15 to 30 minutes of conventional TENS, switching to low-frequency TENS may be advantageous. Brief intense TENS should also be used as an alternative. Again, patients must be cleared for active exercise so that either low-frequency or brief intense stimulation may be safely used.

Pre-TENS treatment evaluation includes measurement of grip and pinch (when appropriate), recording of range of motion, and measurement of joint circumference. The therapist must also understand the cause of each patient's pain. The patient is asked to quantitate subjectively his degree of pain on a scale of 0 to 10, with 10 being the highest degree and 0 being pain free. The therapist examines the involved hand and charts color differences, general posturing of the hand and arm, and any changes in sudomotor activity or hair growth.

Before application of the neurostimulator, patients are given a brief explanation of what TENS is and the theory behind its use. TENS must be presented in a positive manner, but it is important not to promise the patient that it will "cure" his pain. TENS should simply be presented as an adjunct to treatment. For a proper evaluation of TENS, the patient should refrain from taking analgesics 6 to 8 hours before treatment, and the patient should be experiencing pain at the time of treatment.

If the patient complains of pain only in the morning, then that is when treatment time is scheduled. Another, more subtle factor that may influence the success of treatment is whether litigation or a compensation settlement is pending. Consciously or subconsciously, the patient may not be ready to let go of his pain if secondary gain is a possibility.

Electrode placement

A critical factor in the success of TENS is electrode placement. In both conventional TENS and brief intense TENS the paresthesias must be perceived in the area that was previously painful. The patient is asked to locate the distribution of pain by outlining on his arm or shading in painful areas on a diagram. The therapist seeks trigger points by palpation and percussion of the extremity, particularly along the course of the superficial peripheral nerves. When one is looking for specific points for stimulation, it is interesting to note that there is a strong correlation between trigger points, motor points, and acupuncture points.[10,11] If they do not occupy the same location, they are often close enough that one electrode may cover both points. One characteristic all three have in common is a lowered resistance to electrical current.[6] Therefore the therapist should become familiar with the location of motor points, trigger points and acupuncture points in the upper extremity.

Stimulation sites

Some common sites for stimulation of the upper extremity are shown in Figs. 49-4 and 49-5. Good results may also occur when electrodes are placed in corresponding derma-

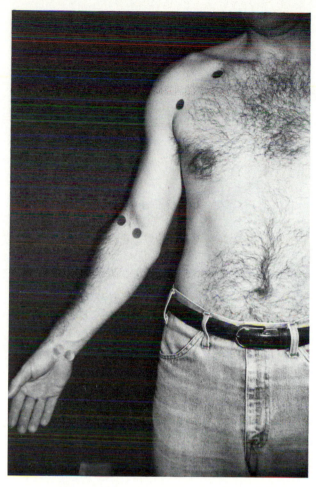

FIG. 49-4. Common sites for TENS, anterior aspect.

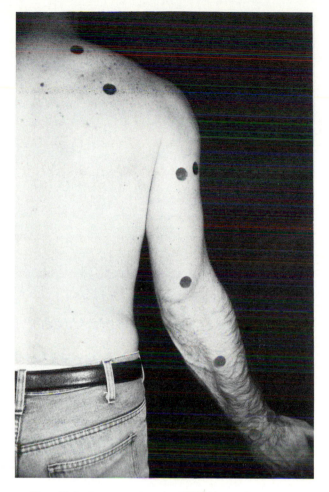

FIG. 49-5. Common sites for TENS, posterior aspect.

tomes or in segmentally related myotomes.[4] According to the literature, the use of TENS should be avoided over carotid sinuses, across the neck, around the eyes, and in the presence of a cardiac pacemaker. Once location of electrode placement is decided upon, the patient is stimulated for 1 hour when conventional or low-rate TENS is being used. Treatment with brief intense TENS should be from 15 to 25 minutes.

Occasionally patients may perceive paresthesias under one electrode of a channel but not the other, a condition that can occur when the area is heavily scarred or there has been damage to the underlying peripheral nerve. In this situation, the electrode may be reduced to one half the size of the remaining electrode. This will increase current density under the smaller electrode.

Patients who complain of diffuse pain over a large area may benefit from having the electrodes placed in an overlapping fashion (Fig. 49-6). In this manner, a greater total area of stimulation is achieved.

Lampe suggests bilateral stimulation if the painful area to be treated has sustained damage to the A fibers, as in a peripheral nerve injury. His suggestion is based on the theory that stimulation of A fibers on the uninjured side would

cross over and produce a relative increase in A-fiber activity, which would then trigger the gating mechanism and block C-fiber input.[7] At the end of the first treatment session, patients are asked to record again the level of pain on a 0 to 10 scale. They are also asked to record the duration of carry-over of pain relief. If pain relief is not achieved, electrode placement should be varied. There is no definite formula for electrode placement according to diagnosis, because each patient and condition will vary. The therapist must be willing to spend time with the patient to achieve optimum electrode placement. The following examples demonstrate electrode placement in two different patients. A patient who has suffered an injury to the median nerve at the wrist may complain of pain at the site of the injury and also of pain that radiates proximally into the axilla and anterior chest wall. Distally, one electrode might be placed over the volar wrist crease, with another electrode placed over the proximal third of the volar area of the forearm (Fig. 49-7). Placement of one electrode proximal in the axilla, and the other over the anterior chest wall has proved beneficial (Fig. 49-8).

Prolonged pain after partial or complete amputation of a finger may be referred along the course of the digital nerve.

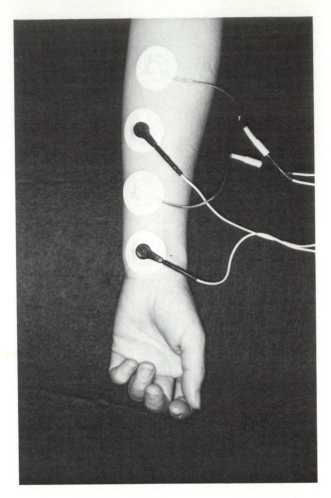

FIG. 49-6. Through overlapping of electrode channels a larger area of stimualtion is achieved.

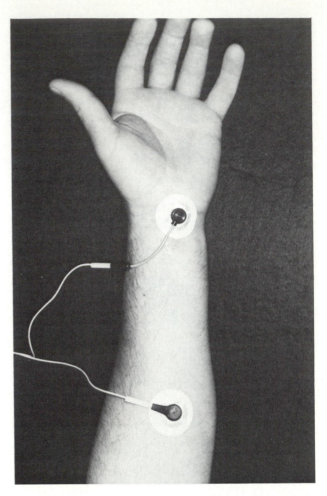

FIG. 49-7. One example of distal electrode placement for patient who has pain resulting from a median nerve injury at wrist.

One electrode is placed in the palm just proximal to the metacarpophalangeal joint of the painful finger. The second electrode is then situated on the dorsum of the hand, also proximal to the metacarpophalangeal joint of the injured digit (Fig. 49-9). Paresthesias should be felt over the amputation stump and along the course of the digital nerves involved. If proximal pain is also present, the second-channel electrodes can be placed either in the axillary scalene area as previously mentioned or over the proximal course of the involved nerve. Although experience may enable the therapist to ascertain in just one treatment session whether TENS will be beneficial to a particular patient, a 2-week trial in the clinic is recommended. This allows enough time for optimal stimulation sites to be located and prevents the patient from experimenting at home on a random basis, which may reduce efficiency. Insurance companies are now willing to reimburse patients for the cost of TENS, but some companies require a 2-week trial before approving the purchase of the device. At the end of the evaluation period, patients obtaining pain relief receive a rental stimulator unit to be used at home for 1 month. Patients who do not achieve pain relief at the end of the 2-week trial are discontinued from this portion of the program.

If the patient is undecided about whether the stimulator is providing pain relief, treatment with TENS is discontinued. The patient is then reevaluated in 3 days. If without the use of the stimulator the patient has experienced an appreciable increase in pain, consideration is given for further treatment with TENS. When the rental stimulator is delivered, the patient is checked out in his proficiency in attaching the electrodes and adjusting the controls.

The patient is instructed initially to use TENS for 1 hour and then to turn off the stimulator but to leave the electrodes in place. He is then told that if he "senses" that pain is returning, he is to use TENS again for 1 hour. The duration of application depends on the severity of the pain, the duration of carry-over, the patient's pain tolerance, and the functional demands placed upon the patient.

SUMMARY

Treatment with the transcutaneous electrical nerve stimulator does not preclude the use of other modalities or procedures. Although some patients present pain as their sole problem, most exhibit edema, decreased joint range of motion, and diffuse hypersensitivity. The purpose of TENS is to decrease pain sufficiently to allow the patient to partic-

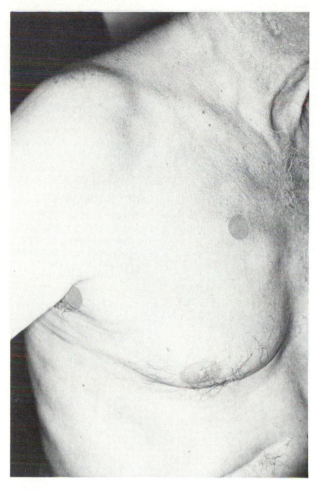

FIG. 49-8. An example of proximal electrode placement.

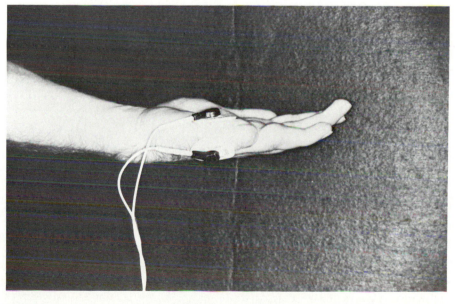

FIG. 49-9. Electrode placement following amputation of little finger. The paresthesias should be felt in amputation stump and along course of digital nerves.

ipate in a complete rehabilitation program and to perform functional activities. TENS should be considered not merely as a modality of last resort but rather as an addition to the treatment regimen of any patient who is experiencing pain severe enough to interfere with his rehabilitation program.

REFERENCES

1. Almay, B.G.L., Johansson, F., von Knorring, L., and others: Endorphins in chronic pain. I. Differences in CSF endorphin levels between organic and psychogenic pain syndromes, Pain **5**:153-162, 1978.
2. Andersson, S.A.: Pain control by sensory stimulation. In Bonica, J.J., Liebeskind, J.C., and Albe-Fessard, D.G., editors: Advances in pain research and therapy, vol. 3, New York, 1979, Raven Press, pp. 569-581.
3. Empi, Inc.: Modulation, 1981, Fridley, Minn.
4. Eriksson, M., and Sjölund, B.: Acupuncture-like analgesia in TNS-resistant chronic pain. In Zolterman, Y., editor: Sensory functions of the skin, 1976, pp. 575-581.
5. Goldstein, A.: Opioid peptides (endorphins) in pituitary and brain, Science **193**:1081-1086, 1976.
6. Gunn, C.C., Ditchburn, F.G., King, M.H., and Renwick, C.J.: Acupuncture loci: a proposal for their classification according to their relationship to known neural structures, Am. J. Chin. Med. **4**(2):183-195, 1976.
7. Lampe, G.: The physical therapists' role in pain management with TENS. In Ersek, R.A., editor: Pain control with TENS, principles and practice, St. Louis, 1981, Warren H. Green, Inc., pp. 40-53.
8. Melzack, R., and Wall, P.D.: Pain mechanism: a new theory, Science **150**(3699):971-979, 1965.
9. Melzack, R.: Phantom limb pain: concept of a central biasing mechanism, Clin. Neurol. **18**:188-207, 1971.
10. Melzack, R.: Prolonged relief of pain by brief, intense transcutaneous somatic stimulation, Pain **1**:357-373, 1975.
11. Melzack, R., Stillwell, D.M., and Fox, E.J.: Trigger points and acupuncture points for pain: correlations and implications, Pain **3**:3-23, 1977.
12. Sjölund, B., and Eriksson, M.: Endorphins and analgesia produced by peripheral conditioning stimulation. In Bonica, J.J., Liebeskind, J.C., and Albe-Fessard, D.G., editors: Advances in pain research and therapy, vol. 3, New York, 1979, Raven Press, pp. 587-592.
13. Sjölund, B., Terenius, L., and Eriksson, M.: Increased cerebrospinal fluid levels of endorphins after electro-acupuncture, Acta Physio. Scand. **100**:382-384, 1977.

BIBLIOGRAPHY

Melzack, R.: The puzzle of pain, New York, 1973, Basic Books Inc.

Lampe, G.N.: Introduction to the use of transcutaneous electrical nerve stimulation devices, Phys. Ther. **58**:1450-1454, 1978.

Santiesteban, A.J., and Sanders, B.R.: Establishing a postsurgical TENS program, Phys. Ther. **60**:789-791, 1980.

Vander Ark, G., and McGrath, K.: Transcutaneous electrical stimulation in treatment of postoperative pain, Am. J. Surg. **130**:338-340, 1975.

VIII
REPLANTATION

50

Surgical aspects of replantation and revascularization

JAMES B. STEICHEN and RICHARD S. IDLER

One of the greatest technologic advances in surgery made this century has been the ability to revascularize complete and incompletely amputated digits and limbs. Many surgeons dealing with extremity injuries are now well versed in the use of the operating microscope and techniques of microvascular surgery. In major replantation centers throughout the world, survival rates of greater than 80% have been reported in series of digital and major limb replanations.[27,50,70,87,96] These excellent survival rates have come about through better surgical skills developed by experience and through refinements in technique, instrumentation, and suture, as well as the development of stringent criteria for acceptable candidates to undergo replantation. Microvascular techniques that were developed through experience with replanation surgery are now being applied to secondary reconstruction in cases of trauma and congenital deformities. The ability to take free composite-tissue transfers of skin, bone, muscle, nerve, toes, digits, and all combinations of the above and to reestablish a blood and/or nerve supply to these tissues has been made possible through experience gained through replantation surgery.[77]

Although replantation surgery has made the transition from the exotic to the commonplace among surgeons, the lay population and the media still focus on the technical feat rather than the functional outcome of replantation. Although advances in techniques of microvascular surgery have enhanced survival of replanted parts, many problems related to the management of other soft-tissue injuries remain, such as the inability to obtain excellent sensory return or tendon gliding after injury. Many major centers that have been actively involved in replantation surgery are now beginning to report their long-term results. The limitations in functional recovery and the problems of secondary reconstruction in replantation patients are becoming apparent. We hope continued refinement in the selection of candidates for replantation can be made so that the best functional results can be provided. Basic understanding of the response to injury of all tissue types is required in order to improve the ultimate function of all patients with hand injuries.

HISTORY OF MAJOR LIMB AND DIGITAL REPLANTATION

Successful experimental major limb replantations were achieved as early as the start of this century by investigators such as Hopfner[17] in 1903 and Carrel and Guthrie[6] in 1906.

This early experimental work was performed on laboratory dogs; it was supplemented by Reichert[68] in 1931, who reported on 52 replants in dogs. Lapchinsky[32] in 1960 reported on follow-up work performed by Soviet investigators during the 1950s on experimental major limb replantation. One significant piece of information to be produced from this work was the importance of limb cooling for limb survival. Snyder[76] in 1960 continued experimental major limb replantation and used a pump oxygenator in an attempt to prolong part preservation. In May 1962, the first clinical major limb replantation was performed by Dr. Ronald Malt.[43] Reports of other major limb replantations rapidly followed—from Ch'en[8] in 1963, Horn[18] in 1964, Shorey and others[74] in 1965, and Williams[94] in 1966. Many replantation centers have continued to perform major limb replantation, mainly of the upper extremity, and the Chinese have accumulated fairly large numbers of major limb replantations and are now beginning to report their long-term follow-up.[55,91]

Before digital replantations could be achieved, the development of the operating microscope and microinstrumentation was necessary. The father of the modern operating microscope is considered to be Nylen, who used the scope experimentally for inner ear dissection in rabbits.[12] Clinical introduction of the operating microscope for middle and inner ear surgery was made in the 1920s by Gunnar Holmgren.[16] Experimental work on vessel anastomoses in dogs with vessel diameters from 0.5 to 4 mm was performed by Seidenberg[71] in 1958. Improvements in magnification and instrumentation by Jacobsen and Suarez permitted successful vascular anastomoses in vessels of 2 mm in dogs and rabbits.[23] The first successful clinical application of small vessel surgery took place in November 1962, when Dr. Harold Kleinert anastomosed a digital artery, revascularizing a partially amputated thumb.[25] By applying techniques of microvascular surgery to other clinical examples, Kleinert was able to demonstrate the feasibility and value of revascularization in upper extremity limb salvage.[24,28] In 1965, Buncke and Schulz reported on their experience with replantation of partial hand amputations in rhesus monkeys, achieving one survival out of nine attempts.[4] In July 1965, Komatsu and Tamai reported the first successful replantation of an amputated thumb after several previous failures.[30] After this, many attempts at digital replantation were made.

By the early 1970s, large series of digital replantations

were reported by O'Brien and Miller,[64] Ch'en,[9] Lendvay,[34] Ikuta,[21] Tsai,[84] and other authors. Continued experimental work was performed during this time to achieve refinements in technique, needles, sutures, and instrumentation. In 1974, O'Brien and Baxter reported on the successful long-term survival of replanted index fingers in stump-tail monkeys, anastomosing vessels of only 0.5 to 0.6 mm.[62] At that same time, Hayhurst and others demonstrated with cooling techniques that successful digital replantation could be performed in monkeys up to 24 hours after amputation.[15] Since the first digital replantation in a human, a wealth of clinical material has been accumulated. This has been supplemented by experimental work in areas such as microscopic changes in vessel anatomy after vessel injury and repair,[1] evaluation of the no-reflow phenomenon,[49] use of intravital stains to identify luminal trauma,[67] and noninvasive techniques of monitoring blood flow.[2] O'Brien in 1977 reported a survival rate of 63% in complete amputations and 80% in incomplete amputations in a series of 103 digits in 74 patients.[56] Recently a number of major replantation centers have reported success rates of greater than 80% after replantation of completely or incompletely amputated digits.[27,50,70,87,96]

REQUIREMENTS FOR REPLANTATION SURGERY

Replantation surgery should be performed only at hospitals with the appropriate equipment and facilities and trained personnel. Although formal replantation centers have not been established in this country, informally several medical centers have established reputations for expertise in replantation surgery. Any center undertaking replantation surgery must have access to emergency transportation systems, particularly if the patient needs transportation over long distances. In digital replantation, because of the absence of muscle tissue, cooling of the part has prolonged the permissible ischemia time. In major limb replantation, however, no more than 6 hours of warm ischemia should elapse, because of the possibility of irreversible muscle death. The primary health care personnel who first manage the potential replantation patient must be educated as to evaluation of appropriate candidates for replantation, initial preparation of the amputated part and stump, appropriate means of transporting the amputated part, and management of associated injuries before and during transit. The replantation center must have the capacity to accept a replantation patient at any time and to initiate immediate treatment. Rapid response to this type of an emergency is facilitated by the creation of a replantation team, with each member having an appropriate job and responsibility. Because replantation surgery frequently involves many hours of operative time, the team approach is beneficial in providing fresh personnel who can be alternated during the course of the procedure. Usually a minimum of two fully trained surgeons is required in order to provide an acceptable replantation service. In large centers where several surgeons are available to function on the team, it is advisable that at least one physician, preferably the one who initiates the procedure, remain throughout the course of the entire operation in order to coordinate the sequence of events. The commitment to replantation surgery

requires the availability of a high-quality operating microscope and well-kept microsurgical instruments. Someone should be available to supervise the maintenance of these items at all times. In addition, an animal laboratory is required so that the surgeons are able to maintain their practical skills and to develop new techniques before their application to humans.

Just as important as the operative care is the postoperative management. Immediately after surgery the replantation patient requires close observation, so that any clinical deterioration in the status of his replanted part can be recognized and appropriate treatment instituted. During this period, other support personnel are necessary to manage problems arising from the sociological and psychological disruption produced by a replantation. Finally, a hand therapy center with therapists fully skilled in the rehabilitation of patients with difficult problems of the upper extremity may be the most important factor in achieving the best functional result possible.

DEFINITIONS

If a part has been *completely* traumatically divided from the body and has lost all vascular supply and all tissue connection, the situation is defined as a *complete* amputation. If there is *any* tissue connection, such as skin, tendon, or nerve, even though all or some of the part's vascular supply is lost and the part would die from avascularity without reestablishment of arterial or venous flow or both, then the situation is defined as an *incomplete* amputation, or a *devascularization*.

The reattachment and repair of the vascular and nonvascular tissues of a completely amputated part are referred to as *replantation*. The repair of the vascular and nonvascular tissues of an incompletely amputated part is termed *revascularization*. Thus the repair and reestablishment of adequate arterial and/or venous flow for both categories is correctly termed *revascularization,* while only the repair and reattachment of parts that are initially completely separate should be defined as *replantation*. This distinction is similar to the distinction between Cognac and brandy; that is, all Cognac is brandy, but not all brandy is Cognac.

INDICATIONS AND CONTRAINDICATIONS IN REPLANTATION SURGERY

In determining whether a patient is a candidate for replantation, one must remember that the goal of treatment is to establish better function in the rest of the injured extremity than would occur if the part were left amputated and the wound closed. This requires return of sensation, adequate skin coverage, a limb free of pain, and the ability to position actively the parts of the limb in a functional manner. Consideration must be given to the type and level of injury, the physiologic age of the patient, his general health, hand dominance, whether the amputation involves single or multiple digits, and the psychological and socioeconomic considerations as well. Many surgeons believe that age is not a major consideration in the evaluation of a patient for replantation.[29,48,86] Systemic disease is not necessarily an absolute contraindication but may influence aftercare and the results.[29] In evaluating the multiply injured hand one must take care to evaluate the hand in light of other possible concurrent injuries to the same or other extremity. In reconstruction of the hand, attempts should be directed toward achieving at least a thumb, the first web space, and two opposable digits.[27] To accomplish this, one frequently needs to be innovative and to improvise by replanting the best parts in their best sites.

Sophistication in technique has made many amputated parts replantable, but from a functional standpoint, this may not be of benefit to the patient. An effort must be made to discuss with the patient the exact magnitude of his injury, the nature of the surgery, the required period of hospitalization, and the rehabilitative program required after surgery. The alternative methods of treatment must be discussed in detail. Consideration must be given to the needs and motivation of the patient. In the end, however, it is the surgeon who must decide whether to proceed with replantation. The surgeon should not be forced into replanting a part that will not be of functional benefit to the patient.

There is general agreement that any patient with a thumb, multiple-digit, or partial-hand amputation should be considered a candidate for replantation (Fig. 50-1). A child with an amputation of any part, even a single digit, is a reasonable candidate for replantation. Replantation of isolated digits distal to the proximal interphalangeal joint is recommended by May,[50] Kleinert,[29] Tamai,[82] and Urban-

iak.[87] They base their support for this view on the fact that functional results are generally good, there is reasonable sensory return without neuromas, which might be present after an amputation, and the operating time is usually less than for a more proximal amputation.

Contraindications to digital replantation and revascularization include severe crush or mangle injuries; injuries at multiple levels in the same digit (Fig. 50-2); medical illnesses that make the patient a poor surgical risk; peripheral vascular disease secondary to diabetes, atherosclerotic cardiovascular disease, and so on; mental instability; and injuries in which individual digits are amputated proximally to the flexor digitorum superficialis insertion (except possibly in females and musicians). Other contraindications to replantation surgery include life-threatening associated injuries, warm ischemia time greater than 12 hours, extreme contamination, and previous injury or surgery to the amputated part. As mentioned, age is not always considered a contraindication to microvascular surgery; replantations have been attempted in patients from ages 10 weeks[86] to greater than 72 years.[69]

Frequently it is not possible to determine whether a part will be acceptable for replantation until it has been appropriately prepared and examined under the operating microscope in the operating room. Two clinical signs that indicate a poor prognosis for successful replantation are the "red-

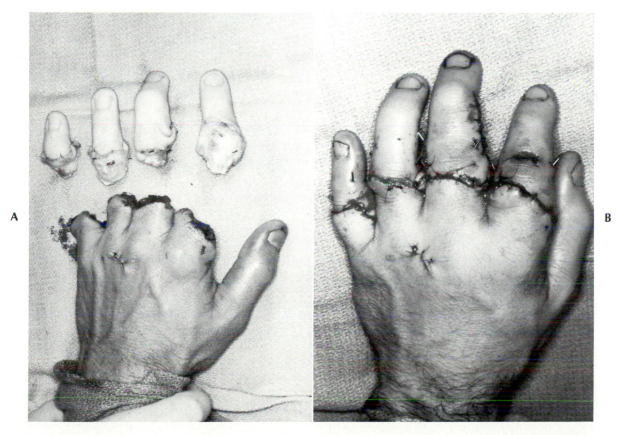

FIG. 50-1. A, Complete amputation of four digits of left hand in a belt and pulley in 25-year-old man. **B,** Replantation with primary repair of all structures of all four digits. *Continued.*

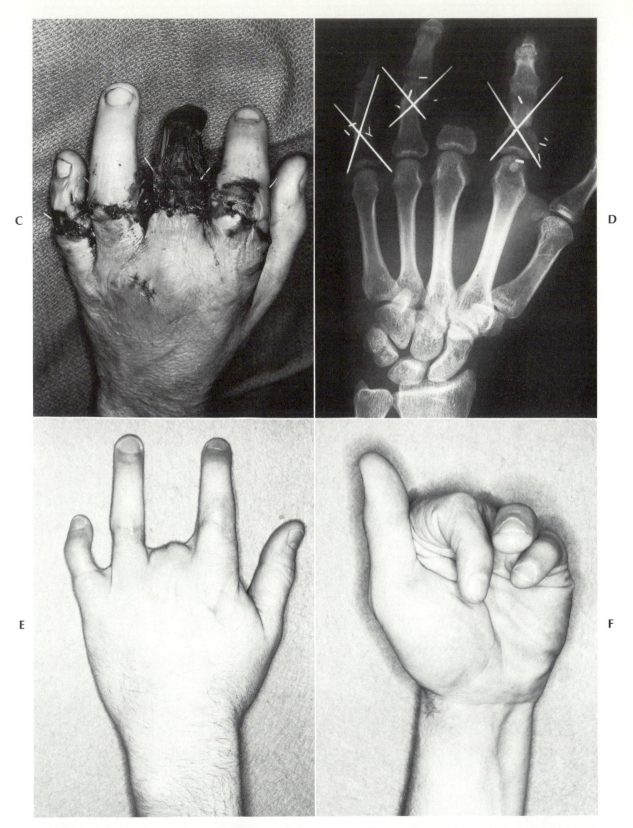

FIG. 50-1, cont'd. C, In immediate postoperative period, long finger developed vascular thrombosis but patient would not consent to surgical reexploration. Digit proceeded to develop avascular necrosis, as shown here 3 weeks after surgery. **D,** Roentgenogram 3 weeks postoperatively showing crossed Kirschner-wire fixation of proximal phalangeal fractures of index and ring and fusion of proximal interphalangeal joint of small finger. **E** and **F,** Result 16 months after replantation. Patient refused secondary capsulotomies and tenolyses to improve range of motion and function.

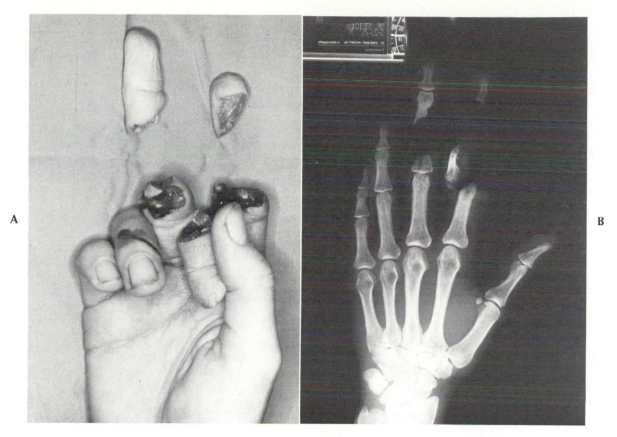

FIG. 50-2. A, Woman, 34 years of age, multilevel amputation of her left index finger and single-level amputation of long finger secondary to a lawnmower injury. **B,** Roentgenogram of injury. Index amputation and devascularization were considered a contraindication to multilevel joint, nerve, and vessel injuries. Long finger was replanted but failed.

line'' sign[28] and the ''ribbon'' sign.[89] The red-line sign, which is visualized on the skin of the amputated part, represents extravasation of blood along a neurovascular bundle, demonstrating a shearing force applied over the length of the neurovascular bundle. The ribbon sign, visualized under the operating microscope, is pronounced tortuosity of the neurovascular bundle secondary to avulsion and represents a relative contraindication to vascular repair requiring resection of the injured length of vessel and vein grafting. Avulsion injuries produce longitudinal trauma to the digital vessels, accounting for the presence of the ribbon and red-line signs. In one series they accounted for 80% of the reoperation rates.[63] Avulsion injuries also carry a poor prognosis because of poor sensory return in avulsed nerves.

Considerations in regard to major limb replantations or revascularizations are similar to those in regard to digital replantation. Although technically major limb replantation may be easier than digital replantation because of the larger size of the vessels, the functional recovery may not be nearly so good, particularly in adults. Pertinent information that is necessary to evaluate in connection with major limb replantation is as follows: age of the patient, occupation, hand dominance, mechanism of injury, associated injury to the other extremities, injuries at other levels of the same extremity, and ischemia time.[47] Children have had the best results in major limb replantation.[44,52] Morrison has sug-

gested an arbitrary upper age limit of 50 years in considering patients for major limb replantation.[52] Sharp amputations occur less frequently in major limb replantations than in digital replantations, but they certainly have a better prognosis than crush or avulsion injuries. Major limb amputations involve higher energy level injuries and subsequently greater soft-tissue injury at the site of amputation. Another factor to consider in major limb replantations is that muscle tissue, which is necessary to make the limb functional, may frequently be traumatically devascularized and crushed. If there has been extensive destruction, devascularization, or contamination of this tissue, then replantation may be contraindicated. Although concomitant injuries in the amputated limb must be taken into consideration, they may be repairable and the limb may be a candidate for replantation. Ch'en has reported on 10 cases involving two-level injury in which limbs were replanted, with six limbs subsequently surviving.[10] Other authors are in agreement that in certain cases two levels of injury of a major limb may not be a contraindication to replantation.[44] However, we believe that in most cases other than those involving children, two-level injury in the same extremity is certainly a contraindication to replantation, because of the poor prognosis for functional return. As with digital replantation, it is not possible to determine before one enters the operating room whether a major limb replantation is possible or indicated. Certainly if arterial flow is established and most of the muscular compartments of the limb are not perfused, replantation should not proceed.

Indications for revascularization are quite straightforward when there is only a loss of circulation or the injuries to other soft tissues are repairable. With devascularization of the multiply injured hand, the considerations in regard to proceeding with surgery are the same as they would be in the case of the same injury with complete amputation. If the decision is made to proceed with surgery, an attempt should be made to reestablish the circulation to all parts of the hand, which will be needed for function or which might be useful in later reconstructive efforts.

DIGITAL REPLANTATION: INITIAL MANAGEMENT

The persons caring for the injured patient at the scene of the accident must be trained to recognize potential replantation candidates. In all cases, the amputated part should be retrieved and brought to the hospital for examination by the physician. Initial care of the amputated part involves placing it in a sponge or cloth moistened with water or a physiologic solution and then placing it in as sterile a container as possible, such as a plastic bag or jar. The plastic bag should be placed in iced fluid in order to reach a chilling temperature somewhere around 4° C. Dry ice should never be used! Care of the amputation site involves topical irrigation with a physiologic solution and attainment of hemostasis with a pressure dressing. It is rare that in digital amputations or amputation of the extremity distal to the wrist that hemostasis cannot be accomplished with the use of a pressure dressing. Appropriate cold preservation of the amputated part is the key to its functional survival; parts appropriately managed have been replanted as long as 37½ hours after the injury. Transportation of the patient and the amputated part from the scene of the accident to a replantation center should be as expedient as possible.

In the emergency room, the patient should be managed with the same care and attention as any other emergency patient. A detailed history should be taken of the accident, so that information is available as to the time of the injury, the mechanism of injury, and whether other injuries were sustained. Other information relevant to making the decision to replant an amputated part consists of the age of the patient, hand dominance, occupation, past medical illnesses, and history of previous injury to the amputated part. A complete physical examination should be performed to establish the patient's ability to withstand lengthy surgery and to determine whether any other injuries that might be life threatening to the patient are present. An x-ray examination should be performed on both the amputated part and the amputation stump. Laboratory procedures of importance include a chest roentgenogram, an electrocardiogram (if the patient is of the appropriate age), hematocrit, urinalysis, prothrombin time, partial thromboplastin time, and type and cross-match for blood. Other laboratory studies may be indicated in specific patients. Before a final commitment is made for replantation, it is important that the patient and his family be informed of the potential surgery, the magnitude of the surgery, the economic considerations involved, the time commitment involved, the potential need for secondary procedures, and a realistic assessment of potential function.

MAJOR LIMB REPLANTATION: INITIAL MANAGEMENT

Accidents producing major limb amputations are usually of a greater magnitude than those causing digital amputations and are therefore more likely to result in associated injuries, which might be life threatening. It is important that these injuries be recognized and managed appropriately. Proper preparation of the amputated limb and expedient transportation of the part is of even greater importance in major limb amputations. The reason is that the more proximal the amputation, the greater the amount of muscle tissue contained in the amputated part. Muscle tissue has a poor tolerance for ischemia, incurring irreversible injury after warm ischemia time exceeds 6 hours. With appropriate cooling of the amputated limb, successful major limb replantations have been performed in China more than 30 hours after the original injury.[7,91] The importance of cooling is that it decreases tissue metabolism, the tissue oxygen requirement, and the production of toxic waste products.

Significant blood loss from the stump after a major limb amputation is more likely to be a problem than after a digital amputation. In most cases, because of retraction of the severed artery into the surrounding soft tissue, hemostasis can be achieved with the use of an appropriately applied pressure dressing.

The use of a tourniquet should be avoided. In rare circumstances of uncontrolled blood loss, it may be necessary to achieve hemostasis by cross-clamping of the offending artery or vein. But this technique should be only rarely contemplated; it may cause more harm than good, since a vital nerve or other tissue may be irreversibly damaged.

In the management of incomplete amputations of either digits or major limbs, care must be taken to align the part appropriately to correct or avoid any kinking of the residual intact tissue. The wound needs to be properly topically irrigated, dressed, and immobilized to prevent any additional injury to the part. Measures must be taken to chill the devitalized part just as if it were completely detached, so that the effects of ischemia are minimized. Perhaps the greatest threat of exsanguination exists in cases of incomplete amputation, since partial arterial injuries will continue to bleed because of their inability to retract into the surrounding soft tissue.

Management of the patient with a major limb amputation upon arrival in the hospital is similar to that of a patient with a digital amputation. It is important that the patient's tetanus status be determined and appropriately updated and that the patient be started on antibiotics prophylactically.

DIGITAL REPLANTATION: SURGICAL MANAGEMENT

An axillary block performed with a long-acting anesthetic such as bupivacaine (Marcaine) is the most appropriate anesthesia for digital replantation and most cases of major limb replantation distal to the elbow. An axillary block is easily and reliably performed by competent anesthesia personnel, it is a rapid form of anesthetic that can be given to a patient even if he has eaten a full meal before his injury, it avoids many of the problems associated with a long general anesthetic, and it provides a sympathetic block to the extremity. A general anesthetic will be required for children and uncooperative adults. It has been recommended that in cases in which a general anesthetic is administered, the anesthetic be supplemented with an axillary block because of its ability to provide long-lasting pain relief after the general anesthesia is over and to provide a sympathetic block.[64,93] Because replantation procedures tend to be prolonged, it is important that the patient be positioned on the operating table in a comfortable position, with sufficient protective padding. It may be necessary to provide a heating blanket, particularly for children, so that core temperature can be maintained at an appropriate level. Intravenous lines are necessary for fluid and antibiotic administration. In some instances, transfusions will be required. In all cases, a Foley catheter should be placed in the bladder for fluid management and to avoid the disruption of the patient needing to void during the procedure. It is important that consideration be given to surgical preparation of other parts of the body in case other tissues, such as skin or veins, are required during the procedure. If it is necessary, the patient can be administered a short-acting general anesthetic for the period of time necessary to take whatever graft tissue may be required.

It is important that all instruments and equipment required for the procedure be available and in working order. This is particularly true of the microvascular instruments, which one should check regularly to ascertain if all are functioning and without damaged parts.

The procedure should begin with inspection of the amputated part. Our procedure is to take the amputated part and gently irrigate it and scrub it with an antibiotic soap such as hexachlorophene or povidone-iodine (Betadine). Once the part has been cleansed, it should be returned to its bed of ice so that it is kept chilled. Attention should be directed first to inspection of the part, particularly if one is uncertain as to whether the quality of the part is such that it can be salvaged. The part should be inspected under high-power loupe magnification or the operating microscope. It should be possible for the surgeon to work on the amputated part while keeping it on a bed of ice, so that the warm ischemia time is minimized. One prepares the amputated part by first identifying and tagging all structures required for repair. If additional exposure is required for finding the neurovascular bundles, lateral midline incisions are made, allowing a volar flap and a dorsal flap to be mobilized. The flexor and extensor tendons are identified and, if necessary, debrided, and a modified Kessler type of repair or other appropriate intratendinous repair using 4-0 synthetic suture is placed into the end of the tendons. Initial bony débridement is performed only to remove contamination and severely comminuted fragments. Dorsal veins are identified and clipped at their most distal ends for later identification and repair. Sometimes it is necessary to explore for volar veins and venae comitantes if adequate dorsal veins are not present.

A two-team approach is utilized at this point, with one team working on the amputated part while the other team begins preparation of the amputation stump site. Once it has been determined by the team working on the amputated part that it is replantable, measures are taken by the second team to prepare the amputation stump to receive the part to be replanted. If the amputation stump is on a digit, lateral midaxial incisions are made in order to achieve exposure of the neurovascular bundles. If the level is more proximal into the palm, zigzag incisions are utilized to obtain additional proximal exposure. At the amputation stump the neurovascular bundles are identified and tagged at their most distal aspect with a clip, with one clip identifying the artery and two clips identifying the nerve. Dorsal veins are identified and tagged. An attempt is made to retrieve the proximal ends of the flexor tendons with minimal trauma to the flexor tendon system. If necessary, additional proximal incisions are made so that the tendons can be retrieved. Once both the flexor and extensor tendons have been retrieved and identified, sutures similar to those described for the amputated part are placed. Bony débridement is again limited to that necessary to eliminate comminution and contamination.

Because of the frequently complex and lengthy nature of the surgery, it is very important that during the procedure, as the parts are being identified, one make a list of the structures that have been identified, describing their condition and their potential for functional utilization.

When confronted with multiple digital amputations, most surgeons would agree that the most important digits should be replanted first. Certainly the thumb takes precedence as the most important digit when it is involved. When possible, each digit should be revascularized individually. This permits the digits awaiting revascularization to remain cool until needed. Occasionally several replanted digits will be connected by skin bridges. Under these circumstances, if it is believed that important lymphatic and venous channels are present within the skin bridge, the digits need to be replanted as a unit, which means that the warm ischemia time may be significant for the last replanted or revascularized finger.

Regarding the order of tissue repair within each digit, we begin with bony fixation, followed by extensor tendon repair, flexor tendon repair, nerve repair, arterial repair, venous repair, and skin closure. There is some controversy as to the exact order of tissue repair, particularly the order of venous versus arterial repair. Investigators such as Phelps,[67] Kleinert,[29] and O'Brien[57] believe that venous repair should be performed before arterial repair. It is their belief that this will minimize blood loss and minimize swelling after revascularization, allowing better skin closure. They have not found that thromboses occur at the site of the venous anastomosis while arterial repair is being awaited and have found no difficulty with multiple deflations and inflations of the tourniquet during other vascular repairs. Those who advocate repair of the artery before that of the vein are surgeons such as Urbaniak[87] and Lendvay.[33] It is their philosophy that early arterial repair diminishes the effects of ischemia on the digit and also may facilitate identification of veins for repair.

Bone shortening

Most investigators believs that bone shortening should be performed not only to eliminate contamination and comminution but also to permit easy approximation of the damaged soft tissues, particularly the neurovascular bundles.* In most cases of sharp amputations of the digit or amputations involving limited local crush, 0.5 to 1 cm of shortening is required; however, this is dictated primarily by the amount of associated soft-tissue injury. Urbaniak also believes that shortening the digit makes it less likely to "get in the way" postoperatively and thus facilitates its function.[87] Others, such as Tupper[85] and Phelps,[67] believe that only a minimal amount of bone shortening should be performed for elimination of contamination or comminution, unless there is a complete segmental defect of all soft tissues. Bone shortening only to eliminate a gap between the neurovascular bundles may also be managed by appropriate vein and neural grafts. When bone shortening is to be performed, it should always, whenever possible, be done on the distal amputated part rather than proximally, to preserve proximal length in case of failure of the replantation or revascularization.

Bony fixation

A number of methods are utilized to achieve bone fixation in replantation surgery. Perhaps the simplest method is use of the single longitudinal intramedullary pin, which is advocated by Urbaniak[86,87] and Lendvay.[33] The advantages of this technique are that it is simple and quick, requires minimal local dissection, provides adequate bone stock for approximation, and allows for rotational adjustment while one is aligning and repairing other soft-tissue structures. Rotational control is provided through repair of the adjacent soft tissues, particularly the flexor and extensor tendons, or may also be supplemented by a second longitudinal wire or an oblique Kirschner wire. Placement of this oblique Kirschner wire should be done before any vascular anastomoses, so as not to jeopardize the vascular repairs in any way. Perhaps the most common method of bone fixation is the use of the crossed Kirschner wire. Other available methods of bone fixation include intraosseous wiring or the combination of Kirschner wires and intraosseous wiring as advocated by Lister,[38] small fragment plates and screws as advocated by Meuli[51] and Tupper,[85] and microscrews as developed by Ikuta and Tsuge.[20] Recently a system of intramedullary screw fixation has been developed independently by Tamai[82] and Irigaray[22] and Yamano.[95] The disadvantage of this system is that it is only applicable to complete amputations and not to incomplete amputations. Leung[37] has recently reported on his experience using autograft or allograft intramedullary bone pegs for fixation. He reported on a series of 25 cases of digital replantation or revascularization and 35 toe-to-hand transfers in which this technique was utilized. He was able to achieve union in all cases and was able to start motion as early as 3 to 4 weeks postoperatively. Bone union was reported as early as 6 to 10 weeks. No supplemental fixation was required, and the technique was useful with fractures and amputations within 0.5 cm of an adjacent

*See references 29, 31, 41, 57, 87, and 92.

joint. Urbaniak, in his series of more than 200 patients with digital replantations, has had a malunion rate of less than 5% and has performed no secondary procedures for nonunion after his method of longitudinal intramedullary Kirschner-wire fixation.[87]

For bone fixation of complete or incomplete amputations through the metacarpal level, Kirschner-wire fixation is usually chosen. For those familiar with small-fragment plate and/or screw fixation, more stable fixation can frequently be achieved with these techniques, allowing earlier mobilization. For amputations through the level of the carpus, proximal row carpectomy with Kirschner-wire fixation may be advised.[45] If substantial damage to either the carpus or the distal radius has occurred, the remaining bony surfaces should be prepared in an attempt to achieve an arthrodesis.

Arthrodesis

When the amputation has taken place near or through the level of the metacarpophalangeal or interphalangeal joint, one must decide whether an arthrodesis needs to be performed. Most surgeons tend to perform arthrodeses of the joint if it is damaged beyond function. O'Brien recommends arthrodesis of the proximal interphalangeal joint of the index finger in a position of 15 degrees of flexion and arthrodesis of the more ulnar digits in approximately 50 degrees of flexion.[57] Phelps advocates proximal interphalangeal arthrodesis at 25 to 30 degrees regardless of the digit and metacarpophalangeal arthrodesis in a position of 30 to 35 degrees of flexion.[67] An alternative to formal arthrodesis, usually performed with crossed Kirschner wires or a tension band technique, is to perform a resectional arthroplasty with the possibility of secondary silicone rubber (Silastic) reconstruction or to perform a primary silicone rubber arthroplasty at the time of replantation.[27] Primary silicone rubber arthroplasty has been performed by investigators such as our group; however, the long-term success of this technique is still not clear. Another innovative technique for management of amputations near or involving the distal or proximal interphalangeal joint is utilization of a polypropylene intramedullary peg, as developed by Harrison. Such intramedullary pegs provide rapid stabilization with minimal shortening. A single peg is available for the distal interphalangeal joint and is preangled at 25 degrees. The proximal interphalangeal pins are individualized to the index, middle, ring, and little fingers and are also preangled, progressing from 20 degrees for the index finger through 50 degrees for the little finger. The ultimate goal of these pegs is to provide sufficient stability to permit early motion of the digit while still leading to an arthrodesis. Harrison in his original report had a clinically stable bony arthrodesis achieved in 5 out of 12 digits and reported no infections or extrusions related to use of the pegs.[14]

Tendon repair

Extensor tendon repair is performed using figure-of-eight or horizontal mattress sutures of 4-0 synthetic braided suture in order to bring about end-to-end approximation of the extensor tendons. Care must be taken that both lateral bands are identified and that these structures are repaired; otherwise one will not achieve adequate extension at the proximal or distal interphalangeal joint.

Flexor tendon repair is performed by reuniting the two ends of the flexor tendon by tying together the ends of the previously placed intratendinous sutures. If the digital amputation is proximal to the insertion of the superficialis tendon, both the profundus and superficialis tendons are repaired. An attempt is made in preparation of the tendons to perform as little débridement as possible—only the amount

necessary to rebalance correct tendon length after shortening. The intratendinous suture may be supplemented by a circumferential suture of 6-0 or 7-0 nylon, if necessary, to achieve a smooth repair. The tendons should be handled as gingerly as possible, just as if one were doing an isolated tendon repair. Tendon adhesions and lack of flexor tendon gliding constitute one of the major postoperative problems after replantation surgery, and probably not enough attention to detail is paid while one is performing repair of the flexor

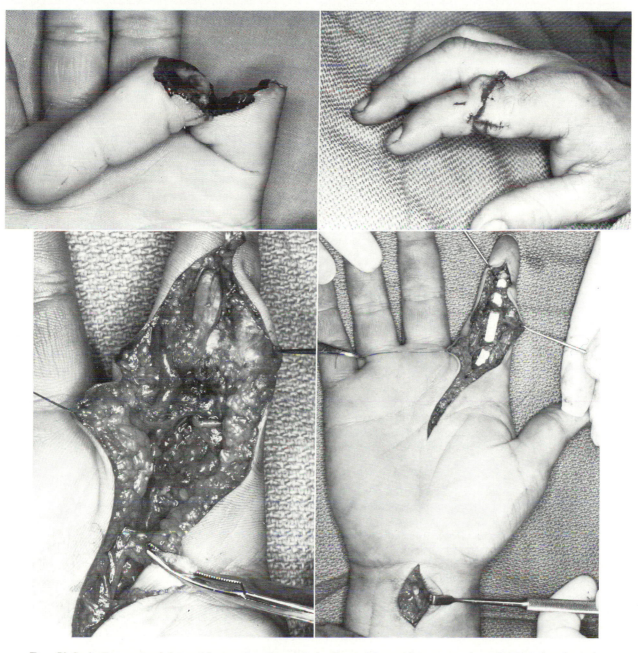

FIG. 50-3. **A,** Power-saw injury with complete devascularization and incomplete amputation of right index finger in 25-year-old butcher. **B,** Revascularization with primary repair of all structures. **C,** Seven months postoperatively, patient had achieved good passive range of motion but no active flexion, and surgical exploration revealed rupture of repaired flexor tendons. **D,** Two-stage flexor tendon reconstruction was performed with insertion of silicone rubber rod followed by later free tendon graft.

Continued.

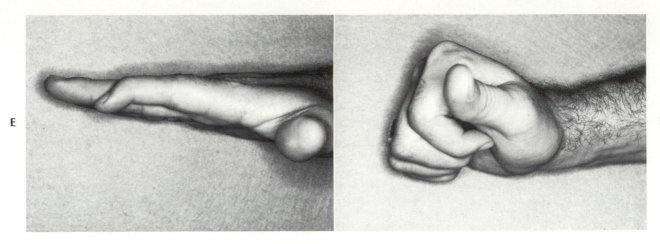

FIG. 50-3, cont'd. **E** and **F,** Final motion as seen 2 years postoperatively, with some remaining cold sensitivity.

tendons (Fig. 50-3). Repair of the flexor tendons may be delayed until after the neurovascular repairs have been performed, because reapproximation of the flexor tendon does tend to put the digit in a position of flexion, which may make subsequent repairs difficult. If the flexor tendon system is not optimal for primary repair, plans should be made for secondary staged tendon reconstruction with silicone rubber rods and tendon grafting.[87] Primary placement of silicone rubber tendon rods has been suggested by Scott,[70] Morrison,[54] and Lendvay.[33,34] Lendvay did report a 20% removal rate after initial placement, but this apparently resulted in no compromise to the digit, and subsequent replacement of the silicone rubber rods without difficulty was possible.

Nerve repair

Many surgeons believe that nerve repair should be performed before arterial repair, because it can be done in a field free of blood. Up to now there is no evidence to demonstrate that ischemia time in the appropriately cooled digit affects the quality of sensory return after primary nerve repair in digital replantation.[13,26,63]

In replantations distal to the wrist, nerve repair is performed with interrupted sutures of 10-0 or 9-0 nylon. The amount of débridement of the nerve required before repair is determined by the nature of the original injury. Using the operating microscope, the surgeon needs to resect the nerve to a level where normal-looking fasciculi with surrounding epineurium are present. It is frequently difficult to identify healthy neural tissue in the acute situation, and especially in avulsion injuries, large defects may be present between two healthy ends of the nerve. For this reason it may be necessary to harvest nerves for interpositional grafting. Available donor sources are the lateral and/or medial antebrachial cutaneous nerves of the forearm, the dorsal sensory branch of the ulnar nerve at the wrist, the sural nerve from either leg, and possibly a digital nerve harvested from a nonreplantable digit. Based on past experience with replantations, primary end-to-end nerve repairs perform much

better than secondary repairs.[70,93] It has not yet been determined, however, that primary nerve grafts perform as well. Secondary nerve repairs are complicated by the tremendous amount of scarring that occurs about the unrepaired neuromas and gliomas, which puts the digit at some risk for potential injury to its repaired blood supply.

Arterial repair

The basic principle of arterial repair is to approximate normal intima to normal intima. With avulsion injuries the extent of longitudinal trauma to the artery may be quite significant, and frequently it is very difficult to identify acutely. An attempt has been made to utilize intravital stains to identify intimal damage, but this has not been consistently accurate.[67] One must closely inspect the vessel under high magnification with the operating microscope to identify any intimal separation from the media or the presence of thrombus formation on the surface of the intima, either of which suggests vessel damage. No arterial repair should be performed under abnormal tension. If the defect created by débridement of the artery is greater than what would permit a primary anastomosis, interpositional grafting must be performed. Ready sources of vein grafts are the volar surface of the forearm and the dorsum of the foot. One should take care to select a vein that is comparable in size to the artery to which it will be interposed. The vein should be reversed from its normal direction of flow so that any valves that may be present in the graft do not obstruct the arterial flow. Care should be taken not to place an interpositional graft that is too long, since it may lead to kinking and subsequent thrombosis. Sometimes it is possible to avoid the use of a vein graft by mobilizing an arterial pedicle from an adjacent normal digit or digit that is not replantable or by crossed arterial repairs within the same digit. In most circumstances, it is the ulnar digital artery that is the largest and most easily repaired in the thumb or the index finger. Most surgeons believe that an effort should be made to repair both digital arteries in the finger so that its vascularity is improved and an insurance policy provided should one of the arterial repairs become thrombosed. Some surgeons have intimated that repairing two digital arteries as opposed to one results in less cold intolerance and better return of sensation; however, there are no data up to now to support either one of these statements.[13,70]

Arterial repairs distal to the level of the wrist are performed with use of interrupted sutures of 10-0 nylon. In preparation of the vessel, minimal adventitial stripping is performed. Only enough adventitial tissue is mobilized to prevent any loose ends of adventitial tissue from entering the vessel lumen. Approximation of the vessel ends for repair is achieved with an approximator microvascular clamp. Some surgeons, such as Urbaniak, believe that these types of clamps should be used only as necessary and that with appropriate bone shortening or appropriate grafts, vessel anastomoses can be performed without the use of the clamps, with hemostasis being achieved at the time of vascular repair by inflation of the pneumatic tourniquet.[87] Urbaniak,[87] Kleinert,[26] and others[81,83] have reported that intermittent inflation and deflation of the pneumatic tourniquet will not lead to thrombosis at the sites of previous vascular anastomoses, either arterial or venous.

One must determine before vessel repair that there is adequate flow through the proximal limb of the artery. One can do this by release of the pneumatic tourniquet or the microvascular clamp, or both, on the proximal limb of the vessel. In a patient with adequate arterial pressure, a digital artery should have enough pulse pressure to generate a stream of blood that reaches beyond the end of the digit and, one would hope, beyond the operative field. If the arterial stream is sufficiently powerful to reach the end of the hand table, we consider this a positive squirt test and a good prognostic sign for flow. Should good flow not be present, one must determine why this is the case. It may be that there is spasm in the proximal artery, which may be relieved with the use of an appropriate topical vasodilator, such as lidocaine or bupivacaine (Marcaine). Sometimes additional adventitial stripping is beneficial, which produces a local sympathectomy. Occasionally one has to pass a fine dilator into the lumen of the proximal vessel to facilitate the removal of an obstructing clot. It goes without saying that atraumatic technique needs to be utilized while one performs the arterial anastomoses. Frequent irrigation of the field with a heparinized Ringer's solution is important, to keep the tissues moist and prevent accumulation from developing on the microinstruments, needles, and suture. Once the arterial repair is completed, the pneumatic tourniquet or microvascular clamp is released and good blood flow should return to the digit. Poor flow may exist initially secondary to vascular spasm. This can be relieved by the use of a topical local vasodilator and by topical irrigation with warm physiologic solutions. Restoration of acceptable blood flow to the finger should result in a digit that is pink and that has good capillary refill. The usual number of sutures necessary for a 1-mm vessel ranges from 6 to 10. It is not unusual to have some bleeding at the anastomotic site after release of the clamps, and one can minimize this by gently wrapping adjacent soft tissue about the anastomosis or using a small piece of background material folded over the anastomosis.

Venous repair

Venous repair is performed in a manner similar to arterial repair, although it is technically more difficult because of the thinner, more friable nature of the walls of the veins. It is necessary to perform a venous repair that unites normal venous intima to normal venous intima. Débridement of the vessel ends must be performed before repair. In most digital replantations, the major veins will be found on the dorsum of the finger, although occasionally only a volar vein or vena comitans will be found for repair. Large gaps between vessel ends are best bridged with vein grafts. No venous repair should be performed under tension. Occasionally it is possible to swing over a venous pedicle from an adjacent digit, although one must do this without jeopardizing the venous drainage of the donor digit. An approximating clamp may be utilized during the venous repair, but great care must be taken to avoid injury to the vessels with the use of this clamp. The recommended ratio of venous to arterial repair is 2:1.[70,87,93] The minimal number of veins repaired per digit should be two.[80] If interpositional venous grafts are necessary to repair the veins without tension, it is important to remember not to reverse the vein graft from its original orientation.

Wound closure

Wound closure at the end of a replantation can be quite difficult, because of several factors. Sufficient skin may not be present because of loss from the original injury or removal with débridement. Local swelling after revascularization may prevent closure. No attempt should be made to close skin under tension. Skin should be loosely approximated so that constriction of the vascular repairs is prevented. Circular wounds can be broken up by Z-plasties. If lateral midaxial incisions have been utilized, no closures of these incisions will be necessary so long as the arterial repairs are appropriately protected by overlying soft tissue. An attempt should be made to provide coverage for any exposed arterial or venous repairs. When this is not possible, split-thickness skin grafts can be applied over vessel repairs.[26,40,64,96] In rare circumstances, there may be indications for performing local flap coverage, such as a dorsal rotation flap or cross-finger pedicle flap, or even for constructing a distant pedicle flap for coverage. The problem with employing such flaps is that should vascular compromise occur during the postoperative period, operative intervention is somewhat hindered by the presence of the flaps.

Thumb replantation

Replantation of a thumb presents several special technical problems. For one thing, preservation of length is the key. Any bone shortening that is being performed in order to achieve soft-tissue approximation should be done on the amputated part, so that should the replantation fail, the patient will still be left with a stump of maximum bone length.

Reestablishing arterial supply to the thumb can be difficult, because of the anatomy of its blood supply and the difficulty involved in positioning the thumb under the operating microscope at the time of repair. Although in 80% of patients, the princeps pollicis artery will arise from the first palmar metacarpal artery, remember that some patients will have a substantial contribution either from the superficial palmar arch or from the first dorsal metacarpal artery.[66] Usually it is necessary to repair the ulnar digital artery, because frequently the radial digital artery of the thumb is quite small and seemingly clinically insignificant. For amputations or revascularizations distal to the midportion of the proximal phalanx, it is usually possible to achieve a primary end-to-end digital artery repair. For more proximal amputations, however, this is frequently not possible, or if large segmental defects are present because of avulsion injuries, vein grafting should be contemplated. Shafiroff has recommended that in these circumstances the distal amputated part be prepared as any other amputated digit is prepared for replantation, with appropriate identification of the neurovascular bundles and preplacement of intratendinous sutures. He then sews any required vein grafts into position to the digital arteries and dorsal veins. The amputated thumb is stabilized and its tendons are repaired. It is now possible to take the previously placed arterial vein graft and to anastomose it into either the dorsal branch of the radial artery or into the superficial palmar arch.[73] In Schlenker's series of thumb replantations, 49 patients underwent primary repair of their digital vessels, but 15 patients required vein grafting for arterial reconstruction. He did this by performing an end-to-side proximal anastomosis with the dorsal branch of the radial artery and then taking the vein graft through the first web to the digital arteries, where either an end-to-end or end-to-side anastomosis was performed with the digital arteries, depending on the size discrepancy between the digital arteries and the vein graft. In no cases in which a distal end-to-end vein-graft arterial anastomosis was performed did the cul-de-sac at the end of the vein graft lead to failure of the replant.[69] Another technique that is sometimes used to provide an arterial supply to the thumb is to mobilize an arterial pedicle, such as the radial digital artery from the index finger, with enough length for anastomosis into the distal digital artery of the amputated thumb.[85] Frequently the radial digital artery of the index finger is quite small, and one may need to take the vascular pedicle from another digit, such as the middle finger. This technique which has been proposed by Lobay, who transfers the ulnar neurovascular bundle of the middle finger to the ulnar neurovascular bundle of the thumb in cases of thumb avulsion. Using this technique, he has been able to increase his survival rate from 54% to 85%. Use of the ulnar digital nerve from the middle finger to provide innervation to the ulnar aspect of the thumb has not improved sensation in the thumb, and in all cases patients have interpreted stimulation of the ulnar border of the thumb as involving the middle finger.[39]

MAJOR LIMB REPLANTATION: SURGICAL MANAGEMENT

From a surgical standpoint, major limb replantations are quite similar to digital replantations. When possible, an axillary block is utilized for upper extremity major limb replantations, although with more proximal amputations a general anesthetic is needed. As with digital replantation, when the patient is being prepared and draped it is important to contemplate the possible need for tissue graft donor sites and to prepare these areas. A team approach is valuable in minimizing ischemia time, with one team preparing the amputated part while the other team prepares the recipient stump.

The major difference between a digital replantation and a more proximal major limb replantation is the presence of muscle. This is a tissue that tolerates trauma and ischemia very poorly, yet its presence and survival are crucial for producing a functioning extremity. The key to achieving a successful major limb replantation is to perform an adequate débridement and to achieve revascularization of the extremity as quickly as possible. It is extremely important that both the amputated part and the amputation stump be examined quite closely as the structures are being identified and tagged. If substantial muscle damage has occurred beyond the point where function will be possible after replantation, the replantation should not proceed. Another important consideration is the status of the nerves, and the mechanism by which the major limb amputation occurred. Although in the young child one can be quite aggressive about major limb replantation, in the adult the presence of nerve avulsion is an ominous sign and needs to be considered in the decision to proceed further with replantation.

In the past, major limb replantation has proceeded first with bone débridement and stabilization. The amount of bone resection is dictated by that necessary to achieve soft-tissue approximation. Resection of as much as 18 cm of bone has been performed in major upper limb replantations. The techniques of bone stabilization that are the most rapid rather than the most rigid have generally been used, in an effort to minimize warm ischemia time. For that reason, the techniques of fixation have usually been simple screw fixation, crossed Kirschner-wire technique, or intramedullary rodding. Recently, Manktelow[46] and Urbaniak[88] have demonstrated that carotid shunts may be placed in both the arterial and venous systems of the replanted major limb, thereby revitalizing the limb and allowing more time to achieve a rigid bony fixation using A-O technique or other methods as preferred by the surgeon. Once bone stabilization has been achieved, attention can then be directed toward removal of the shunts and replacement with a vein graft or primary anastomosis if possible.[46]

The first surgeons having clinical experience with major limb replantations recommended venous repair before arterial repair.[43,46] The reason for this was to prevent major blood loss and to minimize swelling. Most surgeons performing major limb replantation in the United States now recommend arterial repair before venous repair. This allows the limb to be revascularized and to be purged of toxic waste products that have accumulated during the ischemia time. Deaths have occurred in this country after revascularization of major limb replants in which venous repair was performed before arterial repair.[42] Wang, from China, recently reported a series of 91 major limb replantations in which venous anastomosis was performed before arterial anastomosis and had no episodes of complications arising from toxic metabolites after revascularization of the replanted limb. He attributed this to adequate cold preservation of the part before replantation.[91]

When revascularization of the replanted limb has been achieved, it is paramount that all muscle groups be inspected as to their viability. It may be possible that some muscle groups are not adequately perfused, and under these circumstances these muscles should be resected to prevent tissue necrosis and possible severe infection.

Achieving a technically good nerve repair is very important in the success of a major limb replantation, because one is trying to provide a limb that is more functional than a prosthesis. One needs a *sensate* limb with actively movable parts, and this can only be accomplished through reinnervation. One may need nerve grafts to achieve an adequate nerve repair without tension. It may or may not be appropriate to perform a nerve graft as a primary procedure at the time of replantation. If a primary nerve repair or graft is undertaken, one must take care to achieve fascicular alignment.

Muscle repair is performed with absorbable sutures to align the muscle groups. Care should be taken to minimize trauma to the remaining muscular tissue. Adequate muscle tissue must remain in order to make the limb functional. We cannot overemphasize that the key to survival of a major limb replantation is adequate débridement, so that no necrotic muscle or soft tissue is left behind to serve as a potential source of infection. A primary reason for failure of major limb replantations is necrosis and infection.[52,58,91]

In most cases of upper extremity major limb replantation, fasciotomies are indicated in the forearm, carpal tunnel, and intrinsic muscles. In Wang's series of major limb replantations, 65 upper limb replantations were performed and 10 cases of interosseous contracture developed in patients with ischemia times of only 5 to 9 hours.[91]

Skin closure may or may not be possible. Z-plasties and local flaps may sometimes facilitate coverage of vascular and neural repairs. Split-thickness skin grafts may be of great help in achieving wound coverage; in rare circumstances distant pedicle flaps may be utilized, but they are not normally recommended.

POSTOPERATIVE MANAGEMENT

Postoperative management for both digital and major limb replantations begins in the operating room with the application of an appropriate dressing. The purpose of the dressing is to provide protective, comfortable positioning of the extremity. The dressing must be such that it is able to accept drainage from the wounds but at the same time provide protection from external contamination. Maintaining a warm environment for the extremity is important for prevention of peripheral vasospasm from cold exposure. The dressing must be applied in such a way that it does not inflict injury on the replanted part from pressure or constriction. This is particularly true when the dressing becomes soaked with bloody drainage. Although the dressing should not be applied overly tight, it should create a gradient of pressure decreasing distally to proximally to control swelling.

The dressing we apply begins with a nonadherent petrolatum-impregnated dressing that is applied over all wounds but does not overlap. This is followed by fluffed sterile gauze pads that are placed between the fingers and over all exposed wounds. Care must be taken in the placement of any dressing material between the digits, particularly in a digital replantation, so as not to create pressure that might compromise the neurovascular bundles. The fluffed gauze dressing is then supplemented with either foam or polyester fiber (Dacron), and the dressing is completed with a plaster splint applied to one side of the extremity. The plaster splint is held in place with a nontensed elastic bandage.

Postoperative orders should include instructions regarding elevation, antibiotics, anticoagulation, frequency of neurovascular checks, and guidelines outlining circumstances under which the physician should be contacted.

Our recommendation for elevation of digital replantations and distal major limb replantations is to use a sling that gently supports the extremity in an elevated position above the heart, with the elbow flexed between 45 and 60 degrees. Phelps recommends avoiding elevation greater than 30 degrees. He believes that at this point, hydrostatic resistance to flow may jeopardize circulation to the extremity.[67] Care must be taken to watch that the elbow is not overly flexed, which might create obstruction to venous drainage.

An antibiotic in the form of a cephalosporin is begun preoperatively and administered for at least 10 days during the postoperative period. Additional oral antibiotics may be indicated in appropriate circumstances.

During the infancy of replantation surgery, great attention was paid to anticoagulation, based primarily on the results of animal experimentation in which survival was improved with the use of anticoagulants.[15] Initial recommendations were the use of aspirin, low-molecular-weight dextran, dipyridamole (Persantin), and continuous systemic heparinization, with the partial thromboplastin time placed at one and a half to two times normal. It was found that heparinization that was begun intraoperatively frequently lead to significant postoperative bleeding. This was somewhat lessened when heparinization was begun 24 hours postoperatively. As surgical techniques in replantation surgery improved, however, it became apparent that the need for extensive anticoagulation was not necessary. Most surgeons now use primarily aspirin or low-molecular-weight dextran, or both, as protection against vascular thrombosis.[39,50,70] Our regimen is to use 600 mg of aspirin, administered orally twice a day, and 500 ml of low-molecular-weight dextran (LMD) in glucose, given intravenously over 4 hours each day, for 5 to 10 days postoperatively. Some surgeons, such as Bright[3] and Kleinert,[27] still recommend systemic heparinization in replantation of severe injuries or in injuries in which technical difficulties are encountered intraoperatively. For major limb replantation, many surgeons recommend no anticoagulation,[60] although the use of aspirin and LMD is prevalent.

During the immediate postoperative period, the patient is placed on strict bed rest and his activities are limited. An attempt is made to minimize pain and anxiety, because both of these may be factors in producing peripheral vasoconstriction. It is important that the patient be provided with adequate pain medication around the clock as needed during the initial postoperative period. It is important that the morale of the patient be maintained through supportive contacts with the nursing staff and the surgical staff. If sedation is required, chlorpromazine hydrochloride, 25 mg given orally three times a day, is usually recommended, because of its associated vasodilatory effects.

During the initial 24 to 48 hours the patient is not fed, so that should it be necessary to return the patient to the operating room this can be done without delay. Once the patient is started on a diet, he is restricted from caffeine-containing products, and during the entire postoperative time he is in the hospital, he is prevented from smoking.

The greatest risk to the replant during the postoperative period is vascular occlusion, which occurs most frequently within the first 10 days after surgery. Over 80% of vascular occlusions will occur within the first 24 to 48 hours.[53] Close monitoring of the replanted part is essential in order to achieve an early diagnosis of this complication and to take appropriate corrective measures. Attempts have been made to improve on constant monitoring of the replant with the use of devices such as ultrasonic Doppler scanners and digital pulse volume flowmeters. The difficulty with these techniques is that they are not capable of identifying venous obstruction until it has progressed to the point that it begins to compromise arterial function.[3] Constant-temperature probe monitoring has been used effectively by Urbaniak.[88] He uses a three-probe system in which one probe is applied to the replanted digit, one to an adjacent normal digit, and one to the dressing to achieve an ambient temperature. Stirrat[79] reports that normal digital temperature after a replantation is usually 30° to 35° C in the uninjured digit. During the initial postoperative phase, the digital temperature of a replanted digit is frequently greater than that of the normal digit. Thrombosis should be suspected if the temperature of the replanted digit drops more than 2.5° C while the control digit remains unchanged, if the replanted digital temperature drops below 30° C for more than 1 hour, or if the control digit temperature drops below 30° C without an obvious cause. In Stirrat's reported series using temperature monitoring, no replanted digit with a continuous temperature drop below 30° C for more than 12 hours survived.[79]

A healthy replanted digit is warm, it is pinker than a normal digit, and it demonstrates a rapid capillary refill. The pulp of the digit will feel full, with good turgor. Arterial occlusion should be suspected if the digit becomes cool and pale, loses turgor, or demonstrates slow capillary refill. Venous obstruction is usually present if a finger takes on a bluish purple hue, has a drop in temperature, and demonstrates a very brisk capillary refill. Stirrat has been able to correlate these subjective clinical findings with objective temperature changes detected by surface monitoring in replanted digits.[79]

If it is suspected that the digital replant is failing secondary to vascular occlusion, appropriate measures must be taken to correct this. The initial measure is to check the dressing for constriction, usually resulting from hardened blood-stained dressings adjacent to the site of vascular repair. On occasion, adjustment of the position of the arm will improve its circulation. If arterial occlusion is diagnosed, the arm should be lowered below the heart. If venous occlusion is diagnosed, the extremity should be elevated. It is important to rule out diffuse peripheral vascular shutdown as the cause of diminished circulation in the replanted part.

At this point temperature monitoring may be helpful, by allowing identification of a drop in temperature of the normal digits. Diffuse peripheral vascular shutdown may result from inadequate hydration, blood loss, pain, anxiety, offending agents such as caffeine and nicotine, or a drop in core temperature. If conservative corrective measures fail to improve the circulation of the replanted part, the patient should be returned immediately to the operating room for exploration of his neurovascular repairs. Frequently, the administration of a stellate ganglion block (in a nonheparinized patient) and a dressing change will result in a return of normal circulation to the replanted part. Under no circumstances should a major dressing change be performed without the benefit of a stellate block, since digits have been lost secondary to vasospasm occurring during dressing change within the first 3 postoperative weeks. Usually the clinical appearance of the digit and its course of demise give some indication as to whether the obstruction is arterial or venous. The change in blood flow must be diagnosed early, however, because the pale state of arterial occlusion will soon become cyanotic and will then be difficult to distinguish from venous occlusion.

The hospital stay for a replantation is a minimum of 5 to 10 days. After 3 or 4 days of bed rest, the patient's activities are progressively liberalized. The low-molecular-weight dextran is usually stopped after 5 days, but aspirin is continued for a total of 3 weeks postoperatively. Moderate elevation is usually maintained at all times, and dietary and smoking restrictions continue throughout the hospitalization. Phelps has cautioned that the replant must be protected against cold exposure for at least 2 to 4 weeks postoperatively.[67]

A dressing change is not routinely performed until 3 weeks after surgery. At this point, the dressing can be safely removed with minimal concern about vasospasm affecting the viability of the replanted part. At this stage sufficient healing of all involved tissues has taken place to initiate a rehabilitation program. Because open wounds may still be present, continued wound care may be required. Active range-of-motion exercises may be started if there is adequate skeletal fixation. Protective static splinting is performed. By 6 weeks postoperatively, passive range-of-motion exercises may be initiated as well as dynamic flexion and extension splinting, with overnight static splinting. Remember that the replanted part is anesthetic and that passive motion and dynamic splinting should be performed only by persons who are knowledgeable in the use of these techniques and familiar with replantation rehabilitation. Postoperative swelling is common and needs to be managed with appropriate digital and extremity wrapping. Continued elevation remains an important defense against swelling during the rehabilitative phase. Steichen[78] has divided the rehabilitative phase of replantation into three parts. The first 3 weeks represents the immobilization phase. The period of 3 to 6 weeks after replantation represents the early mobilization phase. The period of 6 weeks to 6 months postoperatively represents the late mobilization phase. Others authors, such as Ikuta[19] and Lendvay,[35] advocate the initiation of therapy on the first postoperative day.

In major limb replantations, the emphasis in therapy will

depend on the level of the amputation and the extent of denervation. Distal forearm replantations with functioning proximal muscle bellies will require therapy directed at re-establishment of tendon gliding and active motion of the wrist and more distal joints. In the more proximal major limb replantations, emphasis needs to be placed on maintaining passive motion of the distal joints while reinnervation of the motor units is being awaited.

COMPLICATIONS OF REPLANTATION SURGERY

The most commonly reported complication of replantation surgery and the most common cause of failure in replantation surgery is vascular occlusion.[59,84] Morrison has stated that arterial occlusion is more common than venous occlusion.[53] In the experience of 130 digital replantations in 100 patients reported by Morrison and O'Brien,[53] 49 cases of thrombosis occurred. Thirty-four patients were returned for revision, and at that time, 22 arterial thromboses were documented, six were venous, and six digits were indeterminate. Other investigators, however, believe that venous obstruction is the more common cause of failure in digital replantation. In Leung's series, 20 digital replantations were reported in 10 patients. Venous congestion was found in 11 of 20 patients versus arterial thrombosis in only 6 of 20 patients.[36] Weiland in 1978 reported on a series of 86 replantations performed in 71 patients. In this series, there were 54 unsuccessful replantations, with 68.4% being secondary to vascular thrombosis and 31.4% of undetermined cause. The majority of thromboses were found on the venous side.[92]

The recognition of vascular obstruction has already been discussed. The recommended management, in the event of the failure of conservative measures, is to return the patient to the operating room immediately for exploration. Most surgeons advise complete excision of the failed anastomosis with secondary vein grafting or use of a vascular pedicle brought in from an adjacent normal digit.[41] Salvage after vascular obstruction ranges from 34% in Morrison's series[54] to 50% in Schlenker's[69] series of thumb replantations. Eighty percent of vascular occlusions have been reported to occur within the first 24 to 72 hours after surgery. There have been sporadic cases of vascular failure as late as 12 days.[53,59] If the vascular failure occurs early in the postoperative course or is a catastrophic event, there is a strong indication to return the patient to the operating room for exploration. If, however, the deterioration is gradual and the surgeon believes that his original repair was technically competent, the likelihood of salvage on reexploration is greatly diminished.

The rate of infection is surprisingly small in digital replantations. This has been attributed to the débridement performed before replantation, the frequency of irrigation during surgery, the use of antibiotics intraoperatively and postoperatively, and a loose wound closure. In major limb replantation surgery, infection remains the major cause of failure of the replantation, as well as a devastating complication that potentially can cause death as a result of overwhelming sepsis. The key to avoiding this complication in major limb replantations is thorough débridement of all devitalized soft tissue. If this cannot be performed without

compromising the potential function of the limb, replantation should not proceed. Postoperative bleeding was a more significant complication when heparin was used routinely for anticoagulation. Bleeding can be minimized as a potential complication by meticulous attention to hemostasis before wound closure. It is particularly important that any unsatisfied veins be ligated. Loose wound closure will permit drainage and prevent the accumulation of blood beneath skin flaps. It is important that one apply an appropriate dressing; it must be able to accept any postoperative bleeding without compromising the viability of the replanted part. Isolated instances of digital replantation with only arterial repair and open venous drainage have been reported.[11,72,75] Under these circumstances, it is usually necessary to heparinize the patient and blood loss can run into many units, putting the patient at risk for transfusion complications. It is rare that salvage of a digit is worth the risks inherent in this method, and it is mentioned only to be discouraged.

Postoperative swelling is to be anticipated after replantation, and it is not a complication unless it leads to vascular impairment or compartment syndromes. Compartment syndromes are more likely to occur in major limb replantations. It is important that one keep in mind the possibility of compartment syndromes during the operative procedure, and fasciotomies should be performed routinely. Clinical suspicion of postoperative compartment syndromes can be further documented by the use of the various techniques available for measuring compartment pressures.

Perhaps one final complication that deserves mentioning is an error in judgment that results in replantation of a digit or limb that becomes a liability to the patient. This can be avoided if one adheres to the guidelines developed through previous clinical experience regarding indications and contraindications for replantation surgery. At this time revascularization is technically possible after nearly all amputations, whether complete or incomplete; however, as the Chinese surgeon Ch'en Chung-Wei has stated, "Survival without restoration of function is not success."[5]

Late complications that can occur after replantation include nonunions, malunions, joint stiffness, traumatic arthritis, flexor and/or extensor adhesions, tendon ruptures, neuromas, dysesthesias, and scar contracture.

SECONDARY PROCEDURES

The need for secondary procedures is not uncommon after replantation surgery. In Morrison's review of 130 digital replants in 100 patients, a total of 47 secondary procedures were required among the 96 digits that survived replantation.[54] In Scott's series evaluating digital replantation in 100 patients, over 80% of the patients with surviving replants required secondary surgery, with an average number of operations being 2.6 (range 1 to 4).[70]

The incidence of malunion and nonunion in most replantation series is quite small. Morrison's series contained only one nonunion and 10 malunions, none of which were of clinical significance.[54] In Leung's series, there were two rotational malalignments and one nonunion out of 16 surviving digital replantations.[36] In Urbaniak's series of over 200 digital replantations, his reported malunion rate was less than 5%.[87] If a nonunion or malunion is present and of clinical significance, it must be treated with open-reduction internal fixation and bone grafting. It is important to perform such a procedure, which requires postoperative immobilization, before one proceeds to other soft-tissue reconstruction, which may require movement of the digits for postoperative rehabilitation.

Joints that were partially destroyed in the initial injury and that proceed to deteriorate require either arthrodesis or silicone rubber arthroplasty.

Arthrofibrosis and tendon adhesions can be anticipated in digital replantations through the classic zone 2, or "no-man's-land." Our management of the stiff hand after replantation surgery is to make as many gains as possible through therapy during the first 6 months after replantation. If at that point the patient has plateaued, attention is first directed to the extensor surface of the hand and to the joint capsules. Dorsal capsulectomies and extensor tenolyses of the appropriate digits are performed along with traction tenolyses of the flexor tendons to check the status of the flexores digitorum profundus and superficialis, followed by intensive hand therapy to maintain active and passive motion gained by these procedures. Once an acceptable result is achieved in passive digital flexion after release of the joint capsules and the extensor mechanism, attention is directed to the volar surface of the hand, where flexor tenolyses and volar capsulectomies are performed when indicated. It is our belief, particularly in regard to the replanted digit, that it is quite dangerous to operate on both the volar aspect and the dorsal aspect of the digit simultaneously, because of the severe swelling that follows and the risk of vascular compromise.

Rarely it may not be possible to perform a primary repair of the flexor tendon injuries, and secondary repair must be performed. Surgeons such as Scott,[70] Lendvay,[33,34] and Morrison[54] have suggested or used silicone rubber rods during the primary surgery in reconstruction of the flexor tendon system.

Any injury that results in paralysis of the intrinsic or thenar muscles may require secondary tendon transfers to restore function.

It is recommended that nerve repair be performed primarily whenever possible in replantations or revascularizations. It has been demonstrated in clinical series that the results of primary neurorrhaphy are better than those of secondary repair.[70,93] Attempting to retrieve the nerve endings from the adjacent scar tissue during secondary repair is technically difficult and may place the vascular supply of the extremity in jeopardy. One of the reasons advocated for digital replantation distal to the insertion of the superficialis tendon is that a nerve repair can be performed with less likelihood of painful neuroma formation than an amputation at that same level would produce.[50] Occasionally, disabling paresthesias occurring after replantation will lead to amputation of the digit, as reported by Morrison[54] and Kleinert[26].

Secondary procedures may be required for revision of scar contractures, particularly when linear scars cross the volar surfaces of flexor creases. With major limb replantations and subsequent intrinsic contracture, a tight first web that requires release is not uncommon.[52]

FUNCTIONAL RESULTS IN REPLANTATION SURGERY

Several large replantation centers are now beginning to report long-term results of their replantations. Unfortunately, there is no coordinated list of criteria by which these patients are being judged, and so it is difficult to compare the results of these series. Perhaps the most rigorous criteria put forth in the literature up to now have been those of Kleinert, who believes that functional evaluation of replantations should include sensibility rating, grip strength, range of motion, the presence of cold intolerance and information regarding return to work.[27]

One of the primary goals of replantation surgery is to reestablish sensation in the replanted part. In the series reported by Morrison, 90% of the patients demonstrated two-point discrimination between 4 and 15 mm.[54] O'Brien went so far as to state that the result of sensory return in replantation was as good as simple digital nerve repair.[61] In 1979, Urbaniak reported a series of 187 complete or incomplete amputations. Among the surviving 163 digits, protective sensation was present in 90%, two-point discrimination of 15 mm or less was present in 66%, and two-point discrimination of 10 mm or less was present in 50%.[87] In Scott's series of 38 replanted digits, normal two-point discrimination was believed to be present in 40%, two-point discrimination of 6 to 10 mm was present in 8%, two-point discrimination of 11 to 15 mm was present in 18%, and protective sensation or two-point discrimination greater than 15 mm was present in 34%. In the same series, 55 revascularizations were performed and normal sensation was found in 71% as compared with two-point discrimination of 6 to 10 mm in 24%, two-point discrimination of 11 to 15 mm in 3%, and protective sensation in 2%. Scott's conclusion was that the results of nerve repair in replantation were not as good as in simple nerve repair. Based on his series, he drew a correlation between sensory return, vascularity, age, level of amputation, and the type of injury.[70]

In this series, all patients undergoing replantation complained of cold intolerance, whereas 55% of the revascularization patients complained of cold intolerance. Scott found no relationship between the number of digital arteries repaired and cold intolerance.

Gelberman has examined sensory return in detail in a series of 29 patients with 35 replanted digits. These patients were tested not only for two-point discrimination, but also for constant touch, moving touch, 30 and 250 cps tuning fork perception, heat and cold discrimination, sharp and dull discrimination, and number tracing. Gelberman found that patients with two-point discrimination less than 20 mm were able to perceive the other sensory function tests. In his series, he was unable to find any strong correlation between sensory return and the age of the patient, mechanism of injury, digit involved, ischemia time, or the patency of the ipsilateral artery. Sensory return also did not seem to be dependent on whether one or two arteries were repaired, but was dependent on pulse pressure. Poor sensory return and significant cold intolerance were found in patients whose pulse pressure was less than 70% of that of the normal contralateral digit. In his series, two-point discrimination ranging from 0 to 6 mm was found in nine patients, from

6 to 10 mm in seven patients, from 11 to 15 mm in two patients, and greater than 15 mm in 17 patients. Based on his experience, he also agreed that digital repair in replantation surgery was not as good as simple digital repair.[13] Both Weiland[92] and Scott,[70] in evaluation of sensory return in their series of digital replantations, have stated that the results of primary neurorrhaphy are better than those of secondary nerve repair.

Few studies have given accurate documentation of return of range of motion to replanted digits. Scott in 1981 presented a series of 38 patients with 65 complete digital amputations and 62 patients with 84 incomplete amputations requiring revascularization.[70] Survival rate in his series of complete amputations was 79%, as compared with 97% in the revascularized digits. Average total active motion (TAM) for 21 replantation and revascularization patients was 120 degrees for the digits and 59 degrees for the thumbs. Less than 180 degrees of TAM are considered poor. Eighty-four percent of the fingers were rated as poor, and only 6% were rated as excellent. Total active range of motion was found to be related to the level of injury (being particularly poor in the zone 2 area), nature of the injury (worse with avulsion injuries), age (worse results being obtained in older patients), and concomitant presence of a fracture (in the revascularization group the presence of a fracture decreased the total active range of motion). In Morrison's series of 130 digital replants in 100 patients, joint stiffness was found to be quite common and proximal interphalangeal joint motion averaged 30 to 70 degrees.[54]

It has been stated that the return of function of a replanted part is related to how much it is needed. Scott certainly found this to be true in his series of digital replantations, since isolated digital replants did not achieve significant function.[70] In contrast to this is May's report of digital replantation distal to the insertion of the flexor digitorum superficialis.[50] He reported on 24 digits replanted in 18 patients. The survival rate in this series was 96%, whereas previous survival rates of replant surgery performed at this level were 24% as reported by Tamai[82] and 35% as reported by Morrison.[54] Although all had some degree of cold intolerance, the mean two-point discrimination was 11 mm. Active range of motion at the proximal interphalangeal joint averaged 95 degrees and at the distal interphalangeal joint 9 degrees. Nine of the patients treated were workers, who returned to work in an average of 5.1 months. Among the nine students, return to school was accomplished in 1.7 months. It is intimated in the article that even patients with replantations of the index finger used their replanted digits.[50]

The thumb has been considered the most important digit in priority of replantation; however, the literature contains little information on the functional outcome of thumb replantation. Schlenker[69] reported a series of 51 replantations and 13 revascularizations, with a failure rate of 27%. The failure rate in replantation of the thumb was believed to vary with the nature of the injury and the age of the patient. Among the 47 patients with surviving thumbs, 12 secondary procedures were required, including tenolysis, tendon grafts, tendon transfers, neurolysis, nerve grafting, first web release, interphalangeal arthrodesis, bone grafting for a proximal phalangeal nonunion, and amputation for disabling

hyperesthesias. Twenty-three patients in this series had amputations of digits other than their thumbs, and in five of these, one of the fingers was transplanted to the thumb position. Only three of the five succeeded. Twenty-five patients with surviving replanted thumbs were evaluated in follow-up from 6 months to 3 years after replantation. Two-point discrimination was documented as less than 10 mm in 12 patients and greater than 10 mm in 13 patients. Two of the three heterotopic thumbs were available for evaluation, and in both cases only protective sensation was present. Joint motion was obtained in 14 patients, and the range of motion at the interphalangeal joint was found to average from 10 to 45 degrees and that at the metacarpophalangeal joint from 3 to 32 degrees. Seventy-six percent of the patients employed before their accident returned to work at an average of 7 months after surgery. Among 26 patients interviewed about the function of their thumbs, 10 stated that they used their thumbs more than before, 14 less, and two not at all. The most common reason for decreased use of the thumb was loss of motion. The two patients who claimed that they did not use their thumbs complained of either paresthesias or weakness. Only four of the 26 patients did not complain of cold intolerance. Cold intolerance in this series seemed to be most related to age and not to ischemia time, level of injury, mechanism, or number of vascular repairs.[69]

Few series are present in the literature documenting the functional performance of replantation surgery in children (Fig. 50-4). Van Beek presented a series of eight patients, but presented only case studies and no functional follow-up.[90] O'Brien reported on a series of 31 replantations in children. Four were major replantations, including an incomplete midpalm and forearm amputation and complete leg and foot amputations, and 27 were digital replantations. In this series, all four major replanted parts survived and demonstrated continued growth and return of adequate sensation. The survival rate in the digital replantations and revascularizations was 64.5%. The least successful digit regarding survival was the little finger. Only one out of five replanted little fingers survived. In this series, survival was found to be correlated with age, the level of injury, and the nature of injury. Digital replantation in children less than 2 years of age had a survival rate of only 50%, whereas in children greater than 5 years of age the survival rate was 71%. When two-point discrimination could be documented, it was found to be in the range of 2 to 10 mm. Only four of 16 had normal motion. Seven patients required secondary procedures, including tenolysis, first-web release, secondary tendon repair, tendon graft, and local flaps.[65]

Wang has recently reported on the results of 91 major limb replantations with a success rate of 77%.[91] The age range in his series was from 2 to 55 years. Ischemia time ranged from 4 to 33 hours, with an average ischemia time of 12 hours. Seventy-two major upper extremity replantations were included in this series, 65 of which were successful. Survival was found to be related to the level of injury and mechanism of injury. Replantations after proximal forearm amputations were found to have the worst survival rate. Causes of failure in this series were seven cases of inability to revascularize the limb, nine postoper-

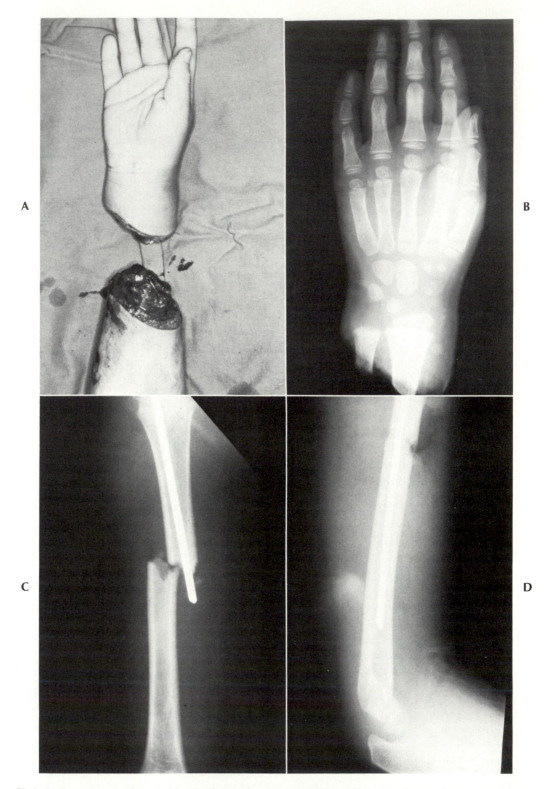

FIG. 50-4. A, Boy, 6 years of age, with complete major upper limb amputation secondary to farm-machinery accident. **B,** Roentgenogram showing level of sharp amputation of right upper extremity. **C** and **D,** Before replanting of right wrist and hand it was necessary to perform an open-reduction internal fixation (ORIF) of open displaced fracture of ipsilateral humerus.

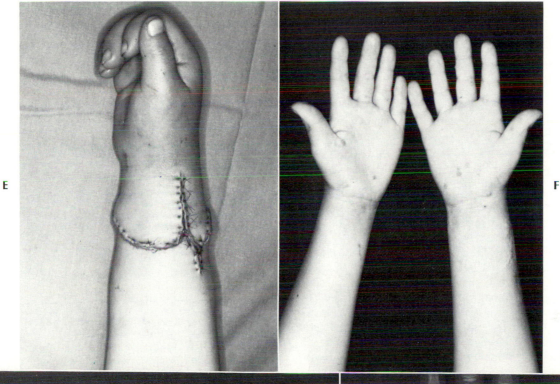

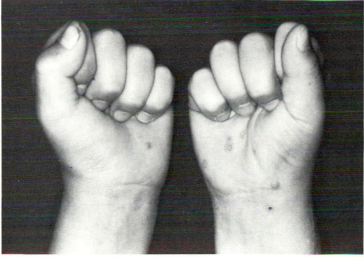

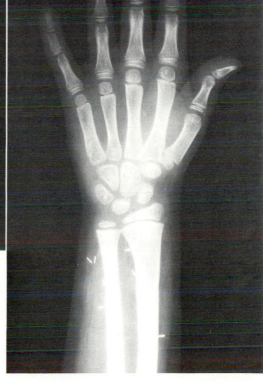

FIG. 50-4, cont'd. E, Replantation was performed, with primary repair of all structures, including revision of laceration to prevent a linear scar contracture with circumferential banding from occurring. F and G, Two and a half years postoperatively, replanted hand shows growth and function similar to normal extremity. H, Roentgenogram taken $2^{1}/_{2}$ years postoperatively shows normal epiphyseal growth.

ative thromboses, and five local complications representing either infection or muscle necrosis. It was reported that venous thromboses were more common than arterial thromboses. Function in these major replanted parts was graded from 1 to 4, or nearly normal to no function. Eighty percent of the surviving replanted limbs were rated as nearly normal or fair in function. Failure to achieve useful function was found to be related to the severity of the initial injury, excessive loss of length, intra-articular fractures, extensive destruction of muscle, irreparable damage to nerves, prolonged ischemia, and inadequate management of soft tissue and bone.[91] Yoshizu presented a series of 99 replantations in 66 patients, which included 20 major upper extremity replantations or revascularizations. The success rate in this series was 92.6%. Evaluation of these major limb replantations demonstrated poor recovery of intrinsic function and only return of protective sensation.[96] Morrison reported on the results of 20 major limb replantations in patients ranging in age from 21 months to 57 years. In this series, there were 16 survivals and four failures. All failures occurred in above-elbow amputations associated with avulsion injuries, diffuse crush, ischemia time greater than normal, or subsequent infection. Among the surviving replanted parts in this series were seven replanted hands and two forearms. In the replanted hands, two-point discrimination was documented between 10 and 30 mm, with an average of 17 mm. All patients wers found to have light touch and protective sensation. On evaluation of the tendon function in the replanted hands, two were found to be nearly normal, five required tenolysis, all but one had intrinsic paralysis and required opposition transfers, and five had first-web contractures. Among the two forearm replantations, two-point discrimination was greater than 20 mm. Tendon function was found to be minimal. One patient was found to have intrinsic contractures.[52]

CONCLUSION

Through technologic advances, surgical experience, and the establishment of reliable criteria for selection of candidates for replantation surgery, most replantation centers are able to achieve success rates of greater than 80% in revascularizing amputated digits and major limbs. As these replantation centers have accumulated their clinical experiences and reported their results, emphasis has evolved from the importance of vascular survival to the establishment of function in the replanted part.

The achievement of the best functional result possible for each patient is dependent on the many factors that have been presented in this review, which has emphasized the nature of the injury to the patient and the surgeon's role in repairing it to the best of his or her ability. The equally important and necessary role of the hand therapist in the patient's rehabilitation is discussed in Chapter 51.

REFERENCES

1. Acland, R.D., and Trachtenberg, L.: The histopathology of small arteries following experimental microvascular anastomosis, Plast. Reconstr. Surg. **60**:868, 1977.
2. Bendick, P.J., Mayer, J.R., Glover, J.L., and Park, H.M.: A photoplethysmographic technique for detecting vascular compromise: a preliminary report, J. Trauma **19**:398, 1979.
3. Bright, D.S., and Wright, S.: Postoperative management in replantation. In American Academy of Orthopaedic Surgeons: Symposium on microsurgery: practical use in orthpaedics, St. Louis, 1979, The C.V. Mosby Co., pp. 83-95.
4. Buncke, H.J., Jr., and Schulz, W.P.: Experimental digital amputation and reimplantation, Plast. Reconstr. Surg. **36**:62, 1965.
5. Buncke, H., Castleton, K.B., Daniel, R.K., and others: Replantation surgery in China: report of the American Replantation Mission to China, Plast. Reconstr. Surg. **52**:476, 1973.
6. Carrel, A., and Guthrie, C.C.: Complete amputation of the thigh with replantation, Am. J. Med. Sci. **131**:297, 1906.
7. Chi Sui-Tan Hospital, Peking, as reported by O'Brien, B.McC.: Microvascular reconstructive surgery, Edinburgh, New York, 1977, Churchill Livingstone, p. 125.
8. Ch'en, C.-W., Chien, Y.-C., and Pao, Y.-S.: Salvage of the forearm following complete traumatic amputation: report of a successful case: Chin. Med. J. **82**:632, 1963.
9. Ch'en, C.-W., as reported by O'Brien, B.McC.: Microvascular reconstructive surgery, Edinburgh, New York, 1977, Churchill Livingstone, p. 156.
10. Ibid.: p. 128.
11. Elsahy, N.I.: Replantation of a completely amputated distal segment of thumb: case report, Plast. Reconstr. Surg. **59**:579, 1977.
12. Gelberman, R.H.: A history of microsurgery. In American Academy of Orthopaedic Surgeons: Symposium on microsurgery: practical use in orthopaedics, St. Louis, 1979, The C.V. Mosby Co., pp. 6-11.
13. Gelberman, R.H., Urbaniak, J.R., Bright, D.S., and others: Digital sensibility following replantation, J. Hand Surg. **3**:313, 1978.
14. Harrison, D.H., and Watson, J.S.: Use of the polypropylene peg for immediate stabilization in digital replantation, J. Hand Surg. **5**:253, 1980.
15. Hayhurst, J.W., O'Brien, B.McC., Ishida, H., and others: Experimental digital replantation after prolonged cooling, Hand **6**:134, 1974.
16. Holmgren, G.: Some experience in surgery of otosclerosis, Acta Otolaryngol. **5**:460, 1920.
17. Hopfner, E.: Ueber Gefässnaht: Gefässtransplantationen und replantation von amputirten extremitäten, Arch. Klin. Chir. **70**:417, 1903.
18. Horn, J.S., and Lond, M.B.: Successful reattachment of a completely severed forearm, Lancet **1**:1152, 1964.
19. Ikuta, Y.: Microvascular surgery, Hiroshima, 1975, Lens Press.
20. Ikuta, Y., and Tsuge, K.: Micro-bolts and micro-screws for fixation of small bones in the hand, Hand **6**:261, 1974.
21. Ikuta, Y., as reported by O'Brien, B.McC: Microvascular reconstructive surgery, Edinburgh, New York, 1977, Churchill Livingstone, p. 156.
22. Irigaray, A.: New fixing screw for completely amputated fingers, J. Hand Surg. **5**:381, 1980.
23. Jacobson, J.H., and Saurez, E.L.: Microsurgery and anastomosis of small vessels, Surg. Forum **9**:243, 1960.
24. Kleinert, H.E., and Kasdan, M.L.: Salvage of devascularized upper extremities, including studies on small vessel anastomoses, Clin. Orthop. **29**:29, 1963.
25. Kleinert, H.E., and Kasdan, M.L.: Anastomosis of digital vessels, J. Ky. Med. Assoc. **63**:106, 1963.
26. Kleinert, H.E., and Tsai, T.-M.: Microvascular repair in replantation, Clin. Orthop. **133**:205, 1978.
27. Kleinert, H.E., Jablon, M., and Tsai, T.-M.: An overview of replantation and results of 347 replants in 245 patients, J. Trauma **20**:390, 1980.
28. Kleinert, H.E., Kasdan, M.L., and Romero, J.L.: Small blood-vessel anastomosis for salvage of severely injured upper extremity, J. Bone Joint Surg. **45A**:788, 1963.
29. Kleinert, H.E., Juhala, C.A., Tsai, T.-M., and others: Digital replantation: selection, technique and results, Orthop. Clin. North Am. **8**:309, 1977.
30. Komatsu, S., and Tamai, S.: Successful replantation of a completely cur-off thumb, Plast. Reconstr. Surg. **42**:374, 1968.
31. Kutz, J.E.: Preparation for replantation. In Daniller, A.I., and Strauch, B., editors: Symposium on microsurgery, St. Louis, 1976, The C.V. Mosby Co., pp. 81-91.
32. Lapchinsky, A.G.: Recent results of experimental transplantation of preserved limbs and kidneys and possible use of this technique in clinical practice, Ann. N.Y. Acad. Sci. **87**:539, 1960.

33. Lendvay, P.: Pursuit of function in digital replantation, In Daniel, R.K., and Terzis, J.K., editors: Reconstructive microsurgery, Boston, 1977, Little, Brown & Co., pp. 168-71.
34. Lendvay, P.G.: Replacement of the amputated digit, Br. J. Plast. Surg. **26:**398, 1973.
35. Lendvay, P.G., as reported by O'Brien, B.McC., and MacLeod, A.M.: Digital replantation. In Daniller, A.I., and Strauch, B., editors: Symposium on microsurgery, St. Louis, 1976, The C.V. Mosby Co., p. 95.
36. Leung, P.-C.: An analysis of complications in digital replantations, Hand **12:**25, 1980.
37. Leung, P.-C.: Use of an intrameduallary bone peg in digital replantations, revascularizations, and toe-transfers, J. Hand Surg. **6:**281, 1981.
38. Lister, G.: Intraosseous wiring of the digital skeleton, J. Hand Surg. **3:**427, 1978.
39. Lobay, G.W., and Moysa, G.L.: Primary neurovascular bundle transfer in the management of avulsed thumbs, J. Hand Surg. **6:**31, 1981.
40. MacLeod, A.M., and O'Brien, B.McC.: Replantation surgery in the upper extremity. In Flynn, J.E., editor: Hand surgery, Baltimore, 1982, The Williams & Wilkins Co., pp. 555-565.
41. MacLeod, A.M., O'Brien, B.McC., and Morrison, W.A.: Digital replantation: clinical experiences, Clin. Orthop. **133:**26, 1978.
42. Malt, R.A., and Harris, W.H.: Replantation of limbs, Advancing with Surgery monograph, Somerville, N.J., 1965, Ethicon, Inc.
43. Malt, R.A., and McKhann, C.F.: Replantation of severed arms, J.A.M.A. **189:**716, 1964.
44. Malt, R.A., Remensnyder, J.P., and Harris, W.H.: Long-term utility of replanted arms, Ann. Surg. **176:**334, 1972.
45. Malt, R.A., Smith, R.J., and May, J.W., Jr.: Replantation of the amputated hand. In Daniel, R.K., and Terzis, J.K., editors: Reconstructive microsurgery, Boston, 1977, Little, Brown & Co., pp. 177-186.
46. Manktelow, R.T.: American Academy of Orthopaedic Surgeons presentation, Feb. 1982.
47. Matsuda, M., Kato, N., and Hosoi, M.: The problems in replantation of limbs amputated through the upper arm region, J. Trauma **21:**403, 1981.
48. May, J.W., Jr., and Gallico, G.G., III: Upper extremity replantation, Curr. Probl. Surg. **17:**634, 1980.
49. May, J.W., Jr., Chait, L.A., O'Brien, B.McC., and Hurley, J.V.: The no-reflow phenomenon in experimental free flaps, Plast. Reconstr. Surg. **61:**256, 1978.
50. May, J.W., Toth, B.A., and Gardner, M.: Digital replantation distal to the proximal interphalangeal joint, J. Hand Surg. **7:**161, 1982.
51. Meuli, H.C., Meyer, V., and Segmuller, G.: Stabilization of bone in replantation surgery of the upper limb, Clin. Orthop. **133:**179, 1978.
52. Morrison, W.A., O'Brien, B.McC., and MacLeod, A.M.: Major limb replantation, Orthop. Clin. North Am. **8:**343, 1977.
53. Morrison, W.A., O'Brien, B.M., and MacLeod, A.M.: Evaluation of digital replantation—a review of 100 cases, Orthop. Clin. North Am. **8:**295, 1977.
54. Morrison, W.A., O'Brien, B.McC., and MacLeod, A.M.: Digital replantation and revascularization: a long term review of one hundred cases, Hand **10:**125, 1978.
55. O'Brien, B.McC.: Replantation surgery in China, Med. J. Aust. **2:**255, 1974.
56. O'Brien, B.McC.: Microvascular reconstructive surgery, Edinburgh, New York, 1977, Churchill Livingstone, p. 171.
57. Ibid.: p. 160.
58. Ibid.: p. 140.
59. Ibid.: p. 169.
60. Ibid.: p. 139.
61. Ibid.: pp. 174-175.
62. O'Brien, B.McC., and Baxter, T.J.: Experimental digital replantation, Hand **6:**11, 1974.
63. O'Brien, B.McC., and MacLeod, A.M.: Digital replantation. In Daniller, A.I., and Strauch, B., editors: Symposium on microsurgery, St. Louis, 1976, The C.V. Mosby Co., pp. 92-97.
64. O'Brien, B.McC., and Miller, G.D.H.: Digital reattachment and revascularization, J. Bone Joint Surg. **55A:**714, 1973.
65. O'Brien, B.McC., Franklin, J.D., Morrison, W.A., and others: Replantation and revascularisation surgery in children, Hand **12:**12, 1980.
66. Parks, B.J., Arbelaez, J., and Horner, R.L.: Medical and surgical importance of the arterial blood supply of the thumb, J. Hand Surg. **3:**383, 1978.
67. Phelps, D.B., Lilla, J.A., and Boswick, J.A., Jr.: Common problems in clinical replantation and revascularization in the upper extremity, Clin. Orthop. **133:**11, 1978.
68. Reichert, F.L.: The importance of circulatory balance in the survival of replanted limbs, Bull. John Hopkins Hosp. **49:**86, 1931.
69. Schlenker, J.D., Kleinert, H.E., and Tsai, T.-M.: Methods and results of replantation following traumatic amputation of the thumb in sixty-four patients, J. Hand Surg. **5:**63, 1980.
70. Scott, F.A., Howar, J.W., and Boswick, J.A.: Recovery of function following replantation and revascularization of amputated hand parts, J. Trauma **21:**204, 1981.
71. Seidenberg, B., Hurwitt, E.S., and Carton, C.A.: Techniques of anastomosing small arteries, Surg. Gynecol. Obstet. **106:**743, 1958.
72. Serafin, D., Kutz, J.E., and Kleinert, H.E.: Replantation of a completely amputated distal thumb without venous anastomoses: case report, Plast. Reconstr. Surg. **52:**579, 1973.
73. Shafiroff, B.B., and Palmer, A.K.: Simplified technique for replantation of the thumb, J. Hand Surg. **6:**623, 1981.
74. Shorey, W.D., Schneewind, J.H., and Paul, H.A.: Significant factors in the reimplantation of an amputated hand, Bull. Soc. Int. Chir. **24:**44, 1965.
75. Snyder, C.C., Stevenson, R.M., and Browne, E.Z., Jr.: Successful replantation of a totally severed thumb, Plast. Reconstr. Surg. **50:**553, 1972.
76. Snyder C.D., Knowles, R.P., Mayer, P.W., and Hobbs, J.C.: Extremity replantation, Plast. Reconstr. Surg. **26:**251, 1960.
77. Steichen, J.B.: The microvascular free groin flap. In American Academy of Orthopaedic Surgeons: Symposium on microsurgery: practical use in orthopaedics, St. Louis, 1979, The C.V. Mosby Co., pp. 279-305.
78. Steichen, J.B., Harmon, K.S., Fess, E.E., and Strickland, J.W.: Rehabilitation of the upper extremity replantation patient. In Hunter, J.M., and others, editors: Rehabilitation of the hand, St. Louis, 1978, The C.V. Mosby Co., pp. 407-414.
79. Stirrat, C.R., Seaber, A.V., Urbaniak, J.R., and others: Temperature monitoring in digital replantation, J. Hand Surg. **3:**342, 1978.
80. Strauch, B., and Terzis, J.K.: Replantation of digits, Clin. Orthop. **133:**35, 1978.
81. Tamai, S.: Multiple digit replantation. In Daniel, R.K., and Terzis, J.K., editors: Reconstructive microsurgery, Boston, 1977, Little, Brown & Co., pp. 172-176.
82. Tamai, S.: Digit replantation: analysis of 163 replantations in an 11 year period, Clin. Plast. Surg. **5:**195, 1978.
83. Tamai, S., Hori, Y., Tatsumi, Y., and others: Microvascular anastomosis and its application on the replantation of amputated digits and hands, Clin. Orthop. **133:**106, 1978.
84. Tsai, T.-M.: Experimental and clinical application of microvascular surgery, Ann. Surg. **181:**169, 1975.
85. Tupper, J.W.: Techniques of bone fixation and clinical experience in replanted extremities, Clin. Orthop. **133:**165, 1978.
86. Urbaniak, J.R.: Replantation of amputated hands and digits. In American Academy of Orthopaedic Surgeons: Instructional course lectures, **27:**15, St. Louis, 1978, The C.V. Mosby Co.
87. Urbaniak, J.R.: Replantation of amputated parts: technique, results and indications. In American Academy of Orthopaedic Surgeons: Symposium on microsurgery: practical use in orthopaedics, St. Louis, 1979, The C.V. Mosby Co., pp. 64-82.
88. Urbaniak, J.R.: Replantation. In Green, D.P., editor: Operative hand surgery, Edinburgh, New York, 1982, Churchill Livingstone, pp. 811-828.
89. Van Beek, A.L., Kutz, J.E., and Zook, E.G.: Importance of the ribbon sign indicating unsuitability of the vessel in replanting a finger, Plast. Reconstr. Surg. **61:**32, 1978.
90. Van Beek, A.L., Wavak, P.W., and Zook, E.G.: Microvascular surgery in young children, Plast. Reconstr. Surg. **63:**457, 1979.

91. Wang, S.-H., Young, K.-F., and Wei, J.-N.: Replantation of severed limbs: clinical analysis of 91 cases, J. Hand Surg. **6:**311, 1981.

92. Weiland, A.J., Villarreal-Rios, A., and Kleinert, H.E.: Replantation of digits and hands: analysis of surgical techniques and functional results in 71 patients with 86 replantations, J. Hand Surg. **2:**1, 1977.

93. Weiland, A.J., Villarreal-Rios, A., Kleinert, H.E., and others: Replantation of digits and hands: analysis of surgical techniques and functional results in 71 patients with 86 replantations, Clin. Orthop. **133:**195, 1978.

94. Williams, G.R., Carter, D.R., Frank, G.R., and others: Replantation of amputated extremities, Ann. Surg. **163:**788, 1966.

95. Yamano, Y., Matsuda, H., Nakashima, K., and others: Some methods for bone fixation for digital replantation, Hand **14:**135, 1982.

96. Yoshizu, T., Katsumi, M., and Tajima, T.: Replantation of untidily amputated finger, hand, and arm: experience of 99 replantations in 66 cases, J. Trauma **18:**194, 1978.

51

Rehabilitation of the patient with an upper extremity replantation

ELAINE EWING FESS

Until recently, total amputation of a body part was considered an unsalvagable situation. However, with the advent of microsurgical techniques and subsequent refinement of surgical equipment, revascularization and replantation procedures have met with increasing success and currently represent accepted surgical methods. Although reattachment of severed parts had been reported earlier in laboratory animals,[12,22,23] the first successful human upper extremity replantation was accomplished by Malt[15] in 1962. Kleinert and Kasdan[8] and Buncke[4] made significant contributions with their work on hand and digital revascularization methods both clinically and experimentally, and in 1965 Komatsu and Tamai[11] successfully replanted a severed thumb, firmly introducing the era of microvascular surgery. Increasing experience identified fundamental requirements for achieving successful viability and function. These included patient factors such as age, general health, physical condition, and motivation; variables of injury involving level and type of amputation, and preservation of essential structures; and ischemia time of the amputated part. Today, many centers throughout the world have the facilities, staff, and expertise to offer successfully replantation as a feasible alternative among surgical reconstructive procedures, reporting overall survival rates up to 96% depending on individual patient circumstances and the level and type of injury.*

The rapid technical advancement of replantation surgery has produced high survival rates, but tissue viability alone does not guarantee acceptable hand function. Playing significant parts, age and level of injury positively correlate with functional capacity, and a decision to pursue replantation must be balanced against the alternatives, with the assurance that the replanted part will provide better function than would the remaining portion of the extremity with or without a prosthetic device. Although controversy exists regarding replantation of single digits (excluding the thumb), there seems to be general agreement with the priorities for replantation defined by Urbaniak,[29] provided that other factors are favorable: (1) thumb, (2) multiple digits, (3) amputation through the palm, (4) child, any part, (5) wrist or forearm, (6) part above the elbow, and (7) individual digit distal to the flexor superficialis insertion.

The hand therapist's role in the management of replantation patients is important both from the aspect of direct therapeutic intervention and in regard to influencing future replantation concepts. In addition to the astute management of the postoperative patient, the therapist's specialized knowledge of assessment techniques can significantly augment the understanding of functional hand use in replantation patients by providing unbiased, numerical data. Based on long-term postoperative results, this information eventually may be used to establish definitive selection criteria for potential replantation patients. The purposes of this chapter are (1) to review therapeutic techniques and methods used in the management of postoperative patients and (2) to discuss current needs and future directions for the field of hand rehabilitation in regard to replantation efforts.

Treatment of replantation patients may be divided into five stages: early healing, active motion, resistive motion, maintenance or further surgical reconstruction, and program assessment. The first four stages involve direct patient contact and are modified to meet the requirements of individual patients, while the fifth stage encompasses analysis and evaluation of techniques, monitoring results, and providing the opportunity to upgrade programs through identification and selection of the methods that were most efficacious.

Communication among the surgeon, the therapist, and the patient is extremely important throughout the entire rehabilitation effort. The therapist must be aware of the medical, surgical, physical, and psychological factors unique to the individual patient, the short- and long-range treatment goals perceived by the surgeon, and specific instructions and information that were given to the patient by the surgical team. Each surgeon approaches the management of replantation patients on a slightly different basis, adhering to fundamental concepts but interjecting changes that reflect personal philosophies. The therapist should have a thorough understanding of both the "routine" course of treatment and the manner in which it is adapted to meet the requirements of the specific patient. This chapter reviews a general rehabilitation approach for replantation patients, emphasizing that the presence of circumstances such as infection, lack of skin coverage, unstable fractures, vascular compromise, unexpected levels of pain, and poor patient cooperation may alter the therapy program considerably.

---

*See references 5, 9, 16-19, 21, 28, 30, and 32.

Patients who undergo elective reconstruction efforts involving transfer of free vascularized grafts to restore thumb or finger function follow rehabilitation programs similar to those of replantation patients, with the exceptions that the donor site must also be treated as a healing wound and preoperative assessment parameters are available, providing better opportunity to define the value of the surgery. Although many options are available, some of the most frequently used transplantation procedures include digit-to-digit, toe-to-thumb, toe-to-hand, and second and/or third toes–to–digits. Removed from the stresses of dealing with acute injury, the surgeon has better opportunity for patient selection and education, resulting in postoperative patients who seem more realistic in their expectations and who exhibit higher levels of motivation than many of the replantation patients do.

The replantation patient differs from patients with other severe injuries in that, instead of selected involvement, all structures at the level of injury are severed, a type of injury requiring specialized microvascular skills and greater operating time for restoration of functional continuity to bone, tendons, vascular structures, nerves, and skin. Once the surgical repairs are completed and vascular patency is established, soft-tissue healing begins, and although controversy surrounds the specific cellular, chemical, and physical responses involved,[14,20,31] inflammation, epithelialization, and collagen synthesis occur first, followed later by fibroplasia and scar remodeling, with collagen-architecture and wound-strength changes continuing over the course of months.

STAGE ONE: EARLY HEALING

Upon arrival in the hospital room, the patient is positioned in bed and the replanted part, immobilized in a bulky nonconstrictive dressing, is placed in neutral or mild elevation. Extremity position may be altered to adapt to problems of venous congestion or arterial inflow, intravenous therapy is given in the uninvolved extremity, and smoking and use of caffeine are prohibited. The patient may be mildly sedated during the first few days to limit activity and to decrease pain and anxiety.

During the early healing stage, vasomotor changes fill the wound with inflammatory exudate containing fibrin strands, protein, and blood cells and forming a semisolid substrate into which, by the third day, fibroblasts move. Concomitantly epithelialization occurs, and within 4 or 5 days the surface of the wound is bridged. As the inflammatory reaction subsides, the epithelial covering thickens, the number of fibroblasts increases greatly, and rapid capillary proliferation is apparent. Fibroblasts, synthesizing collagen, move into the fibrin network, and by a process that is not fully agreed upon, destruction of the fibrin scaffolding takes place. Lasting from a few days to several months, depending on the amount of tissue damage, bacteria, and foreign bodies, the inflammatory phase allows removal of nonviable tissue from the wound and begins the process of physiologic repair. Cellular advancement into the wound space lasts for several weeks.

During the first week to 10 postoperative days, patency of vascular structures is tenuous and must be monitored closely. In addition to its obvious impact on tissue viability, blood flow is believed to relate proportionally to the final functional result of the replant.[3] Cutaneous temperature gauges (Fig. 51-1) provide valuable quantitative data regarding flow parameters, allowing identification of problems and subsequent correctional intervention.[26] Increased sympathetic tone, pain, extremity position, dressing compression, psychologic stress, and local tissue response have been implicated as factors that diminish flow and imperil viability of the replanted part. Aware of the potential problems and their serious repercussions, the hand therapist assumes an active role in monitoring the patient's physical and psycho-

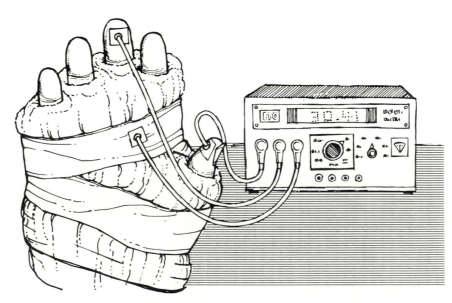

FIG. 51-1. Providing quantitative data about viability of replanted part, a cutaneous temperature gauge monitors early postoperative vessel patency and blood flow.

logical condition, immediately reporting a relative temperature difference between the normal part and the replanted part of more than three degrees Celsius, a drop of several degrees, a temperature less than 30° C, color changes, or a decrease in capillary filling, to the surgical team.

At 2 to 5 days, if the vascular status of the replanted part is stable and with the consent of the surgeon, the patient is allowed out of bed, and active and passive exercise to the joints not immobilized in the dressing may be initiated, including those of the uninvolved extremity. The establishment of an early maintenance range-of-motion program is important in developing a responsible patient attitude and good communication between the therapist and the patient.

Depending on the philosophy of the replantation team and the status of the replanted part; early passive mobilization of tendons may be employed at this time. Traditionally, the replanted part was immobilized for 3 weeks, with early passive mobilization being avoided because of the involvement of both the extensor tendons and the flexor tendons. Recently, however, some centers are using early-motion methods, which are based on work by Duran[6] and Kleinert,[10] for minimizing peritendinous adhesions of flexor tendon repairs in zones 2 and 3. Callahan[5] adapted early passive mobilization techniques to replantation patients by developing an ingenious set of alternately worn splints that control and diminish the tenodesis effect on the reciprocal tendon groups, allowing alternate application of early passive motion to each group of repaired tendons. Implementation of early passive motion usually requires removal of dressings and application of positioning splints. Since removal of an adherent dressing during the early postoperative period may trigger a sympathetic reaction, causing decreased flow and possible loss of the replanted part, it is strongly recommended that dressing changes be done by or under the direct supervision of the surgeon. It should also be emphasized that because of the risk of tendon rupture, early motion techniques are contraindicated in children and unreliable adults.

Education and psychological support of the patient and his family are very important during the first few postoperative weeks. It is a frustrating time for the patient, for in addition to the psychological stress that accompanies major trauma and the confusion of the hospital environment, success of the surgery cannot be guaranteed. Although patients receive specific counseling from their surgeons before and after the replantation procedure, they often misunderstand even the most basic concepts. For example, regardless of counseling, many patients assume that once the dressings are removed, they will have normal use of their hands. The hand therapist is in a unique position to supplement the information provided by the surgeon. Discussions regarding anatomic structures involved, the surgical process of reattaching the amputated part, expected postoperative course, length of hospitalization, and rehabilitation goals and responsibilities help the patient set realistic expectations for himself. Fortunately, successful replantation efforts are becoming more or less routine and earlier problems of sensationalism created by an enthusiastic press are diminishing, allowing patients and staff to proceed without the distractions of zealous reporters and media accounts of miracles.

One never forgets the shock of turning on the local television news program, only to see one's own patient, 6 days after a forearm replantation, happily explaining to a beaming interviewer that he has complete sensation and motion in his fingers!

STAGE TWO: ACTIVE MOTION

By the fourth or fifth week, capillary systems are defined and the number of fibroblasts in the wound is decreased considerably. Collagen fibers increase and become more dense, gradually reconstructing tissue continuity. By 3 weeks the unstressed wound has gained only a small percentage (less than 15%) of its potential strength.[14] The initiation of active motion places tension on the healing structures, increasing tensile strength of the wound and reestablishing relative glide between soft-tissue components. Over a period of months the random collagen fibers will become more oriented and the tensile strength of the wound will continue to increase as scar remodeling takes place.

Once the dressings are removed (10 to 21 days), it is important that one document base-line parameters for range of motion (Fig. 51-2) and sensibility, eliminating the po-

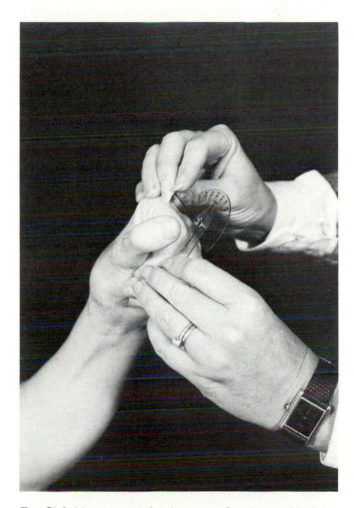

FIG. 51-2. Measurement of active range of motion provides baseline information to which subsequent measurements may be compared.

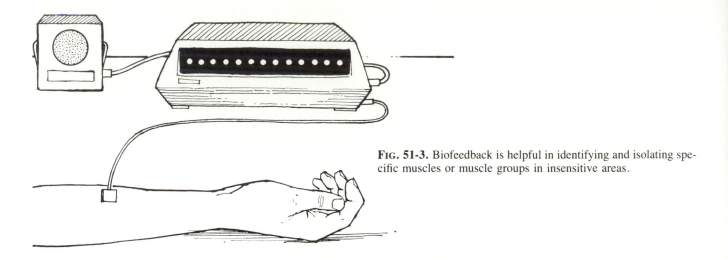

FIG. 51-3. Biofeedback is helpful in identifying and isolating specific muscles or muscle groups in insensitive areas.

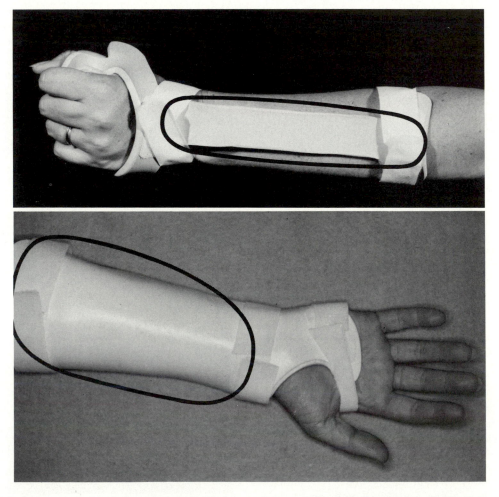

FIG. 51-4. Pressure may be decreased by increasing area of force application. Forearm trough distributes pressure along length of forearm. (From Fess, E., Gettle, K., and Strickland, J.: Hand splinting principles and methods, St. Louis, 1981, The C.V. Mosby Co.)

tential for confusion when assessing gains or losses in the future. Because of the resistive element basic to strength assessment, grip, pinch, and manual muscle-testing measurements requiring use of the replanted part should not be implemented until the repaired structures have sufficient tensile strength to resist loading forces (approximately 8 to 12 weeks). Not involved in the actual surgical procedure, therapists may be freer to be objective in the assessment of replantation patients. Information based on instruments that are accurate and reliable allows the rehabilitation team plan treatment programs, identify changes, and evaluate the effectiveness of treatment techniques and methods. Without quantitative data, therapeutic intervention may be disoriented and ineffective, wasting critical moments in physiologic timing, decreasing rehabilitative potential, and incurring needless expenses to the patient.

Depending on the center[3,16,24,27] and the status of the replant, active motion is initiated from 10 to 21 days after the replantation surgery. Dressings and stitches have been removed, and dorsal or volar immobilization splints are fitted to provide external support to the internally fixed fractures for an additional 6 to 8 weeks. The active motion program must be carefully supervised, especially during the first few weeks when repairs are most vulnerable to rupture. Lacking sensory feedback distal to the level of amputation, the patient is unable to tell how much stress is placed on the repaired musculotendinous units as he actively attempts to move the replanted part. Visual clues combined with nonresistive exercises and activities help the patient learn to monitor motion through the proximal, innervated portions of the extremity. The more proximal the injury, the more problems the patient is likely to experience in identifying and using specific groups of muscles, relying almost entirely on visual clues to monitor the results of his efforts. Biofeedback instruments (Fig. 51-3) are of considerable value to those replantation patients who are unable to isolate and coordinate individual muscles or muscle groups.

When the status of the replant is considered stable, and using body-temperature water, one may use a whirlpool bath to cleanse areas of nonviable tissue, decreasing the length of the inflammatory phase of healing and promoting physiologic repair of the wound. However, unnecessary use of this modality on wounds that do not require débridement should be judiciously avoided because of potential edema problems, which could jeopardize the viability of the replanted part. If the whirlpool bath is used, one should take volumetric measurements before and after each session to closely monitor the effects of dependent position and body temperature heat on the replanted tissues. *Of critical importance is the understanding that application of heat modalities of any kind is contraindicated in tissues with inadequate vascular supply or absent sensation.*[13]

Although many therapists advocate its use, there is no reliable evidence that electrical stimulation will retard muscle atrophy in humans.[25] Additionally, according to method theory, the intensity of muscle contraction with electrical stimulation should be strong and against resistance to achieve maximum benefit,[25] automatically eliminating its use in the active motion stage of rehabilitation of replan-

tation patients because of the potential for rupturing repaired tendons.

Splinting the postoperative replantation patient requires a thorough knowledge of anatomy, kinesiology, and the mechanical principles of splinting, integrated with an understanding of basic splint design, construction, and fit concepts.[7] Because of the severity of the injury, the subsequent multiplicity of structures repaired, and the tenuousness of the replanted part, the hand therapist must anticipate and fully understand the ramifications of splint application. It is of uppermost importance that splints do not obstruct venous return or arterial flow by applying constricting forces or concentrated pressures. Splint design may be altered, better adapting to the requirements of the replantation patient by using components that lessen pressure or change the application of pressures to less critical areas. For example, the choice of a full-length volar forearm trough (Fig. 51-4) instead of a wristband as a base for flexion traction will distribute pressure two thirds the length of the forearm instead of concentrating forces to a small area at the wrist, and in a splint with an extension outrigger, the addition of a lumbrical bar will decrease pressure on the dorsal aspect of the metacarpals (Fig. 51-5). In addition to attaining a congruous fit, one may widen usually narrow splint components such as straps and bars, decreasing splint pressure by enlarging the area of force application. Designs that apply pressure to relatively small areas such as three-point-pressure splints or unyielding circumferential splints such as cylinder casts are contraindicated during the early stages of treatment. As collateral circulation and lymphatic drainage are established, vulnerability of the replant is considerably decreased; however, when new splints are applied, the status of the replanted part should be monitored carefully by both the patient and the therapist.

Splinting during the active motion stage consists in immobilizing splints that are fitted (1) to protect fracture stability, (2) to position proximal joints and diminish tension on repaired tendons, or (3) to protect and position the replanted part between exercise periods and at night. Mobilization splints may also be used to improve passive motion of uninvolved joints adjacent to the replant that developed stiffness during the initial period of immobilization. Because of the tension loads applied to repaired structures antagonistic to those of the splint forces, corrective splinting to joints involved in the replant should be carefully approached on an individual patient basis, with consideration being taken as to time factors, type and tension of repairs, vascular stability of the replanted part, and cooperativeness of the patient. If mobilization splints are used on the replanted part during the active motion stage, the traction used should be minimal, providing very gentle forces, which may be increased as time progresses and tensile strength becomes greater. Attempts to apply forceful traction, either with a splint or manually, should be avoided.!

Pain is not usually a problem during the earlier stages of rehabilitation because repaired nerves have not had sufficient time to regenerate sensory fibers. Although this can be helpful in alleviating patient anxiety during exercise sessions, the anesthetic part should be protected against un-

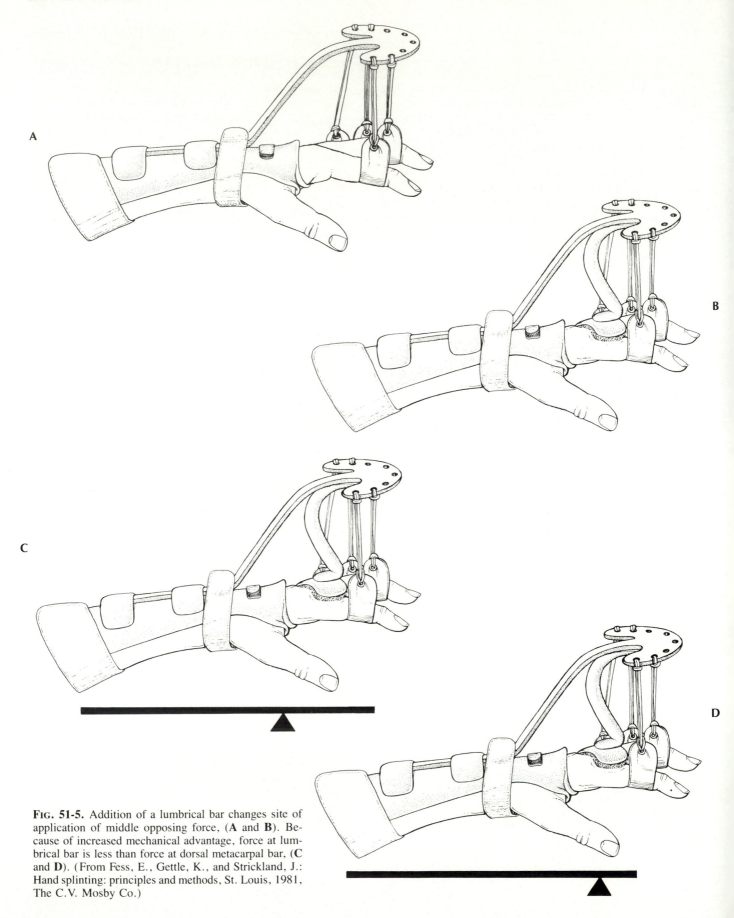

FIG. 51-5. Addition of a lumbrical bar changes site of application of middle opposing force, (**A** and **B**). Because of increased mechanical advantage, force at lumbrical bar is less than force at dorsal metacarpal bar, (**C** and **D**). (From Fess, E., Gettle, K., and Strickland, J.: Hand splinting: principles and methods, St. Louis, 1981, The C.V. Mosby Co.)

intentional overstressing of joints in therapy, and the patient must be cautioned to avoid situations that could lead to decreased flow or venous congestion, such as extremes in temperatures, dependent position, and constrictive clothing.

STAGE THREE: RESISTIVE MOTION

By the sixth postoperative week tensile strength of the wound has increased considerably and will continue to gain strength at a relatively rapid rate through the fourth postoperative month, with approximately 75% of its potential strength being achieved.[14] The fracture sites may be sufficiently healed to allow removal of the Kirschner wires, requiring only small dorsal or volar immobilization splints to provide support for an additional few weeks. Gentle resistive exercises that are gradually increased by graded increments may be added to the existing therapy program, but the patient must be cautioned to avoid lifting heavy objects for an another 2 to 4 weeks, depending, or course, on individual circumstances.

During the first 8 postoperative weeks, considerable physiologic change occurs over a relatively short period of time. This internal environment of plasticity represents a "golden period" in which astute therapeutic intervention may be used to shape and influence positively the eventual functional result. When this most favorable opportunity the patient will have of achieving the full extent of his potential occurs, every effort must be made to use this time advantageously, for these circumstances will not present themselves again. The very process that heals the body becomes simultaneously a friend and a formidable opponent to the rehabilitation team, requiring the surgeon and the therapist to pool their knowledge to create a milieu that effectively alters the reparative process to the patient's benefit. Timed according to the patient's rate of progress, assessment of active and passive range of motion should be carried out on a routine basis, often requiring reevaluation several times a week. Pinch, grip (Fig. 51-6), and individual muscle strength may be measured at approximately 8 to 12 weeks, or whenever the patient is permitted unrestricted use of the replanted part. Based on quantitative values, the treatment program becomes an integrated cycle of evaluation and program modification, being constantly adapted to the individual needs of the patient.

Fortunately, hand rehabilitation specialists have become increasingly more knowledgeable and the era of the modality-dependent patient is rapidly on its way to extinction. Patients know from the beginning that the burden of deriving maximum benefit from therapy is their responsibility and that the surgeon and therapist are available as assistants only. This emphasis on patient independence ultimately produces substantial and measurable rewards through improved motion and hand function. Although the therapist who relies on a multitude of "application modalities" that require no exertion or active participation by the patient may feel personally fulfilled as a provider, nothing can substitute for a carefully planned and exactingly executed program of active motion, augmented by judicious splinting and functional use (Fig. 51-7). Patients must be repeatedly cautioned against relying on therapy sessions as the only time to exercise and are instead instructed to work at home a specified

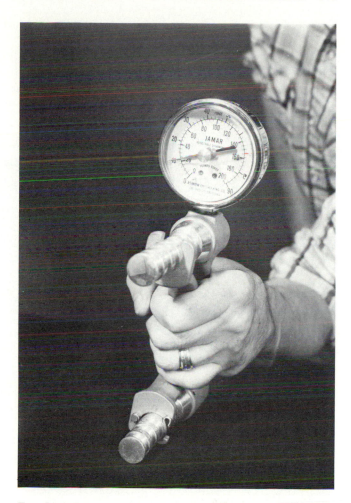

FIG. 51-6. Because of resistive load applied to repaired tendons, grip should not be measured until unrestricted use of replanted part is permitted.

number of minutes per unit of time, such as 15 minutes out of each hour, 30 minutes per every 2 hours, or, for the chronic television viewer, through every commercial!

Requiring less frequent recordings because of the extended time involved in nerve regeneration, sensibility assessment of the replanted part may be carried out on a 4- to 6-week schedule. It is important to monitor several different aspects of sensibility, and in a research environment the testing battery should reflect a representative balance of test instruments that measure the entire spectrum of sensibility including sympathetic response, detection, discrimination, quantification, and recognition parameters. As nerves regenerate, desensitization or sensory reeducation programs may be interwoven with the existing clinic and home exercise routines as needed. Although infrequently a factor, excessive pain may be diminished through the use of a transcutaneous stimulator. However, one should avoid reliance on this modality to control "routine" postoperative pain, eliminating potential problems with gadget distraction and unwarranted psychological dependence on the stimulator.

Splinting regimens continue to be updated to reflect

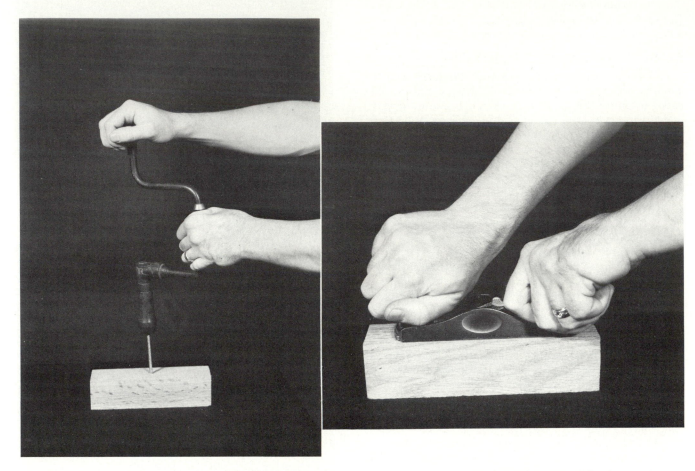

FIG. 51-7. Use of replanted hand in bilateral activities improves active range of motion and gross coordination.

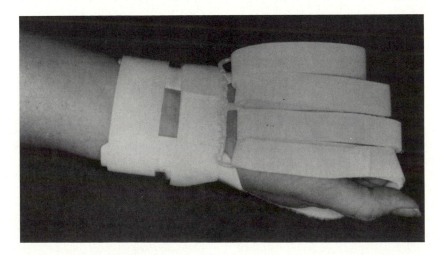

FIG. 51-8. Wrist-band portion of this simple finger flexion splint was widened to decrease pressure on distal forearm. (From Fess, E., Gettle, K., and Strickland, J.: Hand splinting: principles and methods, St. Louis, 1981, The C.V. Mosby Co.)

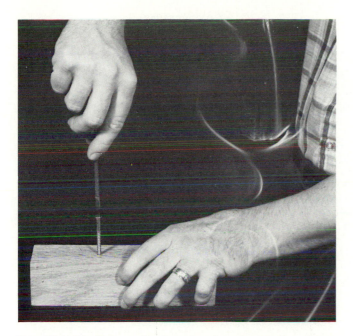

FIG. 51-9. Limited coordination of replanted extremity may necessitate a change in hand dominance.

changing needs of the patient, and greater splint forces (Fig. 51-8) may be used to mobilize joints that have not responded favorably to exercise and more conservative splinting approaches. The slow continuous traction provided by mobilizing splints facilitates collagen realignment and is the key to acquiring and maintaining passive motion in the hand. Rough manual manipulation of joints can create microscopic soft-tissue tears, which begin the reparative process anew, further enhancing scar formation and joint stiffness. As range of motion improves, positional splints that are worn at night or between exercise periods should be reevaluated and altered to maintain the newly achieved motion.

STAGE FOUR: MAINTENANCE AND FURTHER SURGICAL RECONSTRUCTION

Although timing for each tissue type is slightly different, after approximately 5 months soft-tissue structures gain strength slowly through 1 year after replantation, with collagen configuration eventually changing through a remodeling process not fully understood, to closely resemble the specialized architecture of the preinjury tissues[14,31]; that is, collagen in tendon scar begins to resemble that of the uninjured tendon, and peritenon scar is similar to the collagen organization of peritenon. As scar metabolism slows, further reconstructive surgery may be considered to increase function of the replanted part.

By the time the maintenance stage is reached, a more realistic idea of the potential functional capacity of the replanted part is apparent, and the therapy program may be directed toward teaching the patient to use the extremity as an assist (Fig. 51-9) and, if the dominant hand is involved, to changing dominance (Fig. 51-10). Activities of daily living and work evaluations may also be necessary. Although many patients treated in a hand rehabilitation center experience temporary limitation of function, only those with

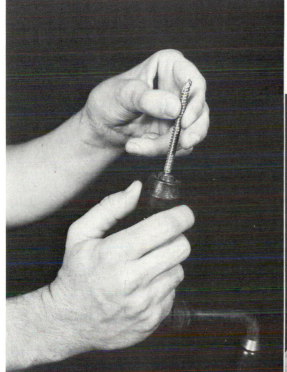

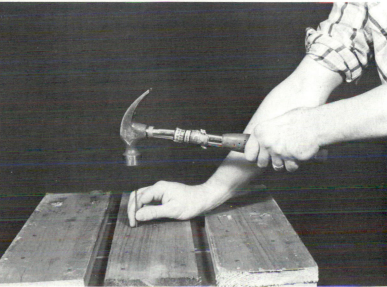

FIG. 51-10. When replantation involves dominant extremity, activities that require fine coordination of uninjured hand are helpful in altering dominance patterns.

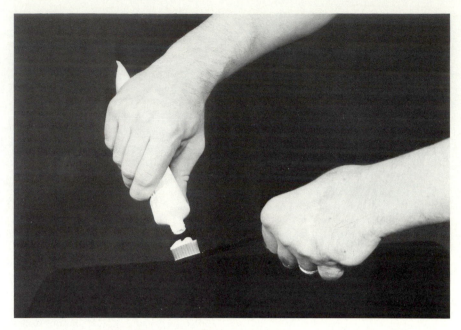

FIG. 51-11. Everyday skills that require bilateral hand use should be assessed to ensure patient independence.

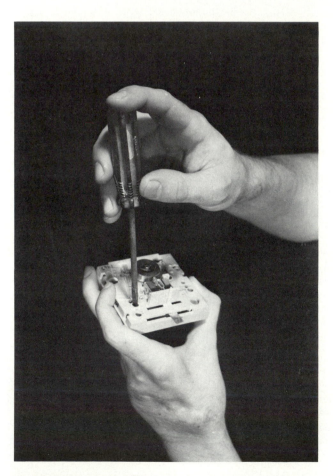

FIG. 51-12. Job skills should be thoroughly evaluated before patient attempts to return to work situation.

major involvement require formal activities of daily living assessment and training. Depending on the extent of injury and the amount of functional recovery, patients who have had replantation of multiple digits, a hand, or a significant portion of an extremity, may need assistance in adapting to those activities of daily living that require use of the hands bilaterally (Fig. 51-11) or use of the replanted hand alone.

The timing and limitations imposed upon the patient's return to work are influenced by many factors, some of which include the extent of injury, presence of secondary complications, the philosophy of the surgeon and rehabilitation center, the attitude of the employer, requirements of the job, stipulations of the third-party provider, and the physical capacity and motivation of the patient. These variables contribute significantly to the way patients are reintroduced into the work force, and each patient has a unique set of circumstances, sometimes necessitating innovative and persistent approaches by the rehabilitation team. Returning to work can be stressful for the patient, especially if the injury occurred on the job. An astute therapist may facilitate the process by communicating closely with the employer, by supporting the concept of return to protected work as soon as daily therapy in the clinic is no longer required, and by preparing the patient both physically and emotionally. On-site visits may provide the therapist with a better concept of job possibilities and the functional requirements they entail (Fig. 51-12). Although each case should be judged individually, a favorable progression of events in an uncomplicated situation is exemplified by return to a one-handed job at 6 weeks after replantation and, if protective sensation is present, return to limited use of the extremity at 3 months. Some patients may require additional formal training to prepare them for alternative employment

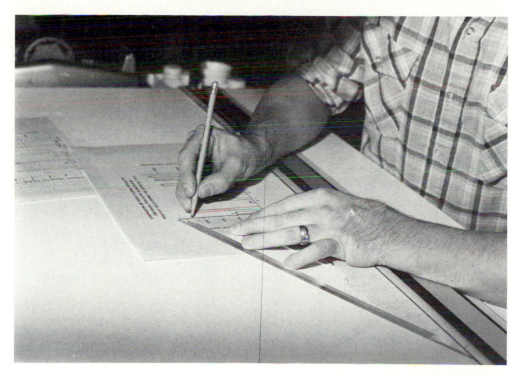

Fig. 51-13. If patient is unable to return to his previous employment, vocational training may be necessary to provide skills that can be adapted to functional capacity of replanted extremity.

that is better suited to their physical capacities (Fig. 51-13).

Although not usually debilitating, cold intolerance of the replanted part is a frequent complaint of patients as they return to their normal life-style routines. More severe during the first year after replantation and sometimes lasting for 2 to 3 years, cold intolerance problems decrease with time as flow patterns increase and become more stable.[3] A cold pressor test may be used for objective comparison of the warm-up times of normal and replanted digits.[2] Commercially available, a battery-powered ''hunter's mitten'' may help the person who experiences considerable discomfort to better tolerate exposure to cold temperatures.

Assessment of range of motion, sensibility, strength, and hand dexterity (Fig. 51-14) play important roles during this stage, providing quantitative data about the patient's ability to maintain what was accomplished during the earlier months of rehabilitation, and definitively identifying functional assets and deficits. These data, combined with information regarding the physical status of the replanted part, allow the rehabilitation team to decide whether further reconstructive surgery, balanced against the inherent risks involved, would significantly enhance composite hand function. General comparisons are drawn between the patient's capacity and previous experience with similar cases and those reported in the literature. If pronounced discrepancies are noted, surgery is seriously considered. For example, if at 6 months the patient continues to exhibit an anesthetic portion of the replant and experience shows that protective sensation should be present, exploration of the nerve in-

volved may be in order; if tendon glide has not been fully established, a tenolyis procedure may produce the final increments of active motion that the patient needs to return to his previous employment; or a tendon transfer may be used to augment limited active motion. The surgeon, therapist, and patient work together to find solutions that will best meet the unique needs of the patient.

If further reconstructive surgery is not feasible and there are active-motion limitations that detract significantly from the patient's ability to use the extremity, consideration of an additional splinting option is appropriate during the maintenance stage of rehabilitation. Dependent on the presence of supple joints, control or functional splinting provides motion that the patient lacks, improving hand coordination and use. These splints, best designed with low-profile outriggers, which permit greater freedom of movement because of reduced bulk (see Chapter 76), are often constructed of more durable materials than the temporary mobilizing or immobilizing splints. Since no splint is ever cosmetically pleasing and patients tend to become gadget resistive with time, standardized hand-function test scores with and without the splint should be carefully compared to ensure that application of a control splint does, in fact, improve coordination and dexterity.

STAGE FIVE: PROGRAM ASSESSMENT

Although often overlooked, program assessment is an essential aspect of patient treatment. By identifying those patients who achieved substantial functional recovery and those techniques that provided consistently superior results,

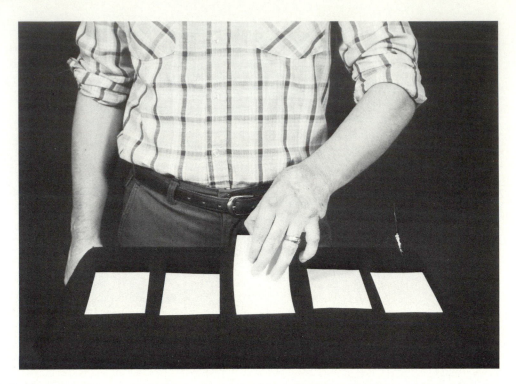

FIG. 51-14. Consisting of seven standardized subtests, the Jebsen Hand Function Test may be used to assess gross hand coordination.

one can comprehensively evaluate replantation programs to ensure quality patient care and contribute to the advancement of professional knowledge. Unfortunately, in coping with the stresses of busy practices, many medical specialists rely on intuition or, at best, educated guesses to assess retrospectively their programs, failing to recognize that critical examination and analysis based on quantitative data could facilitate their efficiency, cost effectiveness, and patient care. Ranging from simple reviews of case histories to complicated studies based on statistical probability limits or correlation coefficients, the methods chosen to evaluate programs should reflect the individual characteristics of those centers involved. The size of the patient population and expertise of the staff, directly affect the parameters of any study that may be undertaken. Although a large center may choose to study more esoteric questions using computer analysis, this approach would be unrealistic for a center that treats two or three replantation cases a year. Program assessment need not be a complicated process, but it does require careful planning to ensure that unnecessary amounts of time are not consumed in information retrieval. The important concept is that a conscientious effort is made to identify important variables and upgrade the program for future replantation patients. Once trends are noted, more sophisticated means of assessing vital questions may be employed.

FUTURE CONSIDERATIONS

The continuing perfection of microvascular techniques and improvement of sucess rates have produced significant changes in the field of hand surgery during the past two decades, providing the surgeon with important options in reconstruction of the severely injured hand. It is toward this continued advancement that those concerned with rehabilitating the replanted hand must strive, for the functional results of replantation efforts have not kept pace with the surgeons' excellent ability to restore viability to reattached parts. Although basic priorities for replantation surgery have been established, much is still unknown about the variables that affect functional capacity. Currently, it is not possible to predict accurately and consistently the return of sensibility, range of motion, or coordination in a replanted extremity.

Through assessment techniques, therapists have the potential to make valuable contributions to replantation concepts. The science of testing and measurement, though firmly established in many other fields, has just begun to be recognized in hand rehabilitation. Many tools currently employed in clinical assessment of patients lack validity and reliability as testing instruments, producing information that is vague or misleading. For example, reports of two-point discrimination return in replanted parts vary considerably, apparently indicating that inconsistencies exist in either patient capacity to regenerate sensory nerve fibers or in the expertise of surgical teams, or both. Recently, however, Bell and Buford[1] presented data that provide a totally different viewpoint of the problem. Using finely tuned transducers and oscilloscopes, they found that there were considerable differences in amount of pressure applied between the one and two points in two-point discrimination tests and that this discrepancy of pressures easily exceeded normal touch-pressure thresholds. Additionally, they noted that even in the hands of experienced hand surgeons and therapists, there were major inconsistencies in amount of pressure applied from examiner to examiner, using skin blanching as a guide to pressure application. This study indicates that serious problems exist with the instrument with which measurements are taken, negatively influencing data collection and professional communication.

The use of hand-coordination tests is frequently reported, but close scrutiny reveals that the majority of these tests are "homemade." Lacking appropriate instrumentation studies, these tests are essentially meaningless. When standardized tests are used, the results are often invalidated because portions of the test were omitted or changed or the test was used as a practice tool in therapy.!

In an age of accountability and scientific advancement, the ability to measure surgical and therapeutic results is extremely important. The lack of understanding of the concepts of tests and instrumentation seriously impedes the advancement of knowledge in any field. Our most immediate and critical challenge is to develop and use test instruments that accurately and reliably assess the many facets of hand function; meeting this challenge requires discipline and quality research. It is the combined knowledge of the surgical and therapy fields that will provide a better understanding of replantation patients and their potential to achieve maximum benefit from rehabilitative efforts.

REFERENCES

1. Bell, J., and Buford, W.: The force/time relationship of clinically used sensory testing instruments, Presented at the thirty-seventh annual meeting of the American Society for Surgery of the Hand, New Orleans, 1982.
2. Bright, D., and Sehayik, R.: Electrophysiology of nerves. In American Academy of Orthopaedic Surgeons: Symposium on microsurgery, St. Louis, 1979, The C.V. Mosby Co.
3. Bright, D., and Wright, S.: Postoperative management in replantation. In American Academy of Orthopaedic Surgeons: Symposium on microsurgery, St. Louis, 1979, The C.V. Mosby Co.
4. Buncke, H., Buncke, C., and Schultz, W.: Experimental digital amputation and reimplantation, Plast. Reconstr. Surg. **36**:62, 1965.
5. Callahan, A.: Replantation: therapist's management, Presentation at Rehabilitation of the hand—'82, Philadelphia, March 1982, Hand Rehabilitation Foundation.
6. Duran, R., and Houser, R.: Controlled passive motion following flexor tendon repair in zones 2 and 3. In American Academy of Orthopaedic Surgeons: Symposium on tendon surgery in the hand, St. Louis, 1975, The C.V. Mosby Co.
7. Fess, E., Gettle, K., and Strickland, J.: Hand splinting principles and methods, St. Louis, 1981, The C.V. Mosby Co.
8. Kleinert, H., and Kasdan, M.: Anastomosis of digital vessels, J. Ky. Med. Assoc. **63**:106, 1963.
9. Gelberman, R., Urbaniak, J., Bright, D., and Levin, S.: Digital sensibility following replantation, J. Hand Surg. **3**:313, 1978.
10. Kleinert, H., Kutz, J., and Cohen, M.: Primary repair of zone 2 flexor tendon lacerations. In American Academy of Orthopaedic Surgeons: Symposium on tendon surgery in the hand, St. Louis, 1975, The C.V. Mosby Co.
11. Komatsu, S., and Tamai, S.: Successful replantation of a completely cut-off thumb: case report, Plast. Reconstr. Surg. **42**:374, 1968.
12. Lapchinsky, A.: Recent results of experimental transplantation of severed limbs and kidneys and possible use of this technique in clinical practice, Ann. N.Y. Acad. Sci. **87**:539, 1960.
13. Lehmann, J., and DeLateur, B.: Diathermy and superficial heat and cold therapy. In Kottke, F., Stillwell, G., and Lehmann, J., editors: Krusen's handbook of physical medicine and rehabilitation, ed. 3, Philadelphia, 1982, W.B. Saunders Co.
14. Madden, J., and Aren, A.: Wound healing: biologic and clinical features. In Sabiston, D., editor: Textbook of surgery: the biological basis of modern surgical practice, ed. 12, Philadelphia, 1981, W.B. Saunders Co.
15. Malt, R., and McKhann, C.: Replantation of severed arms, J.A.M.A. **189**:716, 1964.
16. May, J., Bryant, A., and Gardner, M.: Digital replantation distal to the proximal interphalangeal joint, J. Hand Surg. **7**:161, 1982.
17. Morrison, W., O'Brien, B., and MacLeod, A.: Digital replantation and revascularization: a long term review of 100 cases, Hand, **10**:125, 1978.
18. O'Brien, B.: Microvascular reconstructive surgery, London, 1977, Churchill Livingstone.
19. O'Brien, B., and Miller, G.: Digital reattachment and revascularization, J. Bone Joint Surg. **55A**:714, 1973.
20. Peacock, E.: Wound healing and wound care. In Schwartz, S.I., and others: editors: Principles of surgery, ed. 3, New York, 1979, McGraw-Hill Book Co.
21. Schlenker, J., Kleinert, H., and Tsai, T.M.: Methods and results of replantation following traumatic amputation of the thumb in 64 patients, J. Hand Surg. **5**:63, 1980.
22. Snyder, C., and Knowles, R.: Autotransplantation of extremities, Clin. Orthop. **29**:113, 1963.
23. Snyder, C., and Knowles, R.: Experimental replantation, Plast. Reconstr. Surg. **26**:251, 1960.
24. Steichen, J., Harmon, K., Fess, E., and Strickland, J.: Rehabilitation of the upper extremity replantation patients. In Hunter, J., Schneider, L., Mackin, E., and Bell, J., editors: Rehabilitation of the hand, St. Louis, 1978, The C.V. Mosby Co.
25. Stillwell, G.: Electrotherapy. In Kottke, F., Stillwell, G., and Lehmann, J.: Krusen's handbook of physical medicine and rehabilitation, ed. 3, Philadelphia, 1982, W.B. Saunders Co.
26. Stirrat, C., Seaber, A., Urbaniak, J., and Bright, D.: Temperature monitoring in digital replantation, J. Hand Surg. **3**:342, 1978.
27. Tamai, S.: Twenty years' experience of limb replantation: review of 293 upper extremity replants, J. Hand Surg. **7**:549, 1982.
28. Urbaniak, J.: Replantation of amputated digits and hands. In American Academy of Orthopaedic Surgeons: Instructional course lectures, **27**:15, 1978, St. Louis, The C.V. Mosby Co.
29. Urbaniak, J.: Replantation of amputated parts: technique, results, and indications. In American Academy of Orthopaedic Surgeons: Symposium on microsurgery, St. Louis, 1979, The C.V. Mosby Co.
30. Wang, S., Young, K., and Wei, J.: Replantation of severed limbs: clinical analysis of 91 cases, J. Hand Surg. **6**:311, 1981.
31. Weeks, P., and Wray, R.: Management of acute hand injuries: a biological approach, ed. 2, St. Louis, 1978, The C.V. Mosby Co.
32. Weiland, A., Villarreal-Rios, A., Kleinert, H., Kutz, J., Atasoy, E., and Lister, G.: Replantation of digits and hands: analysis of surgical techniques and functional result in 71 patients with 86 replantations, J. Hand Surg. **2**:1, 1977.

IX

BURNS AND COLD INJURIES

52

Acute care and rehabilitation of the burned hand

ROGER E. SALISBURY, SANDY REEVES, and PHYLLIS WRIGHT

OCCUPATIONAL THERAPY
Splinting

Philosophies vary as to the best time to splint an acutely burned hand, and an increasing number of occupational therapists are no longer splinting immediately after injury. Significant edema usually develops during the first 48 to 72 hours, especially in a large-surface-area burn that requires fluid resuscitation. A splint that is applied immediately upon admission may not fit several hours later. Splints applied with either straps or dressings may become constrictive as swelling increases and must be closely monitored and modified frequently to accomodate larger circumferences. Therefore more emphasis should be placed on keeping the hand well elevated and actively exercising in order to decrease edema and keep joints mobile. The hand should be positioned above the elbow, and the elbow above the shoulder, even if only the hand is burned. This can be accomplished by placing the arm upon pillows or suspending it in an overhead sling or positioning device (Fig. 52-1). If the shoulder or the elbow is also burned, it should also be carefully positioned. The elbow should be positioned in 5 degrees of flexion to prevent hyperextension stress to the joint. The shoulder should be positioned in 90 to 110 degrees of abduction and externally rotated. The shoulder should not be positioned in greater than 110 degrees abduction for extended periods, which could cause injury to the brachial plexus.

After the edema "peaks" the hand should be splinted at the first signs of decreased mobility or skin tightness. Splints should be worn at night and during periods of rest, with the patient's hands being left free during the day. Patients should be encouraged to use their hands and to actively exercise on their own as much as possible. The splinting program should not interfere with activities of daily living. For instance, splints should be removed at mealtime to encourage self-feeding. Patients who lack motivation, who are unable to actively use their hands, or who are beginning to develop contractures in spite of night splinting may need to wear hand splints during daytime periods of inactivity as well.

The burned hand should be splinted in the "antideformity position" rather than the traditional "position of function." The antideformity position will vary, depending on the location and size of the burn. The goal is to position the hand so that the burned surface area is stretched, therefore pre-venting the skin from "drawing" or contracting as it heals. For instance, in circumferential or volar wrist burns the antideformity position of the wrist is 30 to 40 degrees of extension; neutral (0 degrees) is used for dorsal burns. In dorsal hand burns the metacarpophalangeal joints should be flexed as much as possible, with the interphalangeal joints in full extension. The thumb should be abducted fully and slightly extended to preserve the first web space. The antideformity position differs from the so-called position of function in that the latter has more metacarpophalangeal extension and interphalangeal flexion and less thumb abduction and extension (Fig. 52-2). In the case of hand burns to the palmar surfaces only, the most advantageous position may be that of metacarpophalangeal and interphalangeal extension, finger abduction, and thumb extension and abduction, in order to stretch the palmar skin to its maximum. In a circumferential burn, in which there is a potential for both dorsal and volar contractures, it may be advantageous to alternate between the two splint designs, with the patient wearing the antideformity splint during the day and the palmar stretching splint at night.

Low-temperature thermoplastics such as Polyform and Kay Splint are recommended for hand splint fabrication, since these materials are easily reshaped to accomodate changes in edema or increases in range of motion. A strapping material that is soft, washable, nonabrasive, and nonconstrictive, such as Velfoam or Betapile II is recommended.

When a splint is applied over topical antibiotics, it is especially important that the splint be removed, fresh antibiotics be applied, and the clean splint be reapplied, several times per nursing shift. Otherwise the cream will pool under the splint, providing a soupy culture medium in which bacteria may grow. A light gauze dressing over the cream keeps the cream from being rubbed off and helps prevent the splint from sliding distally (which would hold the hand in the position of contracture).

Special splints may have to be designed if peripheral nerve lesions, fractures, or tendon damage were incurred at the time of thermal injury. Early prophylactic splinting can decrease the incidence of secondary deformities and often minimize the number of reconstructive procedures required later in the patient's hospital course. Internal fixation through the burn wound and plaster casting of fractures

585

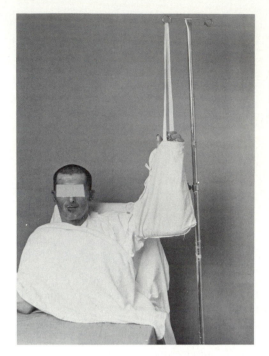

FIG. 52-1. Elevation in a sterile sling is a simple, inexpensive way to reduce hand edema soon after a burn when elbow is uninvolved.

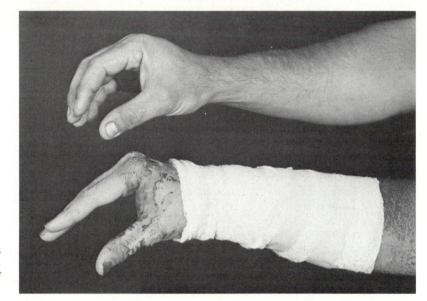

FIG. 52-2. Antideformity position for dorsal burns of hand, *bottom,* has more metacarpophalangeal flexion and interphalangeal extension than position of function, *top.*

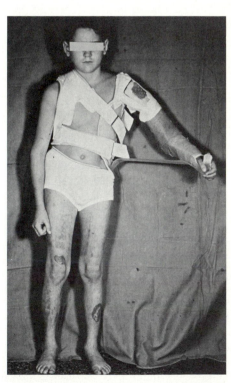

FIG. 52-3. Lightweight Polyform splint provides immobilization for humeral fracture after electrical injury but also allows optimum care of burn wound.

are not recommended, because of potential wound sepsis. Instead, thermoplastic or aluminum splints are employed, because they are sturdy, light weight, easily cleaned, and cover as little of the burn wound as possible while rendering adequate support (Fig. 52-3).

The success of a grafting procedure is often dependent on the quality of intraoperative and postoperative splinting and follow-up therapy programs. Even wounds covered by thick, split-thickness skin grafts may contract, resulting in joint deformity, if appropriate splinting is not initiated promptly and continued until all evidence of skin tightness is gone. Careful preoperative planning between the surgeon and the occupational therapist is necessary, so that both understand what is the desired functional result of the surgery. Although preoperative planning makes it possible for most postoperative splints to be made prior to surgery, often splints must be made in the operating room at the time of surgery, such as in a surgical release of a contracture. In the case of the hand, where no meshed sheet grafts are preferred (for best cosmetic and functional results), immediate and complete immobilization, which allows open treatment of the graft site, is preferred. The size and location of the graft to be treated open will determine the type of postoperative splint to be used. Dorsal hand grafts can be splinted in an antideformity splint, with fingernail traction being used to secure the fingers into the splint (Fig. 52-4). If both the dorsal hand and circumferential forearm and

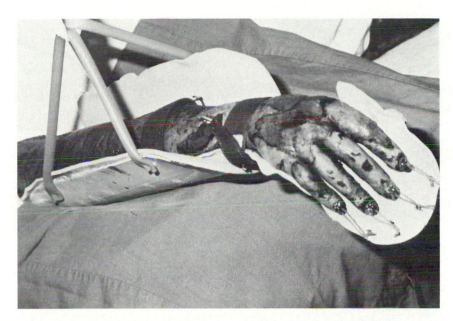

FIG. 52-4. Volar splint with Velcro straps and fingernail traction ensure adequate immobilization to leave grafts without dressings.

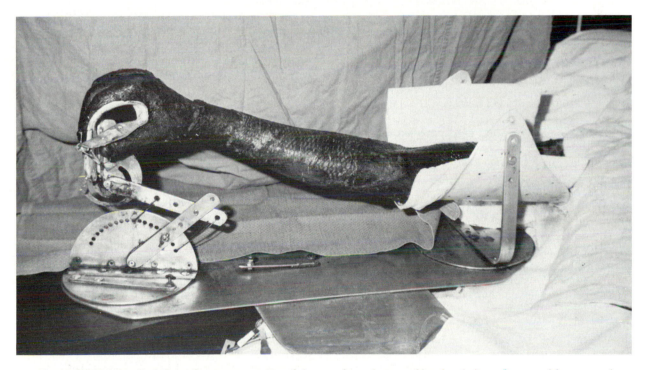

FIG. 52-5. Cobra splint allows for open treatment of sheet grafts to dorsum of hand and circumference of forearm and elbow by immobilizing these graft sites without covering them.

elbow are also being grafted, then a more complicated splint, such as the Cobra splint, may be necessary. The Cobra splint is a mechanically adjustable aluminum and Polyform splint that supports the extremity on the upper arm and volar hand platforms. The patient's hand is held in place with fingernail traction; therefore the Cobra splint is used only with cooperative adults (Fig. 52-5).

After the antecubital fossa has been grafted, one of two splint designs can be used to immobilize the surgical site.

If the graft is being treated open, a posterior elbow splint (with a hole cut into it to avoid pressure to the humeral condyles, olecranon, and ulnar nerves) can be used. If the graft is being treated closed, an anterior elbow splint can be applied over heavy dressings, a technique that not only provides a more stable splint but also protects the graft site from accidental trauma.

Because the postsurgical position of an axillary graft is difficult to anticipate, the splint in such a case is usually

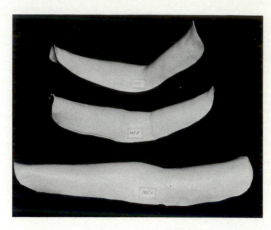

FIG. 52-6. Serial splinting of early elbow-flexion contracture will achieve normal extension with minimal trauma.

fabricated in the operating room. Whether a three-piece airplane splint (for treating the axilla open) or an axillary conformer over heavy dressings is decided upon, caution must be used to avoid splinting the shoulder in more than approximately 110 degrees abduction. As stated earlier, this could cause injury to the brachial plexus as a result of overstretching.

With any of the previously mentioned postoperative splints, it is best to apply the splint in the operating room while the patient is still under anesthesia. This will lessen the chance of disturbing the graft during transfers or when the patient awakes. This is especially important with children, who tend to move around more as they come out of anesthesia.

Splinting may be necessary on a long-term basis in a hand with more serious, deep second- and third-degree burns. Early contractures of the upper extremity can usually be corrected with serial static and/or dynamic splinting techniques. Serial static splinting works best for correcting shoulder-adduction, elbow-flexion (Fig. 52-6), wrist-flexion, and thumb-adduction contractures. It is used in conjunction with an aggressive exercise program. The joint is splinted at the maximum passive range of motion gained during exericse. The splint is modified each time passive range of motion increases. Serial splinting does not increase range of motion but maintains that which is gained through aggressive therapy.

Dynamic splinting exerts a steady force to increase range of motion of the involved joint. It is often used to correct finger contractures, such as in increasing metacarpophalangeal joint flexion, interphalangeal joint extension, or thumb abduction. Dynamic splinting often takes the form of rubber-band traction, in which soft cuff loops are placed over the fingers or clothing hooks are attached to the fingernails with cyanocrylate glue. Longitudinal fingernail traction is often used to maintain metacarpophalangeal flexion and interphalangeal joint extension in a newly burned or recently grafted hand when straps are not able to adequately maintain proper positioning or cross over newly grafted dorsal burns. Fingernail traction also helps control the longitudinal rotation sometimes encountered in laterally or circumferentially burned phalanges. A burned palm may also be spread

open with fingernail traction and a dorsal splint after autografting. Fingernail traction, however, must be done with caution, to ensure that the fingernails are stable and will not pull loose. Also, the fingernail beds may be hypersensitive, making the patient unable to tolerate this technique.

Special care must be taken when deep dorsal finger burns are treated, since the integrity of the extensor mechanism is jeopardized. Unlimited flexion could cause disruption of the central slip and result in a boutonnière deformity. The involved joint, therefore, is exercised only with the distal interphalangeal and metacarpophalangeal joints supported in extension, to prevent stress to the extensor mechanism. The hand is splinted in the traditional antideformity position by means of longitudinal fingernail traction (if possible) when the patient is not receiving wound care or exercise. If the proximal interphalangeal joint is open, however, internal fixation with Kirschner wires may be necessary to maintain immobilization. If a boutonnière deformity is present, the joint should be splinted statically in the more functional position of approximately 40 degrees flexion at all times. It is not uncommon for scar to bridge the central slip defect if the joint is completely immobilized, thus preventing a more severe boutonnière deformity or the necessity for joint arthrodesis.

Pediatric patients pose few special problems except that proper positioning is more difficult to maintain without splinting. They tend to keep their hands in the more comfortable position of deformity (Fig. 52-7). However, a child will often use his hand more spontaneously than an adult with a similar injury. Therefore, although splinting may have to be initiated early, it is important that the child be allowed out of the splint during the day for periods of supervised play to help maintain hand function.

Activities of daily living and hand function

As soon as the patient's condition is stable, he is encouraged to become actively involved in self-care and in activities of daily living. These tasks not only exercise the hands but help prevent deterioration of general strength and endurance. An activities of daily living (ADL) evaluation is performed by the occupational therapist at various stages of the patient's recovery to determine what activities the patient is capable of performing, whether special adaptive devices are needed, and, if they are needed, whether they will be required temporarily or permanently. Before offering help, family members and health care personnel alike are encouraged to allow the patient the chance and the time to try to do a task without assistance, to foster an attitude of self-reliance. Adaptive devices are provided only if absolutely necessary, and each device is removed as soon as the patient can perform the particular task without it.

As soon as the patient is allowed nourishment by mouth, he is expected to participate in self-feeding; this is usually the first ADL task attempted by the patient. Initially, simple adaptive devices, such as a large sponge handle for feeding utensils, may be necessary because of decreased hand range of motion and strength secondary to edema and pain.

The next tasks attempted by the patient are basic hygiene care, such as assisting with bathing, dental hygiene, hair care, and shaving. These activities may also require tem-

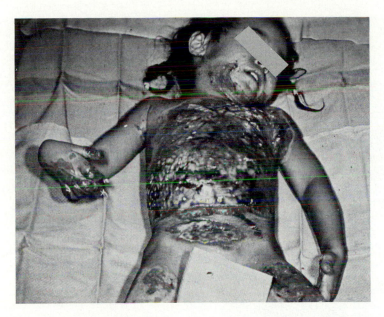

FIG. 52-7. Wrist flexion, metacarpophalangeal hyperextension, and first web space adduction clearly illustrate that child chooses comfortable, not functional, position.

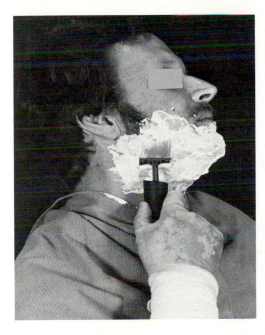

FIG. 52-8. Adaptive devices such as enlarged razor handle for patient with limited grasp increases independence in self-care.

porary assistive devices provided by the occupational therapist (Fig. 52-8). Wound care, application of Ace wraps, and getting dressed are attempted after general endurance and range of motion improves, since these activities require greater joint mobility and general strength. In many cases, job-related tasks or household activities are simulated prior to discharge, so that any difficulties can be anticipated. Any adaptations to tools or work setting can then be provided for or planned for, especially in the case of permanent disability (Fig. 52-9).

During the patient's hospitalization graded activities are provided by the occupational therapist to increase hand strength, joint mobility, and fine motor skills. These activities may range from squeezing a sponge during the first few days to help decrease edema, to working on a selected therapeutic craft activity to increase hand mobility and coordination. Throughout the patient's hospitalization and after discharge, hand function is evaluated with both standardized and nonstandardized techniques in order to monitor changes in joint range of motion, strength, coordination, and sensation (Fig. 52-10).

Scar control

Any deep second- or third-degree burn of the hand has a high potential for hypertrophic scarring, which not only is unappealing cosmetically but also can compromise function. Therefore it is essential that a scar control program be begun as soon as initial healing occurs.

Good basic skin care is taught, including what types of moisturizing lotions and sunscreens to use. Petroleum jelly or oil-based lotions act as moisture barriers and are best used after washing the hand, to seal in moisture already absorbed. These ointments and lotions cannot be used when scar compression garments are being worn. These substances are absorbed into the material, causing a loss of elasticity as well as grease stains. Water-based lotions (which readily rinse off the skin with water alone) add moisture to the skin, but because they do not prevent evaporative water loss, they have to be applied more often. Water-based lotions can be used with scar compression garments without staining them or ruining the elasticity. Moisturizing the skin frequently, especially prior to exercise, increases the flexibility of the skin and helps minimize breakdown, which occurs to a greater degree if the newly healed burns are allowed to become too dry. Avoidance of direct sunlight on the burn is recommended, to prevent sun-

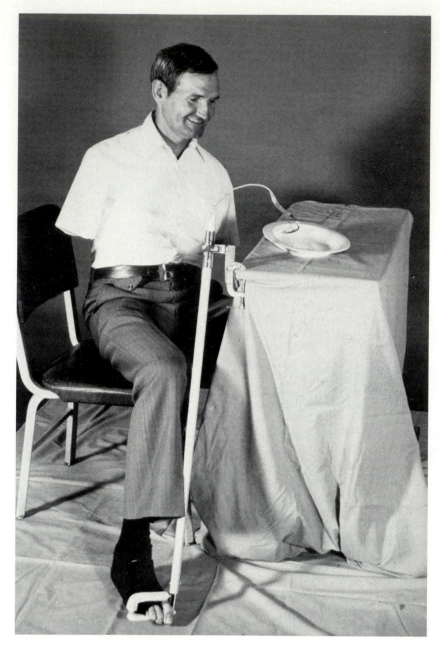

FIG. 52-9. Patient with bilateral shoulder girdle amputations secondary to an electrical injury uses a foot-powered feeding device designed by Larry Smith, Occupational Therapy Adaptive Device Specialist to meet his specific feeding needs.

burn (since a newly healed burn is very sensitive and easily sunburned) and hyperpigmentation. Sunscreen lotions of high numerical rating (the higher the number, the stronger the shielding properties) as well as gloves are recommended until the scars have completely matured.

Scar compression is the primary means of preventing the buildup of hypertrophic scarring. Scar compression garments (such as the Jobskin burn compression garments, by Jobst) should be measured for and ordered prior to discharge, since it may take several weeks for garments to arrive. In the meantime, Isotoner gloves by Aris (with adornments removed and turned inside out so that the seams are outside) serve as practical, temporary, intermediate-stage compression garments; they can be found at most larger department stores. Jobst gloves can be ordered with slant inserts to better compress the dorsal web spaces, but they may also require small Betapile or Velfoam pads between the fingers beneath the glove to prevent dorsal hooding scars. The fingertips of the gloves can be ordered open to allow for sensory input but should be left closed on any finger that has been partially amputated. Volar zippers may be desirable in the wrists of the initial pair of gloves, to increase the ease of application while the newly healed skin is still fragile, so that excessive blistering can be avoided.

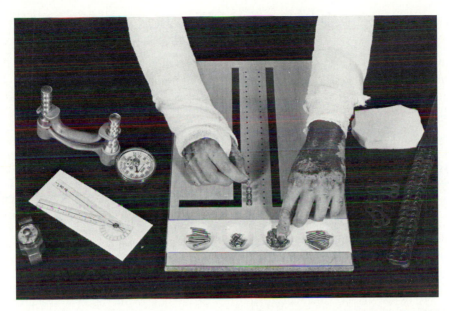

FIG. 52-10. Progress in hand rehabilitation is evaluated by use of standardized tests and completion of functional tasks.

It may also be desirable to order the gloves to come 1½ inches above the wrist so that the dorsal hand and wrist receive better compression, since the elastic band at the cuff does not provide adequate compression. An adequate supply of garments will need to be ordered, since the patient will be required to wear the garments at all times, except during meals and baths, until the scars mature. Maturation takes an average of 12 to 18 months; it is evidenced by a complete fading of the erythema, softening and thinning out of the scars, and an increase in wrinkling and flexibility of the scars.

Certain areas of the hand present special scar problems, which require not only exercise, moisturizing, and compression but also massage to obtain the optimal results in scar control. Scar bands tend to form at the web spaces and palmar surfaces across flexion creases. These areas should be well lubricated with a moisturizing cream prior to massage or exercise. During massage, firm pressure is applied with the fingers, and the skin is manipulated in a circular motion perpendicular to any existing scar band. At the same time, the skin should be gently, passively stretched to increase the skin surface area.

Discharge

Prior to discharge the patient is provided with a written home program, including instructions regarding exercises, splinting, activities of daily living to be performed, and scar control techniques. The therapist's phone number is provided in case unforeseen questions arise prior to the patient's first outpatient visit.

Outpatient follow-up

The patient continues to be seen regularly by the occupational therapist on an outpatient basis for reevaluation in regard to exercise, splinting, activities of daily living, and scar control programs.

Hand function continues to be reevaluated, and adjustments in exercise and splinting programs are made accordingly. When a patient has permanent impairment, the occupational therapist assists the physician in evaluating the patient's current functional level and employment potential and in determining whether he needs to seek a different line of work. A vocational assessment may be performed, with recommendations being made to a vocational rehabilitation or other service agency. The occupational therapist may help the patient to overcome problems that occurred after discharge involving self-care or other activities of daily living, such as cooking, cleaning, and driving. Suggestions for trying new techniques and for arranging the work space more efficiently are made, and, when necessary, self-help devices are provided.

The patient may need to be measured for new pressure garments to accomodate changes in weight or, in the case of children, growth spurts. Special conformers, not previously required, may be necessary under the Jobst garments to maximize compression.

The occupational therapist will continue to follow the patient as an outpatient (or as an inpatient, if reconstruction procedures are necessary) until the scar control program is discontinued and maximum functional results are obtained. This may take years. The quality of the results is directly related to the motivation and active participation of the patient in the rehabilitation process. Therefore the occupational therapist must emphasize the importance of the patient's involvement in the setting of long-term treatment goals. When rehabilitation of the burned hand is complete, it is the patient who should feel the greatest sense of accomplishment.

Physical therapy

The goals that the physical therapist strives to reach are to maintain the patient's range of motion and strength and to work with the occupational therapist and the surgeon in helping the patient to perform activities in daily living independently. If these goals are reached, numerous surgical procedures for contractures and scar release may be unnecessary. To rehabilitate a patient with upper extremity burns successfully, the physical therapy program must begin in the acute stage of burn care and continue for at least 12 to 18 months. The rehabilitation program includes: (1) proper positioning of the burned joints of the upper extremity when they are not splinted, (2) an aggressive exercise regimen, (3) reinforcing independence in activities of daily living, and (4) comprehensive physical therapy follow-up care.

Positioning

The following positions for upper extremity burns are accepted widely as ideal; however, modifications are often necessary because each patient requires "custom" positioning, with the degree and extent of the burn being taken into account.

Shoulder. If good positioning is not maintained, the shoulder tends to contract in adduction and internal rotation. The ideal position is with a minimum of 90 degrees abduction, shoulder girdle retraction, and neutral rotation, especially after grafting of the axilla, when the shoulder is immobilized for 5 to 7 days.

Elbow. Flexion and pronation contractures occur without adequate physical therapy. The ideal position is in complete extension and neutral with respect to pronation and supination.

Hand. If the hand is not positioned properly, the typical burned-hand deformity can develop. It consists of wrist flexion, metacarpophalangeal hyperextension, proximal interphalangeal flexion and distal interphalangeal flexion or extension, thumb adduction, and interphalangeal extension. Thus the correct positioning for a dorsal hand burn is antideformity, approximately 0 to 30 degrees wrist extension, 90 degrees metacarpophalangeal flexion, 0 degrees proximal interphalangeal and distal interphalangeal flexion (depending on depth of burn), and thumb abduction with slight interphalangeal flexion.

• • •

Correct upper extremity positioning must be maintained (with or without a splint) at all times except during exercise periods. If a patient is motivated, works well on his own, and progresses with his range of motion, splinting need be performed only during long periods of rest. All burned upper extremity joints should be positioned and splinted during sleep.

Communication among surgeon, nurse, occupational therapist, and physical therapist concerning surgical procedures is essential to determine: (1) what area will be debrided and/or grafted, (2) where the donor sites will be, (3) what position the patient will be in postoperatively, (4) if any splints will be needed to maintain the desired position, (5) how and by what means the grafted area is to be supported, and (6) what exercises are permitted. Correct positioning immediately after grafting is critical to the maintenance of range of motion, because all movement of the grafted area is contraindicated for approximately 1 week to allow the graft to adhere to the recipient site. During this period of immobilization, contractures could begin.

Exercise management

In the acute stage of burn care, emphasis is on maintenance of range of motion and muscle tone more than on strength; therefore active and active-assistive exercises are utilized for the burned joints. In most instances these exercises are done while the patient is in the Hubbard tank, because the warm water tends to increase the pain threshold and tissue extensibility. Thus most patients move more willingly, and greater range of motion is possible. As eschar separates and peripheral nerves regenerate, exercising becomes extremely painful. It is at this stage that contractures can begin to appear. The proprioceptive neuromuscular facilitation techniques of contract-relax and rhythmic stabilization are helpful in maintaining range of motion during this period.

When a patient is taken to surgery for débridement and/or grafting of his upper extremity, the physical therapist accompanies him because this is an opportunity to fully evaluate the patient's "pain-free" range of motion and to exercise an uncooperative patient thoroughly. Joints are not forced at this time, and care must be taken not to tear contracted soft tissue. Physical therapy is not discontinued totally during the week of immobilization after grafting. The patient should be instructed to do isometric exercises to maintain the tone of the muscles that act on the immobilized joints, including uninjured areas. Active and/or resistive exercises should be continued for the joints not grafted. Ambulation should be reinitiated as soon as possible after grafting.

After the period of immobilization for grafting, splints are removed and gentle active exercises are begun. Gradually, the patient's upper extremity therapy program is augmented to include active-assistive, resistive, and stretching exercises. The uninvolved extremities and joints of the burned upper extremity must not be overlooked. Resistive exercises should be applied to these areas during all stages of rehabilitation when the patient's medical status allows. Individual exercises are planned for the shoulder, elbow, wrist, and hand because the patient with only a burned hand will often "splint" the rest of the extremity in an effort to make himself comfortable.

Exercise should be supervised at least twice a day by a physical therapist. A minimum of seven to ten repetitions of each exercise should be done. The ideal goal of physical therapy is to have the patient moving his burned upper extremity at least every 2 hours. To attain this goal, the patient's own motivation and willingness to follow through with instructions are critical. Giving the patient a list of the exercises he is to do and putting it where he can see it or having him commit them to memory have been helpful in encouraging him to exercise more. An exercise list also informs the nurse and other medical personnel of the exercises and number of repetitions the patient should be doing independently. Other medical personnel and the patient's relatives can reinforce the physical therapist's efforts by encouraging the patient to do his exercises when the therapist is not present. Goniometric measurements should be taken at appropriate intervals to document progression or regression objectively.

The following exercises are specific ones that have proven successful in maintaining or gaining range of motion and strength for the burned upper extremity.

Shoulder exercises

1. Simple overhead pulley allows one upper extremity to stretch the other in shoulder flexion and abduction and elbow extension.
2. Reaching for opposite ear across the top of the head helps maintain shoulder abduction.
3. Wall climbing exercises with the patient facing the wall are for shoulder flexion; with the side to the wall they are for shoulder abduction.
4. Shoulder is abducted while the patient is lying on a bench and holding a small weight in each hand; the arms are abducted as much as possible, with the elbows kept locked in a neutral position.
5. Hold a stick or broom handle while in a supine position, bringing the arms back as far as possible over the head while trying to touch the bed. This exercise stretches the shoulder.
6. Hanging from stall bars stretches tight shoulders and elbows. This is reserved for healed and/or grafted wounds in deep second- or third-degree burns; however, it can be used as a maintenance exercise for shoulder and/or elbows of an unburned or superficial second-degree burned upper extremity.
7. Wand exercises are good for shoulder abduction, flexion, and internal rotation (Fig. 52-11).
8. With hands clasped behind the head, pull elbows together and then spread them out to the side and back as far as possible.

Elbow exercise

1. Holding a small weight while walking stretches the elbow into extension.
2. Patient can stretch his own elbow into extension by placing the burned arm on the edge of a table and using the other hand to push down on the forearm.
3. Simple overhead pulley helps in elbow extension (see shoulder exercises).
4. Hanging from stall bars helps in elbow extension (see shoulder exercises).

After grafting, elbow extension can be maintained only through vigorous exercise and splinting. It is easier to maintain complete elbow extension after grafting than to reduce an elbow flexion contracture. One should not be overly concerned, however, if a patient develops decreased elbow flexion from prolonged splinting in extension, because as he gradually resumes his activities of daily living, elbow flexion returns to normal limits. The same is not true for decreased elbow extension. When an elbow flexion contracture begins, it tends to worsen with time because most activities of daily living demand elbow flexion.

Forearm exercises

1. Tuck the flexed elbow against the patient's side and manually assist it into supination.
2. Turning a doorknob improves supination.
3. Working with a screwdriver enhances supination or pronation.

Wrist exercises

1. Prayer exercise—holding palms together in a prayer position and winging elbows out to the side to form a right angle at the wrist helps maintain wrist extension (Fig. 52-12).
2. Rocking wrist—place fingers on a table and gently rock the wrist back and forth, pushing wrist into ex-

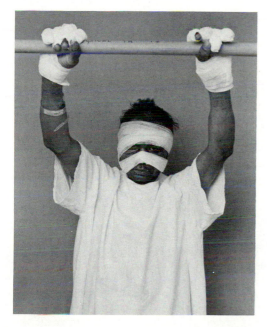

FIG. 52-11. Ward exercises will improve shoulder flexion and increase strength of weak musculature.

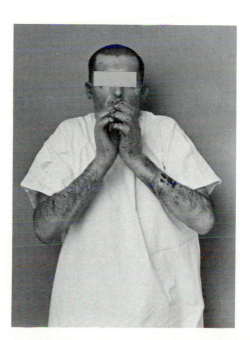

FIG. 52-12. Prayer exercise allows patient to passively stretch his own wrist in extension.

tension. Wrist flexion is achieved by placing the dorsum of the hand on the table and repeating the exercise.

3. Wall push-ups—with hands flat on wall, feet approximately 2 or 3 feet away from wall, and face close to the wall, push chest away from wall with arms, keeping hands flat. This exercise maintains wrist extension.

Hand exercises. The techniques of exercising an acutely burned hand (before grafting) with deep second- and/or third-degree burns are of utmost importance. One must keep in mind the amount of tension placed on the finger extensor mechanism when administering stretching and active-assistive exercises. Pushing fingers into mass flexion to make a fist is dangerous because components of the finger extensor mechanism can slip, split, and be damaged beyond repair. For each individual finger, active-assistive exercises should be performed in the following manner:

1. To accomplish metacarpophalangeal flexion and extension, keep the proximal interphalangeal and distal interphalangeal joints of the same finger blocked in extension.
2. For proximal interphalangeal flexion and extension keep the metacarpophalangeal and distal interphalangeal joints in extension (Fig. 52-13).
3. For distal interphalangeal flexion and extension keep the metacarpophalangeal and proximal interphalangeal joints in extension.
4. Stretch thumb and finger web spaces.
5. For thumb metacarpophalangeal flexion and extension keep thumb interphalangeal joint blocked in extension.
6. For thumb interphalangeal flexion and extension keep metacarpophalangeal joint of thumb blocked in extension.
7. Thumb opposition—assist patient in touching tip of thumb to base of small finger.

8. Fist making—only active, no assistance.
9. Try to touch the tip of each individual finger to palm—only active, no assistance.
10. Rocking weight on fingertips—place fingertips on table and gently rock body weight against them. This helps to check incipient flexion contractures of the finger.

For less extensive burns of the hand—that is, superficial second-degree burns—more aggressive physical therapy can be done. Active-assistive and passive-stretching exercises, if necessary, should be used to maintain range of motion.

After grafting and/or healing, active-assistive fist making should begin with gentle stretching of each finger joint individually. The patient should be encouraged to exercise his hands on his own at least every hour. Using Theraplast or Be-OK Putty is an excellent way to achieve this goal. Theraplast is a flexible substance patients can use independently for exercising their hands; it helps to increase strength and range of motion in the grafted hand. The patient with arthritis of the hands should squeeze foam rubber instead of putty (which is stressful to his joints). By using his burned hands before and after grafting in activities of daily living, the patient is exercising and placing his hands in functional positions.

Follow-up care

Patients with upper extremity burns are discharged with a home exercise program. The period from discharge up to 1½ years after the burn is the most important time. They are scheduled to return at appropriate intervals for evaluation of strength, range of motion, and skin condition. Good physical therapy follow-up care is important because the majority of the healing process takes place at home. Many patients are discharged with normal range of motion, only to return for the first clinic visit with multiple contractures. This problem can be alleviated to a certain extent by intensive follow-up management.

Hypertrophic scars usually make their first appearance after the patient is discharged from the hospital. These scars can be difficult to manage because they can continue to enlarge for 12 to 18 months and if removed surgically they may recur. Antiscar pressure garments have been effective in preventing these unfortunate consequences of burns. Wrapping the burned upper extremity with elastic bandages may help to prevent hypertrophic scars but is not as effective as custom-fitted garments. The patient should be measured for his garments prior to discharge, since it takes approximately 5 weeks for each custom order to be filled. To produce a beneficial result, the garment must be worn continuously except for laundering or if it inhibits the patient during exercise periods.

Because the nurse spends the most time of any member of the burn team with the patient, he or she may facilitate the patient's recovery and rehabilitation. It is the nurse who must ensure that the doctor's orders are carried out, that the hands continue to be elevated, that the splints are worn as they were intended, that the wounds are covered with topical chemotherapy continuously, that the skin grafts do not get dislodged, and that the patient mobilizes the hands continuously. In smaller hospitals, the nurse assumes many of the

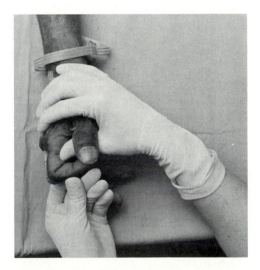

FIG. 52-13. Therapist should support metacarpophalangeal joint in extension while flexing proximal interphalangeal joint, in order to reduce tension on extensor mechanism.

duties described previously for other members of the burn team.

Following skin coverage of the burned hand, it is very tempting to begin reconstruction immediately. Because the character of the healing burn wound changes for more than 6 months after injury, it is wise to delay all but the most immediate problems (such as a severe elbow flexion contracture that obviously cannot be splinted into neutral) and for the burn team to plan an outpatient treatment program for the patient. With proper splinting and an exercise program, strength and muscle mass will increase gradually; skin will soften and become more pliable. After several months, the patient's functional problems will be defined more clearly and definitive surgical reconstruction can be planned.

It is imperative that the burn team act in concert with the vocational rehabilitation counselors, representatives of the insurance companies, rehabilitation nurses, and the patient's family and employer, to achieve meaningful rehabilitation. For instance, in North Carolina in 1975, 46,350 days were lost from work because of burn injuries, at a cost of $2,370,000. Early consultation with the vocational rehabilitation counselor ensures that the patient will have a strong ally when he leaves the hospital and, most importantly, a plan for employment. With unemployment a national problem, it is obvious that an employer may be reluctant to rehire an injured person when he can obtain the services of one with normally functioning hands. The surgeon and the burn team must concentrate all their efforts to achieve a functional result that will allow the patient to resume his previous job or compete for a new one.

BIBLIOGRAPHY

Von Prince, K., and Yeakel, M.: The splinting of burn patients, Springfield, Ill., 1974, Charles C Thomas, Publisher.

Malick, M.H., and Carr, J.A.: Manual on management of the burn patient, Pittsburgh, 1982, Harmarville Rehabilitation Center Educational Resource Division.

53

Remodeling of scar tissue in the burned patient

WANDRA K. MILES

The role of therapy in burn scar management is to maintain and improve function, prevent deformity, and improve cosmesis. Because the survival rate of the burned patient has increased significantly, we are now faced with the challenge of attempting to control scar formation, the major cause of disability. Early excision and grafting, radiation, steroids, ultrasound, pressure, and traction are therapies presently being utilized to manage scar; however, none has proved to be truly effective.[31] Controlled clinical research is greatly needed to determine the effectiveness of any modality being used. This chapter stresses the importance of early management of scar, with emphasis on the most universal methods being utilized: pressure and externally applied traction through splinting.

Scar formation is a natural sequela in the healing process of burned skin. Although it has been observed that scars do diminish with time,[31] motion must be maintained until maturation of the scar has been obtained, to prevent or minimize the necessity for reconstructive surgery. It is important to remember that scarring cannot be prevented; attempting to control it is all that can be done.

CLASSIFICATION OF THERMAL INJURIES

In the burn injury, there are standard classifications to identify depth of injury.[19,20] The superficial, or first-degree burn involves the epidermis and will heal spontaneously with no apparent scarring. In second-degree burns, cell death is confined to the epidermis and upper dermis; these burns demonstrate edema, blister formation, pain, and erythema. If no infection occurs, the skin will heal spontaneously by epithelialization, with good functional ability and cosmesis. Deep partial and full-thickness burns involve damage to the epidermis and corium skin levels. They do not heal spontaneously and require grafting for wound coverage. Deep partial, also referred to as deep second-degree burns, will heal spontaneously with decreased function and poor-quality cosmesis. Full-thickness burns frequently develop contractures and hypertrophic scarring, resulting in major deformity and disability.

WOUND HEALING

Immediately after the thermal injury, significant edema occurs secondary to increased vascular permeability and can result in ischemic necrosis. Macrophage appears in the wound after injury. Its function is to control contamination and to stimulate the presence of fibroblasts.[12,21] These fibroblasts are important in wound healing and in repair of connective tissue because they stimulate collagen synthesis. Myofibroblasts, which have characteristics similar to those of smooth muscle cells, are believed to stimulate wound contraction.[13,21] Baur[3] has reported the presence of fibroclasts, which contain collagen fragments, and myofibroclasts, which contain contracile bundles. It is believed that these cells play a continuing role in the turnover of collagen in wound-healing tissue. They are also believed to contribute greatly to scar formation (Fig. 53-1).

Collagen is the major protein of the body; it is an important element of skin, tendon, ligaments, and bones. It is also the major factor in scar tissue.[21] Since wound healing is generally delayed because of infection and poor nutrition, fibroblasts (myofibroblasts) continue to synthesize dense layers of collagen under the new granulating tissues. As collagen shortens with age, the increased layers produced become very thick and tight, leading to contracture. A contracture has been defined as the shortening of scar causing limitation of joint or skin movement.[20] In Fig. 53-2, A, notice the organized patterns of the normal collagen and in Fig. 53-2, B, the highly disorganized patterns of hypertrophic scar.

HYPERTROPHIC SCARS AND KELOIDS

Once wound coverage has been completed, hypertrophic scars and keloids typically result. Hypertrophic scars have been described as bulky scars that stay within the boundaries of the wound.[20,31] They are frequently found in areas of motion such as the joints. Hunt's[20] has reported that tension along the scar promotes collagen deposits and lessens collagen lysis, resulting in hypertrophy of the skin.

Keloids demonstrate excessive amounts of collagen that no longer conforms to the boundaries of scars; they frequently reach excessive sizes.[20,31] Keloids have a higher incidence in individuals with dark skin, because of increased skin pigmentation.[34] Koonin[26] has hypothesized that increased keloid formation in darker skin appears to be attributable to increased reactivity of melanocytes to melanocyte-stimulating hormones rather than to increased tension on the wound. This viewpoint has been supported clinically,

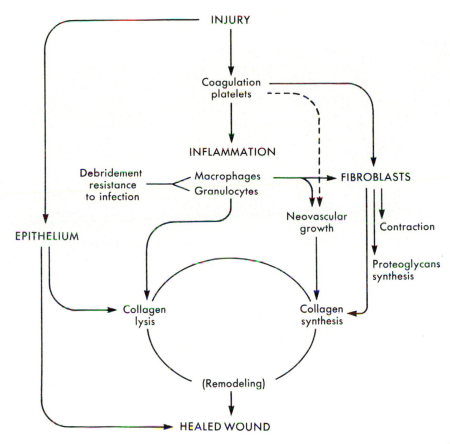

FIG. 53-1. Diagram of wound healing. (Courtesy of Dr. Thomas K. Hunt, University of California School of Medicine, San Francisco.)

since keloids rarely occur on the palms or the soles, where melanocytes are rare.

Keloids in blacks have often been described as very painful. The hyperalgesia appears to be supported by the presence of numerous nerve terminals found in keloids.[34]

Increased histamine levels have also been noted in keloids, and there is evidence that histamine may accelerate collagen formation.[36] This may explain the irritating itching sensations that many persons experience. Studies[9,36] have shown that these symptoms have been reduced or abolished with the use of pharmacologic antihistamine. Topol has presented the question of whether antihistamines would be effective in prevention of keloid recurrence if they were administered after excision.[36] Transcutaneous nerve stimulator (TNS) units and acupuncture have been observed to provide some success in minimizing the itching and burning sensations.

EARLY MANAGEMENT OF SCAR

Hunt[21] has reported that collagen synthesis can begin as early as 7 days after injury and remain rapid for up to 6 months. After 6 months this process slows and continues for 1 to 2 years after injury. Therefore early intervention is imperative for orientation of the collagen fibers being deposited if deformity secondary to scar formation is to be minimized or prevented.

Edema control

During the first 5 days after burns to the upper extremity, it is essential to control edema in order to prevent fibrosis and ischemic necrosis of the intrinsic muscles of the hand.[8,33] One can control edema by elevation, that is, positioning the extremities above the chest level and supporting the arm completely on pillows before the stockinette is secured to intravenous poles. For the upper extremities, stress to the brachial plexus can result if one uses cuffs that support only the humerus of the arms. In addition, if arms are elevated with a stockinette with weight-bearing stress to the olecranon of flexed elbows, numbness can result secondary to pressure to the ulnar nerve.

Compression dressings should not be initiated until vessels begin to regain thier normal permeabilities, which is approximately 5 to 7 days after injury. This can be verified by examination of edema in body areas that were not burned and as well by consultation with the physician. If utilized too early, compression can cause poor venous return with increased capillary pressure, resulting in edema and ischemia.

Motion

Active motion, in conjunction with positioning, is also effective for early control of edema. Simple wiggling of the digits is totally ineffective. The muscle contraction must be

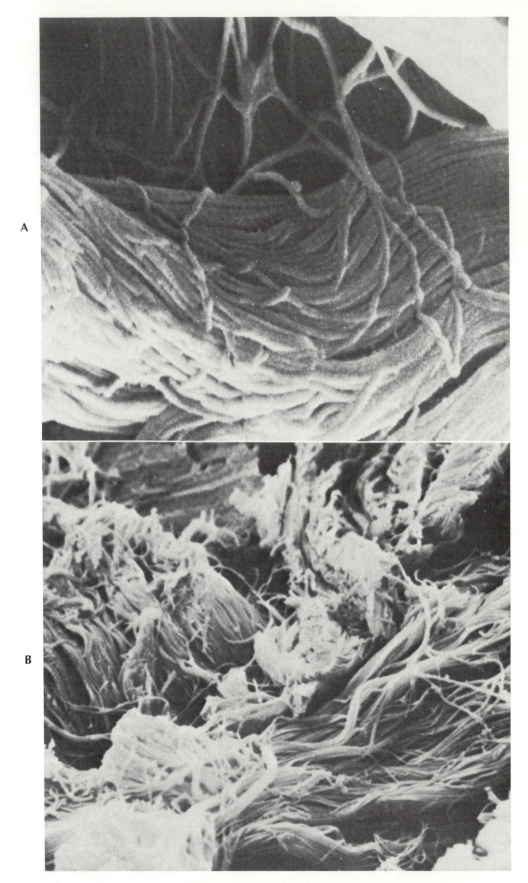

FIG. 53-2. A, Normal skin collagen at 10,000 magnification. Notice uniformity of collagen fibrils. **B,** Scanning electron microscopy of collagen near a rat colon anastomosis. Notice lack of definition and disorganization of new collagen fibrils. (Courtesy Dr. Thomas K. Hunt, University of California School of Medicine, San Francisco.)

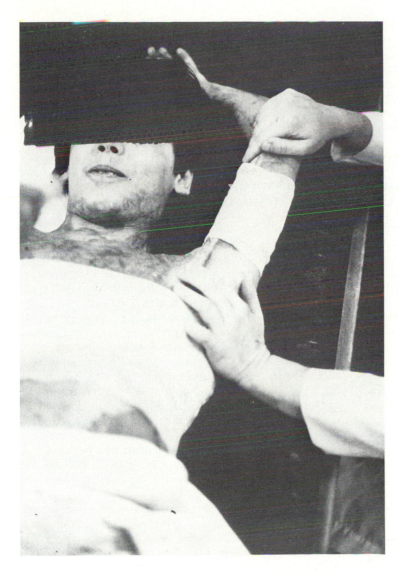

Fig. 53-3. Restriction of forward flexion of shoulder secondary to hypertrophic scar banding in axilla.

forceful to serve as a pumping mechanism to help return venous blood and lymph to the heart.[5] Active motion should be encouraged every 2 hours after removal of support splints and, if possible, during self-care tasks such as feeding. Adaptive devices should be provided as necessary. Exercise sessions should take place during dressing changes, when the therapist can evaluate the skin to determine whether increased edema, eschar, or collagen scar bands are restricting full motion. This analysis should include the assessment as to whether range is being compromised because of inelastic eschar pulling against elastic normal skin, or whether it is newly deposited dense inelastic collagen causing tension. An example of the latter is seen in Fig. 53-3, in which hypertrophic scar banding at the axilla restricts forward flexion of the shoulder.

Forceful and aggressive passive range-of-motion exercise is totally unnecessary to achieve motion and should never be done. Overly aggressive passive ranging constantly reinjures the fragile new tissue by trauma, resulting in an increase of collagen being deposited and consequently more shortening of scar.[22]

Therapy should consist in gentle passive and active assistive stretching exercises to increase motion if needed. It is important to stress to the patient that active motion results in less discomfort than passive. Gently press the scar band with a finger to test the tension of the scar to help judge how much motion should be expected from the patient at his maximum range. If it is as taut as a rubber band, the patient is presently at his maximum range. The range obtained during dressing changes should be maintained in the exercise program at the bedside; therefore dressings should not be restrictive.

TRACTION

Traction provides the opposing force needed to orient the plastic collagen being deposited during the early stages of wound healing and to maintain joint alignment as well. The traction can be accomplished with the utilization of externally applied splints.[1,37] In a study done in 1978 by P.S. Baur,[2] mild continuous traction of 2 pounds was applied to a 65- to 75-degree elbow contracture 122 days after full-thickness thermal injury. The study was done over a 4-week period. The improvement of the elbow by 30 degrees indicated that mild continuous traction accelerates the breakdown of all components of the dermal cells that are maintained in a rigid mat and it helps to reorientate the collagen fibers in normal-like alignment. An analysis of 625 patients done over a 2-year period[18] also demonstrated clinically how externally applied traction and pressure reduced the incidence of contracture and the frequency of reconstructive surgery.

Traction by splinting has four purposes: prevention, correction, immobilization after surgery, and cosmesis.[14] During the acute injury, especially the first 5 days, static splinting is mainly used for support and maintenance of joint alignment. A thorough knowledge of potential deformities is therefore essential for accurate anticipation of problem areas. After a burn injury, patients frequently obtain the position of comfort, which is flexion. If this is allowed, joint stiffness will develop and skin length will shorten upon healing. Therefore every effort must be made to maintain extension, abduction, and rotation of all extremities to prevent severe contractures in the future. The major goal should be to catch the problem early and control it with exercise and close supervision of splinting regimen.

Burns of the entire upper portion of the body can contribute greatly to limitation of upper extremity motion because of skin tension at the neck, chest, and flank. To maintain neck extension and prevent shortening of the skin, the use of pillows must not be allowed. Once the edema has decreased and vessels have regained their normal permeability, a cervical collar can be applied over dressings. Although a thermoplastic splint is effective for support, collars fabricated from Plastizote* or ½-inch Aliplast† are recommended because they mold well to the shape and contour of the neck and are flexible enough to allow some movement. The shoulders and elbows should be splinted only if tightness in range of motion or shortening of the skin in the healing wound is noted. In full-thickness burns with tight eschar, the involved shoulder should be positioned in 90-degree abduction with pillows or foam support secured to intravenous poles with a stockinette. The airplane splint can be utilized if it is difficult to maintain the patient in the necessary position. If elbow extension lacks approximately 20 degrees or greater, an elbow-contoured splint fabricated from Aliplast reinforced with a thermoplastic material is initiated. If a thermoplastic material is used alone to increase extension, it must be watched closely for pressure points because the fit will be slightly altered with each dressing change. The three-point extension splint is also very effective for dynamic traction because it can be easily adjusted in accordance with the patient's progress (Fig. 53-6, A).

In burns to the hand, the wrist is pulled into flexion and the collateral ligaments of the finger shorten.[8] Fibrosis develops secondary to prolonged edema. This results in the metacarpophalangeal joints being pulled into flexion with possible loss of central slip. To counteract this problem, the wrist should be maintained in a 15- to 20-degree extension, metacarpophalangeal joints in approximately 60- to 70-degree flexion with proximal and distal interphalangeal ex-

*Bakelate XL Manufacturers.
†Alimed, Inc., Boston, Mass.

tension and thumb abduction. Prefabricated hand splints can be utilized initially if a therapist is not available immediately. They are generally adequate for superficial burns, but custom splints are needed in full-thickness burns. If the hand is extremely edematous, it must not be forced into the ideal functional position described previously because there is always the possibility of ischemia secondary to loss of capillary integrity. At this time, the splint is used primarily for support when elevated for control of edema. Serial splinting should be initiated approximately 3 to 5 days after injury as edema subsides. It is important to remember that the splint must conform to the person, not the person to the splint.

Because each patient is different, the splinting position should be adjusted accordingly. For example, if the burn is confined to the volar aspect of the hand, the healing tissue will shorten pulling the metacarpophalangeal and the proximal interphalangeal joints into flexion, restricting extension. In such a case, maintaining the metacarpophalangeal joints in flexion as in the splint described earlier will only hasten this process. To prevent this, the patient should be positioned in a palmar and digital extension splint. If there is exposure of the extensor tendons as they cross the metacarpophalangeal and proximal interphalangeal joints, the digit must be splinted in extension, which is the position of rest. The emphasis of splinting at this time is to prevent further destruction of the extensor mechanism until granulation tissue covers the open area. Active motion to maintain tendon glide should be supervised closely during dressing change to prevent rupturing. The tendon must be kept moist with saline soaks during exercise because this prevents the tendon from becoming excessively dry from the heat lamp in the tub room.

To be effective, the splint must be worn continuously and removed only for dressing changes, self-care activities, and supervised exercises. In some cases the splint may need to be removed every 2 to 3 hours to prevent skin maceration. This is especially true for new grafts greater than 1 week after surgery. Generally the splints should be worn during all hours of sleep. It is not unusual for a patient to lose range significantly because the splint was not applied during the night. Once full motion has been regained, traction by splinting must be continued for maintenance as needed until the scar has reached maturity, which is approximately 6 months to 2 years after wound healing.

PRESSURE

In 1968, Fujimori[15] demonstrated the effectiveness of pressure with a soft sponge in the treatment of keloids. He stressed that pressure must be continued until the scar is no longer hyperemic. Studies[25,27,35] on tissue gases in normal dermis in hypertrophic scar have found that pressure of approximately 25 mm Hg is believed to decrease the blood flow to a rapidly metabolizing collagenous tissue. Sloan[35] has shown that the oxygen tension in hypertrophic scar is significantly less than that in normal dermis because of a barrier formed by the collagen nodules. Although hypoxia does not result in increased cell depth in the scar, it does appear to indirectly affect the fibroblast synthesis of collagen. This explains the recurrence of hypertrophy once

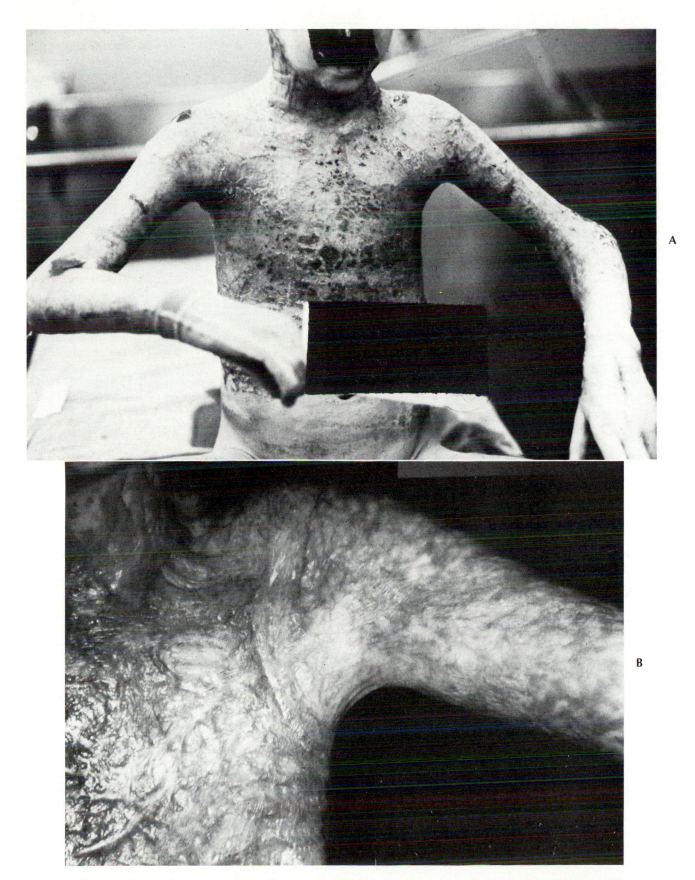

Fig. 53-4. A, Motion of upper extremity is limited as increased tension and webbing of skin at neck, chest, and axilla pulls shoulder into adduction and protraction, elbow into flexion, and wrist into flexion and pronation, with thumb opposition. **B,** Pressure and traction are needed to counteract tension resulting from intense webbing of axilla.

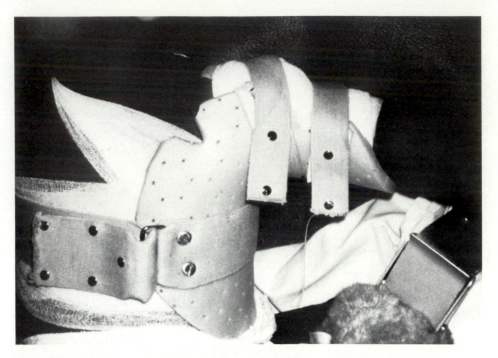

FIG. 53-5. Plastizote reinforced with a thermoplastic material provides the necessary contour pressure with traction needed for webbing in shoulder.

pressure is removed and also suggests the idea that the earlier pressure is applied, the shorter the time period needed for scar maturation.[25]

As with traction, pressure should be applied early during the wound débridement phase and not delayed until complete wound coverage has been obtained. For example, burned web spaces should be packed with gauze incorporated into the dressing as soon as the eschar is debrided.

With distinctly noticeable scar bands of the wound, gauze incorporated into dressings may not be adequate. Rigid external pressure provided by splinting over dressings is needed to help mold the skin to its normal contours and folds. Examine Fig. 53-4 and notice how the shoulders are being pulled into protraction and adduction and the neck into flexion. At this stage, an airplane splint is not recommended, because it does little to control the webbing of the skin in the axilla. The airplane splint is most effective for positioning of shoulders when thick eschar is present or for immobilization of postoperative split-thickness skin grafts, because it places no pressure on the newly grafted skin. Direct pressure provided by a contoured axilla splint fabricated from slightly rigid Plastizote and Aliplast or a rigid thermoplastic material is instead recommended (Fig. 53-5). If Plastizote or Aliplast is used, it can be reinforced with a thermoplastic material if more support is needed. This splint can be applied with elastic wraps in a figure-of-eight pattern across the back to encourage shoulder retraction and for a more uniform and secure fit. This method is also applicable to the elbow, since it can provide specific pressure to the antecubital fossa (Fig. 53-6). T-foam-* or Aliplast-con-

toured inserts can be utilized and secured with elastic wraps or Tubigrip.*

Pressure splints allow active motion, since the material is flexible and encourages spontaneous movements. If necessary, a traction splint should be worn with pressure for maintenance at night. Whatever method is utilized, whether it be pressure or traction to obtain an improvement in range of motion, it is essential that proper assessment of the skin be done to determine the level of increased tension-inhibiting movement.

Pressure can be provided by Tubigrip or elastic wraps until the patient is ready to be measured for custom-fitted pressure garments (Fig. 53-7). Tubigrip is available in low, medium, and high tension. In a study[23] done with 49 patients with average burns of 20% total body area, low-tension Tubigrip (5 to 10 mm Hg) did not appear to apply adequate pressure. The high tension (20 to 30 mm Hg) was observed to cause edema in the distal part of the extremity and was found to be excessively abrasive to newly grafted skin. Medium tension of 10 to 20 mm Hg was found to be most effective. This study also demonstrated that the development of hypertrophy was controlled by the interim use of tubular elastic material.

Custom-fitted pressure garments should be ordered when there are openings no larger than the size of a quarter and the edema appears to be controlled. If garments are forced on fragile skin too early, the friction caused by the material rubbing against the skin can result in blister formation and skin breakdown. A quick test to determine whether a patient with superficial burns needs custom-fitted garments is to

---

*Alimed, Inc., Boston, Mass.

*Seton Products, Ltd., Tubiton House, Oldham, Lancashire, England.

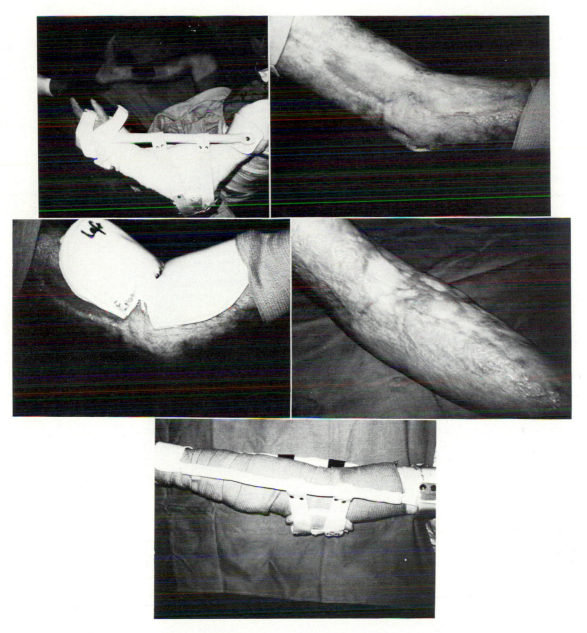

FIG. 53-6. Utilization of three-point extension splint early, followed by Aliplast contour splint after wound healing. Maintenance of elbow extension with combination of pressure and traction.

lightly rub a finger across the uninjured skin and the healed burn wound with eyes closed. If no change in tension of the skin can be detected, scarring probably will not develop.

At this time one should note that, frequently, small open areas remain along the axilla folds and antecubital fossa of the elbow. This delayed wound healing can be attributable to infection or trauma occurring in the fragile collagen gel being deposited by the tension on the newly healed skin with movement. Pressure can also contribute to this problem because the open wound is maintained in a moist environment, resulting in maceration and further delay in healing. Because wound healing always takes priority, therapy in such instances must be modified. If the opening is smaller than the size of a quarter, the area can be padded and garments reapplied. If the opening is larger, custom-fitted pressure garments should be discontinued and dry gauze applied to the open area. Elastic wraps or Tubigrip should replace pressure garments and be removed approximately every 2 hours to allow air to the skin.

It has been observed that many persons cannot tolerate a pressure of 25 mm Hg over certain parts of the body. A variant of approximately 3 to 25 mm Hg is typical.[7] For example, the head average is 6 mm Hg, the sleeve average is 14 mm Hg, and the glove ranges from 30 mm Hg at the distal phalanx to 10 mm Hg at the wrist. The garments should fit snugly but not too tight. It is too loose if one can pinch the material up from the skin. The garments must be replaced every 2 to 3 months to ensure that adequate pressure is being provided, because the elastic property of the material wears out from daily washing. Also, adjustments may be needed for the patient's weight gain or losses. It is important that the garment be worn continuously and be removed only for bathing and skin care. Two pairs should be ordered, one to be worn during the day and the other for night.

Although the pressure garments are custom fitted, they are still unable to provide adequate pressure to the mobile areas of the body such as the neck, breast, axilla, palm, and web spaces of the hand. Therefore the contour splint fabricated from Aliplast and T-foam described earlier can be worn under the pressure garments as needed. The splint utilized in this manner provides adequate support but remains small and flexible enough so as not to inhibit movement because of excessive bulk. This can be accomplished in several ways. For scars to the anterior areas of the chest, it is difficult to maintain sufficient pressure along the sternal notch and under the breast in women. If allowed to hypertrophy, the tension of the scar can pull the shoulder into protraction, compromising shoulder motion. Therefore a

FIG. 53-7. Early management of scar with tubular elastic material.

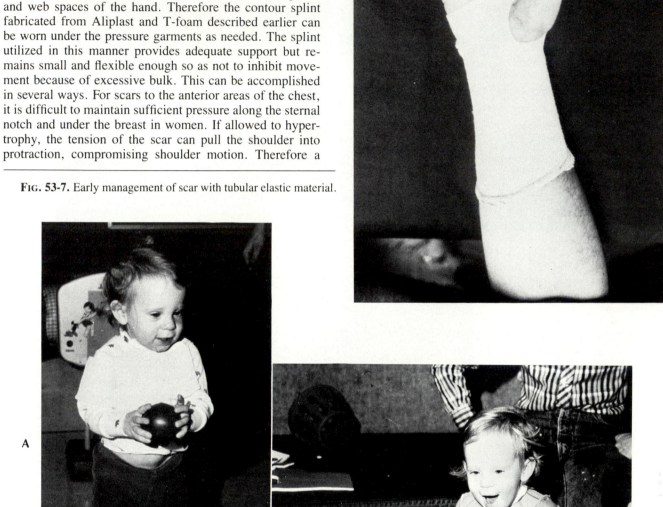

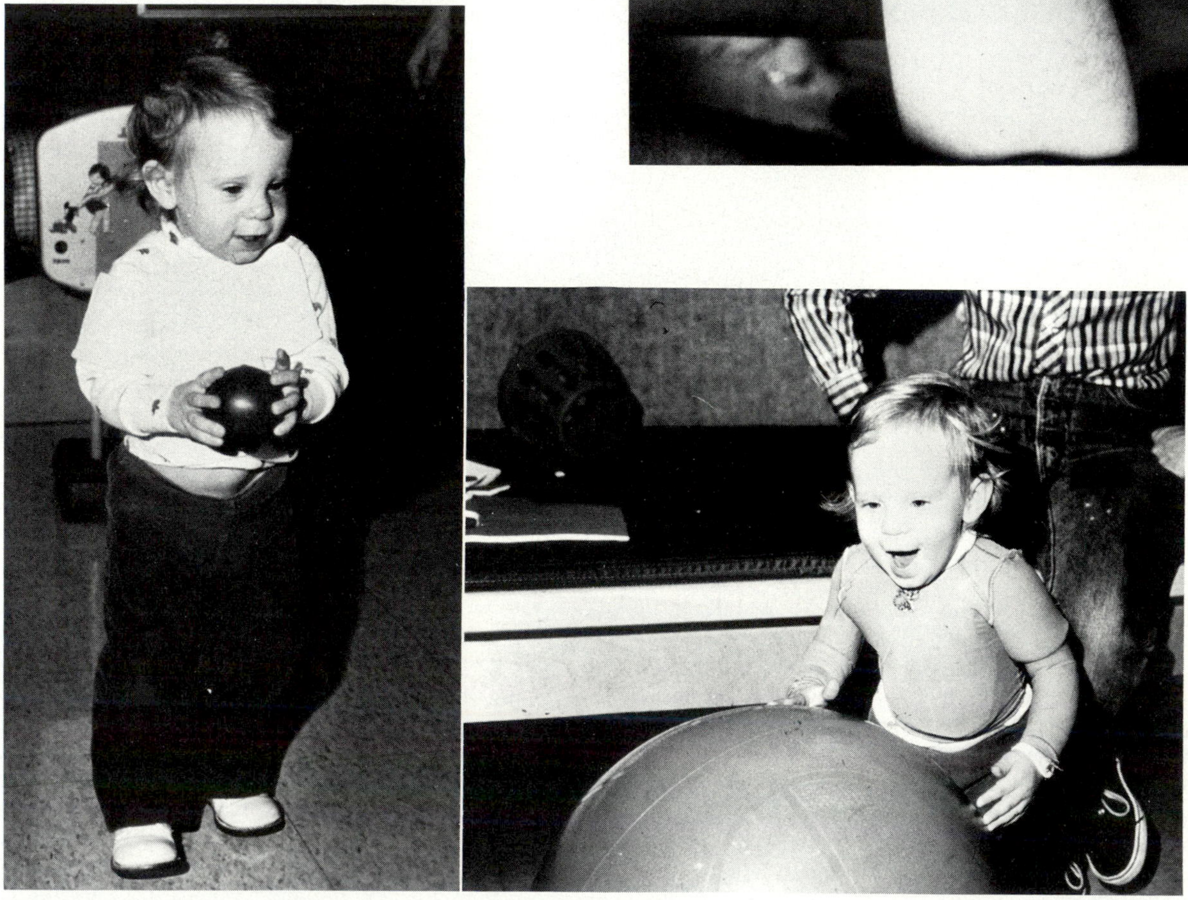

FIG. 53-8. **A,** Application of self-stick soft sponge to T-shirt for scars in anterior part of chest and axilla. **B,** Worn under custom-fitted pressure garments.

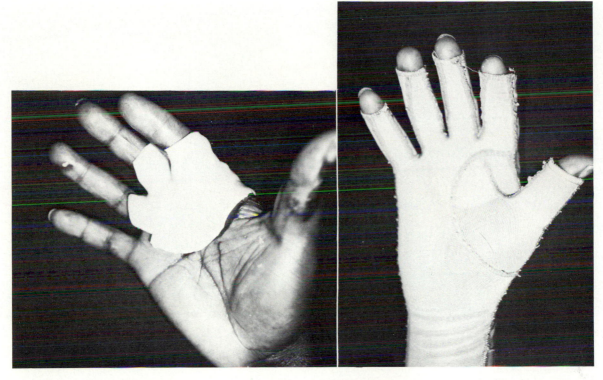

FIG. 53-9. Elastomer is effective for scars to web spaces and palm because it fits securely underneath pressure garment and does not restrict motion.

chest plate fabricated from ¼-inch Aliplast or self-stick soft sponge* applied to a T-shirt[17] that is worn under pressure garments is quite effective (Fig. 53-8).

To maintain the web space of the thumb, ½-inch Aliplast worn under a pressure garment is effective because the thickness of the material holds the thumb into abduction at rest but is flexible enough to allow movement. One fourth– inch Aliplast is recommended it thumb abduction is within normal limits. For the web spaces of the fingers, cotton, Betapile,* Otoform-k,† or Elastomer‡ can be effective, because they mold perfectly to the digits but allow freedom of movement when worn under pressure garments (Fig. 53-9). Elastomer reinforced with the rigid thermoplastic material is also effective in managing palmar scars that pull the digits into flexion, especially at the metacarpal and proximal interphalangeal joints (Fig. 53-10). In severe cases, simple application of elastomer on the scar is not sufficient, because it applies pressure too evenly without any adjustments for normal contours of the skin. Greater pressure that is more specific to the problem can be achieved with a splint that is fabricated from "normal" skin contour. This can be accomplished by a technique that was developed by Paderewski[30] for the face through the fabrication of a positive and negative mold of the scar (Fig. 53-11). An alginate impression of the scar is made from which a plaster mold is fabricated. Once the plaster has set, the scar is chiseled away and sanded smooth. For scars that are greatly elevated,

*Alimed, Inc., Boston, Mass.
†Dreze, Inc., Unna, West Germany.
‡Dow Corning Corp., Midland, Mich.

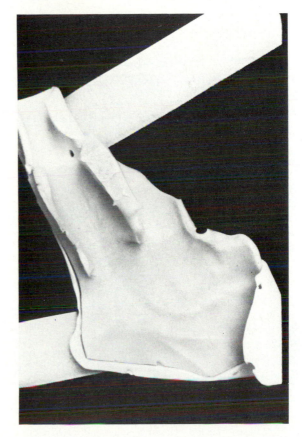

FIG. 53-10. Pressure and traction may be required for significant scarring in palm. Notice outline of palmar scar in elastomer.

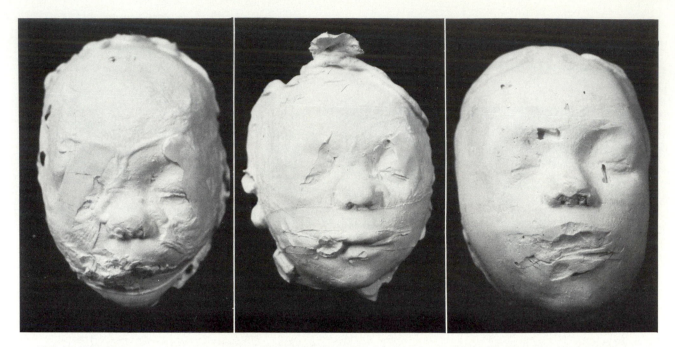

FIG. 53-11. Serial plaster molds taken to demonstrate improvement after use of face mask with pressure garments. Dates of molds are July 1981, January 1982, and June 1982.

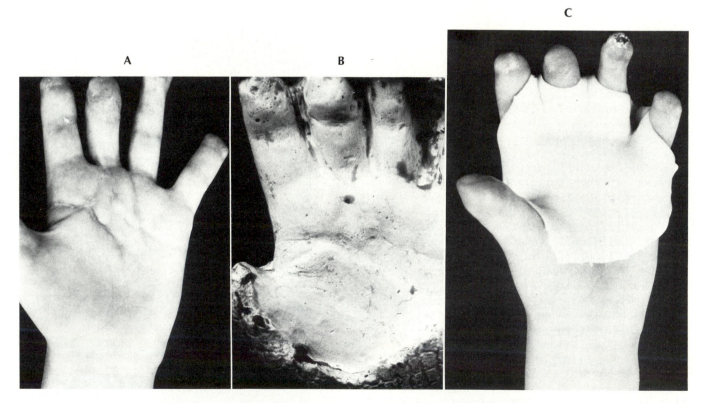

FIG. 53-12. A, Palmar scar after a firecracker explosion to hand required defined and specific pressure. **B,** Positive plaster mold was fabricated, from which scar was chiseled away. Purpose was to obtain normal contour folds and creases of palm. **C,** Final splint fabricated from combination of elastomer and prosthetic foam Q7-4290 by Dow Corning Corporation.

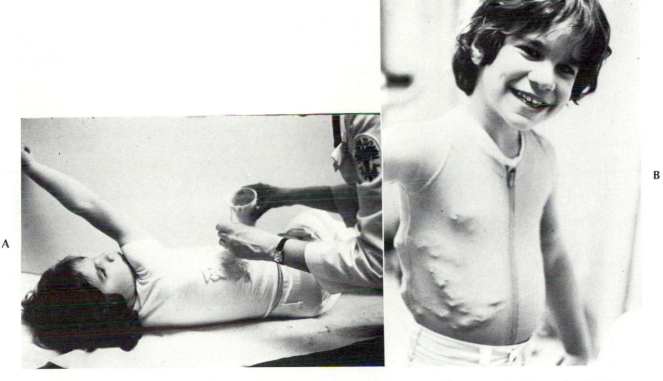

FIG. 53-13. A, Application of silicone rubber mixture to T-shirt for more specific pressure to chest and axilla. **B,** Mixture secured in place with pressure garment.

only part of the scar should be smoothed away, because the change would be too drastic for the splint to fit properly. A cotton stockinette is placed over the plaster mold for additional reinforcement for the silicone rubber mixture of elastomer and prosthetic foam Q7-4290.* This mixture is recommended over the use of elastomer alone because it is stronger material and wears better. After fabrication, the silicone rubber splint should be allowed to air out, and the application of talcum powder will help to diminish the "rubbery" odor. This splint is not only effective for facial scars, but also works well for neck and palmar scars on the hand (Fig. 53-12). Scars on the anterior part of the chest also can benefit from this silicone rubber mixture when applied directly to a T-shirt, which is then worn under the pressure garments[17] (Fig. 53-13). Great care must be taken to prevent skin breakdown by frequent removal of the rubbery Silastic splint to allow air to reach the skin.

Special considerations must always be made for the rapid growth rate of children. Problems frequently occur because the immature healing scar is not elastic enough to expand with the child's growth. For example, the tightness from resistive scars circumferential to the upper torso can restrict full lung capacity resulting in shortness of breath with activity. Also a face-mask pressure garment must be checked frequently because questions have been raised concerning its effect on head growth in the very young and its production

*Dow Corning Corp., Midland, Mich.

of excessive headaches. The younger the child, the faster the growth rate, therefore the more closely he should be followed.

MASSAGE

Massage is important in maintaining mobility by freeing restrictive fibrous bands and in helping circulation.[11] It is also helpful in alleviating the frequently reported itching sensation caused by excessively dry and cracked skin resulting from damage to the sweat glands. Beard[4] has pointed out that massage does appear to stimulate the opening of the sebaceous and sweat glands.

Only very gentle massage should be done to newly healed or recently grafted areas, because the skin is very fragile and friction can result in skin breakdown and blister formation. Greater pressure can be exerted, with the massaging being done with a rotary motion along the scar, as the skin becomes thicker and stronger. Creams that are not water based, such as lanolin, cocoa butter, and lard, are recommended because they are good lubricants and are not rapidly absorbed into the skin. The skin should be massaged a minimum of two times a day. After massage, the excess cream should be removed, and approximately 30 minutes should elapse before pressure garments are reapplied. This will help prevent pimple formation on skin and maintain the elastic quality of the material, which can frequently be damaged because of overaccumulation of oil.

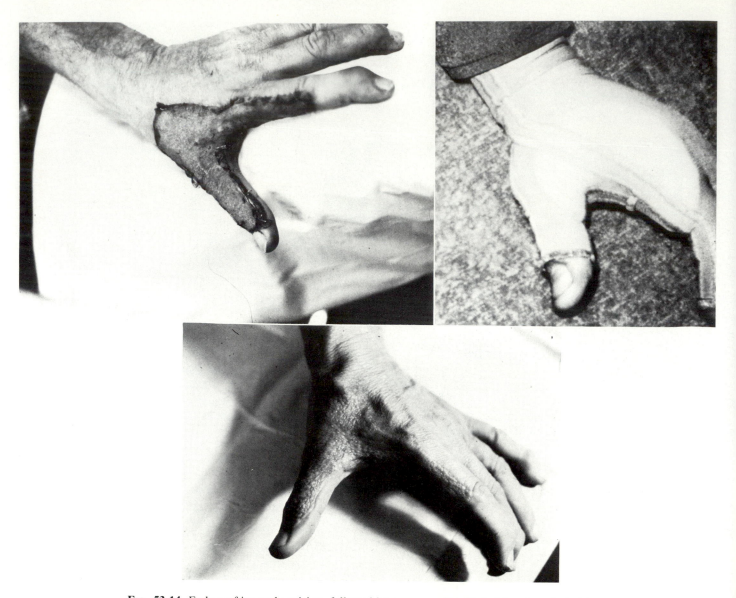

Fig. 53-14. Early grafting and excision, followed by pressure with Aliplast thumb-web stretcher.

SPLIT-THICKNESS SKIN GRAFT

Early excision of eschar and use of split-thickness skin grafts in deep burns appear to decrease the extent of scar formation.[29] Since the skin graft contains flexible dermis and epithelium, the transfer of vasculature from the wound to the graft is quick and the scar tends to remain pliable and supple.[22] Rudolph[32] has found that after a graft is placed there is a rapid rise in the amount of myofibroblast present initially and that it frequently reaches a peak before decreasing. It is his opinion that the skin grafts speed up the process of decreasing the amount of myofibroblast present after its peak synthesis. Unfortunately, early grafting must frequently be delayed because of severe medical complications and infection (Fig. 53-14).

It is crucial to have obtained full range of motion before grafting, because the patient will need to be immobilized for 5 to 7 days after surgery. A splint maintaining the patient in optimal functional position should be applied in the operating room to prevent further loss of motion from shrinkage of the graft site.

STEROIDS

In 1965, Maquire[28] demonstrated successful regression of a keloid through the use of intralesional treatment with triamcinolone. Positive results[16,24] have been reported through the practice of excising small lesions followed by injection of triamcinolone followed by the reapplication of pressure. Cohen[10] has postulated that triamcinolone encourages keloid regression by removing the inhibitory effects of alpha globulins on collagenase. By elimination of the collagenase inhibitors, degradation of collagen is allowed.

Cortisone is generally initiated when the keloid has not responded to conservative management. But if most scars injected with triamcinolone are followed by pressure, it is difficult to determine which factor is actually causing the decrease of scar size.[31] Although controlled studies have been done in which a single scar is injected with triamcinolone on one side with obvious flattening of scar noted, more data are needed to determine its effectiveness accurately.

ULTRASOUND

According to Dyson's[13] work, ultrasound has been demonstrated to increase the rate of protein synthesis and fibroblasts facilitating and encouraging wound healing. It has also been shown to increase the tensile strength of the resulting scar tissue and to cause changes in the patterning of collagen fibers.

In 1953, Bierman[6] presented three case studies of scars treated with ultrasound. One patient had a burn injury to the first dorsal web space. His clinical findings indicated the positive effects of ultrasound in treating scars by the objective increase in range of motion. In 1970, Wright[38] conducted a clinical study of six persons who had developed scar formation from various types of trauma. The scar tissues were treated with ultrasound followed by biopsy specimens and photographs. He concluded that ultrasound may have some effect on keloid or hypertrophic scars treated in the fibroblastic stage with an increase in vascularity. He also noted that ultrasound was unsuccessful in keloids in its later stages when it had developed a great deal of hyalinized connective tissue. He speculated that further experimentation utilizing a larger population with longer treatment periods may produce better clinical results.

Because the studies done with ultrasound so far have been done on a limited population and have not been conclusive, they do indicate that there is a potential use for it. Further research is needed before the true effects of ultrasound on scar tissue can be determined.

SCAR MATURATION

Hypertrophic scars take approximately 6 months to 2 years to reach maturity. Relapse is possible as long as the scar is erythemic.[15] A mature scar should appear less dense to touch, with lessened elevation. Normal coloration should not be expected. Until maturation is achieved, the skin is thin and fragile and must be protected from the sun to prevent blistering. Sun block creams and light covering by clothing are recommended.

If a scar is no longer hyperemic, the purplish or pinkish coloration should be diminished and the scar should not blanch to touch. To assess whether the scar has reached maturity, the patient should discontinue wearing his garment for approximately 1 week to notice any change in the skin. The goal is to obtain a smooth, flat, supple scar.

Reconstructive surgery is usually delayed until the active process of scarring has ceased. However, such surgery may be required earlier in children to accommodate for growth. If surgery is done, pressure must be resumed until scar maturation is complete.

PSYCHOLOGY

Many patients believe that once they have been discharged from the hospital, they are completely healed and everything will return to normal. The early introduction of scar management and the time commitment needed for good results are essential. One must explain the scar-remodeling process fully to the patient to obtain his understanding and full cooperation. One must stress to the patient that he will never have normal skin because he has suffered a major trauma, but one must emphasize that deformity and excessive scarring can be prevented. The patient will need a great deal of support and motivation to comply with treatment requirements. Goals in regard to function should be set high in conjunction with the patient. If the therapist expects less, the patient will do likewise.

SUMMARY

Early introduction of traction and pressure is essential for effectiveness in the remodeling of scar tissue. The goal should be to evaluate the wound and to determine the most effective way to control the scar and maintain motion. Long-term follow-up is essential for the critical assessment of methods presently being utilized. A great deal of controlled research and documentation is still needed in this area, especially clinically, before optimal assessment can be verified.

REFERENCES

1. Abston, S.: Burns in children, Clin. Symp. **28:**3-36, 1976.
2. Baur, P.S., Barratt, G., Linares, H.A., Dobrkovsky, M., de la Houssaye, A.J., and Larson, D.L.: Wound contractions, scar contractures and myofibroblasts: a classical case study, J. Trauma **18:**8-22, Jan. 1978.
3. Baur, P.S., Jr., Barratt, G.P., Brown, G.M., and Parks, D.H.: Ultrastructural evidence for the presence of "fibroclasts" and "myofibroclasts" in wound healing tissues, J. Trauma **19:**744-756, Oct. 1979.
4. Beard, G., and Wood, E.C.: Massage: principles and techniques, Philadelphia, 1981, W.B. Saunders Co.
5. Beasley, R.W.: Secondary repair of burned hands, Clin. Plastic Surg. **8:**141-161, Jan. 1981.
6. Bierman, W.: Ultrasound in the treatment of scars, Arch. Phys. Med. Rehabil. **35:**209-213, April 1954.
7. Blair, K.L.: Prevention and control of hypertrophic scarring and contractures by the application of the custom-made Jobskin Pressure Covers, Toledo, Ohio, 1977, Jobst Institute, Inc.
8. Brown, H.C.: Current concepts of burn pathology and mechanisms of deformity in the burned hand, Orthop. Clin. North Am. **4:**987-999, Oct. 1973.
9. Cohen, I.K., Beaven, M.A., Horáková, Z., and Keiser, H.R.: Histamine and collagen synthesis in keloid and hypertrophic scar, Surg. Forum **23:**509-510, 1972.
10. Cohen, I.K., Diegelmann, R.F., and Bryant, C.P.: Alpha-globulin collagenase inhibitors in keloids and hypertrophic scar, Surg. Forum **27:**61, 1976.
11. Cyriax, J.H.: Clinical application of massage. In Licht, S.: Massage, manipulation and traction, New Haven, Conn., 1960, Elizabeth Licht Publisher.
12. Diegelmann, R.F., Cohen, I.K., and Kaplan, A.M.: The role of macrophage in wound repair: a review, Plast. Reconstr. Surg. **68:**107-113, July 1981.
13. Dyson, M., and Suckling, J.: Stimulation of tissue repair by ultrasound: a survey of the mechanisms involved (abstract), International Symposium on Therapeutic Ultrasound, London, 1981.
14. Evans, E.B., Larson, D.L., Abston, S., and Willis, B.: Prevention and correction of deformity after severe burn, Surg. Clin. North Am. **50:**1361-1375, Dec. 1970.

15. Fujimori, R., Hiramoto, M., and Ofugi, S.: Sponge fixation method for treatment of early scars, Plast. Reconstr. Surg. **42:**322, 1968.

16. Griffith, B.H.: Treatment of keloids with triamcinolone acetonide, Plast. Reconstr. Surg. **38:**202,1966.

17. Grigsby, L.: An approach for applying additional pressure material and maintaining its position under pressure vests in the treatment of pediatric burn patients (abstract), thirteenth annual meeting of American Burn Association, Philadelphia, 1981.

18. Huang, T.T., Blackwell, S.J., and Lewis, S.R.: Ten years of experience in managing patients with burn contractures of axilla, elbow, wrist and knee joints, Plast. Reconstr. Surg. **61:**70-76, Jan. 1978.

19. Hunt, T.K.: Mechanisms of repair and spontaneous healing. In Polk, H., and Stone, H.H., editors: Contemporary burn management, Boston, 1971, Little, Brown and Co.

20. Hunt, T.K.: Fundamentals of wound management in surgery—wound healing: disorders of repair, South Plainfield, N.J., 1976, Chirurgecom, Inc.

21. Hunt, T.K., and Van Winkle, W., Jr.: Fundamentals of wound management in surgery—wound healing: normal repair, South Plainfield, N.J., 1976, Chirurgecom, Inc.

22. Hunt, T.K.: Spontaneous healing of burns. In Fundamentals of wound management in surgery—selected tissues, South Plainfield, N.J., 1977, Chirurgecom, Inc.

23. Judge, J., May, R., and De Clement, F.: Interim use of tubular support bandage as a pressure garment (Abstract), American Burn Association, Durham, N.C., 1982.

24. Ketchum, L., Robinson, D., and Masters, F.: Follow-up on treatment of hypertrophic scars and keloids with triamcinolone, Plast. Reconstr. Surg. **48**(3):256-259, 1971.

25. Kirscher, C.W., and Shetlar, C.W.: Microvasculature in hypertrophic scars and the effects of pressure, J. Trauma **19:**757-764, Oct. 1979.

26. Koonin, A.J.: The aetiology of keloids: a review of the literature and a new hypothesis, S. Afr. Med. J. **38:**913-916, 1964.

27. Larson, D., Abston, S., and Evans, E.B.: Splints and traction. In Polk, H., and Stone, H.H., editors: Contemporary burn management, Boston, 1971, Little, Brown & Co.

28. Maquire, H.C.: Treatment of keloids with triamcinolone acetonide injected intralesionally, J.A.M.A. **192:**325-326, 1965.

29. Montandon, D.: Les problèmes de rétraction tissulaire en chirurgie plastique, Médecine et Hygiène **36:**817-822, 1978.

30. Paderewski, Joseph: Personal communication, Shriner's Hospital for Crippled Children, Burn Institute, Galveston, Texas, 1982.

31. Peacock, E.E., Jr., Madden, J.W., and Triec, W.C.: Biologic basis for the treatment of keloids and hypertrophic scars, South. Med. J. **63:**755, July 1970.

32. Rudolph, R: Inhibition of myofibroblasts by skin grafts, Plast. Reconstr. Surg. **63:**473-480, April 1979.

33. Salisbury, R.E., McKeel, D.W., and Mason, A.D.: Ischemic necrosis of the intrinsic muscles of the hand after thermal injuries, J. Bone Joint Surg. **56:**1701-1707, Dec. 1974.

34. Seghers, M.: Cutaneous pigmentation and keloids, Transactions of the Fourth International Congress of Plastic Surgeons, Rome, 1967, p. 115.

35. Sloan, D.F., Brown, R.D., Wells, C.H., and Hilton, J.C.: Tissue gases in human hypertrophic burn scars, Plast. Reconstr. Surg. **61:**431-436, March 1978.

36. Topol, B.M., Lewis, V.L., Jr., and Benveniste, K.: The use of antihistamine to retard the growth of fibroblasts derived from human skin, scar, and keloid, Plast. Reconstr. Surg. **68:**227-230, Aug. 1981.

37. Willis, B.: The use of orthoplast isoprene in the treatment of the acutely burned child: preliminary report, Am. J. Occup. Ther. **23:**57, 1969.

38. Wright, E.T.: Keloids and ultrasound, Arch. Phys. Med. **52:**208, 1971.

54

Care and rehabilitation of the hand after cold injury

JOHN A. BOSWICK, Jr.

Cold injuries of the hand are infrequent when compared to cuts, crushes, lacerations, and even burns. However, they can result in significant loss of tissue and impairment of hand function. Both loss of tissue and impairment of function can be reduced by timely and appropriate care.

Care should be instituted as soon as possible after injury and be continuous until healing and rehabilitation are complete. In the case of extensive injuries treatment should be directed toward both the systemic response and the local response to injury.

MECHANISMS OF INJURY

The conditions that result in a cold injury can be divided into primary and contributing factors. Primary or basic factors are a low temperature and an adequate exposure time.

One of the most significant contributing factors is wind velocity. It is wind velocity combined with temperature that comprises what is termed ''wind chill factor.'' The time-temperature effect is basic to cold injury, but this may be modified by the time–wind chill effect, since many cold injuries occur in situations where wind velocity is an important consideration.

Increased humidity either in the environment or as increased local wetness will cause a cold injury or increase its significance. This is dramatically demonstrated in persons who have an opening or leak in a glove or boot. Small amounts of moisture may enter without the patient's being aware of it, and several hours later when the glove or boot is removed, the injury will be obvious. This problem is illustrated in situations where there is damage to one extremity caused by a defective boot or glove, and in the other extremity, with intact covering, there is no significant cold injury (Fig. 54-1).

The direct contact of living tissue with cold objects will result in a much more significant cold injury than mere exposure to cold surroundings. Transfer of heat from the skin will occur more rapidly when there is direct contact with metal, glass, or other highly conductive cold materials. This is seen in patients who become comatose or unconscious and sustain a cold injury. An exposed hand will often be in contact with a snowbank, park bench, or the steering wheel of an automobile. The areas in contact with these cold objects usually will be the areas of significant cold injury. This contribution of direct contact or the conduction of heat from living tissue is most pronounced when the cold object is wet, as when a wet glove is in contact with a cold metal object.

Lack of protection can dramatically contribute to a cold injury. However, a minimal amount of protection may prevent a cold injury. The effect of protection or lack of protection relates to the factors of time and temperature and, perhaps, wind velocity. Minimal protection is so important in preventing a cold injury that its value must be emphasized. We have had patients with cold exposure of both hands, one of which was protected by a thin glove and the other unprotected; the protected hand had a mild or perhaps no cold injury, whereas the unprotected hand sustained injury to several digits requiring amputation of several centimeters of tissue. The minimal amount of protection required to prevent a cold injury is unknown. Protection is obviously related to the factors of time, ambient temperature, wind velocity, wetness, and the duration and extent of contact with cold objects.

Other factors may contribute to the severity of a cold injury; one of these is age. There is a strong suggestion that elderly persons exposed to cold sustain a more severe injury than younger persons. Although difficult to document objectively, this may indicate that the younger person is more alert, able to move about, and more likely to detect wet clothing or contact with cold objects. The elderly person is also more likely to have preexisting diseases (arthritis, cardiac disorders, or central nervous system disease) that would prevent him from getting out of the cold.

Decreased vascularity or circulatory impairment has been considered a possible contributing factor to the significance of a cold injury. Persons with arterial or venous disease of the lower extremity appear to have less resistance to cold than those with a normal circulatory system. This observation has been made frequently enough to give a strong clinical impression that it is correct. However, one must note that the natural progress of these circulatory disorders may result in tissue loss without an added cold injury.

In treating a patient with cold injuries of the hand, one should consider several factors before instituting therapy: (1) the general or systemic condition of the patient, (2) the patient's response to the cold injury and the spe-

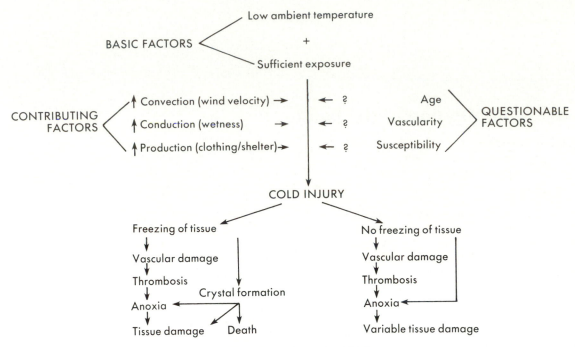

Fig. 54-1. Mechanisms of cold injury.

cific effects of the lowered temperature on other areas of the body, (3) the conditions of the injured tissue at the time of hospital admission, and (4) the extent of injured tissue.

SYSTEMIC MANAGEMENT OF A PATIENT WITH COLD INJURIES

The general care of a patient with cold injuries will depend on the patient's systemic response to the injury and his condition before injury. As the extent of cold injury increases, the likelihood of significant systemic changes such as generalized hypothermia, hypovolemia, acidosis, and hypoxemia increases. In addition, alcoholic withdrawal problems and malnutrition are often present in the patient with cold injuries.

The problem of generalized hypothermia rarely occurs in a patient with cold injuries of only the hands; however, severe cold injuries to the hands commonly occur in patients with generalized hypothermia. Although there is some question about the best technique of rewarming a patient with systemic hypothermia, rapid total body rewarming is generally agreed on as the best technique for local rewarming.

Hypovolemia is a recognized complication of cold injury. Patients with cold injuries involving several extremities that were frozen or cold on admission to the hospital have had hematocrit levels as high as 60%. Since most of these patients had prolonged exposure, dehydration and fluid loss may have played a role in the hypovolemia. The management of this relatively moderate hypovolemia presented no problem. A balanced electrolyte solution in amounts that were twice daily fluid requirements usually corrected the hypovolemia in 24 to 48 hours.

Some degree of acidosis is present in most patients with cold injuries of the hands if the tissue is cold or frozen at the time of admission. The degree of acidosis is related to the extent of injury and to the delay between injury and hospital care. Arterial pH levels as low as 7.16 have been recorded. The initial infusion of 100 to 300 mg of sodium bicarbonate, repeated every 3 to 4 hours, will usually restore the pH to normal in 24 hours.

Decreased arterial oxygen levels occur in patients with cold injuries of the hands when there is cold or frozen tissue. The arterial P_{O_2} in these patients appeared to be lowered in direct relation to the duration of exposure and the decrease in metabolism. Oxygen by mask or nasal catheter restored the arterial P_{O_2} to normal in 8 to 12 hours.

Alcoholic withdrawal symptoms can be a significant problem in the management of a patient with cold injuries. Over 80% of these patients sustain their injury during acute alcoholic intake. If the history or evaluation of the patient suggests alcohol addiction, early treatment is recommended to prevent the development of withdrawal symptoms. The use of sedatives (barbiturates, promazine [Sparine], chloral hydrate, and chlordiazepoxide [Librium]) and antitremor drugs (phenytoin [Dilantin] and magnesium sulfate along with vitamins is the accepted therapy.

Malnourishment is not uncommon in a patient who sustains a cold injury. As soon as possible after injury, adequate dietary intake and supplementary vitamins should be provided. Systemic management should not detract from the early management of the injured tissue. Patients with cold injuries are often seen with tissue that is frozen, cold, blistered, or cyanotic. On occasion gangrenous tissue will be present at the time of admission because of the delay between the time of injury and the time the patient seeks medical care.

MANAGEMENT OF THE HAND AFTER COLD INJURY
Acute care

The immediate or early management of the hand injured by cold depends on the specific condition of the tissue when first seen by the physician who can deliver definitive care. The most severe condition that cold-injured tissue can reach is that of being frozen. Approximately 1% of all patients with a cold injury reach the hospital with frozen tissue. Some of these patients also have generalized hypothermia, that is, a core temperature below 32° C. The management of generalized hypothermia is not discussed in this chapter.

The management of frozen tissue requires not only local treatment but also concurrent system treatment, since rapid rewarming can increase or compound the problem of acidosis. The most effective method of treating frozen tissue in a patient who does not have generalized hypothermia is total body rewarming. After drawing arterial blood for P_{O_2}, P_{CO_2}, and pH determinations, one should insert an intravenous catheter and infuse lactated Ringer's solution with sodium bicarbonate added (100 mEq/500 ml of lactated Ringer's solution). The patient should be placed in a tub or body whirlpool bath with the water at 100° F. Water at 110° F should be slowly added, and after 15 to 20 minutes the skin temperature will usually have been restored to normal. If the patient's skin has not reached near-normal temperature after 20 to 30 minutes, further rewarming should be done cautiously. After rewarming has been achieved, the management of the injured tissue should proceed according to its condition and the progress of the injury.

The management of a patient with a cold injury, where the tissue is cold but not frozen, is the same as that for those with frozen tissue. The time required for rewarming is not so long, and the temperature of the water can be 98° to 100° F, since the cold tissue will not lower the water temperature as rapidly as frozen tissue. After cold or frozen tissue is rewarmed, blistering commonly occurs.

Some patients do not seek hospital care after cold injury until blister formation has occurred, and others not until there is noticeable discoloration or cyanosis. The immediate care of cold-injured tissue that is blistered or discolored is basically the same. The tissue should be kept clean by frequent washings; active exercise should be encouraged; and the limb should be maintained in a functional position. Frequent washings can be accomplished in a variety of ways, depending on the patient's general condition, other injuries, and his ability to cooperate. Whenever possible, patients should be encouraged to wash frequently and move their hands actively through a full range of motion (a full range of motion for the patient with a cold injury of the hands is not the same as that in uninjured hands). One can usually exercise the patient by having him sit in a body whirlpool bath and, with his hands at shoulder-to-face level, wash and actively move his hands. This provides the patient with the opportunity of seeing the hands move and, one would hope, encourages him to increase the amount of active motion each day. As the amount of motion increases, the patient is usually motivated to increase the time and enthusiasm he invests in such a program.

If a body whirlpool bath is not available, the same program can be accomplished at a wash basin. When the feet are involved, they should be kept elevated while the hands are receiving care.

Early débridement of the wounds should be limited to previously ruptured blebs or bullae. Blisters may be present at the time of hospital admission, or they may develop after the rewarming of cold or frozen tissue. In either situation the care is the same. The blebs or blisters are left intact unless they interfere with moving the hand or appear taut (indicating that the pressure might harm the underlying structures), or the blister fluid appears purulent. Primary excision and grafting have no place in early wound care. It is difficult to predict accurately the extent of tissue necrosis. Frequent washings and active motion should be continued until there is optimal healing of the partial-thickness wounds and definite demarcation of full-thickness injuries. This stage of care often extends to 3 or 4 months because the amount of full-thickness injury is often overestimated, and progressive healing requires several weeks. If only the hands are involved, most of the care, starting a few days after injury and continuing until demarcation is complete, can be rendered on an outpatient basis.

After the initial phase of care, it is still important to handle the injured tissue as gently as possible. This philosophy is consistent with the earlier program of frequent washings, gentle active motion, and minimal tissue manipulation. The injured parts should be elevated as much as possible to minimize edema formation, and loose crusts or dead tissue should be removed every 2 to 3 days. This débridement is best accomplished after the hands have been washed, while the tissue is moist and easily separated. The loose tissue is gently trimmed to the point of firm attachment with small tissue forceps and scissors. With this therapy, epithelium regenerates in areas where the wounds are partial thickness in depth; full-thickness wounds will form granulation tissue and require grafting. In deeply injured phalanges that are nonviable, the tissue will tend to contract or shrink. Only after granulation tissue develops between the healed partial thickness and obviously gangrenous tissue is amputation indicated.

Intermediate care and rehabilitation

During the long period from the time a cold injury is sustained until wound closure is obtained by spontaneous healing, skin grafting, or amputation, loss of function and the development of anatomic deformities must be prevented by active and passive exercises and splinting. The role and technique for active motion have been described. Correct positioning of the hands is equally important in preventing complications. The wrist should be in an extended position. Wrist extension is basic in preventing loss of function and the development of anatomic deformities in any program of active hand motion. When the wrist is extended, the metacarpophalangeal joints tend to flex because of the effect of gravity and the increased tension on the intrinsic muscles. The proximal interphalangeal joints are more supple and less likely to develop a flexion deformity, since the pull on the flexor tendons is not so great. When the wrist is allowed to assume a flexed position (a position of rest or comfort), the metacarpophalangeal joints tend to extend or hyperextend causing a compensatory flexion deformity of the interphalangeal joints. A wrist splint may be necessary to keep the wrist extended. This splint should be worn during periods of inactivity and especially at night. On occasion, the wrist extension splint alone will not prevent the development of interphalangeal flexion and thumb adduction deformities. Under these circumstances, the splint should be modified to include an interphalangeal extension device and an extension to abduct the thumb.

SUMMARY

The management of patients with cold injuries of the hands may be extremely simple or relatively complex. The extent of the injury and the systemic response to the cold are the major influencing factors.

In patients with extensive cold injuries, where all or a large portion of more than one extremity is cold or frozen and there has been significant systemic response, treatment should be both systemic and local.

Treatment should be directed toward both the preservation of tissue and the maintenance of function of the damaged part. Minimal daily débridement and late amputations are important guidelines for care.

X

DUPUYTREN'S DISEASE

55

Dupuytren's disease

ROBERT M. McFARLANE and URSULA ALBION

The name of Dupuytren will always be associated with a certain type of flexion deformity of the fingers or toes, because the great French surgeon Baron Guillaume Dupuytren (1777-1835) identified the palmar and digital fascia as the tissue responsible for joint contracture.[2] He demonstrated at autopsy that the flexor tendons were not shortened, as others had suggested. Also, he showed that the skin, although compressed into pits and folds, assumed its normal dimensions when separated from the underlying fascia. Thus he established that the site of disease was the fascia and not the overlying skin or the underlying tendons (Figs. 55-1 and 55-2).

Hueston prefers the term ''Dupuytren's disease'' to that of ''Dupuytren's contracture'' because it broadens one's concept of this condition as a disease process.[5] Joint contracture is but the end result of the process. Much is known about Dupuytren's disease because it is so common. It is of genetic origin, behaving as a mendelian dominant, and occurs primarily in people of northern European origin.[9] It is associated with other diseases, such as epilepsy, diabetes, and alcoholism, and with conditions such as carpal tunnel syndrome and trigger finger. A similar pathologic process occurs in the fascia of the penis (Peyronie's disease) and in the plantar fascia (Lederhose's disease). Clinically it is seen more frequently in males than in females, because the disease appears later in women and is less likely to cause a joint contracture that requires treatment. The disease usually appears in the fifth decade in men and somewhat later in women, although it has been noted in teen-agers of both sexes. The first sign is a nodule that is usually in the palm, near the distal crease and in line with the ring finger.

Although Dupuytren's disease is progressive, it is not possible to predict how rapidly the disease will progress from the first appearance of a nodule to finger joint contracture. The nodule enlarges and others form, and over a period of months or years tendonlike cords form and are readily palpable in the palm and finger. The metacarpophalangeal joint is most frequently contracted. The proximal interphalangeal (PIP) joint may be contracted alone or with the metacarpophalangeal joint. Occasionally the distal interphalangeal (DIP) joint is contracted (Fig. 55-3).

The initial pathologic changes are not known, but early in the course of the disease there is activity of perivascular fibroblasts.[1,11] This cellular proliferation, accompanied by collagen production, accounts for the appearance of the pathognomonic nodule in the palm or the finger. Later, when joint contracture begins, the myofibroblast appears; presumably this cell is responsible for shortening the fascia and thus contracting the finger joints.[1,3] New collagen is produced, and much of it is of type III, which is the type of collagen found in granulation tissue and scar.[7] This leads us to believe that the pathologic changes of Dupuytren's disease are not unique; rather the changes are those of scar contracture. Why this process begins in the hand and progresses for no apparent reason is unknown. Until the pathogenesis of Dupuytren's disease is understood, our methods of treatment remain empirical.

TREATMENT

There is no proved nonsurgical method of treatment. Vitamin E taken orally and the local injection of steroids may cause some change in a nodule. Attempts at stretching the contracting cord in the early stages of joint contracture are uniformly unsuccessful. Other forms of physical therapy, such as ultrasound, are of no benefit. At this time the only way to alter the course of the disease is to remove the diseased tissue surgically.

The presence of a nodule in the palm or digit is not an indication for operation. Frequently the nodule will be tender when first noted by the patient, but almost invariably the tenderness will disappear when the nature of the ''disease'' is explained to the patient. Occasionally, a nodule becomes so large that it is troublesome and excision is indicated. Again, on occasion, the skin of the palm may be involved out of proportion to the degree of joint contracture. The skin may be drawn into pits and folds that are difficult to cleanse and become calloused over the large nodules. In such patients early operation is advised so that the skin can be restored to its previous state.

Most patients are candidates for treatment because of finger joint contracture. The indications for operation are somewhat different at the metacarpophalangeal joint and the proximal interphalangeal joint. It is always possible to correct a metacarpophalangeal joint contracture, regardless of its severity, by an appropriate surgical procedure. The collateral ligaments of the metacarpophalangeal joints are stretched when the joint is in flexion, and therefore there is no restriction to full extension once the offending fascia has

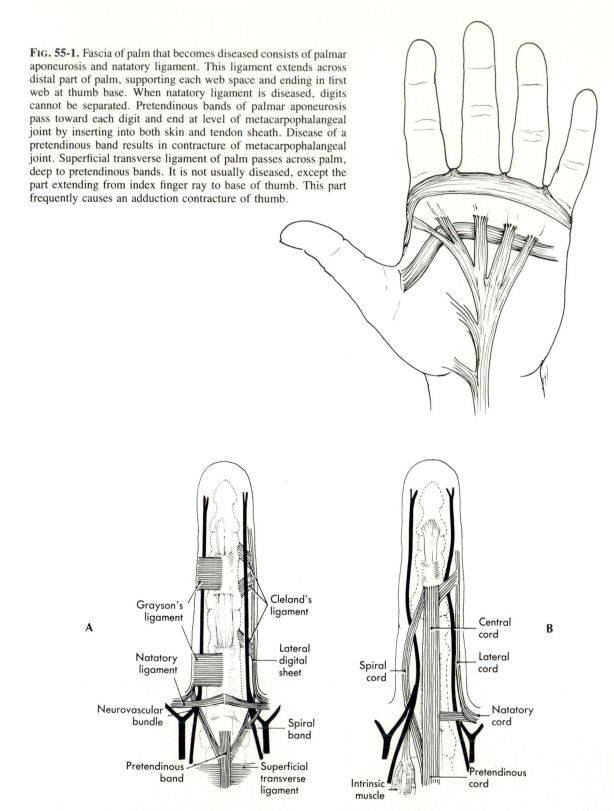

FIG. 55-1. Fascia of palm that becomes diseased consists of palmar aponeurosis and natatory ligament. This ligament extends across distal part of palm, supporting each web space and ending in first web at thumb base. When natatory ligament is diseased, digits cannot be separated. Pretendinous bands of palmar aponeurosis pass toward each digit and end at level of metacarpophalangeal joint by inserting into both skin and tendon sheath. Disease of a pretendinous band results in contracture of metacarpophalangeal joint. Superficial transverse ligament of palm passes across palm, deep to pretendinous bands. It is not usually diseased, except the part extending from index finger ray to base of thumb. This part frequently causes an adduction contracture of thumb.

FIG. 55-2. A, Components of volar digital fascia that may become diseased. **B,** Diagram of diseased cords that are derived from normal fascia. Central, lateral, and spiral cords may occur alone or in combination, and each one causes contracture at proximal interphalangeal joint.

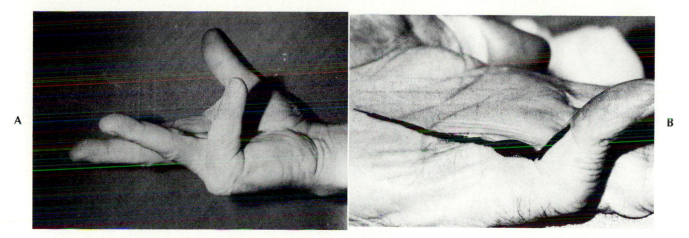

FIG. 55-3. Types of joint contracture. **A,** Contracture at metacarpophalangeal joint only. This patient gained full correction after operation. **B,** Contracture at proximal interphalangeal joint and hyperextension at distal interphalangeal joint. This patient was improved, but not fully corrected, by operation.

been released. For this reason, there is no urgency to operate when the metacarpophalangeal joint only is contracted, because correction is possible at any time. Most patients note some inconvenience or disability with a metacarpophalangeal joint contracture of about 30 degrees, and so this degree of contracture is a reasonable guide to advising a patient when to have an operation.

On the other hand, it is not always possible to correct fully a contracture at the PIP joint.[8] One reason for this is that the collateral ligaments at the PIP joint become shortened in any position of flexion. Release of the diseased fascia may not permit correction of the PIP joint contracture if the contracture has been present for several months. Contracture at the PIP joint of 15 degrees or more is an indication for operation.

Flexion contracture at the DIP joint is not common. It is usually seen in the little finger and may be difficult to correct, for the same reasons that apply to the PIP joint. DIP joint hyperextension is more common and again is most frequently seen in the little finger. It is not attributable to fascial contracture but is compensatory to severe PIP joint flexion.[7] It is difficult to correct even when the extensor tendon is divided.

Disease of the thumb or thumb web is not often of sufficient severity to warrant operation alone. However, contracture in this area should be corrected at the time of operation on other parts of the hand. Tubiana has drawn attention to disease on the radial side of the hand, affecting the thumb, the thumb web, and the index finger, a disease that is aggressive and is often seen in patients with a history of alcoholism.[16] This type of disease, which is uncommon, should be operated upon early and aggressively.

Patients under proper medical control of systemic disease are candidates for operation because the type of anesthetic and operation can be modified accordingly. Patients with a Dupuytren diathesis, which is not common, are likely to have continuing trouble regardless of the type of treatment. Such patients have a strong family history of the disease, which begins at an early age, and show evidence of fibro-

matoses elsewhere than the volar surface of the hand,. Nevertheless, the indications for treatment of these patients are the same as for others. In the same way, patients who are epileptic or alcoholic will not do well with an operation but are still treated according to the state of their disease.

Types of operation

One should distinguish between a type of incision and a type of operation. For example, McCash described a transverse incision in the palm that is left open to heal by second intention.[12] This has nothing to do with what is done to the underlying diseased fascia. King, Exeter, Bass, and Watson described exposure of the fascia by multiple Y-shaped incisions that are converted to V-shaped incisions to make up for the relative shortages of skin.[6] Again this is an adjunct to operation rather than an operation in itself. Incisions should be planned according to the extent of the disease in the palm and the number of digits involved.

Opinions differ about how little or how much fascia need be removed. In the McIndoe operation an attempt is made (through a transverse incision in the palm) to remove all the palmar aponeurosis.[13] This has been called a "radical excision of the palmar fascia." This operation successfully removes the disease in the palm, but hematoma in the palm and morbidity associated with it are common. McCash overcame the problem of hematoma by leaving the wound open, and Skoog did so to some extent by retaining the superficial transverse ligament of the palm.[15]

The antithesis of the McIndoe operation is the subcutaneous fasciotomy of Luck.[10] He believed that because the nodule causes the formation of the contracting cords, only the nodule need be removed. He also believed that in the later stages of disease, when the nodules are not apparent, the contracting cords need not be removed but simply divided. This operation corrects contracture at the metacarpophalangeal joint but does not often correct proximal interphalangeal joint contracture. If the cellular process continues, contracture may recur at both the metacarpophalangeal and proximal interphalangeal joints.

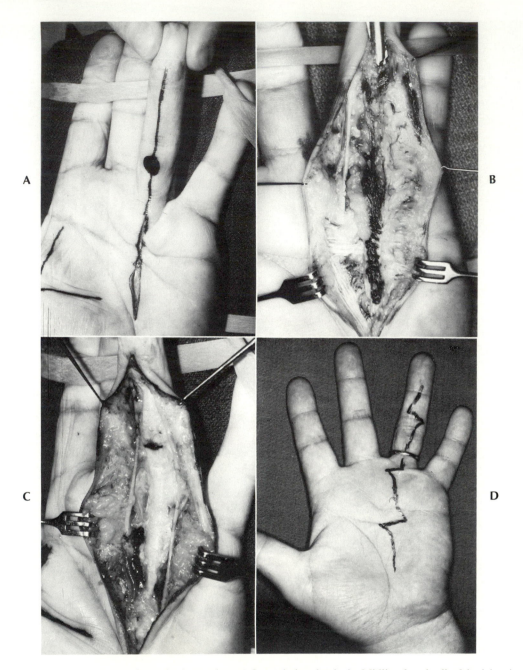

FIG. 55-4. Type of operation performed when only one finger is involved. **A,** Midline longitudinal incision is made from proximal palm to distal crease of finger. **B,** Generous exposure of fascia of palm and finger. **C,** Diseased fascia has been removed. Both neurovascular bundles and flexor tendon sheath between them have been cleared of fascia. **D,** Appearance of hand 8 years later. Longitudinal incision was broken by three Z-plasties to prevent postoperative scar contracture.

Gonzales recommends a limited operation, similar to the fasciotomy of Luck, to minimize the postoperative complications of more extensive procedures.[4] He advocates excision of nodules and incision of cords through transverse incisions. Upon correction of the joint contracture the skin defect is covered with a full-thickness skin graft, thereby holding the ends of the diseased fascia apart.

Radical excision of the palmar fascia is associated with some degree of hematoma formation. If the hematoma is massive, skin loss, infection, edema, and delayed healing will result in prolonged, if not permanent, disability. The patient may not regain either full extension or full flexion of the digits. To overcome this problem, most surgeons have resorted to less extensive dissection in the palm, removing only the diseased fascia (regional fasciectomy). At this stage in our understanding of the disease process this procedure is a good compromise between removal of almost all the palmar aponeurosis, so that recurrence cannot take place, and local incision or excision of a nodule or cord in the

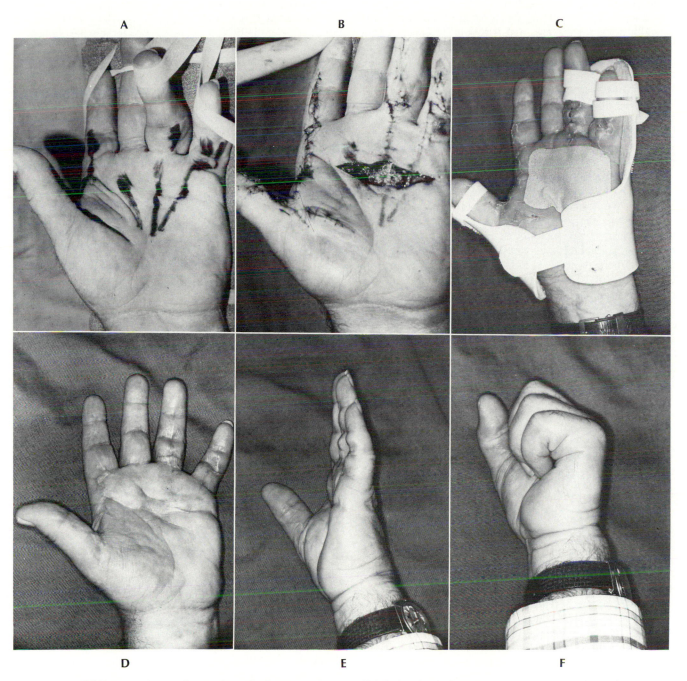

FIG. 55-5. Type of operation performed when more than one digit is involved. **A,** This patient had disease involving pretendinous bands to all five digits as well as disease causing contracture of proximal interphalangeal joints of little, ring, and index fingers. Natatory ligament in thumb web was also diseased, and so patient was unable to fully abduct or extend thumb. **B,** Appearance of hand at end of operation. Longitudinal incisions were made in thumb and index, ring, and little fingers, through which diseased fascia was removed. Incisions were closed by use of multiple Z-plasties. Disease in palm was removed through transverse incision, and this incision was left open. **C,** Three weeks after operation longitudinal incisions were healed. Palmar wound healed in 6 weeks. Patient wore splint most of time for 2 months and at night for another 2 months. **D** to **F,** Appearance of hand 1 year after operation. Wounds are well healed. Patient lacks full interphalangeal extension but has full flexion.

palm on the assumption that interruption in the continuity of the contracting tissue will prevent further contracture. With a regional fasciectomy the surgeon removes only the clinically apparent disease, and it should be clear to both the surgeon and the patient that disease elsewhere in the palm may progress.

As Hueston states, "The only difference between a radical and conservative operation is in the extent of the palmar dissection. Digital dissection will be required for interphalangeal joint deformity in any case."[5] This distinction must be emphasized. The surgeon enjoys a considerable choice of methods of treating disease in the palm, and personal preference or bias may well decide the choice. In the finger, however, a direct approach to the disease is essential both to correct interphalangeal joint flexion contracture and to prevent recurrence of contracture. An understanding of the anatomy of the contracting cords and adequate exposure are essential.[14] To correct a contracture at the proximal interphalangeal joint the exposure should be beyond that joint, at least to the distal crease. Because the distal joint may be involved, it is best to include this area in the original dissection.

Therefore the plan of treatment is to perform a regional fasciectomy in the palm to permit full correction at the metacarpophalangeal joint and also prevent recurrent contracture. In the affected finger a radical fasciectomy is performed to gain maximum correction at the proximal interphalangeal joint and also to remove potentially diseased tissue that can be a source of recurrent contracture. If only one finger is involved, the operation is performed through a longitudinal incision (Fig. 55-4). If more than one finger is involved, a longitudinal incision is used in the finger, but in the palm a transverse incision is used because it provides better exposure (Fig. 55-5).

Postoperative complications

Hematoma, skin necrosis, and infection are a triad of complications that are intimately related. Extensive operations in the palm, followed by closure of the wound, very often result in the formation of a hematoma, which then embarrasses the blood supply to the skin that is already compromised. When the edges of the wound become necrotic, infection is inevitable. The result is swelling and stiffness of the hand. These complications are prevented when the palmar wound is left open. Hematoma is less frequent after limited fasciectomy through longitudinal incisions, but skin necrosis and subsequent infection may occur in the small triangular flaps and Z-plasties and prolong recovery.

The digital nerves and vessels may be damaged intraoperatively because they are often surrounded by the diseased fascia. Severance of both arteries will likely result in loss of the digit unless the arteries are repaired. A severed nerve should be repaired. Observation of the patient overnight in a hospital is desirable.

POSTOPERATIVE MANAGEMENT

On the first postoperative day, the dressing is removed and a static dorsal finger-extension splint is molded of a thermal plastic material. Velcro straps are used to fasten the splint to the hand and to hold the fingers in extension (Fig.

55-5, *C*). The purpose of the splint is twofold. The first purpose is to gain the degree of finger extension obtained at operation. One would hope that this will be full extension, but it is unlikely that more extension will be gained by splinting than that obtained by excision of the diseased fascia. It is important to inform the therapist of whether the finger can be expected to extend fully. The second purpose of the splint is to hold the fingers in maximum extension during the period of wound healing.

Usually the splints are well accepted by the patient and finger extension is easily regained. The patient is instructed to tighten gradually the Velcro straps, extending the fingers within pain tolerance, until the fingers have straightened. The patient is given a goal to work toward—for example, achievement of full finger extension in 2 days. In addition, active exercises are essential to prevent joint stiffness and to regain a full range of motion in the fingers. The splint is worn at all times. The patient is instructed to remove the Velcro straps every hour and to actively or with assistance allow the fingers to fully flex and extend at the metacarpophalangeal and distal and proximal interphalangeal joints. If the patient is to continue these exercises independently at home, it is important that the exercises given are simple and easy to remember. Therefore only complete patterns of motion are stressed—flexion of all fingers to the distal palmar crease and full finger extension. Wrist and thumb exercises may be added if there is any decreased motion. Hand grips and putty can be used to improve grip strength. Progressively resistive exercises to both finger flexors and finger extensors are important in strengthening the hand. Functional activities should be encouraged. When the wounds have healed, hydrotherapy or paraffin wax baths may be used before exercise sessions.

If the fascia has been removed through a longitudinal incision in the palm and digit, the sutures are removed about 10 days after the operation, and the wounds are sufficiently healed in 2 weeks to tolerate most modes of therapy. If more than one digit was involved, the digits are exposed through a longitudinal incision, but a transverse incision is used in the palm. This incision is left open to heal by contraction. The time required for the palmar wound to heal depends on the width of the wound and varies from 3 to 6 weeks after operation. During this time the dressing is changed two or three times each week and the patient wears a splint and is supervised as discussed above. Hydrotherapy is not used until the wound is healed. Fietti and Mackin (see Chapter 56) have described the benefits of whirlpool bath soaks for patients who had an open palm procedure. We have not used this technique as yet but believe that it has merit.

The time required to recover from an operation for Dupuytren's disease is variable. Recovery implies a full range of finger motion. Certainly full flexion should be regained, because almost always patients have full finger flexion preoperatively. Full extension is the goal of treatment, but with severe and long-standing proximal interphalangeal contraction, full extension is unlikely, particularly in the little finger.[8] Most patients will be incapacitated for 6 to 8 weeks. The time required to return to work will depend entirely on the job involved, but a laborer will not likely return to work within 2 months of operation.

Having regained full flexion and maximum extension of

the fingers, the patient is advised to wear a splint at night for about 3 months. The scar contraction that takes place during this time can cause further joint contracture. Many patients do not wear the splint this long, simply because they are satisfied with the correction obtained. As a result, it is not uncommon to see patients 6 months after operation with 10 to 15 degrees more flexion, especially at the proximal interphalangeal joint, than was present under supervised splinting.

SUMMARY

A successful result after operation for Dupuytren's disease requires the cooperation of the patient, the surgeon, and the therapist. An appropriate operation must be designed for the individual patient. Metacarpophalangeal joint contracture can always be corrected, but some residual proximal interphalangeal joint contracture may have to be accepted.

REFERENCES

1. Chiu, H.F., and McFarlane, R.M.: Pathogenesis of Dupuytren's contracture: a correlative clinical-pathological study, J. Hand Surg. **3:**1, 1978.
2. Dupuytren, G.: Permanent retraction of the fingers produced by an affection of the palmar fascia, Lancet, p. 222, 1834.
3. Gabbianni, G., and Majno, G.: Dupuytren's contracture: fibroblast contraction? Am. J. Pathol. **66:**131, 1972.
4. Gonzales, R.I.: Dupuytren's contracture of the fingers: a simplified approach to the surgical treatment, Calif. Med. **115:**25, 1971.
5. Hueston, J.T.: Dupuytren's contracture: the trend to conservatism, Ann. R. Coll. Surg. Engl. **36:**134, 1965.
6. King, E.W., Exeter, M.H., Bass, D.M., and Watson, H.K.: Treatment of Dupuytren's contracture by extensive fasciectomy through multiple Y-V-plasty incision, J. Hand Surg. **4:**234, 1979.
7. Legge, J.W.H., Finlay, J.B., and McFarlane, R.M.: A study of Dupuytren's tissue with the scanning electron microscope, J. Hand Surg. **6:**482-492, 1981.
8. Legge, J.W.H., and McFarlane, R.M.: Predictions of results of treatment of Dupuytren's disease, J. Hand Surg. **5:**608, 1980.
9. Ling, R.S.M.: The genetic factor in Dupuytren's disease, J. Bone Joint Surg. **45B:**709, 1963.
10. Luck, J.V.: Dupuytren's contracture: a new concept of the pathogenesis correlated with surgical management, J. Bone Joint Surg. **41A:**635, 1959.
11. MacCallum, P., and Hueston, J.T.: The pathology of Dupuytren's contracture, Aust. N.Z. J. Surg. **31:**241, 1962.
12. McCash, C.R.: The open palm technique in Dupuytren's contracture, Br. J. Plast. Surg. **17:**271, 1964.
13. McIndoe, A., and Beare, R.L.B.: Dupuytren's contracture, Am. J. Surg. **95:**2, 1958.
14. McFarlane, R.M.: Patterns of the diseased fascia in the fingers in Dupuytren's contracture, Plast. Reconstr. Surg. **54:**31, 1974.
15. Skoog, T.: The transverse elements of the palmar aponeurosis in Dupuytren's contracture, Scand. J. Plast. Surg. **1:**51, 1967.
16. Tubiana, R., and Defrenne, H.: Les localizations de la maladie de Dupuytren à la partie radiale de la main, Chirurgie **102**(12):989, 1976.

56

Open-palm technique in Dupuytren's disease

VINCENT G. FIETTI, Jr., and EVELYN J. MACKIN

In 1831 Baron Guillame Dupuytren presented a patient afflicted with contractures of the fourth and fifth fingers (Fig. 56-1). His accurate description of the palmar aponeurosis as the source of the contracture and his advocacy of treatment by fasciotomy led to the entity's bearing his name[2]. Some 150 years later the cause of this disease remains obscure, the course of the disease unpredictable, and the treatment debated. In Chapter 55 McFarlane and Albion present the characteristics of this disorder and outline the various forms of surgical treatment. In this chapter we describe the open-palm technique.

In Dupuytren's disease, as in any other condition causing a contracture, release of that contracture often results in an insufficient amount of overlying skin for direct wound closure. The classic technique of closure by Z-plasty is often used, with other surgeons preferring to cover skin defects with full-thickness skin grafts. These techniques, though often successful, can be associated with the complications described in Chapter 55. The incidence of wound hematoma and slough of transposed Z flaps in some series of cases is alarmingly high.[1] Because of this, McCash in 1964 advocated leaving the palmar wound open, allowing healing to occur by secondary intention.[3] His series of 43 cases had no hematomas or significant wound complications. It is of interest to note that in Dupuytren's original paper he recommended leaving the palmar incisions open to heal "by granulation."

In the open-palm technique, a transverse incision is mapped out with a marking pencil either in the distal palmar crease (as suggested by McCash) or just beyond. Its length is dictated by the extent of the longitudinal cords, that is, whether only one or multiple digits are involved. On occasion it may be necessary to make a second, more proximal incision parallel to the thenar flexion crease if the diseased cord extends proximally to the base of the palm. The cord is dissected subcutaneously both proximally and distally, with the surgeon deciding on the extent of fasciectomy to be performed. In our patients a limited or subtotal fasciectomy is carried out. A volar Bruner incision is continued onto the involved digits. It may or may not be continuous with the transverse palm incision (Fig. 56-2). Some surgeons prefer multiple transverse "ladder-cut" incisions over the proximal and middle phalanges, but we believe exposure through such incisions is too limited. It cannot be over-

emphasized that adequate exposure is a necessity in Dupuytren's disease, because identifying the neurovascular structures and protecting them from inadvertent injury are of great importance. In the area overlying the proximal phalanx where the diseased longitudinal cord becomes the spiral cord wrapping around the neurovascular bundle these structures may be displaced toward the midline of the digit and "blind" dissection is extremely hazardous.[4]

The dissection is completed, and after hemostasis is achieved, the volar digital incision can be closed directly without flexion to the proximal interphalangeal joint. The transverse palmar wound, however, will now have spread to an oval defect, which cannot be closed without compromising metacarpophalangeal extension (Fig. 56-3). It is therefore left open and covered with Adaptic* and a bulky hand dressing of fluffs and roll gauze. The released digits may be held in full extension in the early postoperative period by means of plaster or thermoplastic splints. Wound healing occurs by marginal epithelialization usually within 4 to 6 weeks, depending on the width of the defect (Fig. 56-4). The open wound allows free drainage, thereby almost eliminating significant hematoma formation. In addition, the lack of tension on the skin is responsible for a dramatic absence of postoperative pain, allowing the patient to exercise in comfort and lessen the chance of digit stiffness.

The patient is usually discharged the morning after surgery and is seen by the therapist on or about the fifth postoperative day. The dressing applied at surgery is removed, and the patient is started on warm whirlpool bath treatment. Betadine† (povidine-iodine complex), an antibacterial agent, is added to the water. In this regard the postoperative management after the open-palm technique differs from that after closure with skin grafts or Z-plasties, when early hydrotherapy would be inappropriate. After the open-palm technique early whirlpool treatment is vital to wound care, both for cleansing the wound and for encouraging early exercise of the hand.

Niederhuber and associates[5] stated that "as an adjunctive modality in the treatment of many types of wounds, the therapeutic whirlpool provides the physiological benefits of heat to promote healing and the atraumatic removal of sur-

---

*Johnson & Johnson Co., New Brunswick, N.J.
†The Purdue Frederick Co., Norwalk, Conn.

624

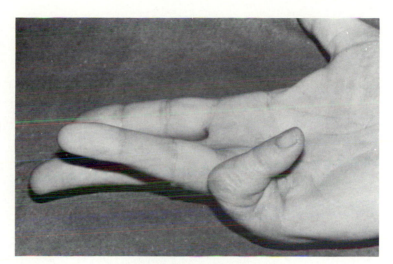

FIG. 56-1. Preoperative flexion contracture of fifth digit.

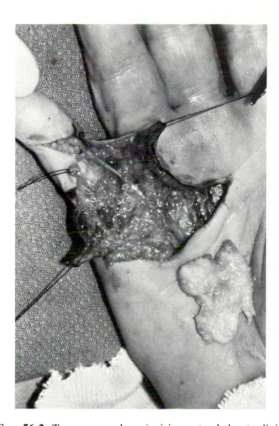

FIG. 56-2. Transverse palmar incision extended onto digit.

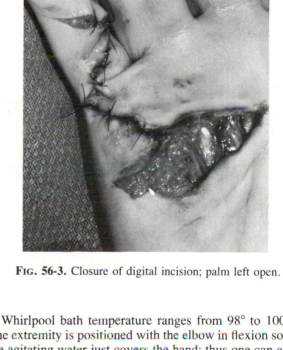

FIG. 56-3. Closure of digital incision; palm left open.

face eschar and exudates where bacteria thrive.'' They found that a combined treatment procedure of whirlpool agitation followed by a clean water rinse was significantly more effective in removing bacteria than a procedure in which the part was not rinsed after removal from an agitated whirlpool bath. In a later study, Bohannon[1] produced further evidence of the value of rinsing contaminated ulcers, wounds, or burns after removal from a whirlpool bath. The whirlpool-rinse procedure is used after the open-palm surgical technique for Dupuytren's disease.

Whirlpool bath temperature ranges from 98° to 100° F. The extremity is positioned with the elbow in flexion so that the agitating water just covers the hand; thus one can avoid a dependent position. Active flexion-extension exercises are initiated. When the whirlpool bath treatment is completed, the patient's hand is rinsed with clean water. A contraindication to a whirlpool bath is edema, which may worsen with the heat of warm water.

Although patients have been informed preoperatively of the specifics of the open-palm technique, they often are

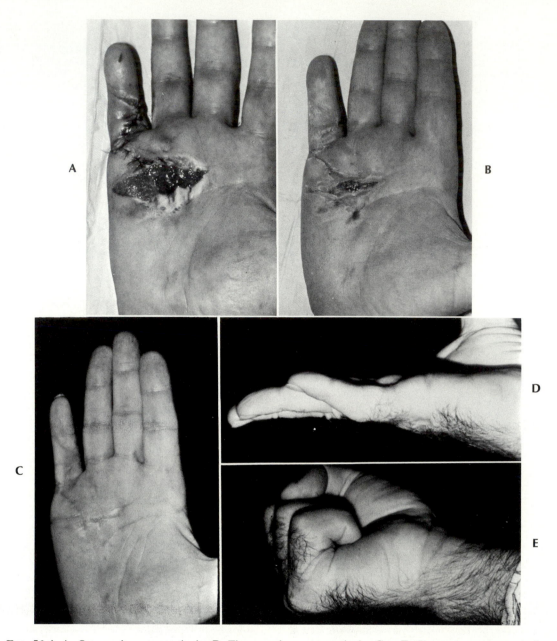

Fig. 56-4. A, One week postoperatively. **B,** Three weeks postoperatively. **C** to **E,** Six weeks postoperatively.

startled at the wound's appearance at the time of the first dressing change. At this time the therapist can be instrumental in reassuring the patient that wound healing will progress over the coming weeks.

The patient is seen two times weekly for therapy. Between appointments the patient soaks the hand at home in a boiled saline solution, prepared with one teaspoon of table salt added to a quart of boiling water. This hypertonic solution is bactericidal. The patient allows the boiling water to cool to lukewarm temperature and then soaks for 10 to 15 minutes three times a day. Active motion is carried out during the whirlpool bath. Home-exercise instructions must always be written and also given verbally to the patient and must be kept simple. The patient is instructed in redressing the

wounds at home in the manner preferred by the surgeon. We have been pleased with Betadine-soaked gauze wrapped with a 5-yard roll, but dry dressings soaked off in the salt solution have also been effective in removing exudate. The critical factor is to keep the granulating wound clean. A small number of patients will develop a superficial infection with an increased amount of daily exudate. Initially we treated this with bacitracin ointment, which must be used sparingly, since it might promote the formation of hypertrophic granulations. We now prefer to manage such infections with saline soaks and dressing changes alone, a minimum of three times daily and more frequently if necessary. Should granulations become exuberant, they respond best to dry sterile dressings or silver nitrate application. If resection into the digit or digits was necessary, the closed digital incision is also bandaged; however, the dressing applied to the digits must not restrict the patient's exercise program, so that full active flexion-extension exercises are possible within the confines of the dressing. A thin piece of gauze cut from a 4 by 4-inch sterile gauze pad, laid over the incision and then covered with a piece of Tubigrip, is very effective when the digital incision is bandaged.

Light, active exercises are started on the first postoperative day, and the program is reinforced when the patient is seen by the therapist.

The active exercise program initiated includes the following:

1. Thumb opposition to each finger
2. Finger blocking (distal interphalangeal flexion with the proximal interphalangeal joint supported and proximal interphalangeal flexion with the metacarpophalangeal joint supported)
3. Flexion of each finger to the distal palmar crease
4. Fist-making
5. Finger abduction and adduction
6. Finger extension
7. Full wrist and thumb range of motion

Severe proximal interphalangeal joint flexion contractures often result in hyperextension of the distal joint. When such contractures are released and pinned at surgery, early active distal interphalangeal joint flexion exercise must be initiated to encourage tendon gliding and distal joint motion.

Gentle passive flexion and extension of all joints is also indicated. Passive motion is facilitated by the heat of warm soaks. Flexion contractures in the palm can be passively stretched by applying gentle pressure to the dorsum of the involved hand with the opposite hand during the soaks. Goniometric measurements of range of motion are recorded during the initial visit to therapy and checked routinely by the therapist. The patient's hand is maintained in a Zimmer* sling, hand-over-heart position, during the first week after surgery, with removal of it only during exercise sessions. During sleep the hand should be elevated on pillows.

As motion improves, one modifies the exercise program by making the exercises more difficult and adding resistance. For example, when finger extension is performed easily, the patient may be asked to cross his fingers, index over long, long over index, long over ring, and so on. One can also make this exercise more difficult, improving finger extension further, by asking the patient to pass a quarter from finger to finger. In some instances the surgeon may not have been able to release a proximal interphalangeal flexion contracture to full extension. It is therefore important for the therapist to know the intraoperative range of motion and the result the surgeon expects postoperatively so that realistic goals can be set.

Although we often hope to gain further extension by means of therapy and splinting, this rarely happens. It is more the case that exercise and the use of splints maintain the extension achieved in the operating room. The regimen of postoperative splinting varies from surgeon to surgeon,

*Zimmer-Rodewalt Associates, Inc., 18 E. Centre Street, Woodbury, N.J. 08096.

and indeed on some patients with minimal disease and pliable skin and in whom good digital extension has been achieved, we have often elected to use no postoperative splint.

In cases in which digital extension was compromised preoperatively, a splint to maintain extension of the digit or digits is fabricated at the first therapy session; it may be a dorsal aluminum extension splint (Fig. 56-5) or a thermoplastic splint.

An aluminum extension splint that maintains the joints at the maximum comfortable range can be easily fabricated. A strip of foam-backed aluminum is cut long enough to extend from the fingertip to the wrist. Two pieces of aluminum (one with the adhesive foam removed) may be fastened together to give added strength to the splint. Velcro straps secure the splint in place. The splint is worn to tolerance during the day and night, with removal only for soaks and exercise. During the day the patient uses gradual pressure to gain full extension of all three joints. When wound healing is progressing and the patient is making good progress in maintaining extension of the joints, the splint may be removed for intermittent periods during the day for activities of daily living (however, the hand still must not be immersed in water other than warm soaks). The extension splint continues to be worn at night until the sixth postoperative month. Wound healing and scar maturation take place over a period of months. During this time extension splinting is vital to a good result. If more than one finger is involved, a thermoplastic splint may be preferred to provide stretch to the palmar and digital scar tissue.

If passive flexion of the proximal interphalangeal or distal interphalangeal joint is needed, the web strap or distal interphalangeal stretcher as described in Chapter 16 may be used. A soft roll of foam may be used to encourage finger flexion even when the palm is open. Gentle squeezing of a foam roll five to 10 times, carried out several times during the day, will improve flexion and grip strength. It should not, however, cause pain or discomfort.

When the wound has healed, lanolin massage of the involved fingers and palm may be given several times a day to soften the tissues of the hand. After the massage, excess lanolin should be removed with a cloth to prevent skin maceration.

Use of putty may also be initiated at this time. Making a "hot dog" from putty, using only the fingers, will strengthen the grip and encourage tendon gliding. Exercises should never be overdone. Squeezing the putty 10 times intermittently during the day is a far better regimen than doing it for 10 or 20 minutes continually, which might result in pain and edema. Putty may also be rolled back and forth by the fingers on a flat surface to improve finger extension.

Occupational therapy is extremely valuable in helping to achieve full function of the hand after Dupuytren's release. While the palmar wound is still open, light pick-up and pinch activities are initiated to encourage active use of the hand. When the wound closes, sustained grip activities, such as woodworking and leatherworking, help regain full flexion and grip strength. Dynamic flexion activities, such as hand-molding ceramics and activities of daily living, also contribute to attaining maximum function.

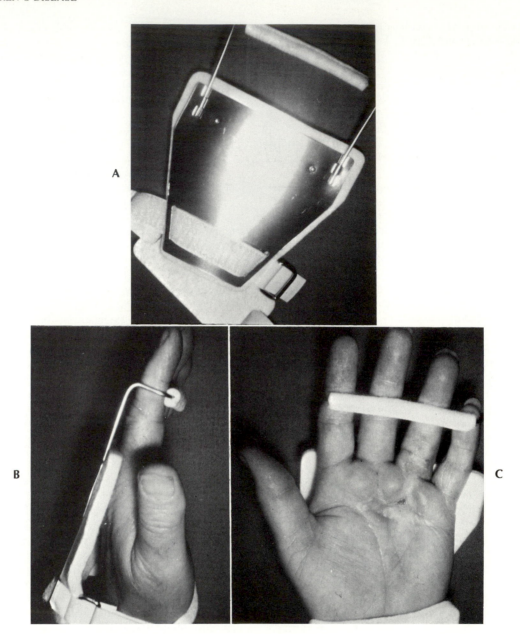

FIG. 56-5. **A,** Bunnell palmar splint. **B** and **C,** Bunnel palmar splint on hand.

The open-palm technique has been used at the Hand Rehabilitation Center in Philadelphia almost exclusively since 1969. In a series of over 200 patients the results both cosmetically and functionally have been gratifying. The incidence of wound complications has been negligible.

REFERENCES

1. Bohannon, R.W.: Whirlpool versus whirlpool and rinse for removal of bacteria from a venous stasis ulcer, Phys. Ther. **62**(3):304-308, March 1982.
2. Dupuytren, G.: Leçons orales de clinique chirurgicale faites à l'Hôtel Dieu de Paris, vol. 1, Paris, 1832, Baillière, p. 1.
3. McCash, C.R.: The open palm technique in Dupuytren's contracture, Br. J. Plast. Surg. **17**:271, 1964.
4. McFarlane, R.M.: Patterns of the diseased fascia in the fingers in Dupuytren's contracture: displacement of the neurovascular bundle, Plast. Reconstr. Surg. **54**:31, 1974.
5. Niederhuber, S.S., Stribley, R.F., and Koepke, G.H.: Reduction of skin bacterial load with use of therapeutic whirlpool, Phys. Ther. **55**:482, 1975.

XI
ARTHRITIS

57

Pathogenesis of arthritic lesions*

ALFRED B. SWANSON

Arthritis is a ubiquitous disease. Almost 100% of the population is susceptible to some form of arthritis, and if an individual lives long enough, he is almost certain to develop one type or another. It is estimated by the United States Public Health Service's National Center for Health Statistics, in a survey conducted in 1966 and 1967, that there are 16.8 million persons in the United States suffering from some form of arthritis. An estimated 3.4 million arthritis victims are completely disabled at any one time. The annual wage loss and medical care costs combined result in a loss to the national economy of approximately $3.5 billion, whereas the total national investment in research and medical education against arthritis in 1968 was only $15 million. Arthritis is considered the second greatest cause of chronic limitation of major activity; heart diseases rank first in limiting activity only by a slight margin. Although arthritis is a crippling disease that seldom kills the patient, no other group of diseases causes so much suffering to so many people for such long periods. Arthritis therefore has great social and economic repercussions.

Disabling work injuries in the United States totaled 2.2 million in 1970, according to the National Safety Council. Arms were involved in 9% of the cases, hands in 7%, and digits in 17%, for a total of 33% of all injuries incurred. Handling objects and falls were the source of more than half of the temporary total disabilities. Motor vehicle accidents accounted for only 4% and machinery accidents for 6% of total temporary disabilities but gave rise to 19% of the permanent partial disabilities. More than half of the injuries to the hand resulted in permanent partial disability. Many of these patients have joint stiffness or destruction, and their rehabilitation is a significant economic, social, and personal problem.

There are many different forms of joint disease, some caused by known etiologic agents and others resulting from unknown etiologic factors. The numerous terms for certain types of arthritis are also confusing. Many classifications of diseases of joints and related structures have been suggested. All have certain disadvantages and remain a controversial problem. For the sake of simplification, clarity,

and unification of terminology, the classification tentatively approved by the American Rheumatism Association has been recommended for general use. Until the etiology of all types of arthritis is known, no grouping can be accurate. The present classifications are based on clinical patterns, pathologic change in the tissues, and etiology when known. The classification accepted by the American Rheumatism Association is shown in the boxed material.

Rheumatoid arthritis is primarily a generalized disease affecting the synovium as its main target, with secondary changes occurring in the articular cartilage. Osteoarthritis is predominantly a disease of the articular cartilage. The main features of the pathogenesis of the lesions occurring in osteoarthritis and rheumatoid arthritis are briefly presented.

RHEUMATOID ARTHRITIS

It is estimated that 3% of the population is afflicted with rheumatoid arthritis, and although it is responsible for only approximately one fourth of the total number of arthritis patients requiring treatment, it is the greatest crippler from the standpoint of severity and prolonged disability.

Rheumatoid arthritis is one of the unsolved enigmas of medicine. It is a systemic disease whose most characteristic lesion is inflammation of the synovial membranes of joints and tendon sheaths. The swelling, redness, heat, and pain occurring in synovial structures in arthritis are based on this inflammatory reaction, which results in damage to joints, supporting soft-tissue structures, and tendons (Fig. 57-1). The inflammatory stage is usually chronic and persistent in two thirds of the cases.

The most widely accepted theory of the pathogenesis of rheumatoid arthritis is that of an immunologic response taking place in the synovial tissues. There are probably two mechanisms involved in the chronicity of the arthritic inflammation. The first is attributable to the initiating, presumably exogenous, antigen; and the second is attributable to development of an autoimmune response to a new antigen from the host tissues. Normally, when a foreign antigen enters the body, it comes in contact with a defender cell, the lymphocyte. The lymphocyte becomes transformed into a larger plasma cell. The plasma cell manufactures antibodies that have surfaces precisely keyed to fit the surfaces of the antigen so that the two can lock together. As antibodies lock in with antigens and immobilize them, a blood sub-

*Text and illustrations taken in part from Swanson, A.B.: Flexible implant resection arthroplasty in the hand and extremities, St. Louis, 1973, The C.V. Mosby Co.

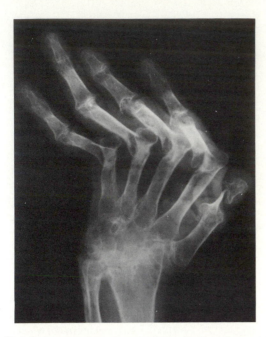

FIG. 57-1. Roentgenogram demonstrating findings in severely involved rheumatoid arthritic hand. There are severe absorptive changes of proximal phalanx of thumb, dislocation of metacarpophalangeal joints, erosive changes in proximal interphalangeal joints, fusions in carpal bones, and subluxation at wrist. Osteoporotic changes are noted.

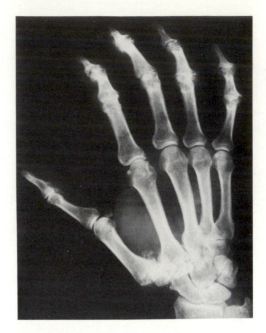

FIG. 57-2. Roentgenogram of hand of 50-year-old woman with primary osteoarthritis. There are severe degenerative changes at first carpometacarpal joint, distal interphalangeal joints, and proximal interphalangeal joints of fourth and fifth digits. Metacarpophalangeal joints and wrist are spared. There is no evidence of osteoporosis.

stance called complement is attracted and combines with them. The three-part combinations formed in this way are called complexes. The scavenger phagocytic cells then engulf the complexes. The phagocytic cells have small sacs called lysosomes that contain enzymes. The enzymes destroy the complexes, thus disposing of the intruder. In rheumatoid arthritis the phagocytic cells become incapable of handling the antigen-antibody-complement complex. Some of the lysosomes escape from the cells and attack the synovium and cartilage of the joints. Destruction of cartilage adds to the requirement for more phagocytic activity to clean up the resulting debris. The phagocytes pour out more of their enzymes and further trigger inflammation. Thus, once triggered, arthritic inflammation becomes self-perpetuating.

The inflammatory synovium forms a pannus, a granulomatous mass that grows over the surface of the cartilage, into and around the tendons, and into ligament attachments. If unchecked, this invasion results in loosening of ligaments, destruction of joint surfaces, and disability of tendons to function, all of which are typical of the advanced rheumatoid process. Every derangement or deformity of the musculoskeletal system seen in rheumatoid arthritis is the result either primarily or secondarily of this synovial invasion.

OSTEOARTHRITIS
Incidence

Osteoarthritis is very commonly seen in adults. Roentgenograms of the hands and feet of persons from 18 to 79 years of age show evidence of osteoarthritic changes in 37.4% of the cases. Approximately 8% of all adults are estimated to have moderate to severe clinical symptoms of osteoarthritis of the hands and feet. In a serial survey of

1000 consecutive autopsies, 72% of the patients showed some osteoarthritic changes of the knee joint, with 9% showing severe changes; 38% had changes of the hip, with 5% showing severe changes; and 22% had changes of the shoulder, with 4% showing severe changes. The prevalence of osteoarthritis rises steeply with age. Approximately 4% of the persons between 18 and 24 years of age are estimated to have some degree of arthritis, whereas nearly 85% of all persons 75 to 79 years of age demonstrate roentgenographic evidence of this condition. In persons less than 45 years old, the prevalence of osteoarthritis is greater in men than in women, suggesting the importance of trauma as an etiologic factor. In the older age groups a larger proportion of women suffer from the disease. The incidence of this condition is not affected by race, geographic location, income, or education. However, the incidence of this disease does appear to be less in certain occupations as compared to others.

Classification

Degenerative arthritis. This more common form is not considered a generalized disease and is usually seen in an increasing percentage of the population as age increases. It most commonly involves the weight-bearing joints and the distal interphalangeal joints of the hand.

Primary generalized osteoarthritis. This form of arthritis usually occurs in middle-aged women and is characterized by roentgenographic evidence of osteoarthritic lesions of the interphalangeal joints of the hand, the carpometacarpal joint of the thumb, the knee and hip joints, the spine, and the metatarsophalangeal joints of the feet (Fig. 57-2).

Nomenclature and classification of arthritis and rheumatism
(tentatively accepted by American Rheumatism Association)*

I. Polyarthritis of unknown etiology
   A. Rheumatoid arthritis
   B. Juvenile rheumatoid arthritis (Still's disease)
   C. Ankylosing spondylitis
   D. Psoriatic arthritis
   E. Reiter's syndrome
   F. Others
II. "Connective tissue" disorders
   A. Systemic lupus erythematosus
   B. Polyarteritis nodosa
   C. Scleroderma (progressive systemic sclerosis)
   D. Polymyositis and dermatomyositis
   E. Others
III. Rheumatic fever
IV. Degenerative joint disease (osteoarthritis, osteoarthrosis)
   A. Primary
   B. Secondary
V. Nonarticular rheumatism
   A. Fibrositis
   B. Intervertebral disc and low back syndromes
   C. Myositis and myalgia
   D. Tendinitis and peritendinitis (bursitis)
   E. Tenosynovitis
   F. Fasciitis
   G. Carpal tunnel syndrome
   H. Others
      (See also shoulder-hand syndrome, VIII E)
VI. Diseases with which arthritis is frequently associated
   A. Sarcoidosis
   B. Relapsing polychondritis
   C. Henoch-Schönlein syndrome
   D. Ulcerative colitis
   E. Regional ileitis
   F. Whipple's disease
   G. Sjögren's syndrome
   H. Familial Mediterranean fever
   I. Others
      (See also psoriatic arthritis, I D)
VII. Associated with known infectious agents
   A. Bacterial
      1. *Brucella*
      2. *Gonococcus*
      3. *Mycobacterium tuberculosis*
      4. Pneumococcus
      5. *Salmonella*
      6. *Staphylococcus*
      7. *Streptobacillus moniliformis* (Haverhill fever)
      8. *Treponema pallidum* (syphilis)
      9. *Treponema pertenue* (yaws)
      10. Others
   B. Rickettsial
   C. Viral
   D. Fungal
   E. Parasitic
      (See also rheumatic fever, III)
VIII. Traumatic and/or neurogenic disorders
   A. Traumatic arthritis (viz., the result of direct trauma)
   B. Lues (tertiary syphilis)
   C. Diabetes
   D. Syringomyelia
   E. Shoulder-hand syndrome
   F. Mechanical derangements of joints
   G. Others
      (See also degenerative joint disease, IV; carpal tunnel syndrome, VG)
IX. Associated with known biochemical or endocrine abnormalities
   A. Gout
   B. Ochronosis
   C. Hemophilia
   D. Hemoglobinopathies (e.g., sickle cell disease)
   E. Agammaglobulinemia
   F. Gaucher's disease
   G. Hyperparathyroidism
   H. Acromegaly
   I. Hypothyroidism
   J. Scurvy (hypovitaminosis C)
   K. Xanthoma tuberosum
   L. Others
      (See also multiple myeloma, XG; Hurler's syndrome, XII C).
X. Tumor and tumorlike conditions
   A. Synovioma
   B. Pigmented villonodular synovitis
   C. Giant cell tumor of tendon sheath
   D. Primary juxta-articular bone tumors
   E. Metastatic
   F. Leukemia
   G. Multiple myeloma
   H. Benign tumors of articular tissue
   I. Others

*From Hollander, J.L.: Arthritis and allied conditions, ed. 8, Philadelphia, 1972, Lea & Febiger, pp. 4-5.

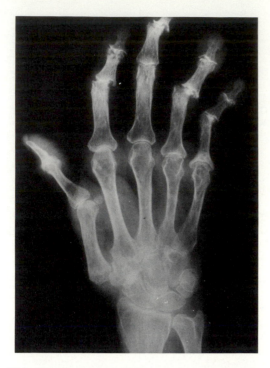

FIG. 57-3. Roentgenogram of 68-year-old woman with erosive osteoarthritis in both hands. Note involvement of first carpometacarpal joint and proximal and distal interphalangeal joints and lack of involvement of wrist joint. There is evidence of erosive changes, moderate osteoporosis, and malalignment of joints.

Erosive arthritis. This disease is characterized by chronic degenerative changes with intermittent inflammatory episodes. It is usually seen in middle-aged women and involves mainly the hands, feet, and cervical spine (Fig. 57-3). The synovium removed from these inflamed joints resembles that of rheumatoid arthritis. However, the predominance of cartilage destruction, juxta-articular erosions, and osteophytic formation without the clinical symptoms of rheumatoid arthritis separates it from this group.

Pathogenesis

The term "rheumatism," invented about 300 years ago, derived from the Greek word *rheuma* (that which flows as a stream or brook), because an increased flow of mucus was believed to be pathogenetic. Since an increased flow of mucus—that is, an increased synthesis of synovial fluid—and a greater increase in degradation of matrix mucopolysaccharide occur in human osteoarthritis, the term may be an accurate description of the pathogenesis of this disease.

The pathogenesis of osteoarthritis has not been thoroughly established. The precise sequence of histologic changes in this condition cannot be reconstructed. Osteoarthritis may be considered a wear phenomenon in which a breakdown of the normal joint characteristics occurs. Consideration of this problem must be given under several headings. The biology of the cartilage and the changes that occur in its degradation; the lubrication of the joint; the reaction of physical factors; and chemical, genetic, vascular, and bone changes are all interrelated factors in the mechanism of joint destruction.

Biology of cartilage. Articular cartilage is a composite material of cellular and extracellular components. The cellular part is the chondrocyte, and the extracellular portion is a matrix consisting of collagen fibers embedded in a mucopolysaccharide (chondroitin sulfate) ground substance. Cartilage is a living, dynamic, ever-changing tissue responding promptly to alterations in activity, environment, nutrition, and trauma. It takes up and expels water freely from the synovial fluid, thus promptly changing as much as 10% of its volume. It proliferates and grows faster with exercise or work, and it shrinks and atrophies with rest and disuse. Articular cartilage is composed of three distinct layers:

1. In the surface layer the collagen bundles are predominantly parallel to the surface. There are small ripples on its surface, so that, actually, the microscopic appearance is one of a rough, undulating surface, which is an important factor for the trapped-pool mechanism in lubrication. This layer also shows the presence of old or degenerated cells that are continuously being exfoliated and shed into the joint.
2. In a thicker elastic layer the collagen fibers are angled intermediately to the articular surface. This layer is responsible for much of the elasticity of the normal hyaline cartilage.
3. The basal layer fixes the cartilage to the subchondral bone plate. It is the growth area where cells divide and multiply. Here the fibers are more or less perpendicular to the articular surface and to the subchondral bone.

Cartilage is peculiar in that it is formed mostly by extracellular material surrounding relatively few cells whose main function is to maintain the composition of this extracellular matrix. Articular cartilage is avascular; approximately the outermost two-thirds zone affected by the early events in osteoarthritis receives its nutrition through exchange of substances between the matrix and the synovial fluid. This exchange is increased by the normal use of a joint; compression of cartilage squeezes fluid out like a sponge, and the matrix draws the fluid back in when the compression is released. Increased compression with continued motion causes thickening of the cartilage and cellular proliferation where mitotic failure is observed. In contrast, when all articular motion is experimentally prevented or when there is no surface-to-surface contact of the joint, the cartilage degenerates, apparently because of a lack of nutrition.

The status of the cartilage, whether healthy, active and growing, or sick, inactive, or aged, can be determined by its histologic appearance. When the cartilage is healthy, there are many large nuclei, often showing mitoses in the basal layer. In the elastic layer, the cells show activity by producing mucopolysaccharides, and there is a larger proportion of matrix to nuclei. The earliest pathologic changes in the cartilage have been described differently by various investigators and include focal swelling of the cartilage matrix, loss of chondroitin sulfate from the superficial layers of the cartilage, proliferation of chondrocytes in a disorderly fashion, a diminution of chondrocytes, fatty degeneration in the matrix, and alteration of the collagen fibrils. These changes probably represent a depletion of ground substance and are seen as cartilage surface irregularities in the form of undulations and fissures.

Gross changes in the articular cartilage have been described as localized areas of softening of the cartilage with flaking of the superficial layers and fibrillation, which represents fissures into the deeper layers. Mechanical abrasion of the fibrillated cartilage takes place with progressive loss of cartilage and exposure of the underlying bone. It may be present in areas of shearing stress on weight-bearing surfaces but also may be seen in nonweight-bearing areas of the joint.

The chondrocytes secrete the macromolecular components. Because the cartilage is avascular, the chondrocytes utilize glucose and other components of the synovial fluid and discharge the waste products of their metabolism into the articular cavity. Cartilage cells must continuously renew the protein-polysaccharide content of the matrix. Irreversible depletion of the matrix and subsequent loss of normal spongelike mechanical properties of the cartilage seriously interfere with the lubrication of the joint.

Lubrication. The diarthrodial joint is a most remarkable mechanical model. There is an extremely low coefficient of friction in this bearing mechanism. Its efficiency in dissipating heat, self-lubrication, and ability to continuously repair itself is remarkable. The basic principles of lubrication known to engineers have been studied in human joints, but the general excellent performance of the normal human joint exceeds the expected conditions. It is important, however, to understand basic concepts of lubrication in bearing surfaces to help explain the osteoarthritic joint and also for consideration in prosthetic joint replacement.

The various types of lubrication include the following.

1. *Fluid-film lubrication* is the development of a film between two opposing surfaces transmitting load.
2. *Hydrodynamic lubrication* occurs when the relative motion of two surfaces draws fluid into the interspace. It is sometimes called the wedge action.
3. *Elastohydrodynamic lubrication* is present when elastic deformation occurs between one or both of the opposing surfaces.
4. *Squeeze-film lubrication* occurs when the opposing surfaces are subjected to a varying load and the lubricating film restores itself before the increased load is again applied.
5. *Boundary lubrication* occurs when the lubrication is governed by the properties of the surface layers of the opposing component.
6. *Hydrostatic lubrication* occurs when the lubricant is supplied under pressure between the surfaces.
7. *Mixed lubrication* is a combination of the various types.

In the human joint the bearing surface is a layer of articular cartilage having an elasticity similar to that of rubber. It is porous, a property that is very important, and the lubricant synovial fluid is contained within a capsule. The surface of the cartilage is undulating, allowing the fluid to be trapped. The fluid-film type of lubrication can also occur because the loading on the joint is intermittent. The elasticity of the cartilage allows elastohydrodynamic lubrication because of the deformation of the substance under contact pressures and the resultant drawing of fluid into the flattened area. There appears also to be a boundary type of lubrication in which the lipid present in the articular cartilage aids the lubricating mechanism by weeping on the surface of the cartilage. This is a type of self-lubricating mechanism.

The normal synovial fluid gets most of its lubricating properties from hyaluronic acid, which is extremely viscous and elastic. In an abnormal joint the synovial fluid loses much of this quality, which in turn affects the lubricating mechanism.

Physical factors. Local physical factors seem to be important in the pathogenesis of lesions. The chemical and morphological alterations occur focally in the joint, and it is likely that mechanical phenomena are important. Loading on a joint surface beyond its tolerance can play a significant role in the eventual disorganization of the joint. The energy absorption function of articular cartilage can be overloaded when joints are unstable; when trauma is repeated, as in certain occupations; when the joint alignment is disturbed by fracture, dislocation, or congenital or developmental defects of the skeleton; or when there is aseptic necrosis of the underlying bone. Shear stresses are more destructive than compressive forces.

Chemical changes that may destroy cartilage include repeated bleeding into the joint, inflammation from infection, and deposition of chemicals such as homogentisic acid in the cartilage in cases of ochronosis.

Genetic factors. Genetic factors clearly influence the incidence of osteoarthritis in human beings and may be related in part to congenital structural factors such as posture, joint alignment, or deformity. The levels of various degradative enzymes and the rate of synthesis and breakdown of cartilage cells at rest or in response to stress could be genetically determined.

Vascular factors. The synovial tissue is the least affected portion of the joint in osteoarthritis. However, in the erosive type of osteoarthritis, an inflammatory type of synovitis is frequently seen; it may be a factor in cartilage destruction similar to that seen in rheumatoid arthritis. Fibrosis of the synovial surface and occasional cartilaginous metaplasia may be seen in advanced osteoarthritis. The inadequate synovium cuts down the normal supply of lubricating synovial fluid (synovia). Inflammatory reaction is seen in late osteoarthritis and is probably related to a foreign body reaction to the cartilaginous debris within the joint. In osteoarthritis there is an increased vascular supply at the level of the juxtachondral blood vessels. This is believed to be a secondary reaction to the degeneration of articular cartilage. A subchondral hyperemia of bone occurs, and vessels may enter the cartilage peripherally or through the subchondral plate. This hypervascularity further weakens the structure of the bone beyond the point where it can withstand compression and shearing forces.

Bone changes. Proliferation of bone in the subchondral zone is most noticeable in areas that have been denuded of cartilage. As the force-dampening effect of the cartilage is lost, bone is subjected to increased strain and responds, in part, by hypertrophy. Cystic lesions, however, may also develop immediately beneath the joint surface, and excessive blood vessel formation occurs around them. These cysts may fill with fluid, and their increased tension may cause peripheral rarefaction of bone and gradual enlargement of the cystic space. There also is remodeling of the bone at the level of the joint surface, which is probably related to bone formation from the calcified layer of the basal portion of the articular cartilage. Severe irregularity of the joint surface may be evidenced in the later stages of this process.

The development of marginal osteophytes is typical of the osteoarthritic process. Some of them protrude into the joint space in the intercondylar areas, and others are present at the periphery of the joint and also at the site of capsular and ligamentous attachments. The formation of osteophytes seems to be governed by the lines of mechanical forces. Osteophytes consist largely of bone and are continuous with

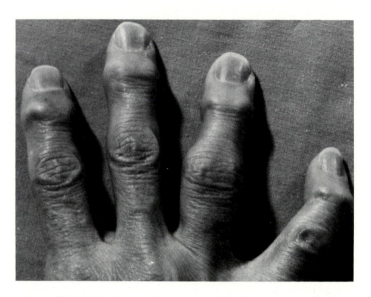

FIG. 57-4. Heberden's nodes are typical finding in osteoarthritis.

the normal bone. They are frequently capped by layers of hyaline cartilage or fibrocartilage, and some investigators have believed that they are caused by a metaplasia of cartilage debris within the joint.

The nature of the physical stresses on distal interphalangeal joints deserves comment since these joints are among the most common sites of osteoarthritic changes, and yet they are not weight bearing. The distal phalanx slides along the middle phalanx on the forces applied in pinch and grasp activities, resulting in great shearing stresses. Osteoarthritic outgrowths into tendon insertions occur at many sites. The extensor tendon inserts at the extreme proximal end of the bone in the distal phalanx. Extension is produced at a considerable mechanical disadvantage. These stresses associated with the degenerative process of osteoarthritis probably contribute to the severe remodeling of the bone with the presence of so-called Heberden's nodes, which is such a typical finding in this condition (Fig. 57-4).

Mechanism of osteoarthritis. In the destruction of the involved joints, there undoubtedly is an interdependence between the wear-and-tear process and the disturbed biologic state of the articular tissues. Mechanical factors of change in the lubrication power of joint fluid, in conjunction with a loss of the smoothness of the cartilaginous surface, gradual decrease of the dampening property of the cartilage, and chemical degradation of the cartilage and fluid joint, result eventually in collapse of the joint surface, with resultant restriction of motion and angulation of the joint. A vicious cycle of deformity is established.

There may be chondrolytic enzymes from the synovial fluid and also from chondrocytes, which break down articular cartilage. Local physical stress may rupture lysosomes in cartilage cells, thus activating proteolytic enzymes. The movement of lysosomes to the cell surface and discharge of their contents externally could induce digestion of extracellular protein polysaccharide. This relationship between the chemical and morphologic alterations found in joints is noted in Fig. 57-5.

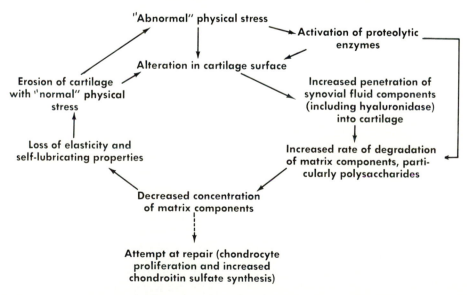

FIG. 57-5. Proposed mechanisms involved in pathogenesis of osteoarthritic cartilage degeneration. (From Bollet, A.J.: Arthritis Rheum. **12:**152-163, 1963.)

The vicious cycle of destruction and repair efforts in a joint has been stated by Trueta as a process that appears to be an attempt to transform a decaying joint into a youthful one, and for this, as in the miraculous rejuvenation depicted in Goethe's *Faust,* a high price must ultimately be paid.

GOUTY ARTHRITIS

The joint lesions of gout are related to the deposition of monosodium urate salts. Aside from the destruction of the articular mechanism by tophaceous deposits, the commonest lesion is of the osteoarthritic type. Urate crystals are deposited not only on and in the surface of the articular cartilage but also in the subchondral cysts, where they constitute the so-called punched-out lesions. These deposits of urate crystals in the articular structures of the hand usually become absorbed after medical treatment. Implant resection arthroplasty has rarely been indicated for gouty arthritis, in our experience.

58

Pathomechanics of deformities in hand and wrist*

ALFRED B. SWANSON

The pathomechanics of deformity in the hand secondary to arthritis relate to the disorganization of the joint and the external forces that are applied to it. Deformities secondary to rheumatoid arthritis are usually more severe than those seen in osteoarthritis. The deformities associated with osteoarthritis are mainly limitation of motion and occasionally angulation. The pathomechanics of deformities associated with rheumatoid arthritis have special significance in treatment.

In the normal hand there is a fine balance between the muscle and tendon system and the architecture of the bones and joints through which they act. If the restraining ligamentous structures of the joints are lengthened by the rheumatoid process, this vulnerable balance is compromised. The normal arch system of the hand is disturbed and the stability and equilibrium necessary for prehension are lost. In the presence of deranged mechanical equilibrium, the use of the hand in daily functional adaptations further compounds the progress of deformity.

An understanding of normal architecture and normal function of the hand is important for the study of pathomechanics and the evaluation of compensatory functional adaptations that become necessary when disability intervenes. A brief outline of the basic architectural considerations is presented for this purpose.

ARCHITECTURAL CONSIDERATIONS

The form of the hand has a certain unique elegance. The skeleton provides the lever arms, the mobile joints, and the stabilizing points around which functional adaptations of the hand take place. A great number of units are compacted into a small area through which greater power and precision can be applied. The arches of this complex enable the digits to bring objects into the hand and control them. The bony architecture of the hand is arranged in three arches: one longitudinal and two transverse. The proximal transverse arch passes through the carpal area, with its center at the capitate bone. The distal transverse arch is developed across the metacarpal heads, its center being the head of the third metacarpal. The fourth and fifth digital rays offer mobility

of the ulnar aspect of the hand around this fixed point. The thumb ray provides mobility around the radial aspect. The digits make up the longitudinal arches, with their apex at the metacarpophalangeal joints. A break in the longitudinal arch system of the digit may result in a collapse deformity of the multiarticulated structure (Fig. 58-1). Stiffness or deformity of the joints will disturb the normal flexion sequence of the digits and create a loss of integrity of this arch system, with resultant disturbance of functional adaptation patterns.

The ligament system of the finger joints is arranged so that stability is provided as flexion occurs. When the joints are in extension, the collateral ligaments are relatively lax. If the digit is immobilized in extension, these ligaments may contract and flexion will be limited. Therefore, when the injured or diseased part is treated, it is important to place the hand in the functional position with the digital joints in a semiflexed position.

The fingers rotate slightly around the third "metacarpal keystone" to converse toward the scaphoid (Fig. 58-2). Only the middle finger lies in a longitudinal axis of its own. Care must therefore be given to align the reconstructed digits according to this convergence; otherwise the fingers may overlap each other in grasping. The ideal result of treatment of any reconstructive problem in the hand would be to obtain mobility, stability, and proper alignment of the lever arm system. This should be the goal of every treatment method.

PATHOMECHANICS OF DEFORMITIES OF HAND AND WRIST IN RHEUMATOID ARTHRITIS

In rheumatoid arthritis the inflammatory synovium forms a pannus. This destructive and invasive granulomatous mass grows over the surface of the cartilage into the ligamentous attachments and into and around the tendons. The result is capsular distension, destruction of cartilage, subchondral erosions, loosening of the ligamentous insertions, impairment of the function of tendons, and, finally, joint disorganization, all of these being typical lesions of the advanced rheumatoid process. Every lesion or deformity of the musculoskeletal system seen in rheumatoid arthritis is the result primarily or secondarily of this synovial invasion, which eventually destroys the normal anatomic relationships. Specific deformities are related to the location and the intensity of this destructive process.

---

*Text and illustrations taken in part from Swanson, A.B.: Flexible implant resection arthroplasty in the hand and extremities, St. Louis, 1973, The C.V. Mosby Co.

638

FIG. 58-1. Bony architecture of hand is arranged in one longitudinal and two transverse arches. In rheumatoid arthritis palmar subluxation of metacarpophalangeal joint causes collapse of longitudinal arch. (Redrawn from Tubiana, R.: Anatomical and physiopathological features. In Tubiana, R., editor: The rheumatoid hand, Group d'Etude de la Main monograph no. 3, Paris, 1969, L'Expansion Scientifique Française.)

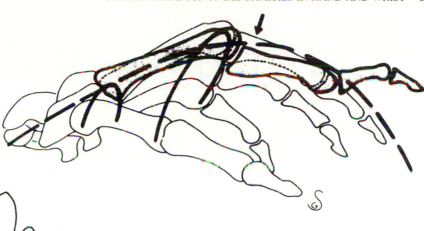

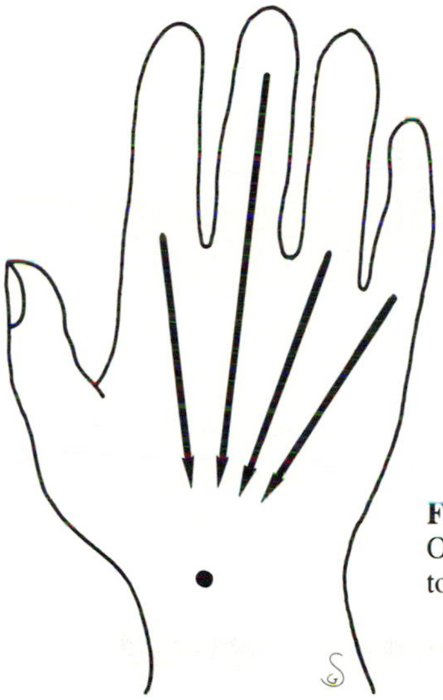

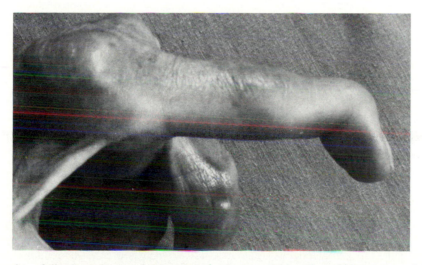

FIG. 58-2. Only middle finger lies in longitudinal axis of its own. Other fingers rotate slightly around third "metacarpal keystone" to converge toward scaphoid.

FIG. 58-3. Loosening of distal attachment of extensor tendon by synovial invasion of joint may result in mallet finger deformity. Isolated mallet finger is uncommon deformity in rheumatoid arthritis.

Distal interphalangeal joint

Synovial invasion of the distal interphalangeal joint resulting in specific deformities is uncommon in rheumatoid arthritis. Loosening of the distal attachment of the extensor tendon may cause a typical mallet, or drop, finger (Fig. 58-3). Loosening of the collateral ligament system, erosive changes in the subchondral bone, and cartilage destruction are aggravated by the daily external forces and may result in instability of the distal joint. The severe absorptive changes occurring in arthritis mutilans may totally destroy the joint in rheumatoid arthritis. Most deformities seen at the distal interphalangeal joint are secondary to the boutonnière or swan-neck collapse deformities.

Proximal interphalangeal joint

The proximal interphalangeal collateral ligament system consists of two parts: an oblique and a vertical component. The oblique component connects the middle and proximal phalanges by a ligament from the head of the proximal phalanx to the side of the middle phalanx. The vertical component, frequently called the accessory collateral ligament, is mainly a system for suspension of the palmar plate and the flexor tendon sheath. The flexor tendons are securely contained within this fibrous tunnel. The extensor apparatus consists of the central tendon, which inserts into the dorsal capsule, and the base of the middle phalanx. It is flanked by lateral tendons of the intrinsic muscles. A synovial pouch from the joint extends proximally beneath the extensor tendons. Another synovial pouch extends proximally between the palmar plate and the underlying bone.

Limited movement of the proximal interphalangeal joint may result from (1) articular causes such as disorganization of the joint and fibrinous adhesions, (2) periarticular causes such as adhesions affecting the attachments of the collateral ligaments, and (3) tendinous causes, arising from involvement of the flexor tendons by hyperplastic synovial tissue, which limits the gliding of the tendon and later forms adhesions.

Collapse deformity, or the buckling phenomenon of the three-joint system of the digit, is seen frequently in rheumatoid arthritis (Fig. 58-4). This disturbance is characterized by hyperextension of one of the joints and reciprocal flexion of the contiguous joints. This zigzag break in the normal flexion-extension pattern of the bony chain is ordinarily prevented by balanced tendon mechanisms and ligament restrictions on hyperextension. The claw, swan-neck, and boutonnière deformities are examples of this dysfunction; the latter two are seen frequently in rheumatoid arthritis. A vicious circle of deforming forces is established. Axially applied forces further aggravate the established deformity.

Boutonnière deformity. The boutonnière, or buttonhole, deformity usually occurs in rheumatoid arthritis through bulging of hyperplastic synovium between the extensor central and lateral tendons. The capsular and bony attachments of the central tendon are weakened, and a relative lengthening of the tendon occurs. The tendon is thus unable to effect normal extension of the middle phalanx. The transverse fibers that connect the lateral tendons to the central tendon are further lengthened by this synovial invasion, allowing the lateral tendons of the extensor apparatus to dislocate in a palmar direction. The lateral tendons are now located below the central axis of the proximal interphalangeal joint and become flexors of the proximal interphalangeal joint. Because the lateral tendons are relatively shortened by their displacement, there is an increased pull on their distal insertion to the distal phalanx, resulting in hyperextension deformity of this joint. Once this collapse deformity is established, it becomes self-perpetuating (Fig. 58-5). The joints may become stiff because of contracture of associated soft-tissue structures, and the proximal interphalangeal joint may become further disorganized and subluxated if the disease process continues.

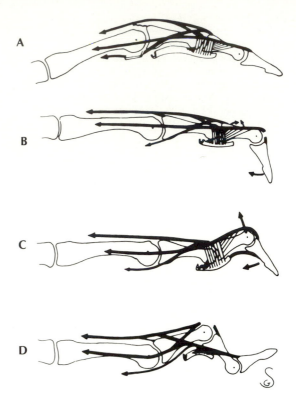

FIG. 58-4. Collapse deformities of three-joint system are often seen in rheumatoid arthritis and are characterized by hyperextension of one of joints, with reciprocal flexion of contiguous joints. Balanced tendon mechanisms and ligament restrictions that normally prevent hyperextension are lost. This shows altered relationship of extensor tendons and bone and joint systems after damage to extensor apparatus. **A,** Normal finger. **B,** Mallet finger. **C,** Swan-neck deformity. **D,** Boutonnière deformity. (Redrawn from Tubiana, R.: The mechanisms of deformities of the fingers due to musculotendinous imbalance. In Tubiana, R., editor: The rheumatoid hand, Group d'Etude de la Main monograph no. 3, Paris, 1969, L'Expansion Scientifique Française.)

The events taking place in the development of the boutonnière deformity in rheumatoid arthritis can be summarized as follows:

1. Capsular distension of the proximal interphalangeal joint
2. Lengthening of the central tendon
3. Lengthening of the transverse fibers
4. Lateral tendon palmar subluxation
5. Increased extensor tendon pull on the distal phalanx
6. Collapse of the three-level system
7. Joint disorganization

Swan-neck deformity. The swan-neck deformity is characterized by hyperextension of the proximal interphalangeal joint and flexion of the distal joint (Fig. 58-6). It probably is caused primarily by a synovitis of the flexor tendon sheath, with restriction of interphalangeal joint flexion. The main function of the long flexor tendon is to flex the interphalangeal joint, especially during the first part of finger flexion. Patients who have flexor tendon synovitis have difficulty initiating or completing interphalangeal joint flexion,

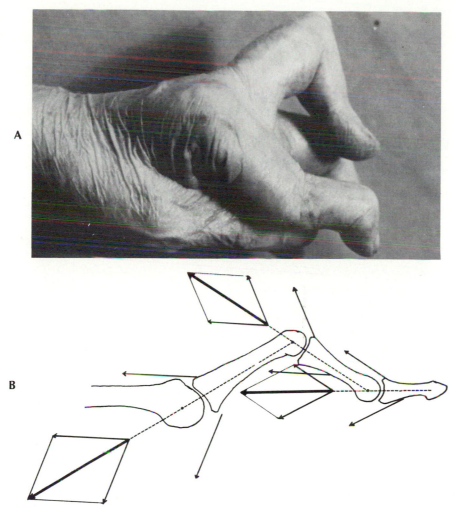

FIG. 58-5. Boutonnière deformity of digits. **A,** In rheumatoid arthritis this deformity usually occurs through weakening of capsular and bony attachments and relative lengthening of central tendon by destructive synovial invasion. Lateral tendons are subluxated palmad. **B,** Once collapse deformity is established, resultant axial forces further aggravate deformity.

either because of pain or because of mechanical restriction of the flexor tendons. The flexor tendons then concentrate most of their power on the metacarpophalangeal joints. This posture of the digit facilitates the pull of the intrinsic muscles to the central tendon across the dorsal aspect of the proximal interphalangeal joint. The failure of proximal interphalangeal flexion therefore gives a greater opportunity for the intrinsic muscles to provide imbalancing forces to the extensor aspect of the joint. The presence of hyperplastic synovium in the proximal interphalangeal joint and its volar pouch further prevents flexion and causes loosening of the attachments of the palmar plate and the accessory collateral ligaments, thus allowing hyperextension of the joint. Treatment programs for this severely disabling deformity must first be directed at the flexor tendon synovitis. Correction of the hyperextension deformity of the proximal interphalangeal joint through readjustment of the balance of the joint system becomes the main problem.

There is a tendency for perpetuation of the collapse deformity by axially directed forces, resulting in further im-

balance of the linked motor system for the chain of joints. As hyperextension deformity is increased, the transverse fibers of the retinacular ligament are stretched out, allowing the lateral tendons to subluxate dorsally, which further magnifies the deforming power through its extensor pull, now located above the center of the axis of rotation of the joint. The oblique retinacular ligaments are stretched, a relative lengthening of the lateral tendons occurs, and the distal interphalangeal joint becomes flexed by the pull of the flexor profundus tendon. Other deforming forces can increase the mechanical advantage of the extensor pull. Palmar subluxation of the metacarpophalangeal joint or the wrist joint, or contracture of the wing-inserted intrinsic muscles secondary to a chronic flexion deformity of the metacarpophalangeal joint, will further accentuate the swan-neck deformity. The failure of the long flexor tendons to flex the proximal interphalangeal joint results in permanent joint stiffness. Further destructive changes result in complete joint disorganization and subluxation.

The events taking place in the development of the swan-

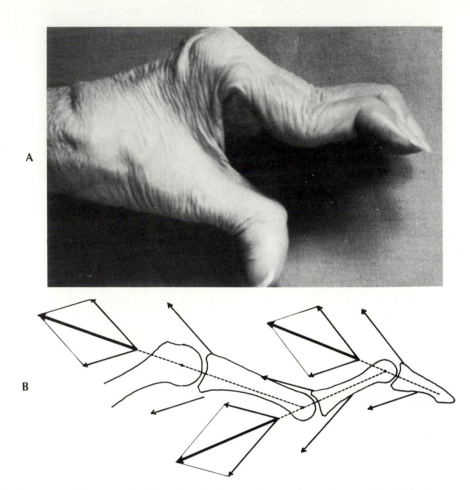

FIG. 58-6. Swan-neck deformity. **A,** This deformity is usually caused, in rheumatoid arthritis, by synovitis of flexor tendon sheaths, which results in restriction of interphalangeal joint flexion. Flexor power becomes concentrated in metacarpophalangeal joint, and in this position intrinsic muscle pull on central tendon is facilitated, resulting in unbalancing of forces to extensor aspect of joint. Hyperextension of middle phalanx on proximal phalanx occurs. **B,** Axially directed forces further aggravate collapse deformity. Lateral tendons become subluxated dorsally above axis of rotation of joint.

neck deformity in rheumatoid arthritis can be summarized as follows:

1. Synovitis of flexor tendon sheath
2. Increased flexion pull on the metacarpophalangeal joint
3. Imbalance to the extensor central slip through the long extensor tendons and the intrinsic muscles
4. Stretch of palmar plate of proximal interphalangeal joint
5. Hyperextension of proximal interphalangeal joint
6. Stretching of transverse fibers of retinacular ligament
7. Dorsal subluxation of lateral tendons
8. Reciprocal flexion of distal interphalangeal joint
9. Joint disorganization

Metacarpophalangeal joint

Deformities of the metacarpophalangeal joint in rheumatoid arthritis are usually manifested by increased ulnar drift and palmar subluxation (Fig. 58-7). The metacarpophalangeal joint is potentially unstable if normal muscle balance is lost or if the restraining structures of the ligament

system are destroyed by rheumatoid disease. The metacarpophalangeal joint differs from the interphalangeal joints in that its movements are not simply flexion and extension movements but also involve some degree of rotation, abduction, and adduction. The metacarpophalangeal joint, because of its complex movements, which are almost constant during functional adaptations of the hand, is subjected to greater stresses. The extensor tendon expansions across the dorsum of the joint are loosely fixed and are vulnerable to disruption. The flexor tendon mechanism and its supporting structures are more complex. The capsule and ligaments of the metacarpophalangeal joint are distended and weakened by the rheumatoid process. Forces generated by the long flexor tendons across the fibrous sheath during pinch and grasp activities may act adversely to produce elongation of the supporting accessory collateral ligaments. The palmad and ulnad displaced flexor tendons produce further deforming forces (Fig. 58-8). The intrinsic muscles, which form a bridge between the extensor and flexor systems and, at the same time, provide direct flexor power across the metacarpophalangeal joint, can become deforming elements once

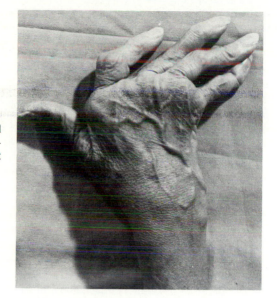

FIG. 58-7. Most common deformities occurring in rheumatoid arthritis are ulnar drift and palmar subluxation at metacarpophalangeal joints. Note swan-neck and boutonnière deformities present in digits.

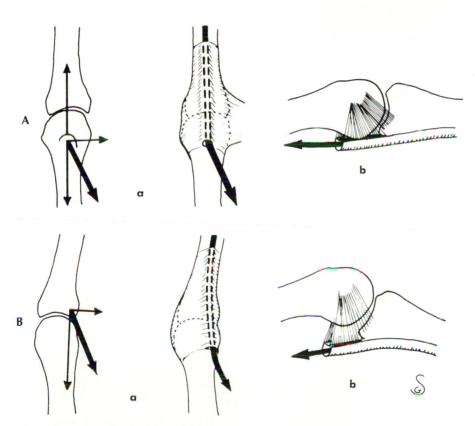

FIG. 58-8. A, Common flexor tendons enter fibrous sheath at an angle, and forces produced by their action have ulnar and palmar component. In normal stable metacarpophalangeal joint, ulnar component has little or no displacement effect, *a*, and resistance of capsule and ligaments prevents displacement of sheath inlet, *b*. **B,** When capsule and ligaments of metacarpophalangeal joint are distended and weakened by rheumatoid process, resistance to these deforming forces is lost. Point of reflection of sheath is displaced distally, ulnad and palmad. Base of proximal phalanx is displaced ulnad, *a*, and palmad, *b*, by action of ulnar component of this force. This mechanism is especially deforming at level of index and middle fingers.

the restraining structures of the metacarpophalangeal joint have been lengthened by the rheumatoid disease. Increased mobility of the fourth and fifth metacarpals is seen frequently in rheumatoid arthritis (Fig. 58-9). It is attributable to ligament loosening at the carpometacarpal joints and to the dysfunction of the extensor carpi ulnaris, as seen in the ulnar head syndrome. The increased breadth of the hand in metacarpophalangeal joint flexion causes ulnad displacing forces to be applied to the extensor tendons through their juncturae tendinum. When the extrinsic extensor tendon across the metacarpophalangeal joint has become displaced ulnad, the balance of the intrinsic extensor tendons is lost. The intrinsic muscles will then further aggravate the tendency toward volar subluxation of the metacarpophalangeal joint and toward ulnar drift of the digits. The normal mechanical advantage of the ulnar intrinsic muscles is greatly increased once the deformity is established. Normally the metacarpal heads are symmetric and present an ulnad slope, especially in the index and middle fingers. The collateral ligaments also show an asymmetry that allows ulnar drift to occur. Wrist deformities and ruptured extensor tendons play a secondary role in further aggravating the metacarpophalangeal joint disturbances. Once ulnar deviation and palmar subluxation have occurred, muscle pull and forces developed in functional activities and by gravity further accentuate the deformity.

The many anatomic and pathologic entities that play a role in creating deformities at the metacarpophalangeal joints are summarized as follows:

1. Normal anatomic asymmetry of second and third metacarpal heads
2. Unequal lengths of ulnar and radial collateral ligaments
3. Wing attachment of ulnar interosseous muscles of the index and middle fingers
4. Forces applied in an ulnar direction on the digits in pinch and grasp activities
5. Postural forces of gravity
6. Hypothenar muscle imbalance to ulnar side of the little finger
7. Attrition of collateral ligaments and bone erosion by the synovitis of the rheumatoid process
8. Stretching of accessory collateral ligaments
9. Synovitis of flexor tendon sheath
10. Subluxation of flexor tendons ulnad
11. Subluxation of extensor tendons ulnad
12. Subluxation of intrinsic tendons volarly
13. Radial deviation and pronation of the wrist
14. Contracture and fixation of intrinsic and extrinsic muscles
15. Associated joint deformities

Thumb ray

The following disabilities are usually seen in the rheumatoid thumb:

1. Postural deformities
   a. Longitudinal collapse deformities
      (1) Boutonnière (primary metacarpophalangeal joint disturbance)
      (2) Swan-neck (primary carpometacarpal joint disturbance)
      (3) Other
   b. Fixed positional deformities
      (1) Adducted retropositioned thumb
      (2) Other
2. Unstable, stiff, or painful joints
   a. Interphalangeal joint
   b. Metacarpophalangeal joint
   c. Carpometacarpal joint
3. Tendon disabilities (contracture, displacement, rupture)
   a. Flexor pollicis longus
   b. Extensor pollicis longus
   c. Extensor pollicis brevis

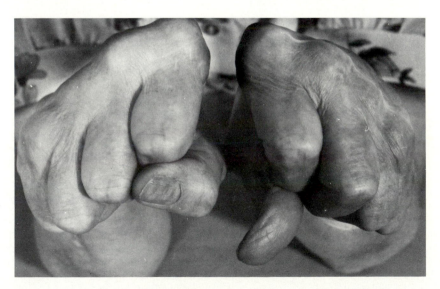

Fig. 58-9. There is increased mobility of fourth and fifth digits in rheumatoid arthritis because of ligamentous loosening at carpometacarpal joints and dysfunction of extensor carpi ulnaris in ulnar head syndrome. Resulting increased breadth of transverse arch can be cause of ulnar displacement of extensor tendons through pull on their juncturae tendinum.

d. Abductor pollicis longus

e. Intrinsics

Boutonnière deformity. The most common collapse deformity of the thumb is the boutonnière deformity. Initially, the joint capsule and extensor apparatus around the metacarpophalangeal joint are stretched out by a synovitis process. The extensor pollicis longus tendon and adductor expansion are displaced ulnad. The lateral thenar expansions are displaced radially in relation to the metacarpophalangeal joint. The attachment of the extensor pollicis brevis tendon to the base of the proximal phalanx is lengthened and becomes ineffective. The ability to extend the metacarpophalangeal joint is decreased and results in a flexion deformity of the proximal phalanx. The long extensor tendon and the extensor insertions of the intrinsic muscles apply all their power to the distal joint and produce hyperextension deformity of the distal joint. Pinch movements further accentuate the deformity, and a vicious circle is established: the more the flexion of the metacarpophalangeal joint, the great-

er the tendency for the interphalangeal joint to hyperextend and the thumb ray to collapse (Fig. 58-10). There is a failure of extension of the metacarpophalangeal joint attributable to loss of power of the extrinsic extensor tendon. In time, as contractures occur, the deformity becomes fixed. Destructive articular changes compound the deformity, and disorganization and subluxation of the joint may occur.

Swan-neck deformity. The swan-neck deformity of the thumb is usually initiated by synovitis of the carpometacarpal joint, followed by stretching of the joint capsule and radialward subluxation of the base of the metacarpal. Abduction becomes painful and a degree of adductor muscle spasm occurs. This imbalance of forces results in an adduction deformity of the metacarpal with contracture of the adductor pollicis muscle.

As abduction of the thumb becomes more difficult, the distal joints are used to compensate for the lack of movement at the base of the thumb. This may result in hyperextension of the interphalangeal joint, but more frequently of the meta-

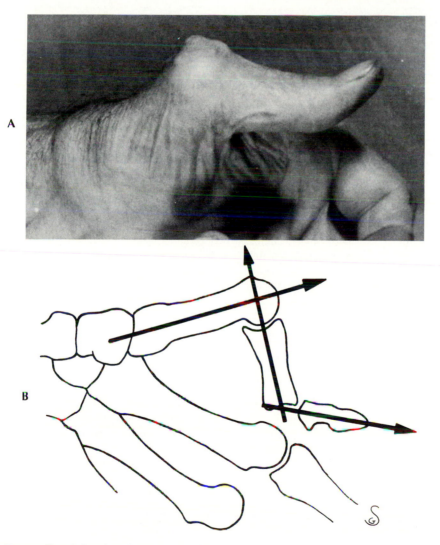

FIG. 58-10. Boutonnière deformity of thumb. **A,** This deformity is common occurrence in rheumatoid arthritis and starts as synovitis of metacarpophalangeal joint. **B,** Pinch movements of functional adaptations accentuate deformity, and vicious circle of deformity is established.

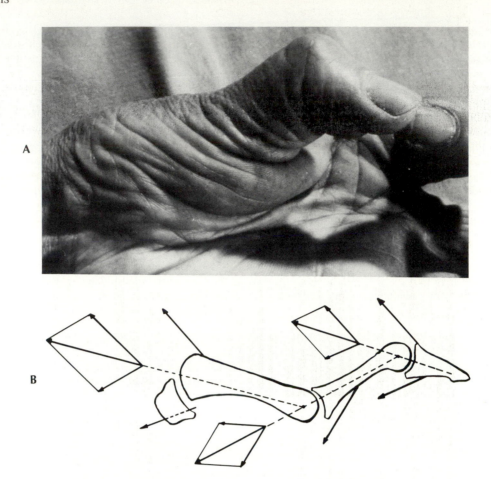

FIG. 58-11. Swan-neck deformity of thumb. **A,** This deformity is usually initiated by synovitis of carpometacarpal joint. It may be accompanied by adduction contracture of first metacarpal joint and subluxation of carpometacarpal joint. **B,** Forces developed in this deformity are self-aggravating. As deformity increases in one segment, it aggravates deformities in other segments.

carpophalangeal joint and adduction of the first metacarpal. A vicious circle of deformity ensues. Further hyperextension of the metacarpophalangeal joint aggravates the adduction tendency of the first metacarpal. This promotes increasing lateral subluxation of the carpometacarpal joint and contracture of the adductor muscle. The interphalangeal joint becomes flexed similarly as in a swan-neck deformity of the finger. The deformity is self-perpetuating, and as it increases in one segment, it is aggravated in associated areas (Fig. 58-11). Occasionally severe erosive changes in the carpometacarpal joint and absorption of the trapezium occur. This decompresses the joint, and the severity of the collapse deformity is decreased.

Adducted retropositioned thumb. The adducted retropositioned thumb deformity is seen in less than 5% of the rheumatoid patients and presents difficult treatment problems. Typically the thumb metacarpal is retropositioned, adducted, and externally rotated. It appears that the deformity is initiated by a synovitis at the carpometacarpal joint. Awkward positioning of the thumb on a flat board during acute illness can result in a permanent deformity. The ability of the extensor pollicis longus muscle to adduct and externally rotate the metacarpal is predominant. Palmar and radial subluxation of the metacarpal off the trapezium

occurs. Consequently the patient has difficulty abducting the metacarpal and may develop an abduction deformity at the metacarpophalangeal joint by stretching the ulnar collateral ligament in grasp activities.

Unstable, stiff, or painful joint. Instability, stiffness, or pain at the interphalangeal, metacarpophalangeal, or carpometacarpal joint may occur as isolated deformities in rheumatoid arthritis, resulting from synovial invasion and erosive changes of the bone or may be seen in association with other deformities (Fig. 58-12). These deformities are accentuated by the forces applied during pinch activities. Gross destruction of the distal joint may occur also in the late stages of the boutonnière deformity.

Tendon disabilities. Tendon disabilities in the rheumatoid thumb may be related to muscle contracture, tendon displacement, adhesions, or ruptures, similar to that seen in the other digits in the rheumatoid hand.

The extensor pollicis longus tendon is the most commonly ruptured tendon in the rheumatoid thumb; this occurs most often within the third extensor compartment in the area of Lister's tubercle. The rupture of this tendon results in a sudden drop of the thumb metacarpophalangeal joint and some loss of extensor power at the distal phalanx. The deformity may be confused with the boutonnière deformity,

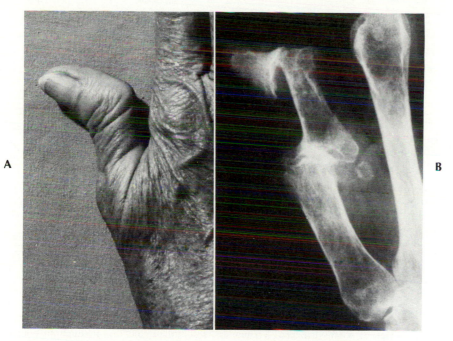

FIG. 58-12. Instability of distal joint of thumb. **A,** Lesions of distal joint of thumb may occur as isolated deformities because of synovial invasion and erosive changes and are accentuated by forces applied during pinch movements. **B,** Roentgenogram showing destruction and subluxation of distal interphalangeal and metacarpophalangeal joints of thumb.

which is also an extrinsic-minus problem; the hyperextension of the distal joint is, however, not so prominent. The lack of extension of the metacarpophalangeal joint is usually associated with less flexion contracture, and, most importantly, the long extensor tendon cannot be prominently palpated on the back of the hand in forced extension and retroposition of the thumb.

Rupture of the flexor pollicis longus is not rare and must be considered in any hyperextended interphalangeal deformity of the thumb. This frequently occurs at the entrance of the digital flexor canal. Careful examination of active flexion will differentiate the hyperextended interphalangeal joint of the thumb from that of the ruptured flexor pollicis longus.

Ruptures of the abductor pollicis longus and extensor pollicis brevis are rare. Disability of the intrinsics usually results from their displacement and secondary contracture caused by synovial invasion and stretching of the dorsal hood of the metacarpophalangeal joint of the thumb. The intrinsic attachment to the dorsal hood is consequently displaced palmad, and this results in a distortion of its normal function.

The wrist

The wrist is the key joint for proper function of the hand. The wrist joints and surrounding soft tissues are frequently affected by rheumatoid arthritis. Roentgenographic evidence of arthritic changes was noted in 65% of the rheumatoid wrists studied. Clinically, pain or loss of movement from associated synovitis was present in an even greater percentage of cases. Involvement may be seen early in the course of the disease in the radiocarpal, intercarpal, or radioulnar joints, or in a combination of these joints.

Typical deformities seen in rheumatoid wrists are flexion, pronation, radial or ulnar deviation, palmar subluxation, and associated dorsal subluxation of the ulnar head. Active flexion and rotation movements of the wrist joint are very important for functional adaptations in the normal hand and even more so when digital disabilities are present.

Anatomy. Flexion, extension, and radial and ulnar deviation movements at the wrist occur in both the radiocarpal and midcarpal joints. The proximal carpal row includes the scaphoid, lunate, and triquetrum bones and links the forearm to the distal carpal row and hand. The scaphoid and lunate bones articulate with facets on the radius and also with the triangular fibrocartilage bridging the radius and ulna. These bones are united by means of interosseous ligaments. The distal row of carpal bones includes the trapezium, trapezoid, capitate, and hamate. These bones are also linked by interosseous ligaments. The articulation between the proximal and distal carpal row forms the midcarpal joint. The volar radiocarpal and dorsal radiocarpal ligaments are extremely important to support the carpal area. The fibers of the volar radiocarpal ligament extends distally and obliquely from the radius, the triangular fibrocartilage, and the styloid process of the ulna (Fig. 58-13). A symmetric pattern is formed by its insertions into the scaphoid, lunate, triquetrum, and capitate bones. Short, deep ligamentous bands connect the trapezium and trapezoid to the scaphoid and the hamate to the triquetrum. The ulnar and radial collateral ligaments provide some lateral wrist stability. The dorsal ligamentous structures are not so dense as the volar ones. The dorsal radiocarpal ligament is connected intimately with the fibrous channels of the digital long extensor tendons located above.

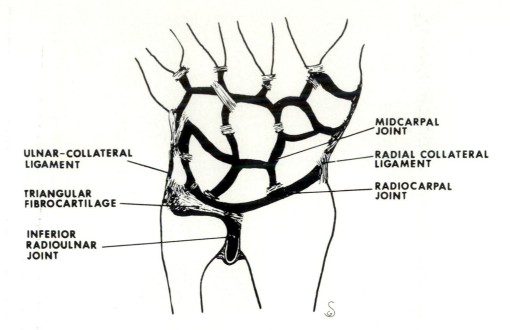

ULNAR-COLLATERAL
LIGAMENT

TRIANGULAR
FIBROCARTILAGE

INFERIOR
RADIOULNAR
JOINT

MIDCARPAL
JOINT

RADIAL COLLATERAL
LIGAMENT

RADIOCARPAL
JOINT

FIG. 58-13. Relationships of wrist ligaments. Triangular fibrocartilage and its important ligamentous attachments between distal radius and ulna are commonly destroyed in early synovial invasion in rheumatoid arthritis, which allows instability of distal radioulnar joint.

Physiology of movements. Ulnar and radial deviation of the wrist occurs mainly at the radiocarpal joint. However, because a bony crest separates the distal radial surface in two concavities and a strong interosseous ligament unites the scaphoid and lunate bones, about 20% of radial deviation movements also arise at the midcarpal joint, mainly around the head of the capitate.

During wrist extension, the first two thirds of movement are principally located at the radiocarpal joint and the last third at the midcarpal joint. In flexion approximately the first half of excursion occurs at the midcarpal level, and the rest at the radiocarpal level. As noted, the scaphoid bone bridges the midcarpal joint. However, from a functional point of view, the midcarpal joint continues distally between the trapezium, trapezoid bones, and adjacent surfaces of the first and second metacarpals; the thumb, trapezium, and scaphoid act as a unit that plays only a small part in midcarpal movements. Motion around the scaphoid takes place in all three body planes: vertically at its proximal pole, horizontally at the distal pole, and coronally at the scaphoid-capitate articulation.

Integrated movements of the radiocarpal and midcarpal joints are made possible by important displacements of the carpal bones. The shape of the proximal carpal row changes in various hand positions, and the shape of the second carpal row becomes modified accordingly. Link systems are present in the hand as they are in the digits. Proper balance of this link system is dependent on the shape of bones and the integrity and tension of their ligaments. Normal functional adaptations and muscle pull apply external strains across the system. However, when the building blocks or their important ligamentous connections are destroyed, the wrist system can no longer tolerate these external forces and collapses into deformities.

Collapse mechanisms. The proximal carpal row represents a link between the region of the forearm and the distal carpal row and hand. If the midcarpal joint becomes unstable, the lunate rotates dorsally and the capitate becomes hyperflexed. The resultant shortening of the long axis of the carpus causes rotation of the scaphoid, which usually is seen only in normal radial deviation. Instability of the midcarpal joint may follow a hyperextension injury of the wrist in which the volar radiocarpal ligaments are partially ruptured and the joint capsule between the capitate, scaphoid, and lunate bones is damaged. In extreme cases of instability the scaphoid dislocates spontaneously and shifts horizontally, so that its distal articular surface points straight forward. Carpal stability is most vulnerable in dorsiflexion and ulnar deviation. Collapse deformity of the wrist can also occur after dislocations of the lunate or loosening of ligaments of the wrist by an arthritic process.

Radiocarpal joint. The multiple-link system of the wrist is disturbed in rheumatoid arthritis as a result of the loosening of ligamentous structures and deformation of bones by the destructive synovitis. In some cases spontaneous fusion will occur before subluxation, and in severe cases a complete dislocation of the wrist may result (Fig. 58-14). Loosening of the ligaments on the radial aspect of the joint is common and will allow an ulnar displacement of the proximal carpal row, resulting secondarily in a radial deviation of the hand on the forearm. The associated subluxation of the distal radioulnar joint causes a loss of stability on the ulnar aspect of the wrist. In some cases loosening of the volar radiocarpal ligament disrupts the longitudinal axis and is followed by a buckling phenomenon. A palmar subluxation of the proximal row on the radius is more common.

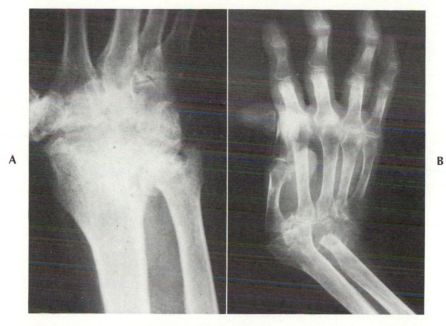

FIG. 58-14. A, Disabilities of wrist joints are very common and are seen early in rheumatoid arthritis. Erosive and cystic changes, collapse of bone, fusion, and subluxation—all may occur in same wrist in either radiocarpal, midcarpal, intercarpal, or distal radioulnar joint. This rheumatoid patient's wrist shows all these roentgenographic findings. **B,** Severe erosive changes occur in radiocarpal joint, with dysfunction of ligaments, absorption of bone, and wrist subluxation, usually with hand deviating palmad and ulnad.

Rheumatoid arthritic changes in the radiocarpal joint are frequent and may be summarized as follows:

1. Erosions in the intercarpal and radiocarpal area, with fusion or fibrosis, or both, and associated stiffness
2. Ulnad shift of the carpus and the radius, which may or may not result in radiad deviation of the hand
3. Palmar subluxation of the carpus on the ulna, with associated absorptive changes in the proximal carpal row
4. Occasional ulnad dislocation of the hand off the radius, which is usually associated with pronounced instability and serious loss of function

Distal radioulnar joint. Rotation is the most important component for adapting the wrist joint to movements of the hand. The distal radioulnar joint is therefore of great importance. Dysfunction of the distal radioulnar joint in rheumatoid arthritis is a common occurrence. Destructive synovitis at this joint sets off a chain of disabilities that impair the normal function of the wrist and hand. Bäckdahl has described this problem very well in his comprehensive essay *The Caput Ulnae Syndrome in Rheumatoid Arthritis.* Approximately one third of our rheumatoid patients undergoing hand surgery had associated distal radioulnar disability, which is characterized clinically by the dorsal prominence and instability of the ulnar head, with increasing weakness of the wrist, pain and crepitation on movement, especially rotation, and decrease of rotation and dorsiflexion, and there may be an increased flexion of the fifth and fourth metacarpals because of the loss of the normal action of the extensor carpi ulnaris, which is displaced palmad, and ruptures of the extensor tendons of the little, ring, and long

fingers, which must be differentiated from the above (Fig. 58-15).

Dysfunction of the extensor carpi ulnaris in this syndrome is an important and frequently ignored problem that can lead to further imbalances in the complex musculoskeletal system disabilities of the rheumatoid hand. Normally the extensor carpi ulnaris acts in dorsiflexion and ulnar abduction of the wrist and helps stabilize the wrist during abduction and extension of the thumb and when the hand is opened for grasp. It also contracts during palmar flexion of the wrist, whereas the other extensors relax. The extensor carpi ulnaris crosses the dorsal surface of the distal ulna to assist in the stabilization of the wrist and to maintain the integrity of the distal radioulnar joint. It helps stabilize the fifth metacarpal through its insertion, and its dysfunction allows greater flexion of the fourth and fifth metacarpals, with secondary deformity and impaired finger function.

As the destructive synovial hypertrophy increases, the ligamentous support of the distal end of the ulna, formed mainly by the triangular fibrocartilage and its ligaments, the ulnar collateral ligament, and the surrounding capsule, undergoes attritional changes; the ulnar head can now dislocate to the line of least resistance dorsally. The sixth dorsal compartment is stretched by the synovial hypertrophy, and the extensor carpi ulnaris is subluxated ulnad and palmad.

Roentgenographic examination may show early dorsal subluxation and erosive changes of the ulnar head and the ulnar notch of the radius. The ulnar head loses its smooth rounded contour and becomes sharp and irregular. The ulnar styloid may become prominent or disappear, or severe absorptive changes of the distal ulna may occur. Extensor

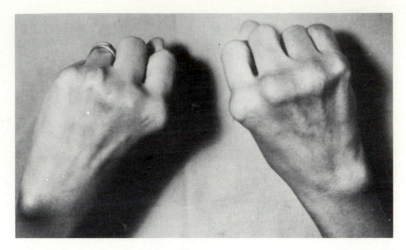

FIG. 58-15. Dorsal subluxation of ulnar head occurs early and commonly in rheumatoid arthritis. It is cause of painful disability that has many functional implications, such as described in ulnar head syndrome.

tendons may rupture over the jagged distal ulna or secondary to attritional changes from the invasive synovitis.

Any involvement through arthritic change or trauma that disturbs the integrity of the bones of the wrist or of their ligamentous support can result in severe functional disability. The problem in reconstruction and rehabilitation of the rheumatoid wrist is to regain stability and at the same time maintain the motion that is so important in functional adaptations of the hand.

The discussion of the pathogenesis of digital deformities in rheumatoid arthritis as given is useful for the surgeon who will be called on to do reconstructive surgery for these problems. We have noted that the changes are secondary to invasive characteristics of the pathologic proliferative synovitis, which distends the joint capsule, destroys ligament and tendon attachments, erodes the joint surfaces, and prevents gliding of the tendons. The disturbed balance of the linked tendon system and the collapse of the skeletal structures further aggravate the deformity.

59

Methods of assessment and management of the rheumatoid hand at the Institute of Rheumatology, Warsaw, Poland

MARIA MUSUR-GRIEVE

The therapist's management of rheumatoid arthritis must take into account the special characteristics of the disease, including its progressive inflammatory nature, the presence of pain, and multiple sites of involvement. Treatment must be dynamic and comprehensive to allow for the constant progress of the disease.

A comprehensive hand rehabilitation program should include the following:

1. Education of the patient regarding the causes of deformity as a result of the disease
2. Instruction in specific exercises, depending on the stage of development of deformities and whether the disease is currently active or in remission
3. Appropriate splinting
4. Education in principles of joint protection
5. Provision of self-help aids to aid joint protection and enable the patient to more easily perform work and other activities of daily living
6. Recommendation for adaptations within the home to enable the patient to live as normally as possible while protecting his joints

The goals of the rehabilitation program can be achieved only through the cooperation of the members of the team: patient, surgeon, rheumatologist, hand therapist, social worker, family of the patient, and others. The final result of a patient's rehabilitation program should be his ability to return to active social life or at least to reach his maximum level of independence.

EVALUATION OF THE RHEUMATOID HAND—A SIMPLE ASSESSMENT

Evaluation of the rheumatoid hand is difficult because of the variety of deformities that may be present and the variability of the clinical picture. The presence of pain will complicate the assessment.

At the Rehabilitation Department of the Institute of Rheumatology in Warsaw, assessment of function of the rheumatoid hand is carried out on the basis of the evaluation of three components of grip[13]:

1. Grasp strength—the ability to hold an object

2. Grip ability—the ability to adjust the fingers to the shape of the object being held
3. Dexterity—the ability to manipulate an object within a certain time period

If necessary, evaluations of sensibility, coordination, and activities of daily living are also carried out. The functional tests are administered by a hand therapist.

When this assessment method was developed at our institute, our aim was to develop a system of evaluating hand function that could be carried out in a busy department. It had to be simple so that equipment used might be easily duplicated. It was important to make the evaluation specific and objective so that the results could be graded and compared. The grading system used enables quick assessment of function before and after treatment.

The evaluation is carried out with the patient sitting comfortably in an adjustable chair at a table, with the elbow flexed at 90 degrees. The evaluation is always done between 11 AM and 2 PM. The patient's general feeling should be neither very bad nor very good; that is, it should be an "average" day for him.

Grasp-strength assessment

Grasp strength is tested with a spring, clockwork dynamometer that has interchangeable handgrips covered with rubber (Fig. 59-1). Cylindric and hook grasps are assessed and recorded as power grips, while pinch is recorded as a precision grip. The patient repeats the test three times by pulling the handgrip with maximum force. The highest value is recorded.

Grip-ability assessment

Grip ability is evaluated with test objects that are cylindric or spheric in shape (Fig. 59-2). The ability to assume cylindric grip, five-fingered pinch, and ball grip is evaluated according to the principle given by Seyfried;[9] that is, adherence of the whole palm and fingers to the test object is scored as 100% grip ability, with each finger contributing 20% of the total grip.

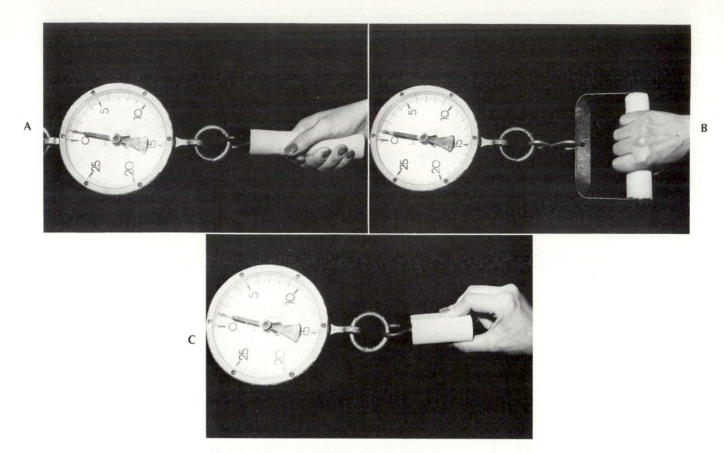

FIG. 59-1. Grasp strength tested with spring clockwork dynamometer that has interchangeable hand grip covered with rubber.

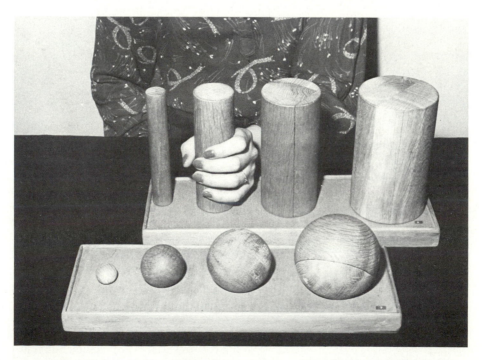

FIG. 59-2. Cylindric and spheric test objects used to evaluate grip ability.

Dexterity assessment

Dexterity is assessed by tests that may or may not incorporate resistance. The dexterity test with resistance requires that the patient turn the knob of a padlock to the right and to the left until it resists. The padlock is of typical dimensions (Fig. 59-3, *A*). When turned, it has a resistance of 1 kg. The test is repeated three times for 10 seconds each time. The largest number of turns made during any of the 10-second intervals is recorded as the score. In the test with no resistance the patient is asked to gather balls that are 1.8 cm in diameter and to throw them into a hollow in the testing board. The balls are arranged in five rows of six balls each, set 4 cm apart (Fig. 59-3, *B*). One ball is picked up at a

time and thrown. The test is repeated three times for 10 seconds each time, and the maximum number of balls thrown into the hole within 10 seconds is recorded as the score.

In the dexterity test without resistance, the patient is instructed to put scattered matches one after another into a box (Fig. 59-3, *C*). The test is performed three times for 10 seconds each time. The maximal amount of matches put into the box within 10 seconds is considered to be the score.

•   •   •

While one is carrying out this functional test, pain is an important factor that must be taken into account and scored: mild pain is indicated by '' + ,'' moderate pain by '' + + ,'' and severe pain by '' + + + .''

A method of comparing the findings was worked out. The mean value found in the control group was considered

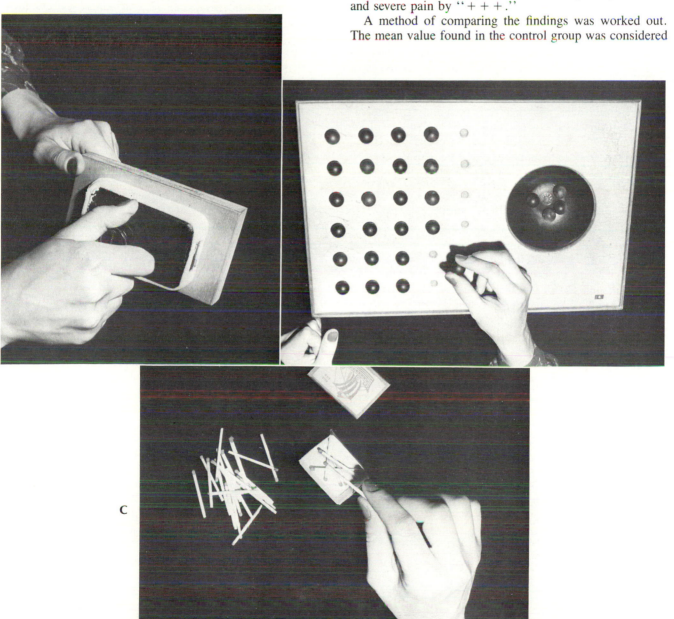

FIG. 59-3. Dexterity assessment. **A,** With resistance. **B** and **C,** Without resistance.

to be the norm. The results were expressed in points. The range of points obtained, called the functional index, was established for each of the three parameters, that is, grasp strength, grip ability, and dexterity. Nine hundred points represents the average values of function in a healthy hand, where 300 points are contributed by grasp strength (three grasps, 100 points each), 300 points are contributed by grip ability (three kinds of grip, 100 points each), and 300 points are contributed by dexterity (100 points for each subtest).

Four degrees of hand function were established according to the total number of points obtained by the patient,[8] as follows:

I 701 to 900 points
II 601 to 700 points
III 501 to 600 points
IV Up to 500 points

This numerical scale allows for comparison of results obtained in a rheumatoid hand with a norm and allows for assessment of improvement or deterioration in the hand within the particular parameters of grip and in general.

Various groups of patients with rheumatoid arthritis were examined with this functional test, including 220 patients from the Institute of Rheumatology, 60 patients from the Disabled Men's Cooperatives,[1,5] and 24 young people suffering from juvenile rheumatoid arthritis.[10] Results of these tests provided information about the capability of the rheumatoid hand.

Capability of rheumatoid arthritic hands

Grasp strength in rheumatoid patients is about one third of grasp strength in healthy people, because of deformities and pain. Correlation of strength with the radiologic stage has shown the dependence of strength on the latter. The strength of hands with radiologic changes characteristic of Steinbrocker's radiologic stages I and II[15] was essentially different from that characteristic of radiologic stages III and IV (Table 59-1). The grasp strength of the rheumatoid hands in stages I and II decreases to 50% of that exhibited by those in the control group and in stages III and IV decreases

to 21% of the strength in the control group. In view of these findings a practical conclusion can be drawn: work requiring even slight hand strength may be undertaken only by the rheumatoid arthritic patient with changes characteristic of radiologic stages I and II. The patient with changes characteristic of stages III and IV should not be involved in work that requires grip strength.

Grip ability in the rheumatoid hand becomes limited as pathologic changes within the hand advance. Ability to grasp is most influenced by the thumb. The larger the cross section of the object to be grasped, the greater the difficulty in grasping. A spheric object with a diameter of 50 mm or a cylindric object with a diameter of 35 mm was found to be most favorable for grasping. Assessment of results of the dexterity test in rheumatoid patients shows that manipulatory operations are performed most skillfully when resistance is not required. This finding suggests an important conclusion concerning the employment of the rheumatoid patient. A job that consists in carrying small, light objects that are to be sorted, placed, or assembled within a small work area can be recommended for the rheumatoid arthritic patient. However, a job requiring manipulation with hand wheels, knobs, or handles, even if they offer a small resistance of 1 kg, is inadvisable for these patients. In general, the dexterity of rheumatoid arthritic patients amounts to 75% of that found in the control group.

Capability of hands in juvenile rheumatoid arthritis

The hands of young patients 15 to 18 years of age were tested, and the results obtained were compared with those found in a control group of young people of the same age. The patient group consisted of 6 boys and 16 girls, and the control group consisted of 30 boys and 30 girls. Comparative analysis showed that the grasp strength in patients with juvenile rheumatoid arthritis amounted to 63%, grip ability to 91%, and dexterity to 82% of the respective values found in healthy hands. It has been found that the parameters of hand grip are evidently dependent on the advancement of

TABLE 59-1. Classification of rheumatoid progression

Stage	Roentgenologic signs	Muscle atrophy	Extraarticular lesions (nodules, tenovaginitis)	Joint deformity	Ankylosis
I	Osteoporosis, sometimes no destructive changes	0	0	0	0
II	Osteoporosis; slight cartilage or subchondral bone destruction may be present	Adjacent	May be present	0	0
III	Osteoporosis; cartilage destruction bone destruction	Extensive	May be present	Subluxation; ulnar deviation and/or hyperextension	0
IV	Same as III with bony ankylosis	Extensive	May be present	Same as III	Fibrous or bony ankylosis

From Steinbrocker, O., Traeger, C.H., and Batterman, R.C.: J.A.M.A. **140**:659-662, May-Aug. 1949.

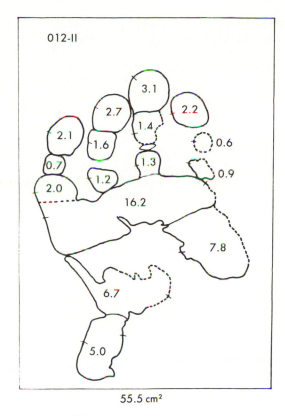

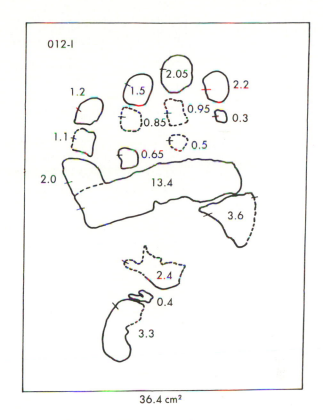

FIG. 59-6. Contourgrams of two palm prints made during squeezing of 50 mm diameter cylinder with maximum strength.

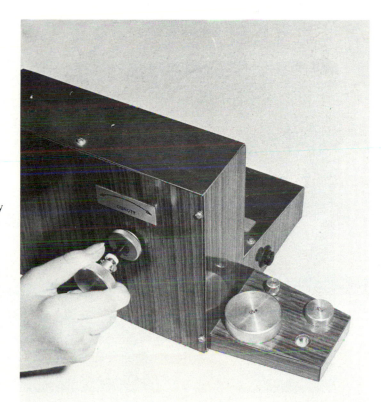

FIG. 59-7. Dexterimeter used for dexterity tests in patients with rheumatoid arthritis.

rected, decreased grip strength, and limited mobility. Radiologically these hands fall into Steinbrocker's stages II and III.[15]

Specific problems observed
1. Joint instability
2. Imbalance of extensor and flexor forces. Most often extension is decreased and there is a tendency toward flexion contracture of the fingers.
3. Collateral ligament contracture resulting in a decrease in flexion of the metacarpophalangeal joints. The contraction of these ligaments is manifested by the decrease of finger abduction with simultaneous limitation of flexion.[7]
4. Beginning of intrinsic muscle contracture
5. Initiation of visible deformities, such as ulnar drift, swan neck, and boutonnière
6. Limited mobility in the thumb joint
7. Lesions and pain within the wrist greatly affecting the function of the whole hand

General aims of treatment
1. Maintenance of range of motion and muscle strength
2. When limitation of flexion occurs simultaneously with a decrease of finger abduction, abduction stretching should be begun, followed by active assistive abduction and finally active abduction-adduction movements (Fig. 59-8). Only when abduction motion is obtained can flexion of the metacarpophalangeal joints be performed.
3. Maintenance and improvement of mobility in all thumb joints and particularly the carpometacarpal joint
4. Maintenance of range of motion and, of paramount importance, stability of the wrist joints
5. Maintenance of the transverse arches to decrease both ulnar deviation and swan-neck deformities. During exercise, the resistance should be appropriate to the hand-strength ability. Recommended exercises are those that use sponges of different shapes and sizes (Fig. 59-9), especially a ball-shaped sponge, which when adjusted to the hand arches prevents joint dislocation (Fig. 59-10). Exercise that requires the use of force on the finger pulp should be applied with caution; otherwise, in the case of unstable joints, such exercise may intensify the deformities.
6. Functional splints, resting splints, splints to stabilize joints, and splints to correct deformities are very important in this group.
7. Provision of adaptive equipment to help prevent deformities and allow for greater independence in work and activities of daily living (Fig. 59-11)
8. Patient education regarding the prevention of further deformities, joint conservation, use and maintenance of splints, and use of adaptive devices
9. Education of the family regarding the patient's needs and to what extent he requires assistance, as well as how to encourage him to be independent and how to adapt the home to his illness

Because of the coexistence of various deformities not only in each patient but also in each particular finger, an exact analysis of each hand of each patient should be done. Then, taking into consideration "general aims" for this group, one can work out a hand therapy program dependent on the patient's needs and deformities. Exercises performed while the splints are on the hand are suggested to help the patient get used to the splints and to encourage him to use them in

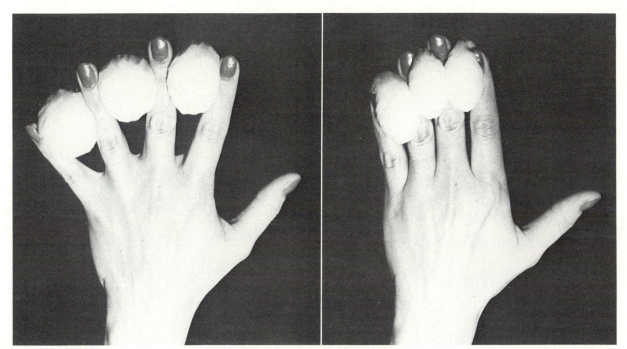

Fig. 59-8. Abductive and adductive exercises with use of ball-shaped sponges.

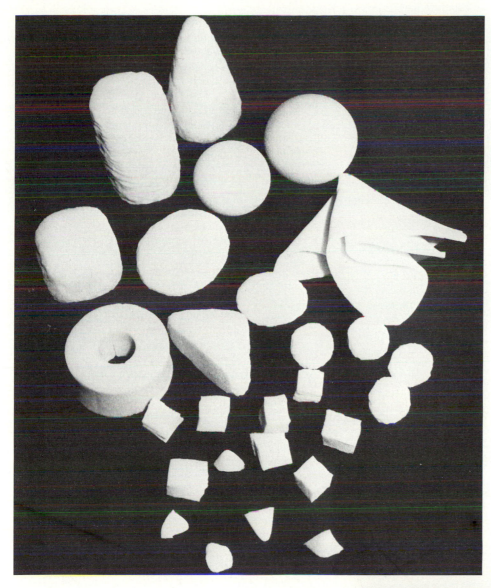

FIG. 59-9. Variety of shapes and sizes of sponges used to exercise hand.

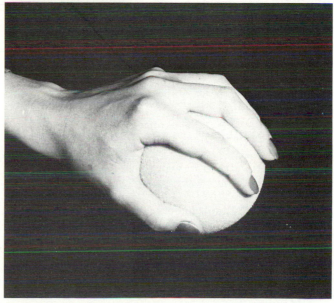

FIG. 59-10. Ball-shaped sponge adjusted to hand arches to prevent joint dislocation.

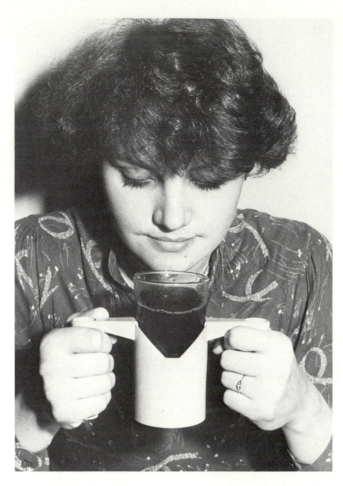

FIG. 59-11. Glass holder designed for use by patient with rheumatoid arthritis.

activities of daily living and work activities to stabilize the joints and to minimize deforming forces on the joints.

Group III

Group III is characterized by the presence of visibly established hand deformities that can be corrected passively. The impairment of hand function is advanced. The breakdown of hand arches is evident, as is the progression of destructive processes in the whole hand. Radiologically these hands belong in Steinbrocker's stage III.[15]

Problems observed

1. Joint instability of the digits and thumbs, resulting in difficulty in grasp and limited grip strength
2. Limited mobility of the carpometacarpal joint of the thumb, resulting in overcompensation in the remaining thumb joints and also causing hypermobility leading to inversion
3. Lesions and contractures of the hand intrinsic muscles, leading to difficulty in adjusting the hand to an object
4. Various deformities, unequally advanced in each particular finger
5. Lesions, instability, and contractures within the wrist, having a profound effect on the function of the whole hand

General aims of treatment

1. Improvement of mobility in the carpometacarpal joint of the thumb. In case of a strong tendency to stiffness in this joint, a resting splint should favor opposition for maximum function. Surgical intervention is frequently necessary in such a case.
2. Maintenance of maximum flexion and extension of all joints of the fourth and fifth fingers and good stability in the thumb and second and third finger joints. The necessary range of motion in metacarpophalangeal and proximal interphalangeal joints of the second and third fingers is 45 to 60 degrees, to enable manipulation (Fig. 59-12).
3. Correction of existing deformities
4. Maintenance of wrist joint stability
5. Use of appropriate splints to attempt to avoid progression of deformities
6. Proper selection of assistive devices for activities of daily living, with a view to each particular patient's deformities.
7. Patient education regarding the use of the self-help devices, joint protection, energy conservation, and how to live with his disability
8. Education of the family regarding the above

As in group II, it is necessary to make a thorough analysis of the hand deformities and to recognize the patient's needs before a hand therapy program is worked out.

Group IV

Group IV is characterized by the presence of deformities that cannot be corrected by conservative treatment. Radiologically these hands belong in Steinbrocker's radiologic stages III and IV.[15] Surgical treatment is usually necessary.

General aims of treatment

1. Patient education regarding independence in activities of daily living and, if necessary, use of self-help devices
2. Exercise to maintain/increase digital extension to maximize grip opening
3. Increase in grip strength
4. Splinting of an unstable joint
5. Education of the patient's family

• • •

From the practical and therapeutic points of view it was necessary to divide the rheumatoid patients into four groups according to the severity of the deformities. The activity of the disease is as well a very important factor. When a very high activity is manifested in the hands, as evidenced by swelling, local rise in temperature, and pain, resting splints are suggested, and carefully performed passive exercises are carried out in short sessions several times during the day. At a moderate activity level of disease, active exercises without resistance should be performed several times a day. The activity of the disease and the severity of the deformities should be decisive factors in working out the hand therapy program and determining its intensity for each particular patient.

The importance of teamwork and the necessity of for-

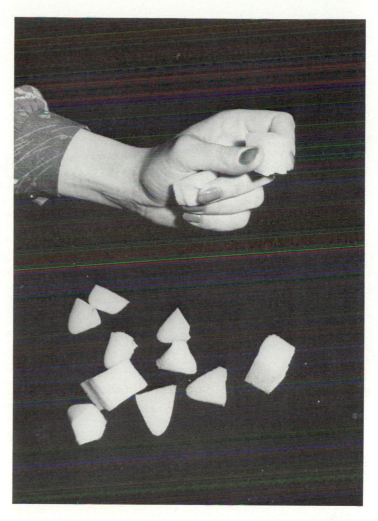

FIG. 59-12. An exercise to increase ability to manipulate small objects requires the patient to pick up small sponges with the thumb and index finger and transfer them to the third, fourth, and fifth fingers.

mulating an appropriate home program for the patient cannot be emphasized enough in regard to obtaining good results.

Splinting

It should be stressed from the beginning that the indiscriminate use of splinting on a rheumatoid hand may be of great harm to the patient instead of help. The decision to splint should be thoroughly analyzed, and if splinting appears to be indispensable, the choice of splint can be properly made only by use of a functional approach when one is analyzing the hand.

Seyfried[14] introduced four functional degrees of ulnar deviation:

1. Ulnar deviation of fingers visible, patient's active correction possible
2. Patient unable to correct the deviation actively, yet when helped (either with the other hand or by another person) can keep his fingers in a corrected position
3. Only passive correction possible
4. Deformity stabilized, even passive correction impossible

In fact, the above classification can be applied to other hand deformities. This classification suggests the following indications for splinting: With the first degree of ulnar deviation, the patient should be taught how to correct the deviation without any help. If given a splint to correct the deformity, the patient usually does not use it. With the fourth degree of ulnar deviation, if the deformity is already fixed and there is no chance for improvement, splinting should not be used because it will unnecessarily raise hopes. Splinting is most appropriate for the second or third degree of ulnar deviation. The best results can be expected with the second degree.

When applying these indications to the previously presented four groups of patients in hand therapy, one can observe that the splinting is most applicable for the groups II and III. With patients of group II, deformities can be successfully prevented, whereas with the group III patients it is only possible to check the progress of the deformities. Splinting should be treated as one of the components of the general hand therapy program.

Conclusions

The hand therapy program described was implemented in the Rehabilitation Department of the Institute of Rheumatology in Warsaw with 50 patients during a period of 1½ to 2½ years.[11,12] The illness had lasted for one-half year to 30 years, and patients were between 18 and 67 years of age. Patients stayed in the institute from 2 to 4 weeks and when discharged continued the program at home. Hand function before and after the treatment program was assessed by use of the functional tests described.[8] The effectiveness of treatment was individually estimated with the use of a five-point scale, as follows: "significant improvement," "improvement," "unchanged," "deterioration," and "substantial deterioration." An improvement of greater than 20% over the baseline value obtained from the first examination was considered to be a "significant improvement," while an improvement of 20% to 10.1% was considered "improvement." When either improvement or deterioration was observed in first and second examinations of patients in groups I and II did not exceed 10%, the status was regarded as "unchanged." "Deterioration" meant a worsening of 10.1% to 20% in comparison with the starting value. Deterioration over 20% was considered to be "substantial deterioration."

Taking into account the overall values of grasp strength, grip ability, and dexterity, the research group ascertained that, out of 100 hands tested, in 69 hands grip function remained unchanged, 10 showed improvement, and eight had significant improvement of 23.4% to 66.1%. Deterioration occurred in 10 hands, and substantial deterioration occurred in 3 hands. The results concerning hand strength were most differentiated, oscillating between improvement and deterioration. It is worth noting that 35 hands had improved strength.

In 80% of the patients either improvement or deterioration took place symmetrically and simultaneously in both hands.

When one considers the progressive character of the disease, the results achieved—69% of hands being unchanged in grip function and 18% showing improvement—can be regarded as positive.

REFERENCES

1. Boreczek, G.: Occupational work of the severely disabled rheumatoid patients employed at Disabled Men's Cooperative, master's thesis, Poland, 1979.
2. Flatt, A.E.: The care of the rheumatoid hand, St. Louis, 1974, The C.V. Mosby Co.
3. Flatt, A.E.: Salvage of the rheumatoid hand, Clin. Orthop. **23**:207-219, 1962.
4. Gąsiorowska, E.M.: The influence of morning stiffness on basic parameters of rheumatic hand functions (English abstract), Reumatologia, vol. 13, no. 2, 1975.
5. Konieczna, T.: Vocational rehabilitation of the rheumatoid patients, master's thesis, Poland, 1981.
6. Łukaszewska, M., and Szcześniak, D.: The influence of the wrist stabilisation on the finger muscles strength in rheumatoid hands, master's thesis, Poland, 1981.
7. Musur, M.T., Pągowski, S., and Seyfried, A.: Analysis of mechanical causes of limitation of hand gripping ability in rheumatoid arthritis (English abstract), Reumatologia **16**(1):37-40, 1978.
8. Musur, M.T., and Seyfried, A.: Therapeutic rehabilitation of patients with rheumatoid arthritis and impaired hand functions (English abstract), Reumatologia **18**(4):410-415, 1980.
9. Musur, M.T., Seyfried, A., Frączek, J., and Kwasniewska, B.: Distribution of power on the fingers in cylinder grip, Proceedings of the IXth International Congress WCPT, Stockholm, 1982.
10. Polisiakiewicz, A., and Zagórowicz-Polisiakiewicz, A.: Hand function evaluation in juvenile arthritis, master's thesis, Poland, 1981.
11. Sadowska-Wróblewska, M., and others: Methods for evaluation of the morphotic and functional state of the hands in rheumatoid arthritis cases, Reumatologia **18**(4):405-408, 1980.
12. Sadowska-Wróblewska, M., Garwolinska, H., and Musur, M.: Evaluation of the dynamics of morphotic and functional changes in the hands of R.A. patients who had two years of therapeutic rehabilitation (English abstract), Reumatologia **18**(4):417-422, 1980.
13. Seyfried, A., and Pągowski, S.: Die Prinzipien der Behandlungsrehabilitation der pcP Hand, Orthopäde, vol. 263-65, 173.
14. Seyfried, A.: An own explanation of the mechanism of ulnar deviation of the hand in the course of rheumatoid arthritis, Reumatologia **7**(3):239-245, 1969.
15. Steinbrocker, O., Traeger, C.H., and Batterman, R.C.: Therapeutic criteria in rheumatoid arthritis, J.A.M.A. **140**:659-662, May-Aug. 1949.
16. Wójtowicz, A.: Dexterity in R.A. patients, master's thesis, Poland, 1981.

60

Joint protection program

MARGARET S. CARTER

In the treatment of rheumatoid arthritis, patient education is the area of primary responsibility for both the physician and the therapist. A joint protection program, to educate the patient about internal and external forces that stress the joint, should be an integral part of each patient's treatment.

The primary emphasis of joint protection is on positive measures to protect the joints, conserve energy, and preserve function during performance of activities of daily living. Patients that most benefit are those in the early stages of rheumatoid arthritis, presurgical patients, and those who have had reconstructive surgery. Self-help catalogs, information from the local branch of the Arthritis Foundation, and reputable local sources for adaptive devices should be made available at each session. Another effective approach is to ask patients to keep a daily diary of their activities and to note what activities are difficult to perform and create the most obvious stress on their joints. This personal information from the patient can then be reviewed with him on an individual basis over the length of his treatment time (refer to Chapter 63).

The first principle of joint protection is *preservation of muscle strength and joint range of motion,* achieved through performance of the activities of daily living. For individual problems or maintenance of specific motions, a directed active-exercise program can supplement self-care skills.

The second principle is *prevention of positions of deformity in the hands* by reduction of external forces on the joints, avoidance of patterns of ulnar deviation and reduction of internal joint stresses by avoidance of a strong grip, full flexion of the fingers, and a strong lateral pinch. For example, the patient is taught to substitute lateral pinch with a tripod or gross grasp when possible. Motions of the hand are encouraged to be in the direction of the thumb whenever possible. Small-handled tools can be built up to prevent a tight grip.

The third principle is *utilization of the strongest joint available for the job.* A purse with a small handle held by tightly flexed fingers can be changed to a shoulder purse. Adaptive equipment (such as a car door opener) can be substituted for push or pull motion with the most delicate or painful joints. When a patient is lifting, several joint systems can be employed at the same time to redistribute forces.

The fourth principle is *employment of each joint in its most stable anatomic and functional plane.* Awkward motions, such as using the hands to pull the body weight out of a chair, create joint stress and must be altered.

The fifth principle is *maintenance of muscle balance and correct patterns of motion.* Good posture and full utilization of intrinsic-extrinsic muscle groups prevent imbalance, reduce effort, minimize joint strain, and prevent fatigue. When flexing the fingers, one should begin the motion at the small joints of the fingers. When extending the fingers, one should begin the motion at the metacarpophalangeal joint level.

The sixth principle is *adaptation of tasks requiring static positioning of the joints.* Muscle fatigue, joint wear, and ligament strain are produced by a sustained activity. Periodic rest and joint range of motion must be interspersed in such activities. For example, when writing, one should put down the pencil every 10 minutes to place the entire upper extremity through range of motion. Many forms of adaptive equipment are available to reduce or totally eliminate sustained grasp (for example, a card holder). Activity aids should be presented to the patient as a preventive measure, if possible, before joint deformities have occurred.

The seventh principle is *elimination of activities that cannot be halted immediately if they prove to be beyond a person's ability to complete.* Activities that tire the muscles, thus dangerously straining the joint capsule and ligament, need to be adapted (such as use of a kitchen cart to transport heavy, hot, or breakable items).

The eighth principle is *application of scientific management principles to each task.* Scientific management embodies work simplification and time and motion economy. Correct use of the body, convenient arrangement of the work place, and appropriate selection of tools and equipment can alter extrinsic forces on the joints. The kitchen or work area can be arranged to minimize needless waste of energy by convenient placement of items.

The ninth principle is *respect of pain.* The patients are advised to learn to distinguish a level of "discomfort" that ceases during rest from "pain" that persists for several hours after completion of an activity. Activities producing pain must be modified or eliminated if necessary.

The effectiveness of a joint protection program is directly related to the manner in which it is presented to the patient. A visual program (slides) that specifically covers the correct manner in which to perform activities, supplemented by a detailed handout for home, is only the beginning. The therapist is suggesting the alteration of habits of a lifetime. Individual counseling, open discussion with other patients, and frequent reinforcement of joint protection principles are necessary.

Providing the patient with the means to assist in preventing deformity (in early disease) or recurrence of deformity (after reconstructive surgery) is a responsibility of the therapist that is just as essential as an exercise or splinting program. It is hoped that by providing the patient with an educational tool to modify joint stress, the therapist will enable him to enjoy a more satisfying life-style in which the activities of daily living can be dictated by the person and not by the disease.

ACKNOWLEDGMENTS

We wish to acknowledge Jay Cordery for her research in 1965 on joint protection. Her work is the basis for our joint protection program. We also wish to acknowledge John Madden and Gloria DeVore for their assistance in helping us to set up our metacarpophalangeal implant arthroplasty program in 1974.

BIBLIOGRAPHY

Brattström, M.: Principles of joint protection in chronic rheumatic diseases, Lund, Sweden, 1973, Student Literatur.

Buchanan, L., and Swanson, A.B.: Home exercise program for patients with Silastic finger joint implants (Swanson design), Orthopedic Reconstructive Surgeons of Grand Rapids, Michigan, 1975.

Cordery, J.C.: Joint protection—a responsibility of the occupational therapist, Am. J. Occup. Ther. 19:285-293, 1965.

Flatt, A.E.: Care of the rheumatoid hand, ed. 3, St. Louis, 1974, The C.V. Mosby Co.

Hakstian, R.W., and Tubiana, R.: Ulnar deviation of the fingers: the role of joint structure and function, J. Bone Joint Surg. 49A:299-316, 1971.

Linscheid, R.L., and Dobyns, J.H.: Rheumatoid arthritis of the wrist, Orthop. Clin. North Am. 2:649-655, 1971.

Madden, J.W., DeVore, G., and Arem, A.J.: A rational postoperative management program for metacarpophalangeal joint implant arthroplasty, J. Hand Surg. 2:358-366, 1977.

Shapiro, J.S., Heijna, W., Nasatir, S., and others: The relationship of wrist motion to ulnar phalangeal drift in the rheumatoid patient, Hand 3:68-75, 1971.

Smith, R.J., and Kaplan, E.B.: Rheumatoid deformities at the metacarpophalangeal joints of the fingers, J. Bone Joint Surg. 49A:31-47, 1967.

Swanson, A.B.: Flexible implant resection arthroplasty in the hand and extremities, St. Louis, 1973, The C.V. Mosby Co.

Zancoli, E.: Structural and dynamic bases of hand surgery, Philadelphia, 1968, J.B. Lippincott Co.

61

Postoperative rehabilitation programs in flexible implant arthroplasty of the digits

ALFRED B. SWANSON, GENEVIEVE de GROOT SWANSON, and JUDY LEONARD

A successful arthroplasty should be stable, mobile, durable, retrievable, and free from pain. The postoperative care and rehabilitation program are of great significance for the quality of the final result of the arthroplasty. Individual variations presented by patients, especially in the "complex hand" problem, demand the greatest mastery of the many factors involved.

The use of flexible materials as an adjunct to resection arthroplasty provides a new and different approach to joint reconstruction—it allows us to take an easier and safer alternative in helping nature build her own new joint system through the resection arthroplasty concept.

FLEXIBLE IMPLANT ARTHROPLASTY: CONCEPTS

The flexible implant resection arthroplasty concept can simply be expressed by the following:

Bone resection + Implant +

Encapsulation = New functional joint

The finger joint silicone elastomer intramedullary stemmed implant is a flexible hinge that acts as an internal mold, around which a new capsuloligamentous system develops (Figs. 61-1 and 61-2). One of the most important functions of a flexible implant is to maintain internal alignment and spacing of the reconstructed joint while early motion is started, with the implant acting as a dynamic spacer. Early guided motion is essential in promoting the development of a new, functionally adapted fibrous capsule. That collagen formation and development can be guided is a basic concept to be understood by the surgeons who would undertake arthroplasty procedures. In the early stages of healing, the orientation and tension of the developing capsule are extremely important. In fact, the immediate postoperative positioning and the control of joint movement during the first 6 to 8 weeks after reconstruction by dynamic splinting and therapy are as important as surgery itself. In the postoperative course, the implant continues to act as a dynamic spacer to support the important fibrous capsule and maintain the integrity of the new joint space. We have named this important phenomenon the "encapsulation process."

The stems of the flexible implant are included in the encapsulation process; the fact that the implant is not fixed to the bone increases the life of the implant because forces developed around the implant on flexion and extension movements are not concentrated in one particular area but, rather, are spread over a broader section. The distribution of forces of stabilization of the implant over a broad area with a low-modulus material (softer than bone) also decreases interface problems because the bone is less likely to react at the juncture with the implant if the forces are within the strain tolerances of the bone.

In finger joint arthroplasty, the encapsulation phenomenon offers further advantages. Early mobilization can and should be started to ensure a greater eventual range of motion to the joint. The implant can find the best position with respect to the axis of rotation of the joint; a rigid implant would not have this advantage. The capsuloligamentous structures around any flexible implant can be reconstructed to improve the stability, alignment, and durability of the implant; revision procedures to further reinforce or release the capsule and ligaments when necessary are easily performed. Because the implant stems are not firmly attached to the bone, replacement of an implant for either infection, fracture, or subluxation is a simple procedure. Furthermore, if a fracture of an implant develops or removal becomes necessary, the joint can continue to function adequately as a simple resection arthroplasty. In case of fracture, the implant continues to function by maintaining the joint and the integrity of the capsular space; in case of implant removal, the implant has fulfilled much of its mission as a spacer to support the development of the capsule-ligament system.

Because the tissue reaction after surgery alters the physical properties of the host tissues by destroying or replacing their normal structures with scar, an understanding of wound healing reactions and scar formation form the biologic basis for reconstructive surgery of the hand. It seems appropriate in this chapter to review some of the basic concepts of tissue reactions that are so important to achieve a good result.

BIODYNAMICS OF SCAR FORMATION

A general sequence of events occurs after surgery on a joint. Within minutes the wound space is filled with clotted blood, and the components of the acute inflammatory reaction become manifest: white blood cells leave the confines

665

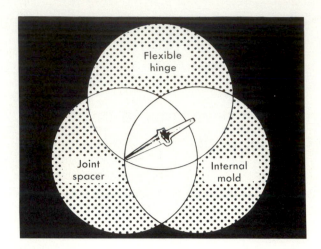

Fig. 61-1. Function of finger joint implant as flexible hinge, internal mold, and joint spacer can be represented in this Venn diagram. Insertion of implant assists nature in development of more predictable and reproducible resection arthroplasty, which has proved to be pain-free, stable, mobile, and durable. (From Swanson, A.B.: Flexible implant resection arthroplasty in the hand and extremities, St. Louis, 1973, The C.V. Mosby Co.)

of the vascular walls and accumulate in the wound, fixed tissue macrophages become mobile and active, and a pronounced vasodilatation occurs with accompanying local edema. Injured tissue components and dead cells are removed by phagocytosis. If there has been limited tissue damage, the inflammatory phase is completed quickly.

Within hours of wound closure, the epithelial cells of the basal layer of the skin at the wound edge begin to migrate centrally and completely cover the open surface of the wound within 36 to 48 hours. During the first few days, local cells present within the confines of the wound and identifiable as fibroblasts by their content of large amounts of rough endoplasmic reticulum begin to divide rapidly and migrate into all areas of the wound space. Fibroblasts gradually replace all but a few mononuclear white blood cells.

Although collagen fibers form the bulk of mature scars, fibrils are not apparent microscopically until the fourth or fifth day. Once fibrils begin to form, however, the wound space is rapidly filled with randomly oriented collagen fibers that increase in size and abundance during the first 3 or 4 weeks. Newly synthesized collagen fibers link all portions of the wound within a three-dimensional network of collagen fibers. As the content of scar collagen becomes more abundant, wound cellularity decreases. Fibroblasts, isolated within the collagen network, gradually lose most of their characteristic rough endoplasmic reticulum and become fibrocytes. By the third week, the rate of accumulation of scar collagen is greatly decreased, and the total amount of collagen in the scar becomes stable.

The cohesive forces between the epithelial cells, fibroblasts, and endothelial cells give some strength to the wound during the first few days of healing. These forces, however, are weak, and wounds may be easily disrupted. A rapid gain in tensile strength begins with the appearance of collagen fibrils, and wound strength increases as collagen becomes more abundant. It usually reaches clinical adequacy in 3 weeks.

As noted by Madden and Peacock, early in fibril formation collagen molecules are held together by hydrogen bonds and other weak physical forces. If tension is applied to new aggregates, fibrils are ruptured easily. With time, however, newly formed fibers demonstrate a sharp increase in tensile strength. As fibrils mature, the weak intermolecular forces are supplemented by the formation of covalent bonds, the strongest union between atoms. Ultimately, collagen fibers become giant polymers, each molecule being linked to its neighbor by these strong covalent bonds.

Aggregation and covalent bonding produce a strong flexible fiber that can be woven into many different tissue patterns. The quantity of scar collagen, the anatomic configuration of the fibers, and the density of inter- and intramolecular covalent bonding determine the physical characteristics of the reconstructed joint capsuloligamentous system.

Remodeling of scar tissue

All wounds undergo remarkable changes in color, firmness, and bulk. A well-healed wound 2 months after initial injury bears little resemblance to the same wound 1 year later. The measurable physical properties of incised and sutured wounds as to strength also change slowly over prolonged periods of time. Collagen gains strength rapidly during the first 3 to 4 weeks but continues to gain strength at a steady rate for 12 months or longer. Alterations in scar architecture are most striking as the scar collagen becomes oriented in parallel bundles. This physical weave of collagen fibrils and the parallel orientation of collagen fibers are the most effective configurations to resist longitudinal stresses.

All the factors that control the morphology of remodeling of scar tissue are not known. Age plays an important role in the remodeling of scars; younger patients tend to remodel scar tissue more rapidly than older ones. The total amount of randomly oriented scar collagen present in a wound also affects remodeling; larger amounts of scar collagen limit

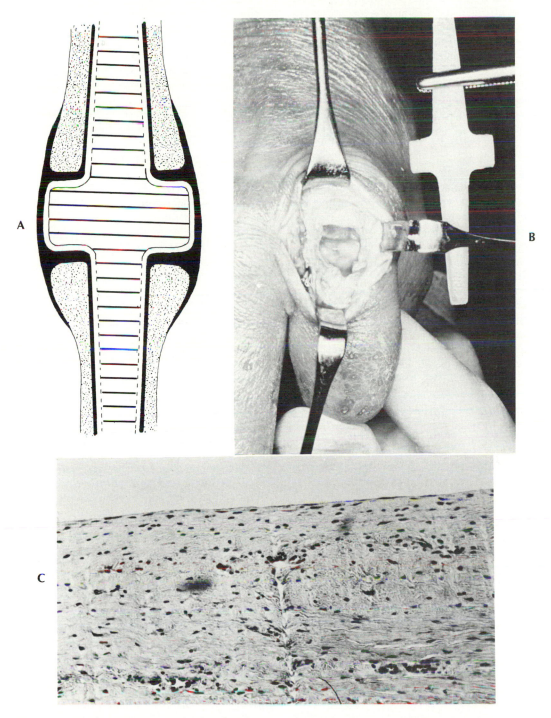

FIG. 61-2. Fixation by encapsulation. **A,** Formation of new capsuloligament system that totally surrounds implant and stabilizes its position. **B,** Implant removed from second metacarpophalangeal joint 1 year postoperatively for purposes of capsulotomy and lipid analysis of implant in prospective research study. Note capsular formation around implant and into intramedullary stems that represents internal mold. **C,** Microscopic sections of capsular specimen in **B** showing organized longitudinal arrangement of collagen fibers, which is not unlike ligament tissue. Single-cell mesothelial lining is noted in upper portion of specimen, which was adjacent to silicone implant. (From Swanson, A.B.: Flexible implant resection arthroplasty in the hand and extremities, St. Louis, 1973, The C.V. Mosby Co.)

effective remodeling. The remodeling changes that occur at a later period may be insufficient to reestablish proper scar morphology if the collagen deposition was too great. For this reason, old previously remodeled scar tissue, present within a new wound, has detrimental effects on the remodeling of the new wound and should be removed during the reconstructive procedure. This is especially important in posttraumatic cases.

Physical forces such as longitudinal stresses and shearing forces acting on the scar-containing area play an important role in the remodeling of collagen tissue. The precise relationship between tension and scar remodeling, however, remains obscure. During the remodeling of bone, electrical field forces generated by deforming tissue play an important role in the organization of collagen fibrils and bony spicules. These same forces may be at work in soft-tissue healing but have not been clearly demonstrated to date. The biologic condition of the tissues at the time of surgery also plays an important role in scar remodeling. There are also significant differences among individuals in their capacity to deposit and remodel collagen.

The deposition and remodeling of collagen around the joint and the implant provide the reconstructed joint with a proper balance of mobility and stability and are of obvious importance to the finger joint reconstruction. The implant acts as an internal mold around which the collagen is deposited and further continues its role in acting as an internal spacer to maintain the integrity of the joint space.

The proper control of scar formation by appropriate rest, protection, and properly applied tension forces during the postoperative period is the basis of the rehabilitation program. It would appear that motion must be started early and continued until the collagen reaction is stabilized. In our experience, early motion must be started within the first week after surgery, and exercises must be continued for at least 3 months in the average patient.

Remodeling of the cut bone end

Bone remodeling occurs from a constant interplay between bone absorption and bone formation. An optimum amount of stress is necessary for production of a satisfactory degree of osteogenesis, which will not occur if the stress is too little or too great. The remodeling of the cut bone ends in an arthroplasty is dependent on both mechanical and biologic considerations. The palmar edge of the sectioned bone end is the most susceptible area. Compression and shear-loading forces, exceeding biologic and mechanical tolerance, will cause bone absorption. The condition of the bone affected by the arthritic process, rough handling and drill burning, fracturing of the bone edges, stripping of the periosteum containing its blood supply, or excessive reaming of its endosteal surface are all important factors that affect the eventual strength of the cut bone end and its resistance to the loads applied to it. Mechanical factors are not solely responsible for bone absorption; biologic factors affected by nutritional and vascular changes are also important in bony response. This especially is true in the active rheumatoid patient.

The following are factors that will help assure a proper remodeling of the bone at the arthroplasty site: (1) correction of subluxating forces to decrease the shear-loading stresses at the interface between the implant and the bone; (2) limiting the amount of flexion at the joint (In our experience, 70 degrees of flexion would appear to be functionally and mechanically ideal. This is especially important if the bone stock is inadequate or too thin.); (3) obtaining more collagen formation around the joint to limit the mechanical stress of increased flexion and also to absorb some of the deforming forces applied to it; (4) appropriate operative technique; (5) the mechanical characteristics of the flexible implant as to its softness and stress loading are important; and (6) the proper postoperative care and rehabilitation program. Bone modeling should be carefully evaluated by serial roentgenographic studies in the postoperative period. A long-term study of bone-remodeling phenomena around flexible implants at the metacarpophalangeal joint was carried out. This study showed the bone-remodeling process to occur as a newly formed cortical bony shell around the implant stems and thickening of the metacarpal and phalangeal metaphysis. Thickening of the phalangeal midshaft was present. A decrease of the metacarpal midshaft was noted early after surgery and remained permanent; this was related to the surgical reaming. It was concluded that the clinical durability of this procedure was linked in part to the favorable biologic effect of this implant at the bone interface.

Our long-term retrieval studies have shown that the flexible hinge implant arthroplasties have stood up well through the years: the durability of the range of motion, the implant, and the host interface tissue is very good. One of the interesting radiographic observations is the maintenance of the shape of the bone where the implant has been used as compared to the simple resection arthroplasty. The implant apparently maintains the anatomic shape of the bone end, and the remodeling process that usually results in shortening and narrowing and spike formation after simple resection arthroplasty does not occur in the presence of the implant.

BASIC OPERATIVE AND EARLY POSTOPERATIVE CONSIDERATIONS

Variations of the arthritic involvement presented by many patients demand special consideration of all factors involved. Reconstructive procedures of weight-bearing joints of the lower extremity that will require walking with crutches, should precede upper extremity reconstruction. Excessive manual labor and awkward hand weight bearing, such as seen in some crutch walkers, should be avoided after surgery. If crutch walking cannot be avoided, special platform type of crutches should be used. Multiple reconstructive procedures must be appropriately staged. Tendon repair and synovectomy of tendon sheaths should be done 6 to 8 weeks before joint reconstruction in the rheumatoid hand. However, if the extensor tendons are ruptured and the metacarpophalangeal joints are dislocated, arthroplasty of the metacarpophalangeal joints is done before tendon repair. In swan-neck deformity, arthroplasties of the metacarpophalangeal and proximal interphalangeal joints are done at the same stage. However, in boutonnière deformity, it is preferable to reconstruct the proximal interphalangeal joint before the metacarpophalangeal joint. Any tendon imbal-

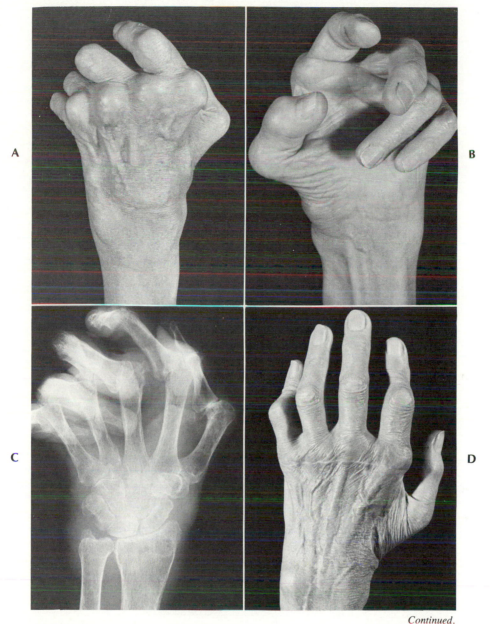

Continued.

FIG. 61-3. Flexible implant resection arthroplasty of metacarpophalangeal joint in a rheumatoid hand. **A to C,** Preoperative views showing classic findings of rheumatoid deformity in hand with severe subluxation of metacarpophalangeal joint, deviation and lack of extension of fingers, ulnar subluxation of extensor tendons, and deformity of thumb. **D to G,** Clinical appearance of roentgenogram of same hand 2 years after flexible implant resection arthroplasty of all five metacarpophalangeal joints. Note improved appearance of hand with good correction of deformities. Patient remains pain free and has functional range of flexion and extension.

ance or bone and joint malalignment must be corrected; otherwise, it will affect the long-term result of joint replacement. Precise anatomic dissection, adequate soft-tissue release, respect for gliding surfaces, prevention of edema, and early guided movement in functional planes are essential for good results in arthroplasty procedures (Fig. 61-3).

As noted, wounding of any part of the body results in a vascular reaction and edema. This reaction can result in scar formation, which in turn can cause stiffness. From the early stages of treatment, every measure should be taken to decrease, if not prevent, unnecessary residual stiffness. Stiff-

ness in the hand is in itself a difficult reconstructive problem. Contracture of the elbow and shoulder joints can result in severe loss of function by preventing the hand from being properly positioned in space. Knowledge and strict application of certain basic principles of hand care are therefore essential to avoid these complications. These include proper operative dressing, immobilization in a functional position, postoperative elevation, early motion, and exercises.

Constrictive dressings and passive movements should be avoided. Proper elevation of the hand and extremity will enhance venous return and decrease the escape of fluids into

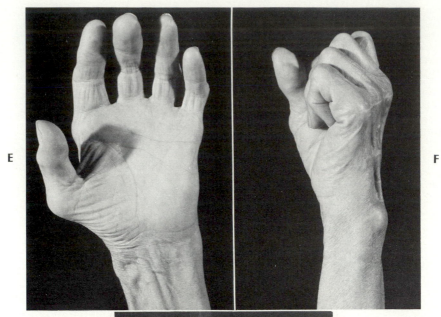

E

F

G

FIG. 61-3, cont'd. For legend see p. 669.

the interstitial spaces of the injured parts, thus reducing edema. Slings should not be worn when the patient is in the upright position because they may prevent use of the extremity. Early motion is also important to maintain muscle length, reduce edema, prevent ligament contracture, prevent adhesions of tendons and other gliding surfaces, and maintain hand architecture. Motion should be encouraged not only distally but also at the level of the wrist, elbow, and shoulder joints to avoid sympathetic dystrophy and maintain mobility. The rheumatoid patient usually has already some loss of motion and some functional impairment. He should be frequently examined for new loss of mobility of the elbow and shoulder, for even a few degrees of loss of abduction and external rotation may signal an impending shoulder-hand syndrome. Circumduction exercises of the shoulder and active movements of the digits, especially with the hand

elevated, if done early and continued throughout the treatment program, will avoid many of the disastrous effects seen in improperly treated patients. Specific exercises for the reconstructed part must follow an organized and supervised regime.

The flexible implant acts as an internal splint that separates the incongruous bone ends; once the released ligaments and scar have healed, they will stabilize the joint in a fashion similar to the function of normal ligaments. As with simple resection arthroplasty, if motion is restricted during the healing phase, there will be poor mobility. The greatest challenge in postoperative rehabilitation of finger joint arthroplasty is to maintain a proper balance between good healing of the surrounding scar tissue and at the same time apply proper amounts of tension across the scar to obtain the desired range of motion. Controlled motion during this pe-

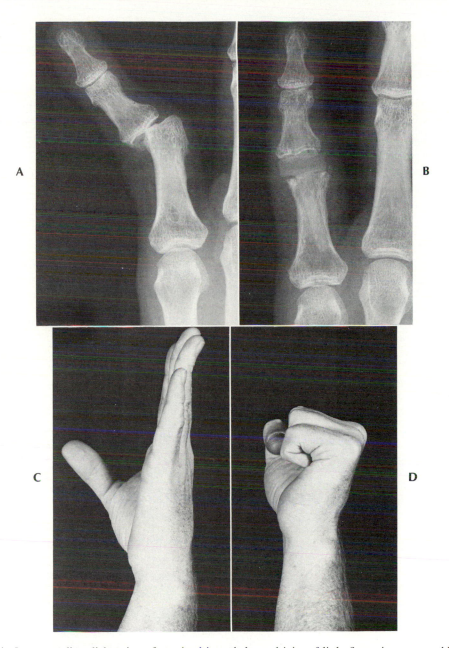

FIG. 61-4. A, Long-standing dislocation of proximal interphalangeal joint of little finger in young, athletic male. **B,** Roentgenogram showing excellent position and tolerance of implant 3 years postoperatively. **C** and **D,** Patient recovered full use of his hand with excellent flexion and extension.

riod will train the new capsule to have sufficient looseness for flexion and extension and sufficient tightness in the mediolateral plane for rotation and angular stability. An adjustable dynamic splint is therefore necessary to guide the motion of the joint in desired planes and to prevent recurrent deformity during the early postoperative course. Scar formation will vary according to the joint involved, the type of surgery performed, and the differences in the collagen reaction in each patient. It is therefore the responsibility of the operating surgeon to control the process when he can by providing a well-organized and preplanned rehabilitation program for his patients. The patients receive specific instructions and are regularly coached through their exercises

in the early postoperative period. They are instructed to sit comfortably, to stabilize the proximal joints, including the shoulder, elbow, and wrist, and to concentrate the movement at the reconstructed joints. Using mirrors can be most helpful in assisting the patient's self-evaluation of his degree of movement. Once the sutures are removed, we encourage the patients to precede their exercises with an oil or lotion massage. The follow-up should be meticulous and include objective measurements of the patient's progress. This is as important to the final result as the surgical procedure. To fail to understand these basic facts is to miss the opportunity of the pleasure of a complete success (Figs. 61-3 and 61-4).

DYNAMIC SPLINT

We have designed a splint to facilitate early postoperative motion in our patients who have undergone finger joint implant resection arthroplasty. Its use has greatly improved the anatomic and functional results. The splint prevents undue stretching of associated reconstructed tendons and ligaments and also assists the digital extensors and flexors, which are frequently weak because of long-standing deformity, accompanying tenosynovitis, and fibrosis. The dynamic splint has three major functions: (1) to provide complete and adjustable correction of residual deformity; (2) to control motion in the desired plane and range; and (3) to assist flexor and extensor power, ensuring an adequate alternation of complete extension and flexion ranges of movement in the joint.

The basic splint for the finger joint arthroplasty is a dorsal splint that provides a stable base for outriggers and support for the weak or deficient wrist. The splint is available in three basic sizes.* Three transverse straps are attached to the basic dorsal splint and are made of malleable metal to be easily adjusted to the shape and size of the patient's forearm; adjustable Velcro straps are attached to these malleable transverse straps to hold the splint in position. Two Velcro straps are placed around the forearm, and a narrow Velcro strap is placed across the palm; the latter has a palmar pad to help maintain the arches of the hand and prevent rotation of the splint. A transverse bar to which finger slings are attached is fitted onto a dorsal arm. The position of the transverse bar can be adjusted in all three planes. The finger slings are of soft plastic with multiple perforations and are connected to the transverse bar with rubber bands. Short radially placed outriggers may be added for correction of the pronation deformity often present in the index and middle fingers of rheumatoid hands. A longer bar can be used for thumb abduction. All of these outriggers are attached with thumb screws.

When weakness of the flexors is present, specific measures must be taken to ensure flexion of the joint through an adequate range of motion. Available devices are discussed later.

METACARPOPHALANGEAL JOINT POSTOPERATIVE PROGRAM
Goals and special considerations

The results of an organized postoperative program for these patients are so much better than those of any other method that all attempts should be made by the surgeon to provide this type of care for his patient. It is extremely useful to have the adjustable dynamic splint available preoperatively for patients undergoing metacarpophalangeal joint implant resection arthroplasty to avoid any delay in its application.

The ideal motion to be obtained after implant resection arthroplasty at the metacarpophalangeal joints would provide adequate flexion of the ulnar digits, allowing the surface of their pulps to touch the palm at the distal palmar crease for adequate grasp of smaller objects. Full flexion of the

*Swanson Postoperative Hand Splint, Orthopaedic Division, Parke Davis and Co., 74 N.E. 75th St., Miami, Fla. 33138.

index and middle fingers is less critical for grasping because these digits are mainly used for pinch activities. A degree of spreading of the fingers into abduction, especially of the index finger, is important. Full extension at these joints is also important for performance of normal hand activities and maintenance of the balance of the distal joints. Chronic flexion deformity of the metacarpophalangeal joints can further aggravate hyperextension tendencies at the proximal interphalangeal joints. Pronation deformity of the index finger and occasionally the middle finger can be a problem in the rheumatoid hand and can, to some degree, be corrected in the postoperative program.

Patients who have normal proximal interphalangeal joints frequently will not gain the full expected range of motion at the metacarpophalangeal joint after arthroplasty because they will rather flex the proximal interphalangeal joint during their exercise program and thus their metacarpophalangeal joints will be relatively immobilized. To help localize all flexion forces at the metacarpophalangeal joints in these patients, we recommend taping small padded aluminum splints on the dorsum of the proximal interphalangeal joints during exercise periods for the first 3 or 4 weeks after surgery. This seems to improve the range of motion obtained after this surgery. Occasionally, in the presence of associated swan-neck deformity, temporary Kirschner-wire fixation of the proximal interphalangeal joints can also be used for the same functional purpose.

Splint fitting and early postoperative treatment

The voluminous conforming operative hand dressing is left on until the postoperative swelling has decreased, usually in 3 to 5 days. The dynamic splint is applied over a lightly padded dressing after removal of the postoperative dressing. If the splint is not available, one may still obtain guided early motion by applying a lightweight, short arm cast fitted with outriggers and similar rubber band slings.

The dorsal wrist splint with a ¼-inch felt pad placed between the forearm and the splint, should be applied loosely enough so that it is not constrictive and yet tightly enough so that it does not rotate on the forearm and hand. If there is a tendency toward continued swelling, the limb may still be elevated with the wrist supported in extension against an intravenous infusion stand. Active exercises in the elevated position may then be carried out.

The rubber band slings are placed on the proximal phalanges to guide the alignment of the digits into the desired position. The pull of the slings in the radial direction will usually require adjustment to prevent recurrent ulnar drift. The tension of the rubber bands should be tight enough to support the digits and yet loose enough to allow 70 degrees of active flexion; this is especially true of the little finger, which may have weak flexion power (Fig. 61-5). The splint may require adjustment once or twice a day in the early postoperative course.

The thumb outrigger is usually applied in all cases because of the tendency for the patient to bring the thumb over the fingers on flexion. This movement should be avoided because the pressure applied by the thumb to the index finger would be in the ulnar direction, thus aggravating the tendency toward ulnar drift deformity.

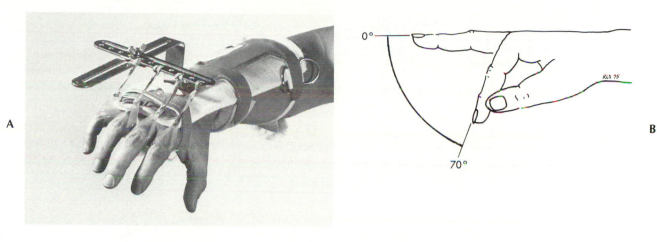

FIG. 61-5. **A,** Finger slings of dynamic splint are placed on proximal phalanges to assist metacarpophalangeal joint extension and guide alignment of digits. Slings are adjusted to pull from radial side to prevent ulnar deviation. Padding underneath splint with lightweight dressing or dorsal strip of felt may be necessary. **B,** Ideal goal of rehabilitation program is to obtain full extension to 70 degrees of flexion. Rubber bands should be loose enough to allow 70 degrees of flexion at metacarpophalangeal joint, especially of little finger. If flexion strength is weak, slings must be removed periodically to allow full range of motion.

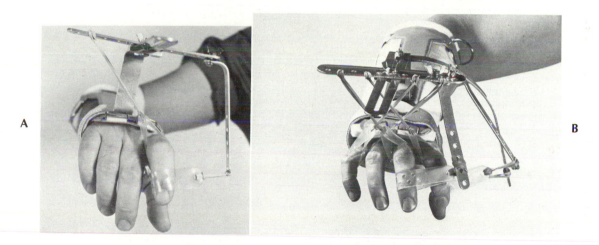

FIG. 61-6. **A,** Method of using combined pull of two slings on one digit to form couple-producing supinatory torque force without interfering with flexion and extension movements. This technique can be used to assist in correction of pronation deformity, which is often seen in index and middle fingers in rheumatoid hands. **B,** Dynamic splint with all outriggers attached for correction of ulnar drift, rotation deformity of index and middle fingers, and to control abduction of thumb.

If there is a tendency toward medial rotation (pronation) in the index or middle fingers, additional outrigger bars are applied to provide a rotation force at the metacarpophalangeal joint according to the concept of a force couple; a force couple is defined as two equal and opposite forces that act along parallel lines, and it is obtained by applying the loops to the digit that shows a tendency for pronation, as shown in Fig. 61-6. A rubber band sling is fitted from an additional outrigger to the distal phalanx of the digit showing a pronation tendency. This combined pull of two slings forms a coupling that produces a torque force in the direction of supination on the digit without interfering with flexion and extension movements.

The extension portion of the splint is worn continuously day and night for the first 3 weeks, alternating with specific flexion measures as required and discussed later. The flexion exercises in the splint with the extension slings in position are carried out, starting at 3 days postoperatively, both actively and passively (with no more than 2 pounds of force) on an hourly basis (Fig. 61-7). The ideal goal of 0 degrees of extension to 70 degrees of flexion is constantly stressed. The patient is seen at least three times by the physician or the therapist during the first week, and the splint is carefully readjusted as necessary. Only exceptionally, if there is considerable flexor weakness of the little finger with adequate extensor stability, can the extension sling be removed from this digit during the exercise periods.

During the second and third weeks, the extension portion

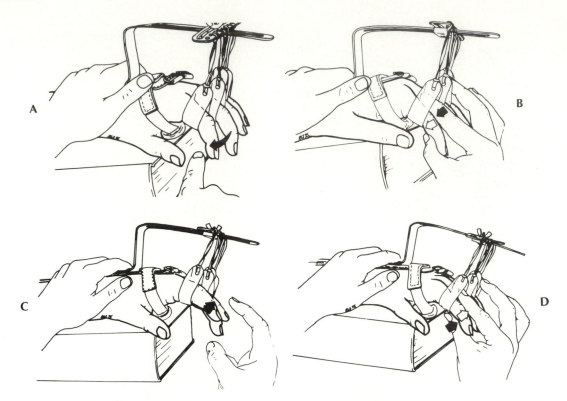

FIG. 61-7. Flexion-extension exercises for metacarpophalangeal joint. **A** and **B,** Active and passive flexion exercises are carried out in the splint starting at 3 days postoperatively. No more than 2 pounds of force should be applied to assist passive flexion. Arm is positioned on a firm surface to help stabilize proximal joints and allow movement of digits. Proper adjustment of tension of rubber bands is essential to allow full range of motion. Extension portion of splint is worn continuously for first 3 weeks. **C** and **D,** Active and passive extension exercises are carried out in splint.

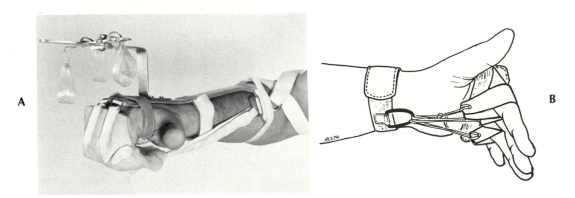

FIG. 61-8. Passive flexion devices that can be used starting at 3 weeks postoperatively. **A,** Flexion cuff in place to passively assist flexion of joints. Velcro strap pulls to radial side and may be used by patient to gradually increase stretching effort. Figure-of-eight elbow strap should be used to prevent distal migration of brace. **B,** Finger slings placed on proximal phalanges are attached to loop of special Velcro wrist strap or to strap of dynamic splint to provide flexion traction.

of the splint is also worn continuously day and night. If there is severe flexor weakness and good extension, the extensor slings can be removed 1 to 2 hours a day to achieve greater active flexion of the metacarpophalangeal joints. If the patient appears not to be obtaining 70 degrees of flexion, several measures can be taken. Should most of the motion be occurring at the proximal interphalangeal joints, these joints may be splinted in extension as previously described

(p. 672), to help localize the flexion force at the metacarpophalangeal joints. The rubber bands may be lengthened to decrease the extension force applied.

At 3 weeks any residual flexor weakness should be energetically treated. The flexion cuff may be worn 1 to 2 hours twice a day to flex passively the metacarpophalangeal joints in conjunction with active flexion exercises. As this cuff is used, the figure-of-eight elbow strap should be applied to prevent distal migration of the splint (Fig. 61-8, *A*). In the presence of adequate extension the preferred flexion traction method consists in placement of finger slings on the proximal phalanges and attachment of them volarly to the loop of a special Velcro wrist strap or to that of the dynamic splint (Fig. 61-8, *B*). If the distal and proximal interphalangeal joints are stable, dressmaker hooks can be glued to the fingernails with a cyanoacrylate adhesive. Individual rubber bands are than attached from the loop of the special wrist strap to the nail hooks similarly as described for the proximal interphalangeal joints. A small Band-Aid is applied over the hooks for increased patient comfort between exercise periods. These traction methods give better control on the alignment and desired amount of flexion pull for each individual finger. The methods are especially useful and can be started during the early postoperative course in certain cases presenting severe preoperative stiffness or flexor weakness with adequate extensor mechanism. In these difficult cases one can reach a functional compromise by sacrificing a few degrees of extension.

The extension portion of the splint is usually worn at night only, starting on the fourth postoperative week for another 3 weeks. In a few cases where there is a persistent extensor lag or a tendency for flexion contracture or deviation of the digits, continued part-time support by use of the splint must be prescribed for several more weeks or even months. The patient should follow a continued exercise and stretching program for 3 months postoperatively to maintain the movement obtained in the earlier phase. After this time the final range of motion will have been established.

Collagen maturity and scar contracture vary from patient to patient. The associated tendon deficiencies also vary; therefore the use of the splint in the postoperative period requires tailoring and careful follow-up by the operating surgeon or therapist, or both. The patient's progress is evaluated by measurement of the range of motion with accurate goniometer readings; one observes the movements of the digits without the splint to be sure that the patient is getting the desired result. The reconstructed joints start tightening up during the second postoperative week and will be quite tight by the end of 3 weeks. If the desired range of motion has not been obtained by 3 weeks, it will be difficult to gain further improvement in motion.

THUMB METACARPOPHALANGEAL JOINT

Postoperative care for the thumb metacarpophalangeal joint implant arthroplasty differs from that previously described. The goal of this procedure is to obtain adequate stability with limited motion ranging from approximately −10 degrees of extension to 25 degrees of flexion.

At the time of surgery a 0.045-inch Kirschner wire is carefully passed longitudinally through the fingertip into the flexor tendon sheath for temporary internal fixation of the distal and metacarpophalangeal joints; this wire is left in place for 2 to 3 days or until the postoperative swelling has sufficiently decreased to allow circumferential bandaging of an external splint. At that time a padded aluminum splint extending distally to the end of the thumb and proximally to the wrist is taped dorsally for 4 to 6 weeks (Fig. 61-9). No special exercises are prescribed after splint removal ex-

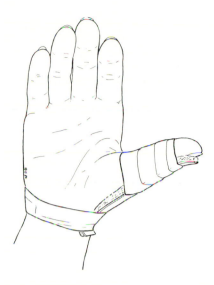

FIG. 61-9. Dorsal thumb extension splint extending distally to end of thumb and proximally to wrist.

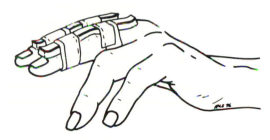

FIG. 61-10. Taped-on padded aluminum splint to hold digits in extension is worn as night splint or continuously, depending on degree of extensor lag present (described further in text). Same splint may also be applied slightly to ulnar or radial side of digit to correct associated angulation deformities.

cept normal functional adaptations. Forceful activities should be avoided for 6 to 8 weeks postoperatively.

PROXIMAL INTERPHALANGEAL JOINT POSTOPERATIVE PROGRAM

The type of postoperative care for the proximal interphalangeal joint varies with the preoperative deformity and the surgical reconstruction. There are three basic situations: (1) reconstruction of a stiff proximal interphalangeal joint, (2) reconstruction of a swan-neck deformity, (3) reconstruction of a boutonnière deformity.

When the implant arthroplasty has been performed for a *stiff proximal interphalangeal joint*, active movements of flexion and extension should be started within 3 to 5 days after surgery. The ideal range of motion after this surgery is 0 degrees of extension to 70 degrees of flexion. Small, taped-on padded aluminum splints to hold the digit in extension are worn mainly as night splints and may be used for several weeks postoperatively, depending on the degree of extensor lag present (Fig. 61-10). The same splint may also be applied slightly to the ulnar or radial side of the dorsum of the digit to correct any associated angulatory deformity. Active flexion and extension exercises can be performed with a variety of exercise devices such as those described later in this chapter.

If one needs to do so, the distal interphalangeal joint may be temporarily pinned with a Kirschner wire to concentrate the action of the flexor profundus at the proximal interphalangeal joint. There are almost always a few degrees of extension lag in these types of cases.

If the implant resection arthroplasty of the proximal interphalangeal joint has been done for a *swan-neck deformity*

in association with a tendon reconstruction procedure, a padded taped-on aluminum splint is usually placed on the digit after the postoperative edema has subsided. The joint is immobilized in 10 to 20 degrees of flexion, and the splint is left on for 10 days until the exercises are begun. It is important to obtain at least 10 degrees of flexion contracture of these joints in order to prevent recurrent hyperextension tendencies. Unless the central slip has been released, there may be an imbalance of the joint in favor of extension. During the healing phase the digit should be held in the

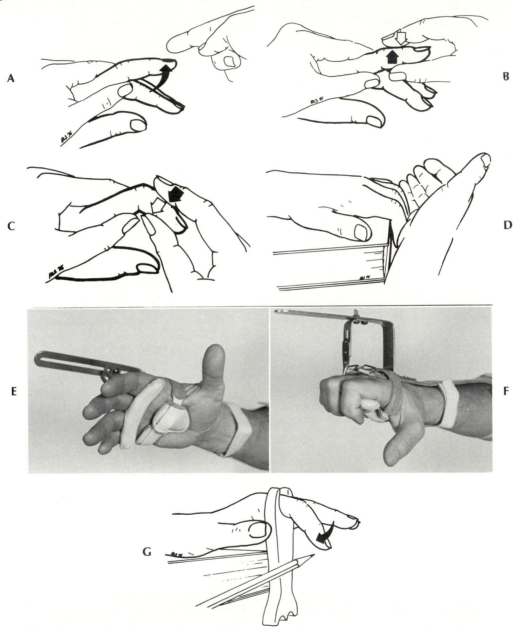

FIG. 61-11. Flexion and extension exercises for proximal interphalangeal joint. **A** and **B**, Active and passive extension exercises are carried out while stabilizing proximal phalanx. **C** and **D**, Passive flexion exercises can be carried out with opposite hand while proximal phalanx is stabilized either over edge of book by assistant, or with dowel. **E**, Reverse lumbrical bar can be used to support proximal phalanges and eliminate motion of metacarpophalangeal joints during flexion exercises. Note palmar pad used to maintain transverse arches of hand and assist in preventing rotation of brace. **F**, Flexion of proximal interphalangeal joints over reverse lumbrical bar. Flexion cuff can be applied to gently force flexion if it appears to be necessary. **G**, We designed "finger crutch" to help support proximal phalanx in extension during flexion exercises.

flexed position with the aluminum splints at least on a part-time basis. To obtain adequate correction of the swan-neck deformity, one must not let the distal interphalangeal joint remain in too great a flexion, and this may require pinning in 0 degrees of extension. The metacarpophalangeal joint should be supported in extension with the rubber band slings of the splint or with the reverse lumbrical bar. After the second week gentle passive flexion exercises of the proximal interphalangeal joint can be started if it appears necessary.

If the implant resection arthroplasty procedure has been done to correct a *boutonnière deformity,* it is important to maintain the extension of the proximal interphalangeal joint and to allow flexion of the distal interphalangeal joint. The reconstruction of the extensor mechanism should be protected for approximately 10 days with an extension splint applied after the postoperative swelling has decreased. The aluminum splint, in this situation, should immobilize only the proximal interphalangeal joint in extension for 3 to 6 weeks, depending on the degree of extension lag present. The distal joint should be allowed to flex freely. Active flexion and extension exercises are usually started from 10 to 14 days after surgery in alternation with the use of the extension splint, which should be worn at night to hold the proximal interphalangeal joint in extension until the position of the joint is stable. This may require 10 weeks.

A Kirschner wire passed into the flexor sheath through the fingertip can be used as a temporary internal splint for immobilization of either the distal interphalangeal or prox-imal interphalangeal joints. A 0.035-inch wire is very carefully passed into the flexor sheath through the fingertip distally to proximally; the wire should touch the palmar aspect of the proximal end of the proximal phalanx and is left in place for several days or until the postoperative swelling has decreased sufficiently so that splints with circumferential bandaging can be used.

Exercises for the proximal interphalangeal joint can be carried out actively and passively, with care always being taken to support the metacarpophalangeal joint in extension. This can be done with the opposite hand, over the edge of a book, or with a variety of orthotic devices (Fig. 61-11). Extension of the metacarpophalangeal joints can be supported with the reverse lumbrical bar attached to the dynamic splint or to a special wrist splint. Passive flexion at the proximal interphalangeal joints can then be obtained with the flexor cuff or with rubber band traction to fingernail hooks. A dowel can also be used to support the metacarpophalangeal joints (Fig. 61-12, *B*). One can carry out passive stretching of flexion contractures of the proximal interphalangeal joint by blocking hyperextension of the metacarpophalangeal joint with the lumbrical bar and applying extension force to the middle phalanx with the extension rubber band slings of the dynamic splint (Fig. 61-12, *C*). We have developed a small "finger crutch" that we have used in a similar fashion to the Bunnell wood block to support the proximal phalanx during exercises; this is made of ¼-inch plywood or hard rubber material.

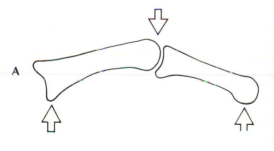

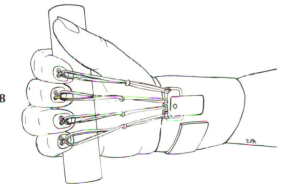

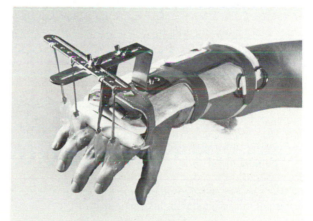

FIG. 61-12. A, Passive stretching of joint requires use of three-point principle of pressure application. **B,** An extremely efficient method of obtaining passive flexion of proximal interphalangeal joints after arthroplasty. Dowel provides support to proximal phalanges and limits motions of metacarpophalangeal joints. **C,** Splint can be adjusted to stretch proximal interphalangeal joints in extension with lumbrical bar in normal position for cases of flexion deformities. This adaptation of splint should not be used after metacarpophalangeal joint arthroplasty because it may produce a palmad subluxation of base of proximal phalanx.

DISTAL INTERPHALANGEAL JOINT POSTOPERATIVE PROGRAM

Treatment of the distal interphalangeal joint must be considered in reconstructive procedures of the proximal interphalangeal joint, especially if it is deformed. In reconstruction of a stiff proximal interphalangeal joint, the distal interphalangeal joint may be temporarily pinned with a Kirschner wire to concentrate the action of the flexor profundus at the proximal interphalangeal joint. These pins can be removed after approximately 3 weeks.

In reconstruction of a swan-neck deformity, the distal interphalangeal joint may also be temporarily pinned in a neutral position if a severe flexion deformity of the joint is present. This will localize the flexion forces at the proximal interphalangeal joint and help the recovery of movement.

In the reconstruction of a boutonnière deformity, one should release the distal interphalangeal joint, if in severe hyperextension, by sectioning the lateral tendons over the middle phalanx or by relatively lengthening the lateral tendons. Flexion exercises specifically located at this joint are important to recover movement of this joint and also to help correct the imbalance of the proximal interphalangeal joint.

POSTOPERATIVE PROGRAM FOR COMBINED PROCEDURES

Patients who present a "complex hand" show involvement at multiple joint levels. Knowledge of hand function and of surgical principles is essential for selection of the proper timing of surgical procedures. As a rule, the proximal joints are given priority in the surgical and rehabilitation program. In combined involvement of the metacarpophalangeal and proximal interphalangeal joints of the same digit, the metacarpophalangeal joint should receive priority. However, the goals and principles of each reconstructive method at each specific level are always respected so that a balance of functional motion is obtained.

If two different involvement levels are presented in separate digits of the same hand, the above principles apply as described in the following example: metacarpophalangeal joint reconstruction of the index and long fingers and proximal interphalangeal joint reconstruction of the ring and small fingers for boutonnière deformities. The described protocol for metacarpophalangeal joint arthroplasty is followed for the index and long fingers; the described postoperative protocol for a boutonnière deformity is followed for the ring and small fingers. In this case, however, we would favor including the ring and small fingers in the slings of the dynamic splint to provide a balanced tension within the hand.

If reconstruction of the metacarpophalangeal and proximal interphalangeal joints of the same digit is carried out at the same seating, such as that seen for the swan-neck deformity, the described postoperative program for each level and specific deformity is followed, giving priority to the metacarpophalangeal joint.

In all cases and even more so in these complex cases, it is critical that oral and written instructions be given clearly and that the patient understands his responsibility.

OTHER MODALITIES OF POSTOPERATIVE TREATMENT

General physical and occupational therapy modalities should be considered in most patients; however, if such modalities are not available, most patients can be managed by the surgeon.

Some simple heat applications may be of benefit in the postoperative course after complete wound healing. We occasionally will use paraffin or contrast baths for their heating and analgesic benefits. The methods for these baths are described in the following.

Paraffin bath for the hands

This bath requires four cartons of paraffin and one 10-ounce bottle of baby oil.
1. Put these materials in a large can or double boiler. Heat slowly to melting point, approximately 100 to 110° F.
2. Dip hand in quickly to 2 inches beyond the wrist, keeping hand over can; repeat 12 times or until ¼ inch of wax remains on hand.
3. Wrap the paraffin-covered hand for 15 minutes with plastic or waxed paper and a large bath towel. Exercise fingers with wax on.
4. Remove paraffin by stripping it off while holding the hand over the can.
5. Massage and exercise warm fingers. Elevate the arm if the hand is swollen. Wear gloves to maintain the heat, especially if going outdoors in cold weather.

This bath may be repeated two or three times a day. There should be no open wounds or unusual swelling of tissue or skin reaction.

Contrast bath for the hands

1. Sit at the side of a sink that has a mixing faucet to regulate hot and cold water.
2. Run the faucet at moderate speed, mixing hot and cold water to a temperature of approximately 105° F.
3. The hands should be placed under the water. Active flexion and extension movements of the fingers with the hands together in a wringing-of-the-hands movement should be done.
4. The hot water should be used for 4 minutes; switch to cold water for 1 minute, hot water for 4 minutes, cold water for 1 minute, hot water for 4 minutes.
5. The hands are then dried and a small amount of hand lotion can be rubbed into the skin.

Active exercises

The patient may increase the range of motion and the strength of the reconstructed joints through a variety of exercises over devices such as the Bunnel block or modifications thereof, cylinders of progressive sizes, or a variety of special hand-exercise devices that are commercially available. These devices should maintain the architecture of the hand and should not force the digits into deforming positions (Fig. 61-13). To be efficient, they must support the bone proximal to the reconstructed joint to obtain the best mechanical advantage; with these goals in mind, we devised a

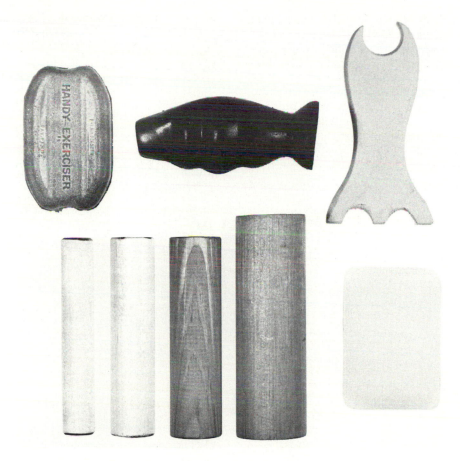

FIG. 61-13. Variety of exercise devices used to increase joint range of motion and strength. *Top (left to right),* Rubber modified Bunnel block; ''finger gripper'' shaped to maintain proper anatomic position of digits and arches of hand; ''finger crutch'' designed to help support proximal phalanx during flexion exercises of proximal interphalangeal joint. *Bottom (left to right),* Progressively sized wooden dowels; plastic modified Bunnel block.

''finger-gripper'' exercise device. Isotonic movements in which joint movement accompanies the exercise effort are important for the gliding mechanism of the joint. Isometric exercises, as in grasping around a solid object or therapy putty, are especially good for muscle strengthening. The use of progressively smaller objects to grasp, such as various sizes of wood dowels, is an excellent way of obtaining an improved range of motion.

It is advisable for the patient to use his hand protectively during the early postoperative phase. The postoperative rehabilitation program must be continued for at least 3 months after surgery because of the tendency of these previously stiffened joints to tighten up. It is best to discontinue the exercises gradually, rather than abruptly, and it is wise to follow a weekly self-evaluation of the range of motion. After this, the patient can safely use his hand for activities of daily living and vocational skills. However, the patient should continue to exercise and splint as necessary for up to 1 year after surgery.

A very cooperative patient following a good rehabilitation program can obtain an excellent range of motion using the implant resection arthroplasty method.

Stretching of contractures

Most contractures around joints can be progressively stretched by application of splints or plaster casts, which slowly elongate the tissues without causing the secondary reactions after overzealous movements that tear the collagen. If bone adhesions are not involved in the contracture, diligent stretching by repeated applications of splints can be of benefit.

Manipulation

Manipulation of joints to correct contracture deformities is usually not indicated. Gentle progressive stretching is preferred. Occasionally, if the contracture has not been long established, gentle manipulation of the joint with or without anesthesia may achieve better positioning of the joint. We have used this technique very infrequently in our practice. If a manipulation is done, temporary fixation in the corrected position is usually indicated.

Rehabilitation techniques are highly individualized with each reconstructive surgeon. A physical therapist and occupational therapist and other trained personnel, when available, can be of assistance in carrying out postoperative therapy programs. However, they require close supervision by the surgeon to properly adhere to his prescribed program. An understanding of the basic concepts of the flexible implant resection arthroplasty and the development of good rapport with the patient can allow the operating surgeon to obtain ideal results from this method.

BIBLIOGRAPHY

Madden, J.W., and Peacock, E.E., Jr.: Studies on the biology of collagen during wound healing: dynamic metabolism of scar collagen and remodeling of dermal wounds, Ann. Surg. **174:**511-520, 1971.

Madden, J.W., Arem, A., and DeVore, G.: A rational post-operative management program for metacarpophalangeal implant arthroplasty, J. Hand Surg. **2**(5):358-366, 1977.

Swanson, A.B.: A flexible implant for replacement of arthritic or destroyed joints in the hand, N.Y.U. Interclin. Inform. Bull. **6:**16-19, 1966.

Swanson, A.B.: Flexible implant resection arthroplasty in the hand and extremities, St. Louis, 1973, The C.V. Mosby Co.

Swanson, A.B.: Flexible implant arthroplasty in the hand, Clin. Plast. Surg. **3:**141-157, 1976.

Swanson, A.B., and de Groot Swanson, G.: Bone remodeling phenomena in flexible (silicone) implant arthroplasty in the hand: long-term study, Kappa Delta Award Lecture, 49th Annual Meeting of Orthopaedic Surgeons, New Orleans, Jan. 21-26, 1982, Orthop. Rev. **11**(7):129, 1982.

Swanson, A.B., and de Groot Swanson, G.: Joint replacement in the rheumatoid metacarpophalangeal joint. American Academy of Orthopaedic Surgeons: Symposium on Total Joint Replacement of the Upper Extremity, A. Inglis, editor: American Academy of Orthopaedic Surgeons: St. Louis, 1982, The C.V. Mosby Co., pp. 217-237.

Swanson, A.B., de Groot Swanson, G., and Leonard, J.: Postoperative rehabilitation program for flexible implant arthroplasty of the fingers. In American Academy of Orthopaedic Surgeons: Symposium on Total Joint Replacement of the Upper Extremity, Inglis, A. editor: St. Louis, 1982, The C.V. Mosby Co., pp. 238-254.

Swanson, A.B., and Netter, F.H.: Reconstructive surgery in the arthritic hand and foot, Ciba Clin. Symp. **31**(6), 1979.

62

The rheumatoid thumb

EDWARD A. NALEBUFF and CYNTHIA A. PHILIPS

The bad news is that rheumatoid arthritis frequently involves the all-important thumb, resulting in significant deformity and functional loss. The good news is that it is possible to understand the various deformities and to carry out both nonsurgical and surgical treatment to prevent and correct them, with restoration of function. Disruption of the normal thumb biomechanics often leads to significant loss of the patient's ability to carry out activities of daily living. Such activities as buttoning of clothing or the manipulation of small objects is greatly diminished if the patient lacks either control or stability of the thumb joints. Before embarking on a discussion of our current treatment program, we will review the most common thumb deformities and determine the factors that lead to their development.

DEFORMITIES OF THE RHEUMATOID THUMB

The deformities encountered in the rheumatoid patient are varied and are the result of changes taking place both intrinsically and extrinsically to the thumb. Synovial hypertrophy within the individual thumb joints not only can lead to destruction of articular cartilage, but also can stretch out the supporting collateral ligaments and joint capsules. As a result of this, each joint can become unstable and react to the stresses applied to it both in function against the other digits or as a result of the deforming forces of the extensor or flexor tendons acting upon it. A number of years ago one of us (E.N.)[5] proposed a classification in which the deformities were divided into three types. The type I deformity was believed to be the most common and was characterized by metacarpophalangeal joint flexion, distal joint hyperextension, and metacarpal abduction. Others have called this the "Boutonnière deformity" of the thumb,[12] which is confusing because the flexion deformity in this thumb deformity is at the metacarpophalangeal joint rather than at the proximal interphalangeal joint as in a digit. The usual sequence of events leading to this particular deformity is as follows: Synovitis of the metacarpophalangeal joint stretches out the extensor mechanism made up of the extensor pollicis brevis and extensor pollicis longus tendon. After this, the proximal phalanx tends to subluxate volarly or assumes a flexed position. Although the patient may maintain passive extension, there is an inability to extend the joint actively. As a compensating mechanism, the patient will abduct the first metacarpal and hyperextend the distal

joint. This hyperextension of the distal joint and the flexion of the metacarpophalangeal joint as well is accentuated when pinch forces are applied to the thumb. This particular deformity is best described as an "extrinsic-minus" deformity (Fig. 62-1). As stated above, the most common site for the initial change is at the metacarpophalangeal joint, and it is the lack of extrinsic extensor power that starts the sequence of events. Not only can this be the result of changes occurring at the joint level itself, but also a rupture of the extensor pollicis longus at the wrist level can lead to the same deformity (Fig. 62-2). Although this particular deformity of the thumb most commonly originates at the metacarpophalangeal level with the distal joint hyperextension being a secondary factor, the reverse can also occur. As a result of stretching of the volar plate of the distal joint or rupture of the flexor pollicis longus tendon, the distal joint hyperextension can be primary, with metacarpophalangeal joint flexion being secondary (Fig. 62-3). In these patients the metacarpal abduction is usually not a significant factor. Therefore, when faced with a patient presenting with a type I deformity, one should evaluate not only the extensor tendons controlling the metacarpophalangeal joint but also the flexor tendon controlling the distal joint in order to determine the primary site of imbalance.

In the original classification of thumb deformities, deformities of type II and type III were described.[5] In both of these instances the original alteration was at the carpometacarpal joint level with subluxation of the first metacarpal, which then assumed an adducted position. In some of these patients the metacarpophalangeal joint and interphalangeal joint assumed positions identical with the type I deformity in that the metacarpophalangeal joint was flexed and the distal joint was hyperextended. This particular combination of metacarpal adduction with metacarpophalangeal joint flexion and distal joint hyperextension (type II) (Fig. 62-4) is not common and assumes importance only in that it should be recognized as different from the type I deformity because of the metacarpal adduction. A much more common sequence of events after carpometacarpal joint subluxation and metacarpal adduction is metacarpophalangeal joint hyperextension and distal joint flexion (type III) (Fig. 62-5). This deformity is the opposite of the common type I deformity in all respects. It has been called a "swan-neck deformity" of the thumb, but since the hyperextension is at the meta-

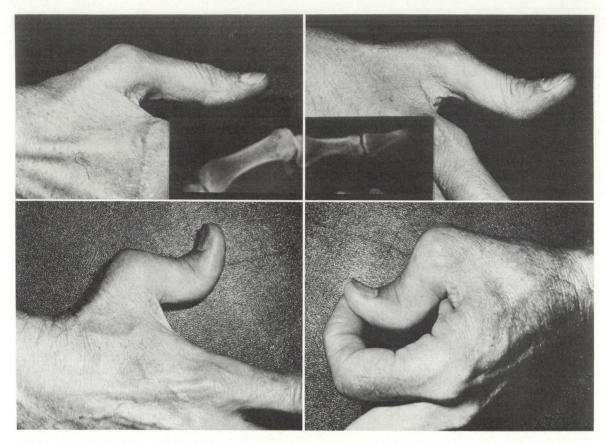

FIG. 62-1. Development of the common type I thumb deformity with early metacarpophalangeal flexion. Roentgenogram shows associated volar subluxation of joint. *Lower left,* Metacarpal abduction and distal joint hyperextension, as patient tries to straighten thumb. Deformity is accentuated with pinch, *lower right.*

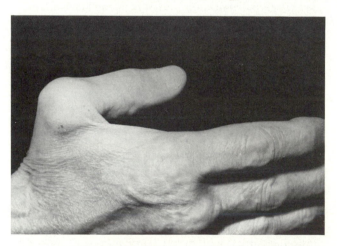

FIG. 62-2. Metacarpophalangeal joint flexion deformity of thumb secondary to rupture of extensor pollicis longus tendon at wrist.

carpophalangeal joint rather than the proximal interphalangeal joint, it is a confusing term and we believe should be avoided in classifying thumb deformities. At first, the metacarpophalangeal joint hyperextension is passively correctable. In fact, with time the range of metacarpophalangeal joint flexion diminishes and ultimately the joint is fixed in either a straight or hyperextended position. Any attempt to correct the type III deformity requires the first metacarpal to be abducted. If the carpometacarpal joint is subluxated, abduction can often only be accomplished by surgery. With restoration of metacarpal abduction the metacarpophalangeal joint hyperextension deformity may correct itself, but if fixed hyperextension persists, this joint must also be treated, either by arthrodesis, tenodesis, or capsulodesis in a flexed position.

Since our original description of these three thumb deformities, we have encountered a number of patients with deformities that at first glance appear similar to the type III deformity but originate at the metacarpophalangeal joint level. The most common of these, which we call type IV (Fig. 62-6), is the result of stretching out of the ulnar collateral ligament of the metacarpophalangeal joint as a result of synovitis. As the proximal deviates laterally at the metacarpophalangeal joint level, the first metacarpal secondarily assumes an adducted position. After this, the first dorsal interosseous and adductor muscles are shortened and the web space between the thumb and index finger becomes contracted. Although the first metacarpal is adducted in these patients, there is no subluxation at the carpometacarpal joint. The key to treatment with this deformity is to restore stability to the metacarpophalangeal joint in a corrected

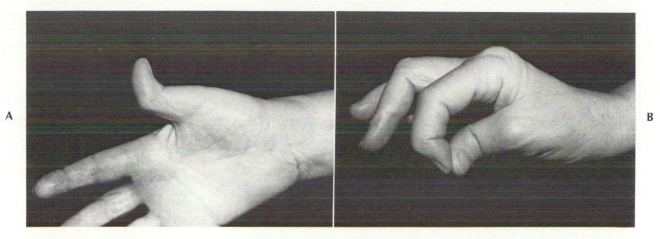

FIG. 62-3. Type I thumb deformity secondary to distal joint hyperextension. **A,** Hyperextension of distal joint, as result of stretching out or rupture of volar plate. **B,** Accentuation of deformity with pinch.

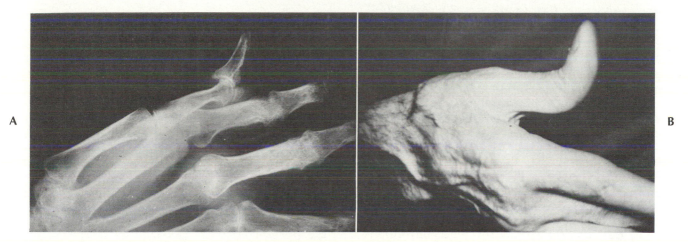

FIG. 62-4. The uncommon type II thumb deformity with metacarpal adduction and metacarpophalangeal joint flexion and distal joint extension. **A,** Metacarpal adduction at carpometacarpal joint. **B,** Clinical appearance of thumb.

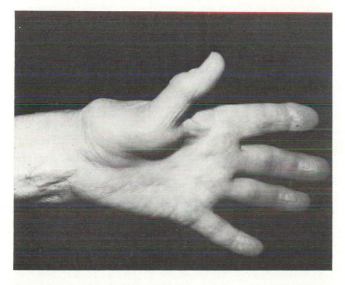

FIG. 62-5. Type III thumb deformity—metacarpal adduction with metacarpophalangeal joint hyperextension and distal joint flexion. Initial step in this deformity is subluxation of carpometacarpal joint.

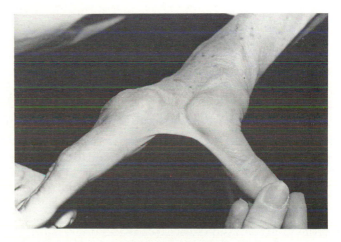

FIG. 62-6. Type IV deformity demonstrates adducted metacarpal with abduction of metacarpophalangeal joint. Initial stage of this deformity is stretching of ulnar collateral ligament. Metacarpal adduction and tight web space are secondary.

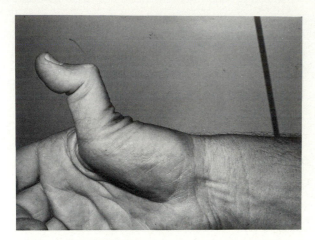

FIG. 62-7. Demonstrates type I deformity with hyperextension of metacarpophalangeal joint secondary to stretching of volar plate. Metacarpal adduction in this case is secondary to metacarpophalangeal hyperextension. Carpometacarpal joint is preserved.

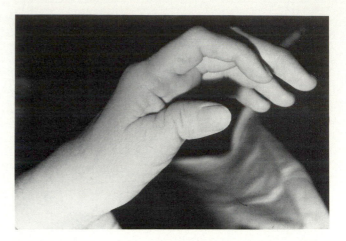

FIG. 62-8. Type VI thumb deformity showing collapse with loss of bone substance. In this particular case, major bone loss involves area adjacent to interphalangeal joint.

position and to release the first web space contracture. A Z-plasty of the skin in the first web space may be needed. Surgery is ordinarily not necessary at the carpometacarpal joint level. Another thumb deformity, type V, should also be recognized. There are patients in whom the major deforming factor is instability or stretching out of the volar plate of the metacarpophalangeal joint of the thumb. As a result of this, the metacarpophalangeal joint hyperextends and the distal joint assumes a flexed position (Fig. 62-7). In these patients, however, the first metacarpal bone need not assume an adducted position and the carpometacarpal joint is usually not involved. This particular deformity is best treated by stabilization of the metacarpophalangeal joint either by a fusion or a capsulodesis in a flexed position. These five thumb deformity patterns are the result of imbalances occurring between the various joints of the thumb. One can see that in each of these cases the alteration of posture at one level has an affect upon the adjacent joint. However, there is another type of thumb deformity, type VI (Fig. 62-8), which should be mentioned in which the major element is a collapse or loss of bone substance.[7] Patients with arthritis mutilans develop thumbs that become quite short and are characteristically unstable with what appears to be abundant skin in relationship to the underlying skeleton. Although this condition can be isolated at the thumb level, it is ordinarily associated with similar difficulties in the other digits.

The six patterns of thumb postures described above unfortunately do not exhaust the deformities one encounters in rheumatoid arthritis. It is possible, for example, for the patient to stretch the supporting structures of a joint causing either a flexion, extension, or lateral deformity. However, instead of the adjacent joint assuming the opposite posture, it may assume an abnormal position secondary to a tendon rupture. Thus a patient might present with hyperextension of both the metacarpophalangeal and proximal interphalangeal joints or in fact flexion at both levels. When patients are encountered with adjacent joints deformed in the same direction, it usually implies that a combination of factors

have brought this about. The examiner should check each individual joint for instability and also the controlling tendons for their integrity.

EVALUATION OF THE THUMB

Although it is of value to recognize the various thumb deformities and gain an understanding of their development, it is still necessary in each case to evaluate the individual joints of the thumb in order to determine appropriate therapy. One should, of course, not limit the evaluation to the thumb but instead assess the whole hand and upper extremity joints, since the thumb does not act in isolation in the hand function. Our evaluation ordinarily includes a recording of the active and passive ranges of motion, pinch strength, and grip strength as well as a functional status of the hand. Ranges of motion are recorded with a goniometer. Grip strength is recorded with a Jamar Dynamometer, and pinch strength is recorded with a standard pinch meter. Normal grip strength varies with age and sex. However, a normal grip strength for a man is around 100 pounds.[2] We have found that a grip strength of at least 20 pounds is necessary to perform most daily activities. One must keep in mind that many people with rheumatoid arthritis have grip strengths far below this functional level. Pulp, lateral, and three-jaw chuck pinch are also tested. Although grip strength is, of course, important, pinch strength has a particular application when one is assessing self-care skills. These include holding eating utensils, buttoning clothing, writing, and manipulating small objects for precision grip. Normal pinch strength ranges between 15 and 20 pounds.[2] We have found that a pinch strength of 5 to 7 pounds is necessary to accomplish most daily activities. Many rheumatoid patients have less than this. Therefore they encounter considerable difficulty in accomplishing even simple activities.

Functional assessment is also done as part of our examination. We use the Moberg pickup test to evaluate dexterity[4] (Fig. 62-9). We may also use other objective tests such as the Purdue Peg Board Test if the situation merits

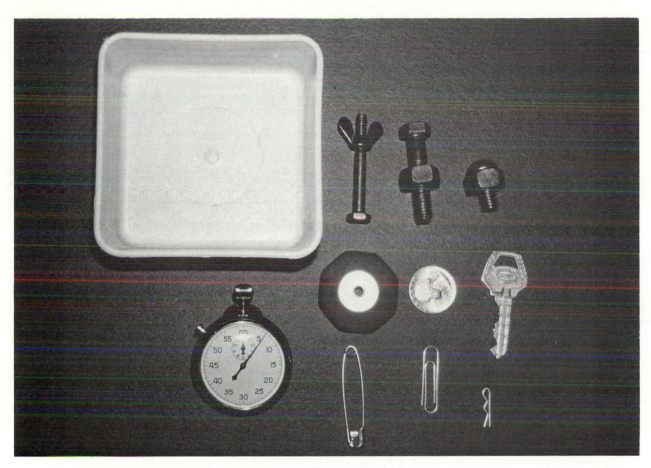

FIG. 62-9. Materials used to perform Moberg pickup test. Nine objects of varying shapes and sizes are used. Patient picks these objects up and places them in basket, first with eyes open and then with eyes closed. Stopwatch is used to record speed.

additional testing. In more complex cases we may use the Jebsen Hand Function Test.[1]

The types of deformities encountered and the mechanism of these deformities have been previously discussed. Initially they are passively correctable. At this stage, the goal of hand therapy is to help maintain joint mobility and to help protect the joint through splinting and joint protection procedures. When the carpometacarpal joint becomes involved, the synovitis stretches out the joint capsule. As stated previously, this stretching can lead to joint subluxation or dislocation, with the metacarpal assuming an adducted position. The goal of therapy at this joint is to help prevent the adduction contracture and to maintain a functional range of motion. To accomplish this goal, we fabricate a carpometacarpal joint splint to maintain the thumb web space and to stabilize and protect the carpometacarpal joint. The splint extends distally to the interphalangeal joint level and proximally past the carpometacarpal joint to a level reaching the middle or proximal area of the forearm (Fig. 62-10). In this way, the carpometacarpal joint has good stabilization and the metacarpophalangeal joint can be maintained in a corrected position. We advise patients to wear this splint at night. They are also encouraged to wear the splint during the day as much as possible while performing functional activities. Patients are instructed to remove the splint at least

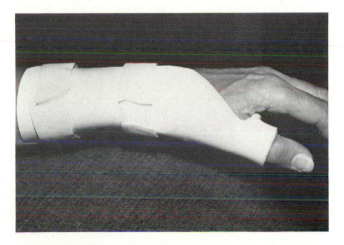

FIG. 62-10. Splint used for stabilizing the carpometacarpal joint. This is used both for relief of pain and as a protective device for patients with carpometacarpal involvement.

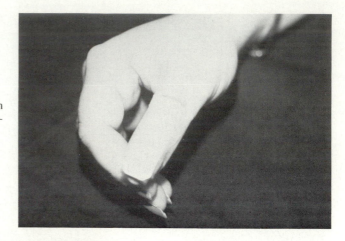

FIG. 62-11. Interphalangeal joint protected with aluminum foam splint during activities. This is used when patient shows involvement at that joint.

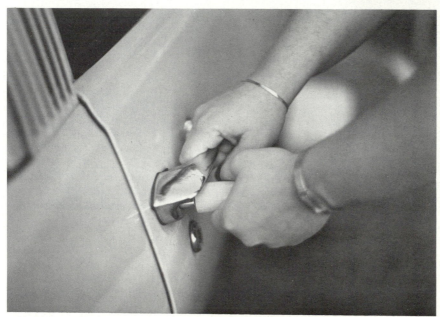

FIG. 62-12. Patient using dowel to open car door to minimize force to joints of thumb.

FIG. 62-13. Patient wringing out a dishcloth in a way that decreases stress to thumb, wrist, and other digits.

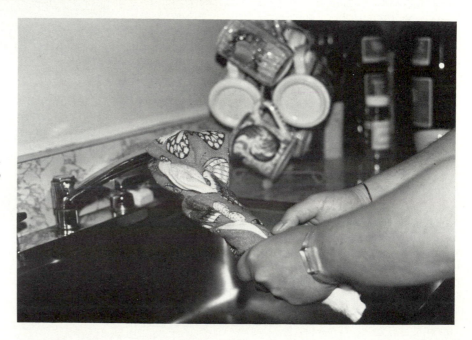

three times a day to take the thumb through a gentle range of motion. In our experience, a short opponens splint is not effective in stabilizing and positioning the carpometacarpal joint of the thumb.

In cases where the metacarpophalangeal joint is involved, the goals are to prevent the deformity from becoming fixed and to help protect the joint from external forces that can produce further joint damage and deformity. One way this can be accomplished is through the use of a small splint for the metacarpophalangeal joint. One can do this by taping an aluminum foam splint to the metacarpophalangeal joint or by fabricating a metacarpophalangeal splint from a thermoplastic material. Since immobilizing one joint can cause added stress to adjacent joints, the therapist must watch for signs of increased synovitis or pain in these areas. The splint is worn during the functional activities and removed several times a day for range-of-motion exercises.

The interphalangeal joint can also be protected by the use of an aluminum and foam splint taped to the joint (Fig. 62-11). This provides both stability and protection to the interphalangeal joint. If this joint becomes unstable, splinting helps to improve pinch while the person is awaiting corrective surgery. These small splints should be changed frequently to prevent any skin maceration.

One of the most important aspects of treatment is to teach the patient techniques of joint protection. The joints of the thumb are subject to great external stresses during activities of daily living. When the joints are swollen with synovitis, they are even more vulnerable to these outside forces. Therefore we instruct patients in general joint protection principles and specifically those that will minimize stress to the joints and soft-tissue structures of the thumb. Special devices are recommended for use during certain activities. One of the most stressful activities for the thumb is the opening of a car door. A piece of dowel that can be kept in the patient's pocket or purse can be used for car doors with a push button. The patient uses the dowel to push the button rather than placing the strain on the thumb (Fig. 62-12). There are also commercially available car-door openers. Turning a key can also be both stressful and difficult for patients with severe thumb involvement. A commercially available key holder can be used or a device can be fabricated using thermoplast materials. One tries to provide a greater surface area for grip. This will reduce the stress to the thumb and the index finger as well. We also advise patients to use built-up pens or large-diameter pens, which are available in stationery stores, to help minimize the stress to the thumb when writing. It takes less strength for the patient to stabilize the large-diameter object. Patients may find felt-tip pens easier to use because of reduced friction on the paper. Eating and other utensils can also be built up to reduce the external forces not only on the thumb but on the whole hand. We encourage patients to use as many lightweight utensils as possible. Activities such as wringing out clothes or a washcloth can put a great deal of strain on the wrist and thumb, particularly the carpometacarpal joint. This stress can be reduced by wrapping the cloth around the water faucet rather than twisting it with the hands. The cloth is wrapped around the water faucet and then is squeezed rather than twisted (Fig. 62-13). Certain repetitive activities such as the use of

scissors are particularly stressful to the carpometacarpal joint and should be avoided as much as possible. We also advise patients to limit knitting and crocheting. These activities often lead to increased pain in the thumb and to symptoms of carpal tunnel syndrome. These activities also keep the hand and wrist in very poor positions, actually the position of deformity.

These suggestions for alteration of activities in daily living and the use of splints can afford these patients considerable relief. They may also slow the progression of deformity. However, surgical therapy is often the final treatment to correct the deformity, provide stability, and relieve pain.

SURGICAL TREATMENT

Despite the fact that there are various deformities affecting the thumb leading to bizarre alterations in posture at multiple levels, the surgical procedures that are applicable are more determined by the joint involved than by the specific type of deformity encountered. For this reason, we discuss the surgical procedures commonly performed at each joint level rather than discussing the individual deformities and their specific treatment.

INTERPHALANGEAL JOINT

The terminal joints of the thumb can, as a result of stretching of supporting structures, assume either a flexed, extended, or laterally deviated position. Flexion and extension deformities at this level can result from ruptures of the extensor or flexor pollicis longus tendons. In these particular instances restoration of tendon function is attempted if the articular surface and supporting structures of the joint are intact. In the case of loss of extensor power, the tendon usually ruptures at the wrist level. With retraction of the muscle it is ordinarily not possible to carry out end-to-end tendon repairs, and restoration of extensor pollicis longus function is ordinarily achieved by transfer of the extensor indicis proprius to the extensor mechanism over the metacarpophalangeal joint of the thumb.[6] In evaluating extensor tendon ruptures of the thumb affecting the distal joint one must check the extensor apparatus both at the wrist level and at the metacarpophalangeal level where local ruptures can also be encountered. Because of the strong flexor power that is present with the intact flexor pollicis longus tendon, any extensor repair should be splinted for at least 5 weeks before one encourages active motion with force. The ruptures of the flexor pollicis longus tendon are quite common in the rheumatoid patient. The most frequent site of rupture is at the volar aspect of the wrist in the region of the carpal scaphoid[8] (Fig. 62-14). A portion of the scaphoid bone ordinarily erodes through the volar joint capsule and acts as a sharp edge against which the flexor tendon ruptures. When faced with a patient who has lost active flexion of the distal joint of the thumb, which is usually in a hyperextended position, one should assume that the tendon rupture is at the wrist level. In those instances in which the distal joint of the thumb is irregular or unstable so that restoration of active motion does not seem worthwhile, one might consider stabilizing the joint by bony fusion. However, if the diagnosis of flexor pollicis longus rupture has

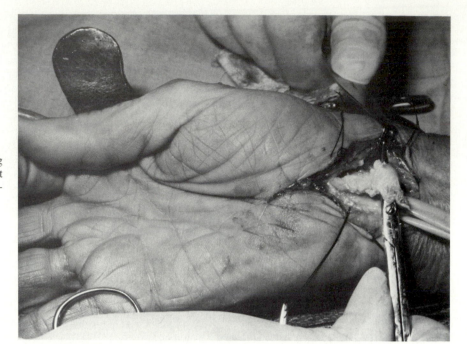

FIG. 62-14. Volar view of wrist, demonstrating rupture of flexor pollicis longus tendon at wrist. This is an attrition rupture on bony spicule of scaphoid.

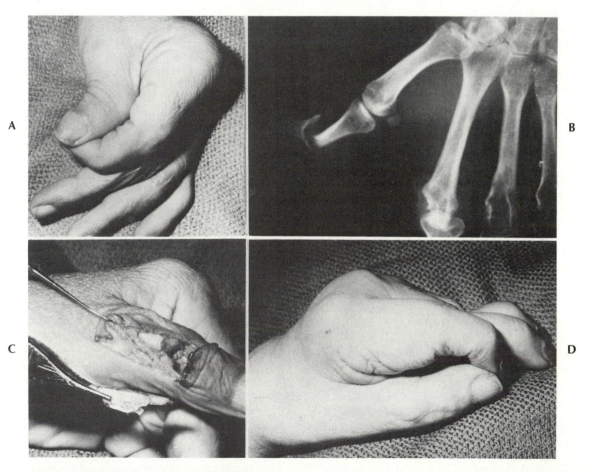

FIG. 62-15. Surgical treatment for unstable thumb with collapse deformity. Bone graft used to restore length. **A,** Preoperative pinch with collapse. **B,** Roentgenogram showing loss of bone substance. **C,** At surgery, bone graft prepared for insertion. **D,** Postoperative pinch stability restored.

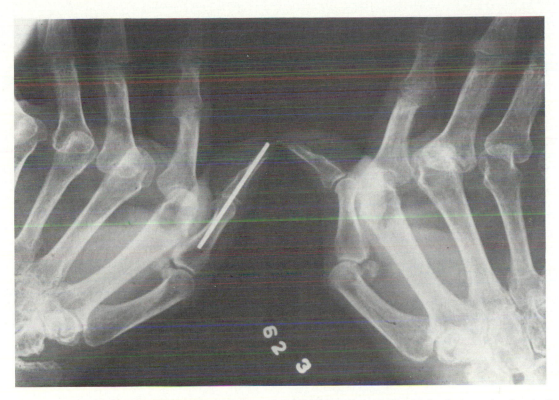

FIG. 62-16. Roentgenogram showing correction of type I thumb deformity with distal joint fusion using longitudinal Kirschner wire. Thumb on opposite hand demonstrates untreated type I thumb deformity.

been made, it is suggested that the volar aspect of the wrist also be explored with removal of any bone spicule in the carpal region. If this is not performed, the adjacent flexor tendons of the index finger are in jeopardy and, if left untreated, would sustain the same fate of spontaneous rupture. When one attempts to restore flexor pollicis longus function, it is also unusual to be able to carry out an end-to-end repair. Short "bridge" tendon grafts have been found useful, and in other patients tendon transfers using the superficial flexor of the ring finger can be carried out. In those patients in whom the joint is grossly unstable with or without intact extrinsic tendons, one should seriously consider an arthrodesis. Fusion of the terminal joints of the thumb does not cause significant functional loss and in fact improves the patients ability to pinch objects with force. Fusion at this level often makes it possible for one to correct rotation deformities of the thumb by putting the terminal joint in a slightly flexed and pronated position. In patients with the collapse type of deformities, the use of supplemental bone grafts is required not only to achieve fusion but also to restore length (Fig. 62-15). The most common fixation technique for interphalangeal joint fusion in the rheumatoid thumb is the use of a longitudinal Kirschner wire that is kept in place for at least 8 weeks (Fig. 62-16). An external aluminum splint can be used to protect the joint allowing mobility at the metacarpophalangeal level. In patients in whom volar instability is present but the joint surface is intact one could consider a flexor tenodesis using one half of the flexor pollicis longus attached distally to the proximal phalanx.[8,12] Arthroplasties for interphalangeal joint involve-

ment in the rheumatoid thumb are rarely indicated, because they do not provide good lateral stability.

METACARPOPHALANGEAL JOINT

The surgical procedures found useful about the metacarpophalangeal joint in the rheumatoid patient include synovectomy, extensor pollicis longus rerouting, arthrodesis, arthroplasty, and capsulodesis. Synovectomy is advisable in those patients in whom the joint is chronically swollen and whom x-ray evaluation reveals that the joint surfaces are still well maintained. When synovectomy is performed for the rheumatoid thumb, one often encounters a stretching out or elongation of the extensor mechanism. In these cases, it is advisable to carry out some shortening of the extensor mechanism followed by splinting so that the rapid onset of a flexion deformity is prevented. In patients in whom a flexion deformity has occurred but passive extension is still possible, a reinforcement of the extensor forces to the metacarpophalangeal joint can be performed. A number of techniques have been advised, but one of us (E.N.)[5] has been pleased with the use of an extensor pollicis longus rerouting procedure, in which the long extensor tendon is rerouted through the dorsal capsule of the joint to provide additional extensor force at this level. When this procedure is done, the intrinsic muscles of the thumb, the flexor pollicis brevis and abductor pollicis brevis, act as extensor forces for the distal joint (Fig. 62-17).

For the metacarpophalangeal joint that is grossly unstable or in which the articular cartilage has been destroyed one must choose between arthrodesis or arthroplasty. For those

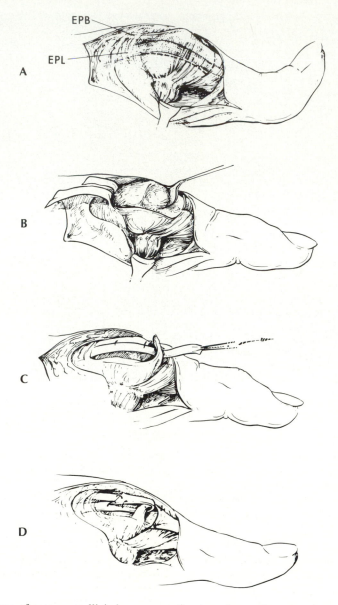

EPB

EPL

A

B

C

D

FIG. 62-17. Technique of extensor pollicis longus rerouting to restore active extension to metacarpophalangeal joint.

patients with flexion deformities it is possible to correct the deformity by resection of a portion of the adjacent joint surfaces and insertion of a Swanson flexible implant.[10-12] This procedure is ordinarily supplemented by a reinforcement or shortening of the extensor mechanism (Fig. 62-18). Patients undergoing arthroplasties at this level ordinarily are not started on early motion. It is important to splint these thumbs in almost full extension for 4 to 5 weeks before allowing unrestricted motion. We tend to limit the use of the implant arthroplasty at the metacarpophalangeal level to those patients having flexion deformities. In patients with hyperextension deformities arthrodesis of the metacarpophalangeal joint in a slightly flexed position is advisable. We are reluctant to insert a flexible implant in these patients because of the lack of volar stability. When one is

performing an arthrodesis of the metacarpophalangeal joint of the thumb, the position to strive for is 15 degrees of flexion, 5 degrees of abduction, and 20 degrees of pronation (Fig. 62-19). For fixation we usually use two crossed Kirschner wires. Supplementary bone grafts are advisable if there has been some previous bone collapse or loss. It is important in these patients to start early postoperative interphalangeal joint motion, because there is a possible risk of the extensor mechanism becoming adherent at the fusion site. Fusions of the metacarpophalangeal joint in slight flexion to correct the hyperextension deformity are particularly important. By fusing the metacarpophalangeal joint in slight flexion one takes considerable strain off of the carpometacarpal joint. This is particularly important in those patients who have undergone or will require an arthroplasty at that level. In

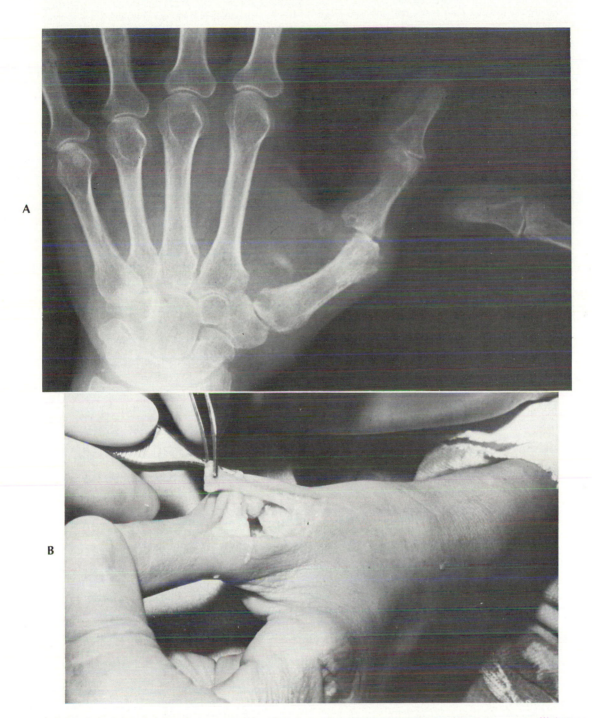

FIG. 62-18. Type I thumb deformity treated with arthroplasty of metacarpophalangeal joint and extensor pollicis longus rerouting procedure. **A,** Roentgenogram of subluxation of metacarpophalangeal joint showing much irregularity and loss of bone substance. **B,** Appearance at surgery with resection of joint before insertion of prosthesis and reattachment of extensor pollicis longus.

Continued.

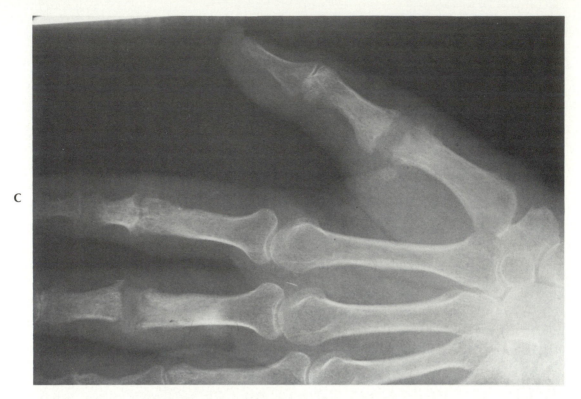

FIG. 62-18, cont'd. C, Postoperative correction of deformity with Swanson flexible implant arthroplasty in place.

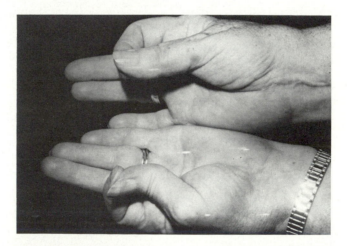

FIG. 62-19. *Right hand,* Correction of type I thumb deformity with arthrodesis of metacarpophalangeal joint. *Left hand,* Preoperative appearance with collapse of thumb on pinch.

patients with full flexibility of the metacarpophalangeal joint but a tendency to assume the hyperextended position, one can carry out a capsulodesis to maintain the joint in approximately 15 degrees of flexion.

At the carpometacarpal joint the surgical procedures performed include various types of arthroplasties and in specific instances arthrodesis. Because rheumatoid arthritis commonly affects multiple joints, it is ordinarily not advisable to fuse the carpometacarpal joint. Subsequent involvement at the metacarpophalangeal joint level requiring fusion would leave the patient with very little mobility. An exception to this rationale is the patient with lupus erythematosus.[9] In this condition, articular cartilage seems to be spared, and the major problem is an instability with subluxation of the joints. Therefore arthrodesis of the carpometacarpal joint can provide a solid foundation for the thumb. However, in most cases surgical treatment of the carpometacarpal joint implies some form of arthroplasty. Because carpal involvement is common in rheumatoid patients the trapezium implant commonly utilized in degen-

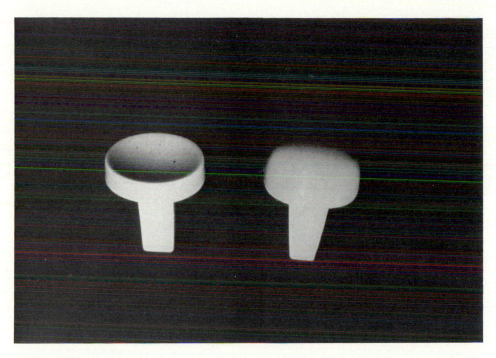

FIG. 62-20. Two types of prostheses used for hemiarthroplasty at base of thumb. *Left,* Concave prosthesis. *Right,* Convex condylar prosthesis.

erative arthritis is not used in these patients. The type of arthroplasty we commonly carry out at the carpometacarpal joint level in the rheumatoid arthritic patient is a resection arthroplasty in which bone is removed in order to allow the first metacarpal to assume an abducted position. Soft-tissue interposition using a piece of tendon is often helpful.[3] In other patients a hemiarthroplasty using either a concave or convex hemiprosthesis (Swanson) with a single stem inserted into the first metacarpal has been found to be worthwhile.[12] (Fig. 62-20). It is important after any carpometacarpal joint arthroplasty in the rheumatoid patient to maintain the thumb in a position of abduction for approximately 5 to 6 weeks before starting motion. As stated in the discussion of metacarpophalangeal joint surgery, it is imperative that one not leave a hyperextended metacarpophalangeal joint when performing an arthroplasty at the carpometacarpal joint level. If the metacarpophalangeal joint is allowed to collapse into hyperextension, the forces are quite strong to adduct the first metacarpal, leading to subluxation of any implant.

POSTOPERATIVE HAND THERAPY

Hand therapy is instituted very early in the postoperative management and is important in rehabilitating these patients. The therapy after thumb reconstruction is geared toward the functional use of the thumb. Periodic postoperative assessments are done to monitor the patient's progress. Postoperatively the thumb is immobilized for approximately 6 weeks. During this immobilization we encourage the patient to perform range-of-motion exercise of the other digits to prevent stiffness.

When the splint is removed, active and active-assistive range-of-motion exercises are started. These include circumduction, abduction, and opposition exercises. Initially, warm-water soaks may be helpful when one is initiating motion. Dexterity activities are then introduced into the program. The functional use of the thumb is gradually increased as tolerated by the patient. Increasing the program too rapidly can cause pain and increased swelling and should be avoided. However, if this should occur, the thumb must be rested before the therapy program is resumed.

After metacarpophalangeal arthroplasty of the thumb, immobilization is maintained for 5 weeks to ensure capsular healing. The goal is to provide a stable, pain-free joint for pinch. After the immobilization period, active and active-assistive exercises are started. Dexterity activities are introduced gradually over the next few weeks. Our goal is not to achieve a large range of motion, but enough to be functional. One does not need a great deal of metacarpophalangeal motion to have good hand dexterity and pinch strength. In fact, this joint has a wide variation in range of motion in the normal population.

In many cases other hand-reconstructive procedures may be done at the time thumb reconstruction is undertaken. Naturally one must keep that in mind when planning the patient's treatment program.

SUMMARY

Although the thumb is frequently involved in rheumatoid arthritis, causing significant function loss as well as pain and deformity, much can be done both nonsurgically and surgically to alleviate the condition and restore function to the patient.

REFERENCES

1. Jebsen, R.H., Taylor, N., Trieschmann, R.B., Trotter, M., and Howard, L.: An objective and standardized test of hand function, Arch. Phys. Med. **50:**311-319, June 1969.
2. Kellor, M., Kondrasuk, R., Iverson, I., and Hoglund, M.: Technical manual hand strength and dexterity tests, Minneapolis, 1971, Sister Kenny Rehabilitation Institute.
3. Millender, L.H., Nalebuff, E.A., Amadio, P., and Philips, C.: Interpositional arthroplasty for rheumatoid carpometacarpal joint disease, J. Hand Surg. **3**(6):533-541, Nov. 1978.
4. Moberg, E.: Objective methods of determining functional value of sensibility in the hand, J. Bone Joint Surg. **40:**454-466, 1958.
5. Nalebuff, E.A.: Diagnosis, classification and management of rheumatoid thumb deformities, Bull Hosp. Joint Dis. **29:**199, 1968.
6. Nalebuff, E.A.: The recognition and treatment of tendon ruptures in the rheumatoid hand. In American Academy of Orthopedic Surgeons: Symposium on Tendon Surgery in the Hand, St. Louis, 1975, The C.V. Mosby Co., pp. 255-269.
7. Nalebuff, E.A., and Garrett, J.: Opera-glass hand in rheumatoid arthritis, J. Hand Surg. **1**(3):210-220, Nov. 1976.
8. Nalebuff, E.A., and Millender, L.H.: Reconstructive surgery and rehabilitation of the hand. In Kelley, W.N., and others: Textbook of rheumatology, Philadelphia, 1981, W.B. Saunders Co., pp. 1900-1920.
9. Nalebuff, E.A., Dray, G., Millender, L.H., and Philips, C.: The surgical treatment of hand deformities in systemic lupus erythematosis, J. Hand Surg. **6**(4):339-345, July 1981.
10. Swanson, A.B.: Silicone rubber implants for replacement of arthritic or destroyed joints in the hand, Surg. Clin. North Am. **48:**1113-1127, 1968.
11. Swanson, A.B.: Flexible implant arthroplasty for arthritic finger joint, J. Bone Joint Surg. **54A:**435-455, 1972.
12. Swanson, A.B.: Flexible implant resection arthroplasty in the hand and extremities, St. Louis, 1973, The C.V. Mosby Co.

63

Preoperative assessment and postoperative therapy and splinting in rheumatoid arthritis

GLORIA L. DeVORE

In this chapter I discuss the method of patient selection for implant arthroplasty and the postoperative splinting and therapy employed at Hand Therapy Associates, Inc., in Tucson, Arizona. This protocol has evolved over 10 years in the evaluation and diagnosis of hundreds of patients. We believe it contributes greatly to our excellent results and satisfied patients.

In the development of the following evaluation techniques, we know that some portion of each aspect of the process must be utilized to some degree but the exact amounts are controlled and adjusted by the patient, the surgeon, and the therapist—the team. We seldom see rheumatoid arthritic patients in the beginning stages of their diseases; instead, most of them are referred to us when they are in the last stages of deformity.

PHILOSOPHY

In order that you understand our approach to upper extremity reconstruction for the rheumatoid hand, I will present the manner in which we approach the patient: The surgeon might ask, "How can I help you, Ms. Jones?" The answer almost invariably is, "I have arthritis and I would like you to fix my hands." Surgeon: "What is the problem with your hands, Ms. Jones? Where would one start to fix your hands?"

In looking at the hands (Fig. 63-1, *right hand*), you can appreciate the problem that confronts the surgeon. Before him are 24 finger joints, six thumb joints, and two wrists, all badly needing reconstructive surgery.

The question then becomes, "Where would one start?" From the viewpoints of the surgeon and therapist, many possibilities for surgical reconstruction exist. But would our viewpoints answer for the patients the questions of what and where their primary problems are located?

We start to help the patients define their problems by having them participate in a complex evaluation, which includes the following questions: In which joints are the problems located? Am I having difficulty because of pain, power, or position?

The following printed diary instructions and examples are reviewed and given to the patients. They are asked to keep diaries for at least 1 week.

Diary instructions

The purposes of this diary are:
1. To increase your awareness of yourself
2. To increase awareness regarding your particular disability

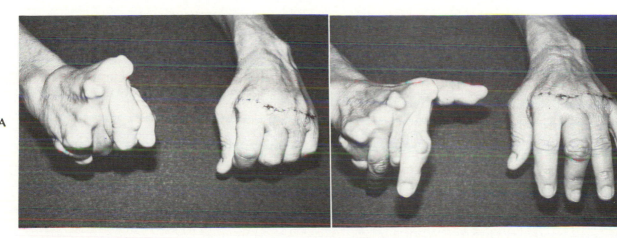

FIG. 63-1. **A,** Patient making a fist, 3 weeks after metacarpophalangeal implant anthroplasty on left hand. **B,** Patient extending fingers. Notice improved appearance of left hand. Surgery was performed on right hand 3 months later.

3. To aid us in accurate diagnosis and management of your disability
4. To make *you* an active participant in diagnosis and management of your disability

Before we get into the specifics of your diary, please begin by listing:

1. Current and past medications. Give frequency and doses of *current* medications only (example: Clinoril, 100 mg 4× daily).
2. Surgeries. List surgeon, operative date, and the procedure.
3. Wish list. Pretend your doctor and your therapist have a magic wand and are able to grant you three wishes as we begin to discuss your problems.

We hope this diary will raise your level of consciousness about yourself. As you complete your diary, you will discover many things about your hand that you have not been aware of previously. By doing this, your awareness and understanding will increase. All of this will be of great help to you, your doctor, and your therapist.

As you go through your daily routines and you come across activities that you used to do but are now unable to accomplish, or have difficulty accomplishing, write them in your diary under "Activity." Break the activity column into three components:

1. Pain
2. Position
3. Power

If you experience *pain,* list it in the pain column. A check (✔) is not enough. We need *location* of the pain and a description of what the pain feels like—the more adjectives used the better. If you become confused about a particular joint, just place your hand on the attached diagram and then identify the joint.

Next, think about the activity and decide if you are unable to accomplish the task successfully because you cannot *position* your hand correctly *on* or *around* the object. List the joint and the position that you are having difficulty achieving. Again, if you get confused about the name of the joint, place your hand on the diagram.

And last, ask yourself if your inability or difficulty in accomplishing the task is a result of lack of *power* or of *strength,* or both. In this column, you may simply place a check (✔). However, if you would like to make a comment, please do so.

You may construct your chart like the one below. The results of your diary may vary with each activity. There is no need to list activities twice. Please identify the hand in which you are experiencing the problem.

Read the examples carefully.

Bring your diary with you when you come to us for your functional evaluation. Your therapist will review your activities with you.

If you should have any questions, please feel free to call us.

Activity	Pain	Position	Power
Holding a coffee mug	MP joints of fingers and CMC joint of thumb	Can't grab cup with MP joints—extend ulnar deviation	Because of ulnar drift and position
Opening or unscrewing pill bottle or lids	Right wrist—ache MP joints MP joint of thumb	Can't grasp because of ulnar drift and inability to tightly flex MPs and PIPs	No power because of inability to position
Combing hair	Shoulder—ache and tight Elbow—same Wrist—same	Unable to lift shoulder, flex elbow, and extend wrist, hold brush simultaneously	Yes, because of position and pain
Lifting pan off stove	Wrist and CMC joint of thumb—burning, pulling, dull ache	No problem	Yes, because of pain and weakness
Using keys for door or car—turning or twisting motion	MP joint (index, long) CMC and MP joints of thumb and wrist	Can't pinch hard enough with thumb, index, and long	Yes, limited by position and power
Writing	MP joint of all fingers, carpal area, and ulnar burning, pulling	_____	Maintaining position is difficult

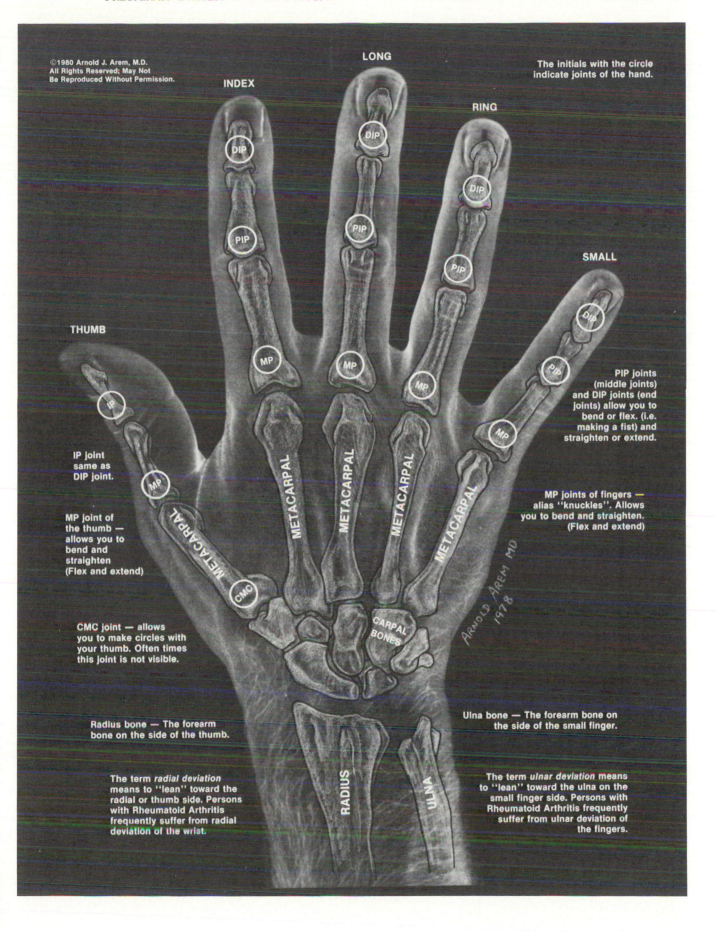

©1980 Arnold J. Arem, M.D.
All Rights Reserved; May Not
Be Reproduced Without Permission.

The initials with the circle
indicate joints of the hand.

LONG

INDEX

RING

SMALL

DIP

DIP

DIP

PIP

DIP

PIP

PIP

DIP

PIP

THUMB

MP

MP

MP

IP

PIP

PIP joints
(middle joints)
and DIP joints (end
joints) allow you to
bend or flex. (i.e.
making a fist) and
straighten or extend.

MP

IP joint
same as
DIP joint.

MP

MP joint of
the thumb —
allows you to
bend and
straighten
(Flex and extend)

METACARPAL

METACARPAL

METACARPAL

METACARPAL

MP joints of fingers —
alias "knuckles". Allows
you to bend and straighten.
(Flex and extend)

CMC

Arnold Arem MD
1978

CMC joint — allows
you to make circles with
your thumb. Often times
this joint is not visible.

CARPAL
BONES

Radius bone — The forearm
bone on the side of the thumb.

Ulna bone — The forearm bone on
the side of the small finger.

RADIUS

ULNA

The term *radial deviation*
means to "lean" toward the
radial or thumb side. Persons
with Rheumatoid Arthritis
frequently suffer from radial
deviation of the wrist.

The term *ulnar deviation* means
to "lean" toward the ulna on the
small finger side. Persons with
Rheumatoid Arthritis frequently
suffer from ulnar deviation of
the fingers.

The patients return to the clinic with their completed notes, and the functional evaluation is performed in one and sometimes two periods. It should be noted that functional evaluations are not limited to the upper limbs; the diaries can be used for various problems involving the entire body.

FUNCTIONAL EVALUATION
History

Extensive histories of the patients are first taken so that a data base and the patients' attitudes toward their chronic disease can be established. Included are medications, past and present progress of the disease, other medical problems, and present home setting. It is of great importance that patients become aware of their position on the team. Patients must come to understand that all future decisions that are made regarding their care must be made with their understanding and commitment and that they hold the ultimate responsibility for their own care.

As we continue to gather our data base, range-of-motion (ROM) and ulnar drift measurements are taken for all joints in both upper extremities. This is done for objective documentation of their status on that date.

Joint protection

To continue the evaluation, we use questions clustered around broad topics. Inevitably, joint protection becomes a topic of conversation. A patient facing the therapist across the table will eventually rest his head upon his hand, with the fingers being pushed off into ulnar deviation. This provides a perfect opening to discuss the best physiologic and mechanical way to rest the head on the hand without causing further damage.

We then ask for demonstrations of how patients get up from their chairs. Many patients are no longer at a stage where even the most widely accepted standards can be utilized in getting up from a chair. A trial-and-error session must take place to provide a way of getting them to their feet without causing undue forces in the wrong direction, especially if any type of joint replacement is to be considered. This is always a difficult task, because these established habit patterns are very difficult to change, and it is sometimes too traumatic to try.

Muscle testing

Muscle testing and evaluation of tendon continuity are performed carefully. We believe there must be evidence of muscle contraction in all muscle groups surrounding a joint being considered for possible replacement. Tendon rupture always changes the complexity of reconstruction and serves as an indicator of the extent of the disease process on the tendons. We have observed clinically that when one tendon has ruptured, patients are in great danger of further ruptures. A discussion now takes place regarding the synovial linings around the tendon sheaths. We explain that early in the disease a synovectomy with removal of the diseased tissue acts as a deterrent to tendon rupture.

Further discussions about the anatomy of the dorsal surface of the wrist, the volar surface of the wrist, the metacarpophalangeal joints, and the proximal interphalangeal joints are carried out. We point out differences between dorsal and volar compartments. Many times patients believe their problems are isolated only in the dorsa of their hands, because of the obvious deformities. We explain to them that significant hidden volar problems often exist.

We find it easier for patients to understand the involved anatomy when we use a plastic skeleton of the wrist. We demonstrate how the tendons on the volar surface are trapped, along with the median nerve, in the carpal tunnel by the transverse carpal ligament. Dorsally the tendons are all held in place by a wide band, the extensor retinaculum (retinaculum extensorum). Under this band, the tendons are surrounded by sheaths so that they glide back and forth.

Sensation

Sensation is tested by light-touch sensory testing, with the right and left hands being compared. We ask about being awakened at night by the hands going to sleep. We go into further detail regarding the volar compartment and discussion of the median nerve, which often gets compressed by the hypertrophic synovium, which cannot be seen as readily on the volar surface as on the dorsal surface. On many occasions, we find that the sensory problems are not at the wrist at all but are much more proximal, often in the neck. This is tested by having the patient assume the position that causes the paresthesia.

By this point in the evaluation, patients are beginning to have more understanding of their complex problems and can speak with us regarding the progression of their disease in terms other than a decrease in their sedimentation rate.

Exercises

Only very specific exercises are given in our clinic. Some patients who have had arthritis for over 20 years are still trying to do the same exercise program they were given when the disease was first diagnosed. As a consequence of this experience, we are unwilling to give patients three pages of by-the-number exercises. We believe we can do this only when we are assured of being able to follow the patients and only if we can design a program when the exercises are active and under direct control of the patients.

Flatt has stated that joint range without sufficient muscle control is of no value and leads to joint instability. Our clinical observation bears this out. Can you visualize patients continuing to do finger exercises of thumb-to-finger-tips opposition when every metacarpophalangeal joint is subluxated and intrinsic tightness is already severe? Many patients continue to try to do radial exercises when structurally it is no longer possible.

There are two mobility plans we are willing to give patients that, if they should continue for 20 years, would keep them much more functional and make for a better life-style. One is the overhead-pulley exercise for shoulders, with a piece of adaptive equipment that we make in our clinic. The other is hip abduction. Hip abduction mobility over the years becomes crucial; many patients in the process of their evaluation talk to us about the loss of this motion.

Sometimes at the end of the assessment, patients come

to the realization that their problems are not in their hands as they suspected, but that the lack of power and position are due to shoulder pain and immobility.

We have all experienced the often-repeated story of inability to get the hands where they need to be to carry out the tasks required (such as dressing or taking care of toilet needs). This is a shoulder problem and not a hand problem.

Diary assessment

Now we come to the special part of the evaluation, the diary, examples of which follow.

Wish list—J.M., early forties, pipe salesman in construction industry

Would like to wear gloves.
Would like to put baseball glove on left hand.
Would like to pass baseball or football with sons.
Would like to be able to use a hammer, screwdriver, or any tool in the proper manner.
Would like to hold a gun to hunt and a fishing rod to fish.
Would like to be able to shake hands. When I try now the other man's grip hurts my knuckles.

Diary excerpt—B.M., 59-year-old woman, retired teacher

In a public restroom, unable to open door after it was unlocked. Had to knock to get out.

Turning on T.V., had to use both hands to hold remote control unit in proper position to punch on program.

In looking at recent photographs, I notice I always try to hide my hands; however, they usually show anyway and their deformity. A more "normal" appearance would be pleasing to me.

Writing this is bad for me psychologically. I was never aware of so many dreads and difficulties. I didn't know I was having such a hard time as I was busy and happy. Now, I look for trouble. Habitually, I have always just gone along doing the best I could and ignoring most difficulties. I really don't like being made so acutely aware.

Diary excerpt—B.Q., 44-year-old woman, not employed

When applying hair spray, I am unable to use any type or size of bottle except a 4 oz nonaerosol. Anything larger I am unable to reach the back of my head. The sides and front of my hair I can manage with the spray quite easily, but in spraying the back, I am holding a mirror in one hand to see the back of my head. Not only do my fingers and wrists not work normally or in the way I wish them to, but pain and stiffness in my shoulders also limit my ability in that area.

While shopping I need to use both hands to pick up items. Any item I am unable to reach because it might be too high or in an otherwise difficult position, I am not at all bashful about asking a stranger for help in reaching it for me.

I always keep ice cubes in a milk carton in the freezer; that makes it easier and saves time. When drinking a glass of ice tea, I must lift the glass with both hands. It is impossible to lift with only one hand.

Actually, I believe I have more strength in my hands than people would ever believe from looking at them, that is, a lot of power for certain jobs. On the other hand, for another type of job, no strength at all. No strength to remove a lid from a jar but enough strength to put one on tightly. My husband wonders how I am able to get the lid on his thermos so tight.

Diaries come to us in many different forms; sometimes they read like novels. Initially, many patients complain bit-terly at having to enter into this process actively. They do not like to concentrate on their problems and have spent many years trying not to notice their disabilities. What they are really telling us is, "I do not want to be bothered; you make the decision." The diary exercise forces them to define the problems as presented in Fig. 63-1. The diary helps them focus on many insidious problems that they have stopped thinking about and that they no longer consider problems. Now, the norm is any way that they can get the job done. They will tell us they can do everything they ever did. They have forgotten the long-ago episodes of painful synovitis and entrapment of the flexor tendons, leading to early development of swan-neck deformities and the inability to grasp objects firmly.

It does not matter whether the result will be a surgical procedure or whether patients come to the realization that the more significant problems are in their feet, knees, hips, shoulders, elbows, wrists, neck, or hands, because they can now start to make choices. Patients then begin to become active participants in their programs. Unfortunately, sometimes the choice is not to be bothered any further with the details of the arthritis.

As part of their diaries, the patients make "wish lists," in which they record in order of importance their wishes regarding their hands and upper extremity function. In evaluating these wishes, I invariably notice that never first on the list but second or third is that patients would like their hands to look better. Number one usually has to do with the area in which patients feel most frustrated in hand function—that is, the ulnar drift, which reduces all hand-position functions and contributes to deformity of other joints and reduces their power as well. As diary items are reviewed, a continuous teaching situation occurs. Patients are shown an easier way of performing the functions, and we go over the adaptive devices that are available and might help with their particular problems. We never suggest adaptive devices unless the patients have brought them to our attention. The clinic offers to obtain the appropriate devices if the patients can see that the devices might help their problems. After many years in rehabilitation, it is obvious to us that patients accept suggestions for devices much better if they believe the ideas are their own. Therefore we acquaint patients with the devices and leave the choices up to them.

Diary descriptions are converted into medical terms. For example, an observation might be that a patient has difficulty putting on pajamas because of an inability of one of the shoulders to get into the sleeve. This is defined in relation to pain or position and is listed by the therapist under shoulder problems. The next item might be a problem in switching on lamps. This is translated into a key-pinch problem, which has to do with position and which is due to ulnar drift, volar subluxation, and Z-deformity of the thumb. This is listed under hand problems.

After we have gone through a patient's diary, converting the problems into medical terms and listing them under the classifications feet, knees, hips, shoulders, elbows, wrists, hands, and neck, we see which classification contains the largest number of problems. Some patients eliminate them-

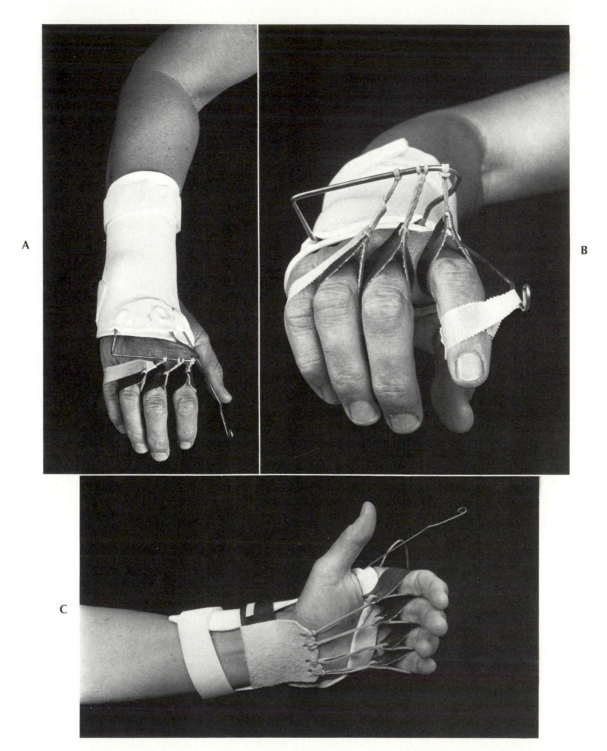

FIG. 63-2. A, Dynamic splint with extension outrigger. Notice that there is no padding and small finger is taped to ring finger. **B,** Dynamic splint with small finger taped using Dermicel tape to ring finger and outrigger for pronation or supination problems. Microfoam tape, which stretches, controls pronation or supination of index and long fingers but allows flexion and extension. **C,** Splint with flexion bands.

selves from the program in this way. Many times a patient realizes it is not his hands that need to be fixed and that are causing all his problems. Perhaps, it is an edematous knee, a painful hip, or even a shoulder without proper range of motion that prevents him from being able to carry out most functions. However, having gone through the laborious task of maintaining a diary, a fair number of patients are able to reach the conclusion that they need more stability either in their metacarpophalangeal joints or in their wrist to rid themselves of pain and perhaps gain more power.

The surgeon or the therapist could have outlined the program quite nicely without involving patients to this degree. However, our team finds it difficult to make the above-described decisions for the patients. We prefer to utilize this procedure as an effective way to involve them actively in their care. Since they are the most important members of the team, the patients must assume their part of the responsibility. They must understand that although the surgeon can give the potential for good hand function and the therapist can supervise, teach, and splint, the patients are the ones responsible for all the hard work.

POSTOPERATIVE GOALS AFTER IMPLANT ARTHROPLASTY

Let us consider the rationale for implant arthroplasties and the use of silicone rubber implants. There are two goals regarding postoperative care to consider: (1) development of scar for stability and (2) development of scar for allowing motion. The patients must understand that the implants are not joints but only spacers that prevent the two raw ends of bone from rubbing together. We hope the patients are beginning to understand that the remnants of their joints will be gone and that *all* stability will then be gone as well. Until the areas develop scars around the implants, they will continue to be unstable and may fall off into ulnar deviation when the patient tries to move the joints.

How are we to accomplish our two goals? We demonstrate to the patients how they will be given the potential for stable motion in the proper plane and that it is up to them and the therapist to develop flexion and extension while not allowing any lateral motion.

Splinting

Our first goal, stability, will be assured by splints that are made especially for the patients on the fifth postoperative day, when they come out of their bulky hand dressings. Some centers utilize commercially available splints for this aspect of the program, but we believe universal splints do not suffice in many cases because they do not accommodate the residual deformities in rheumatoid patients and are cumbersome. Our splints (Fig. 63-2) are molded from one of the many thermoplastic materials on the market. The splints are cut from this material with patterns that usually look like that in Fig. 63-3. The three areas that usually deviate from this basic pattern and need to be modified on any splint depend on the patient's thumb (Fig. 63-3, *1*), the location of the suture line (Fig. 63-3, *2*), and the length of the forearm (Fig. 63-3, *3*). To the dorsal surface of this splint (Fig. 63-3, *2*) a welding rod (3/32 inch diameter) outrigger

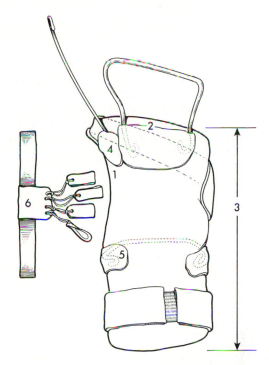

FIG. 63-3. Dynamic splint with low-profile extension outrigger and flexion band. *1*, Thumb area—splint accomodates thumb deformities. *2*, Distal edge of splint should not hit on suture line; area of attachment of extension welding rod (3/32 inch diameter) outrigger. *3*, Length of forearm—splint should cover two thirds of forearm. *4*, Outrigger—use 1/16-inch-diameter welding rod for pronation and supination problems. *5*, Flexion rod outrigger for patients with "stiff" arthritis. *6*, Flexion band, made from Velcro and moleskin.

is added. This wire should be bent in such a way as to be low profile and yet hold the fingers in the proper position, that is, 10 degrees of radial deviation and just holding, not pulling, into extension to compensate for ulnar motion when the patient flexes hard. If patients have pronation or supination problems, a smaller piece of welding rod (1/16 inch diameter) can be attached to the radial side of the splint to help control this (Figs. 63-2, *B*, and 63-3, *4*).

The height of the outrigger should be such that a number 10 rubber band through the finger loop is just the right tension to hold the finger in proper alignment. The small finger does not get a finger loop or rubber band because it obliterates the distal palmar arch and becomes stiff much faster than the other digits do. It is simply taped to the ring finger (Fig. 63-2, *A*). Padding should not be used as a substitute for a proper splint fit. I believe that clinically this splint, as described, will provide stability with no lateral motion for the 6 weeks the patient is required to wear the splint. At the end of 6 weeks, we start to wean the patient from the splint during the day and have him continue to wear it at night in either flexion or extension, depending upon the particular requirement, for a full 3 months. We make this determination based on the total active motion (TAM) recorded on the measurement sheets.

The second goal to be accomplished during this 6-week period is to mold or stress the scar in a flexion and extension plane to remodel the scar dynamically to allow motion in flexion and extension. Weekly measurements are taken, with the therapist's goal being to develop at least a 90-degree total passive motion (TPM) at the metacarpophalangeal level and a 70-degree total active motion. If the patients do well with the program and our two goals are met during their first 2 weeks of daily therapy, the visits to the clinic over the next 4 weeks are greatly reduced.

The dynamic-flexion part of the splinting program is started anywhere from 10 to 21 days postoperatively. This judgment is based on the TPM and TAM measurements. Also of primary consideration is whether patients have "stiff" or "floppy" arthritis. Those having stiff arthritis start the flexion bands earlier, and those with floppy arthritis sometimes never need flexion bands. This band is worn initially 1 to 2 hours each day, and the time is increased until the patients can stay in the band during sleep. They then wear extension bands during the day to allow for activities of daily living and flexion bands at night. The flexion band can be attached in two ways: (1) by a volar welding-rod outrigger (Fig. 63-3, 5) for attachment of the loops and bands to provide the proper angle of pull for those with stiff arthritis, or (2) when bridging is not necessary, by Velcro strap and moleskin (Fig. 63-3, 6). If patients have enough TPM to utilize the Velcro straps, it is much more comfortable for them and can be adjusted proximally or distally by attachment of a Velcro holder (Fig. 63-3, 5) to the splint. One begins resistive extension exercises when the flexion band is initiated, by having the patient extend the fingers against the rubber band.

Rehabilitation and management

Therapy requires a time commitment from the patient because the procedure takes about 2 hours daily to complete. In therapy we use moist heat in the form of hydrocollator packs (hot packs) so that the positions of the fingers are always under control. This takes about 15 to 30 minutes. After this, massage and passive range-of-motion exercise are carried out simultaneously. *No lateral motions are allowed.* We strive to obtain at least a 90-degree TPM during these sessions so that the patients will end up with a 70-degree TAM.

If the patients have difficulty of any sort, such as edema, excessive stiffness, or more pain than expected, they are treated in short sessions several times during the 2-hour period.

After the splint is back in place, we work on active long extensor gliding through the dorsal scar.

The home exercise program is of the utmost importance during the period of joint capsule formation. Active flexion and extension exercises within the dynamic splint, with the finger loops in place, are carried out on an hourly basis. Flexion exercises are performed in an intrinsic-plus position, maintaining interphalangeal extension and metacarpophalangeal flexion so that the flexion force is concentrated at the metacarpophalangeal joints. Should most of the force be occurring at the proximal interphalangeal joints, the joints may be immobilized with removable small dorsal aluminum splints or plaster casts. Immobilization of the proximal interphalangeal joints localizes the force at the metacarpophalangeal joints, thereby increasing active metacarpophalangeal flexion.

Patients are shown how to activate their extensor tendons in an intrinsic-minus position, extending the metacarpophalangeal joints while maintaining the interphalangeal joints in flexion.

In addition to the active flexion and extension exercises in the dynamic splint, patients perform passive flexion and extension exercises demonstrated by the therapist.

At 6 weeks, when daytime splinting is discontinued, the patient may begin resistive flexion exercise using putty.

CONCLUSION

The procedures described in this chapter have proved to be clinically successful in the accomplishment of the goals as originally outlined: (1) the surgeon gives the patient the potential for good motion, (2) the therapist provides instruction and splinting, and (3) the patient provides the hard work.

With this understanding, the therapist and the patient return to the surgeon's office, and the results of the functional evaluation are discussed with the surgeon. Included are the decisions reached by the patient regarding what he believes needs to be "fixed." The unwritten contract and time commitment to the program are complete.

BIBLIOGRAPHY

Arem, A., and Madden, J.W. Effects of stress on healing wounds. I. Intermittent non-cyclical tension, J. Surg. Res. **20:**93-102, 1976.

Flatt, A.E.: Care of the rheumatoid hand, ed. 3, St. Louis, 1974, The C.V. Mosby Co.

Madden, J.W., Arem, A., and DeVore, G.: A rational postoperative management program for metacarpophalangeal implant arthroplasty, J. Hand Surg. **2**(5):358-366, 1973.

Swanson, A.B.: Flexible implant arthroplasty in the hand, Clin. Plast. Surg. **3:**141-157, 1976.

XII

HEMIPLEGIA AND TETRAPLEGIA

64

Rehabilitation of the upper extremity after stroke

ROBERT L. WATERS, DOROTHY J. WILSON, and ROSEMARIE SAVINELLI HECKER

Rehabilitation of the upper extremity after a stroke involves a careful evaluation of the patient's motivation, cognition, motor control, peripheral sensation, and sensory integration. The goals of both surgical and nonsurgical therapy are to maximize functional use of the upper extremity and to prevent contractures or pain caused by spasticity. Treatment always includes therapy to prevent contractures whether the potential for use of the arm or hand is present or not.

The largest portion of spontaneous neurologic recovery in the stroke patient occurs within the first 2 months. This enables an early prediction of whether therapy should be directed toward rehabilitation of the patient's affected upper extremity as an assist in bilateral tasks or whether treatment will be to prevent pain and contracture while the patient is being taught to function one-handed.

EVALUATION

The patient's cooperation with the assessment of function is dependent on his ability to translate the therapist's communication into action. To determine the difference between a communications impairment and a physical or cognitive impairment, all tests are first performed on the normal side. Communication with the patient should be conducted at a level that produces the most accurate responses. For example, some patients cannot understand spoken communications but will respond to written communication or gestures. Other patients will respond to simple phrases but not to complex sentences. The speech therapist can determine the optimum method of communication.

Cognition and communication

Cognition is one of the most important factors in determining upper extremity function. It determines the ability of the patient to profit from a rehabilitation program. The patient must be capable of following simple verbal or pantomimed instructions and have sufficient memory ability to retain what is taught. If problem-solving ability, memory, organization, and attention span are severely impaired, the patient may not function well enough to learn one- or two-handed skills. Most stroke patients without bilateral cortical involvement have sufficient cognition to learn routine independent self-care activities. The ability to learn and retain new skills must be assessed over several sessions with the patient. Only then can one determine whether the patient is educable and therefore a rehabilitation candidate.

Sensation and sensory perception

The final steps in sensory perception occur in the cerebral cortex where basic sensory data are integrated into more complex sensory phenomena. If the cerebral infarct involves the entire sensory cortex, the patient will respond to touch and pain. However, the more complex aspects of sensation (shape, texture, point localization, proprioception, and so on) will not be present. If such a patient has intact motor function, observation and questioning his family will reveal that he may use the hand on request, using the eyes for visual sensory feedback, but he will not spontaneously use the affected extremity unless he has a task that can only be performed with two hands.

Sensory evaluation should measure proprioception and two-point discrimination.[13] These are accurate tests of the patient's ability to receive and interpret sensory information for function (Fig. 64-1). Object identification is often difficult to use as a test in stroke patients because of their motor inability to handle objects and determine texture and shape.

Hemiplegic patients will not use their affected hand unless proprioception is intact and they can discriminate between two points applied simultaneously to the fingertips less than 1 cm apart.[1] The exception is the extremely motivated patient with an important task to perform that can only be performed with two hands. These patients use the eyes for sensory feedback and have intact visual perception.

Even slight sensory deficits limit the use of the affected extremity to assist in performing functional tasks because the patient will have persistent problems performing fine manipulative tasks.

Stroke patients may also have other sensory-integration problems: distorted perception of sensory input, interpretation of that input, and integration of the input with the available motor control to perform purposeful tasks. These deficits are manifested by lack of kinesthetic awareness of body parts, the relation of these parts to each other, and their position in space. Inability to organize and sequence motor acts and denial or neglect of the affected extremities are other higher sensory deficits.

Kinesthetic awareness may be checked by positioning of the involved arm in space while the subject looks toward his intact extremity. The patient is then instructed to duplicate the same posture on the uninvolved side. Patients who spontaneously use their involved hand as an assist without visual feedback can duplicate the posture of the

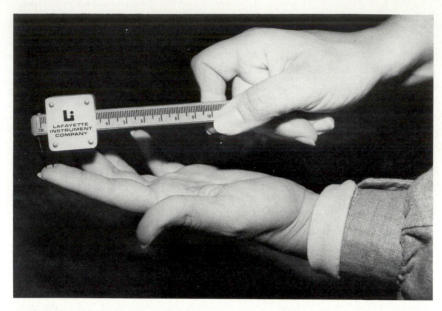

FIG. 64-1. Two-point discrimination is one of the sensory tests used to determine patient's ability to interpret sensory input.

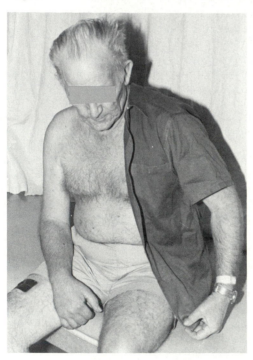

FIG. 64-2. Patient with right hemiplegia unsuccessfully attempting to put on shirt because of an inability to organize and sequence activities.

pencil tools to identify likely areas of functional problems to observe. Observation of motor tasks that require sequential planning and execution of individual motions should be included in the sensory-integration evaluation (Figs. 64-2 and 64-3).

Ataxia is often present when severe sensory loss is present, even when the eyes are used for visual feedback. Assessment of speed and precision during motor acts and the patient's ability to cross midline or change direction should also be included in the sensory and perceptual evaluation. Sensory integrative deficits greatly influence the patient's rehabilitation because they interfere with the motor performance of the normal limb as well.

Vision

Evaluation of vision identifies problems of visual perception and the effects of these aberrations on the patient's functional ability. Visual acuity should also be tested.

Homonymous hemianopsia often occurs after a stroke; the patient is unable to see objects placed on his affected side. This impedes function because the patient is unable to see one half of what is in front of him (Fig. 64-4). Most patients learn to compensate by turning the head. Even when homonymous hemianopsia is not present, the patient may have distortions of verticality or visual inattention in the contralateral visual field.

Balance and body handling

Use of the upper extremities depends on trunk stability, balance, and body-handling skills. Trunk stability is important for upper extremity use and is a prerequisite for sitting and bed activities (Fig. 64-5). Most hemiplegic patients with unilateral involvement recover sufficient balance and body-handling skills for independent sitting activities within 6 weeks of the onset of the stroke if placed on a rehabilitation program.

involved extremity within a few degrees at the shoulder, elbow, forearm, wrist, and metacarpophalangeal joints.

Perceptual deficits are best evaluated by observation of the patient's attempts to perform functional or purposeful tasks. Some screening tests of visual perception, such as foreground-background discrimination, rotation of forms in space, and eye-hand coordination, are useful paper-and-

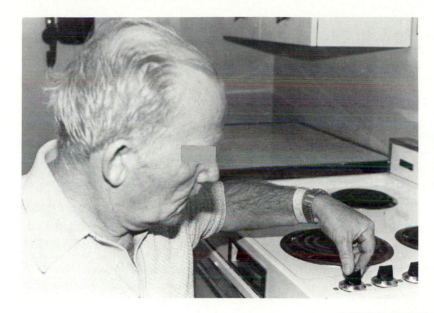

FIG. 64-3. Observation of patient's behavior during kitchen evaluation allows therapist to determine if patient is safe and able to use good judgment while operating stove.

FIG. 64-4. Patients with homonymous hemianopsia frequently ignore food on half of tray, unless they are trained to compensate for this problem.

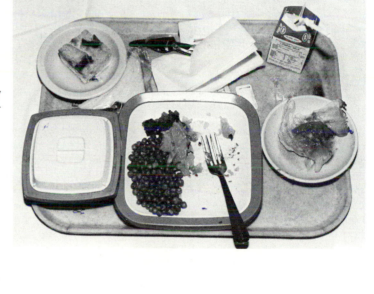

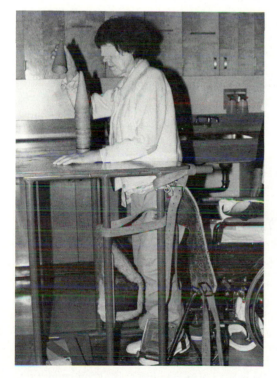

FIG. 64-5. Development of standing balance and body-handling skills is an important prerequisite for obtaining functional use of the upper extremities.

Motor control

The patterned synergistic movements and abnormal reflexes in the stroke patient represent the failure of cortical regulation of normal subcortical responses. John Hughlings Jackson first recognized the hierarchic organization of the nervous system. The spinal reflexes comprise the basic organizational unit. Supraspinal reflexes involving the midbrain and medulla modify the excitability of the spinal reflexes. The cerebral cortex provides the versatility and precision of willed movement and can act directly on the anterior motor neurons through the corticospinal pathways or indirectly through the extrapyramidal system. Several recent reviews detail the role of these mechanisms in the central nervous system–damaged patient.[9,11,14,16]

Return of functional use of the hand and arm depends on the type of volitional movement present. Normal use of the upper extremity requires versatile and precise motion. The accomplishment of routine tasks requires a wide variety of normal upper extremity movements at all joints.

An understanding of the flexion and extension synergy patterns is necessary for assessment of the hemiplegic patient's motor control. Impairment of motor control in stroke patients can be manifested in minimal loss of fine motor control, motion of the extremity only in pattern movements, or complete paralysis of the extremity.[18] The most common flexion synergy in the arm is abduction, extension and external rotation of the shoulder, elbow flexion, forearm supination, and flexion of the wrist and fingers. The most common extension pattern is forward flexion, adduction and internal rotation of the shoulder, extension of the elbow, forearm pronation, and extension of the fingers and thumb. The actual posture of the limb and exact movements vary considerably among patients, since these movements themselves produce secondary stretch-reflex responses.[21]

Return of voluntary motion in the completely paralyzed limb first occurs as flexion of the shoulder, followed by flexion of the elbow, wrist, fingers, and, last, supination of the forearm.[18] At that time, any movement of the affected extremity causes simultaneous flexion at all joints. Flexor spasticity is greatest at this period. If recovery stops at this stage, the patient will develop contractures if the joints are not passively extended daily in a direction to counteract flexion forces.

By the time the flexor synergy includes the wrist and fingers, extensor motion at the shoulder and elbow has usually occurred. At this point there is a wait of several seconds between the order to execute muscle movement and the time contraction or relaxation occurs. The ability to flex all joints of the upper extremity selectively without invoking a total flexor synergy response usually returns first at the shoulder and elbow. Once selective extension has been reestablished, there is a notable reduction in flexor spasticity as well as improvement in speed and precision of flexor motor control.

Simultaneous flexion and extension of all fingers occurs before the ability to selectively flex and extend one finger only. The index and middle fingers are usually the first to acquire this ability. Thumb opposition, when first performed, is done with the thumb opposed to the side of the index finger (key pinch). Last, the thumb can be opposed to the tips of each finger. Complete selective motion may return as well as normal speed and control and normal reflexes.

The preceding events can be summarized as follows: In the flaccid limb joint, flexor spasticity develops before voluntary flexion. Voluntary motion in the mass flexor synergy pattern occurs before the development of extension in the mass extensor synergy. Selective flexion precedes selective extension, and the amount of flexor spasticity varies with the quality of extensor control. Usually both pattern and selective motion begin at proximal joints and are later acquired at distal joints.

Most hemiplegics will not use their affected hand as an assist unless recovery has reached the stage where selective finger or thumb extension is present without simultaneous extension of the elbow in a mass extensor synergy. When recovery is arrested at a level where pattern movements meet upper extremity demand and some selective extension in the fingers or thumb is present, but incomplete because of mild flexor spasticity or myostatic contracture, the surgeon can improve function by lengthening the flexors to increase active extension.[15,19]

Posture and tone

Reaction of the muscles of the hemiparetic upper extremity to quick (phasic) stretch by the therapist is used to determine the extent of spasticity. The response may be graded as no abnormal response (none), a palpable response that does not block continued passive motion (minimal), a response that blocks passive motion but can be overcome by slow, steady tension (moderate), or a response that produces block to further passive motion that cannot be overcome (severe). The exaggerated flexor response to stretch represents a failure of normal cortical inhibition. When that response is present, there is also a failure of the normal relaxation action of the flexors during extensor movements (reciprocal inhibition) directly and indirectly interfering with the strength, speed, and range of extension. Clinically, the amount of flexor spasticity is inversely proportional to the amount of extensor control. Repetitive voluntary flexion and extension increases the amount of spasticity.

The precision and speed of normal hand function makes the least degree of spasticity conspicuous. Even minimal spasticity is associated with loss of fine motor control. If spasticity is moderate or severe, contractures of the elbow, wrist, and fingers will occur if the patient is not placed on a preventive therapy program. Also, functional use of the hand is not possible when moderate spasticity is present in the fingers or thumb. Some patients with moderate flexor spasticity may manually open the hand with their intact extremity and then grasp objects to perform activities that can only be performed two-handed.

The influence of body position on the posture and tone of the hemiplegic upper extremity should be determined. The tonic labyrinthine reflex arises from end organs in the inner ear and is activated when the head is in the upright position. This reflex activates the fusimotor fibers in the muscle spindle, increasing the excitability of the stretch reflex. Thus flexor spasticity is greater when the subject is sitting or standing than when supine. Proprioceptive righting reflexes involving the position of the neck, trunk, and limbs also influence spasticity and the voluntary response. For example, patients with limited wrist and finger extensor strength may have greater electromyographic activity during a voluntary contraction if the shoulder and elbow are extended rather than if they are restricted in flexion.

Range-of-motion

Range of motion (ROM) is evaluated by the muscle response to slow stretch. The joint is slowly extended over a period of several minutes. This is to avoid the velocity-sensitive components of the muscle spindle that are responsible for causing the monosynaptic phasic stretch reflex. Even when the extremity is extended slowly, some tonic activity may persist. Differentiation between what is presumed to be myostatic contracture and persistent muscle activity can be determined only after anesthetic block of the peripheral nerves and examination of the patient under anesthesia.

Most patients require minimum active ranges of joint motion to perform tasks. Minimum functional shoulder range should be flexion to 100 degrees, abduction to 90 degrees, external rotation to 30 degrees, and internal rotation to 70 degrees. The elbow range of motion should be flexion to 120 degrees and extension to 30 degrees. The forearm should have full pronation and 60 degrees of supination. The wrist should extend to −30 degrees, and the fingers should have at least −30 degrees of metacarpophalangeal and proximal interphalangeal flexion. The thumb should abduct to 30 degrees and have full interphalangeal extension.

NONOPERATIVE TREATMENT

Once evaluation has been completed, a treatment program is planned. The first objective in treating the spastic upper extremity is to prevent contracture. Proper extremity positioning, exercises, and electrical stimulation (of the extensor muscles) may be used. Now that most patients receive early therapy aimed at preventing contractures, severe deformities at the shoulder, elbow, and wrist are seen only in the neglected patient.

Most hemiplegic patients can be taught to do exercises using their unaffected arm and hand to passively move the joints of the affected extremity. This important task must be performed by family or nursing personnel if the patient is unable to do it himself. If the exercises are done properly, an adequate amount of joint range can be maintained. Range-of-motion exercises should be performed slowly to prevent triggering the stretch reflex and aggravating spasticity. They should be performed only within the patient's pain-free arc of motion, since pain also increases spasticity.

Assistive equipment can be used to position the upper extremity to help prevent contractures and support the shoulder. The reason for positioning is that spastic muscles are extended but not subjected to sudden changes in position that trigger the stretch reflex and aggravate spasticity. Muscles then become adjusted to the new position. Brief periods should be scheduled when the upper extremity is not positioned for mobilization and hygiene.

An overhead suspension sling attached to the wheelchair is used for patients with adductor or internal rotator spasticity of the shoulder. Leather straps rather than springs are suggested to counteract excessive mobility, which may trigger the stretch reflex. An alternative is an arm trough attached to the wheelchair (Fig. 64-6). When using this device, one should support the wrist by a splint if a flexion deformity is present.

It is usually not possible to maintain the wrist in a neutral position with a hand splint when wrist flexion spasticity is severe. With minimal to moderate spasticity, either a volar or a dorsal splint can be used. The splint should not extend to the fingers if finger flexor spasticity is severe. Splinting the fingers in extension fails when spasticity is severe be-

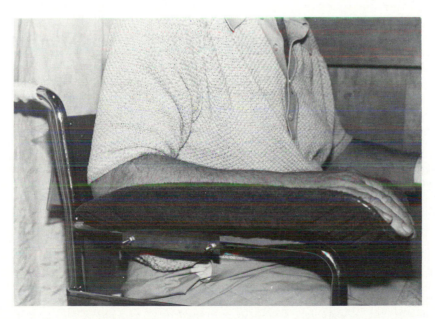

FIG. 64-6. Arm trough is one alternative for supporting affected upper extremity when patient is in wheelchair.

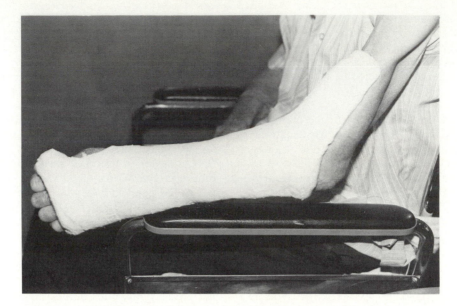

FIG. 64-7. Drop-out cast with posterior half of humeral cylinder removed to allow future elbow extension range.

cause sensory contact on the fingers or palm may provoke spasticity or elicit the grasp response, causing the fingers to jackknife out of the splint.

Serial casts are often helpful in the neglected patient with flexion contractures of the elbow, wrist, or fingers. Correction of flexion contractures of the elbow is obtained by a drop-out cast applied to the extremity in maximum extension. The posterior half is removed above the elbow to allow for further extension (Fig. 64-7). Until maximum range of motion has been achieved, the cast is changed weekly.

Electric stimulation may be used to correct or prevent flexion contractures of the wrist and hand.[6] Electrodes are applied cutaneously over the extensor muscles of the wrist and fingers, and these muscles are cyclically contracted. Follow-up of patients receiving stimulation shows that not only can contractures be prevented and extensor muscles strengthened, but mild flexion contractures can be corrected.

The shoulder deserves special attention. A variety of different factors may contribute to shoulder pain, glenohumeral subluxation, shoulder-hand syndrome, spasticity, central pain, degenerative changes about the shoulder, and referred pain resulting from cervical spondylosis. If early range-of-motion exercises within the pain-free arc are performed and the extremity is properly positioned with a sling to reduce subluxation, severe or chronic pain at the shoulder is rarely seen. When pain is present, patients should be examined to determine if the shoulder pain is related to degenerative changes and can be treated by methods such as aspirin and localized steroid injections. Methods to increase control of musculature that help hold the head of the humerus are also indicated when subluxation is present. Each of these techniques is successful with some patients; however, none is reliable for all patients. The exception is the patient with pain of central origin; no specific treatment is available for this cause of pain. These patients require positive psychologic reinforcement, and the use of narcotics should be avoided.

Edema

Edema contributes to joint contracture in the nonfunctional, flaccid upper extremity. The shoulder-hand syndrome is a common cause of pain and swelling in stroke patients. Elevation is the most important method of preventing and controlling edema. The extremity should be supported by a sling while the patient is ambulating and by overhead suspension while he is in a wheelchair. Intermittent or continuous positive pressure can be externally applied by pressure machines such as the Jobst. Although not as effective, an edema mitt that is applied directly to the edematous hand has the advantage of giving positive pressure to the hand while one is walking.

Motor-sensory reeducation

Facilitatory techniques to increase motor control depend on the amount and type of control present and the length of time since the stroke. What is perceived as a rapid performance of a complex motor act only occurs after practice and the development of motor engrams. Although the normal person can easily learn to activate and control the discharge frequency of individual motor units, the time interval for perception and motor response is sufficiently prolonged (300 meters per second) so that even during slow movements a person can consciously control only two or three motions at a time. This is readily apparent when a person attempts to perform a new, unpracticed movement; he becomes aware that he cannot regulate multiple motions. Just as a normal person learns new motor tasks, it is possible for stroke patients to increase the strength and precision of the motor response impaired by stroke and learn new patterns of motor behavior.

Hemiplegic patients who have made some spontaneous neurologic recovery and who are seen within the first 6 weeks after a stroke may benefit from therapy directed to elicit motion.[7] Motion may be elicited by strong muscular contractions of the uninvolved extremity. Rapid tapping,

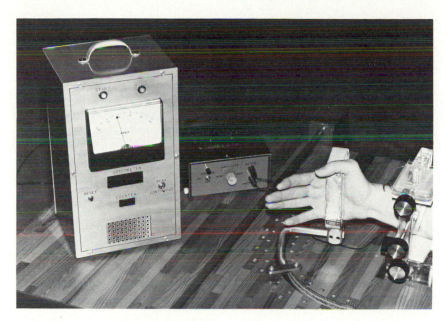

FIG. 64-8. Combination of electrical stimulation and biofeedback is used to increase motor control and strength of wrist extension of hemiparetic upper extremity.

vibration, or electrical stimulation of the muscle belly may also activate the voluntary response. These techniques are usually not indicated for patients who are more than 6 weeks after a stroke and who still have no voluntary motion.[2,3,6,8,12]

Patients with some limited motion may profit from techniques that strengthen or improve existing motor control. Weak selective motion can be strengthened by treatment and equipment that assist active motion once it has been initiated by the patient. As the patient progresses, increased extremity strength and precision are gained through use of exercise or recreational activities.

Patients with primitive synergistic motion who begin to develop some selective movement are often restricted by moderate spasticity. Upper extremity function may be improved by inhibiting spasticity with treatment that depends on body and limb positioning, equilibrium and balance reactions, proximal joint stability, and equipment designed to inhibit the influence of specific spastic movements.

Improved motor performance has been reported after biofeedback training.[1a] During this training electromyography is usually used to detect muscle contraction. In this instance the signal is amplified and displayed via audio and visual signals, and the patient is instructed to maximize this response.

Functional electric stimulation (FES) facilitates motor recovery in the stroke patient. Electric stimulation of the extensors increases muscular strength and inhibits spasticity in the antagonistic flexor musculature. After stimulation of the wrist and finger extensor muscles, voluntary extension is temporarily improved in some patients.[1,10] By electrically contracting the muscle, the patient becomes more aware of the actual sensation of muscle contraction and is better able to initiate a motor command. Also, afferent pathways from peripheral sensory receptors in skin, muscles, tendons, and joints are stimulated, and such stimulation may increase excitability of the anterior motor neurons.

Biofeedback and functional electric stimulation have been combined in an experimental program at Rancho Los Amigos Hospital to maximize elbow, wrist, and finger extension in hemiplegic patients. A goniometer attached to the affected wrist provides audio and visual biofeedback in proportion to the amount of extension. Electric stimulation is then used to complete extension once the patient's maximum has been attained (Fig. 64-8).

Once a patient has recovered sufficient motion, an activity program incorporating functional gains is begun. The essence of the therapy program becomes practice and repetition to develop motor engrams enabling functional use of the extremity. The methods for retraining the upper extremity can be exercise, recreation, or craft activity. The appropriate approach is based on the muscles or muscle groups involved and whether the patient's control is localized at a specific joint or if the lack of control is caused by an absence of strength in the total extremity.

Simple tasks need to be broken down into several steps. These steps are taught separately and then gradually combined into the single task (Fig. 64-9).

Training in daily-living activities

Routine self-care activities such as dressing and feeding are basic skills for every person. Home and community skills such as cooking, cleaning, marketing, and driving are considered to be higher level tasks that are evaluated and training implemented when appropriate (see Fig. 64-3). The goal of rehabilitation is to achieve the highest possible level of self-care, home, and community skills.[22]

SURGICAL TREATMENT OF THE FUNCTIONAL UPPER EXTREMITY

Surgery to improve extension of the wrist, thumb, or fingers is performed when there is a restriction of extension caused by mild spasticity or myostatic contracture. The fol-

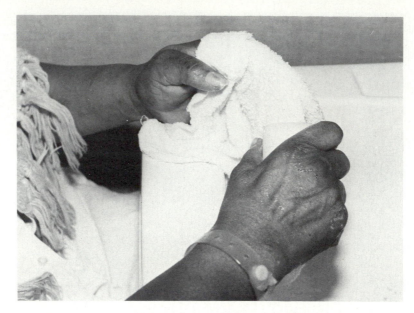

FIG. 64-9. Use of any improved control in hemiparetic hand should be incorporated immediately into the performance of basic self-care tasks.

lowing general rules will help the surgeon select hemiplegic patients who will reliably benefit from surgery.

1. Nine months have elapsed after the stroke, and the patient has intact cognition and is well motivated.
2. Selective extension is present at the fingers or thumb.
3. The patient already spontaneously uses the hand for some functional activities, even if only as a passive paperweight.
4. Proprioception is intact and two-point discrimination is less than 10 mm at the palm or fingertips.
5. The patient has no fixed joint contractures.

Local anesthetic block of the median or ulnar nerves is used to differentiate spasticity from contracture. It is also used as a preoperative demonstration of whether the patient will benefit from surgery. If restriction of extension is attributable to spasticity, improved extension will occur after the block.

Extensor strength is often temporarily greater after local anesthetic block of the median nerve. Extensor strength commonly improves for several months after flexor tendon lengthening. This leads to the conclusion that spastic flexors not only act directly to mechanically restrict extension but indirectly through neurologic pathways to inhibit the extensor anterior motor neurons. Clinically the surgeon can generally count on increased extensor strength and increased active range of motion after flexor tendon lengthening in the spastic patient.

Fingers

Active finger extension, restricted by mild spasticity or contracture, may be improved by flexor tendon lengthening. Surgical release of the flexor pronator origin has been advocated in the past as a method of treating spastic wrist and finger flexion deformities.[4] This procedure requires extensive dissection; in our experience, supination deformity has often resulted, and lengthening of the individual flexor tendons has proved to be a more reliable procedure.

Myostatic contracture shortens the active range of muscle excursion. Lengthening of spastic flexor tendons results in partial loss of voluntary flexor strength and contractile range. Because of these factors, overlengthening of the flexor tendons resulting in a loss of flexion range and strength is the most common surgical error. The amount of tendon lengthening performed is determined preoperatively. The tendon is lengthened only one half of the length necessary (usually 1 to 1.5 cm) to extend the finger from the point of restriction of the voluntary extension to full extension.[15,19] The surgeon should resist the temptation to perform further lengthening.

Passive extension of the fingers often reveals that only the sublimi appear to restrict motion. However, lengthening of the sublimi alone often uncovers restrictive spasticity in the profundi. Accordingly, both tendons are lengthened an equal amount.

Either fractional lengthening or multiple Z-plasties of the individual tendons are performed (if only one or two fingers are involved) (Fig. 64-10).[19] The hand is splinted for 3 weeks after surgery. A vigorous hand rehabilitation program after removal of the splint is essential to a successful result. Therapy is scheduled for 1 to 2 hours a day, 5 days a week for a minimum of 2 weeks. The program includes functional electrical stimulation of the wrist and finger extensors and gentle passive range of motion to the wrist and finger flexors. Treatment is progressed to include active exercises and activities that maximize wrist and finger-extension response and full grasp of the hand.

Fixed contracture of the proximal interphalangeal joints may be present in long-standing deformities. If so, surgical release is performed at the time of flexor tendon lengthening. After a dorsal longitudinal incision is made, the skin is retracted laterally on either side of the proximal interphalangeal joints to expose the collateral ligaments, volar plate,

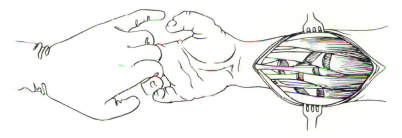

FIG. 64-10. Fractional lengthening is performed by making one or two transverse cuts in the flexor tendon proximal to the most distal insertion of muscle fibers on same tendon. Surgeon extends fingers to obtain desired amount of lengthening. Underlying muscle fibers preserve continuity. (From Waters, R.L.: Upper extremity surgery in stroke patients, Clin. Orthop. **131**:30-37, 1978.)

and flexor sheath, which are contracted. The proximal attachments of the collateral ligaments and volar plate are released and the flexor sheath is excised. If the skin on the volar surface now restricts extension, Z-plasty is performed. The proximal interphalangeal joint is transfixed with a Kirschner wire at 25 degrees of flexion for 3 weeks to prevent subluxation.

Thumb

Patients with voluntary key pinch between the thumb and side of the index finger commonly have restricted extension because of spasticity in the adductor pollicis or flexor pollicis longus muscles. The contribution of the adductor pollicis is assessed by anesthetic block of the ulnar nerve. If improved extension occurs after the block, the patient will benefit from adductor release. The adductor pollicis tendon is released distally. Significant loss of lateral pinch strength or late metacarpophalangeal instability has not been seen after this procedure.

When the interphalangeal joint of the thumb flexes during thumb extension, the flexor pollicis longus is restricting terminal extension. The flexor pollicis longus is lengthened in the forearm one half the amount necessary to extend the thumb from the position of restriction of voluntary extension to full extension (usually 1 cm). Stability is ensured by fusing the interphalangeal joint. Commonly, adductor release, flexor pollicis longus tendon lengthening, and interphalangeal joint fusion are performed at the same time.

Fusion of this joint is indicated also in patients with paresis of the flexor pollicis longus and hyperextension at the interphalangeal joint hindering pinch.

Wrist

Patients with shortening of the wrist flexors, because of spasticity or myostatic contracture, may also have shortening of the finger flexors. Before a decision is made to lengthen the wrist flexor tendons, it is important to determine whether the patient will still be able to extend the fingers if only the wrist flexor tendons are lengthened and be unable to extend the fingers if wrist flexion deformity is corrected. To do this, the wrist is manually held in the corrected position. If satisfactory finger extension is still present, wrist flexor tendon lengthening can be performed safely.

It is important to determine which wrist flexor tendons to lengthen. Manual palpation usually reveals the flexor carpi ulnaris is active during attempted hand opening. Anesthetic block of the ulnar nerve, which innervates the flexor carpi ulnaris, determines to what extent this muscle hinders wrist extension. If satisfactory wrist extension occurs after the block, only this tendon is lengthened. If wrist extension is still inadequate after the nerve block and the palmaris longus and the flexor carpi radialis are taut on palpation, these should be lengthened as well.

When excessive flexor spasticity is present at both the wrist and fingers preventing functional use, lengthening of both sets of tendons is performed. Once again, it is important to lengthen the tendons only one half the amount necessary to correct the wrist and fingers to a neutral position.

We have not found it advisable to transfer the flexor tendons to the wrist extensors in stroke patients. Electromyograms of the wrist flexors reveal different patterns of abnormal phasic activity. There are no guidelines to determine how to secure the transferred tendon under the proper amount of tension. If secured too tightly, wrist hyperextension will occur or wrist flexion may be restricted preventing release. Fortunately, stroke patients with selective finger extension have sufficient strength to extend the wrist if the wrist flexors are lengthened.

Postoperative treatment

After lengthening of the spastic flexor tendons, the patient is placed in a short arm cast with hand included for 3 weeks after surgery. The cast and sutures are then removed, and an anteroposterior splint is made at that time. If the patient has active finger flexion, one can cut away the volar portion of the cast over the fingers to allow active flexion while protecting against overstretching.

The therapy program at this time consists of cyclic functional electric stimulation to finger and wrist extensors for 30 minutes twice a day, with the patient attempting to extend the wrist and fingers actively through as much range as possible with the stimulation. It may be necessary to stimulate the wrist and fingers separately so that a good extensor response is obtained. In addition to extensor stimulation, passive range of motion is performed to maintain the range of wrist and finger flexion.

When the patient is able to complete the full available extension ranges actively, stimulation is discontinued and active finger and wrist extension exercises are initiated. Grasp and release activities with various-sized blocks and pegboards of graded sizes are used. The patient is progressed to theraplast exercises when muscle power is F⁺ and can take some resistance, usually within 6 weeks postoperatively. At this time also, passive range of motion into extension can be initiated, if needed, without damage to the surgical site being imposed.

Once strength and range are regained, the patient is instructed and encouraged to incorporate his new release abilities into all upper extremity functional tasks.

SURGERY IN THE NONFUNCTIONAL UPPER EXTREMITY

Surgery in the nonfunctional upper extremity is indicated to correct flexion deformities of the hand, elbow, or shoulder that cause pain or prevent adequate hygiene.

Hand

The temptation to release all finger and wrist flexors should be resisted; the wrist may become hyperextended and dislocated dorsally if extensor tone was unmasked after surgery.

When severe wrist and finger flexion deformities are present, the sublimis to profundus transfer is an excellent method of achieving the flexor tendon lengthening necessary to obtain correction.[5] Through an incision on the volar aspect of the forearm, all the sublimis tendons are divided distally and all the profundus tendons are divided proximally. The proximal end of the sublimis is sutured en masse to the distal end of the profundus. Sufficient lengthening is allowed so that the wrist and fingers can be extended to neutral position without tension. Unless finger flexion deformities are long-standing and the skin is contracted on the volar surface, fixed contracture of the finger joints can be corrected by gentle passive manipulation. Passive manipulation should not be performed in the functional hand, since it results in greater postoperative edema and stiffness than what occurs after surgical release. The wrist flexors and flexor pollicis longus may be lengthened through the same incision.

When excessive finger flexion is present without wrist flexion, a sufficient flexor tendon lengthening can be obtained by fractional tendon lengthening. As in the case of the funtional hand, usually only the sublimis tendons appear tight on passive stretch of the fingers; however, the profundus tendons should be lengthened as well. Lengthening of the sublimis alone will unmask spasticity in the profundus tendons, preventing satisfactory correction.

When finger flexion deformity is present, the intrinsic muscles are commonly spastic. If surgical attention is directed only to the flexor tendons, the fingers will assume an intrinsic-plus posture after surgery. Evidence of intrinsic spasticity is sought preoperatively by examination of the thumb. If the adductor pollicis is spastic, the intrinsic muscles of the fingers also may be presumed spastic. Neurectomy of the motor branch of the ulnar nerve performed at the time of flexor tendon lengthening will improve the cosmetic appearance of the fingers and relieve adductor spasticity of the thumb as well. Conspicuous intrinsic atrophy is not a problem and is obscured by slight edema and sub-

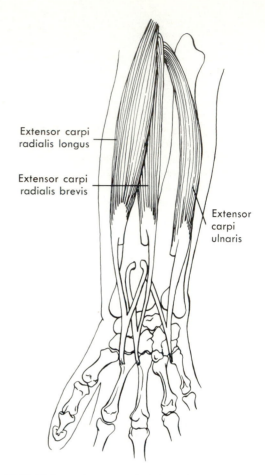

FIG. 64-11. Wrist extensor tenodesis is performed by securing one half of the extensor carpi radialis longus, extensor carpi radialis brevis, and extensor carpi ulnaris to radius. Remaining portions of wrist extensor tendons are left intact. (From Waters, R.L.: Upper extremity surgery in stroke patients, Clin. Orthop. **131:**30-37, 1978.)

cutaneous fat, which is present in most nonfunctional hands if the patient is well nourished.

Because some patients lack extensor tone, the wrist may remain in a flexed position because of gravity after flexor tendon lengthening if the forearm postures in a pronated position. A wrist splint may be prescribed or extensor tenodesis performed at a second operation. The three wrist extensors (extensor carpi radialis brevis, extensor carpi radialis longus, extensor carpi ulnaris) are divided longitudinally and one half of each tendon inserted through two holes in the dorsum of the radius (Fig. 64-11). The wrist is protected in a splint in 20 degrees of dorsiflexion for 8 weeks after surgery.

Elbow

Most stroke patients receive early range of motion therapy after a stroke, and elbow flexion contractures are not common. It is common for the elbow to assume a flexed posture while the patient is walking, and it may bounce up and down because of clonus. Patients will purposefully slow their walking speed to decrease clonus. Musculocutaneous neurectomy will improve cosmesis and eliminate clonus. The loss of elbow flexion strength is not important, since nearly all stroke patients with excessive elbow flexion have nonfunctional hands. Since the brachioradialis is innervated by the radial nerve, which is left intact, some elbow flexion will persist after surgery. The loss of musculocutaneous sensation is not bothersome to the hemiplegic patient.

When elbow flexion contracture is present, lengthening of the biceps tendon alone will not significantly improve elbow flexion deformity and attention must be directed to the brachialis muscle as well. X-ray examination is performed to ensure that heterotropic bone is not present. Myostatic contracture is differentiated from spasticity by anesthetic block of the musculocutaneous nerve (axillary nerve block) or by examination of the patient at surgery. If there is less than 75 degrees of fixed deformity, musculocutaneous neurectomy is performed. Residual deformity is corrected after surgery by dropout or serial casts.

Musculocutaneous neurectomy is performed through a longitudinal incision extending distally from the tendon of the pectoralis major in the interval between the short head of the biceps and coracobrachialis muscles. This incision can be extended proximally or distally if further exploration to locate the nerve is required. A 1 cm segment of nerve is excised.

In the long-standing elbow flexion deformities, if the amount of fixed deformity is more than 75 degrees, release of the elbow flexor muscles is performed instead of musculocutaneous neurectomy. Surgery is performed through a lateral incision over the origin of the brachioradialis. After release of the origin of the brachioradialis, the biceps tendon and brachial muscle are divided. About 45 degrees of correction is obtained before excessive tension is placed on the brachial artery or median nerve, which are usually also shortened. However, further correction is obtained postoperatively by serial casting.

Shoulder

As at the elbow, passive range-of-motion exercises begun immediately after a stroke prevent severe contractures, which usually only occur in the neglected patient. Once a common deformity, it is now rare.

Surgical release is indicated when spastic contractures cause severe pain or prevent axillary hygiene.

Four muscles are responsible for adduction and internal rotation contractures of the shoulder. These are the pectoralis major, subscapularis, latissimus dorsi, and teres minor.[23] To determine which muscles contribute to the deformity, one abducts the arm and rotates it externally. All but the subscapularis are clinically palpable. If, with the arm at the side, the humerus resists external rotation, the subscapularis may be presumed to be spastic as well.

Surgery is performed through an incision over the insertion of the pectoralis major tendon. The pectoralis major and subscapularis are released and also the teres major and latissimus dorsi if the latter muscles were tight preoperatively.

The range-of-motion program initiated immediately post-

operatively by the therapist and continued after hospital discharge by the patient or his family is essential to the success of the surgery.

REFERENCES

1. Baker, L., Yeh, C., Wilson, D., and Waters, R.L.: Electrical stimulation for hemiplegic patients, J. Am. Phys. Ther. Assoc. **59**(12):1495-1499, 1979.
1a. Basmajian, J.V., Kukulka, C.G., Naraflan, M.G., and others: Biofeedback treatment of foot-drop after stroke compared with standard rehabilitation technique: effects on voluntary control and strength, Arch. Phys. Med. Rehabil. **56**:231-236, 1975.
2. Bobath, B.: Adult hemiplegia: evaluation and treatment, London, 1970, William Clowes & Sons, Ltd.
3. Bobath, B., and Cotton, E.: A patient with residual hemiplegia and his response to treatment, J. Am. Phys. Ther. Assoc. **45**:9, 1965.
4. Braun, R.M., Mooney, V., and Nickel, V.L.: Flexor-origin release for the pronation-flexion deformity of the forearm and hand in the stroke patient, J. Bone Joint Surg. **52A**:907-920, 1970.
5. Braun, R.M., Vise, G.T., and Roper, B.: Preliminary experience with superficialis to profundus tendon transfer in the hemiplegic upper extremity, J. Bone Joint Surg. **56A**:466-472, 1974.
6. Brunstrom, S.: Movement therapy in hemiplegia: a neurophysiological approach, New York, 1970, Harper & Row, Publishers, Inc.
7. Caldwell, C., Wilson, D.J., and Braun, R.: Evaluation and treatment of the upper extremity in the hemiplegic stroke patient, Clin. Orthop. **63**:69, 1969.
8. Flanagan, E.M.: Methods for facilitation and inhibition of motor activity, Am. J. Phys. Med. **46**(1):1006-1011, 1967.
9. Fugl-Meyer, A.R. In Buerger, A.A., and Tobis, J.S., editors: Neurophysiologic aspects of rehabilitation medicine, Springfield, Ill., 1974, Charles C Thomas, Publisher.
10. Gracinin, F., and Dimitrijevic, M.R.: Application of functional electrical stimulation in rehabilitation: The use of reflex mechanisms in reeducation of mobility, Praha, 1969, Blanea.
11. Kottke, F.J. In Buerger, A.A., and Tobis, J.S., editors: Neurophysiologic aspects of rehabilitation medicine, Springfield, Ill., 1974, Charles C Thomas, Publisher.
12. Knott, M., and Voss, D.E.: Proprioceptive neuromuscular facilitation: patterns and techniques, New York, 1956, Harper & Row, Publisher, Inc.
13. Moberg, E.: Criticism and study of methods for examining sensibility in the hand, Neurology **12**:8-19, 1962.
14. Mooney, V.: A rationale for rehabilitation procedures based on the peripheral motor system, Clin. Orthop. **63**:7-13, 1969.
15. Perry, J., and Waters, R.L.: Surgery. In The American Academy of Orthopaedic Surgeons: Instructional course lectures **24**:40, St. Louis, 1975, The C.V. Mosby Co.
16. Perry, J., Giovan, P., Harris, L.J., and others: The determinants of muscle action in the hemiparetic lower extremity (and their effect on the examination procedure), Clin. Orthop. **131**:71-89, 1978.
17. Reference deleted in proofs.
18. Twitchell, T.E.: The restoration of motor function following hemiplegia in man, Brain **74**:443-480, 1951.
19. Waters, R.L.: Upper extremity surgery in stroke patients, Clin. Orthop. **131**:30-37, 1978.
20. Reference deleted in proofs.
21. Wilemon, W.K., DePaoli, F., Caldwell, C., and Perry, J.: Hemiplegic upper extremity posture and tone analysis. Paper presented at American Academy of Orthopaedic Surgeons Meeting, San Francisco, March, 1971.
22. Wilson, D.: Adult hemiplegia: a treatment guide for occupational therapist, unpublished guide, Downey, Calif., 1968, Rancho Los Amigos Hospital.
23. Zarins, B.: Evaluation of the painful shoulder in hemiplegia using EMG. In Orthopedic Seminars, Downey, California, Rancho Los Amigos Hospital **V**:459-462, 1972.

65

Helpful upper limb surgery in tetraplegia*

ERIK MOBERG

A NEW APPROACH

More can now be accomplished by reconstructive surgery to help the victims of cervical spinal cord lesions increase function of their upper limbs than is generally believed. My opinion is derived from experience with a total of approximately 200 handgrip reconstructions and elbow extensor transfers (Fig. 65-1), with additional knowledge of about half this number of similar cases operated on by surgeons I have instructed.

Very important work in this field should not be forgotten.[3-6, 9-15, 25] Only the following names are mentioned here: Freehafer, Lamb, Lipscomb, Nickel, Perry, and Zancolli. Important unpublished work by McDowell[14] must also be mentioned. In two earlier papers of mine, important facts, which cannot be fully repeated here, are discussed.[16-18,22]

The results are limited and it is of paramount importance not to give rise to unrealistic expectations. But from the other point of view, one should remember what Sterling Bunnell said: "If you have nothing, a little is a lot." It is no wonder that in most centers for tetraplegia, reconstructive surgery has been almost a forbidden field, no doubt because trials have sometimes given rise to a loss instead of a gain.

To get results, first of all a *new basic approach* seems required, including:

1. A new concept of physiology for gripping function[6,18,22]
2. A useful way to examine sensibility, because this factor is so important in the evaluation[16,18]
3. A new classification[17,18]
4. A new aim for gripping function[17,18]
5. A new functional follow-up treatment method

Of course adequate hand surgical skill and resources are required just as other basic training. Poor results can be expected if:

1. The patient is for one or another reason bedridden when examined or treated.
2. The patient does not want surgery or is mentally too inactive.

3. The patient has not yet fully understood his prognosis and not accepted the fact that wheelchair conditions will continue for a lifetime.
4. The remaining motor activity is of abnormal *quality*. However, spasticity in some of the muscles is not always a contraindication.
5. There is lack of adequate nursing facilities for tetraplegics.
6. The surgeon in charge cannot direct all details himself, starting with the examination and ending with the follow-up treatment.

If conditions are adequate, in my opinion and experience some help can now be offered to at least 60% to 70% of all tetraplegia cases. This number can probably be raised beyond the figure mentioned. Already it is time to make surgery a *routine* part of tetraplegia treatment. This, however, requires a surgeon at each center with time enough and sufficient interest to lead all this work. It is clearly inadequate to perform this surgery without specially trained staff for the follow-up treatment. One should start with the simpler cases, with arms here classified as good (OCu:2)[17] or a bit better, and then gain experience and advance slowly.

New concept of physiology for gripping function.[22] The motor area has always been regarded as the predominant part of grip function. If sensibility has been mentioned at all, it has been in regard to so-called feedback function. This mistake has dominated the literature on the tetraplegic hand, just as it is still dominating prosthetic work. Now the problem must be put into proper perspective. Every useful motor grip is just a response to *afferent* impulses, coming from cutaneous sensibility, vision, or the auditory system. Man has to learn his gripping functions the hard way, by training. During the act of learning, a person gets his computer system, the unconscious system, provided with a program, which enables him to perform ordered activities and even very complicated activities with *skill and speed* and leaves his conscious mind free for other purposes. Now, afferents from muscles, tendons, and perhaps joints do not signal to the conscious mind and are therefore useless as afferents for learning. Their impulses are "private to the muscles"[6] but very important for the trained system's computer function. Tetraplegic extremities that are operated on need to learn new functions, and so afferent impulses to the *conscious* mind are required. The majority of these come

*This work was supported by a grant from Greta and Einar Askers Stiftelse, Göteborg, and made possible through the cooperation of University Departments of Surgery and Rehabilitation in Göteborg, Copenhagen, Helsingfors, and Stockholm. It was followed up by me during a stay as visiting professor at the University of California (Irvine), at Rancho Los Amigos Hospital, Downey, and Veterans Administration Hospital, Long Beach, California.

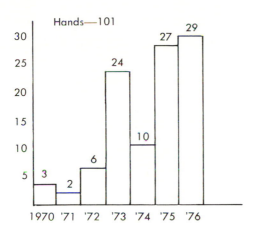
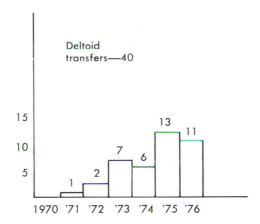

FIG. 65-1. Number of reconstructions performed up to 1976. Total personal experience up to June, 1983: surgery on 143 hands and 73 elbow extensor constructions.

from tactile gnosis through the skin if this function is preserved (in about 50%). Vision is almost the only source of afferent impulses if tactile gnosis is lost but also helps very much in cases where it is preserved. Very few impulses come from other sources.

Another most important factor here is proprioception. The control of position, motion, and power load is, to a great extent, dependent on cutaneous stimulation. What part the joints play in this respect must be regarded as unknown. Proprioception must be understood and checked in tetraplegia surgery.[18]

Useful way to examine hand sensibility. Because tactile gnosis is the only quality of sensory function that can "put an eye" on the fingers to let them know what they are doing and where they are, the majority of current tests for sensibility are useless here. For example, pinprick, cotton wool test, figure writing, tests for temperature, and tests for the difference between sharp and blunt must be totally abandoned. The Weber two-point discrimination test, performed in the modern version with an instrument made of a 0.9 mm paper clip wire and applied with not more than 10 gm of pressure is the only one I have found of value. Because the skin provides proprioception, the same method is useful for determining the absence or the presence of this function. This factor can be evaluated segment for segment in a digit, and the result can be given numerically. Worse than 10 to 12 mm means that neither tactile gnosis nor proprioception is present in adequate quality. But even if present on only one of two gripping surfaces, a useful grip, though less precise, can result.

Classification. Without an adequate classification no comparison between results and no scientific discussion are possible. Therefore my classification does not consider the injury level in the cord or whether the lesion is complete or incomplete, it simply records what function is present. As 50% of all tetraplegics have important differences between their two upper extremities, every patient is given one classification for the right and one for the left upper extremity. The afferent impulses that are most important head the grouping: hands that must rely on only *ocular* afferents

belong to group "O." If they also have *cutaneous* afferents of enough quality, their group is "OCu."

Each of these groups are divided according to the number of muscle groups of grade 4 or better, including and distal to the brachioradialis. Thus a hand with tactile gnosis at least on the thumb pulp and having the brachioradialis and the radial wrist extensors in function with grade 4 power would be classed as OCu:2, while an arm with insufficient sensibility for tactile gnosis and only brachioradialis in function with grade 4 would be classed as 0:1.

Of 321 arms classified according to this system, 12% belonged to 0:0, 24% to 0:1, 16% to OCu:1, 27% to OCu:2, and only 8% belonged to the OCu:3 group. Only 6.5% were better than this. Other groups existed but were very small. First from the OCu:3 group a majority of the extremities had useful triceps function. The figures given are from my own experience in Scandinavia and in the United States. In some countries much fewer high-level cases are coming to reconstructive work, which of course means that on the average more complicated hand reconstructions with better results can be performed and fewer elbow extensor transfers are needed. The higher-level cases, however, are the ones for whom surgical reconstruction is most needed.

A difference of two or three neurologic levels between the two arms, or between sensory and motor level in the same arm, is not uncommon.

New concept for restoration of gripping function. Previously the aim here was to provide two- or three-point pulp pinch against the thumb as well as opposition and finger flexion. This requires a lot of motor function, and therefore only a few tetraplegics could be offered surgery. Only a minimum of motors is required for key grip, and therefore I try to restore this capability. If only a grade 3 wrist extensor is available or can be obtained through the transfer of the brachioradialis, a useful grip is achievable. The tetraplegic does not have to pick up needles or small objects but needs to handle his utensils for eating or to perform other simple activities.

Follow-up treatment. Follow-up treatment requires more

brain work than hand work. It is easy, unfortunately, to undo the surgical work with "routine" physiotherapy. This is especially the case with the elbow extensor procedure.

All exercise must be *active*. No passive tension produced by the human hand is permitted. A variety of splints is used.

Especially in elbow extensor cases, my rule, based on experience, is that the temptation to speed up recovery of flexion is great and all can be lost if this is done. Only extension of the elbow is trained, never flexion, and flexion should not be permitted to advance more than 10 degrees a week. Therefore at least 4 months should elapse from surgery to the moment when the hand can again come up to the mouth. Another method[27] for elbow extensor construction claims much shorter rehabilitation time, but in my hands the gain has been only moderate.

THE HAND

Should surgery be performed on one or both hands? With which hand should one start? In my experience there is no doubt about the answers to these important questions. If only ocular afferents can be relied on, only *one* hand can be given an independent grip. The first hand operated on should always, even in cases with enough afferents for surgery to both hands, be the hand that is presently the leading one. Should surgery begin with the elbow or with the hand? If surgery to both is planned, I always try to start with the elbow extension operation. If, as was done earlier, we began with the hand and it started to become useful after surgery, immobilization after the elbow procedure took away this already appreciable gain for several months. This was a most tiresome period for the patient.

But there is another point of view[20] that makes starting with the elbow important. The brachioradialis muscle, for example, when used to reinforce the wrist extensors or to act as a finger flexor, needs an antagonist to act properly. When no triceps is present, this means that surgery must start with the elbow extensor.

One important principle is that no surgery should impair function that is already present, especially not the ability to transfer or to handle wheelchairs. Nor should the hand be less useful for human contact. Therefore every surgical procedure should be reversible. If the patient wants to return to his peroperative condition, it should be possible to do so. This means that rarely should an arthodesis be performed in a finger without a previous test with a temporary Kirschner-wire tenodesis.

When good active wrist extension exists in tetraplegic patients, good finger flexion can be restored in more cases than was previously believed. Such flexion is usually achieved through the transfer of the extensor carpi radialis longus. But this can be done only if the brevis is strong enough to act alone as a good wrist extensor. This power has to be evaluated through open exposure in local anaesthesia. If the brevis can lift 5 kg, it is good enough.

Several cases have been seen, where this examination was not performed before a transfer and the patient lost wrist function. The risk of a late contracture when finger flexors without extensors are constructed must always be remembered.

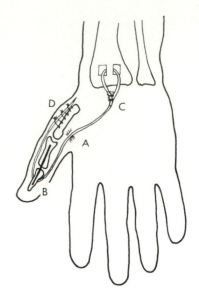

FIG. 65-2. Basic procedures for key grip.

BASIC SURGICAL PROCEDURE

My basic surgical procedure, recommended for the majority of tetraplegic hands, consists in using the preserved wrist extensor system as the basis for a flexor hinge key grip, with the thumb gripping against the radial side of the flexed index finger. If the wrist extensors are paralyzed, it is necessary to transfer the brachioradialis to the extensor carpi radialis brevis. The next steps (Fig. 65-2) are *(A)* release of the flexor pollicis longus tendon from the annular ligament over the metacarpophalangeal joint so that bowstringing and increased power are created, *(B)* stabilization of the distal thumb joint with a longitudinally inserted 2-mm Steinmann pin, *(C)* tenodesis of the flexor pollicis longus tendon to the distal end of the radius with loop fixation through bone windows, and *(D)*, if necessary, tenodesis of the long thumb extensors over the metacarpal shaft to reduce joint flexion if the metacarpophalangeal joint has passive flexion beyond 40 degrees.

After completion of these procedures, the thumb flexor tenodesis will bring the thumb pulp in a broad pinch against the radial side of the index finger when the wrist is dorsiflexed. When the wrist, by gravity, moves into flexion, the thumb releases (Fig. 65-3).

OTHER SURGICAL PROCEDURES

In addition to the basic procedures just mentioned, a number of other procedures and variations can be indicated,[20,21,28-29] some of which are resection of the extensor retinaculum at the wrist to permit bowstringing and thereby increase wrist extensor power, transfer of the brachioradialis to the abductor pollicis longus to get active thumb abduction, transfer of the same muscle to the extensor pollicis brevis or a rerouted extensor pollicis longus to get similar function, and sling procedures to get a brachioradialis to act not only as a wrist extensor but also as a weak pronator when this function was lost.

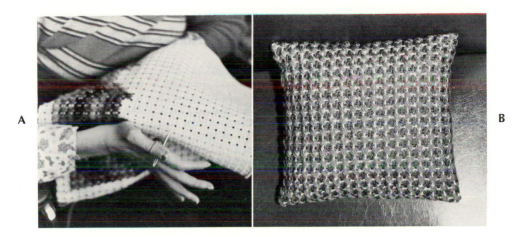

FIG. 65-3. A, Key grip with needle. **B,** Result of needlework performed with key grip hand.

In patients with lower cord level lesions where more muscles are available, tactile gnosis and proprioception are often normal. In these patients the approved reconstruction of the hand will be similar to that after a trauma. But even in cases with higher-level lesions the Zancolli "lasso" operation[28] can help to counteract hyperextension in the metacarpophalangeal joints.

Resection of nerves to spastic muscles to let functional muscles overcome resistance is sometimes useful. In very few cases wrist fusion is of value to reduce a difficult flexion contracture, but never to get more muscles for transfer.

All procedures must be modified and combined with respect to the results of a careful individual examination. Useful evaluation sheets are shown on pp. 720 and 721. Of course, very often many more details must be examined and recorded. The aim must be, except for the small group (6% to 8%) with lower-level lesions, to concentrate all available resources in one single strong action. To list all that is lost and attempt to substitute for too many functions is unrealistic and can lead to disappointment. One must not forget that functional loss in tetraplegia is far beyond that which a superficial examination will reveal. This is especially true in the sensory area.

Plaster fixation is an important part of the surgical procedure. Pressure sores must be avoided, and the correct position for the different parts must be found along with the right moment chosen for removal of the plaster splint. Usually after 3 weeks, the plaster splint can be removed and active training started. The surgeon must direct the aftercare with all the attention to detail it requires. Of course, when inexperienced, neither he nor anyone else has the necessary training. But he will, as I have had to do and am continuing to do, learn from his patients. Tenodeses are apt to slacken in the postoperative period, and so they should be put in a bit on the tight side. If at surgery the flexor pollicis longus tenodesis produces a steady grip with the thumb pulp against the side of the index finger when the wrist is brought to 5 degrees of extension, tension is adequate.

In tetraplegics one has the impression that tendons used in grafts and in tenodeses more easily elongate than in sim-ilar surgery performed in other patients. This is especially the case in deltoid transfers for elbow extension where it takes at least 3 months before they can withstand moderate resistance.

IMPROVEMENT OF ELBOW EXTENSION

An elbow extensor of moderate power can be obtained by transferral of the independently innervated posterior part of the deltoid to the triceps tendon with the help of free tendon grafts from the toe extensors.[17,20] It seems useful to give some technical details of this operation, which, in contrast to the hand reconstructions, can be standardized.

Surgical procedure. Using a long, curved incision over the posterior part of the deltoid, one exposes the posterior margin of this muscle and from there the rest of the distal two thirds of the muscle can be mobilized. It is possible to palpate a line of separation between the anterior and posterior portions, through which one can proceed to the humerus. From under the posterior margin of the deltoid a curved pair of scissors can be brought in close to the humerus under the muscle and out through the separation line. From this location it is easy to free the muscle, first distally with its fibrous insertion and later bluntly in the proximal direction. Great care must be taken not to harm the innervation. The muscle must be freed sufficiently to allow about 3 cm of distal elongation when the muscle is gently pulled. Careful hemostasis is necessary during this procedure because many circumferential vessels cross the field.

Usually three toe extensor tendons are used as grafts. The Brand stripper can be used to remove these tendons from the foot. The proximal ends of the tendon grafts are interlaced back and forth through the distal part of the deltoid and sutured to the fibrous tissue here. They are brought down in a wide subfascial canal to the triceps tendon, which is exposed through a small incision, and interlaced here; then they are brought up again to the deltoid and interlaced and fixed for the second time. During the placement of the graft, the arm should be at about 40 degrees of abduction from the body and the elbow fully extended so that the right tension is obtained. To avoid rupture of the junctures when

Australia, Finland, France, Japan, Scotland, Spain, Sweden, Switzerland, and the United States.

SUMMARY

By the establishment of realistic goals, important functional improvement can be offered through surgery to a large number of tetraplegic patients.* The procedures described, being reversible, can be offered without fear of reducing these patient's already limited function. Careful attention to all the details of evaluation, selection, surgery, and aftercare is essential to success.

The field is in rapid development now. See also recent articles (January to May, 1983) in *The Hand, The Journal of Hand Surgery,* and *The Journal of Bone and Joint Surgery* (British).

---

*See references 1, 2, 6-8, 12, 19-21, 23, 24, 26, and 29.

REFERENCES

1. Bryan, R.S.: The Moberg deltoid-triceps replacement and key-pinch operations in quadriplegia: preliminary experiences, Hand **9:**207, 1977.
2. DeBenedetti, M.: Restoration of elbow extension power in the tetraplegic patient using the Moberg technique, J. Hand Surg. **4:**86, 1979.
3. Freehafer, A.A., Vonhaam, E., and Allen, V.: Tendon transfers to improve grasp after injuries of the cervical spinal cord, J. Bone Joint Surg. **56A:**951, 1974.
4. Freehafer, A.A.: Flexion and supination deformities of the elbow in tetraplegics, Paraplegia **15:**221, 1977-1978.
5. Freehafer, A.A.: Determination of muscle-tendon unit properties during tendon transfer, J. Hand Surg. **4:**331, 1979.
6. Granit, R.: The functional role of the muscle spindles: facts and hypotheses, Brain **98:**531-556, 1975.
7. Hentz, V.R., and Keoshian, L.A.: Changing perspectives in surgical hand rehabilitation in quadriplegic patients, Plast. Reconstr. Surg. **64:**509, 1979.
8. House, J.H., Gwathmey, F.W., and Lundsgaard, D.K.: Restoration of strong grasp and lateral pinch in tetraplegia due to spinal cord injury, J. Hand Surg. **1:**152, 1976.
9. Lamb, D.W.: The management of upper limb in cervical cord injuries. In Proceedings of a Symposium held in the Royal College of Surgeons of Edinburgh, June 7 and 8, 1963, London, 1963, Morrison & Gibbs, Ltd.
10. Lamb, D.W., and Landry, R.: The hand in quadriplegia, Hand **3:**31-37, 1971.
11. Lamb, D.W., and Landry, R.M.: The hand in quadriplegia, Paraplegia **9:**204-212, 1972.
12. Lamb, D.W.: Current situation in the management of the upper limb in tetraplegia, Int. Rehabil. Med. **1:**135-137, 1979.
13. Lipscomb, P.R., Elkins, E.C., and Henderson, E.D.: Tendon transfers to restore function of hands in tetraplegia, especially after fracture-dislocation of the sixth cervical vertebra on the seventh, J. Bone Joint Surg. **40A:**1071-1080, 1958.
14. McDowell, C.: Personal communication, Richmond, Va., 1976.
15. McDowell, C.L., Moberg, E., and Smith, A.G.: International conference on surgical rehabilitation of the upper limb in tetraplegia, J. Hand Surg. **4:**387, 1979.
16. Moberg, E.: Criticism and study of methods for examining sensibility in the hand, Neurology **12:**8-19, 1962.
17. Moberg, E.: Surgical treatment for absent single-hand grip and elbow extension in quadriplegia, J. Bone Joint Surg. **57A:**196-206, 1975.
18. Moberg, E.: Reconstructive hand surgery in tetraplegia, stroke and cerebral palsy: some basic concepts in physiology and neurology, J. Hand Surg. **1:**29-34, 1976.
19. Moberg, E.: Editorial, Hand **9:**205, 1977.
20. Moberg, E.: The upper limb in tetraplegia: a new approach to surgical rehabilitation, Stuttgart, 1978, Goerge Thieme Verlag.
21. Moberg, E.: A report from the Committee on Spinal Cord Injuries, 1980, Paraplegia **19:**386-388, 1981, International Federation of Societies for Surgery of the Hand.
22. Moberg, E.: The role of cutaneous afferents in position sense, kinaesthesia, and motor function of the hand, Brain **106:**1-19, 1983.
23. Moberg, E., and Lamb, D.W.: Surgical rehabilitation of the upper limb in tetraplegia, Hand **12:**209, 1980.
24. Moberg, E., and Nigst, H.: Kongressbericht: Internationale Arbeitstagung in Edinburgh über chirurgische Rehabilitation der oberen Extremitäten der Tetraplegie, Handchirurgie **11:**255, 1979.
25. Nickel, V.L., Perry, J., and Garrett, A.L.: Development of useful function in the severely paralyzed hand, J. Bone Joint Surg. **45A:**933-951, 1963.
26. Smith, A.G.: Early complications of key grip hand surgery for quadriplegia, Paraplegia **19:**123, 1981.
27. Pita, L., and Castro, A.: Personal communication, Göteborg, Sweden, 1978.
28. Zancolli, E.A.: Functional restoration of the upper limbs in traumatic quadriplegia. In Structural and dynamic bases of hand surgery, Philadelphia, 1968, J.B. Lippincott Co.
29. Zancolli, E.A.: Surgery for the quadriplegic hand with active, strong wrist extension preserved: a study of 97 cases, Clin. Orthop. **112:**101-113, 1975.
30. Zrubecky, G.: Operative und konservative Wiederherstellung einer Greifform von Schlaf gelähmten Händen bei Halsmark-geschädigten, Handchirurgie **4:**71-79, 1972.

XIII
BIOFEEDBACK

STRATEGIES

By a system of trial and error, various teams have worked out differing strategies. For example, our former team at Emory University[3] approached the upper limb and hand somewhat differently from the way our present team at McMaster University does.[6] The following is for guidance, not dogma.

Shoulder region

We have been able to decrease and often eliminate subluxation by remobilizing the shoulder girdle and shoulder joint, using the knowledge of normal shoulder function.[4] We did this by giving the patient feedback from the upper part of the trapezius for elevation, middle part of the deltoid for abduction, and its anterior part for flexion. These muscles are easily monitored and give the patient an accurate picture of the movement desired. Feedback from the scapular muscles (which seems ideal) can be confusing to the patient because it is difficult to imagine contracting an obscure muscle, such as the serratus anterior. By gaining control and strength, the patient also gains the scapular movements necessary to allow smooth movement.

Initiating activity in the upper part of the trapezius can be first learned by various easy procedures. After applying the electrodes over the muscle belly, the therapist may ask the patient to shrug both shoulders while looking in the mirror. Resistance given in the uninvolved shoulder often elicits activity in the involved muscle, which is made obvious by the feedback equipment. Although movement may not be apparent, the feedback should be emphasized and used as a guide until enough strength is gained to produce overt movement of the shoulders.

The middle of the deltoid is easily monitored for training of abduction. The therapist's taking the arm through abduction several times will give the patient a good idea of the movement to be learned. If either the patient is unable to understand the movement or the extension synergy dominates attempts at abduction, the goal-oriented approach may be helpful, such as having the patient put his elbow on the arm of the chair.

To monitor the anterior part of the deltoid, the electrode placement must minimize pickup of activity from either the middle deltoid or the pectoralis major nearby. Flexion seems to be the most difficult for patients. Placing and holding the patient's other hand on the affected shoulder allows the patient to concentrate on moving the elbow. The arm can be passively brought into shoulder flexion and the patient asked to hold that position. By monitoring the anterior deltoid the therapist encourages the patient to assist with the affected arm and can reinforce the early appearance of new activity.

The pectoralis major muscle is a strong component of the extension synergy. It often becomes hyperactive and restricts the passive range of motion. Its frequent recruitment when the patient flexes or abducts at the shoulder interferes with the gaining or greater range of motion. With electrodes placed over this muscle, the patient is instructed to maintain electrical silence in it because both passive and active movements are carried out at the shoulder.

If the only way the patient can initiate activity in the target muscle is by bringing in the synergy, then initially the synergy is tolerated until the target muscle is strengthened. The patient must then learn to separate the voluntary contraction of the specific muscle from the synergy by increasing the sensitivity of the biofeedback apparatus. This permits feedback before the synergistic movements occur.

Elbow region

Electrodes placed over the triceps brachii will usually pick up activity from the flexors and vice versa, unless the electrodes are placed very close together. Control of spasticity of the flexors of the elbow can usually be taught to the seated patient with electrodes over the biceps. The elbow is positioned so that the flexors are quiet, and then the elbow can be passively moved into extension while the patient tries to maintain electrical silence in the flexors. Initially the electromyograph sensitivity should be set so low that there is very little feedback for the patient to reduce. The speed of the passive movements can be gradually increased as the patient gains control of the spasticity. For complete control, the patient must be able to relax both the biceps and brachioradialis.

With a satisfactory electrode placement, one can elicit flexor activity by resisting flexion of the uninvolved elbow or by placing the hand close to the patient's mouth (that is, elbow flexion) and having him attempt to hold it there while the therapist gently extends the elbow. Holding the patient's hand so that the forearm is supinated seems to inhibit the tendency toward elbow extension. If he tends to go into the extension synergy, active elbow flexion can be enhanced by the therapist's holding the forearm in supination.

Wrist and fingers

Flexor spasticity of the wrist and fingers often interferes with effective extension. Collectively the wrist and finger flexors are easily monitored, and a wide electrode placement during initial training through passive stretch is wise. To reduce forearm flexor spasticity, one follows the same course as for the elbow. First the limb should be positioned so as to quiet the flexors. The patient then tries to maintain relaxation during passive extension of the wrist and fingers. Once this skill is acquired, he is taught to perform the passive movement using his uninvolved hand, with emphasis on feeling the difference in resistance because the feedback indicates different amounts of spasticity. As he performs the passive extension, not only is he learning an effective method of practicing the targeted relaxation at home (without any feedback apparatus), but he is also learning to isolate the activity of one arm from the other.

After the patient has mastered control of the spastic flexors, the next task is to maintain relaxation during active extension. A standard vibrator may be used here to facilitate the extensors without causing interference to the biofeedback electrodes over the flexors. The patient also should be instructed to help raise the wrist and fingers, because vibration is not usually enough stimulation to effect movement of the joints. Initiating extension can be attempted in one of two ways. The most direct is to place electrodes over the extensors and have the patient attempt extension or try to hold the extended position. The feedback generated as a

Digital goniometer. Two-joint finger goniometers allow for feedback of two joints in flexion and extension, one in flexion and one in extension, as when a person tries to overcome intrinsic tightness (Fig. 67-13). This particular device also has incorporated into it a meter calibrated to coincide with degrees of motion for further feedback.

With a single-joint goniometer the pow[er] enough to fit in a shirt pocket (Fig. 67-14 cable may be taped to the arm for convenien[ce] plugs into the power pack. On all the ele[c] devices the threshold knobs are calibrated Ten patients who had metacarpophalang[eal]

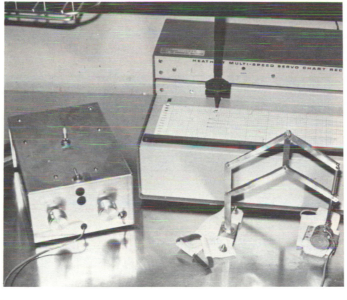

FIG. 67-12. Dynamic wrist goniometer also plugs into strip chart recorder, which graphically measures motion.

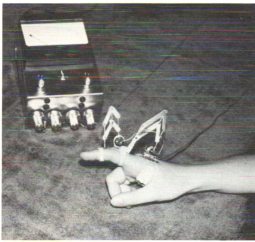

FIG. 67-13. Two-joint finger goniometer allows for feedback of two joints in flexion and extension or one in flexion and one in extension, as when one tries to overcome intrinsic tightness. This particular device also has incorporated into it a meter calibrated to coincide with degrees of motion for further feedback.

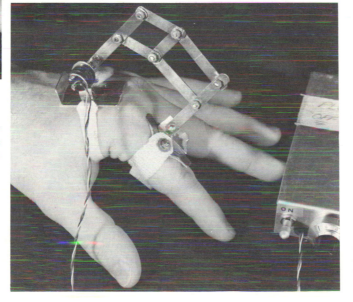

FIG. 67-14. Single-joint goniometer. Power pack is small enough to fit in shirt pocket. Electrical cable may be taped to arm for convenience. Earphone plugs into power pack.

result of the extensor muscle group activity can be used as encouragement until visible movement occurs. With thin patients care must be taken with electrode placement because "cross talk" of muscle potentials from the flexors can be picked up and display a "false" feedback; this reinforces the wrong response from the patient. Very close electrode placement over the extensors can help to prevent or reduce this problem.

The flexors can be monitored to help the patient learn extension. Often as the patient attempts extension, the first muscle response is flexion. After the patient has mastered control of the flexors through stretch, he is asked to attempt active extension or to hold the extended position without bringing in the flexors. In this case the feedback is used as negative reinforcement.

Initiating finger extension is often difficult for the patient, partly because of the dominance of the flexors. One way to work on finger extension is to combine it with wrist extension, to take advantage of any mass extension response that may take place. Electrode placement over the extensor digitorum will usually pick up some wrist extensor activity because of the proximity of the muscles. Interference from the wrist extensors can be minimized by careful placement and use of the stretch reflex to ensure that the extensor digitorum is being monitored.

A useful strategy to elicit mass extension is to have the hand flat on a firm pillow. With the forearm stabilized at the wrist to prevent elbow flexion, cutaneous stimulation in the form of brushing is given to the dorsum of the hand and finger, and the patient is instructed to raise his hand and fingers straight up off the pillow. This strategy requires the patient to extend the wrist past neutral; the intense effort on the part of the patient coupled with the cutaneous stimulation may be helpful in bringing in the finger extensors.

The above strategy requires that the flexors be well relaxed and not dominant during attempts at extension. For those patients who do not demonstrate a great deal of control, the following strategy might be more useful. The forearm is placed in the neutral position between supination and pronation. The patient's wrist and fingers are flexed completely, and the therapist's hand covers the patient's hand. The patient is instructed to attempt to open up his hand—to push his fingers into the therapist's overlying fingers. The therapist will need to stabilize the wrist to prevent extension at that joint. This position reduces the tendency to go into flexion because the flexors are as slack as possible; the extensors are put on maximum stretch to facilitate their activation.

The thumb

Electrode placement over the muscles of the thumb must be very close together. Optimal electrode placement can be confirmed by use of the stretch reflex of specific muscles. One can usually minimize extraneous activity by positioning the hand, such as maintaining the neutral position to minimize activity from the pronator quadratus. With surface electrodes it is very difficult to isolate the extensor pollicis brevis from the abductor pollicis longus. When one is first teaching the patient to initiate activity from these thumb muscles, either movement is acceptable. Once the patient

has control of one movement, it is usually easier to attempt the other. The proper position of the hand helps the patient gain the proper movement; the neutral position tends to assist thumb extension, while the supinated position tends to assist abduction. Good control of the thumb flexors is essential to prevent attempts at extension or abduction from being diverted to the flexors.

To assist in abduction, one places the electrodes over the area of the abductor pollicis longus and "scratches" the thenar eminence area over the abductor pollicis brevis. This helps stimulate the brevis and give the patient an idea of which direction to try to move the thumb. Spasms can be put to good use when one is working with the thumb, since appropriately placed electrodes will pick up activity of a muscle spasm. The muscle can often be set off into a spasm by repeated quick stretches. One should have the patient relax the spasm and then quickly reactivate the muscle before he forgets which muscle it was he controlled by relaxation. This has worked with thumb extension and abduction. Another strategy along the same line is to bring in the muscle through a reflex response, such as quick supination and pronation of the forearm several times, ending in supination to recruit the thumb extensors. The patient can be instructed to first relax the muscle and then quickly reactivate it, or he can be asked to assist the reflex at the appropriate time.

Movement artifact (electrical interference caused by gross movements of electrodes and wires) may interfere with the training session because of the amount of movement involved. This problem can be minimized if the electrodes are placed in such a manner as to allow the wires to be secured to a part of the arm that is fairly stable. The therapist can best judge where to secure the wires after working with this strategy a few times.

The thenar eminence can be monitored with widely spaced electrodes when one is teaching a patient to isolate thumb and finger movements. The patient is instructed to maintain silence in the thumb muscles while attempting finger movements. Visual reinforcement can be used while the patient moves the thumb and tries to keep the fingers relaxed.

CONCLUSION

As noted earlier, the combined behavioral–physical therapy approach is more comprehensive than current standard physical therapy approaches, and it appears to be superior in retraining hand function in the brain-damaged person. The integrated behavioral and physical therapy methodology is still semi-experimental and being developed. Our intuition that it is superior to our previous standard methods of upper limb retraining appears to have been justified by pilot studies. The method is designed to take full advantage of the concepts of motor skill acquisition, cognitive behavioral therapy, and electromyographic feedback. Great importance is placed on the patient recognizing that it is he who possesses the ability to make the arm and hand functionally active.

The therapist initially teaches the patient the elements of motor skill acquisition. Cognitive strategies and electromyographic feedback allow the patient and the therapist to from a priori reasoning, that feedback goniometers help patients to exercise and work with activities more effectively.

Electronic motion feedback goniometers

Electrokinesiologic tracking (motion) devices are gaining more and more popularity in treating upper extremity trauma. Feedback goniometers have calibrated threshold settings, which allow the therapist to set multiple goals for the patient of very small increments of motion. They incorporate several forms of feedback such as visual (single light, multiple displays of lights), auditory (beeps, variable pitch sounds), or combinations of the above. Very small, lightweight, plastic goniometers using extremely simple electronics have been created to reduce cost and make it ex-

tremely simple for the therapist accessibility of materials for fa locale.

Wrist goniometer. The use o the flexion and extension arc (Fig to be helpful in a variety of situat in carpal fractures, and after wr

Dynamic wrist goniometers g tion (Fig. 67-11). Goniometers c feedback and a beep for auditor ensure that the person does not for an unobtainable goal. Two one for each light. The dynamic be plugged into a strip chart rec sures the motion (Fig. 67-12).

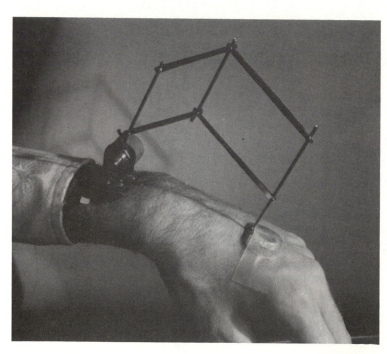

FIG. 67-10. Wrist goniometer adherence.

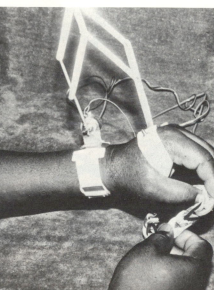

FIG. 67-11. Dynamic wrist goniometer.

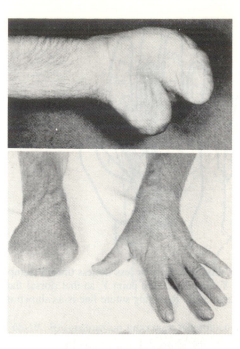

FIG. 68-23. Case H.G. Amputation, by power saw, of all digits through proximal phalanges, leaving a mitten hand but no thumb cleft. By a plastic maneuver and removal of the index metacarpal, a thumb cleft ¾ in. deep was constructed. It opened ¾ in. and closed against the hand. Patient could write and hold objects. Limited facility can be combined with the use of a prosthesis. (From Bunnell, *Surgery of the Hand*, 3rd ed., Lippincott, Philadelphia, 1956, by permission.)

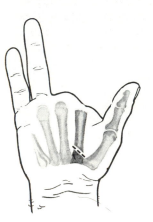

FIG. 68-24. Operative procedure for loss of the second and third digits. Excision of the second metacarpal, but with retention of the third, furnishes easy apposition for the sound thumb.

remnant of the thumb to work against (Fig. 68-22). Preservation of the broad tip of the third metacarpal is particularly desirable when a complete thumb remains (Fig. 68-24).

The range of motion of a normal thumb extends from a position at the side and slightly back of the hand, with the nail at right angles to the palm, through a wide ellipse toward the volar aspect until it is opposite the fingers, the nail being

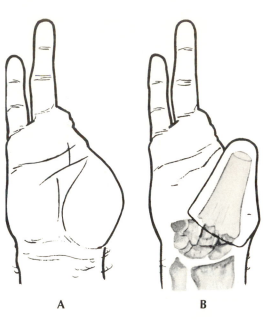

A   B

FIG. 68-25. Surgical construction of a new "thumb." **A,** Poorly functioning partial hand retaining digits four and five only. **B,** Serviceable partial hand made by constructing new "thumb" with pedicle and bone graft. Function is apt to be better than if a prosthesis were applied.

then parallel to the palm. In the latter position, the thumb is available to participate with the fingers in grasping large objects. The motion is effected by the ten muscles, long and short, that control the thumb. In paralysis of the median nerve, in injury to the thenal muscles, in stiffness of the carpometacarpal joint of the thumb, or in flexion contracture on the dorsum of the web, normal range of motion of the thumb is lost. If the other parts of the hand are mobile, the ability to appose the thumb can readily be provided by a simple tendon transfer that draws the thumb toward the pisiform bone and pronates it. When this is not possible, the thumb may be held permanently in a useful position by a bone graft at the base of the first metacarpal.

When a thumb is closely bound to the rest of the hand by scar, it can be spread away by excising the scar tissue and cutting across the cleft from a point opposite the hinge of the first two metacarpals on the dorsal side to the corresponding point on the volar side. The thumb is spread to the side and front of the hand, and the large denudation of skin is covered either by a large diamond-shaped free skin graft or, better, by a pedicle graft from the abdomen. In three weeks, pedicle grafts are detached from the abdomen and laid smoothly on the hand.

Although the thumb stump remaining after amputation through the metacarpophalangeal joint usually is not very serviceable, it may be built out by pedicle and bone graft. If a thumb is amputated proximal to the metacarpophalangeal joint, it should in any case be built out longer. If the thenar muscles and the stub of the metacarpal remain intact, the thumb will be quite movable. A short thumb is a good thumb. Various motions, such as apposition, extension, and flexion, may be furnished it by tendon grafts.

In the case of total loss of the thumb, a new one can be

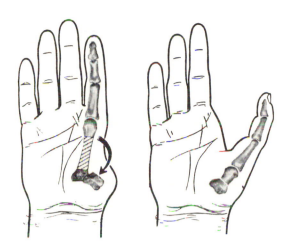

FIG. 68-27. Pollicization of index finger.

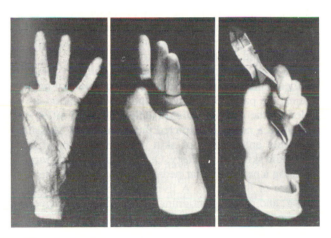

FIG. 68-28. Case H.W.W. First (1929) physiological reconstruction of thumb by pollicizing remains of the index finger. Metacarpal lashed to trapezium, nerves and vessels carried over, and all tendons and muscles connected up. ''Thumb'' had strong motion and normal sensation and was well positioned. Patient worked well as a carpenter for 20 years. Superior to prosthesis. (From *Surgery, Gynecology, and Obstetrics,* by permission.)

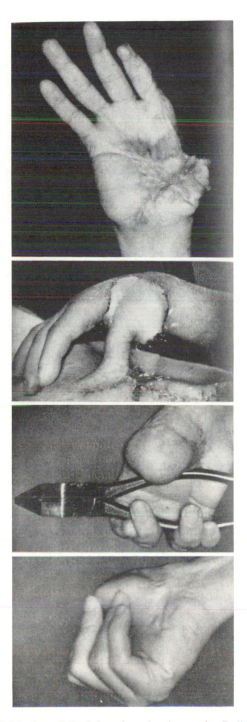

FIG. 68-26. Case C.B. Injury from hand grenade. Pedicle graft covered the thumb, and arthrodesis was done on the trapezium by a graft from the ilium. Abduction was furnished index finger by a proprius tendon graft. A very useful hand resulted. No prosthesis needed. (From Bunnell, *Surgery of the Hand,* 3rd ed., Lippincott, Philadelphia, 1956, by permission.)

supplied in various ways. The simplest approach is to raise a tube pedicle from the abdomen, attach the pedicle to the hand, and place in it a bone graft from the iliac crest (Figs. 68-25 and 68-26). Although this expedient gives sensation, it does not provide much stereognosis. Nevertheless, a reconstructed thumb is apt to be very serviceable and con-

siderably better than a prosthesis. The graft should be grounded on some other bone rather than connected by a joint. It may be placed on the carpus to make a pad in the base of the palm, or it may be placed on the trapezium or on the stub of the metacarpal.

The requirements of a new thumb are three in number: motion, sensation, and proper placement. The best new thumbs are made by pollicization of a finger, preferably the index finger but sometimes the long finger. Often, as part of the injury, the index finger is already somewhat shortened. In such a case, the finger, or a portion of suitable length, is transferred together with a bridge of skin and with its nerves, blood vessels, and tendons intact (Figs. 68-27 and 68-28). It may even be transferred on a neurovascular

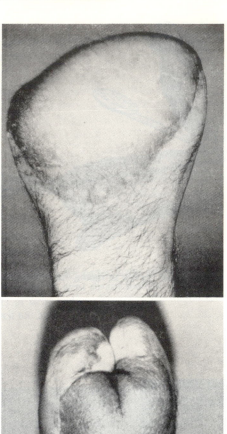

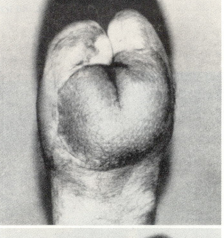

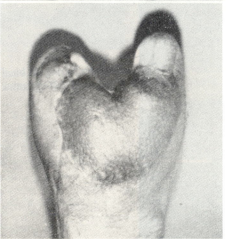

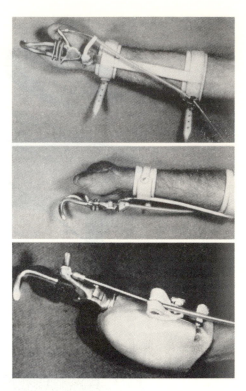

FIG. 68-37. Case E.E. *Left, top to bottom:* Right hand pulled into hay chopper. Dèbridement and abdominal pedicle. Later a two-digit hand was made with a tendon T operation for prehension and a spread of 1½ in. *Right, top and middle:* A prosthesis which enabled the hand to work against a hook. This was discarded because it was too unstable. *Right, bottom:* A prosthesis made by Robin-Aids Manufacturing Company, Vallejo, Calif., that was very satisfactory. It preserved residual wrist motion and could be removed when fine digital motions were required.

for elbow disarticulation,[1,3,5] the polycentric elbow joint for below-elbow cases,[1] the variable-ratio step-up hinge for the very short below-elbow case,[1] the flexible cable units to allow pronation and supination for the very long below-elbow and wrist-disarticulation cases,[8] and the elbow-coupled shoulder joint for shoulder-disarticulation amputees.[7]

For the arm amputee, these devices help to carry the terminal device (hook of artificial hand) to a place of usefulness, The *Manual of Upper Extremity Prosthetics*[11] gives a full account of these and other devices that comprise a full armamentarium for upper-extremity amputees. But the case of the partial hand amputation is not included.

Prosthesis for one-digit hands

For most practical purposes, loss of one or more distal phalanges does not require application of a prosthesis. Nevertheless, there are exceptions. An accomplished violinist, losing the distal phalanx of even one string finger, for example, is incapable of managing the strings properly. This could mean an occupational change for such a person. A good prosthetic replacement may enable him to continue his occupation. The same occasionally occurs with an organist, a pianist, a typist, or other person in any occupation where finger dexterity means the difference between success and failure. A suitable prosthesis for such a case can be made using thin stainless steel for the socket and extension framework and then dipping the device in flexible vinyl plastic to form the tip cushion and finger build-up. The socket

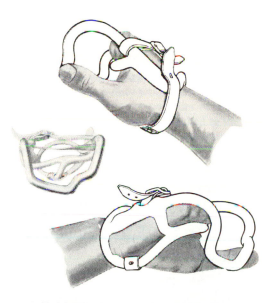

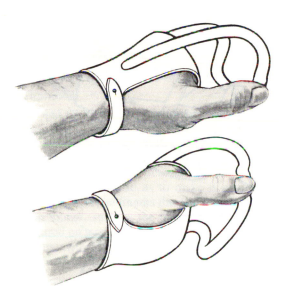

FIG. 68-38. Prosthesis for loss of all the fingers at, or slightly distal to, the metacarpophalangeal joint line. Metal ring, covered with vinyl plastic, is so shaped as to furnish one large hook, representing the index finger, and one small one, representing the little finger. Thumb works against ring throughout the range of the carpometacarpal articulation. (Courtesy Robin-Aids Manufacturing Company, Vallejo, Calif.)

FIG. 68-39. Prosthesis for transmetacarpal amputation. Socket may be of leather, molded plastic, or hammered stainless steel. Metal ring, covered with vinyl plastic, is shaped to simulate fingers, as in Fig. 68-38. (Courtesy Robin-Aids Manufacturing Company, Vallejo, Calif.)

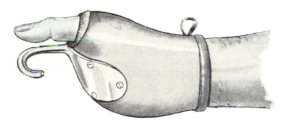

FIG. 68-40. Simple prosthesis for loss of most of the palm but with retention of the thumb. Wrist and hand stump are encased in a socket to which is attached a single stainless-steel hook. The hook may be used by itself or as a member for apposing the thumb.

portion may be split along one side to allow it to expand and contract, thus ensuring snugness of fit.

For amputation of all of the fingers at the metacarpophalangeal joint, or approximately half an inch distal thereto such that the volar crease of the metacarpophalangeal joint remains, a 1/8-in. rod framework of stainless steel can simulate the socket while leaving a maximum amount of exposed palm for traction and sensation (Fig. 68-38). The distal portion of the framework is bent to simulate the finger tips, the little-finger side being curved to form a hook for pulling or lifting and the index side shaped to appose the thumb as would the first two fingers in three-jaw-chuck prehension.[4] This arrangement provides for prehension between the simulated index finger and the remaining thumb. A similar appliance can be made for an amputation proximal to the metacarpophalangeal joint, but in such a case the remainder of the hand must be fitted with a plastic, metal, or leather socket for attachment to the formed rod (Fig. 68-39). The notable disadvantage is the coverage of surfaces otherwise capable of sensation. In both instances, the rod

framework is dipped in flexible vinyl plastic to provide a surface with adequate traction.

Fig. 68-40 shows a single stainless rod curved in hook fashion and mounted to a stainless-steel plate, which in turn is attached to a molded hand and wrist socket. The hook is so positioned as to give apposition to the thumb, and the thumb is exposed to utilize its capability for sensation. This single hook, being small and smooth, allows easy entry into pockets and other tight places.

Since the thumb is the most important single digit of the hand, it would seem a sound principle not to involve it as a motor for powering other mechanisms. A collar around the thumb would appear to diminish tactile surface, and any mechanical linkage would seem to lessen mobility and dexterity. In general, wrist flexion-extension provides a far more desirable motor with less hindrance to function. But these principles have only general applicability and are not specific. For certain special needs, a thumb-powered mechanism may be desirable. In any individual case, the selection of equipment must be left to the mutual judgment of the

69

Restoration of thumb function after partial or total amputation

JAMES W. STRICKLAND

Perhaps no problem has challenged the armamentarium of the hand surgeon more than restoration of function after partial or total amputation of the thumb. Numerous technical advances in reconstructive surgery of the upper extremity have resulted from ingenious efforts to design procedures that would return function to this important part. This chapter is an attempt to sort out and identify the most effective of these procedures and to indicate their application based on the experience of the author. Although most of the important contributions are referenced, specific historical documentation and detailed considerations are beyond the scope of this discussion.

RECONSTRUCTIVE CONSIDERATIONS

The functional requirements of the thumb include adequate sensation, enough length and mobility to oppose the other digits, joint stability to allow strong function without collapse, and freedom from pain.[104] Careful consideration of each of these factors is important to the surgeon when one is planning a reconstructive procedure after thumb injury.

With regard to thumb length, there is some controversy as to the amount of thumb shortening that may be permitted before a significant impairment of function occurs.[30] It would appear that at least 2 cm of proximal phalanx is the minimum effective length of the thumb[146] and that amputations occurring through the distal one third of that phalanx will function quite well with no need for surgical lengthening or web space–deepening procedures.[47,138,141,169] Thumb loss at the base of the proximal phalanx or through the metacarpophalangeal joint results in a residual stump that is inadequate for many pinching and grasping functions.[143]

A restored or reconstructed thumb with minimal sensory perception is of little functional value, and every effort must be made to provide satisfactory tactile sensation and stereognosis at the time of primary thumb repair or reconstruction.* Before a patient will consistently use the thumb after an injury, the thumb must have painless skin that is resistant

to normal usage and sensation that is at least protective and preferably of near-normal quality.[169] The use of magnification and better instrumentation for nerve repair has increased the quality of sensory regeneration after nerve interruption, and the use of neurovascular island pedicle techniques and other methods of transferring innervated skin has greatly improved the hand surgeon's ability to restore sensation in thumb salvage or reconstruction.

The position and mobility of the thumb are also of considerable importance. If it is not in the correct anatomic area where it can be brought into position to oppose the adjacent fingers or to grasp objects, it will not carry out any useful function.[24,119,146,165] Although motion is not necessarily required at the metacarpophalangeal or interphalangeal joints, thumb function is dependent on carpometacarpal joint motion for rotation away from or toward the palm.[24,67,119,146] If an immobile post must be created, it is important that it be positioned in near-full abduction-opposition so that the other mobile digits can be flexed to meet it. It is also important that the three thumb joints are sufficiently stable to provide strong resistance without collapse.

Numerous procedures for salvage and reconstruction of the badly injured thumb have been described, and an excellent historical review of many of these techniques is provided by Littler.[103,104] Unfortunately, very little attempt has been made to define the specific indication for these techniques or to consider which procedures are most applicable in certain circumstances. Factors that must be taken into consideration when one is planning a restorative effort include age, sex, occupation, hand dominance, and the specific desires of the patient. One must acknowledge that not all patients require or desire elaborate reconstructive procedures and that many will adjust to the loss of thumb length, particularly when good contralateral hand function is present. When reconstruction is desirable, however, the exact level of thumb loss is probably the most important single factor in determining the proper procedure to be selected.[6,115,143,167,169] In this chapter I discuss injury and amputation of the thumb at various levels with indications as to the procedures that would appear to best provide restoration of the functional requirements at each level.

---

*See references 23, 24, 67, 119, 146, 165, and 169.

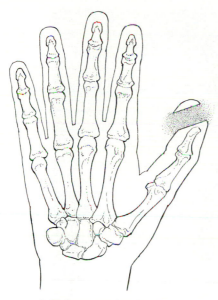

Guillotine amputation of thumb tip

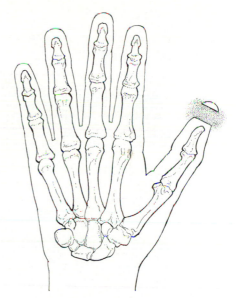

Partial amputation of distal phalanx

PARTIAL AMPUTATION OF THE DISTAL PHALANX

As with distal phalangeal injuries of other digits, a wide assortment of avulsion and amputation injuries may occur in the thumb. Reparative considerations in this area include the need for good, painless skin and subcutaneous tissue with satisfactory sensory perception. Procedures for accomplishing these goals vary depending on the amount and depth of tissue loss.

Guillotine amputation of thumb tip

Small transverse loss of skin and subcutaneous tissue from the terminal aspect of the distal phalanx may be managed by free skin grafts, lateral triangular advancement flaps,[49,93] or the V-Y advancement technique.[4] The advantages of small split-thickness skin graft on this type of lesion lie in its high percentage of successful "take" and the ultimate contractility of the graft, which results in a minimal defect with near-normal sensation.[29,159]

Oblique avulsion of thumb pad

Larger avulsions of the thumb pad involving approximately 50% of the volar portion of the distal phalanx are well managed by the advancement of a large volar flap containing the neurovascular structures, with or without proximal skin release and grafting.[88,113,137] This technique has the advantage of bringing well-innervated volar thumb skin distally to resurface the pad lesion and restoring near-normal sensory perception with durable skin and subcutaneous tissue.

Avulsion of entire volar pad of thumb

When the entire volar surface of the distal phalanx of the thumb has been avulsed, free grafting will provide inadequate long-term coverage, and the volar advancement tech-

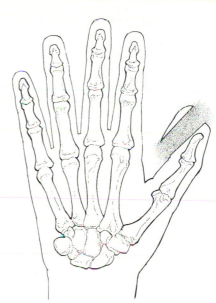

Oblique avulsion of thumb pad

nique becomes technically difficult. A cross-finger flap designed from the proximal phalanx of the index finger will often provide the best coverage of this type of injury with satisfactory skin and subcutaneous tissue and the expectation of a satisfactory sensory recovery* (Fig. 69-1). The primary use of a neurovascular island pedicle flap may occasionally be indicated[161] and other more elaborate procedures, including the use of the tip of the fifth finger,[172] a one-stage advancement rotational flap combination,[84] or the use of a flag flap,[81] increase the degree of difficulty with little improvement on the reliable performance of a cross-finger pedicle flap.

*See references 5, 37, 72, 109, 125, 136, 138, 142, and 160.

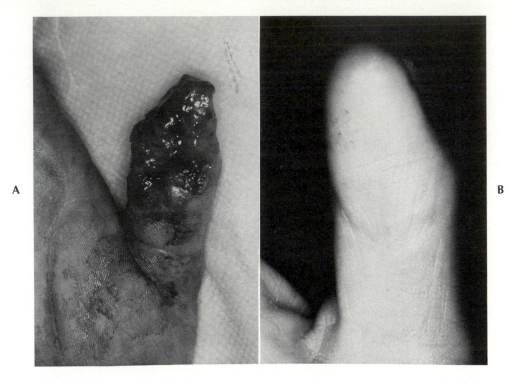

FIG. 69-1. A, Avulsion of entire volar pad of thumb. **B,** Thumb appearance 6 months after resurfacing with cross-finger flap from dorsum of proximal phalanx of index finger. Sensory perception is adequate.

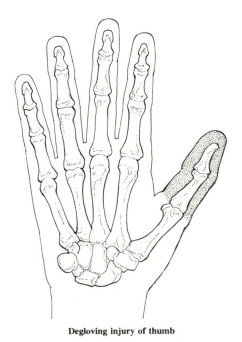

Degloving injury of thumb

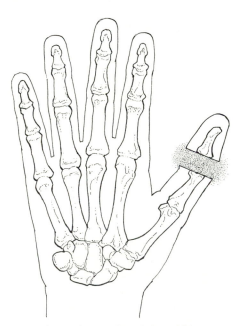

Amputation near interphalangeal joint

DEGLOVING INJURIES OF THE THUMB

The occasional degloving injury to the thumb with loss of all skin and subcutaneous tissue is a major reconstructive challenge. The importance of thumb function would preclude amputation in this type of injury, and because revascularization of the denuded skin is only occasionally suc-

cessful using microvascular techniques, it is necessary to resurface all or part of the thumb and in most instances to provide sensory input. The use of a tubed abdominal pedicle flap followed by the addition of a neurovascular island pedicle flap taken from the long and ring fingers appears to be the best method of restoration after deglovement.[143,146] It is usually necessary to remove the distal phalanx to achieve

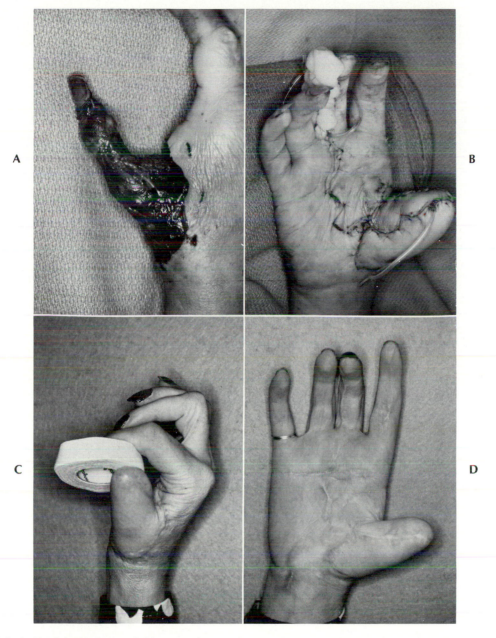

FIG. 69-2. **A,** Total deglovement of skin, subcutaneous tissue, and neurovascular bundles from thumb. **B,** Resurfacing of thumb after amputation of distal phalanx with tubed groin flap and neurovascular island pedicle taken from ulnar side of long finger. **C** and **D,** Appearance of thumb at 1 year after defatting procedure. Function and sensation were good. (Courtesy Dr. James B. Steichen.)

the correct length, and it should be emphasized that the ability to provide sensory perception to the resurfaced thumb is the critical factor in returning it to a satisfactory functional state. The neurovascular island pedicle transfer, as described by Moberg and Littler[99,100] and extended by others,* has become an extremely important technique in the armamentarium of the hand surgeon, particularly as an adjunct in reconstructive procedures in which no other method of sensory restoration is possible. In the degloved thumb that has been resurfaced by an abdominal pedicle flap, the island

pedicle technique has proved to be of great value (Fig. 69-2).

Avulsing thumb injuries may result in the loss of large amounts of skin and soft subcutaneous tissue without total deglovement. Resurfacing in these situations may be accomplished by the use of free grafts or, when the transfer of sensory innervated skin is necessitated, local tissue flaps based on the first web space,[109] neurovascular island pedicles, or the transfer of sensory innervated cross-finger flaps.[1,11,55] Particularly in those cases in which there has been longitudinal loss of the entire volar thumb with its neurovascular structures, the use of a large cross-finger pedicle flap that carries a sensory branch of the radial nerve

*See references 75, 121, 144, 158, and 166.

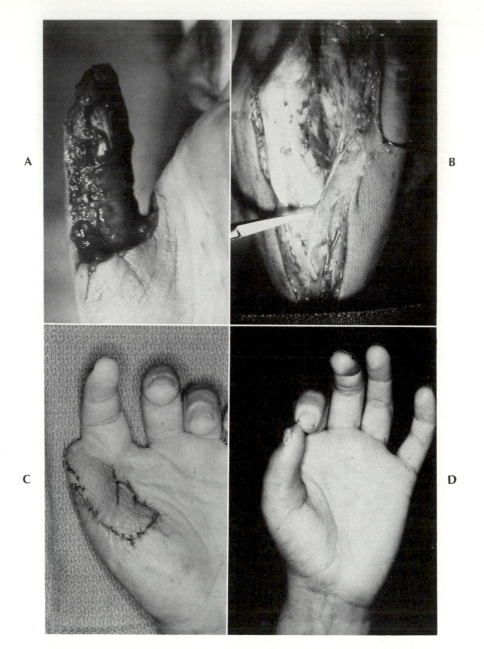

FIG. 69-3. Longitudinal avulsion of entire volar thumb. **A,** Avulsion of entire volar thumb caused by removal of circumferential pipe. **B,** Use of sensory innervated cross-finger flap from second metacarpal and index finger. Scissors point at nerve branch within flap. **C,** Appearance of transferred sensory innervated cross-finger flap at time of detachment (3 weeks). **D,** Satisfactory resurfacing with excellent motion and sensation at 9 months.

has proved effective (Fig. 69-3). An alternative technique should be the use of a remote pedicle flap (chest, abdomen, or arm) with the addition of a neurovascular island pedicle flap.

AMPUTATION NEAR THE INTERPHALANGEAL JOINT

It has already been shown that amputation distal to, through, or just proximal to the interphalangeal joint is consistent with satisfactory length for nearly all thumb functions. The requirements after amputation at this level are

that the resulting stump be left pain free with good sensation. The best procedure to achieve that goal is primary amputation closure with minimal additional shortening. It is important that that closure be carried out with good amputation principles, including the careful identification and proximal resection of the digital nerves.[35,46,74,111] On occasion, the use of a small dorsal skin graft will be necessary when the obliquity of the amputation has resulted in sufficient dorsal skin loss that bone shortening would be necessary for amputation closure using local skin (Fig. 69-4).

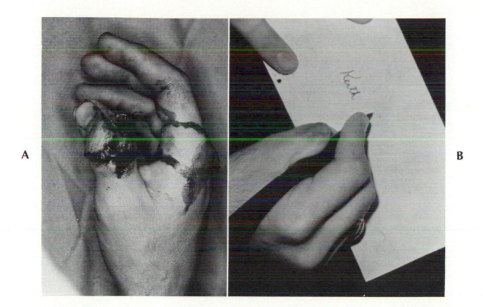

FIG. 69-4. Amputation at interphalangeal joint. **A,** Near-complete amputation through interphalangeal joint of thumb with loss of significant dorsal skin. **B,** Appearance of thumb 4 months after dorsal resurfacing with split-thickness skin graft to prevent necessity of further shortening.

REPLANTATION OF THE AMPUTATED THUMB

The rationale for attempting replantation after thumb amputation is undeniable. A successful replant with the recovery of at least protective sensation will prove more functionally satisfactory than any other type of thumb-reconstructive technique, even with some shortening and the loss of motion at both the metacarpophalangeal and interphalangeal joints. It is, therefore, important that the possibility of thumb replantation be recognized in emergency care facilities so that transfer of patient and part to a microvascular replantation center can be facilitated as quickly as possible.

The requirements for replantation of an amputated thumb include sharp severance with minimal avulsion or crushing in a patient in the proper age group. It is important that the part be cooled and that transfer to a microvascular center be carried out within a few hours. The replantation team will proceed with the sequential repair of the phalangeal bone, flexor pollicis longus, extensor pollicis longus, digital nerves, at least one digital artery, several digital veins, and the skin. Extended hospitalization with careful observation of the replanted thumb and anticoagulation are often necessary, but the long-term functional result after successful replantation will justify this additional effort (Fig. 69-5). Numerous reports of successful thumb replantations have appeared,* and there can be no doubt that it is the procedure of choice for amputations proximal to the interphalangeal joint when the proper requirements are met.

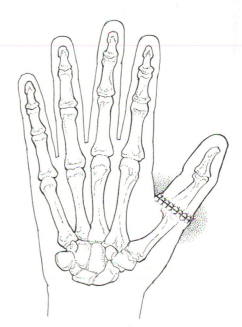

Replantation of amputated thumb

*See references 16, 79, 91, 92, 154, and 174.

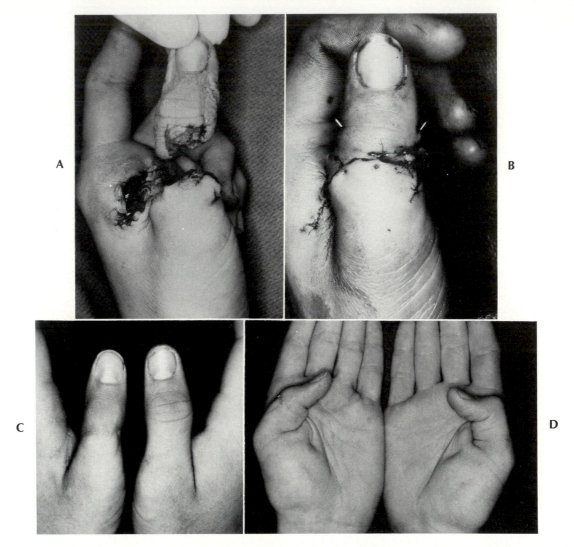

FIG. 69-5. Replantation of amputated thumb. **A,** Complete amputation through proximal phalanx. **B,** After replantation. **C,** Appearance of thumb, *left,* at 6 months. **D,** Thumb at 6 months demonstrating satisfactory flexion. Sensation and strength were good.

AMPUTATION THROUGH THE MIDPROXIMAL PHALANX

When unsalvageable amputations occur at the midprox-imal phalangeal level, satisfactory thumb function can usu-ally be achieved by procedures designed to deepen the first web space and create an adequate thumb index cleft. These procedures have been called "phalangization" and utilize methods that deepen the interdigital cleft so that the first metacarpal and remaining proximal phalanx are relatively lengthened. This may be achieved by a simple Z-plasty,[23,50] by a four-flap Z-plasty technique,[177] by free skin grafts, by dorsal rotational flap techniques,* or by the use of remote pedicle flaps. The indications for these techniques vary ac-cording to the amount of thumb web contracture, the mo-bility of the first metacarpal, and the condition of the web-space skin and muscle.†

The simple or four-flap Z-plasty techniques are adequate to achieve web-space deepening when the first metacarpal is mobile and there is no muscle contracture[23,50,177] (Fig. 69-6). Occasionally the injury that has resulted in thumb loss through the proximal phalanx will also result in con-siderable adjacent tissue injury with a poorly surfaced thumb remnant and a tight contracture of the first web space. In these instances a rotational flap technique has been effective in providing deepening, mobilization, and partial resurfac-ing of the metacarpal-phalanx unit. This phalangization technique employs sequential division of all restraining skin, muscles, scar, and capsular adhesions and can result in a very satisfactorily functioning thumb unit[14,100,131,155] (Fig. 69-7).

*See references 14, 100, 131, 152, and 155.
†See references 3, 13, 14, 50, 60, 73, 77, 97, 98, 105, 114, 123, 152, and 171.

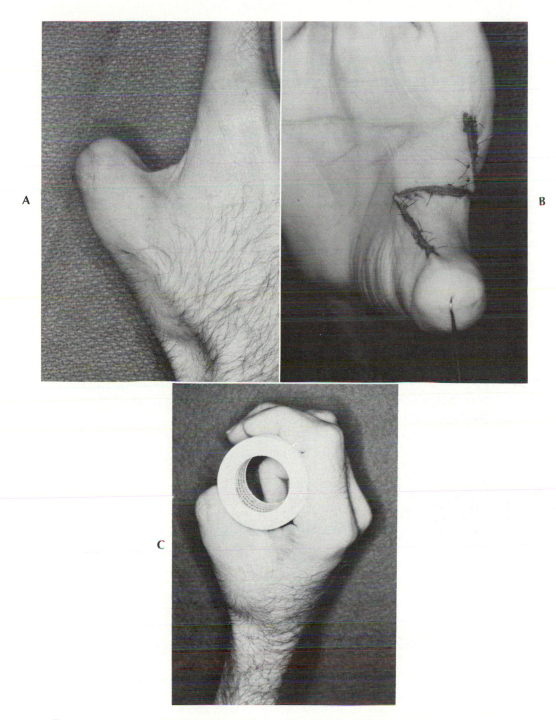

FIG. 69-6. Z-plasty deepening of first web space. **A,** Limited thumb-index cleft after amputation through distal proximal phalanx. **B,** Thumb web deepening using simple Z-plasty. **C,** Improved grasping function at 6 months.

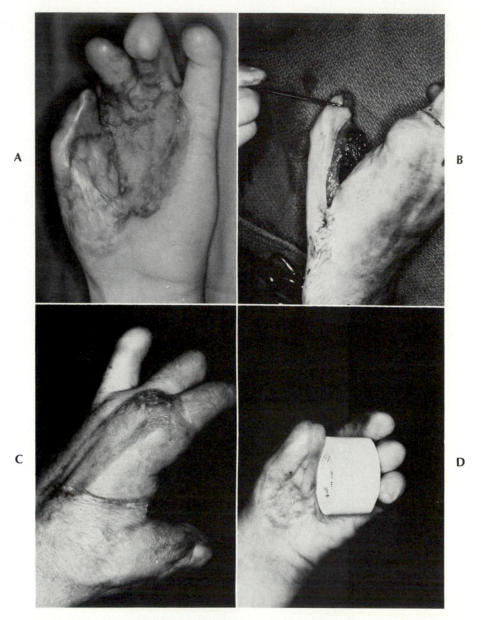

FIG. 69-7. Phalangization of badly damaged metacarpophalangeal unit. **A,** Tightly contracted metacarpal and proximal phalanx with poor skin coverage after crush burn. **B,** Mobilization of metacarpal and division of contracted web, excision of poor skin and scar, and recession of first dorsal interosseous and adductor pollicis muscles. **C,** Proved abduction of phalangized thumb at 4 months. **D,** Improved grasp and pinch at 4 months.

AMPUTATION NEAR THE METACARPOPHALANGEAL JOINT

When unsalvageable thumb amputation occurs near the metacarpophalangeal joint, the resulting stump is inadequate to carry out many of the important functions of the thumb.[143,149] In these instances added length of 1 to 2 cm is required with the transference of satisfactory sensory perception.

In the acute injury, autograft techniques may be used with skin and subcutaneous tissue removed from the amputated part. The remaining thumb, consisting of bone and tendon, is either replaced primarily or preserved in an abdominal pocket and reattached after several weeks or months. Reconstruction is then carried out in a manner similar to that described for the degloved thumb. Although this procedure is not widely used, several authors have considered it worthwhile and have emphasized that when the thumb is cleanly amputated but cannot be replaced, the autograft technique can provide a very satisfactory return of thumb function.*

When the deformity created by the loss of the thumb at the metacarpophalangeal joint level is already in existence, reconstruction may be carried out by pollicization of an adjacent injured or partially amputated digit or by the use of a "cocked-hat flap." Other alternatives include the use of osteoplastic reconstruction techniques involving the use of a bone graft covered by a tubed pedicle flap and the addition of an island pedicle flap or pollicization of the middle and distal phalanges of the normal ring finger.[61,70,95,104]

Because injuries that result in the loss of the thumb quite often involve destruction of adjacent digits, it is occasionally possible to transfer part of the injured digit or metacarpal to the base of the proximal phalanx or the first metacarpal in order to add length and sensory perception.* Careful planning before making this composite tissue transfer is necessary so that sensation can be preserved and the vascular status of the transferred digit ensured. When the second or third metacarpal stump is transferred, the cosmetic appearance of the reconstructed thumb may be somewhat bulbous, but the functional improvement resulting from this lengthening procedure can be substantial, and the patient is usually satisfied[28,30,32,33] (Figs. 69-8 and 69-9).

The use of the "cocked-hat flap" as originally suggested by Gillies[59] is also a reconstructive possibility when the thumb amputation is at the metacarpophalangeal joint level, and an adjacent injured digit is not available. This procedure, which involves local mobilization of skin and subcutaneous tissue from the dorsum and lateral aspects of the first metacarpal to cover a length of iliac bone graft up to 2½ cm, provides a useful increase in thumb length with at least protective sensibility.† Although some authors have found the procedure disappointing,[90] it has proved beneficial provided that close attention to the details of the technique are carried out (Fig. 69-10).

The technique of first metacarpal lengthening that has been described by Matev[107,108] would also have application for thumb loss at the metacarpophalangeal joint level. Continued investigation of these lengthening techniques may prove them to be safer, more reliable, and more esthetically pleasing than either the transfer of an injured adjacent digit or the "cocked-hat" technique.

---

*See references 56, 59, 70, 124, 139, 143, 144, 146, 148, and 176.

*See references 20, 38, 57, 62, 63, 87, 97, 98, 119, 131, 143, 149, and 165.
†See references 58, 79, 143, 146, 150, and 167.

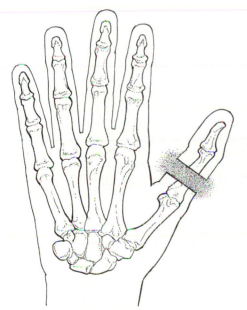

Amputation through midproximal phalanx

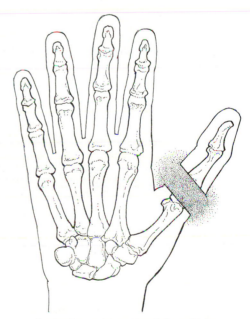

Amputation near metacarpophalangeal joint

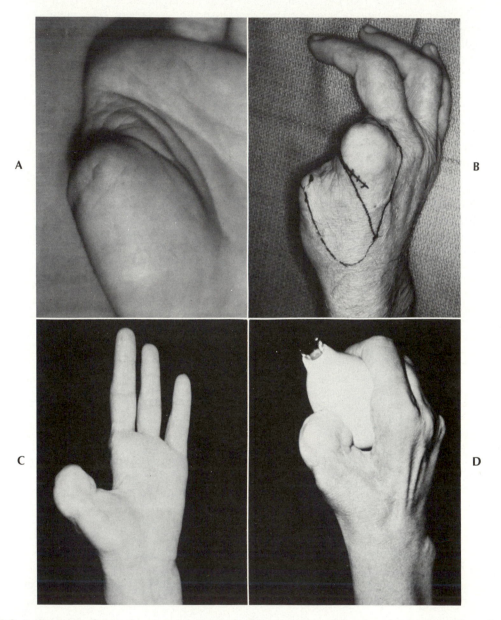

FIG. 69-8. Pollicization of second metacarpal stump. **A,** Old amputation of thumb and index finger through metacarpophalangeal joints. **B,** Incisions outlined for pollicization of index stump to first metacarpal. **C,** Appearance of transferred index metacarpal at 6 months. **D,** Excellent restoration of pinch and grasp after this transfer.

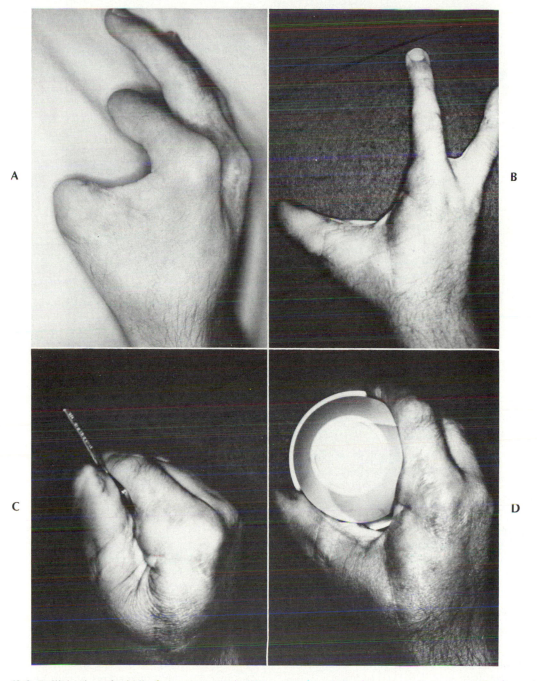

FIG. 69-9. Pollicization of middle finger remnant. **A,** Old amputation of distal thumb, index ray, and distal two thirds of long finger. **B,** Nine months after transfer of proximal phalanx of long finger. **C,** Satisfactory pinch. **D,** Satisfactory grasp.

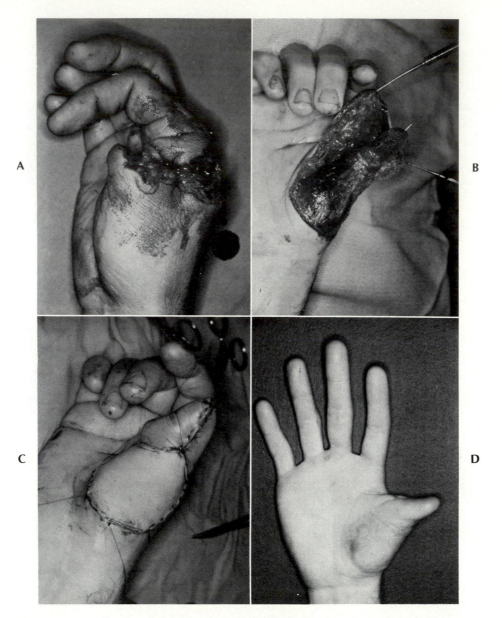

FIG. 69-10. A, Power-saw amputation of thumb at metacarpophalangeal joint with concomitant injury to the index finger. **B,** First metacarpal lengthening utilizing 2 cm of iliac bone graft and local flap from dorsal radial aspect of first metacarpal. **C,** Appearance of lengthened metacarpal unit at conclusion of surgery with full-thickness skin graft resurfacing of donor area. **D,** Satisfactory functional improvement at 6 months.

AMPUTATION THROUGH THE DISTAL ONE THIRD OF THE METACARPAL

When the thumb amputation has occurred through the distal one third of the first metacarpal, an additional 2 to 4 cm of length are necessary in order to achieve satisfactory thumb function. Again, the need for restoration of adequate sensory perception is important and pollicization of an adjacent injured digit is the best procedure. In the absence of such a digit for transfer, osteoplastic thumb reconstruction utilizing a bone graft, tubed abdominal pedicle flap, and an island pedicle flap would become the best method of restorative surgery.

As with thumb loss at a more distal level, the use of an injured digit, whether it be intact or partially amputated, to add length with sensation is an excellent procedure after amputation through the distal first metacarpal. Despite the fact that the joints or tendons of the transferred digit may not be functional, the added length and sensory perception will result in a substantial improvement in function. Joint stabilization procedures may be indicated, and great care should be taken to ensure near-normal thenar muscle function and first metacarpal rotation. The techniques of transfer are similar to those of pollicization of a normal digit, and the same attention to preservation of the neurovascular structures is mandatory (Fig. 69-11).

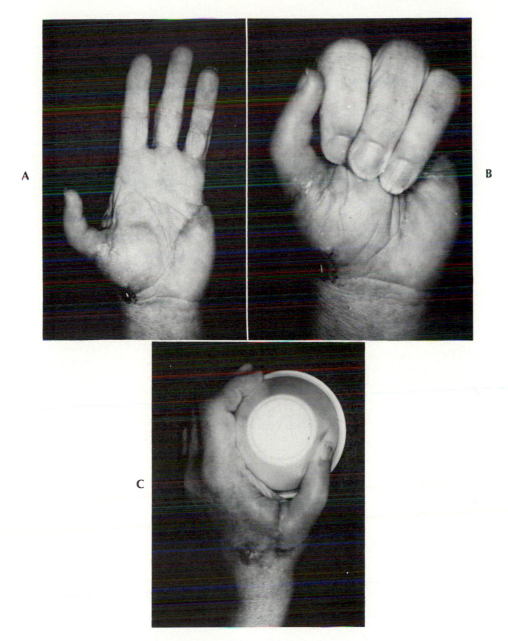

FIG. 69-11. Pollicization of small finger. *A*, Forty-seven-year-old woman 2 months after pollicization of poorly functional finger to first metacarpal stump. **B**, Satisfactory pinch. **C**, Satisfactory grasp.

With the advent of refined and predictable microneurovascular techniques, other method of transfer of digits or metacarpals from an otherwise irreparably damaged hand to the opposite hand may occasionally be indicated. Although the clinical circumstances favoring this type of reconstruction are admittedly rare, the result may be quite satisfactory.[15,157]

Osteoplastic thumb reconstruction has been carried out by use of various techniques since it was first attempted (but apparently aborted) by Nicoladoni[126] in 1897. Although there were many reports of successful thumb reconstruction before 1955 using bone graft and tubed pedicle flap tech-

niques,* the results of these techniques were generally considered to be unsatisfactory because they failed to provide adequate sensory perception to the reconstructed thumb and because there was usually significant resorption of the bone graft inside the pedicle. After the suggestions of Moberg[116,118] and Littler[99,100] that neurovascular island pedicle transfer be incorporated in osteoplastic reconstruction of the thumb, many surgeons have developed techniques

---

*See references 2, 6, 7, 9, 40, 45, 63, 64, 106, 126, 127, 132, 133, 135, 140, 150, 162, and 173.

that have proved to be considerably more successful.* Some authors continue to believe that this multiple-staged techniques has questionable merit[118,131,151] and the problem of resorption of the bone graft that compromises the long-term result of this procedure still exists (Fig. 69-12). Nevertheless, osteoplastic techniques have regained popularity as a method of thumb reconstruction at this level when the other fingers are normal or too badly damaged to be transferred and the first metacarpal has satisfactory rotation.[103] It is interesting to note that there have been several reports of

---

*See references 1, 23, 29, 31, 39, 48, 72, 75, 96, 104, 110, 120, 130, 131, 144, 148, 156, 158, 166, 167, and 170.

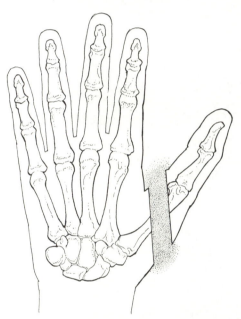

Amputation through distal one third of metacarpal

osteoplastic procedures since 1955 not utilizing neurovascular sensory transfer.[12,90]

As osteoplastic reconstruction has been modified over the years, the number of stages and the time interval required to complete the thumb reconstruction have been reduced, with most techniques now requiring two stages.[39,110,120,144] Although the tibia[7,106] or the clavicle[2,40,110] have been used as the source of bone graft, iliac bone is believed to be the best type of graft for this reconstruction. Unfortunately, no graft source seems to be free of the tendency toward gradual resorption. The tubed pedicle flap has in most instances been raised from the abdomen or groin, with some surgeons preferring a deltopectoral flap[120] or an inframammary flap.[7,40] Flaps taken concomitantly with the removal of iliac crest[12,48] or clavicle bone[110] may speed union and decrease resorption.[48] The use of a sensory innervated cross-finger flap in this type of reconstruction[1,96] has also been advocated rather than the use of a neurovascular island flap,[115] and various other ingenious procedures often utilizing local flaps have been described.[130,148,168]

An excellent technique of osteoplastic repair consists in a reconstruction as described by Reid[1,44] and emphasized by DeOlveira.[39] It consists in adding an iliac bone graft 2 to 4 cm in length to the distal metacarpal stump, followed by the application of a thin, tubed pedicle flap usually from the upper abdomen. On occasion it may be possible to salvage intact phalangeal bone from the amputated part of sufficient length to use as a bone graft with the hope that there may be less tendency for resorption. The length of the grafted bone should not exceed the level of the normal thumb interphalangeal joint or it will be too long to function effectively. At 3 weeks the tubed pedicle is detached and a neurovascular island pedicle flap, usually from the ulnar side of the long finger, is immediately implanted in the desired tactile area of the bone tube extension. The extended neurovascular flap technique[75,158] is utilized and provides an

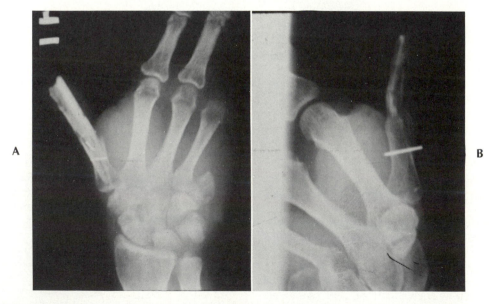

FIG. 69-12. Resorption of bone graft and remote pedicle flap. **A,** Appearance of fibular bone graft 2 months after osteoplastic reconstruction utilizing upper abdominal tubed pedicle flap. **B,** Appearance of same graft at 18 months.

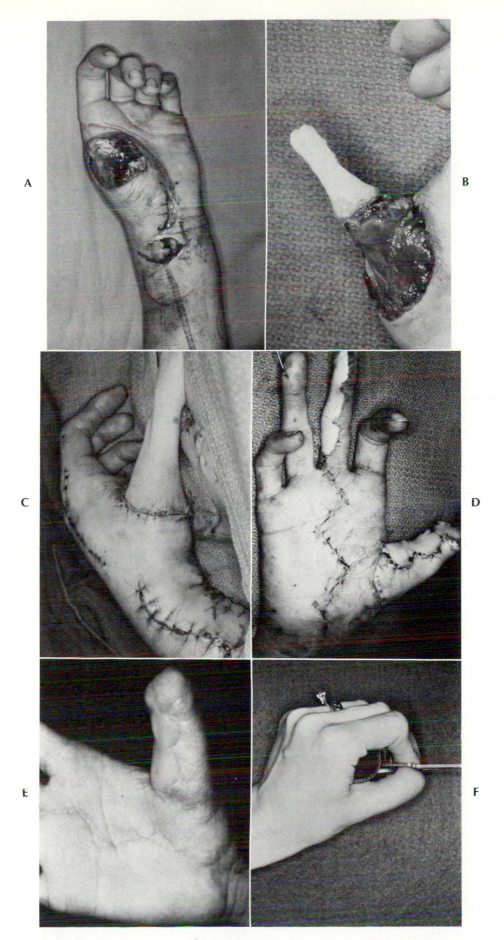

Fig. 69-13. Osteoplastic reconstruction of thumb. **A,** Traumatic amputation of thumb through distal first metacarpal. **B,** Bone graft using preserved proximal phalanx and amputated thumb. **C,** Application of upper abdominal, thin, tubed pedicle flap. **D,** Transfer of neurovascular island pedicle flap from ulnar aspect of long finger at time of pedicle flap detachment (3 weeks). **E,** Appearance of thumb unit at 6 months. **F,** Satisfactory pinch and grasping function at 6 months.

adequate area of sensory perception for both pinch and grasp functions. In this manner there has been a rapid and effective restoration of thumb length and sensation, with the patient able to resume functional activity within 6 to 8 weeks in most instances (Fig. 69-13).

The sacrificing of a normal digit to achieve thumb function may occasionally be indicated after amputation at the distal first metacarpal level, although, when a mobile first meta-carpal with satisfactory thenar muscle and basilar joint function is present, osteoplastic reconstruction would seem a more logical alternative.

AMPUTATION THROUGH THE PROXIMAL TWO THIRDS OF THE METACARPAL

When amputation of the thumb involves loss of the entire thumb and the majority of the first metacarpal, a procedure designed to provide total thumb reconstruction is required. Because the required length of the reconstructed thumb will usually be in excess of 5 cm and the mobility achieved in a short first metacarpal stump may be limited, osteoplastic reconstructive procedures are probably not indicated. Pollicization of an injured or partially amputated digit would remain as the procedure of choice, with pollicization of a normal digit, usually the index finger, as an alternative. Transfer of the great toe may be occasionally considered in those patients who are poor candidates for pollicization procedures.

The use of adjacent injured digital structures for thumb reconstruction remains applicable for amputations with a shorter first metacarpal stump. Because of the frequent loss of basilar joint rotatory motion, it is desirable for the transferred digit to have at least some motion, preferably at the metacarpophalangeal joint, that can provide some power flexion in the thumb position (Fig. 69-14). Even if little or no motion is present in the injured digit, careful attention to positioning can allow it to function as a satisfactory post against the remaining digits.

The pollicization of a normal finger into the thumb position before the advent of neurovascular transfer techniques was an extremely difficult and hazardous operation, requiring the mobilization of large tissue segments, with the ultimate performance of the transferred digit often being marginal by present standards.* In some instances abdominal flaps were used to fill the cleft left by the digital transfer,[41] while in other techniques tendons and nerves were not joined.[171] The first true pollicization of an index finger, utilizing neurovascular dissection and transfer techniques, was carried out in 1949 by Gossett,[61] with similar pollicization of the long finger being carried out shortly thereafter by Hilgenfeldt.[70] Since that time the procedure has been modified with technical considerations emphasized by Littler,[97-99] Harrison,[68,69] and others.† Although most authors have tended to favor the index finger as the digit to be transferred, the use of the long finger,[70,83] ring finger,‡ and

Amputation through proximal two thirds of metacarpal

even the small finger[89] have been advocated by some surgeons. In recent years careful consideration of the fundamental priorities and technical considerations to restore muscle balance, proper length, and the correct rotation have been emphasized.* In addition, the contribution of surgeons carrying out pollicization in congenital absence of the thumb has added further modifications of the technique for use after traumatic thumb loss.[17,43,67,94,179]

The pollicization of a normal finger on the stump of the first metacarpal has the advantages of being a one-stage procedure that maintains at least some functional joint motion and has near-normal sensation and vascularization.[170] I have been satisfied with the use of the index finger for pollicization employing the technique described by Littler[102] (Fig. 69-15).

Surgical efforts to transfer a finger from the opposite hand[85,86] or toes to replace a thumb have been occasionally carried out since Nicoladoni's first toe-to-hand transfer in 1900.[127] Before the advent of predictably successful microvascular anastomoses, the staged transfer of a toe (usually the big toe) to the hand was extremely difficult and fraught with complications. Although hand function may have been improved by this transfer, the technical difficulty, cosmetic appearance, poor sensation, and marginal performance of the transferred part served to prevent this method of reconstruction from becoming popular.† After the experimental work of Buncke,[18] Cobbett,[36] Buncke,[19] O'Brien,[129] and Tamai[164] have successfully described and refined procedures for the free transfer of the great toe to the thumb position with vessel, nerve, and tendon repairs.

At the present time toe-to-thumb transfer should be reserved for patients who are poor candidates for other re-

---

*See references 6, 38, 41, 80, 83, 119, and 171.
†See references 10, 18, 22, 25, 54, 89, 95, 111, 134, 151, and 167.
‡See references 25, 54, 95, 151, and 167.

---

*See references 68, 69, 102-104, and 111.
†See references 8, 27, 31, 32, 34, 52, 59, and 178.

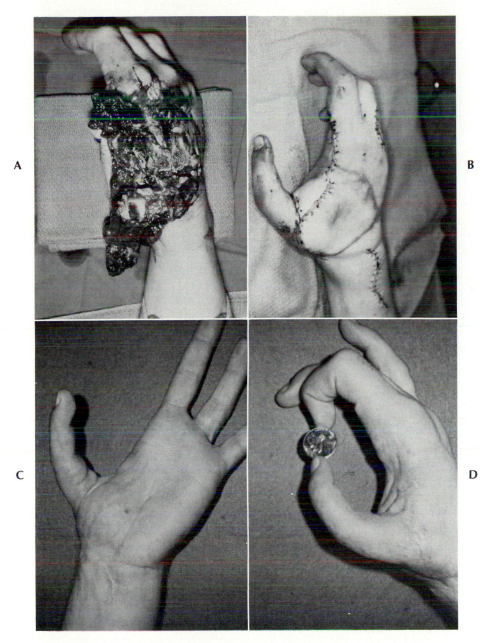

FIG. 69-14. Pollicization of injured index finger. **A,** Mutilating injury resulting in thumb amputation and destruction of second metacarpal and extensor tendons. **B,** Appearance of hand at 2 months after abdominal pedicle resurfacing and pollicization of damaged second metacarpal-index finger ray. **C,** Appearance of hand at 3 years. **D,** Ability to carry out fine pinch and strong grasp.

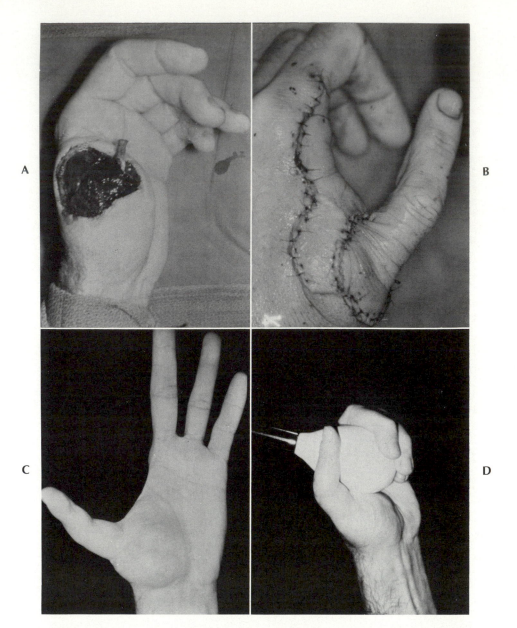

FIG. 69-15. Pollicization of normal index finger. **A,** Complete amputation of thumb through midfirst metacarpal. **B,** Pollicization of index finger. **C,** Appearance of pollicized index finger at 1 year. **D,** Satisfactory function of pollicized index finger.

constructive techniques and are of the proper mental and physical status for the prolonged procedure and subsequent rehabilitation. The procedure should only be carried out by trained microvascular teams, and the patient should be aware of and in agreement with the possibility of failure that would compound the thumb amputation by loss of the great toe. The technique of O'Brien[129] simplifies the procedure by allowing for transfer of the great toe on the dorsalis pedis artery and dorsal veins, obviating the necessity for the difficult plantar dissection of vascular structures (Fig. 69-16). Perhaps as microvascular skills improve and more centers are established, and the repugnance for this procedure on the part of reconstructive hand surgeons diminishes, toe-to-thumb transfer will increase in popularity and take its place as an important reconstructive possibility after thumb loss.

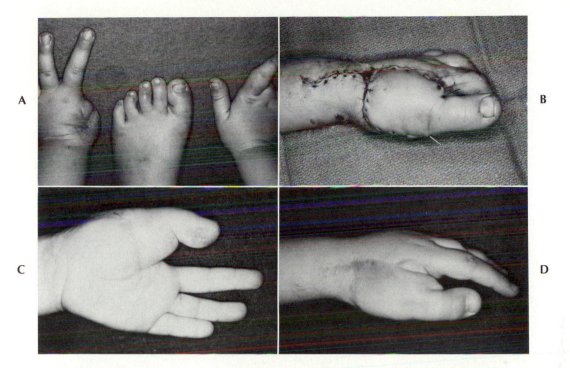

FIG. 69-16. Toe-to-thumb transfer. **A,** Loss of thumb and index finger in left hand of child with appearance of child's left foot and badly injured right hand also shown. **B,** Immediately after transfer of left great toe to thumb position. **C,** Appearance of transferred toe at 8 months. **D,** Appearance of toe at 8 months with satisfactory pinch, grasp, strength, and sensation. (Courtesy Dr. James B. Steichen.)

LOSS OF THUMB AND ALL DIGITS

The occasional amputation of the thumb and all digits results in a catastrophic functional loss to the hand. The reconstructive surgeon faced with this deformity must assess the possibility of restoring two opposable rays with strong motion in at least one. Techniques that provide length by the addition of bone grafts and insensitive abdominal flaps usually provide little long-term functional improvement and should be generally condemned. When there are phalangeal remnants present, it may be possible to phalangize mobile metacarpal segments with satisfactory strength and sensation to accomplish crude pinch and grasp functions.[115] These procedures have varied from phalangization of the first metacarpal,[13] to "reverse pollicization" of the second metacarpal to the first metacarpal,[44] to clefting operations between the first and third metacarpals with removal of the second or second and third metacarpals.[63] By utilizing these or similar techniques,[23,66,112,131] one can hopefully achieve a wide enough cleft for an opening and closing pincer function (Fig. 69-17).

Technical considerations for phalangization procedures include removing enough metacarpal and often distal carpal row to provide a satisfactory cleft and at the same time attempting to preserve as much adductor and abductor pollicis function as possible to ensure the mobility of the first metacarpal ray. In those patients with no phalangeal remnants or short metacarpal segments, the procedure may often prove technically impossible. Although small increments of length may occasionally be gained by interpositional or add-on grafting, usually with use of portions of the metacarpals

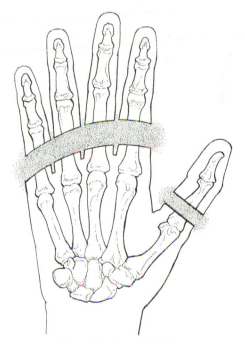

Loss of thumb and all digits

excised to create a cleft, the results may prove disappointing if one cannot ensure a satisfactory midray space, opposable strength and motion of at least one ray, and satisfactory sensory perception on the opposing sides of the pincer.

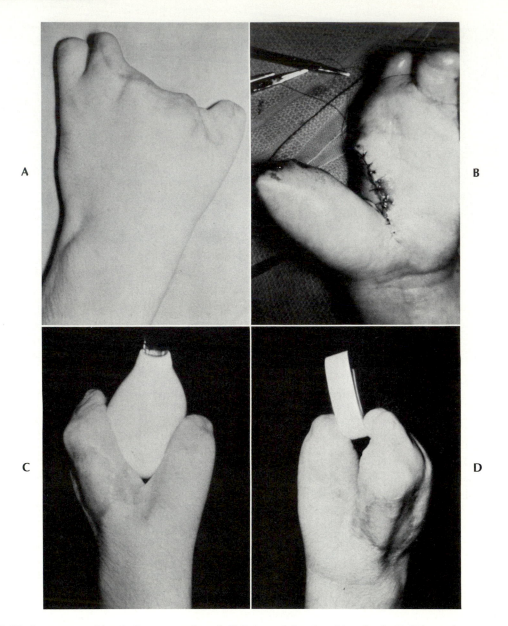

FIG. 69-17. Appearance of hand after amputation of all digits and thumb, with only short phalangeal remnants present over first, second, and fifth metacarpals. **B,** Immediately after phalangization of first metacarpal with midhand clefting permitted by excision of second and majority of third metacarpals and trapezoid. **C,** Appearance of hand at 6 months with satisfactory grasping function. **D,** Appearance of hand at 6 months demonstrating pinch.

DISCUSSION

One may note from this chapter that there are many esoteric and technically difficult procedures available for the reconstruction of thumb function after partial or total loss. Emphasis has been placed on a careful evaluation of the functional requirements necessitated at each level of thumb amputation, and procedures that best meet those requirements are suggested (Fig. 69-18). A genuine consideration of the specific desires of each patient is mandatory, and it is the obligation of the reconstructive surgeon to explain in detail the realistic goals of each restorative procedure and the possible complications. A sufficient time interval after

thumb amputation should elapse before any secondary reconstructive procedure is undertaken in order for the patient to adjust to the hand function necessitated by thumb loss so that he may knowledgeably participate in decisions relating to reconstruction. Finally, it should be emphasized that these procedures require not only a cooperative patient but a highly skilled hand surgeon familiar with intricate reconstructive procedures of this nature and, one would hope, the availability of hand rehabilitation unit to aid in the restoration of thumb function after surgery. Any compromise in these basic considerations will almost inevitably lead to disappointing results.

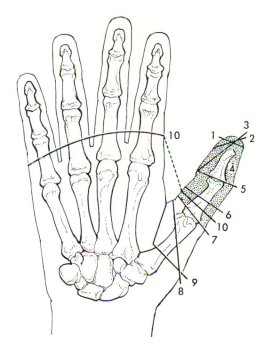

FIG. 69-18. Diagrammatic summary of best procedures for thumb loss at various levels. *Level of thumb loss: 1,* Guillotine tip; *2,* oblique avulsion; *3,* entire volar pad; *4,* deglovement; *5,* interphalangeal joint; *6,* midproximal phalanx; *7,* near metacarpophalangeal joint; *8,* distal one-third first metacarpal; *9,* proximal two-thirds first metacarpal; *10,* thumb and digits. *Best reconstruction procedures: 1,* Split-thickness graft; *2,* volar advancement flap; *3,* cross-finger flap; *4,* tubed flap and neurovascular island pedicle flap; *5,* primary closure; *6,* web deepening; *7* (a), pollicize adjacent injured digit, (b) "cocked-hat" flap, (c) first metacarpal lengthening; *8* (a) pollicize injured digit, (b) osteoplastic reconstruction; *9* (a) pollicize injured digit; (b) pollicize normal digit; (c) toe transfer; *10,* phalangization of first metacarpal.

CONCLUSION

The surgeon dealing with the patient whose hand performance is severely impaired by partial or complete loss of the thumb, and in whom a reconstructive effort is indicated, must decide from a wide variety of surgical possibilities. Careful consideration must be given to the level of amputation with an understanding of the specific requirements for satisfactory reconstruction that are necessitated at each level. Proper length, position, mobility, stability, and, above all, sensory perception must be achieved without sacrificing significant function from other areas of the hand or body. An attempt has been made to describe the best procedures for each level of thumb amputation, with the recognition that a number of other factors may play an important part in the ultimate restorative decision.

REFERENCES

1. Adamson, J.E.: Sensory rehabilitation of the injured thumb, Plast. Reconstr. Surg. **40:**53-57, 1967.
2. Albee, F.: Synthetic transplantation of tissue to form a new finger with restoration of function of the hand, Ann. Surg. **69:**379, 1919.
3. Arana, G.B.: Phalangization of the first metacarpal, Surg. Gynecol. Obstet. **40:**859, 1925.
4. Atasoy, E., Loakimidis, E., Kasdan, M.L., Jutz, J.E., and Kleinert,

H.E.: Reconstruction of the amputated finger with a triangular volar flap, J. Bone Joint Surg. **52A:**921-926, 1970.
5. Barclay, T.L.: The late results of finger tip injuries, Br. J. Plast. Surg. **8:**38, 1955.
6. Barsky, A.J.: Restoration of the thumb by transplantation, plastic repair and prosthesis, Surgery **23:**227-247, 1948.
7. Beardsley, J.M., and Zecchino, U.: Reconstruction of thumb, Am. J. Surg. **71:**825-827, 1946.
8. Blair, V.P., and Byars, L.T.: Toe to finger transplant, Ann. Surg. **112:**287, 1940.
9. Blake, H.E.: Notes on the reconstruction of the thumb, Br. J. Plast. Surg. **1:**119-122, 1948-1949.
10. Bowe, J.J.: Thumb construction by index transposition, Plast. Reconstr. Surg. **32:**414-424, 1963.
11. Bralliar, F., and Horner, R.L.: Sensory cross-finger pedicle graft, J. Bone Joint Surg. **51A:**1264-1268, 1969.
12. Broadbent, T.R., and Woolf, R.M.: Thumb reconstruction with contiguous skin-bone pedicle graft, Plast. Reconstr. Surg. **26:**494-499, 1960.
13. Brown, H., Welling, R., Sigman, R., Flynn, W., and Flynn, J.R.: Phalangizing the first metacarpal, Plast. Reconstr. Surg. **45:**294-297, 1970.
14. Brown, P.W.: Adduction-flexion contracture of the thumb—correction with dorsal rotation flap and release of contracture, Clin. Orthop. **88:**161-168, 1972.
15. Brownstein, M.L.: Thumb reconstruction by free transplantation of a damaged index ray from the other hand—a case report, Plast. Reconstr. Surg. **60(2):**280-283, 1977.
16. Bruner, J.M.: Salvage of the "all-but-amputated" thumb, Plast. Reconstr. Surg. **14:**244-248, 1954.
17. Buck-Gramcko, D.: Pollicization of the index finger: method and results in aplasia and hypoplasia of the thumb, J. Bone Joint Surg. **53A:**1605-1617, 1971.
18. Buncke, H.J., Buncke, C.M., and Schulz, W.P.: Hallux-to-hand transplantation, utilizing micro-vascular anastomoses, Br. J. Plast. Surg. **19:**332, 1966.
19. Buncke, H.J., McLean, D.H., George, P.O., and others: Thumb replacement: great toe transplantation by microvascular anastomosis, Br. J. Plast. Surg. **26:**194, 1973.
20. Bunnell, S.: Physiological reconstruction of a thumb after total loss, Surg. Gynecol. Obstet. **52:**248, 1931.
21. Bunnell, S.: Opposition of the thumb, J. Bone Joint Surg. **20:**269-284, 1938.
22. Bunnell, S.: Digit transfer by neurovascular pedicle, J. Bone Joint Surg. **34A:**772-774, 1952.
23. Bunnell, S.: The management of the nonfunctional hand—reconstruction vs. prosthesis, Artif. Limbs **4:**76-102, 1957. (See Chapter 68 of the present book for reprint.)
24. Bunnell, S.: Reconstruction of the thumb, Am. J. Surg. **95:**168-172, 1958.
25. Butler, M.B.: Ring-finger pollicization (with transplantation of nail bed and matrix on a volar flap), J. Bone Joint Surg. **46A:**1069-1076, 1964.
26. Byane, M.B., and Clarkson, P.: Traumatic amputations of the fingertips. In Flynn, J.E., editor: Hand surgery, Baltimore, 1966, Williams & Wilkins Co.
27. Chandler, R., and Clarkson, P.: A toe-to-thumb transplant with nerve graft, Am. J. Surg. **95:**315-317, 1958.
28. Chase, R.A.: An alternative to pollicization in subtotal thumb reconstruction, Plast. Reconstr. Surg. **44:**421, 1969.
29. Chase, R.A., and Laub, D.R.: The hand, therapeutic strategy for acute problems, Curr. Probl. Surg. **27:**June 1968.
30. Chase, R.A., Milford, L.W., Goldner, J.L., Flatt, A.E., and Smith, R.J.: In thumb repair, is length most crucial? Mod. Med., pp. 75-79, Aug. 20, 1973.
31. Clarkson, P.: On making thumbs, Plast. Reconstr. Surg. **29:**325-331, 1962.
32. Clarkson, P., and Furlong, R.: Thumb reconstruction by transfer of big toe, Br. Med. J. **2:**1332-1334, 1949.
33. Clarkson, P.W.: Reconstruction of hand digits by toe transfers, J. Bone Joint Surg. **37A:**270-276, 1955.
34. Clarkson, P.W., and Chandler, R.: On making thumbs, Plast. Reconstr. Surg. **17:**393, 1956.

35. Clifford, R.H.: Evaluation of three methods of finger tip injuries, Arch. Surg. **65:**464, 1956.

36. Cobbett, J.R.: Free digital transfer (report of a case of transfer of a great toe to replace an amputated thumb), J. Bone Joint Surg. **51B:**677-679, 1969.

37. Curtis, R.M.: Cross finger pedicle flap in hand surgery, Ann. Surg. **145:**650, 1957.

38. Cuthbert, J.B.: Pollicization of the index finger, Br. J. Plast. Surg. **1:**56, 1948.

39. DeOlveira, J.C.: Some aspects of thumb reconstruction, Br. J. Surg. **57:**85-89, 1970.

40. Dial, D.E.: Reconstruction of thumb after traumatic amputation, J. Bone Joint Surg. **21:**98-100, 1939.

41. Dunlop, J.: The use of the index finger for the thumb: some interesting points in hand surgery, J. Bone Joint Surg. **5:**99, 1923.

42. Dykes, E.R.: Reconstruction of the thumb, Hawaii Med. J. **26-27:**33-35, 1966-1968.

43. Edgerton, M.T., Snyder, G.B., and Webb, W.L.: Surgical treatment of congenital thumb deformities (including psychological impact of correction), J. Bone Joint Surg. **47A:**1453-1474, 1965.

44. Elsahy, N.I.: Reverse pollicization of thumb reconstruction, Hand **63:**233-235, 1974.

45. Esser, J.F.S.: Island flaps, N.Y. J. Med. **106:**264, 1974.

46. Flatt, A.E.: The care of minor hand injuries, St. Louis, 1963, The C.V. Mosby Co.

47. Flatt, A.E.: An indication for shortening of the thumb (description of technique and brief report of five cases), J. Bone Joint Surg. **46A:**1534-1539, 1964.

48. Finseth, F., May, J.W., and Smith, R.J.: Composite groin flap with iliac-bone flap for primary thumb reconstruction, J. Bone Joint Surg. **58A:**130-132, 1976.

49. Fisher, R.H.: The Kutler method of repair of finger tip amputations, J. Bone Joint Surg. **49A:**317, 1967.

50. Flynn, J.E.: Adduction contracture of the thumb, N. Engl. J. Med. **254:**677-686, 1956.

51. Flynn, J.E., and Burden, C.N.: Reconstruction of the thumb, Arch. Surg. **85:**56-60, 1962.

52. Freeman, B.S.: Reconstruction of thumb by toe transfer, Plast. Reconstr. Surg. **17:**393-398, 1956.

53. Freiberg, A., and Manktelow, R.: The Kutler repair for fingertip amputations, Plast. Reconstr. Surg. **50:**371, 1972.

54. Garcia-Velasco, J.: Thumb reconstruction using the ring finger, Br. J. Plast. Surg. **26:**406-407, 1973.

55. Gaul, J.S.: Radial-innervated cross-finger flap from index to provide sensory pulp to injured thumb, J. Bone Joint Surg. **51A:**1257-1263, 1969.

56. Gillies, Sir H.: Autograft on an amputated digit, a suggested operation, Lancet **1:**1002, 1940.

57. Gillies, Sir H., and Cuthbert, J.B.: Operation for pollicization of an index finger, Medical Annual, 202, Bristol, 1943, John Wright & Sons Ltd.

58. Gillies, Sir H., and Millard, D.R.: The principles and art of plastic surgery, Boston, 1957, Little, Brown & Co.

59. Gillies, Sir H., and Reid, D.A.C.: Autograft of the amputated digit, Br. J. Plast. Surg. **7:**388, 1955.

60. Gordon, S.: Autograft of amputated thumb, Lancet **2:**823, 1944.

61. Gosset, J.: La pollicisation de l'index, J. Chir. (Paris) **65:**403, 1949.

62. Graham, W.C.: Reconstruction of the thumb, N.Y. J. Med. **49:**49-50, 1949.

63. Graham, W.C., Brown, J.B., Cannon, T., and others: Transposition of fingers in severe injuries of the hand, J. Bone Joint Surg. **29:**998, 1947.

64. Greeley, C.P.W.: Reconstruction of the thumb, Ann. Surg. **124:**60-70, 1946.

65. Guermonprez, F.: Notes sur quelques résections et restaurations du pouce, Paris, 1887, Passelin.

66. Haas, S.L.: Operation for the loss of all fingers of both hands, Am. J. Surg. **36:**720, 1936.

67. Harrison, S.H.: Restoration of muscle balance in pollicisation, Plast. Reconstr. Surg. **34:**236-240, 1964.

68. Harrison, S.H.: Pollicisation in cases of radial club hand, Br. J. Plast. Surg. **23:**192-200, 1970.

69. Harrison, S.H.: Reconstruction of the thumb. Proceedings of the Second Hand Club, 1956-1957. Brentwood Essex, 1975, Westbury Press.

70. Hilgenfeldt, O.: Operativer Daumenersatz, Stuttgart, 1950, Ferdinand Enke Verlag.

71. Holevich, J.: A new method of restoring sensibility to the thumb, J. Bone Joint Surg. **45B:**496-502, 1963.

72. Hoskins, H., and Curtis, R.M.: Versatility of cross-finger pedicle flap, J. Bone Joint Surg. **41A:**778, 1959.

73. Howard, L.D.: Contracture of the thumb web, J. Bone Joint Surg. **32A:**267-273, 1950.

74. Howard, L.D., Jr.: Plastic procedures in hand surgery, 1963, Manual Distributed at Instructional Courses Lectures American Academy of Orthopaedic Surgeons.

75. Hueston, J.: The extended neurovascular island flap, J. Bone Joint Surg. **18:**304-305, 1965.

76. Hughes, N.C., and Moores, F.T.: A preliminary report on the use of a local flap and peg bone graft for lengthening a short thumb, Br. J. Plast. Surg. **3:**34-39, 1950-1951.

77. Huguier, P.C.: Replacement du pouce par son métacarpian, par l'agrandissement du premier espace interosseux, Arch. Gen. Med. **1:**78, 1874.

78. Hydroop, G.L.: Transfer of a metacarpal with or without its digit for improving the function of a crippled hand, J. Plast. Reconstr. Surg. **3:**533, 1948.

79. Ikuta, Y., Watari, S., Kubo, T., and others: The reattachment of severed fingers, Hiroshima J. Med. Sci. **22:**131, 1973.

80. Iselin, M.: Reconstruction of the thumb, Surgery **2:**619, 1937.

81. Iselin, F.: The flag flap, Plast. Reconstr. Surg. **52:**374-377, 1973.

82. Jeffrey, C.C.: A case of pollicisation of the index finger, J. Bone Joint Surg. **39B:**120-123, 1957.

83. Jepson, P.N.: Transformation of the middle finger into a thumb, Minnesota Med. **8:**552, 1925.

84. Joshi, B.B.: One-stage repair for distal amputation of the thumb, Plast. Reconstr. Surg. **45:**613-615, 1970.

85. Joyce, J.L.: A new operation for the substitution of a thumb, Br. J. Surg. **5:**499-504, 1917-1918.

86. Joyce, J.L.: The results of a new operation for the substitution of a thumb, Br. J. Surg. **16:**362-369, 1928-1929.

87. Kaplan, I.: Primary pollicization of injured index finger following crush injury, Plast. Reconstr. Surg. **37:**531-535, 1966.

88. Keim, H.A., and Grantham, S.A.: Volar-flap advancement for thumb and finger-tip injuries, Clin. Orthop. **66:**109-112, 1969.

89. Kelleher, J.C., and Sullivan, J.G.: Thumb reconstruction by fifth digit transposition, Plast. Reconstr. Surg. **21:**470-478, 1958.

90. Kelly, A.P.: Subtotal reconstruction of the thumb, Arch. Surg. **78:**582-585, 1959.

91. Kleinert, H.E., Kasdan, M.L., and Romero, J.L.: Small blood vessel anastomosis for salvage of severely injured upper extremity, J. Bone Joint Surg. **45A:**788, 1963.

92. Komatsu, S., and Tomai, S.: Successful reimplantation of a completely cut-off thumb, Plast. Reconstr. Surg. **42:**374-377, 1968.

93. Kutler, W.: A new method for finger-tip amputations, J.A.M.A. **133:**29, 1947.

94. Laico, J.: Total reconstruction of a thumb in a thumbless hand, J. Phillipine Med. Assoc. **30:**381-387, 1954.

95. Letac, R.: Pollicization of the ring finger, J. Int. Coll. Surg. **22:**649, 1954.

96. Lewin, M.L.: Sensory island flap in osteoplastic reconstruction of the thumb, Am. J. Surg. **109:**226-229, 1965.

97. Littler, J.W.: Subtotal reconstruction of the thumb, Plast. Reconstr. Surg. **10:**215-226, 1952.

98. Littler, J.W.: The neurovascular pedicle method of digital transposition for reconstruction of the thumb, Plast. Reconstr. Surg. **12:**303-320, 1953.

99. Littler, J.W.: Neurovascular pedicle transfer of tissue in reconstructive surgery of the hand, J. Bone Joint Surg. **38A:**917, 1956.

100. Littler, J.W.: The prevention and correction of adduction contracture of the thumb, Clin. Orthop. **13:**182-192, 1959.

101. Littler, J.W.: Neurovascular skin island transfer in reconstructive hand surgery, Edinburgh, 1960, E. & S. Livingstone, Ltd.

102. Littler, J.W.: Digital transposition. In Adams, J.P., editor: Current practice in orthopaedic surgery, vol. 3, St. Louis, 1966, The C.V. Mosby Co.

103. Littler, J.W.: On making a thumb: one hundred years of surgical effort, J. Hand Surg. **1**:135-51, 1976.

104. Littler, J.W.: Reconstruction of the thumb in traumatic loss. In Converse, J.M., editor: Reconstructive plastic surgery, vol. 6, ed. 2, Philadephia, 1977, W.B. Saunders Co.

105. Lyle, H.M.: Deformity of the hand—formation of a new thumb from the stump of the first metacarpal, Ann. Surg. **76**:121-125, 1922.

106. Maltz, M.: Reconstruction of thumb, Am. J. Surg. **58**:429-433, 1942.

107. Matev, I.B.: First metacarpal lengthening for thumb reconstruction, Ortop. Travmatol. **6**:11-14, 1969.

108. Matey, I.B.: Thumb reconstruction after amputation at the metacarpophalangeal joint by bone lengthening, J. Bone Joint Surg. **52A**:957-965, 1970.

109. McFarlane, R.M., and Stromberg, W.B.: Resurfacing of the thumb following major skin loss, J. Bone Joint Surg. **44A**:1365-1375, 1962.

110. McGregor, I., and Simonetta, C.: Reconstruction of the thumb by composite bone-skin flap, Br. J. Plast. Surg. **17**:37, 1964.

111. Metcalf, W., and Whalen, W.P.: Salvage of the injured distal phalanx—plan of care and analysis of 369 cases, Clin. Orthop. **13**:119, 1959.

112. Michon, J., and Dolich, B.H.: The metacarpal hand, Hand **6**:285-290, 1974.

113. Millender, L.H., Albin, R.E., and Nalebuff, E.A.: Delayed volar advancement flap for thumb tip injuries, Plast. Reconstr. Surg. **52**:635-639, 1973.

114. Minkow, F.V., and Stein, F.: Phalangization of the thumb, J. Trauma **13**:648-655; 1973.

115. Miura, T., Yoshitake, K., and Nakamura, R.: Reconstruction of the mutilated hand, Hand **8**:78-85, 1976.

116. Moberg, E.: Discussion of paper. In Brooks, D., editor: Nerve grafting in orthopaedic surgery, J. Bone Joint Surg. **37A**:305, 1955.

117. Moberg, E.: Aspects of sensation in reconstructive surgery of the upper limb, J. Bone Joint Surg. **46A**:117, 1964.

118. Moberg, E.: Discussion. In Reid, D.A.C.: Policization—an appraisal, Hand **1**:31, 1969.

119. Moores, F.T.: The technique of pollicisation of the index finger, Br. J. Plast. Surg. **1**:60-68, 1948-1949.

120. Morgan, L.R., and Stein, R.: Method for a rapid and good thumb reconstruction, Plast. Reconstr. Surg. **50**:131-133, 1972.

121. Murray, J.F., and Gavelin, G.E.: The neuro-vascular island flap, J. Bone Joint Surg. **49A**:1285, 1967.

122. Murray, R.A.: The injured or abnormal thumb: recommendations for treatment, South. Med. J. **52**:845-850, 1959.

123. Mutz, S.B.: Thumb web contracture, Hand **4**:236-246, 1972.

124. Nemethi, C.E.: Reconstruction of the distal part of the thumb after traumatic amputation, J. Bone Joint Surg. **42A**:375-391, 1960.

125. Nichols, H.M.: Manual of hand injuries, ed. 2, Chicago, 1960, Year Book Medical Publishers, Inc.

126. Nicoladoni, C.: Daumenplastik, Wien, Klin. Wochenschr. **10**:663, 1897.

127. Nicoladoni, C.: Daumenplastik und organischer Ersatz der Fingerspitze (Anticheiroplastik und Daktyloplastik), Arch. Klin. Chir. **61**:606, 1900.

128. Nicoladoni, C.: Weitere Erfahrungen über Daumenplastik, Arch. Klin. Chir. **69**:697, 1903.

129. O'Brien, B. McC., Macleod, A.M., Sykes, P.J., et al.: Hallux-to-hand transfer, Hand **7**:128, 1975.

130. Orticochea, M.: Reconstruction of the thumb using two flaps from the same hand, Br. J. Plast. Surg. **24**:345-350, 1971.

131. Peacock, E.E., Jr.: Reconstruction of the thumb. In Flynn, J.E., editor: Hand surgery, Baltimore, 1966, The Williams & Wilkins Co.

132. Petersen, N.: Plastic reconstruction of the thumb, S. Afr. Med. J. **17**:137-138, 1943.

133. Pierce, G.W.: Reconstruction of thumb after total loss, Surg. Gynecol. Obstet. **45**:825-826, 1927.

134. Pohl, A.L., Larson, D.L., and Lewis, S.R.: Thumb reconstruction in the severely burned hand, Plast. Reconstr. Surg. **57**:320-328, 1976.

135. Polonsky, B.: Reconstruction of a missing thumb, S. Afr. Med. J. **23**:812-814, 1949.

136. Porter, R.W.: Functional assessment of transplanted skin in volar defects of the digits, J. Bone Joint Surg. **50A**:955, 1968.

137. Posner, M.A., and Smith, R.J.: The advancement pedicle flap for thumb injuries, J. Bone Joint Surg. **53A**:1618-1621, 1971.

138. Pringle, R.G.: Loss of distal thumb need not be severe disability, Injury **3**:211-217, 1972.

139. Prpić, I.: Reconstruction of the thumb immediately after injury, Br. J. Plast. Surg. **17**:49, 1964.

140. Rank, B.K.: Reconstruction of opposition digits for mutilated hands, Aust. N.Z. J. Surg. **17**:172-188, 1947-1948.

141. Ratliff, A.H.C.: Amputations of the distal part of the thumb, Hand **4**:190, June 1972.

142. Reid, D.A.C.: Experience of a hand surgery service, Br. J. Plast. Surg. **9**:11, 1956.

143. Reid, D.A.C.: Reconstruction of the thumb, J. Bone Joint Surg. **42B**:444-465, 1960.

144. Reid, D.A.C.: The neurovascular island flap in thumb reconstruction, Br. J. Plast. Surg. **19**:234, 1966.

145. Reid, D.A.C.: Pollicisation—an appraisal, Hand **1**:27, 1969.

146. Reid, D.A.C.: Thumb injuries, Hand **2**:126-129, 1970.

147. Riordan, D.C.: In Milford, L., editor: The hand, St. Louis, 1971, The C.V. Mosby Co.

148. Robinson, O.G., Jr.: Primary reconstruction of the thumb using amputated part and tube pedicle flap, South. Med. J. **66**:1025-1029, 1973.

149. Sallis, J.G.: Primary pollicisation of an injured middle finger, J. Bone Joint Surg. **45A**:503, 1963.

150. Sanders, G.B.: Reconstruction of the thumb, Am. J. Surg. **83**:347-351, 1952.

151. Sels, M.: Present methods of reconstruction of the amputated thumb, Plast. Reconstr. Surg. **32**:672, 1963.

152. Sharpe, C.: Tissue cover for the thumb web, Arch. Surg. **104**:21-25, 1972.

153. Shaw, M.H., and Wilson, I.S.P.: An early pollicisation, Br. J. Plast. Surg. **3**:214-215, 1950-1951.

154. Snyder, C.C., Stevenson, R.M., and Browne, E.Z.: Successful replantation of a totally severed thumb, Plast. Reconstr. Surg. **50**:553, 1972.

155. Spinner, M.: Fashioned transpositional flap for soft tissue adduction contracture of the thumb, Plast. Reconstr. Surg. **44**:345-348, 1969.

156. Stefani, A.D., and Kelly, A.P.: Reconstruction of the thumb: a one-stage procedure, Br. J. Plast. Surg. **15-16**:289-291, 1962-1963.

157. Steichen, J.B., and Strickland, J.W.: Successful pollicization of thumb from irreparably damaged hand to opposite hand, 1977. (Unpublished.)

158. Storvik, H.M.: The extended neurovascular island flap in thumb reconstruction, Scand. J. Plast. Reconstr. **7**:147-149, 1973.

159. Strickland, J.W., and Dingman, D.L.: Avulsions of the tactile finger pad: an evaluation of treatment, Am. Surg. **35**:756-761, 1969.

160. Sturman, M.J., and Duran, R.J.: Late results of finger-tips injuries, J. Bone Joint Surg. **45A**:289, 1963.

161. Sullivan, J.B., Kelleher, J.C., Baibak, G.J., Dean, R.K., and Pinker, L.D.: The primary application of an island pedicle-flap in thumb and index finger injuries, Plast. Reconstr. Surg. **39**:488-492, 1967.

162. Szlazak, J.: Total reconstruction of the thumb, Plast. Reconstr. Surg. **8**:67-70, 1951.

163. Tajima, T.: Treatment of open crushing type of industrial injuries of the hand and forearm: degloving, open circumferential, heat-press, and nail-bed injuries, J. Trauma. **14**:995-1011, 1974.

164. Tamai, S., Hori, Y., Tatsumi, Y., and Okuda, H.: Hallux-to-thumb transfer with microsurgical technique: a case report in a 45 year old woman, J. Hand. Surg. **2**:152-155, 1977.

165. Tanzer, R.C., and Littler, J.W.: Reconstruction of the thumb (by transposition of an adjacent digit), Plast. Reconstr. Surg. **3**:533-547, 1948.

166. Tubiana, R., and Duparc, J.: Restoration of sensibility in the hand by neurovascular skin island transfer, J. Bone Joint Surg. **43B**:474, 1961.

167. Tubiana, R., Stack, H.G., and Hakstian, R.W.: Restoration of prehension after severe mutilations of the hand, J. Bone Joint Surg. **48A**:455-473, 1966.

168. Uzelac, O.: Reconstruction of the thumb: another possibility, Br. J. Plast. Surg. **23:**85-89, 1970.

169. Verdan, C.: The reconstruction of the thumb, Surg. Clin. North Am. **48:**1033-1061, 1968.

170. Verdan, C., Tubiana, R., Harrison, S.H., and Littler, J.W.: Transactions of the Third International Congress of Plastic Surgery, Washington, D.C., 1963, p. 25.

171. Verrall, P.J.: Three cases of reconstruction of the thumb, Br. Med. J. **2:**775, 1919.

172. Watman, R.N., and Denkewalter, F.R.: A repair for loss of the tactile pad of the thumb, Am. J. Surg. **97:**238-240, 1959.

173. Weckesser, E.C.: Reconstruction of the distal portion of the thumb, Ohio State Med. J. **44:**602-603, 1948.

174. Weiland, A.J., Villarreal-Rios, A., Kleinert, H.E., Kutz, J., Atasoy, E., and Lister, G.: Replantation of digits and hands; analysis of surgical techniques and results in 71 patients with 86 replantations, J. Hand Surg. **2:**1-12, 1977.

175. White, W.F.: Fundamental priorities in pollicisation, Br. J. Bone Joint Surg. **52B:**438-443, 1970.

176. Wilson, J.B.: The autografting of an amputated thumb, Transactions of the Third International Congress of Plastic Surgery, Washington, D.C., p. 1012.

177. Woolf, R.M., and Broadbent, T.R.: The four-flap Z-plasty, Plast. Reconstr. Surg. **49:**48-50, 1972.

178. Young, F.: Transplantation of toes for fingers, Surgery **20:**117-123, 1946.

179. Zancolli, E.: Transplantation of the index finger in congenital absence of the thumb, J. Bone Joint Surg. **42A:**658-660, 1960.

70

Prosthetic and adaptive devices for the partial hand amputee

JILL G. WHITE and BRENDA C. HILFRANK

Patients who suffer an injury that results in the partial amputation of a hand need not be resigned to the loss of a functional hand as well. Through the use of a partial prosthesis, which provides a restoration of prehensile patterns so that the patient can maximize use of the remaining hands or digits, a patient may regain functional use of the hand. The fabrication and fitting of this prosthesis, whether it is functional or cosmetic, is an important part of the overall management program for partial hand amputees.

A prosthesis has been defined by *Webster's Medical Dictionary* as an "artificial substitute for a missing body part used for functional or cosmetic reasons or both." Evidence of attempts to replace the functions of the hand and arm has been found dating back to the second Punic War (218-201 B.C.)[7] As stated above, a prosthesis can be functional or cosmetic. A functional prosthesis can be thought of as a "tool," since it is used as an extension of the hand to perform a specific task, much in the way a hammer is used to drive a nail.[1] A cosmetic prosthesis provides an esthetically acceptable hand, although without motion it cannot be truly natural looking.

At this time there is no such thing as a truly artificial hand, although there are numerous total hand prostheses available that are either functional (hook) or cosmetic. The fitting of a prosthesis for a subtotally amputated hand is more complex than the fitting for a complete hand amputation. With the subtotal amputation, the shape of the stump and the function of the remaining digit or digits must be considered. Other important factors are general function, specific tasks, and the patient's individual needs.

CLASSIFICATION OF AMPUTATIONS

Normal prehensile patterns allow the hand to be divided into two functional units. The radial unit is composed of the thumb, index finger, and long finger and is responsible for precision manipulation. The ulnar unit, made up of the long, ring, and small fingers, gives the hand its power grasp. When a portion of the hand has been amputated, normal prehensile patterns are disturbed. The prosthesis for the partial hand amputee is designed to help the patient complete one or more prehensile patterns.

When considering the function of the hand and its units, we believe it more useful to classify amputations by function than by level. The classification system presented here has been described by Robert W. Beasley.[2]

Transverse amputations

Transverse amputations may occur at any level. For example, they may involve one or several digits or may involve the palm. Selection of a partial hand prosthesis will vary with the level and number of digits affected. Loss of one digit (except the thumb) rarely requires a functional prosthesis. A functioning partial finger also may be sufficient to complete prehension without the aide of a functional prosthesis, although a cosmetic prosthesis may be considered.

Radial amputations

Amputation of the thumb or index finger, or both, is considered a radial amputation. Precision manipulation is lost when the thumb has been amputated. A prosthetic opposing post is extremely useful in helping to provide this prehensile pattern (Fig. 70-1, *A*).

Ulnar amputations

When an ulnar amputation occurs, (Fig. 70-1, *B*) there is a loss of the power grasp unit. The patient no longer is able to grip objects with force against the palm. Prosthetics helpful for this partial hand may include a "scoop"-shaped device, which substitutes for the ulnar digits that ordinarily would have held an object to the palm. This "scoop" can be devised to incorporate the palm only, or even incorporate the wrist for stability. Several scoops of different sizes may be necessary to accommodate the various objects commonly used by patients at home and work.

Central amputations

Central amputations involve the central digits, the long and ring fingers. In most cases prosthetics for cosmesis only are appropriate (Fig. 70-1, *C*).

PATIENT SELECTION

In considering a particular patient as a candidate for a prosthesis, several conditions should be examined. Most importantly, the patient should be able to use his hand more effectively with a device than without it. He also must be sufficiently motivated to want to regain the use of his hand. The device should be presented as a tool, and the patient should know that the device may be very specialized in its use. The degree of specialization will vary, depending on the needs of the patient. For instance, a manual laborer may

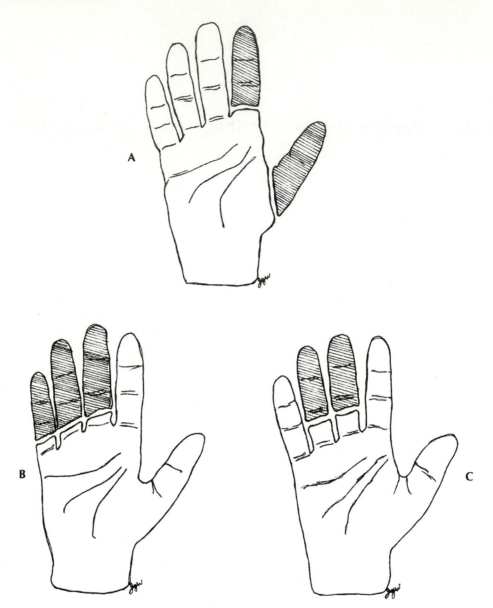

FIG. 70-1. A, Radial amputation. **B,** Ulnar amputations. **C,** Central amputations.

require a heavy-duty "tool," while a receptionist may require a cosmetic prosthesis. Cosmesis versus function should be discussed with the patient, and the patient should understand that a particular prosthesis or adaptive device that is suitable for work may not be appropriate for home use. The patient may want the option of having a prosthesis designed for each. The patient must be willing to accept the prosthesis as a helping device. The therapist also should recognize that a patient's acceptance or rejection of such a device could be influenced by such nonmedical concerns as socioeconomic and cultural backgrounds.

The stump surfaces should have adequate soft-tissue coverage with good subcutaneous padding to withstand the pressure of a prosthesis. Sensibility is also important. The stump should be examined carefully for neuromas, which would not allow the patient to tolerate the pressure of a prosthesis. If any areas of dysesthesia or other sensory dysfunctions

are present, a preliminary desensitization program is appropriate.

All assets of the involved upper extremity should be maximized. Mobility of the remaining digit or digits and the entire upper extremity should be improved. If the amputation has been long-standing, the patient may well have held his hand in his pocket and developed stiffness and atrophy of his entire arm. In this case, a program of splinting and exercise should be developed. Strengthening is also initiated when muscular atrophy is present. A progressive resistive exercise program is helpful and the patient is encouraged to use his hand with the temporary device for functional activities.

FABRICATION

Several prostheses providing a functional post have been described.[3-8]

We will discuss the subject of a temporary device that can be fabricated to evaluate the effectiveness of a partial hand prosthesis before its final fabrication.

This testing device is fabricated as a prototype of the permanent prosthesis. It can be used to help evaluate the need for such a prosthesis and to help assess the patient's functional capabilities with and without a prosthesis. It can also be used to aid in the design of the permanent prosthetic device by allowing one to determine the best post position for precision pinch and to test the post's height and position for maximum strength. Thus it allows experimentation with as many revisions as necessary for the design of the best possible device for the individual patient, utilizing material readily available to the therapist in a clinical setting.

For treatment purposes, the device is valuable because it allows the patient to begin such activities as stump accommodation to a prosthesis and practice with a prosthesis while waiting for the permanent device. The temporary or testing device can also be incorporated into the total exercise regimen for strength and range of motion by allowing the patient to perform specific tasks and exercises using the involved hand. The patient may also get a psychological boost by being able to use his hand again to some degree.

Equipment and supplies

1. Hydrocollator or frying pan
2. Heat gun
3. Scissors, bandage, or splinting
4. Paper towels
5. Pencils
6. Splinting material (for example, Kay-Splint, Polyform)
7. Velcro (hook and pile)
8. Foam rubber padding
9. Lotion

Importance of using the proper material

When fabricating the testing device, select a pliable thermoplastic material that will contour well to the receiving surface. This material also must be lightweight for comfort, strong and durable for wear and tear, and washable for good hygiene. Such material is required because of possible changes in both the post and the socket.

Making the pattern for the socket

On a paper towel, trace the volar and dorsal aspects of the hand from the wrist crease to the distal palmar crease. Combine these two pieces so that there is one piece surrounding this portion of the hand. The proximal and distal aspects of the pattern must not interfere with mobility of the wrist or remaining digits, or interfere with sensation. If the wrist is to be included, the pattern should extend two thirds the length of the forearm.

Molding the socket

The most important part of molding the socket is the provision of a precise contour to the receiving surfaces of the stump. There must be no area of increased pressure that will cause skin breakdown, especially if there is decreased sensibility or a bony prominence. When vulnerable areas are recognized, there are ways to avoid them—for example,

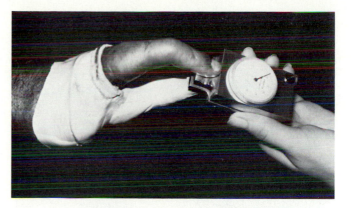

FIG. 70-2. Height is adjusted for maximal pinch strength, which can be measured with a pinch gauge.

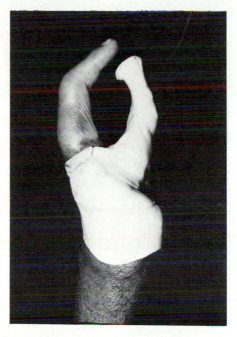

FIG. 70-3. Prototype is molded from a pliable thermoplastic material that contours well to the receiving surfaces.

by placing a doughnut foam pad over the area or by doming the material.

Making the other components

When molding the opposing post for a radial amputation, one rolls a rectangular piece of splinting material into a solid tube. The tube is shaped into a modified C shape formed from the base so that its strength will be increased.

The configuration should be positioned so that its distal portion allows maximal pulp contact with the post. The height is adjusted for maximal pinch strength, which can be measured with a pinch gauge (Fig. 70-2). The tip of the post should be flattened to provide enough friction for manipulation of objects; for example, foam rubber padding can be added to the tip to aid in reducing slippage. The shape and size of the post will be determined by the individual patient and his specific needs (Fig. 70-3).

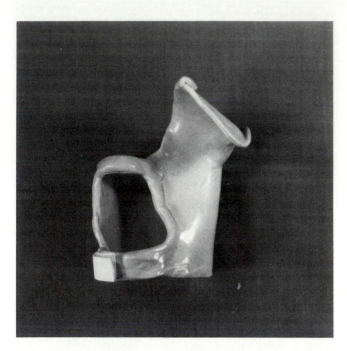

FIG. 70-4. For ulnar amputation a scoop-shaped device is fabricated.

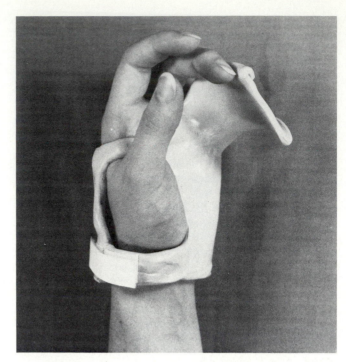

FIG. 70-5. Scoop is positioned as fingers would grasp in slight flexion.

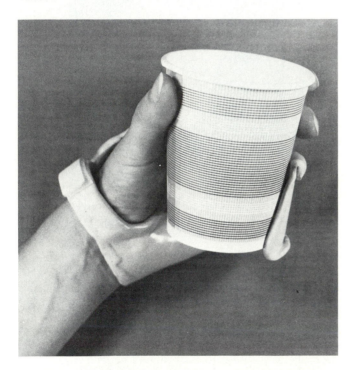

FIG. 70-6. Volar aspect is molded in concave shape to allow for grip.

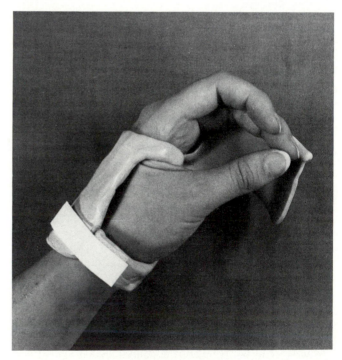

FIG. 70-7. Velcro strips can be used to assure a snug fit.

For the ulnar amputation a scoop-shaped device is fabricated (Fig. 70-4). The length of the scoop is directly proportioned to the length of the remaining digits. The scoop is positioned as the fingers would grasp in slight flexion (Fig. 70-5). The volar aspect is molded into a concave shape to allow for grip (Fig. 70-6). The thumb should be able to oppose the distal aspect of the device. The device should

allow full motion of the thumb. But the size again is dependent on the general use. The device can incorporate only the palm or may include the wrist for stability.

Fasteners may or may not be needed with this device. Under ideal conditions the opposable post's socket will fit so snugly on the hand that no fasteners would be required. At other times, as when the ulnar aspect may be cut to allow the prosthesis to slip over the hand, Velcro fasteners will be needed to ensure a snug fit. In the case of the scoop-shaped device, a slit is made along the radial aspect at the base of the thumb to allow the prosthesis to slide over the thumb. Velcro fasteners close this gap, assuring a secure fit (Fig. 70-7). If the prosthesis incorporates the wrist, usually two Velcro closures are necessary.

Assessment

When assessing the device and the patient's response to it, one must evaluate several aspects. The socket must be comfortable or the patient will not wear the device. There must be no pressure areas or discomfort when the patient has developed a tolerance to the prosthesis.

Initially the patient wears the prototype for short periods, but as the patient adjusts to this prosthesis, the wearing time is gradually increased. If the patient has been made a spare device, he should alternate between the two devices. He should practice using the device for both work and activities of daily living and report any problems or special needs to the therapist so that the prototype can be perfected before the permanent device is made. Any revisions that need to be made can be done quickly at the clinic during a patient's regularly scheduled treatment session.

Finally, has the patient accepted this device? That is, does he readily use the prosthesis to improve his function and believe that he has a better hand with the device than without it?

ADAPTIVE AND ASSISTIVE DEVICES

There are many adaptive and assistive devices on the market that can aid a patient in achieving maximal independence in various everyday activities. However, the more complex the device, the less willing a patient is to experiment; therefore the therapist should recommend a simple device. The patient's activities of daily living and social situation (with and without the functional prosthesis) should be examined thoroughly, and once the individual problems are identified, specific product recommendations can be made. Many one-handed adaptive devices are especially useful to a partial hand amputee. The injured hand can serve as a helping hand in assisting and stabilizing any such device. These devices fall under several categories: *self-care products,* such as Rocker knives with long, curved blades, electric razors, and suction-based brushes that can be stabilized; *homemaking devices,* such as suction-feet cutting boards with stainless steel nails for holding and assisting in preparing and cutting vegetables, and nonslip rubber mats; *communications equipment,* such as push-button telephones, electric typewriters, and wider pens and pencils; and *avocational items,* such as cardholders and sewing and needlepoint stands.

In addition to these special products, many everyday utensils and tools already present in the patient's home can be adapted for use. In most cases the adaptations are simple, usually involving the wrapping of a layer of tubular foam, rubber foam, or Betapile around a tool to provide a better grip. For instance, handles can be built up to make them easier to grasp and to reduce slippage. Scraps of splinting materials also can be valuable in building up keys, pens, paint brushes, hammers, and so on.

Periodic reevaluation of the need for these assistive, adaptive devices is important. As the patient becomes more confident in his ability to use his prosthesis, this dependence on special devices may lessen, and everyday utensils, with certain modifications, will replace specialized utensils.

ILLUSTRATED EXAMPLE

A 58-year-old, right-handed machine operator sustained traumatic amputation of his thumb and transmetacarpal amputations of his left index, long, and ring fingers. Surface coverage was obtained initially by skin grafting. The patient received no further treatment or therapy after hospital discharge.

Five months later the patient was referred to a hand surgeon. On evaluation a severe flexion contracture was present at the proximal interphalangeal joint of the remaining small finger. This measured 80 degrees initially. The metacarpophalangeal joint was limited both actively and passively in flexion, and there was minimal active motion at the distal interphalangeal joint. An intensive therapy program was initiated. Serial casting was effective in gaining nearly full extension of the proximal interphalangeal joint. A strengthening program for all the musculature of the left upper extremity was established. Regaining tendon glide and mobility of the metacarpophalangeal and distal interphalangeal joints was also chosen as a goal of therapy. The one-digit hand is unable to grasp or pinch without a device that provides an opposable post for prehension patterns (Fig. 70-8). Therefore a prototype for a functional prosthetic device

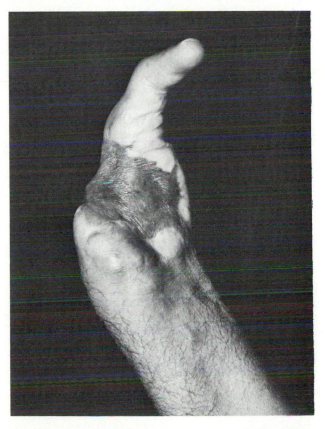

FIG. 70-8. One-digit hand is unable to grasp or pinch without a device that provides an opposable post for prehension patterns.

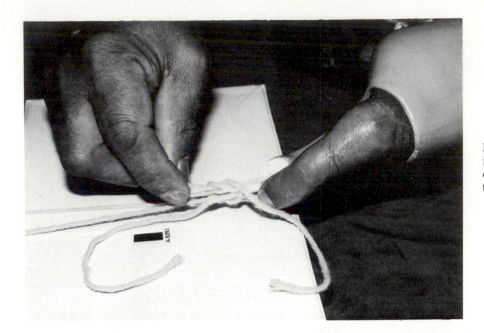

FIG. 70-9. Permanent prosthesis is fashioned from prototype to enable patient to complete activities of daily living such as tying a bow.

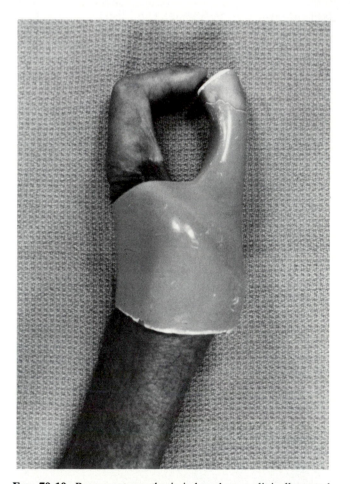

FIG. 70-10. Permanent prosthesis is based on a clinically tested prototype.

was fabricated. The patient immediately reported a more functional left hand and a greater independence, especially in activities of daily living, when using the device (Fig. 70-9). With the prototype being used as a positive mold, a permanent prosthesis was fabricated (Fig. 70-10). The patient also has been provided with a cosmetic prosthesis, which he uses only with "dress clothes."

CONCLUSION

Management of the partial hand amputee is a challenging problem. Fitting and fabricating the appropriate prosthesis is part of the complete management program. Each patient's amputation, particular needs, and remaining assets must be carefully evaluated so that the prosthesis will provide maximal benefit. Both the functional and cosmetic requirements of each partial hand amputee must be considered. A clinical testing device (fabricated in the clinic by the therapist) is helpful for evaluation of a particular prosthesis. The hand therapist can play a large role in evaluating, designing, and fabricating prosthetic and adaptive devices for the partial hand amputee.

REFERENCES

1. Beasley, R.W.: Hand injuries, Philadelphia, 1981, W.B. Saunders Co.
2. Beasley, R.W.: Management of upper limb amputations, Orthop. Clin. North Am. **12**(4):767-768, Oct. 1981.
3. Bunnell, S.: The management of the non-functional hand reconstruction vs. prosthesis, Artif. Limbs **4:**76-102, 1957. (See Chapter 68 of the present book for reprint.)
4. Smith, R., and Dworecka, F.: Treatment of the one digit hand, J. Bone Joint Surg. **55A:**113-119, Jan. 1973.
5. Swanson, A.B.: Restoration of hand function by the use of partial prosthesis, J. Bone Joint Surg. **45A:**276-283, 1963.
6. Tubiana, R., Stack, H.G., and Hakstian, R.W.: Restoration of prehension after severe mutilations of the hand, J. Bone Joint Surg. **48B:**455-473, Aug. 1966.
7. Wilson, A.B., Jr.: Some observations on upper extremity prosthetics. In Murdock, G., editor: Prosthetic and orthotic practice, London, 1969, Edward Arnold Publishers Ltd.
8. Wynn Parry, C.B., and others: Rehabilitation of the hand, London, 1966, Butterworth & Co. Ltd.

71

Esthetic hand prosthesis: its psychological and functional potential

JEAN PILLET

To lack beauty
Is not to be ugly:
Ugliness is displeasing
To the eye.

(PATIENT REFERRING TO HIS STUMP)

When we started making our first esthetic prostheses in the 1950s, everyone—surgeons, physicians, and therapists—viewed them as being a beautiful accomplishment but, at the same time, as rather an extravagance that an amputee could permit himself so long as he did not actually use it. Their attitude was in fact that since the prosthesis was inert, insensitive, and nonfunctional it could only be likened to a mere gadget.

Thirty years have gone by, and more than 5000 amputees have been fitted with esthetic prostheses. It is therefore appropriate to review these patients to ascertain which kinds of patients require an esthetic aid and to evaluate the psychological and functional potential of this type of prosthesis. For the sake of clarity this study has been limited to unilateral distal amputees.

It is always difficult for surgeons and therapists to realize that certain patients have need of an esthetic aid, since these professionals mainly come into contact with the recent amputee, a severely handicapped person to whom they wish to give functional help. However, the futures of such persons are poorly known. In addition, surgeons and therapists quite often have no experience whatsoever with agenesis patients, because such patients never have been physically injured and have not required their assistance.

ATTITUDE OF THE UNILATERAL DISTAL AMPUTEE

After amputation, the amputee experiences a major functional handicap. He believes in the miracles of surgery and the possibilities of prosthesis. It is a period of illusions, but progressively the amputee adjusts to reality during the period of fitting, reeducation, and vocational rehabilitation. It is a period mixed with hope and frustration during which doctors, therapists, and psychologists all have important roles to play.

Some amputees become invalids, never being able to accept their amputations. They hide their stumps and refuse to use them. They wear their functional prostheses but do not make use of them, as if the mere presence of the prostheses justified their behavior. Others accept their amputations only too well—they are delighted to be helped and to be treated as children, and their attitude reflects a psychological need.

Contrary to this small group, the majority of amputees get down to the business of leading a normal life. They reintegrate with their families and society and are able to do so because they have succeeded in making a realistic assessment of their disabilities. They very rapidly make full use of their remaining capabilities. In conjunction with the stump the remaining hand becomes increasingly skillful, to the amazement of not only immediate family members but also the amputee himself.

Thus one may say that for certain amputees it is the unesthetic aspect of the stump rather than the functional handicap that is the inhibiting factor and that causes the amputee to blame his amputation for his failures. Such transfer of blame clearly exists, and most amputees suffer from it. No functional prosthesis is going to eliminate it. Most patients finally grow accustomed to their physical impairments, learning to disregard them and even to forget about the function that has been lost. However, even this group may feel for a long time, and perhaps forever, esthetic frustration like that experienced by the congenital amputee.

THE UNILATERAL DISTAL CONGENITAL AMPUTEE AND HIS PROSTHETIC REQUIREMENTS
Functional needs

In my experience unilateral distal congenital amputees almost never ask spontaneously for a functional prosthesis. In the very rare exceptions encountered, it was relatively easy to discern the influence of parents or family practitioners, both equally misinformed.

When one is treating a congenital amputee, it is frequent and almost normal to commit a dual error by considering him as a disabled person and by wishing to fit a functional prosthesis.

It is our reasoning that is wrong concerning such a person.

801

He is not a true amputee but rather has an imperfect development on account of a congenital deformity. He has established his own perception of his body, which differs from our perception of it. He sees himself as being complete and normal. This mistaken reasoning whereby we imagine ourselves to have undergone an amputation as we try to "put ourselves in his shoes" is not exclusive to normal people. Congenitally deformed persons themselves are astonished when people with more pronounced deformities than theirs are able to carry out the same tasks as they, and even just as quickly and just as well.

To suggest fitting a functional prosthesis for a patient with unilateral agenesis, however perfect the prosthesis may be, is tantamount to encumbering a normal person with a third hand. In fact, that was the very reaction of such a patient whom I asked why he did not have a functional prosthesis. "Doctor," he said, "What would you want with a third hand?"

Congenital unilateral amputees are therefore disabled, but essentially in our eyes only. Whatever their ages, they manage all activities of daily living without any prostheses. For each need they use a technique that differs from ours. Naturally they have some frustration from not being able to do certain things, and this varies from one person to another. As among normal people, there are lazy and also clumsy agenetics, and giving them insensitive functional prostheses will make not them any more dexterous.

In the sixteenth century, Ambroise Paré reported seeing "an armless man do almost all the things any one else could do with his hands."

Esthetic needs

Unlike the amputee, an agenetic person is not submitted to the initial emotional shock of losing a hand. Only gradually does he come to realize that he is not like other people. This discovery comes rather late, between the ages of 6 and 8 years. The realization is not spontaneous, but rather the work of those around him. As long as the child is confined to the family circle, he usually is unaware of his anomaly. This protective phase is, however, critical. Those who use their stumps very little or awkwardly are invariably found to have had abnormal upbringings, cut off from others by ill-advised parents who hid them and helped them to do everything. This misapprehension condemns those unfortunate children to suffer from a dual moral and physical handicap.

Generally speaking, awareness of their anomaly begins when children start school. Their school friends show their curiosity. They begin to fear medical checkups and gym.

Finally, the hurdle of adolescence is most important. A young person often tends to blame his malformation for all his teen-age troubles.

The congenital amputee considers himself from the outset as being normal from a functional point of view, but he suffers from being different. We find these patients to have the same esthetic need felt by the amputee who has had a traumatic or surgical loss.

ESTHETIC IMPORTANCE OF THE HAND

The esthetic prosthesis fulfills a deep-rooted need of both the agenetic person and the amputee: to wish to go unnoticed and have two hands like everybody else. That is the whole problem. It demonstrates the importance of the beauty of the hand.

One must understand that for some patients the hand not only is a functional tool but also possesses expressive beauty: the appearance of the stump may seriously inhibit adaptation. For such patients the hand is the bearer of trophies; it emphasizes the beauty of a gesture, the gracefulness of a movement.

The manner in which esthetics is perceived varies from one person to another and from one ethnic group to another. Our patients, for example, are mostly of Latin origin. Very few come from Britain or Germany, and even fewer are Scandinavian. We have tried to determine whether the same pattern is encountered in the United States. The Latin and Anglo-Saxon peoples differ in their perceptions of the esthetic importance of the hand. With the intermingling of ethnic groups over many generations attitudes have become attenuated, but they have never quite disappeared. The problem is quite different in the case of amputees in the Middle East. My opinion is that some request an esthetic prostheses in order to become whole once more.

The distribution of our patients fitted with prostheses according to the level of amputation is shown in Table 71-1.

The distribution of our prosthesis patients between agenesis and traumatically acquired amputations is also interesting, with the percentages being more or less equal for the arm and forearm but with a decisive preponderance of traumatic cause in the hand proper (Table 71-2).

TABLE 71-1. Level of amputation of patients fitted with prostheses

Level of amputation	Percentage of patients
Arm	5
Forearm	30
Total hand	15
Metacarpal bone	20
Fingers	30

TABLE 71-2. Cause of amputation in patients fitted with prostheses

Level of amputation	Agenesis (%)	Trauma (%)
Arm/forearm	50	50
Total hand	45	55
Metacarpal bone	10	90
Fingers	3	97

ESSENTIAL CHARACTERISTICS OF ESTHETIC PROSTHESES

To be of real and lasting benefit, esthetic hand prostheses must be technically of high quality, matching well in details to the individual patient (Fig. 71-1). This is especially true for fingers, because they are viewed alongside normal fingers and thus generally require preparation of expensive molds for each person. Fingernail details are especially important; the nails must be fabricated of hard, translucent materials, be inlaid in the prosthesis, and be able to accept lacquer without problems (Fig. 71-2). The material must accept permanent pigmentation to correspond to normal skin color but not be stained by ordinary materials such as newsprint (Fig. 71-3). It must be strong and flexible and resistant

to hardening and burning (Fig. 71-4). A lack of all of these qualities has been the reason for the failure of the commonly used polyvinyl chloride prosthesis. Satisfactory material should be translucent like skin and approximate the texture and fine details of skin. The material must not be irritating or incite dermatologic reactions. It must be able to be readily repaired if damaged (Fig. 71-5).

Fixation of the prosthesis must be secure, comfortable, and simple. If the materials are supple, like reinforced silicones, and the fitting is perfect, attempts at removal create a negative pressure that must be broken, or removal is impossible even with very short sockets.

In areas of wide variations in climate, each patient should have two prostheses, one with its color adjusted to the av-

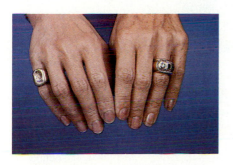

FIG. 71-1. Well-worn but fine esthetic, custom-fabricated prosthesis is compared with normal hand. Prosthesis must be of high quality to be of much benefit. (From Pillet, J.: Orthop. Clin. North Am. **12**(4):961, 1981.)

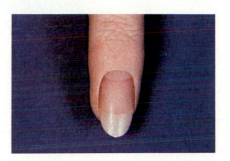

FIG. 71-2. This fingernail was carefully fashioned to match those of corresponding normal hand and inlaid for perfection. Such fingernails can be polished, if desired, like normal fingernails. (From Pillet, J.: Orthop. Clin. North Am. **12**(4):961, 1981.)

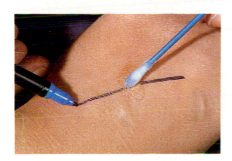

FIG. 71-3. Ink does not stain the silicone prosthesis and is readily removed with a moist applicator. (From Pillet, J.: Orthop. Clin. North Am. **12**(4):961, 1981.)

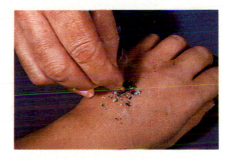

FIG. 71-4. Silicone prostheses are not subject to ordinary thermal damage. (From Pillet, J.: Orthop. Clin. North Am. **12**(4):961, 1981.)

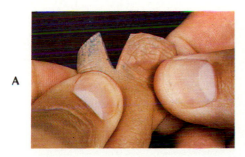 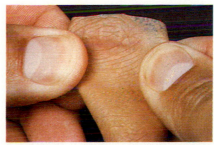

FIG. 71-5. **A,** Tear in thin proximal end of a fine silicone finger prosthesis. **B,** Repair of tear cannot be detected. Small tears in a silicone prosthesis can be perfectly repaired, but mutilation requires replacement. (From Pillet, J.: Orthop. Clin. North Am. **12**(4):961, 1981.)

erage winter pigmentation and the other to the summer. This does not increase the total cost, because two prostheses will wear twice as long as one. Also, this plan provides a prosthesis to be worn if the other needs repairs.

FUNCTIONAL POTENTIAL OF ESTHETIC PROSTHESES

The first objective of the esthetic prosthesis is purely psychological. It is to restore the appearance sufficiently close to normal to eliminate to a high degree the stigma associated with the disfigurement. Often the severity of disfigurement is more in the mind of the patient than real, but this is not important, for it is in fact on the basis of the patient's inerpretation that behavior will be predicated. There is little relation between the degree of actual physical loss and the psychological weight each individual patient will give to it and the degree it will influence performance. The man who finds himself unable to take his hand from his pocket, even though it is very "functional," may be as handicapped as if it were lost. Thus, in a global sense of function, the esthetic prosthesis may be beneficial even if it at times introduces some restriction of the prehensile capability of remaining parts. In allowing use of a stump that the amputee considers too repulsive to expose and use, the

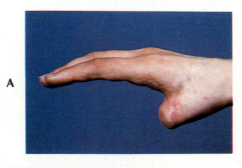
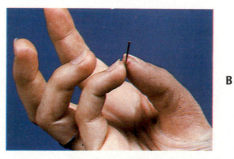

FIG. 71-6. A, Patient had a thumb amputation through base of proximal phalanx. **B,** Esthetic and functional improvement with a prosthesis. Thinness of silicone prosthesis permits reasonably good sensibility through it. (From Pillet, J.: Orthop. Clin. North Am. **12**(4):961, 1981.)

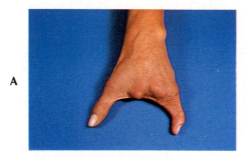
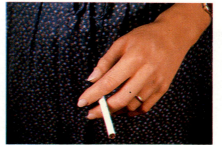

FIG. 71-7. A, Patient suffered from unesthetic appearance. **B,** Silicone prosthesis that is nearly identical to normal contralateral hand resolved problem of self-consciousness and improved function. Prosthesis is very thin over thumb to preserve both sensibility and mobility. Single finger is placed in ring-finger position in prosthesis for best relation to thumb for prehension. Satisfactory prosthetics for subtotally amputated hand present most difficult problem and challenge in prosthetic fabrication. (From Pillet, J.: Orthop. Clin. North Am. **12**(4):961, 1981.)

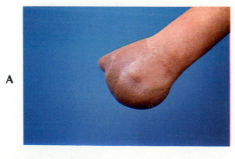
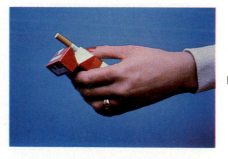

FIG. 71-8. A, From prosthetic point of view, transcarpal amputation is same as amputation through wrist or lower forearm. **B,** Passive total hand prosthesis can be "loaded" to offer some useful assistance aside from removing social stigma of loss. (From Pillet, J.: Orthop. Clin. North Am. **12**(4):961, 1981.)

prosthesis may well improve overall function.

Sometimes the prosthesis may be indicated in conjunction with surgical efforts by which an effective pinch mechanism has been restored but with which the part remains too grotesque for public presentation. The patient continues to amputate it mentally and keeps it constantly bandaged to preclude use. Covering the reconstructed part with a thin, flexible prosthesis of high quality may provide the essential element to realizing the most from the reconstruction, by giving it a socially acceptable presentation.

In the incompletely amputated hand the passive esthetic prosthesis can often provide an essential physical part against which remaining parts can oppose. This part may lengthen a short thumb (Fig. 71-6), or it may be a stable thumb post against which remaining mobile digits can work. Since potential combinations are innumerable, fitting such a hand with the optimal prosthesis is most difficult and demands the greatest ingenuity but often is also the most rewarding (Fig. 71-7). Fabrication of these prostheses is made possible by the availability of tough, thin, strong, flexible new materials with which good mobility and useful skin sensibility can be preserved. Occasionally, function will be improved just by the protective effect of covering a tender stump to free the injured person from fear of using it. Often the prosthesis can be useful for holding light objects that are placed in it, even though it is totally passive (Fig. 71-8).

Obviously, psychological improvements and improvements in physical capacity both contribute to a better rehabilitation potential for the amputee. When a professional activity involving frequent contacts with the public has been interrupted, the esthetic prosthesis often is the key to returning to the employment for which the patient is already prepared. When retraining is required, the prosthesis broadens greatly the number of vocational possibilities that one can realistically consider.

ESTHETIC PROSTHESES FOR CHILDREN

If the stump does not have a pinch mechanism, fitting of a prosthesis may be carried out at a very early age—usually between 6 and 18 months. However, there are often skin-related problems before 18 months.

If the stump has a useful pinch mechanism, the prosthesis will be functionally more bothersome than useful. In these circumstances it is preferable to postpone fitting until the child has attained adolescence, at which time he will be more motivated.

Sometimes, however, it is necessary to fit a child with a prosthesis if the parents are suffering from psychological trauma. In such cases, it is the parents we are treating through the child. This is not a very conventional approach.

ESTHETIC PROSTHESES FOR BILATERAL AMPUTEES

Physical impairment is so great for the bilateral amputee that it overshadows the esthetic concern, but such a concern is in fact not diminished in these patients. Benefits may be derived in the bilateral amputee by fitting one side with an esthetic prosthesis, but the need for sensibility of a part on at least one side precludes useful bilateral fitting.

PROSTHETIC CONSIDERATIONS ACCORDING TO LEVEL OF AMPUTATION
Loss of fingernail only

The appearance of a finger cannot be good if the fingernail has been lost. Fabrication of a fingernail of good likeness is not a problem, but secure fixation to the digit remains difficult. If there is partial nail loss with a trouble-free remnant remaining, cementing to this can be very satisfactory, but cementing to skin is a consistent failure. When a nail fragment exists, the prosthetic nail needs to be made to conform to it.

Commercially available nails are tedious to apply, fit imperfectly, are easily broken, and rarely have a natural appearance. Surgical fixation of fingernails, as with formation of a skin-lined pouch, is unsatisfactory, having a poor appearance with frequent cellulitis and skin complications. The only method yet available for secure fixation of a normal-looking fingernail involves covering the entire distal phalanx with a very thin prosthesis like a thimble, but the disadvantages are obvious. Secure fixation remains a problem without a good solution.

Phalangeal amputations

Satisfactory prosthetic fitting of the finger requires a minimum stump length of 1.5 cm. It should be tapered with pain-free healthy skin coverage. A smaller size than that of the corresponding normal part is desirable. Skin should not be loose and redundant. Sometimes in borderline situations sufficient length for secure fixation can be gained by surgical recession of the interdigital webs.

The proximal end of the prosthesis is feathered to a thin edge without pigmentation, making the break in skin relatively inconspicuous. When the juncture lies over the proximal phalanx, use of an ordinary ornamental ring perfectly disguises the juncture, except in the case of the thumb. In the latter case, if a better disguise of the juncture is desired, it is best achieved if one wears a small skin-colored Band-Aid or medical tape, as if covering an ordinary minor scratch.

Prosthetic fitting of the middle or ring finger when the stump is too short for secure fixation can sometimes be achieved by suspension, with ornamental rings worn on the adjacent digit, but the arrangement is complicated and fixation is less than secure.

The firmness and flexibility of the prosthesis depend on the functional needs. If the proximal interphalangeal joints of the fingers are present, the prosthesis is made very flexible at this level to allow motion. If amputation is through the proximal phalanx, the prosthesis is stiff and semicurved in opposition to the thumb, for prehension. Individual fitting of all four fingers is feasible if the stump is of adequate length for secure individual fixation; otherwise a glove is required, usually with the thumb exposed if it is in good condition, so that one of the opposing parts has good sensibility. Obviously, the number of possible physical combinations is almost as great as the needs of individual patients, all of which must be given most careful consideration if the best solution is to be offered (Figs. 71-9 and 71-10).

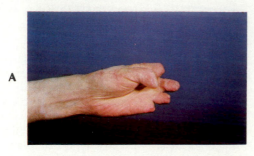
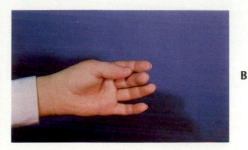

FIG. 71-9. **A,** Hand of chemical engineer severely burned in an industrial accident. **B,** Total hand prosthesis is both esthetic and functional. Prosthesis replaces missing fingers and covers hand scars. It permits opposition of thumb to the other fingers, whereas it was difficult without prothesis. Patient has been wearing his prosthesis daily for the past 6 years, from morning until night, both at work and at home.

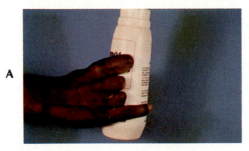
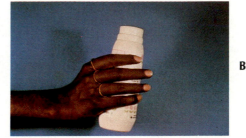

FIG. 71-10. **A,** Several digit amputations. **B,** Prostheses lengthen fingers and facilitate prehension.

Metacarpal amputations

Metacarpal amputations can be transverse, central, or oblique (in a direction such that the thumb, or alternatively the small finger, is preserved). In the case of transverse amputations, the prosthesis is essentially a total hand.

When only a portion of the thumb remains, it is generally covered with a total hand prosthesis that extends the length of the thumb to normal and provides it with a natural-looking fingernail. In such a case the prosthesis is made very thin in appropriate areas to allow free motion of the thumb remnant and sensibility through the cover. The fingers are made firm in a semiflexed position to serve as opposition parts for the mobile thumb.

When a normal thumb has been preserved, one has the option of using a complete glove prosthesis made very thin on the part covering the good thumb or allowing the thumb to protrude freely through the glove. The latter method presents the problem of disguising the opening in the glove, but for most activities it is so functionally superior that it generally is recommended.

When a useful small finger remains after an oblique metacarpal amputation in which all or most of the thumb is lost, it is best that the second metacarpal be surgically resected and the small finger fitted into the ring finger of the prosthesis. This not only is more functional, with the single finger having a better working relation to the thumb post, but also allows the prosthesis to be fabricated to the exact size of the other hand.

A prosthesis with a small finger long enough to slip over the remaining small finger must be conspicuously larger than the other hand; thus a good esthetic result is precluded. Placing the small finger in the ring finger of the prosthesis solves this problem with no disadvantage.

When a metacarpal amputation is central, involving index, middle, and ring fingers, such as that often resulting from a punch press, both thumb and small finger are preserved. Functionally, it is best to leave both thumb and small finger protruding from the prosthesis if they are normal. This presents little problem for the small-finger juncture, since it can be naturally disguised with an ordinary ring. Also, leaving the thumb and small finger exposed avoids the problem of having to make the prosthesis appropriately thin over these parts (Fig. 71-7).

Prosthetic fitting of partially amputated hands is a most difficult problem. The variety of physical problems encountered is enormous, and potential solutions must be carefully weighed against the needs of the patient, which are almost as variable. The absence of any perfect solution gives rise to a great variety of possibilities that one must carefully consider.

Amputations through the wrist or more proximal levels

Patients with amputations through the wrist or more proximal levels have strong indications for total hand prostheses, and the prosthetic problems chiefly involve the best socket

FIG. 71-11. A, Traditional fiberglass. **B,** New materials and techniques have made possible fabrication of prosthetic sockets, even for shoulder disarticulations, that are light, soft, flexible, and secure. These improvements in sockets represent a major step in progress with prosthetics.

A

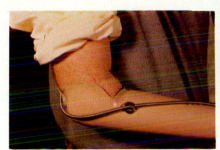

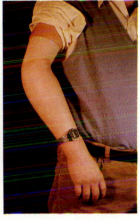

B

arrangement. When amputation is through the carpus, the prosthesis is made thin over the palm area, so that useful sensibility can be readily transmitted.

With wrist disarticulation it is desirable that the patient be able to take advantage of the sensibility of the long stump. Only in rare instances will this degree of shortening be obvious or visually disturbing.

New materials and techniques, in contrast to the traditional fiberglass, have made possible fabrication of prosthetic sockets that are light, soft, flexible, and secure, even for shoulder disarticulations. Those for amputation distal to the shoulder usually require no straps for completely reliable fixation. These improvements in sockets represent a major step advancement in prosthetics (Fig. 71-11).

ACCEPTANCE AND UTILIZATION OF ESTHETIC PROSTHESES

A review of our patients revealed a high percentage of continued utilization of their esthetic prostheses in general. This may in part reflect considerable selectivity in patients fitted, those without strong motivation usually being detected and rejected at the outset. All were unilateral amputees. Most of the patients were found to fall into a well-adjusted group, which in turn could be subdivided into two subgroups. Some put on their prostheses each morning and removed them only for sleep, making the devices much a part of themselves. Others treated their prostheses much as clothing, wearing them regularly when out of the home but being frequently without them within the confines of the family circle.

A small number were found to have established peculiar attitudes toward their prostheses, but all still had a need for them. A few wore their prostheses day and night, removing them only for skin care. Others kept them available but in fact wore them only rarely—for special occasions such as holiday celebrations or family events. A very small group never wore their prostheses but refused to give them up, keeping them in readiness "in case of an emergency."

There seems to be little difference in utilization between patients with amputations and patients with agenesis. The highest satisfaction was in the age group of 15 to 40 years. The quality of the prosthesis was a major factor as one would expect, as it is primarily esthetic in purpose.

Finally, if the prosthesis is set aside, that may not imply failure of the prosthesis, but rather the excellent effects of psychological treatment. The patient gives up his prosthesis because he has returned to a normal life. He has been cured; he no longer requires taking his medicine, and so he just stops. All we have done is simply aided him to come through a difficult period of his life.

CONTRAINDICATIONS TO ESTHETIC PROSTHESES

An absolute contraindication to the provision of an esthetic prosthesis would be a patient without motivation or one with unrealistic expectations as to what the device is expected to accomplish.

There are also patients in whom borderline indications for fitting exist. These patients will seek an esthetic prosthesis despite the fact that such a device may be uncomfortable, result in significant functional loss, or even achieve a poor esthetic result. For example, with disarticulation of several digits, the prosthesis must cover the hand completely for adequate fixation. Attempts at fixation in short stumps can result in trophic skin changes that will make the prosthesis unbearable. Even with stumps long enough for good fixation, several digital prostheses on the same hand reduce its sensibility as well as its gripping functions. When there are bulky or badly aligned stumps, esthetically pleasing prostheses may not be constructable without prior surgical revision. It should also be noted that in bilateral amputations an esthetic prosthesis should be provided only on one side.

SUMMARY

A high-quality esthetic prosthesis can be equally helpful to an amputee and to a patient whose loss is attributable to agenesis. Restoring near-normal appearance improves a patient's function in a global sense, enabling him to better utilize what he has in the complex socioeconomic environment of today's mobile society. The esthetic prosthesis often also gives some prehensile assistance, providing an opposition part for remaining digits or thumb.

The needs of each patient must be carefully considered, and the prosthesis must conform to the high standards of quality outlined. Its use is primarily for the unilateral amputee who is making a good adjustment to the loss, with realistic expectations.

72

Fabrication of an early-fit prosthesis

LORETTA M. MAIORANO

A useful development in the management of upper extremity amputees is the fabrication of an early-fit prosthesis by the therapist or prosthetist in the operating room or shortly thereafter. Such a prosthesis is fabricated to improve the amputee's acceptance of a prosthesis and to encourage bilateral use of his extremities.

In the past, the patient with an upper extremity amputation frequently learned to compensate for loss of his limb by unilateral use of his extremities long before he was fitted with a definitive prosthesis. The early-fit prosthesis helps in reduction of edema,[1,2] pain, and uncomfortable phantom-limb sensation by early contact of the stump with the rigid socket.[1,2]

Materials used in fabrication of an early-fit prosthesis
1. Terminal device with either voluntary opening or voluntary closing hook
2. Triceps pad
3. Flexible elbow hinges
4. Housing cross-bar assembly
5. Inverted-Y suspensor strap
6. Figure-of-eight harness
7. Friction wrist unit with anchor straps
8. Base plate
9. Housing
10. Standard cable
11. Retainer
12. Triple swivel terminal
13. Stockinette
14. Polyester fluff
15. 4-inch elastic plaster bandage
16. 3-inch standard plaster bandage

Equipment needed (Fig. 72-1)
1. Nipper
2. Crimper

FABRICATION AND APPLICATION OF THE HARNESS

1. Rivet the cross-bar leather to the center of the triceps pad (Fig. 72-2).
2. Rivet the flexible elbow hinges to the distal end of the triceps pad (Fig. 72-3).
3. Rivet two small buckles to either end of the proximal end of the triceps pad.
4. Burn three holes in each end of the inverted-Y strap so

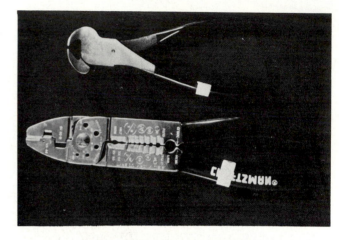

FIG. 72-1. Nipper and crimper.

that it can be placed through the buckle at the proximal end of the triceps pad (Fig. 72-4).
5. Attach the single end of the inverted-Y suspensor strap to the O ring of the Northwestern ring harness.
6. Place the harness on the patient and adjust it so that the O ring is located on the unamputated side of the midline and just below the C7 vertebral body.

SOCKET FABRICATION

1. At surgery, a sterile adhesive gauze is placed over the amputation site, followed by a light sterile dressing. If socket application is not done in the operating room and the wound is healed, a light dressing is applied as a buffer for the end of the stump.
2. Place polyester (Dacron) fluff over the distal end of the stump as a buffer between the stump and the rigid plaster socket (Fig. 72-5).
3. Measure and cut a single stockinette 2 inches longer than the length of the amputated forearm. Stitch one end of the single stockinet. Place this over the stump and Dacron with the seam side out.
4. To form the rigid plaster socket to the stump, wrap one roll of 4-inch elastic plaster in a figure-of-eight manner distally to proximally. For a snug fit, elastic plaster is preferred over nonelastic plaster because it can be

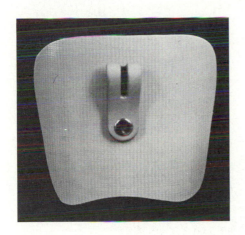

FIG. 72-2. Cross-bar leather riveted to triceps pad.

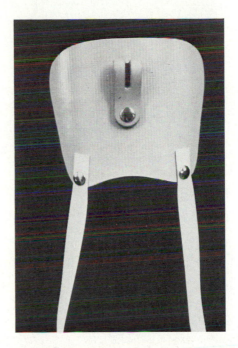

FIG. 72-3. Elbow hinges riveted to triceps pad.

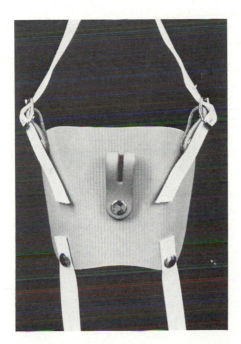

FIG. 72-4. Ends of inverted Y strap buckled to triceps pad.

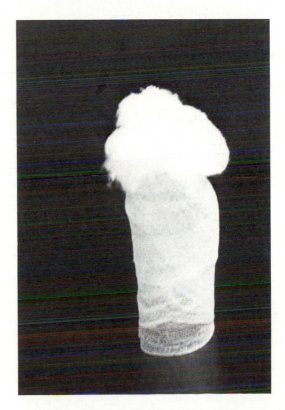

FIG. 72-5. Dacron fluff over dressing.

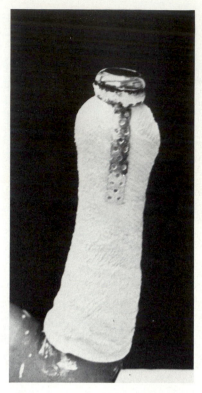

FIG. 72-6. Wrist unit with anchor straps.

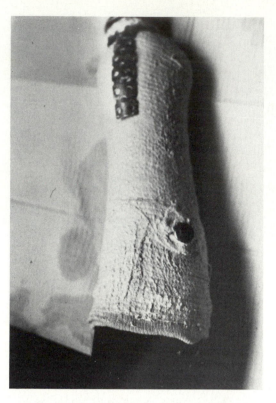

FIG. 72-7. Base plate secured to socket.

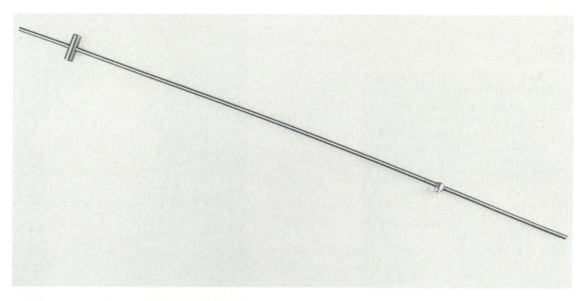

FIG. 72-8. Retainer and cross bar screwed to housing.

stretched when wet and contracts as it dries. Shape the socket by applying pressure to the anterior and posterior surfaces of the forearm.

5. When the plaster is dry, place a wrist unit with anchor straps over the socket (Fig. 72-6). If the amputation is at midforearm or shorter, an extension piece must be added to the socket. Do this by adding a paper cup over the plaster socket and wrapping plaster to incorporate

this cup into the forearm. The wrist unit would be added to this extension piece as above.

6. As an anchor for the housing, the base plate is secured to the lateral proximal forearm section of the socket by nonelastic plaster (Fig. 72-7).

7. A roll of 3-inch nonelastic plaster is wrapped onto the socket proximally to distally to secure the elbow hinges, base plate, and the wrist unit.

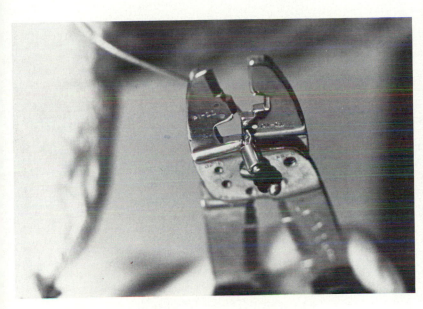

FIG. 72-9. Ball terminal crimped to cable.

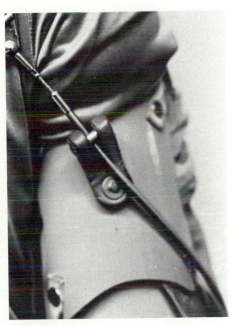

FIG. 72-10. Cross-bar assembly.

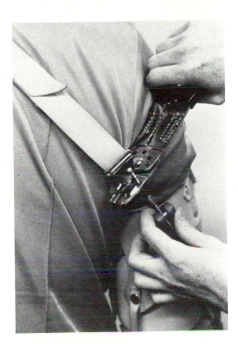

FIG. 72-11. Hanger crimped to cable.

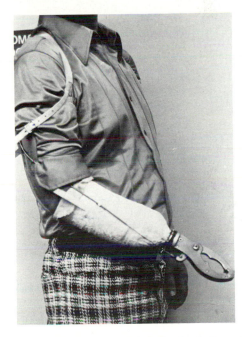

FIG. 72-12. Activation of terminal device by ipsilateral forward flexion of shoulder.

APPLICATION OF CABLE AND TERMINAL DEVICE

1. Screw the retainer to the distal end of the housing and the cross bar to the proximal end of the housing (Fig. 72-8).
2. Thread the control cable through the metal housing.
3. Crimp the ball terminal to the distal end of the cable (Fig. 72-9).
4. Attach the cable and the housing to the socket by fitting the retainer into the base plate.
5. Attach the cable in the housing to the triceps pad using the cross-bar assembly (Fig. 72-10).
6. Crimp the hanger to the proximal end of the cable (Fig. 72-11).
7. Attach the hanger to the control strap of the figure-of-eight harness.
8. Screw the terminal device into the wrist unit and attach it to the cable by the triple swivel terminal.
9. To ensure proper functioning of the terminal device, the patient is observed as he performs ipsilateral forward flexion of the shoulder (Fig. 72-12). If the terminal de-

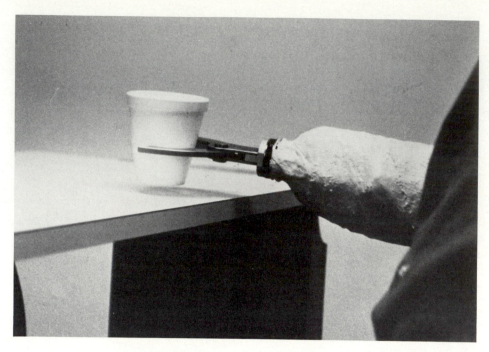

FIG. 72-13. Picking up a Styrofoam cup.

vice does not open or close fully, adjustments must be made in the length of cable or the harness, or both.

EARLY PROSTHETIC TRAINING

Ipsilateral-shoulder forward flexion activates the terminal device. The patient performs various control drills to develop a good feel for the amount of muscle activity necessary to operate the terminal device. Drills include the following:

1. Opening and closing the hook in different body positions, as at the mouth or waist, above the head, and at floor level.
2. Picking up objects of different sizes by opening the hook just wide enough to accommodate the object; opening it too wide wastes energy.
3. Picking up objects of different densities and making sure he maintains the object's shape by maintaining appropriate tension on the cable (Fig. 72-13).

DISCUSSION

From October 1979 to October 1982, 16 patients were fitted with an early-fit prosthesis. There were 14 men and two women, ranging in age from 19 to 56. One of the women completely rejected any functional prosthesis and was fitted with a cosmetic hand. Of the remaining 15 patients, two were lost to follow-up. Thirteen patients were reviewed; six of these patients had been fitted with myoelectric prostheses in addition to conventional prostheses. At the time of this

review, all the patients were questioned in regard to wearing patterns, work status, and phantom pain.

Eight patients stated that they wore prostheses all day, and three wore prostheses for up to 6 hours a day. Two patients were not fitted with definitive prostheses because of lack of funds.

Six patients had returned to work, five to the same job and one his own business, which he just started. Two patients had retired, and one patient had returned to school. Of the remaining four, three of the patients' cases were in litigation.

Of the 13 patients questioned, only two had phantom pain, although most had some degree of phantom sensation of the hand and fingers.

SUMMARY

An early-fit prosthesis can help to improve the amputee's acceptance of a prosthesis and to encourage bilateral use of his extremities. An early-fit prosthesis can also help in reduction of edema and pain.

REFERENCES

1. Burkhalter, W.E., Mayfield, G., and Carmona, L.S.: The upper-extremity amputee: early and immediate post-surgical prosthetic fitting, J. Bone Joint Surg. **48A**(1):46-51, 1976.
2. Jacobs, R.R., and Brady, W.M.: Early post surgical fitting in upper extremity amputation, J. Trauma **15**(11):966-968, 1975.

73

Management and prosthetic training of the adult amputee

BONNIE L. OLIVETT

Throughout history there have been reports of humans designing replacements for amputated hands. Certainly the loss of a hand has been and will continue to be a great catastrophe to the individual person in society, since the functional and esthetic losses are potentially devastating. The rehabilitative problem today is that these two concepts—that is, function and esthetics—may be incompatible, a situation that probably accounts for the fact that there is no simple answer as to the "best prosthesis" to satisfy all needs.

It is the purpose of this chapter to discuss the functional value and use of the conventional prosthesis with the adult acquired amputee. The importance of an early fit and prosthetic training will be stressed, since this will enhance the amputee's use of the prosthesis functionally.

HISTORY OF UPPER LIMB PROSTHETICS

In 1958, the Smithsonian Institution reported the discovery of a skull dating back about 45,000 years. It was deduced that the skull belonged to a person who must have been an upper extremity amputee, because of the appearance of the teeth, which seemed to have been used functionally to compensate for the loss of a hand.[22]

From the Middle Ages come written accounts along with paintings and museum pieces showing soldiers being fitted with artificial limbs to be worn in battle. The first recorded use of an artificial hand involved the Roman general Marcus Serquis. He reportedly lost his hand during the Second Punic War (218-201 B.C.), and subsequently instructed his armorer to fit him with an iron hand to be clamped onto his shield during battle. Possibly of similar design was the Alt-Ruppin hand, made of iron (Fig. 73-1), which was recovered along the Rhine River in 1863. This hand, along with other artificial limbs of the fifteenth century are on display at the Stibert Museum in Florence, Italy.[22]

Ambrose Paré, who lived during the sixteenth century, can be credited with the most significant contributions to amputation surgery and prosthetics.[19] Paré designed and manufactured ingenious devices that expressed his interest in rehabilitating the amputee. His drawings of the hand and upper extremity prostheses were technically described in his *Dix Livres de la Chirurgie* in 1564. No volitional control was used in his prostheses, which utilized the principles of articulated joints (Fig. 73-2).

Peter Baliff, a Berlin dentist, designed in 1818 the first below-elbow prosthesis, which was operated by harness-controlled pull cords. Also reported during the nineteenth century were various assistive devices for upper extremity amputees, such as a sponge clamped onto a tray and a nail brush fastened upside down. These devices were described by Captain George Derenzy in 1822, after he lost his right arm near the elbow.

The first split-hook terminal device was developed in 1912 by D.W. Dorrance. He designed this hook in an attempt to replace the function of his own amputated hand. Although this hook has been refined, the original version is still used in prosthetics today because of its simplicity and durability.

It was not until after World War II, which produced great numbers of amputees, that an organized attempt was undertaken to produce functional, lightweight, yet inexpensive, prostheses. This impetus, along with the commercial development of plastics, created major advancements in prosthetic fitting for the upper extremity amputee.

INCIDENCE OF AMPUTATION

Approximately 43,000 major amputations occur yearly in the United States.[17] Of the 311,000 amputees reported in the United States in 1970 by the National Center for Health Statistics, 32% involve the upper extremity. There is a peak between 20 and 40 years of age, with nearly 90% of all the upper extremity amputations resulting from trauma.[1-3] The injuries are equally divided between the right and left sides; however, males outnumber females 4 to 1.[1-3] Possibly, the higher incidence of injuries in males is attributable to the hazards of physical vocational and avocational work in which men engage. According to the *Newsletter of the Amputee Clinics*, October 1972, only 50% of the amputees fitted continued to wear their prosthetic limbs.[5]

PROSTHETIC ADVANCEMENTS

Unfortunately, we all are subject to some rather unrealistic expectations about current prostheses because of the sensationalism of the media. Certainly the field of prosthetics is making greater strides than ever before with the use of external power, myoelectric controls, and sensory feedback systems. Because many of these components and designs are being researched, availability in the United States remains limited.

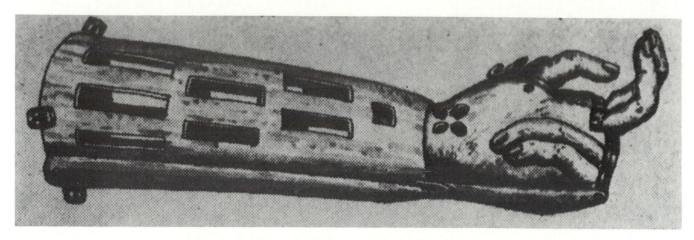

Fig. 73-1. Alt-Ruppin hand, recovered along Rhine River in 1863.

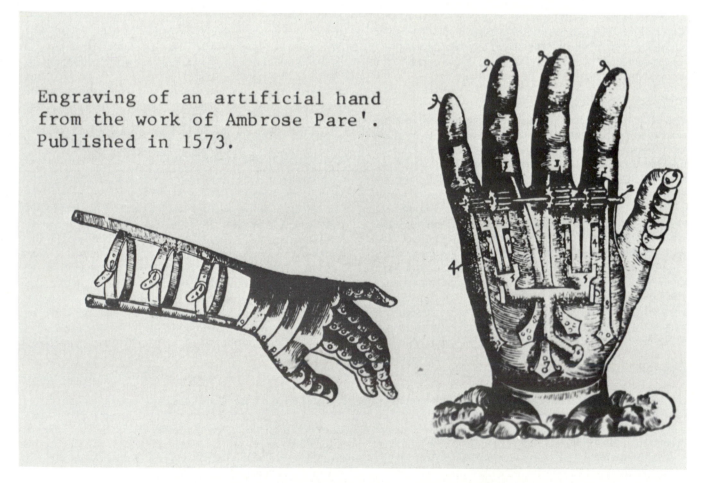

Engraving of an artificial hand
from the work of Ambrose Pare'.
Published in 1573.

Fig. 73-2. Prosthetic hand with articulated joints designed by Ambrose Paré.

Many powered components and designs developed between 1955 and 1970 did not satisfy needs sufficiently to even warrant commercial production.[18] Prosthetic systems using external power and supplementary sensory feedback systems are primarily available in the United States today through major prosthetic research centers, such as Northwestern University, U.C.L.A., Rancho Los Amigos Hospital in Downey, California, Southwestern Research Institute in San Antonio, Texas, and the Veterans Administration Prosthetics Center in New York.

The consensus of several researchers is that myoelectrically controlled prostheses have no significant functional advantage over the standard cable-controlled system and even with sensory feedback the performance is no better and may only reach a level equal to the conventional cable-operated prostheses.[12] Although new materials and techniques have made available passive cosmetic devices that are meeting very high standards, these devices fall short of the ideal goals of motion and sensibility.[17] As Beasley states, "It is important to dispel the concept of the artificial hand, for such will probably never exist."[4]

CONVENTIONAL METHODS

The conventional prosthesis continues to play an important role in the field of prosthetics because of availability and ease of maintenance and upkeep. According to Burkhalter,[8] "The vast majority of upper limb amputees still use standard and conventional components that are activated by body powered control."[8]

PREOPERATIVE CARE

Although preparation of the patient before the amputation is not always possible, there are cases when the patient knows in advance that an amputation is inevitable. It is helpful to show the patient what an artificial limb looks like and to begin making him aware of what function can be anticipated. It is also important to convey if possible, the functional limitations of the prosthesis.

Range of motion and strength of the upper extremity should be assessed bilaterally, if the patient's condition is stable. The general condition of the patient should be noted and his intellectual, psychological, social, vocational, and avocational needs appreciated so that one may begin planning the patient's prosthesis.

POSTOPERATIVE CARE

The period of early postoperative care is one of the most crucial phases. During this time the attitudes of the patient are in flux and his reactions can be dealt with most effectively. The early postoperative goals are to maintain range of motion and strength while preventing the development of contractures and assisting in the conditioning of the stump. Elevation of the stump should be encouraged in order to prevent edema, thereby decreasing pain.

Frequent active exercises may generally begin 24 hours after surgery, along with gentle assisted stump range-of-motion exercise within the patient's tolerance. The use of exercises will help to improve circulation, while increasing strength, which according to Friedman[10] helps prevent

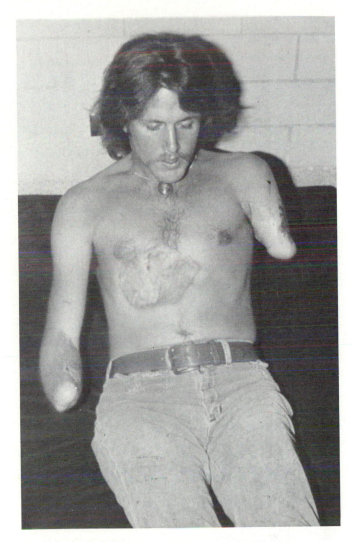

FIG. 73-3. Sit-ups for generalized conditioning.

"alienation" of the muscles of the stump after the trauma of amputation. Resistive exercises of the stump are contraindicated until the muscles are well healed.

As the general condition of the patient improves, strengthening exercises include exercises for the trunk and upper extremities, such as sit-ups, one-arm push-ups, and pivot-prone exercises (Fig. 73-3). Barbells, pulleys, and Theraband are also effective modalities for strengthening (Figs. 73-4 and 73-5).

The patient is encouraged to care for himself and to assist with the dressings and bandaging if soft compressive dressings are used (Fig. 73-6). Postural awareness must be emphasized, because all amputees have the tendency to carry the stump side higher or lower than the other shoulder until they have regained the sense of balance. Certain pieces of adaptive equipment may be useful, including a suction-cup brush (Fig. 73-7) and a one-handed knife (Fig. 73-8), along with instructions for tying shoelaces with one hand.

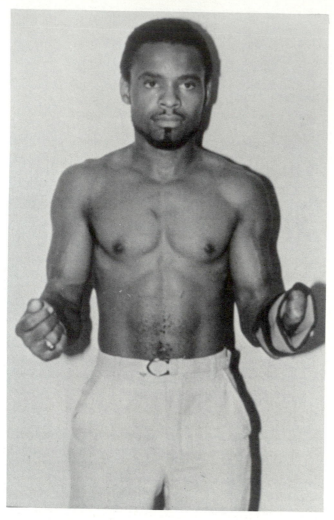

FIG. 73-4. Cuff weights used for upper extremity strengthening.

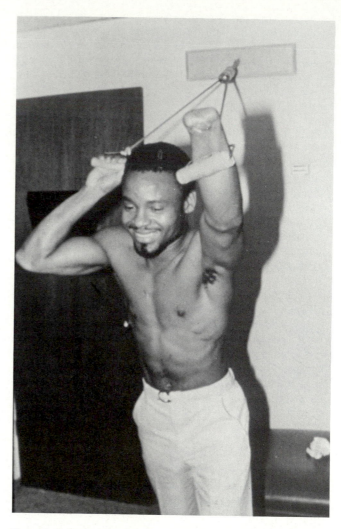

FIG. 73-5. Pulleys used for range of motion and strengthening.

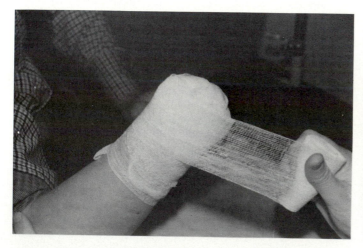

FIG. 73-6. Patient applying dressing, using oblique, distal-to-proximal figure-of-8 configuration.

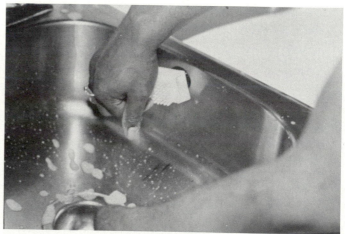

FIG. 73-7. Suction-cup brush for cleansing hand and fingernails.

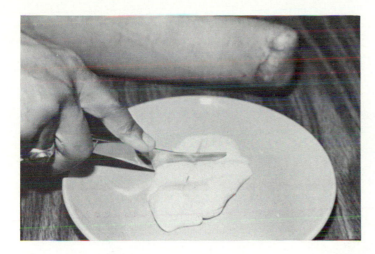

FIG. 73-8. Rocking knife used for one-handed cutting while patient awaits prosthetic fitting.

FIG. 73-9. Immediate fit with a cast applied in shape of Münster below-elbow socket.

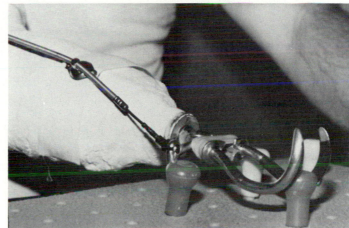

DOMINANCE CHANGE

If the dominant hand is amputated, a change in hand dominance is strongly recommended. The normal limb with sensation will be more useful for fine manipulation. One-handed activities that help develop coordination and dexterity during dominance change are copper tooling, painting, or writing.

PREPROSTHETIC MANAGEMENT

An immediate or early fitting is recommended and is especially valuable to the trauma-induced amputee.[10] If an immediate fit is used, the below-elbow amputee should have a cast applied in the shape of the Münster below-elbow socket (Fig. 73-9) but constructed higher than the Münster socket to utilize the humeral condyles to assist with suspension. The above-elbow amputee should have a socket constructed in the shape of a shoulder spica.

For the bilateral amputee, I recommend fitting one side with a functional prosthesis and placing a rigid total contact plaster cast on the other side to reduce pain and edema.[13]

A temporary or mock-up prosthesis fabricated from thermoplastic materials may be useful when there are postsur-

gical complications or if fitting may be delayed while one is awaiting scar maturation. A prosthesis of this type is used for early training and to provide early function (Figs. 73-10 and 73-11).

Another benefit of the immediate postsurgical fit is that surgeons have become more aware of early functional restoration of the amputee, thus directing the emphasis away from the surgery itself and toward a return of function.[6]

CONTRACTURES

A joint contracture is a complication that is occasionally inevitable because of the posture of the stump during healing. A slow, steady stretch might be useful while one is attempting to correct a contracture. However, stretching, using the technique of inhibition of antagonist muscles through proprioceptive neuromuscular facilitation, is generally more effective. The use of thermoplastic night splints, such as a three-point splint at the elbow (Fig. 73-12), may help avoid or reduce a contracture. Serial casting might also be utilized to help reduce a contracture. Serial casting might also be utilized to help reduce a contracture.

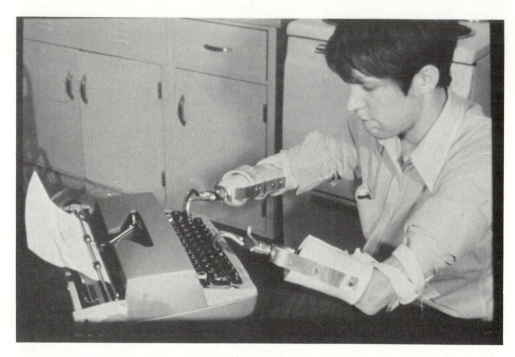

FIG. 73-10. Temporary thermoplastic prosthesis may be useful for early training and function.

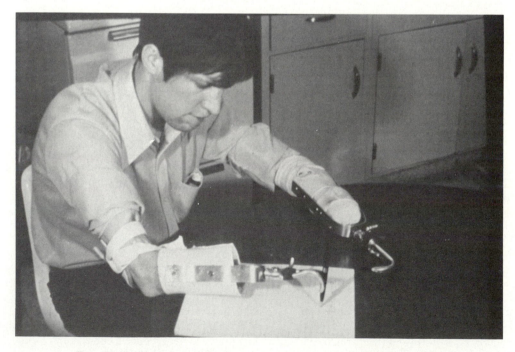

FIG. 73-11. Mock-up prosthesis may be used for early function and training.

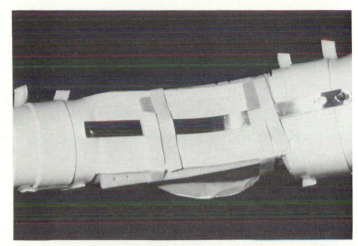

FIG. 73-12. Three-point splint may help avoid or reduce an elbow flexion deformity.

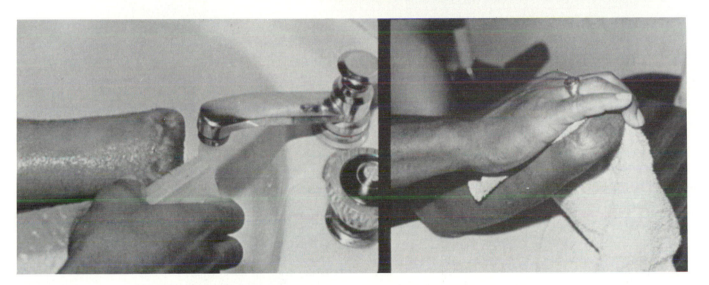

FIG. 73-13. Early desensitization techniques being used to reduce paresthesias.

PREPARATION AND CONDITIONING OF THE STUMP

The adult traumatic or acquired amputee will always experience phantom sensations, the ability to perceive cortical images of the lost limb. Some of these sensations may be disagreeable,[9] such as "pins and needles," "cramping," "twisting," or "burning" sensations. Although the upper limb phantoms are stronger and longer lasting than those of the lower limb, they tend to be more annoying than painful.[16]

My experience has been that early desensitization techniques greatly reduce these paresthesias and help prepare the limb for the prosthetic socket. Patients generally respond first to deeper pressure such as brushing and massage (Fig. 73-13) to help soften and stretch adherent scarring. As the stump becomes desensitized, lighter touch such as tapping, vibration, and working with textures are all helpful modalities (Fig. 73-14). The use of physical agents, such as cold, electrical muscle stimulation, and transcutaneous nerve stimulation, can also help diminish phantom sensations.

Tensor bandages may be prescribed to help reduce edema and promote stump shrinkage to prepare the contour of the

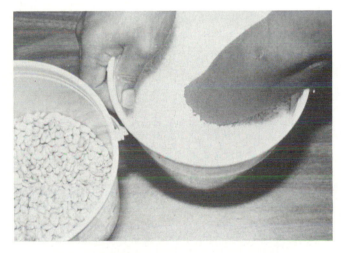

FIG. 73-14. Modalities used for desensitization.

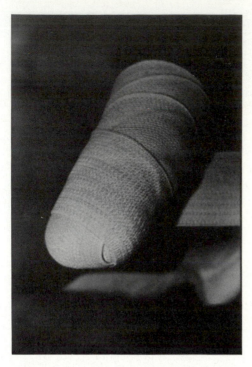

FIG. 73-15. Tensor bandages provide constant compression to promote shrinkage.

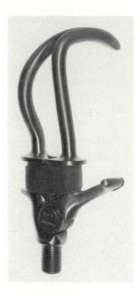

FIG. 73-16. Left voluntary-opening hook-type terminal device. (Courtesy Hosmer/Dorrance Corp., Campbell, Calif.)

stump for prosthetic fit. A constant distal-to-proximal, oblique, figure-of-eight compression is used. Since it is difficult to establish and maintain proper pressure, frequent reapplication of the bandages is recommended (Fig. 73-15).

PROSTHETIC COMPONENTS
Terminal devices

Terminal devices are designed for prehension. There is a wide variety available. Some are designed and shaped to look like a hand with one or more movable fingers, and some are designed as two-fingered devices with a hook type of configuration (Fig. 73-16). The terminal device must be suited to the person according to his psychological, vocational, and avocational needs. A hook is recommended if bilateral skills requiring manual dexterity are desired.

Cosmetically, prosthetic hands are superior to hooks (Fig. 73-17) and may be preferred by the individual in a socially oriented vocation. The hands may be active or passive terminal devices. Functionally they are a poor comparison to the hook. The functional and cosmetic hands are commonly covered with a polyvinyl chloride glove, which tends to be sensitive to sunlight, temperature, dyes, and chemicals. Recent use of polymers of dimethyl siloxanes has shown better results, because they are not altered by temperature appreciably and are more resistant to soiling.[14]

Voluntary-opening hooks are prescribed more frequently than any other terminal device, because of their mechanical simplicity and ease of operation.[11] The Hosmer/Dorrance name is associated with a wide range of voluntary-opening hooks. These terminal devices may be prescribed with canted fingers to permit better visualization and manipulation

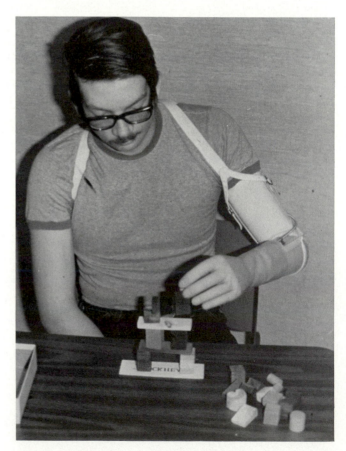

FIG. 73-17. Prosthetic training with a Dorrance functional hand.

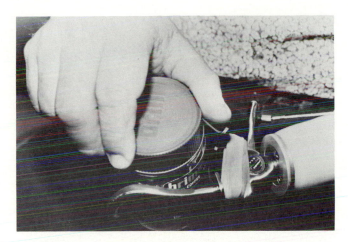

FIG. 73-18. Lyre-shaped fingers help grasp and hold rounded objects.

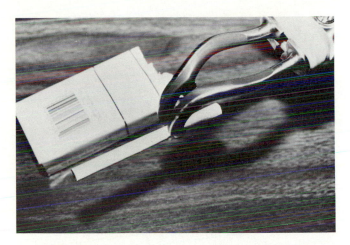

FIG. 73-19. Voluntary-opening hooks permit easy visualization for manipulation of small objects.

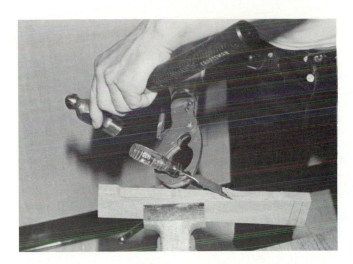

FIG. 73-20. Use training with Prehensile Hand.

of small objects, or they may be lyre shaped, making it easier to grasp or hold rounded objects (Figs. 73-18 and 73-19). Optional neoprene linings provide increased friction while holding objects. The force of prehension is determined by rubber bands placed at the base of the hook fingers. As a general rule, each band produces approximately 1 pound of prehensile force.

Voluntary-closing hooks allow the prehension force to be increased progressively by increasing tension, enabling the amputee to adopt a force suited to the object being handled. A clutch or locking mechanism is generally used if a grasp is required for a long period of time. The APRL hook (Army Prosthetic Research Laboratories) is of this type; however, it is seldom prescribed, because of its mechanical complexity, fragility, and cost. The Prehensile Hand developed by Therapeutic Recreation Systems (2860 Pennsylvania Ave., Boulder, Colo. 80303) has been designed as a voluntary-closing device (Fig. 73-20). This invention is different from the APRL hook, because its prehension is obtained by the muscle power of the user. The advantages of

this terminal device appear similar to those of the voluntary opening heavy-duty terminal devices designed for holding, grasping, chiseling, or using carpentry tools and manipulating long-handled implements, such as shovels and rakes.

Wrist units

A wrist unit connects the terminal device to the prosthetic forearm and provides pronation and supination to the user. The most common unit is the wrist friction unit, which consists of a nylon washer that provides a friction hold during prepositioning (Fig. 73-21). A minimum space of 6 cm is required for placement.

The wrist flexion unit has the same friction feature as the wrist friction unit; however, it allows three positions of flexion: neutral, 25 degrees of flexion, and 50 degrees of flexion. This unit is essential for the bilateral amputee to enable him to work the terminal device close to his body (Fig. 73-22).

The quick-change wrist unit allows a quick change of the terminal device. This unit is not commonly recommended because it wears poorly.

Hinges

The use of flexible or rigid elbow hinges is a form of suspension and part of the transmission of power for the wrist disarticulation or below-elbow amputee. Rigid hinges provide torsional stability at the elbow against the rotational stress of the prosthesis.

Elbow units

The standard elbow unit is an internal multiple-locking unit that is manufactured by Hosmer/Dorrance Corporation. This unit allows 5 to 135 degrees of flexion with 11 locking positions of the forearm (Fig. 73-23). The locking mechanism is controlled through the suspension system. A minimum space of 8 cm is required for the use of this unit.

The external unit, which is an outside-locking elbow, is designed for the long above-elbow or elbow disarticulation amputee (Fig. 73-24). The disadvantage of this unit is its bulkiness, which often damages clothing.

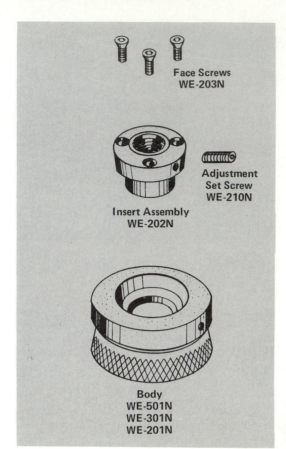

Face Screws
WE-203N

Adjustment
Set Screw
WE-210N

Insert Assembly
WE-202N

Body
WE-501N
WE-301N
WE-201N

FIG. 73-21. Constant-friction wrist unit. (Courtesy Hosmer/Dorrance Corp., Campbell, Calif.)

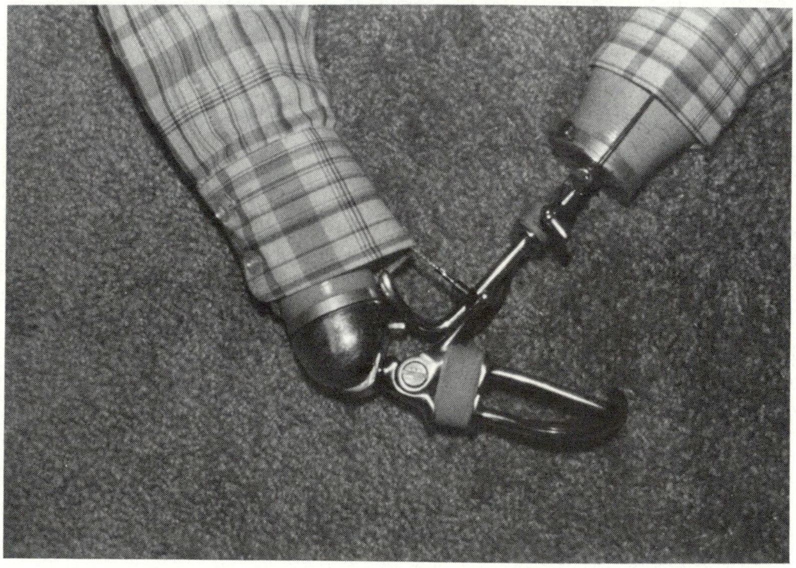

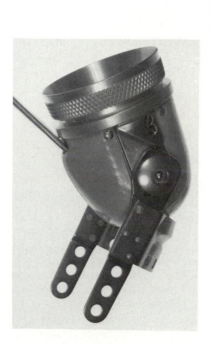

FIG. 73-22. Wrist flexion unit being activated by a bilateral amputee.

FIG. 73-23. Internal multiple-locking unit.

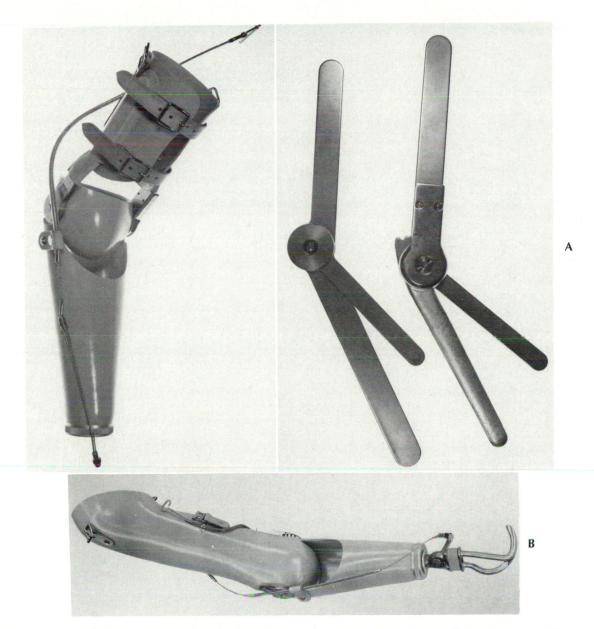

FIG. 73-24. A, Rigid, stump-activated locking hinge for very short below-elbow amputee. **B,** Outside-locking hinges used in elbow unit designed for elbow disarticulation and transconylar levels of amputation. (Courtesy Hosmer/Dorrance Corp., Campbell, Calif.)

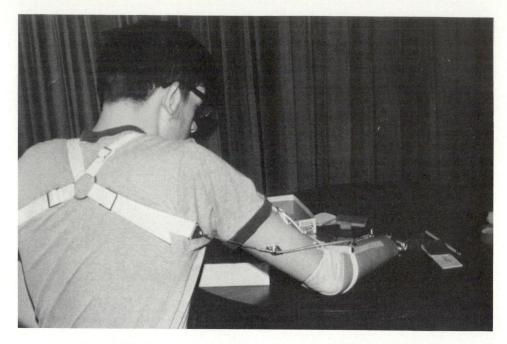

FIG. 73-25. Figure-of-eight harness worn by a below-elbow amputee.

Harness and control systems

The figure-of-eight harness is most commonly used to suspend the conventional body-powered prosthesis and control the terminal device, since it is the least bulky and provides good control (Fig. 73-25). The disadvantage of this type of harness is the pressure exerted on the axilla of the opposite extremity. If the amputee must lift heavy loads or perform strenuous activities, a shoulder-saddle type of harness or chest strap may be better tolerated (Fig. 73-26).

The cable is used to provide the force necessary to operate the terminal device. The Bowden cable is used for the below-elbow amputee. It consists of an inner tension cable and an outer housing. The housing maintains a constant length regardless of the motion involved. A dual-control cable is a split-housing cable that activates the forearm lift or the terminal device, or both, depending on whether the elbow lock is in the locked or unlocked position. If the elbow is unlocked, the forearm will lift when tension is placed on the cable. When the elbow is locked, the terminal device will open as tension is applied to the cable. This control system is used for the above-elbow and elbow disarticulation amputee.

Socket

The socket is the most important component of the prosthesis. It must provide support, stability, and comfort. Almost all upper extremity sockets are total contact and double-walled to provide better control and proprioception. The internal wall is contoured to fit the stump, following the principle of total contact. The external wall is contoured to match the normal limb. For a detailed review of the upper limb prosthetic systems, the suggested reading is Chapter 9 of *Atlas of Limb Prosthetics*.[7]

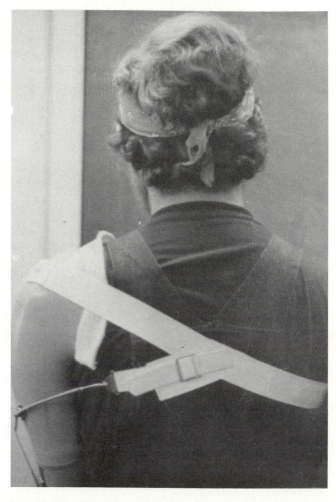

FIG. 73-26. Chest strap worn by a very short above-elbow amputee.

AMPUTEE REHABILITATION

As far back as 1918, Mayer stated that the "greatest educator of the stump is the artificial limb itself."[15] The point he was stressing so long ago was that early fitting is highly recommended whenever possible. Emphasized by Slocom[20] is the placing of the amputee "back into the normal life of his community." This goal can only be realized when the patient has a satisfactory and durable stump, a well-fitted and properly constructed prosthesis, and very diligent training in the use of his prosthesis. All these factors are interdependent and require a healthy attitude on the part of the amputee toward his disability. The "psychological" health of the patient is of utmost importance.[10]

PROSTHETIC CARE AND HYGIENE

When prosthetic training commences, the use of a T-shirt is recommended to avoid irritation from the harness. Later the use of a T-shirt is optional. Women might prefer using Kleinerts Short Sleeve Garment Shields, number 1206, manufactured by Kleinerts, Inc. (Kutztown, Pa. 19530).

Stump socks generally are preferred by the upper extremity amputee because they help absorb perspiration and give a sense of warmth and padding. A clean sock should be applied daily. The importance of daily stump hygiene must be stressed in order to avoid skin infections and irritations. The prosthetic socket should also be wiped clean daily, and the harness washed when soiled. Two harnesses should be supplied so that one can be laundered while the other is being worn.

EVALUATION AND CHECKOUT

The appearance, comfort, and function are evaluated when the prosthesis is received. It should closely match the color and contour of the normal limb, and the socket must be smooth with the edges slightly rolled away from the patient's skin. The length of the prosthesis is correct if the tip of the terminal device ends at the tip of the thumb on the remaining limb while the prosthesis is hanging at the patient's side.

All movable parts must function smoothly permitting maximal range of motion. The patient's ability to open the terminal device is examined at different levels of the body. There should be no sharp bends in the cable, and it should slide in and out of the casing smoothly. The control-system efficiency is a measurement to determine the amount of force lost between the terminal device and the harness. Although there are minimum standards set by the prosthetic and orthotic schools, I have found that this efficiency can be increased more than 80% with the use of a Teflon-lined cable.

The points that have been mentioned here are the major areas of importance when a new prosthesis is evaluated. For complete and detailed evaluations on prosthetic efficiency and mechanical checkout, various forms are recommended and may be obtained through Northwestern University, through New York University (Prosthetic-Orthotic Center), or in Santschi's *Manual of Upper Extremity Prosthetics*.[21]

CONTROLS TRAINING

Controls training teaches the patient to be aware of the body motions necessary to operate the prosthesis. The per-

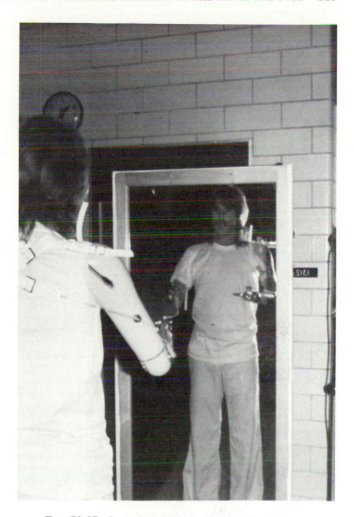

FIG. 73-27. Controls training and postural awareness.

son being trained needs to appreciate the difference between muscular contraction, holding, and relaxation, both for motion and stabilization. Training should take place in front of a mirror (Fig. 73-27) because this helps the patient develop correct posture and also a proprioceptive awareness of the limb without looking directly at the prosthesis.

With the below-elbow amputee the power is transmitted for one purpose only, prehension. A single-control system using humeral flexion is the major power source used to operate the terminal device, with the opposite shoulder acting as a stabilizer.

For the above-elbow amputee, power is transmitted to substitute for prehension, forearm motion, and elbow function. A dual-control system using humeral flexion is the major power used to operate the terminal device and forearm. The major source of body power used to operate the elbow lock is humeral extension and scapular abduction.

FUNCTIONAL TRAINING
Use

Once the controls become smooth and natural and the body-controlled motions become barely perceptible, functional application commences. Activities requiring grasp

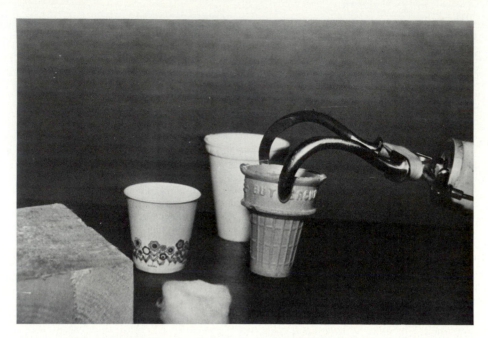

FIG. 73-28. Various weights and textures are employed for grasp and release training.

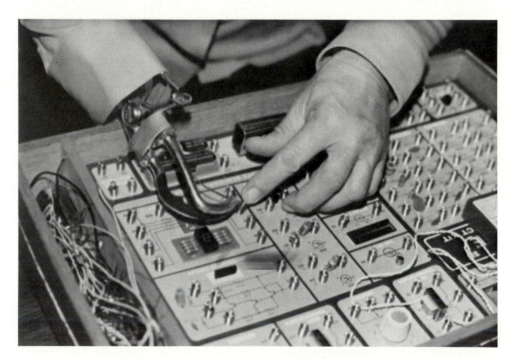

FIG. 73-29. Use training to improve speed, coordination, and dexterity.

and release of objects are employed, and the objects used are of various sizes, weights, and textures (Fig. 73-28). During this time close attention is given to the correct pre-positioning of the terminal device to minimize unnecessary and awkward positions. As the ability to grasp and release objects improves, repetitive drills and activities are utilized to achieve speed, coordination, and dexterity (Fig. 73-29).

Activities of daily living

The concept of functional training is geared toward a problem-solving approach in which the patient is guided through an activity with different methods being used to determine which method is easiest and most comfortable.

The amputee will learn to develop sensory feedback through the harness, since a part of the training is learning

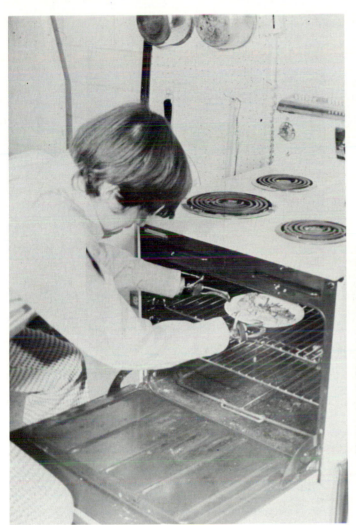

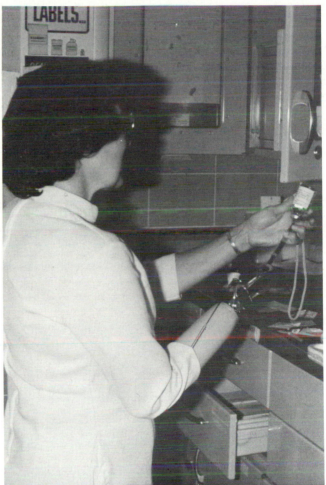

FIG. 73-30. Functional training to improve household skills and independence.

FIG. 73-31. Vocational skills are included in functional training.

how much tension should be exerted to hold onto varied objects. The bilateral amputee is trained to use the longer limb with better motion as the dominant extremity.

The aim of treatment is for the patient to become as self-sufficient as possible in all aspects of daily living, including personal hygiene, eating, dressing, and household tasks (Fig. 73-30). This area of training is pursued until the patient feels confident in his abilities. The more he is able to do for himself, the more successful will be his emotional and physical rehabilitation.

Social, avocational, and vocational skills are important aspects of training (Fig. 73-31). Sports activities with or without the use of the prosthesis are encouraged (Fig. 73-32). Special adaptive equipment may be necessary to pursue a special interest (Fig. 73-33).

Modifications in clothing may be required, as well as prosthetic adaptations and special devices, as in driving (Fig. 73-34) or the use of hand tools (Fig. 73-35). Once the patient has become proficient in daily living, he should

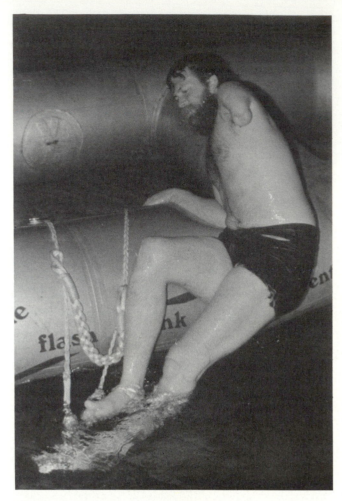

FIG. 73-32. Certain sports without the use of the prosthesis are encouraged.

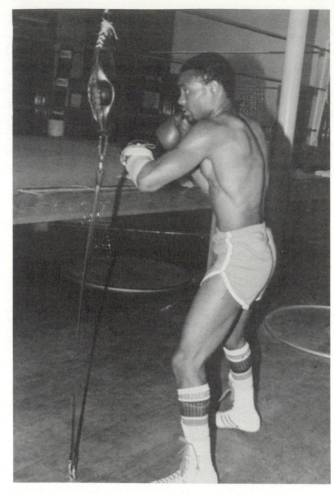

FIG. 73-33. Adaptive equipment may help patient pursue a special interest.

be rechecked at periodic intervals for assessment of the prosthetic fit and its continued ability to function to capacity. This is particularly important during the first year.

CONCLUSION

Historical accounts suggest that when an artificial device is designed to replace a lost limb, the primary goal of both the designer and the amputee is to restore the function of that limb. Although there have been many recent advancements in the field of upper extremity prosthetics, there still is no prosthesis that is capable of simultaneously duplicating the function, sensibility, and cosmesis of the human hand.

According to Beasley,[4] "90% of the activities of daily living can be accomplished with one normal hand." This

fact may account in part for the high percentage of upper extremity amputees who discard their prostheses. No doubt, the prognosis is influenced by the level of amputation, the quality of the stump, the quality of the prosthetic fit, and the quality of training. Certainly, the prognosis is also influenced by the social needs and the psychological adjustment of the patient. Success is more likely achieved if the patient is given a full appreciation of the limitations of the prosthesis both functionally and cosmetically. Once the limb is fitted, training should include the establishment of the desire within the patient to make the effort required to accept the prosthesis as a functional part of himself. The skill with which the patient is trained may well be the difference between acceptance and rejection of the limb.

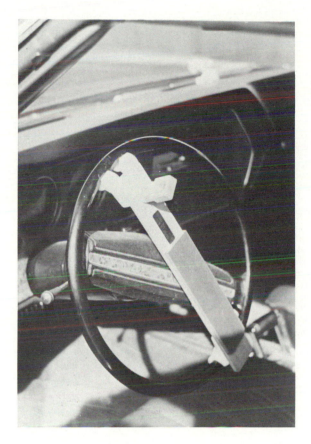

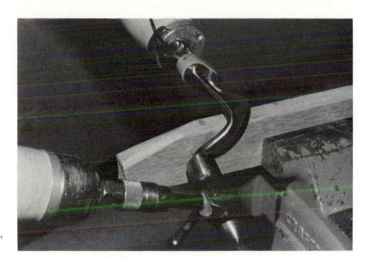

FIG. 73-34. Adaptive driving aid. (Mobility Products & Design, Inc., 709 Kentucky St., Vallejo, Calif. 94590.)

FIG. 73-35. Adaptive Ampu-Tool set. (Wright & Filippis Inc., 19326 Woodward Ave., Detroit, Mich. 48203.)

REFERENCES

1. Baumgartner, R.F.: Management of bilateral upper limb amputees, Orthop. Clin. North Am. **12:**971, 1981.
2. Baumgartner, R.F.: Active and carrier-tool prosthesis for upper limb amputation, Orthop. Clin. North Am. **12:**961, 1981.
3. Baumgartner, R.F.: The surgery of arm and forearm amputations, Orthop. Clin. North Am. **12:**805, 1981.
4. Beasley, R.W.: General considerations in managing upper limb amputations, Orthop. Clin. North Am. **12:**743, 1981.
5. Burgess, E.M.: Current status of immediate post-surgical prosthetics, Newsletter of the Amputee Clinics **4:**11, 1972.
6. Burgess, E.M.: General principles of amputation surgery and post-operative management. In American Academy of Orthopaedic Surgeons: Atlas of limb prosthetics, St. Louis, 1981, The C.V. Mosby Co.
7. Burgess, E.M.: Principles of amputation surgery in upper limb. In American Academy of Orthopaedic Surgeons: Atlas of limb prosthetics, St. Louis, 1981, The C.V. Mosby Co.
8. Burkhalter, W., Hampton, F., and Smeltzer, J.: Wrist disarticulation and below-elbow and shoulder disarticulation and forequarter amputation. In American Academy of Orthopaedic Surgeons: Atlas of limb prosthetics, St. Louis, 1981, The C.V. Mosby Co.
9. Frazier, S.H., and Kolb, C.C.: Psychiatric aspects of pain and the phantom limb, Orthop. Clin. North Am. **1:**481, 1970.
10. Friedman, L.W.: The surgical rehabilitation of the amputee, Springfield, Ill. 1978, Charles C Thomas, Publisher.
11. Fryer, C.: Upper limb prosthetic components. In American Academy of Orthopaedic Surgeons: Atlas of limb prosthetics, St. Louis, 1981, The C.V. Mosby Co.
12. Körner, L.: Afferent electrical nerve stimulation for sensory feedback in hand prostheses: clinical and physiological aspects, Orthop. Scand. Suppl. **178:**52, 1979.
13. Kritter, A.E.: The bilateral upper extremity amputee, Orthop. Clin. North Am. **3:**397, 1972.
14. Law, H.T.: Engineering of upper limb prostheses, Orthop. Clin. North Am. **12:**929, 1981.
15. Mayer, L.: The orthopedic treatment of gunshot injuries, Philadelphia, 1918, W.B. Saunders Co.
16. Omer, G.: Nerve, neuroma and pain problems related to upper limb amputations, Orthop. Clin. North Am. **12:**751, 1981.
17. Pillet, J.: The aesthetic hand prosthesis, Orthop. Clin. North Am. **12:**961, 1981.
18. Peizer, E.: Research trends in upper limb prosthetics. In American Academy of Orthopedic Surgeons: Atlas of limb prosthetics, St. Louis, 1981, The C.V. Mosby Co.

19. Rang, M., and Thompson, G.: History of amputations and prostheses. In Kostuik, J., editor: Amputation surgery and rehabilitation: the Toronto experience, New York, 1981, Churchill Livingstone, Inc.
20. Slocum, D.B.: An atlas of amputations, St. Louis, 1949, The C.V. Mosby Co.
21. Santschi, W.R.: Manual of upper extremity prosthetics, ed. 2, 1958, University of California Press.
22. Wilson, A.B.: The modern history of amputation surgery and artificial limbs, Orthop. Clin. North Am. **3**:276, 1972.

BIBLIOGRAPHY

Barcome, D.F., and Eickman, L.: Prosthetic management of high bilateral upper limb amputees, Orthop. Prosthes. **34**:22, 1981.

Bender, L.F.: Prostheses and rehabilitation after arm amputation, Charles C Thomas, Publisher. Springfield, Ill., 1974.

Burgess, E.M.: Immediate postsurgical prosthetic fitting: a system of amputee management, Phys. Ther. **51**:139, 1971.

Clippinger, F.W., Avery, R., and Titus, B.: A sensory feedback system for an upper-limb amputation prosthesis, Bull. Prosthet. Res. **10**:247, 1974.

Derenzy, G.W.: Enchiridion: or a hand for the one-handed, London, 1822, Underwood, Publisher.

Edwards, J.W.: Orthopaedic appliance atlas, Vol 2. Ann Arbor, Mich., 1960, American Academy of Orthopedic Surgeons.

Ficarra, B.I.: Amputations and prostheses through the centuries, Med. Rec. **156**:94, 1943.

Graupe, D., Beer, A., Monlux, W., and Magnussen, I.: A multifunctional prosthesis control system based on time series identification of EMG signals using microprocessors, Bull. Prosthet. Res. **10**:4, 1977.

Harris, R.: Common stump problems. In Kostuik, J., editor: Amputation surgery and rehabilitation: the Toronto experience, New York, 1981, Churchill Livingstone, Inc.

Harris, R.: Principles of amputation surgery. In Kostuik, J., editor: Amputation surgery and rehabilitation: the Toronto experience, New York, 1981, Churchill Livingstone, Inc.

Hunter, G., Kennard, A., Burt, W., and Heger, D.: The upper limb amputee: experience of the Workman's Compensation Board of Ontario Amputee Team. In Kostuik, J., editor: Amputation surgery and rehabilitation: the Toronto experience, New York, 1981, Churchill Livingstone, Inc.

Kato, I.: Trends in powered upper limb prostheses, Prosthet. Orthot. Int. **2**:64, 1978.

LaBlanc, K.P., and Mason, C.P.: The VAPC functional elbow orthosis, Orthop. Prosthet. **34**:13, 1980.

Marshall, M.: 1981. The upper extremity in children. In Kostuik, J., editor: Amputation surgery and rehabilitation: the Toronto experience, New York, 1981, Churchill Livingstone, Inc.

MacDonald, J.: History of artificial limbs, Am. J. Surg. **19**:76, 1905.

Mason, C.P.: Practical problems in myoelectric control of prosthesis, Bull. Prosthet. Res. **10**:39, 1970.

Mital, M., and Pierce, D.: Amputees and their prostheses, Boston, 1971, Little, Brown & Co.

Northmore-Ball, M., Heger, H., and Hunter, G.: The below-elbow myoelectric prosthesis, J. Bone Joint Surg. **62**:3, 1980.

Prior, R., and Lyman, J.: Electrocutaneous feedback for artificial limbs: summary progress report (Feb. 1, 1974–July 31, 1975), Bull. Prosthet. Res. **10**:3, 1975.

Prior, R., and Lyman, J.: Supplemental sensory feedback for the VA/NU myoelectric hand: background and preliminary designs, Bull. Prosthet. Res. **10**:170, 1976.

74

Myoelectric prosthesis: prescription and training

LORETTA M. MAIORANO and JAMES M. HUNTER

The below-elbow amputee represents the largest group in the upper extremity amputee population.[2] A myoelectric prosthesis offers these patients high cosmesis, freedom from harnessing, and superior pinch when compared to the voluntary-opening hook of the conventional prosthesis.[2] By definition, a myoelectric prosthesis uses residual stump muscles to control the terminal device. More specifically, surface electrodes placed over selected muscles monitor electrical output from those muscles and deliver signals to an amplifier and processor and finally to the direct motor of the terminal device. Myoelectric prostheses are available for above- and below-elbow amputees from 2 years of age through adulthood. The purpose of this chapter is to describe currently available myoelectric control systems, criteria for patient selection, advantages and disadvantages of myoelectric control, and preprosthetic and postprosthetic training in use of the myoelectric prosthesis.

HISTORY

The first myoelectrically controlled prosthesis was introduced by Carl Reiter in 1948.[2] Since this prosthesis preceded the era of transistors, the control unit was relatively large in size (about the size of a shoe box) and was attached to the prosthesis by an electrical cord. The control unit was bulky.

In 1961 Kabrinsky[2] used the newly developed transistors to design the first Russian myoelectric controlled prosthesis. His control unit was twice the size of a cigarette pack and had to be worn on a belt around the waist.[2] Kabrinsky's work generated interest in other countries and research geared toward improvement in reliability, miniaturization, and less power-hungry circuitry was begun in England, Canada, Austria, Germany, Italy, and the United States.[2]

In 1964, the first commercially available myoelectric system outside the USSR was manufactured in Vienna by Viennaton according to the design of Zeman.[2]

In 1967, the firm of Otto Bock introduced their Myo-Bock System.[2] In Canada at about the same time, Scott and Sauter fitted the first three-state control system in which one muscle controls opening and closing of the myoelectric hand to a child patient at the Ontario Crippled Children's Centre in Toronto.

In 1970, proportional controlled systems were introduced by Lo'zach in Montreal and Childress in Chicago. In a proportional controlled system the speed of the hand is regulated by the intensity of the muscular contraction.

Most below-elbow myoelectric control systems are two-state systems using two muscles for the control of two different functions, such as hand opening and closing. Generally, the wrist extensors are chosen to command opening of the hand and the wrist flexors to command closing of the hand.

Research and technological developments in the field continue. At present there are three myoelectrical control systems currently available in the United States. Two of these systems are designed for wear by adults, and the third system was designed for the child amputee.

CURRENTLY AVAILABLE SYSTEMS

Myoelectric systems currently available in the United States are as follows.

Veterans Administration, Northwestern University (VANU)

The VANU System was conceived by Childress of Northwestern University and sponsored by a Veterans Administration contract. This is a proportional system in which the speed of the hand is regulated by the intensity of the muscular contraction. A grip strength of up to 25 pounds can be generated. Hand function is limited to a three-point pinch. The hand is motored by a 12-volt battery, which is housed in the distal part of the forearm (Fig. 74-1, A). The weight of the hand is 2.4 pounds. Motor noise is considered to be a disadvantage of this system especially in an otherwise quiet room. An advantage of this system is ruggedness and durability. The terminal device is available in one size only, adult male, which has a length of 7¾ inches. Because of the length of the hand and the location of the battery in the distal socket, this system is appropriate for a stump that terminates 3 or more inches proximal to the wrist.

Otto Bock System

The Otto Bock System is a digital system in which hand speed cannot be controlled. A three-point pinch strength up to 20 pounds is possible. The terminal device weighs 1 pound, 3.5 ounces. The mechanics of this system are smooth and quiet and embody advanced engineering. The system is powered by a 6-volt removable rechargeable battery,

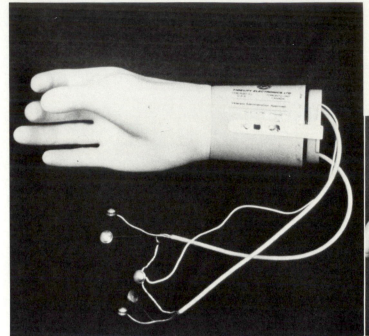

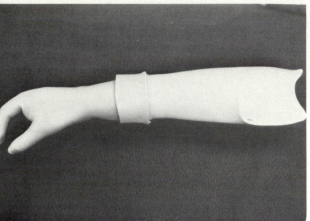

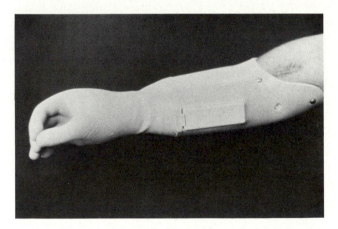

FIG. 74-2. Otto Bock Myoelectric System with removable batteries.

which is housed on the volar surface of the forearm (Fig. 74-2). The location of the battery on the forearm allows for accommodation of all lengths of below-elbow amputation stumps. The hand comes in four sizes: standard adult male, extra-large male, adult female, and adolescent. An interchangeable myoelectric hook (Greifer, Fig. 74-3) is available for either right or left hand. This system is available to prosthetists who have undergone training in the Otto Bock System. Current developments with this system include myoelectric control of supination and pronation for the amputee whose level is in the proximal half of the forearm.[4]

Swedish Hand

The Swedish Hand is a digital control system. The terminal device is powered by a 6-volt battery. The system is designed for children 2½ to 8 years of age, and two hand sizes are currently available. This system is the first to offer practical fitting for the child amputee. Refer to Chapter 75.

COMPONENTS OF THE BELOW-ELBOW MYOELECTRIC PROSTHESIS

Regardless of individual differences in design, each currently available myoelectric system includes the following components:

1. An intimately fitting forearm socket fabricated from a laminated resin of polyester or acrylic and a suspension system. Socket suspension for the patient with a wrist disarticulation is achieved by use of the epiphyseal flares. For other levels of below-elbow amputation, suspension is supracondylar. (See Fig. 74-1, *B.*)
2. Surface-contact electrodes. These electrodes are precisely placed in the proximal segment of the socket to lie over a selected area of muscle mass (Fig. 74-4).
3. A wrist connection unit that may be controlled manually or electrically depending on the needs of the patient.
4. A motor that is located in the hand or hook.
5. Rechargeable battery and battery charger.
6. Terminal device that may be either a myoelectric hand with three-point pinch or interchangeable myoelectric hook.

CRITERIA FOR PATIENT SELECTION

A potential myoelectric wearer must be intelligent and motivated, and have the kinesthetic skills to isolate muscular contractions of the command muscles. The patient must also be realistic in his expectations of the functioning of the

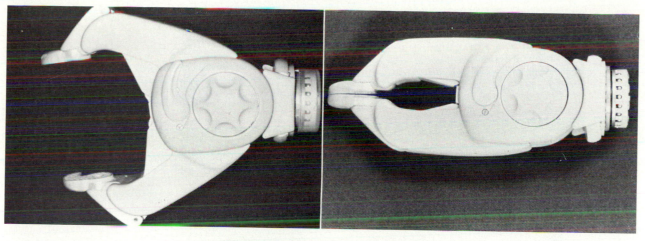

FIG. 74-3. Greifer myoelectric hook.

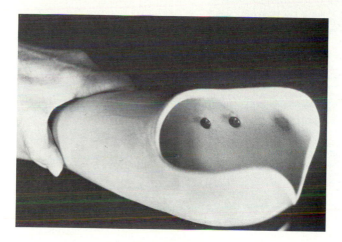

FIG. 74-4. Socket with surface electrodes.

prosthesis. He must appreciate the limitations and the capabilities of the prosthesis and must not expect it to be "bionic."

PREPROSTHETIC TRAINING

Preprosthetic training includes active and passive range-of-motion exercise for joints proximal to the amputation site, and strengthening of remaining muscles. Weight lifting with graduated cuff weights is included in the home program. Isometric training of the potential command muscles is essential.

Edema control is facilitated through an immediate, or early-fit, conventional prosthesis fabricated at the time of amputation or shortly after. The socket is changed as the circumferential measurement of the stump decreases (refer to Chapter 72). The patient is also given an elasticized stockinette to be worn when not wearing the prosthesis.

APPROPRIATE TIME FOR FITTING A MYOELECTRIC PROSTHESIS

Most potential myoelectric wearers are fitted with a temporary conventional prosthesis in the operating room or within 4 to 6 days after injury using a plaster socket. This allows for early acceptance and training in the use of a prosthesis (refer to Chapter 72). Circumferential measurements of the muscle bellies of the proximal forearm and of the distal end of the stump are taken weekly. When these measurements have stabilized for 3 to 4 consecutive weeks, the patient is ready for fabrication of the myoelectric prosthesis. Generally this occurs at about 4 to 6 months after amputation.

An immediate myoelectric fit has been accomplished by the surgeons at Emory University School of Medicine. The VANU System was used because the location of the battery is in the distal part of the forearm.

ELECTRODE PLACEMENT

The site chosen for electrode placement should be free of skin grafts and scar and should be located over a motor point. Optimum site for electrode placement is facilitated by the use of a myotester (Fig. 74-5), a biofeedback device that electronically measures the intensity of the muscle contractions.[5] The myotester is used as a training unit before surgery for the elective amputee who is to be provided immediately with a myoelectric prosthesis, and it is also used as a training unit for future potential myoelectric users soon after amputation while the sensation of the phantom hand is still present and can be used to advantage to help the patient isolate command muscles.

The myotester has two search electrodes, a ground, two indicating meters, and two gain controls that can be made more or less sensitive to the electrical signals generated by the command muscle. These dual controls allow simultaneous monitoring of signals from two different sites.

Before using the myotester, the patient is shown the motions necessary to control the myoelectric prosthesis, that is, tensing the wrist extensors to command opening of the hand and tensing the wrist flexors to command closing of the hand. He then practices these motions with his sound hand and attempts to duplicate the muscular contraction on the amputated side by moving his phantom hand. These motions are repeated several times with interim periods of relaxation. When the patient has adequately familiarized himself with the command motions, the myotester is used

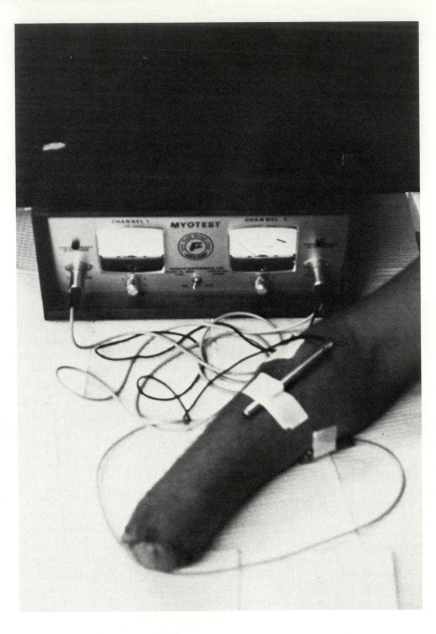

FIG. 74-5. Myotester.

to search for the optimum site for electrode placement. Generally this site lies directly over the motor point of the muscle. Adequate power to control the myoelectric prosthesis requires that the myopotential be at least 0.4 milliamps as measured on the myotester with a gain set at 5.

One test motion should be evaluated at a time. When the patient can adequately perform both test motions individually they are monitored together. He practices alternating the contractions of the two muscles, relaxing the antagonist while the agonist is contracting.

TRAINING THE PATIENT IN THE USE OF THE MYOELECTRIC HAND

The patient is taught the component parts of the prosthesis: socket, myoelectric hand or hook, electrodes, and battery units.

Stump socks are not worn over the area of the stump with which electrodes make contact. Before applying the prosthesis, the patient moistens the area of the arm where the electrodes make contact and flexes the elbow at least 90 degrees to facilitate donning of the socket. Frequently it is necessary to use a stockinette or sheer nylon stocking placed over the stump and threaded through the pull hole at the side of the distal end of the socket to pull the stump into the intimately fitting socket. Initial wearing time to condition the stump is 2 to 3 hours a day. The terminal device must be turned off when the prosthesis is donned and doffed to prevent draining of the battery.

The patient is instructed to recharge the unit every evening. The prosthesis is removed during the recharging process.

The socket of the prosthesis should be wiped daily with a damp cloth. The patient can wash his prosthetic hand but must not submerge the entire prosthesis.

The patient is advised that the hand looks most natural at rest when the fingers are open about one fourth of an

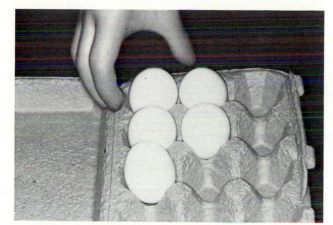

FIG. 74-6. Picking up objects of different densities.

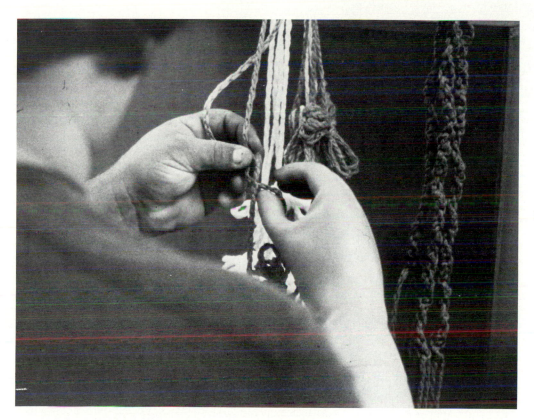

FIG. 74-7. Bilateral activities.

inch. This has a further advantage of preventing the fingertips from being pressed flat under constant load and also prevents the patient from sending "close" signals when the hand is already closed.[3]

The motions necessary to activate the myoelectric terminal device are the same as those practiced when one is using the myotester; that is, tensing of the wrist extensors commands opening of the hand and tensing of the wrist flexors commands closing of the hand. Initial exercises and training are therefore simply opening and closing of the terminal device by contraction of the correct command muscles.

When the patient has mastered grasp and release, he prac-

tices this skill on different-sized objects. Next, he must learn to pick up objects of different densities, making sure not to deform the shapes of the objects (Fig. 74-6). Bilateral activities (Fig. 74-7) are used to integrate the prosthetic arm with the normal arm. Activities of daily living, including dressing, feeding, and other tasks, are also incorporated into the patient's therapy program (Fig. 74-8).

It has been observed that as patients gain experience in the use of the myoelectric prosthesis they begin to demonstrate some element of sensibility feedback. It appears that the loss of real sensibility feedback is in part overcome by kinesthetic feedback. The combination of visual cues, the sound of the micromotor, and proprioceptive feedback

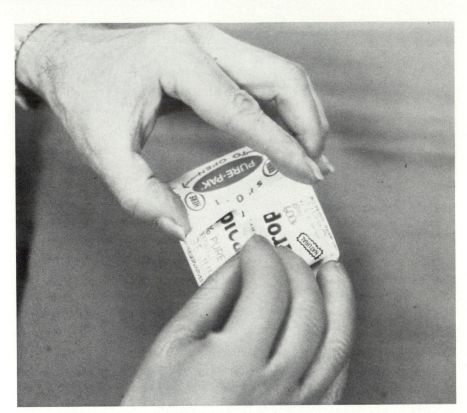

FIG. 74-8. Activities of daily living.

combine to further enhance the patient's skill in using the prosthesis. The therapist should encourage the use of these cues in the patient's prosthetic training.

MYOELECTRICS IN THE PROSTHETIC PROGRAMS OF INDIVIDUAL PATIENTS

Although myoelectric prostheses have many advantages, including cosmesis, lack of harnessing, and greater pinch power, they do have some disadvantages, including inability to be used in water, spontaneous activation of the terminal device from outside electrical interference, such as high-voltage lines and automatic color television changers. Therefore it is frequently appropriate to provide the patient with a conventional prosthesis and a myoelectric prosthesis according to his life-style and occupational needs. The following case examples will demonstrate the interaction between the myoelectric and conventional prosthesis for several patients.

B.N. is a 22-year-old right-handed accounting student who sustained an injury of his left hand and forearm in June 1979 while working at a summer job. The injury necessitated an ablation of the hand at the wrist level and grafting of the volar middle-to-distal forearm. Because of the need for grafting, an early-fit prosthesis was not applied. The patient received a definitive conventional prosthesis with a voluntary-opening hook and interchangeable hand 4 months after amputation. Myoelectric fitting with the Otto Bock hand with styloid suspension was provided 18 months postoperatively when the Otto Bock System became available locally.

Presently the patient is still a student and wears his myo-electric prosthesis approximately 10 to 12 hours per day. He finds it useful to switch to his conventional prosthesis with the hook for such manual activities as car work, cooking, and yard work, because these activities require a terminal device that can withstand "dirty work" and work around hot materials.

L.C. is a 51-year-old right-handed carpenter who sustained an injury to the left hand in February 1981 while at work. The injury resulted in an amputation at wrist level. He was fitted with an early-fit conventional prosthesis 1 month later. He received a definitive conventional prosthesis with voluntary-opening utility hook and interchangeable hand 3 months postoperatively. He then went on to receive an Otto Bock myoelectric hand and a Greifer (hook) 9 months postoperatively. He returned to work as a carpenter 1 year postoperatively. He states that he wears a prosthesis during all waking hours. He finds the conventional prosthesis most useful for heavy work, such as framing a house, and uses his myoelectric Greifer (hook) for trimming the house. During hot weather in the summer he is more comfortable in the conventional prosthetic socket because the myoelectric prosthetic socket has a tendency to slip off the forearm because of increased perspiration while he is working, since no stump sock is worn with the myoelectric prosthesis. He uses his myoelectric hand strictly for dress.

B.B. is a 26-year-old right-handed male who sustained an amputation of the right hand at wrist level in July 1980 while at work. He was fitted with an early-fit conventional prosthesis 1 month later. He received a definitive prosthesis with a prehensile hand (voluntary-closing hook) and interchangeable hand 3 months postoperatively. He was provided with an Otto Bock myoelectric hand in March 1981. He returned to his same job as a laborer in August 1981. He states that at work he uses his conventional prosthesis, since he works with water, and that he uses his myoelectric prosthesis for dress.

In a study by the Toronto Workmen's Compensation Board Hospital and Rehabilitation Centre, 43 patients with below-elbow amputations who had been fitted with myoelectric prostheses were reviewed. All these patients had been previously fitted with conventional prostheses with a hook terminal device. There were 39 men and 4 women in this study. It was found that the use of the myoelectric prosthesis was related to the patient's work and that most myoelectric users had office jobs. Patients stated that the myoelectric hand allows better sensory feedback because of the intimate fit of the socket and the necessary isometrics of the stump musculature to control the prosthesis. These patients also stated that the myoelectric hand feels more like a part of them.[1]

SUMMARY

A myoelectric prosthesis offers the below-elbow amputee freedom from harnessing, superior cosmesis, and the possibility of improved grip strength as compared to a conventional prosthesis. Most patients who have been fitted with a myoelectric prosthesis find it most useful for light bilateral activities and for dress occasions and find the conventional prosthesis more advantageous for heavier work. The myoelectric prosthesis allows the patient better sensory feedback, and myoelectric wearers state that the prosthesis feels more like a part of them than their conventional prosthesis does.[1]

REFERENCES

1. Northmore-Ball, M.D., Hagger, H., and Hunter, G.A.: The below elbow myoelectric prosthesis: a comparison of the Otto Bock myoelectric prosthesis with a hook and functional hand, J. Bone Joint Surg. **62B**:363-367, Aug. 1980.
2. Sauter, W.F.: Fitting consideration and approaches for myoelectric and microswitch controlled upper extremity prostheses, Presented at Contemporary Issues in Upper Extremity Amputation and Prosthetic Function, April 30-May 2, 1981, Houston Center for Amputee Services, Houston, Texas.
3. Sauter, W.F.: Powered upper extremity prosthetics: dos and don'ts, Myoelectric Services, Rehabilitation Engineering Department, Ontario Crippled Children's Centre, Toronto, Ontario.
4. Sauter, W.F.: Personal communication, Ontario Crippled Children's Centre, Toronto, Ontario, Nov. 1982.
5. Operating instructions, Fidelity Mini Myotest MTM-1 for VANU, American Myoelectric Hand System.

75

Prosthetics for the child amputee

LORETTA M. MAIORANO and JAMES E. SWEIGART

In this chapter, our main focus will be on the child with a partial hand deficiency or with below-elbow limb deficiency; we will concentrate on the CAPP terminal device for the conventional below-elbow prosthesis, the Swedish myoelectric hand for the below-elbow limb-deficient child, and the opposition post for the partial hand deficiency. These children are generally fitted with appropriate prostheses when sitting balance has been established, usually at 6 to 7 months of age. At this age, the parents are an integral part of the prosthetic team. They have a major responsibility for the child's acceptance and use of the prosthesis. They must be informed as to what is available and appropriate for their child at the present time and what they have to look forward to in the future.

CAPP TERMINAL DEVICE

The CAPP terminal device, which is fitted to a conventional prosthesis, was designed and developed at the Child Amputee Prosthetic Project (CAPP) at the University of California in Los Angeles (Fig. 75-1). Its shape is neutral so that it can be used on either the right or the left side. It is made of plastic preflexed and shaped to blend with the forearm in a continuous flowing line.[4] The terminal device has a wide palmar face with a frictional resilient cover made of Kraton* so that one may hold objects without requiring extensively strong pinch or concern for critical object positioning.[5] The shell of the terminal device is made of Delrin.† The frictional covers are injection molded and shaped to extend over the outer edges of the shell so as to provide friction for gross stabilizing activities. Full opening at the tips of the terminal device is 2¾ inches, which is between the opening of the two child-size Dorrance voluntary-opening hooks, number 10, which opens to 2¼ inches, and number 99, which opens to 3 inches. Presently there are two springs available to control strength of prehension. The spring with regular tension is most frequently used; however, a soft spring is used with infants or with children who have difficulty opening the terminal with the regular spring.

The child with the congenital below-elbow absence of

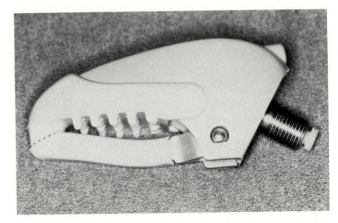

FIG. 75-1. CAPP terminal device.

the forearm is fitted with a conventional prosthesis at about 7 months of age. This prosthesis consists of a forearm socket made of laminated nylon or polyester resin, a harness or humeral cuff as a means of suspension, and a CAPP terminal device. If the residual forearm is short, the forearm section would consist of a double-walled construction with the inner wall fitting the distal end of the stump. A long stump requires a single-walled forearm section in order to match the overall length of the unaffected side. Different from the adult amputee, the infant may present problems in fitting because of the lack of well-defined bony prominences and an overall chubby build. Many times a full harness with a cable to the terminal device may be required to suspend the prosthesis even though the child will not be able to activate the terminal device. Suspension of the prosthesis for these infants may be a figure-of-eight with a Northwestern ring, figure-of-nine, or a simple type of suspension for the unactivated terminal device where single-pivot elbow hinges are attached to a humeral cuff. The object is to use the simplest means of suspension.

In the early months a prosthesis acts as an extension of a congenitally deficient extremity. The child will accept its daily application and incorporate the prosthesis into his body image. The parents are integral in early prosthetic training; while playing with the child, the parent opens the terminal device and places a toy in it. The child pulls the toy out of the terminal device and then will try to open it with his

*Thermoplastic rubber made by Shell Oil Co., Inc., Houston, Texas.
†Thermoplastic produced by E.I. du Pont de Nemours & Co., Wilmington, Del.

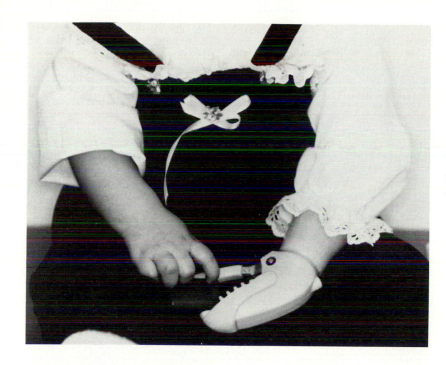

FIG. 75-2. Placing a toy in terminal device with other hand.

other hand (Fig. 75-2) or mouth while he places a toy into it.

Provided that there is general acceptance of a prosthetic plan by the parents, the prosthesis is activated when the child shows an interest in operation of the terminal device and attempts to place objects in it by opening it with his sound hand. This generally occurs at 18 to 24 months of age when more skilled shoulder movements are evident.[2] At this age training is possible because of increased understanding, attention span, and cooperation of the child.[2] The child is treated in a sunny, moderate-sized room with minimal distractions, preferably in the morning or after a nap when he is rested. Initial therapy involves passive range of motion with the prosthesis on. The child observes the terminal device opening and imitates this motion. Activities involving picking up objects above shoulder level are good activities to initiate terminal device opening. Developmentally appropriate activities encouraging bilateral use of the extremities are initiated, such as playing with pop beads, sewing cards, and Tinkertoys. The therapist should find out what special interests the child has and incorporate them in therapy.[2] The therapist sits in front of the child and places toys in the midline. Activities are changed every few minutes because attention span wanders. Short rest periods are allowed between activities. Therapy treatment time depends on the age and attention span of the child. Activities of daily living are also encouraged at this time. The parent is invaluable in continuing therapy at home; generally it is important to have the parent present during the therapy visit at which time a change or addition of activities is discussed.

CAPP terminal device no. 1 is now available from Hosmer/Dorrance Corporation and may be used for the child with a long elbow congenital deficiency by routing the cable for opening on the dorsum of the CAPP terminal device as opposed to running the cable through the center bolt, a technique that is used for short below-elbow congenital deficiencies.[5] The activating cable is braided Dacron 130-pound trolling fishing line.

MYOELECTRICS

Myoelectrically controlled hands are presently available for children 2 to 9 years of age, in addition to the already available myoelectric hand for adolescents and adults. The hand for children that is shown in Fig. 75-3 is available from Steeper (Roehampton, England).

A prosthesis with supracondylar suspension is fabricated for below-elbow limb-deficient children. The electronics of the hand are housed within the hand itself.[6] A 6-volt rechargeable battery may be placed within the socket or mounted externally depending on the length of the residual limb and the age of the child. Most children who have been fitted with a myoelectric prosthesis also have a conventional prosthesis for "dirty" or "water" play. The myoelectric prosthesis is quite reliable, but it must be properly cared for. The cosmetic glove must be replaced if it is torn, to prevent dirt from getting into the motor of the hand. An intimate fit of the socket with the residual limb is necessary for the electrodes to make consistent contact with the command muscles for hand opening and closing. This will necessitate many changes of the inner socket during the growing years as the stump grows in length causing loss of electrode contact with the command muscles.

To evaluate a child's myoelectric potential, a myoelectric hand, battery, electrode cables, and electrodes can be utilized. The electrodes are taped over the muscle belly of the wrist flexors and extensors, and the child is told to open (Fig. 75-4) and close the myoelectric hand (Fig. 75-5). Initially the gain control for amplification of the myoelectric signal is set high to allow for immediate positive feedback.[6] As the child becomes adept at opening and closing the hand,

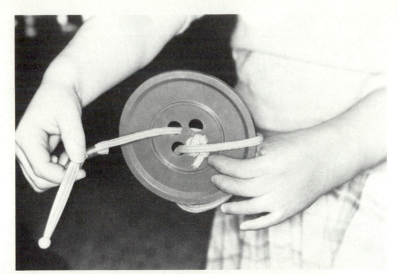

FIG. 75-3. Myoelectric hand holding large toy button.

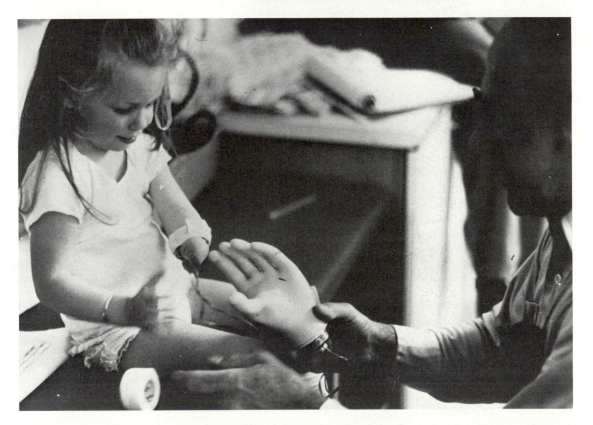

FIG. 75-4. Opening test of myoelectric hand.

the gain control is lowered to avoid outside electrical interference. It is believed that the myoelectric application should be done at a very early age. Children teach themselves to open and close the hand in a very short period of time after its application.[6] When fitted early, the child more readily incorporates the hand into his body image.

Several children 2½ years old have been successfully fitted with myoelectrically controlled prostheses at the Ontario Crippled Children's Centre in Canada. These patients did not immediately become prosthetic superperformers, but because they were given a chance to grow up with my-

oelectrically controlled prostheses, they became much superior users and demonstrators than any of their peers who switched to myoelectric prostheses as teen-agers.[3]

OPPOSITION POST

"The ideal prosthesis is one which restores both motor and sensory function of the missing limb. The usual upper extremity prosthesis provides prehension while sacrificing sensory feedback."[7] Children with congenital deficiencies of the limb, either transcarpal, transmetacarpal, or mono-digital, have been provided with an opposition post against

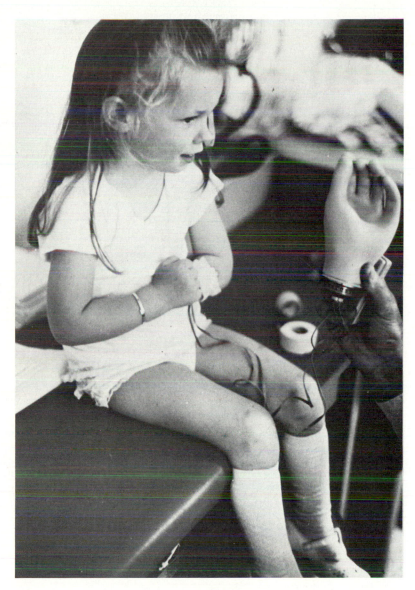

FIG. 75-5. Closing test of myoelectric hand.

which the remnant hand can flex to grasp an object without loss of sensory feedback. Over the years the opposition post has taken many shapes and forms.[1] The simplest one consists of a piece of aluminum slightly smaller in area than the volar surface of the hand remnant (Fig. 75-6). This aluminum pad is covered with Plastizole* and attached to a volar bar that extends approximately halfway up the forearm. To this bar is attached two bands that encircle the wrist and forearm at approximately 180 degrees.

The opposition post can also be made of Nyloplex,† a transparent thermoplastic formed over a positive mold of the child's hand remnant. One can provide friction surface by gluing a piece of industrial belting to the plastic post. This type of construction is cosmetically superior to the aluminum band type (Fig. 75-7).

The opposition post is often useful for specific applications in school or play and then later in work. It has been

our experience that a child may reject it at some point in his development, particularly in adolescence, and come back to it several years later when he recognizes a specific use for it in his trade or occupation.

Several years ago, the Child Amputee Prosthetic Project developed a CAPP multiposition post. This CAPP post consists of a plastic bracelet and a projectile post, which are hinged at the wrist (Fig. 75-8). The post can be manually placed at any of three positions in relation to the palm to hold different-sized objects.[5] The activating mechanism of the CAPP multiposition post is cast in stainless steel. It is made in two sizes and has a manual push button for right- or left-hand operation. The multiposition post is appropriate for children 7 years of age and older and offers them more versatility because of the ability to adjust its position to pick up different-sized objects.

SUMMARY

Children are different from adults; they are not scaled-down adults and present their own set of values. Children

---

*Liquid vinyl plastisol manufactured by Barley-Earhart Co., Portland, Mich.

†Thermoplastic acrylic plastic manufactured by Rohm & Haas Co., Inc., Germany.

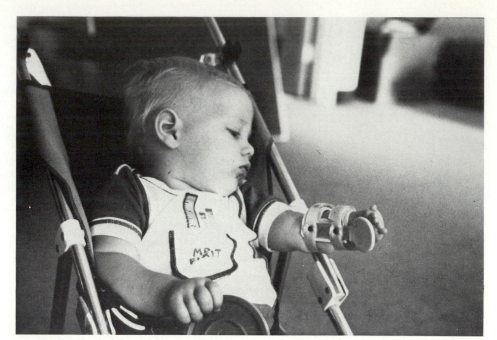

FIG. 75-6. ''Simple'' opposition post.

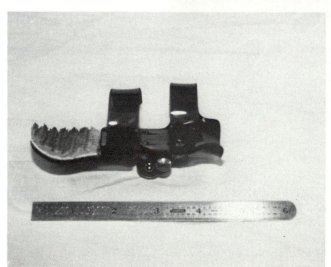

FIG. 75-7. Opposition post with friction surface.

FIG. 75-8. CAPP multiposition post.

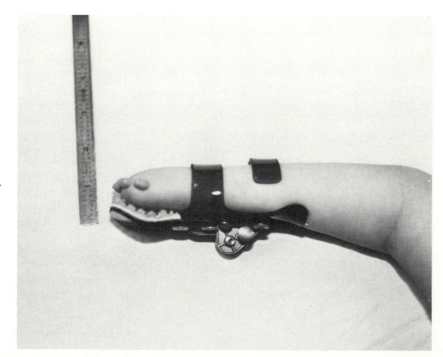

respond more readily to any form of treatment that is helpful to them, and they do not place so much emphasis on appearance or what other people think. The child who is fitted early with the appropriate prosthesis will accept its daily application and incorporate it more readily in his body image. The initial fiting of the prosthesis should be done when sitting balance has been established.

REFERENCES

1. Bryant, M., Donohue, J., Hunter, J., and Sweigart, J.: A prosthesis to restore opposition in children with congenital absence of the hand, Interclinic Information Bulletin **17**(6):5-10, 1979.
2. Patton, J.: Management of the juvenile amputee, Northwestern Medical Course Notebook. Symposium on Contemporary Issues in Upper Extremity Amputation and Prosthetic Function, Sponsored by Baylor College of Medicine, Department of Physical Medicine and Rehabilitation Research and Training Center, No. 4, National Institute of Handicapped Research, April 30–May 2, 1981, Houston Center for Amputee Services, Houston, Texas.
3. Sauter, W.F.: Myoelectric and microswitch controlled upper extremity prosthesis, Presented at Symposium on Contemporary Issues in Upper Extremity Amputation and Prosthetic Function, April 30–May 2, 1981, Houston Center for Amputee Services, Houston, Texas.
4. Shaperman, J.: The CAPP terminal device: a preliminary clinical evaluation, Interclinic Information Bulletin **14**(2):1-12, 1975.
5. Shaperman, J., and Sumida, C.T.: Recent advances in research in prosthetics for children, Clin. Orthop. Rel. Res. **(148)**:26-33, May 1980.
6. Sörbye, R.: Myoelectric prosthetic fitting in young children, Clin. Orthop. Rel. Res. (148):34-40, May 1980.
7. Swanson, A.B.: Congenital limb deficits: classification of treatment, Clin. Symp. **33**(3):1-32, 1981.

XV
SPLINTING

76

The forces of dynamic splinting: ten questions before applying a dynamic splint to the hand

PAUL W. BRAND

A dynamic splint is one that achieves its effect by movement and force. It is a form of manipulation. It may use forces generated by the patient's own muscles or externally imposed forces using rubber bands or springs.

Whenever passive movement and manipulation of the hand are used, there is a danger that too much force will be used by a surgeon or therapist who is anxious to get results in the limited time available at the clinic. The result is often that the patient has pain; the hand gets swollen, and the short-term gain in mobility is followed by long-term stiffness. We prefer to encourage active exercise and work-related movements because these are controlled by the patient who keeps within the limits of pain. Brain-hand reflexes and coordination, which are essential to real hand health are restored.

However, in many cases, it is not possible to achieve a full range of motion by active exercises alone. They may need to be replaced or supplemented by a dynamic splint. Sometimes active movements are used during the day, and then a splint is worn at night. However, even in such cases the splint may have the same bad results as manipulation of the hand unless the surgeons and the therapists exercise stern discipline to ensure that the forces they impose are well controlled. Too little force will do no good. Too much will do harm. *How much is just right?*

To obtain consistently good results from dynamic splinting, I believe that we have to develop a whole new approach. We have to measure, and we have to calculate. It is not enough to say "rubber-band traction" or "not too much force" or "be gentle." We have to be quantitative. Pharmacology would still be in the dark ages if we continued to prescribe a handful of this medicine or a mouthful of that. We now use milligrams and milliliters. So in terms of force on the hand, we must use units. Then we can begin to compare results, and we shall begin to develop a science. Most books and articles about splints are concerned with design. I want to deal only with measurements and objectives here.

We first must realize that a splint by its very presence on the hand is doing harm. It is inhibiting the free movement and use of the hand. It is only justified if the specific good that it will do compensates for the general harm and restriction.

Thus the first step is to define the object of the dynamic splint for the specific hand we are dealing with and for the specific joint or joints that we want to mobilize or modify. Then we need to ask ten questions in relation to the forces we propose to use: (1) How much force? (2) Through what surface? (3) For how long? (4) To what structure? (5) By what leverage? (6) Against what reaction? (7) For what purpose? (8) Measured by what scale? (9) Avoiding what harm? (10) Warned by what signs?

HOW MUCH FORCE?

In most dynamic hand splints the force is provided by rubber bands or steel springs. At the present time these are not marketed for our profession with information about force or tension. Orthodontists use graded rubber bands, but these are too small for our purpose. Thus each therapist or splint-maker has to purchase rubber bands and springs in batches that appear uniform and then test them for tension. A simple stress-strain diagram should be prepared for each batch to be a guide for future use. I use five points on a curve from 100 to 500 gm and measure the length of the band as it hangs with each of those five weights hooked one by one into its end. Fig. 76-1 shows the curve for one of our rubber bands. If a dynamic splint requires a pull of 200 gm from an outrigger 6 cm from the finger, a quick glance across our graphs will show which band we should use and how far we should stretch it. At the time it is applied we can check the tension with a spring scale (Fig. 76-2).

In most dynamic splints there will be a range of movement that will result in lengthening and shortening the rubber band or spring. Thus the tension will change. This too should be noted. For example, when Dr. Harold Kleinert has done a primary suture on a severed flexor tendon, he likes to use a rubber band from the fingernail to a wrist band. The purpose of this is to hold the finger flexed when it is at rest and to allow the patient to extend his finger against the tension of the rubber band by using the extensor muscles. The rubber band should be strong enough to pull the finger back into flexion without the use of the flexor muscle-tendon unit. For such a purpose, I would use a rubber band that was 5 cm long at rest (no tension) that would have a tension of 200 to 300 gm at 15 cm length.

If one is using a spring-steel wire that exerts force at right

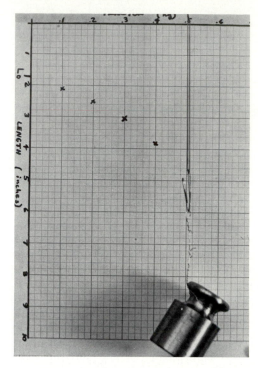

FIG. 76-1. Rubber band being tested by hanging succession of weights from its end and marking its length on force-elongation curve.

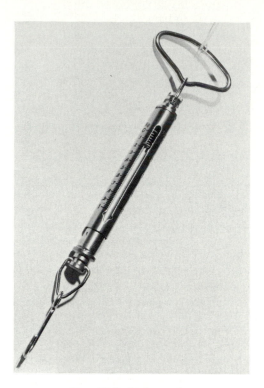

FIG. 76-2. Spring scale.

angles to its length, this may be calibrated ahead of time with a similar stress-strain curve or may be checked after it is in position by pulling it with a spring scale through the same range that it will act on the finger.

Thus in many cases the question "How much force?" is answered by two figures—for example, 250 gm when the finger is extended and 50 gm when the finger is flexed.

To many surgeons and therapists such figures will be meaningless because they have not used them before and do not know what 100 gm feels like. If so, it is time to start to learn. Check a tension that "feels right" on the hand and then measure how much tension there is by using a spring scale.

THROUGH WHAT SURFACE?

Every applied force may be presumed to act on the bones or on the musculoskeletal system. However, it has to act *through* the surface of the body. Often the limits on the amount of force we can use are set more by what the skin can stand than by what the joint can accept. Most forces in a hand splint are applied through a sling around a finger and most are quite comfortable at the time they are applied. However, as time passes, they become uncomfortable and finally painful because of ischemia from pressure. This is probably the commonest cause of patients discarding a splint or becoming "uncooperative." If they were more cooperative, they would keep the splint on all night (taking pain-killing medication) and come to the doctor the next day with gangrene under the sling.

Both the ischemia and the pain are caused by *pressure* not just by force. Pressure is force divided by area. Thus a

given force may be safe if the sling is wide, and unsafe if it is narrow.

A good general rule is that if a force is to be applied continuously, it should not result in a pressure of more than 50 gm/cm². This is about the same as 35 mm Hg, which is within the margin of safety for long-term pressure on soft tissues. Note that 35 mm Hg is higher than actual capillary pressure, but capillaries in normal tissue can withstand higher pressures.[1] Thus a 200 gm pull needs a 4 cm² area of sling. All 4 cm² should take equal pressure. If the sling includes curved areas that take oblique stress, it would be better to have 6 cm². This, in old terminology, means that 8 ounces of pull need a full square inch of sling.

A special danger from pressure occurs when a sling becomes tilted. Perhaps the finger changes its angle because the whole splint is loose. Now the same force acts only on the *edge* of the sling. The actual effective surface of the sling may now be less than a quarter of what it was, and so the pressure is multiplied by four. Result—the patient becomes "uncooperative" or else endures pain.

Pressure is relatively unimportant if it is intermittent. It is the sustained pressure that keeps the blood supply from the skin. This is what hurts and then kills the skin.

FOR HOW LONG?

Time is important in two respects—the total time the splint is on the hand, and the time that the actual force is pressing on the tissues. If the force only acts in certain positions or when certain muscles pull against it, it is intermittent and the question of ischemia may not arise. If there is any risk from continuous pressure, it is better to use the splint for only 4 or 5 hours at a time and then remove it and look at the skin to see if a flush of reactive hyperemia, or a "hot spot," indicates that the skin has been short of blood. If all is normal, the splint may be worn for gradually longer periods of time.

If the object of the splint is to lengthen a scar or to stimulate the development of free loose skin where previously tight skin has limited joint motion, then time has another kind of importance.

We sometimes speak of "stretching" skin or scar. Stretch is a passive action that results in the elongation of elastic elements in skin, scar, or ligament. Every bit of elongation of tissue that is accomplished by *stretch* will shorten again when the force is relaxed. When a rubber band is pulled, it becomes longer. It is "stretched." When the pull is relaxed, it returns to its old length. If it is pulled harder, it may break. It is the same with living tissue. The immediate lengthening of tight skin that is produced by pulling will be lost when it is relaxed. If it is pulled too hard, microscopic ruptures in the tissue result in inflammation and later scar formation. The last state may then be worse than the first.

The real true lengthening of any living tissue results from the activity of living cells as they constantly take up and absorb old tissues and lay down new tissues. Old collagen is absorbed; new collagen is laid down in new patterns responsive to new needs. Cells in the skin multiply and proliferate in response to need. Our responsibility is not to try shortcuts by "stretching" or breaking the old tissues but to *stimulate* the living cells to do the work. We do this by keeping the tissues in a physical state that demonstrates the need. The cells will then sense the need and will make changes to meet that need.

The best way to do this is to keep the tissues *constantly* in a state of mild tension. The optimum state requires less tension than most of us use, but it needs to be maintained longer than most of us do. A good test is blanching of the skin. If we pull so hard that the skin begins to blanch, that is too much tension for the stimulation of optimal growth. The tension should be maintained for many hours every day for maximum efficiency. I often prefer to use cylindric plaster casts reapplied every day to hold the joint in its daily fresh optimal position. However, a good dynamic splint that exercises fairly constant tension is nearly as good and involves fewer visits to the therapist. However, it is of no use unless it is kept in position almost 24 hours a day.

TO WHAT STRUCTURE?

In dealing with stiff joints we have to determine what the limiting structures or tissues are. If we decide that the tissues all around the joint are tight and inflexible, the patient probably should not be in a splint except for pain or inflammation. He should be exercising freely and using his hand. However, if the tissues are free on one side and tight on the other, a corrective splint may be of value. Even so, it is good to know which is the target tissue.

On the flexor side of a proximal interphalangeal joint, for example, tight skin or connective tissue will probably remodel with constant tension. An adherent tendon or volar plate, however, may not respond. A good general test is to pull the finger gently toward extension. If it comes to a slow stop and if the skin blanches a little on further attempted movement, this suggests the skin may be short; the prognosis for improvement with a splint is good. If the joint moves freely to a certain point and then stops dead, the prognosis for conservative treatment is poor, and splinting may be a waste of time.

BY WHAT LEVERAGE?

When it is determined which structure or layer around the joint is in need of lengthening, it is possible to visualize the problem in terms of levers around the axis of the joint. The axis of movement of most joints of the hand is at about the midpoint of the head of the proximal bone. Thus, if the palmar skin of the proximal interphalangeal joint is tight, it may be about 1 cm from the axis of the joint in an adult male. Thus, if a sling is placed 3 cm down the finger and hooked up to a force of 250 gm to pull the finger straight, the leverage will be 3 to 1, and the skin will experience a tension of 750 gm (Fig. 76-3, *A*). If the skin is bowstringing across the joint, it will be farther from the joint axis and will have a longer lever arm. It will be more difficult to get an effective tension to it without producing pressure effects under the sling.

We use the term "mechanical advantage" to express the ratio between the length of the lever through which force is applied and the length of the lever arm through which the force is delivered. In the case of hand splinting this is commonly a number between 2:1 and 5:1. We use the *length* of the finger or hand to *apply* the force, and half the *thickness* of the finger or hand to *deliver* the force. When muscles are moving the fingers from inside the hand, they have very small mechanical advantages because they use levers related to finger thickness to apply their force and have to move levers related to finger length to deliver the force. Thus their ratios are inverted and are commonly 1:5. This is why active exercises are safer than passive movements. They use small leverages and are less likely to do violence to the tissues.

I do not seriously suggest that the mathematic ratios of leverages must be worked out on paper every time a dynamic splint is applied. I do not seriously suggest that the mathematic ratios of leverages must be worked out on paper every time a dynamic splint is applied. I do suggest that it is good to work it out sometimes as an educational exercise, and that it should be *thought about* every time. Once a therapist starts to think in terms of leverages and mechanical advantages, he or she is much less likely to make the mistake of overstressing or understressing the key tissues we are trying to modify.

AGAINST WHAT REACTION?

"To every action there is an equal and opposite reaction." Newton knew about this 300 years ago, but we forget it every day. We make a sling to spread the pressure on a finger where we pull, but we forget that the *pull* on the finger results in a *push* on the hand. In the reaction, as well as in the primary action, the damage is done most often by pressure rather than by force. Pressure is force divided by area. Our areas are too small, and so our pressures are big. Consider a simple and common example. A finger has a proximal interphalangeal joint that is stiff in flexion and a

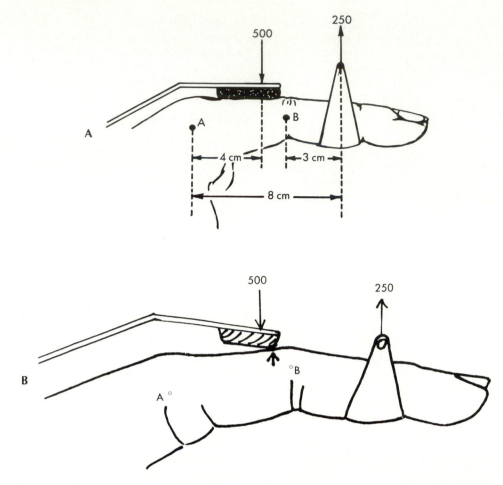

FIG. 76-3. A, Diagram of finger subjected to force of 250 gm through sling 3 cm from axis, *B,* of interphalangeal joint. Proximal segment of finger is held in flexion by felt pad, which is 4 cm from axis, *A,* of metacarpophalangeal joint. This pad receives thrust of 500 gm to balance force on sling; 500 gm × 4 cm = 250 gm × 8 cm. **B,** Same finger as in **A** but because proximal part of hand was not supported, whole finger has tilted. Now only edge of felt pad presses on finger, creating high pressure.

metacarpophalangeal joint that is freely mobile. A splint is applied to provide traction in a dorsal direction to result in tension on the palmar side of the proximal interphalangeal joint. Using our previous figures, the dorsal pull is 250 gm at 3 cm from the axis of the proximal interphalangeal joint, resulting in a 750 gm tension on the volar skin.

How much force will be needed as a *reaction* or stabilizing force to hold the proximal phalanx steady so that the distal force can act on the proximal interphalangeal joint? If no other force is applied, the finger would *hyperextend* at the metacarpophalangeal joint where it is not stiff and the proximal interphalangeal joint would not benefit.

So, *how much?* I find that most therapists and orthotists assume that the *reaction* force should be the same as the *action* force, that is, in this example it would be 250 gm. If you pull north with 250 gm, you can balance it by pushing south with 250 gm. Right? Wrong! Think about leverages and moments. The proximal interphalangeal joint is stiff and will not move much. The movable joint is the metacarpophalangeal joint. The 250 gm force is applied 3 cm

distal to the proximal interphalangeal joint, which means it is about 8 cm distal to the metacarpophalangeal joint. Thus its moment for extending the proximal interphalangeal joint is 750 gram-centimeters, but for the metacarpophalangeal joint it is 250 × 8 gm-cm = 2000 gm-cm. Now to oppose that moment at the metacarpophalangeal joint, 2000 gm-cm is needed in the opposite direction. If the restraint on the dorsal surface is placed 4 cm distal to the metacarpophalangeal joint, 500 gm of force will be exerted on the restraining pad to balance the moment of 2000 gm-cm: 500 × 4 = 250 × 8. So it takes double the force on the proximal phalanx to balance the force farther down the finger (Fig. 76-3, *A*).

Splintmakers commonly use a flat bar across the proximal phalanges to balance a sling around the fingers. A sling spreads the force around the fingers; a flat bar presses only on the dorsum.

Furthermore, the volar side of the finger is soft and compliant, while the dorsal side is bone and skin. This is why both the pain of a splint and the damage from the splint are

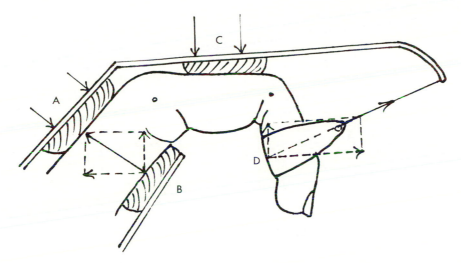

FIG. 76-4. Vector diagram to show how both horizontal forces and vertical forces need to be balanced. Whereas in Fig. 76-3, *A,* sling was pulling dorsally, here it pulls obliquely because interphalangeal joint is flexed. Vector diagram of force of sling, *D,* shows that horizontal vector is double dorsal vector. Thus felt pad, *C,* which balances dorsal force, will not take much force. However, feld pad in palm, *B,* must be capable of considerable horizontal restraint. It also has dorsal vector, which keeps hand snug against pad, *C,* and prevents tilting shown in Fig. 76-3, *B.* Pad *A* has no force to exert or absorb. It is there to stabilize against *B* and prevent unexpected shifts of position of hand as a whole.

more common from the dorsal reaction bar than from the pull on the volar side.

Recognizing how common dorsal problems are, most orthotists and therapists take care to use a broad plate and have it padded. However, the breadth of the plate is of no significance if the finger does not remain in total contact with it. The elastic pull on the finger, failing to straighten the proximal interphalangeal joint, may use the reaction bar as a fulcrum and tilt the finger upward and the metacarpophalangeal joint downward, resulting in the finger pressing only on the edge of the plate. *Result?* The force becomes concentrated on a narrow edge: small area = high pressure = pain or gangrene, or both (Fig. 76-3, *B*).

The way to prevent all this is to think ahead and think in numbers, leverages, moments, and axes. Also, use snug total contact fitting for the proximal support of the hand so that the proximal phalanx cannot move in relation to the hand or the splint (Fig. 76-4).

FOR WHAT PURPOSE?

It has already been stated that before a splint is prescribed, there must be a definition of its specific object. In such a definition it is necessary to bear in mind the harm that comes to the whole hand and perhaps to the patient's own will to recover by keeping him tied up for a long time in a splint. Thus a typical statement of objective might read ''to overcome the flexion contracture of the proximal interphalangeal joints of the index and middle fingers and to restore full passive range of motion. The splint may be judged useful as long as 10 degrees of improvement are being recorded per week.''

MEASURED BY WHAT SCALE?

The introduction of specific objective criteria that are time related should ensure that splints are discontinued as soon as their job is done or as soon as they have stopped contributing to total improvement.

In other cases the criteria may be related to muscular strength, reeducation, or some other factor. However, some way should be found to link it to a scale of numbers that may be periodically checked and graphically recorded. Both the therapist and the patient should use the graph and share in the evaluation of the progress and of the value to the patient of the objective that has been chosen.

AVOIDING WHAT HARM?

In addition to the general frustration and harm that comes from confinement in an obtrusive splint, there are sometimes specific problems that arise. These are different for different patients and for different diseases and splints. This is why it is good to pause at the beginning and ask oneself what possible harm could come to *this* hand from *this* splint. One example is when too much force is used to mobilize a stiff joint. The result is inflammation of the periarticular tissues followed by swelling and subsequent increased stiffness. Another example is in rheumatoid arthritis when a dynamic splint applies force distally on the fingers to extend stiff metacarpophalangeal joints. Frequently, there is already some degree of volar subluxation of these joints and a tight volar plate. Distal force will then angulate the finger backwards at the metacarpophalangeal joint without true gliding of the joint. This results in intense pressure on the dorsal lip of the proximal articular surface of the phalanx, which presses into the head of the metacarpal because this is now the fulcrum of this abnormal movement. Finally, the lip wears away and complete subluxation ensues. This common problem can only be prevented if the therapist and the patient understand how the joint works and are warned never to try to extend a subluxating joint by external force unless the force is applied *close to the joint* at the base of the finger,

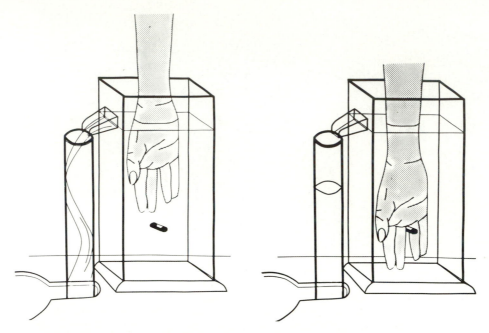

FIG. 76-5. Water displacement volumeter. (Details of this may be obtained from the Rehabilitation Branch, PHS Hospital, Carville, Louisiana 70721.) (From Brand, P.W.: Surgical treatment of primary deformities of the hand. In McDowell, F., and Enna, C.D., editors: Surgical rehabilitation in leprosy, Baltimore, 1974, The Williams & Wilkins Co.)

where it will stimulate gliding at the joint not just angulation.

A third problem is that the presence of a big splint sometimes results in the disuse of other, previously normal, joints. These may then become stiff. This is especially true in elderly, arthritic, and apprehensive patients.

Prevention consists in being forewarned and in the institution of regular range-of-motion exercises to all joints that might be affected.

WARNED BY WHAT SIGNS?

When potential dangers are identified, all members of the team need to be alerted to the signs that might indicate the beginning of actual harm.

I like to have a graphic record of hand volume and joint temperatures for problem hands. A water-displacement, hand volumometer gives a quick record of changes in hand volume (Fig. 76-5). Volume goes up when patients keep their hands hanging down or when the hand gets inflamed from excessive use of force. A simple skin thermometer or thermistor probe may be used to keep a record of temperature differentials between a given joint and a contralateral normal joint. Rising temperatures suggest inflammation. Low temperatures may sometimes be associated with sympathetic dystrophy. A careful inspection of the surface of the hand and the feel of the hand by the sensitive palm of the therapist will often pick up redness or swelling or hot spots. A very important modality is the changing reaction of the patient who has been educated and alerted to the potential benefits and problems of any treatment method. The patient experiences a constant feedback that is more significant than some artificially contrived biofeedback apparatus. His or her brain adds up and analyzes a stream of information from skin, joint, and muscle and integrates it with an awareness of personal priorities. The subconscious mind, more flexible and better programmed than any computer, comes up with an evaluation of a splint that should be taken seriously by any physician or splintmaker. We may be specialists treating a single limb with a scientific instrument, but we must be guided by the whole individual—body, mind, and spirit—who has to decide the extent to which he is prepared to place his whole person at the service of one of his digits and restrict his whole freedom and activity to improve a single joint.

The art of a therapist is to remain poised and flexible, responsive to the input of science and technology on the one side and to the human values of a patient on the other. This is a challenge that is constantly different and keeps us constantly alert. You are a hand therapist and spend your time adjusting rubber bands? Look higher! You are in the business of rebuilding human lives.

REFERENCE

1. Daly, C.H., and others: The effect of pressure loading on the blood flow rate in human skin. In Kenedi, R.M., and Cowden, J.M., editors: Bed sore biomechanics, Strathclyde Bioengineering Seminars, London, 1976, The Macmillan Press Ltd.

77

Principles and methods of splinting for mobilization of joints

ELAINE EWING FESS

Although significant advances have been made in materials and techniques during recent decades, application of external devices to alter upper extremity deformity is not a contemporary concept. Early descriptions of hand splints emanate from the mid-1600s (Fig. 77-1), and surprisingly the primitive appearance of many of these appliances belies a relative sophistication of design. Obvious predecessors to current splints, these inventions often provided serial adjustment in tension through mobilizing forces applied with leather strings, chained loops, or metal screws.

Today's thermoplastic materials facilitate the construction and fitting phases of splint preparation, but these technological advancements have not automatically led to better understanding of splint design and use. Far too often a splint is exactingly reproduced from a picture without an understanding of the underlying pathologic conditions of the hand and the realistic goals expected of the splint and without utilization of the principles of mechanics, design, fit, and construction that must be correctly applied to achieve effective results. Unfortunately, this "cookbook" approach to splinting often ends in frustration, failure, and undue expense for the patient. Of paramount importance is the understanding that there are no rote splinting solutions to combatting pathologic conditions of the hand. Splints must be individually created to meet the unique needs of each patient, as evidenced by designs that incorporate the variable factors of anatomy, kinesiology, pathology, rehabilitation goals, occupation, and psychological status.

PURPOSES AND CLASSIFICATION OF MOBILIZING SPLINTS

Mobilizing splints may be used to correct existing deformity through application of gentle forces that gradually cause collagen realignment, tissue growth, and concomitant increased passive range of motion; or they may substitute for lost active motion, thereby enhancing functional use of the hand. Requiring full passive joint motion, control or substitution splints are often fabricated of more-durable, less-adjustable materials because of their expected length of use (Fig. 77-2). If full joint excursion is not present, a different type of splint is necessary to first decrease existing deformity. Splints designed to improve passive joint motion are usually temporary and should be constructed of materials that are easily altered, because of recurring configuration changes that must be made as range of motion improves.

By selecting an inappropriate design option, one can create a splint that is ineffective or that actually contributes to the existing pathologic condition. Control splints frequently do not incorporate the type of forces necessary to alter fixed deformity; conversely, correctional splint designs may temporarily impede functional use of the hand (Fig. 77-3). It is therefore imperative that a splint design accurately reflect the purpose for which the splint is intended.

Historically, splints have been classified according to purpose of application, configuration, power source, material, and anatomic site. One of the most commonly used classification systems was that of grouping splints according to inherent mechanical characteristics, resulting in two major subdivisions. Static splints had no moving components and were used to provide support and immobilization, while dynamic splints employed traction devices such as rubber bands, springs, or cords to apply corrective forces to stiffened joints. However, with the advancement of splinting experience and knowledge, the value of using "static" splints to improve range of motion through consecutive configuration changes was recognized and the limitations of this classification method became increasingly apparent.

Based on three independent variables, (1) splint forces and the planes in which they occur, (2) the anatomic site of emphasis, and (3) the primary kinematic goal of the splint, a descriptive classification system provides a more definitive means of grouping splints. Splints are described in terms of these three variables, which in essence consist of the "how," "where," and "why" of splint design and application. The first of the three variables is the complexity of the forces used within a given splint; in this regard splints can be divided into simple, compound, and complex categories. The second variable is the anatomic site to which the mobilizing forces are directed—thumb, index proximal interphalangeal joint, ring metacarpophalangeal joint, and so on. The third variable is the intent or kinematic direction of the splint—in other words, flexion, extension, rotation, or abduction. A simple finger flexion splint applies a similar mobilizing flexion force to all joints incorporated in the splint (Fig. 77-4), while a compound proximal interphalangeal flexion splint utilizes a series of differing forces to simultaneously control and mobilize the sequential joints of the digit, with the primary mobilizing force of the splint directed toward flexion of the proximal interphalangeal joint (Fig. 77-5). Simple and compound splints are designed to

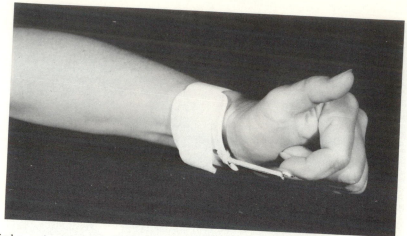

FIG. 77-4. Classified as a simple finger flexion splint, the traction device exerts a similar mobilizing force on the three successive digital joints. (From Fess, E.W., Gettle, K.S., and Strickland, J.W.: Hand splinting: principles and methods, St. Louis, 1981, The C.V. Mosby Co.)

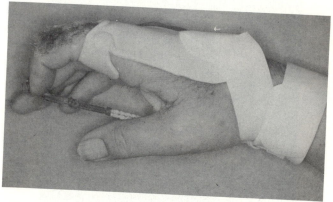

FIG. 77-5. The normal metacarpophalangeal joint is immobilized in this compound proximal interphalangeal flexion splint, allowing the flexion force to be directed to the proximal interphalangeal joint. (From Fess, E.W., Gettle, K.S., and Strickland, J.W.: Hand splinting: principles and methods, St. Louis, 1981, The C.V. Mosby Co.)

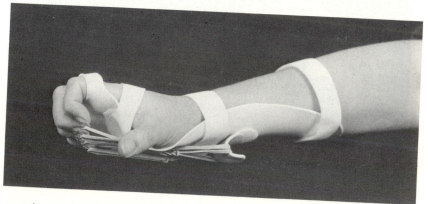

FIG. 77-6. This complex interphalangeal flexion splint controls the positions of the wrist and metacarpophalangeal joints in addition to providing mobilizing forces to the interphalangeal joints. (From Fess, E.W., Gettle, K.S., and Strickland, J.W.: Hand splinting: principles and methods, St. Louis, 1981, The C.V. Mosby Co.)

improve articular and capsular motion, but because they do not control the wrist, they do little to effect extrinsic tendon excursion. Providing an additional level of control to the open upper extremity kinetic chain, complex splints control wrist motion and therefore may be used to increase passive glide of extrinsic tendons in addition to digital joint motion (Fig. 77-6).

A descriptive splint classification based on well-defined categories that accurately and reliably groups and defines the seemingly endless array of splints is fundamental to the continued development of splinting knowledge and professional communication. This method of classification also allows the splint designer considerable latitude for creating splints that meet the unique needs of patients. Types of forces, materials, surface of application, and splint configurations are options that are left to the discretion and creativity of the person designing and fitting the splint. Latitude is important if splinting is to advance beyond the "cookbook" stage and be used to its full potential as a viable and integral aspect of hand rehabilitation.

PRINCIPLES OF MOBILIZATION SPLINTING

There are basic rules that apply to all phases of splint preparation regardless of the purpose of application and ultimate splint configuration. These principles define fundamental elements that contribute to the creation of an effectively working splint that is comfortable, durable, and cosmetically acceptable, and that successfully meets individual patient requirements. Failure to incorporate these principles may result in splints that are eventually discarded because they are uncomfortable and ineffective or, worse, splints that, if worn, cause additional damage to the hand through pressure sores, attenuation of ligaments, compression or distraction of joint surfaces, or inappropriate application of forces to healing structures. The decision to apply

mobilizing forces to an injured or diseased hand is a serious consideration; it should involve close communication between the physician, the therapist, and the patient. It is important that the goals of fitting a splint be realistic and that all those involved thoroughly understand and accept the responsibilities of such an endeavor.

Mechanical principles

Because splinting consists in external application of forces to the extremity, an understanding of basic mechanical engineering concepts is an essential prerequisite to the design, construction, and fitting of all hand splints. One may control or diminish pressure from the splint on the extremity by widening the area of force application and by increasing the mechanical advantage of lever systems. Clinically, this means that splints that are longer and wider are more comfortable, and a contiguous fit of narrow components and over bony prominences is of paramount importance (Fig. 77-7). Elimination of the translational component of an applied force by maintenance of a 90-degree angle of approach to the segment being mobilized (Fig. 77-8) is also of utmost importance when one is designing and fitting splints. This allows the full magnitude of the rotational force to be directed toward correcting the joint deformity and excludes force components that cause compression or distraction of the articular surfaces. Additionally, understanding of torque and the integrated effects of reciprocal parallel forces allows identification and control of the magnitude of corrective and stabilizing forces as they relate to the placement of specialized splint parts. The relative degree of passive mobility of successive joints also plays an important role in splint design. If mobilizing forces are dissipated at normal or less involved joints, the potential for increasing passive motion of stiff joints within the same longitudinal segment is diminished considerably. Splints

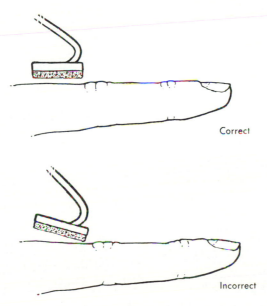

Correct

Incorrect

FIG. 77-7. To reduce pressure, narrow splint components should be carefully fitted to achieve contiguous contact between splint part and hand. (From Fess, E.W., Gettle, K.S., and Strickland, J.W.: Hand splinting: principles and methods, St. Louis, 1981, The C.V. Mosby Co.)

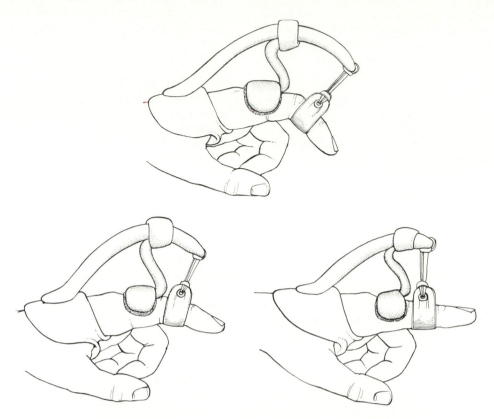

FIG. 77-8. As arc of motion improves, adjustment of outrigger is necessary to maintain 90-degree angle of pull. (From Fess, E.W., Gettle, K.S., and Strickland, J.W.: Hand splinting: principles and methods, St. Louis, 1981, The C.V. Mosby Co.)

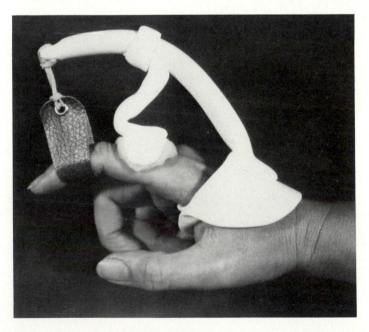

FIG. 77-9. A compound splint allows the mobilizing force to be directed to a single joint when relative joint motion is dissimilar along the digital ray. (From Fess, E.W., Gettle, K.S., and Strickland, J.W.: Hand splinting: principles and methods, St. Louis, 1981, The C.V. Mosby Co.)

therefore must be designed to apply corrective forces to only those joints that lack passive motion (Fig. 77-9). Finally, for a more effective method of increasing splint durability than the retrospective trussing of layers of plastic, one may increase material strength by designing contour into the splint. Mechanical principles determine splint effectiveness, comfort, and durability and should be carefully incorporated into the design, construction, and fitting phases of splint preparation.

Design principles

The principles of design may be divided into two basic groups—general considerations and specific considerations. General principles incorporate broad concepts that result in a splint that is practical for both the patient and the therapist, while the more specific guidelines are concerned with the unique pathologic conditions exhibited by individual patients. Factors such as age, ability to accept responsibility, independence, and occupational demands contribute to the overall design of a splint, as do anticipated utilization time and prescribed exercise regimens. Splints should allow maximum function and sensation and should be as simple in design and appearance as possible. Construction time should also be within reason. Specific principles of design encompass concepts that individualize splints to the existing requirements of pathology, anatomy, and kinesiology. Is the splint intended to substitute for absent active motion, or is it designed to correct existing deformity? Will elastic or inelastic forces be more effective? What splint components are required to control which joints, and what type of mobilizing forces will provide the greatest potential for increasing passive motion of stiff joints? Which mechanical principles should be utilized to increase effectiveness, comfort, and durability? These and many other questions must be anticipated and answered before design concepts reach the finality of pattern construction.

Component designing lends an organized and rational approach to creating splints that meet individual patient needs. Problems are identified and splint parts are mentally assembled to control or diminish the projected pathologic situation. This approach requires that the designer be fully cognizant of the uses and ramifications of each splint component. For example, low-profile outriggers have been shown to lose adjustment more quickly than do high-profile outriggers (Fig. 77-10). This however, is a viable concept only if one is dealing with correctional forces. If the purpose of a splint is to substitute for active motion, full passive joint motion is a prerequisite and the need for sequential adjustments to accommodate motion improvements is nonexistent. Low-profile outriggers are appropriate design options for control or substitution splints because sequential adjustments are not needed. Conversely, high-profile outriggers provide longer increments of near 90-degree angle of pull than do the low-profile designs, indicating that for correctional splints the higher design option will require fewer adjustments as improvements in motion are gained. Whether this is an important concept in the designing of a correctional splint is entirely dependent on the patient's capacity to return to the clinic for adjustments and the time demands of the therapist's case load.

Splint designing should never be approached in a rote or routine manner. Although patients may present with similar diagnoses, the pathologic conditions presented are unique, as are the patient's intellectual and emotional capacities to deal with injury and dysfunction. One must approach each case anew in order to attain maximum rehabilitation potential, using splints designed efficaciously, realistically, and practically for all those involved.

Construction principles

Observing proper construction principles and selecting equipment and methods appropriate to the materials utilized will help to ensure the durability, cosmesis, comfort, and usefulness of the finished splint. Splint corners should be

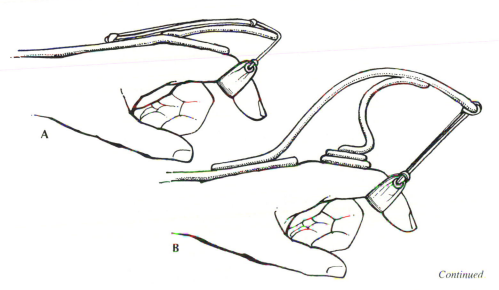

Continued

FIG. 77-10. Schematic representations of low-profile outrigger (**A**) and high-profile outrigger (**B**). Comparison of low- and high-profile outriggers indicates that as passive motion improves, the high-profile design maintains a better angle of pull without adjustment than does the low-profile design (**C** and **D**).

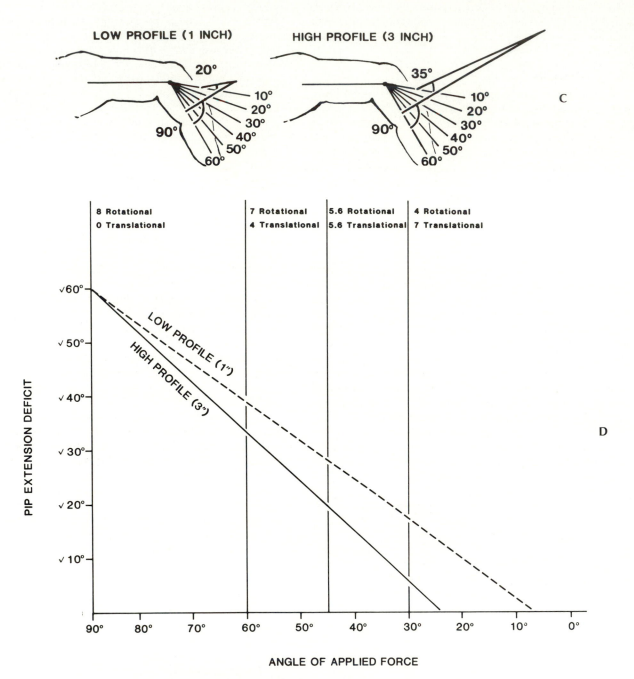

LOW PROFILE (1 INCH)

20°

90°

10°
20°
30°
40°
50°
60°

HIGH PROFILE (3 INCH)

35°

90°

10°
20°
30°
40°
50°
60°

C

| 8 Rotational | 7 Rotational | 5.6 Rotational | 4 Rotational |
| 0 Translational | 4 Translational | 5.6 Translational | 7 Translational |

PIP EXTENSION DEFICIT

√60°
√50°
√40°
√30°
√20°
√10°

LOW PROFILE (1″)
HIGH PROFILE (3″)

90° 80° 70° 60° 50° 40° 30° 20° 10° 0°

ANGLE OF APPLIED FORCE

D

Fig. 77-10, cont'd. For legend see p. 859.

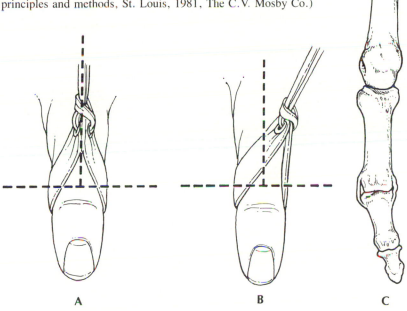

FIG. 77-11. To avoid attenuation of a collateral ligament because of unequal force application (**C**), a mobilizing force should be applied in a direction that is perpendicular to the rotational axis of the joint (**B**). **A,** Correct alignment. (From Fess, E.W., Gettle, K.S., and Strickland, J.W.: Hand splinting: principles and methods, St. Louis, 1981, The C.V. Mosby Co.)

A　　　　　　　　　　B　　　　　　　　　　C

uniformly rounded, edges smoothed, joined surfaces stabilized, rivets finished, and straps and padding secured. Mechanical principles should be analyzed and incorporated to enhance durability and comfort, and careful adherence to safety precautions when one is working with splinting equipment is important. The equipment and the type and temperature of heat should be selected to meet the demands of the splinting material used. Failure to adhere to construction guidelines may result in splint disuse because of patient discomfort, lack of acceptance, or splint breakage from mechanical failures, all of which represent loss of time and needless expense for both the patient and the members of the rehabilitation team.

Principles of fit

Fitting principles may be divided into four groups—mechanical, anatomic, kinesiologic, and technical. Mechanical factors include utilization of forces that are perpendicular both to the bone being mobilized and to the axis of joint rotation (Fig. 77-11). When traction is applied simultaneously to several joints within a digit, care must be taken to ensure that the pull is perpendicular to the rotational axis of each joint. Additionally, pressure reduction through contiguous fit and application of lever systems in fitting splint components is important. Anatomic factors encompass the use of skin creases as guidelines for splint boundaries, identification and adaptation to bony prominences, support of longitudinal and transverse arches, understanding of ligamentous stress, and proper alignment of splint and anatomic joint axes. A hand in motion presents a multiplicity of dif-

fering external configurations and internal muscle dynamics as it moves through various planes. Kinesiologic considerations, which include kinematic and kinetic principles, are very important to splint design and fitting phases. Splint parts must be fitted to allow motion, and they must be placed appropriately to control or augment motion, depending on individual requirements. Technical considerations emphasize efficiency and include developing patient rapport, developing work skills, and adapting methods to the materials used. A splint must be continually reevaluated to ensure a proper fit. As the hand heals and motion improves, one must recognize changes that occur and for which appropriate adaptations must be incorporated into the splint. Failure to do so will invariably render the splint less effective, impeding the advancement of the rehabilitation process.

CONCLUSION

Mobilizing splints play an important role in the rehabilitation process of the diseased or injured hand. These splints may provide correctional or substitutional forces and are designed and fitted according to specific requirements unique to each patient. It should also be emphasized that splinting programs should be augmented with appropriate exercise routines and activities that encourage functional use of the extremity. Splints alone do not produce the active motion necessary for hand use. It is the astute combination of passive motion, provided through splinting endeavors, and active exercise programs that forms the foundation for hand rehabilitation techniques and that allows the patient to return to a productive life-style.

78

Spring-wire splinting of the proximal interphalangeal joint

JUDY C. COLDITZ

HISTORY

The proximal interphalangeal joint is vulnerable to injury, since it lies midway between the long lever arms of the proximal and middle phalanges. Its tight anatomic construction and intricate anatomy are unforgiving of forces crossing it in any plane but the normal flexion or extension. Residual flexion contracture of the proximal interphalangeal joint is a frequent complication after phalangeal fractures, proximal interphalangeal joint dislocation, volar plate injury, flexor tendon repairs, chronic boutonnière deformity, partial or complete tear of a collateral ligament, or major hand trauma resulting in edema and immobilization.[2,6,8] The powerful flexor tendon system with its efficient pulley system is far more effective in gaining flexion of the proximal interphalangeal joint than the primarily intrinsically powered dorsal hood mechanism is in gaining extension. The last range of full proximal interphalangeal joint extension can be gained most effectively by a gentle prolonged stretch to the tissues toward full extension in order to reestablish the balance of motion. Proximal interphalangeal joint splinting is effectively achieved by a low-profile spring-wire splint incorporating only the finger, as first described by Capener.[4,5] This is a splint of a three-point design with spring coils lying at the axis of the proximal interphalangeal joint laterally (Fig. 78-1). This design is frequently referred to as the Capener splint,[7,9-12] and many commercially available splints using the lateral coil are sold as "Capener" splints. Bunnell illustrates the use of both clock-spring splints and spring-wire splints to extend proximal interphalangeal joint flexion contractures.[3] Wynn Parry illustrates in detail the construction of spring-wire finger splints after Capener but describes the spring as being used primarily for resistance for finger flexion after flexor tendon repair or for full-time wear for immobilization in extension, as with a boutonnière deformity.[11] The gauge of wire, the increasing diameter of the coils, and the number of coils described by Wynn Parry provide a lower tension than the technique described below. The technique described below is of greater ease and speed of construction than the soldering of tin as described by Wynn Parry. The splint described is designed with the goal of correcting mild flexion deformities of the proximal interphalangeal joint.

CUSTOM SPLINTING

The advantage of the custom-made splint over the commercially available splint is obvious in that the length of the splint can be made to exactly match the length of the available lever arms and the coils can be located at the exact axis of the joint. Additionally the dorsal piece lying over the proximal phalanx can be of maximum size, and it ends exactly at the axis of the proximal interphalangeal joint (Fig. 78-1), thus distributing pressure well on the dorsum of the finger, where there is little natural padding. The Velcro strap on the volar aspect of the distal end of the middle phalanx offers the patient adjustability of the tension so as to keep it within comfortable tolerance. Since the resting position of the splint force arms is at 0 degrees of extension, this design does not have the danger of hyperextending the proximal interphalangeal joint, as the reverse knuckle bender can. The use of spring wire eliminates the fatigue factor one encounters with the rubber band outrigger systems, and therefore the splint is effective for long-term use without adjustments.

The lateral coil system is effective only for flexion contractures of approximately 45 degrees or less, since a severely contracted finger will provide a counterforce that is at a right angle to the dorsal splint piece and thus the splint itself slips distally, being ineffective in gaining proximal interphalangeal joint extension. If clinical examination of a flexion contracture slightly greater than 45 degrees reveals a springy joint that responds to passive stretch, one can perhaps begin with the spring-wire design with realistic anticipation of early gains. The spring can be fitted initially so that the force arms of the splint rest in a somewhat flexed position, decreasing the tension being applied on the joint. At the next therapy visit it is often possible to bend the wire up to the 0-degree resting position, because the tolerance to the force has increased. In cases of severe long-standing flexion contractures of the proximal interphalangeal joints, one needs to devise a molded splint base with outrigger arms in order to provide effective extension force.

Not only does this three-point design provide an efficient extension force, but also by its low profile design it is easily tolerated by the patient. It allows movement of the meta-

862

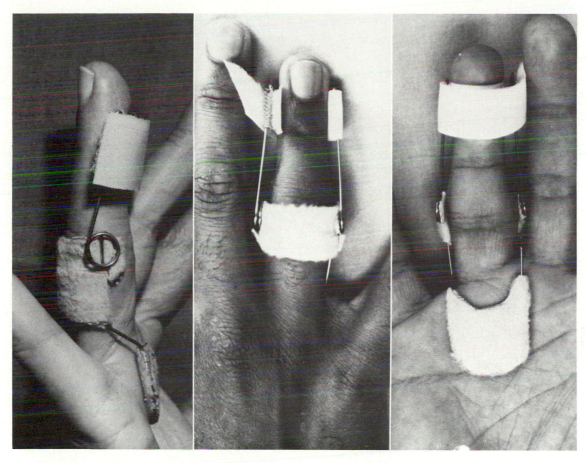

FIG. 78-1. Multiple views of low-profile spring-wire splint for proximal interphalangeal joint extension.

carpophalangeal joint of the splinted finger and does not impede motion of the other fingers. The size of the splint allows it to be carried in the pocket for easy and frequent application. Two splints may be worn on adjacent fingers (Fig. 78-2), but if three fingers are involved, a hand-based splint with outrigger system is recommended for ease of application, removal, and diminished bulk between the fingers.

Patients frequently state that the wearing of the splint offers a distinct relief to the tight feeling within the joint, and they demonstrate an eagerness to wear the splint. For these reasons this splint is considered to have a high rate of patient compliance. For the experienced therapist it requires no longer than 10 minutes to construct.

INSTRUCTIONS FOR WEAR

As with any dynamic splinting program the forces applied must be tolerable over an extended period of time in order to effect permanent alteration of the collagen formation. With a weaker extensor mechanism, as opposed to a stronger flexor system, it is important to instruct the patient that after use of the splint the flexion deformity will recur. Explain to the patient that this is a normal phenomenon and that a period of stretch may gain full extension but that it will not

yet have permanently relieved the tightness of the tissues. Patients who have full flexion of the proximal interphalangeal joint are frequently instructed to wear the extension splint at night and are advised to observe how long it is after removal of the splint before the deformity recurs. If it recurs during the waking hours, the patient is then instructed in regard to periods of wear during the day, with the splint being removed for flexion exercises. Instruct the patient that the goal is to be able to maintain full extension for longer and longer periods when the hand is out of the splint. When only a slight lag develops after a full day out of the splint, it is appropriate to go to a routine of night splinting only. These instructions vary depending on the nature and extent of the injury and whether flexion range is also limited and flexion splinting and/or exercises need to balance off the extension force. Only an experienced hand therapist can evaluate the balance of motion and the amount of tightness and devise an appropriate splinting schedule.

CONSTRUCTION OF SPLINT
Materials

The materials used for the construction of the spring-wire splint are readily available (Fig. 78-3).

FIG. 78-2. Two spring-wire splints can easily be tolerated on adjacent fingers.

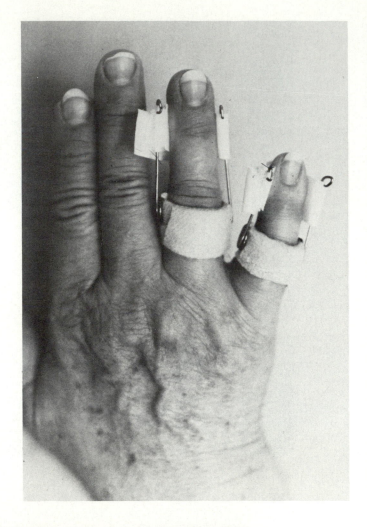

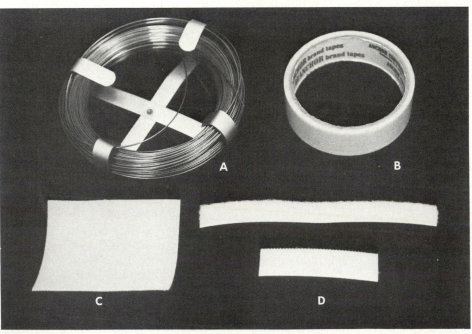

FIG. 78-3. Materials for spring-wire splint include, *A*, spring-steel piano wire; *B*, 1-inch filament tape; *C*, adhesive moleskin; and *D*, Velcro loop and pile.

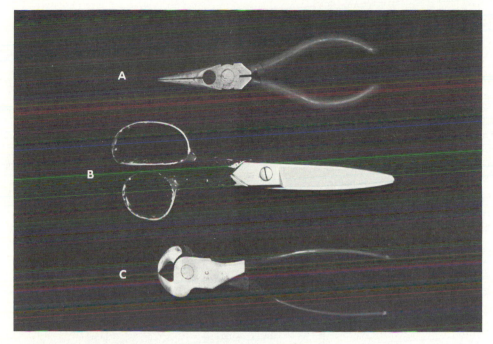

FIG. 78-4. Tools required for making spring-wire splint include, *A*, flat-jawed needlenosed pliers; *B*, leather scissors; and *C*, end-cutting nippers.

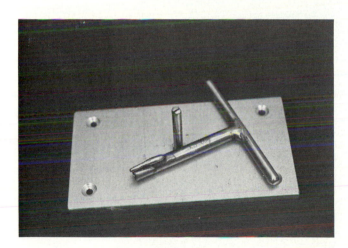

FIG. 78-5. Special jig for turning coils for spring-wire splint.

Spring-steel wire of 17.0 gauge (0.039 inch in diameter) is recommended and may be obtained from a local piano tuner or a piano supply company. One-pound coils (approximately 248 feet) are available and allow easy procurement of an appropriate length of wire. Spring steel has an inherent resistance to deforming forces and therefore must be overbent in order to obtain the desired shape. Avoidance of sharp bends will prevent the wire from snapping.

Filament tape used for packaging is used to cover the wire superstructure and may be obtained from any office supply company. A 1-inch width is most workable for this technique, and it is important that no substitutions be made, because the filaments provide the necessary strength for long-term durability.

Adhesive-backed moleskin, available from splinting or surgical suppliers, is used to cover the filament tape for both its padding and cosmetic effect.

Velcro fasteners are used for the distal strap, with the adhesive-backed hook providing easy attachment of the strap to the wire and the Velcro loop providing the strap itself. Velcro that is half an inch wide provides the least waste for this technique.

Tools

As with any technique it is the correct tool that creates ease and efficiency in the construction (Fig. 78-4).

Firmly constructed flat-jawed needlenosed pliers are necessary to bend the resistant spring steel. Smooth or round jaws allow rotation of the wire. Six- or 8-inch flat-jawed needlenosed pliers with teeth are recommended. Wire-cutting pliers called "end-cutting nippers," which have a broad cutting area, are helpful, since the last step of construction requires cutting of the wire where it is inaccessible to the cutting jaws on the needlenosed pliers.

Sharp scissors with short blades so as to be effective in cutting at the tip of the scissors are necessary for easy trimming and cutting in the small tight areas. Leather shears are excellent for this purpose.

The coil for the spring wire is effectively turned by the use of a special jig (Fig. 78-5) fashioned after the design illustrated by Wynn Parry.[11] Use of the jig allows one to turn a tight and compact coil, which is difficult when attempted manually with pliers. The dimensions of the jig are specifically for the 17-gauge wire used for the proximal interphalangeal joint splint, although the jig may be used for other splint designs. The jig dimensions may be obtained from me, or the jig itself may be obtained commercially.*

Procedure

1. Cut a length of 17-gauge piano wire approximately 14 inches in length.
2. Form a ∪-shape in the wire by holding the wire with the pliers and bending the wire gently with the fingers. Keep the wire and the pliers moving back and forth to create a smooth-curved shape (Fig. 78-6).
3. After the initial curve is made in the wire, it will retain

*Available from Roylan Manufacturing Co., P.O. Box 555, Menomonee Falls, Wisc. 15215.

the curved shape. With the fingertips apply a force to bend the wire in the direction opposite the resting curve. Slide the fingertips down the wire while applying this force to straighten the wire (Fig. 78-7).

4. Working on the volar aspect of the finger, measure the wire shape and adjust it so that it is slightly wider than the width of the finger (Fig. 78-8). It is important at this stage and throughout the splintmaking that the wire be parallel in all planes. At this stage it should lie evenly on a flat surface.
5. With the wire ∪-shape positioned on the volar aspect of the finger and the curve resting at the distal palmar crease level, mark the point of the wire just distal to the finger-web space (Fig. 78-8).

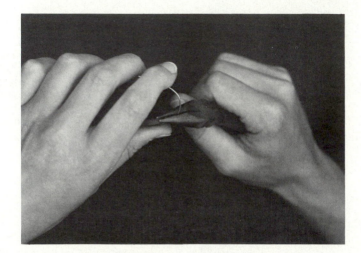

FIG. 78-6. Step 2. Bending initial curve.

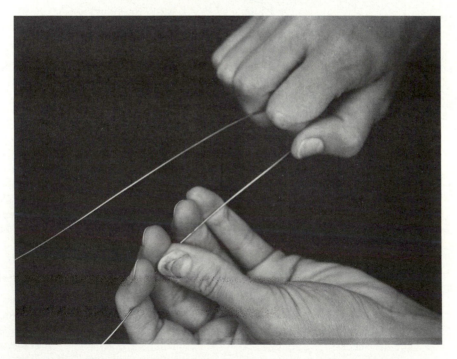

FIG. 78-7. Step 3. Straightening wire ends, making ∪ shape of wire.

6. Bend the wire at a 60-degree angle so that it is between the fingers. Pay special attention to the finger webs, and measure carefully on both the radial and ulnar aspects, since they differ on each finger. Hold the wire with the wide part of the jaws of the pliers, and bend the wire sharply at the edge of the pliers by applying force with the fingers (Fig. 78-9).

7. Bend the wire again at a 60-degree angle so that it now lies in a position midlaterally on the finger. Again check to be sure the wire is parallel (Fig. 78-10).

8. Replace the splint on the volar aspect of the finger, and mark the location of the axis of the proximal interphalangeal joint. One easily determines the axis by locating the apex of the middle volar finger crease.

9. Place this point of the wire in the middle of the slot in the jig base (Fig. 78-11). Place the jig handle over the jig base, and while maintaining a downward pressure on the wire, turn two complete revolutions (Fig. 78-12). It is important during this procedure to hold the splint superstructure with a bit of torque so that the coil is turned at exactly a 90-degree angle to the axis of the parallel wires. Since the wire superstructure cannot rest directly under the coil being turned, the coil will not be parallel unless this torque is applied (Fig. 78-12). It is important to remember that for extension splinting of the proximal interphalangeal joint the coil is always turned toward the volar aspect of the finger.

10. Replace the splint with one coil turned on the volar aspect of the finger, and mark the remaining axis location (Fig. 78-13).

11. Repeat step 9 to turn the second coil (Fig. 78-14).

12. Pad the base of the splint by wrapping six to eight layers of filament tape around the curved area. Trim it with scissors to fit the shape of the wire curve, and cut out a curved shape between the beginning of the coil and the bend of the wire that goes down at the finger-web space (Fig. 78-15).

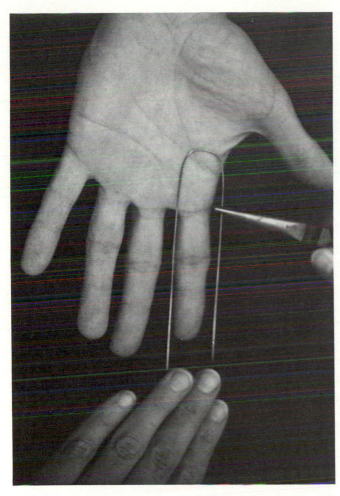

FIG. 78-8. Step 4, measuring width of splint superstructure, and step 5, marking location of bend to carry wire to lateral aspect of finger.

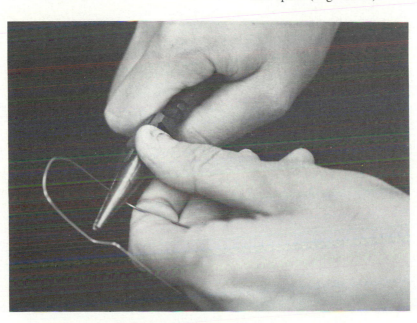

FIG. 78-9. Steps 6 and 7. Bending wire at 60-degree angles.

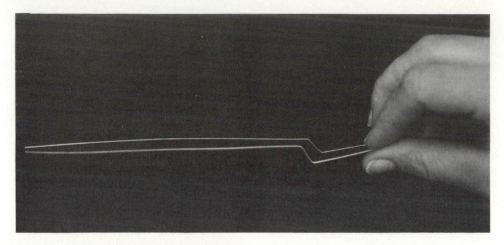

FIG. 78-10. Steps 6 and 7. Lateral view of parallel wire superstructure.

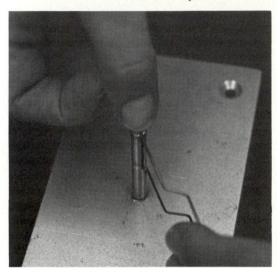

FIG. 78-11. Step 9. Placement of joint axis location in center of jig slot.

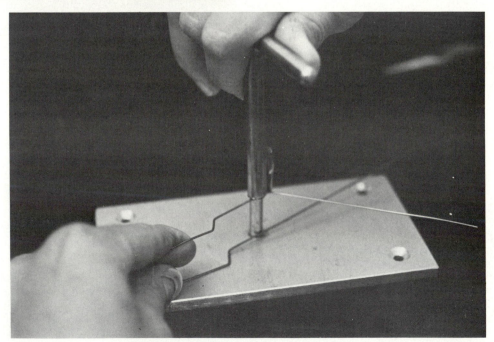

FIG. 78-12. Step 9. Turning initial coil.

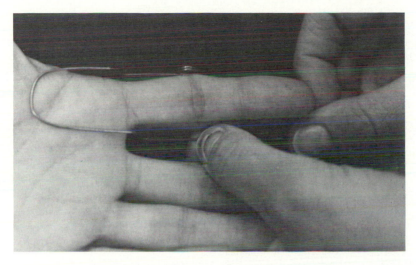

FIG. 78-13. Step 10. Marking second joint axis location.

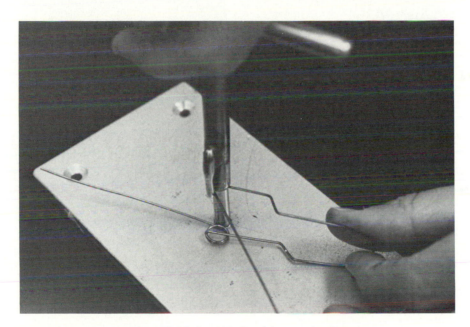

FIG. 78-14. Step 11. Turning second coil.

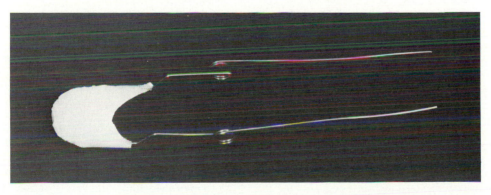

FIG. 78-15. Step 12. Covering proximal area with tape padding.

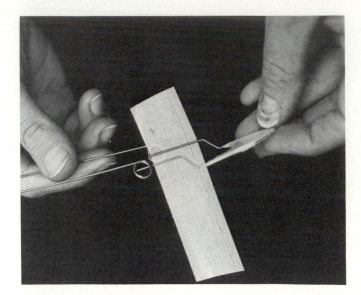

FIG. 78-16. Step 13. Applying dorsal hood piece.

FIG. 78-16. Step 13. Applying dorsal hood piece.

FIG. 78-17. Step 13. Applying dorsal hood piece.

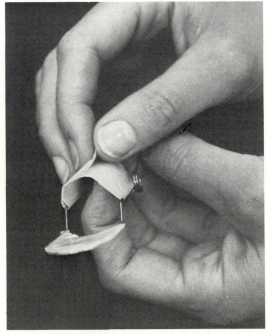

13. Slide the tape under the coil, with the sticky side of the tape toward the splint (Fig. 78-16). Wrap tape around the opposite side, and once again ease it under the coil. The nonsticky side of the tape should lie against the skin of the finger. Fit the splint on the patient's finger, and adjust the length of tape so that the coils lie exactly in the midlateral position of the finger, at the proximal interphalangeal joint axis. After adjusting the length of the tape, attach it to itself securely (Fig. 78-17).

14. Replace the splint on the finger, locating coils at the axis of the joint. Slide a piece of adhesive-backed Velcro hook (½ by 1½ inches) between one side of the finger and the lateral wire, with the sticky side toward the wire (Fig. 78-18). Fold the Velcro over the wire at the level of the distal interphalangeal joint crease. Adhere the Velcro to itself, making sure that the unit is pointing volarly.

15. Apply a ½ inch by 4- to 5-inch piece of Velcro loop to the Velcro hook on the side touching the volar aspect of the finger. Take this piece of Velcro up dorsally between the finger and the wire, and loop the Velcro over the wire, carrying it volarly again to adhere to the Velcro hook (Fig. 78-19). The Velcro thus forms a sling under the finger and allows adjustability, since the sling length can be determined by the amount of pull exerted on the length of the Velcro loop.

16. With the splint still on the finger, mark the wire at the point where the splint should end (Fig. 78-19). The point should be just distal to the distal interphalangeal joint crease, since the strap should lie directly under the distal interphalangeal joint.

17. Remove the splint and turn a tight coil around the end of the needlenosed pliers at the point marked for the end of the splint (Fig. 78-20). Make sure to have a few inches of wire to work with, because it will make the

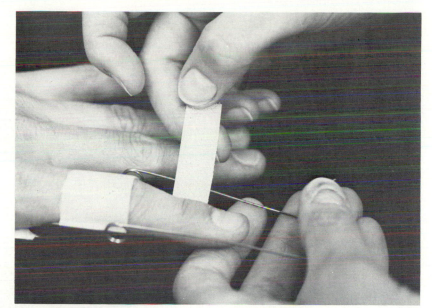

FIG. 78-18. Step 14. Applying Velcro hook.

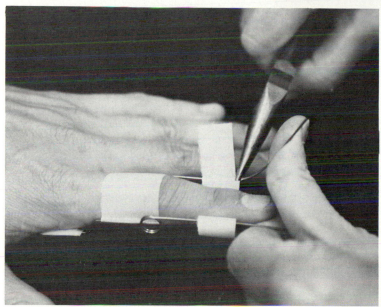

FIG. 78-19. Step 15, Applying Velcro loop to complete strap, and Step 16, marking end of splint.

FIG. 78-20. Step 17. Making end coil.

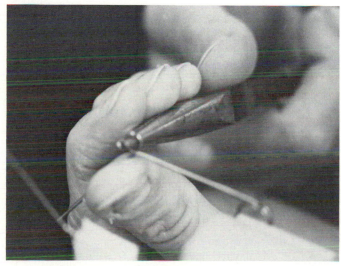

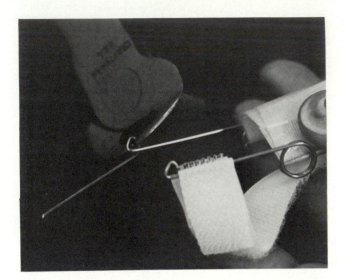

Fig. 78-21. Step 17. Cutting end coil.

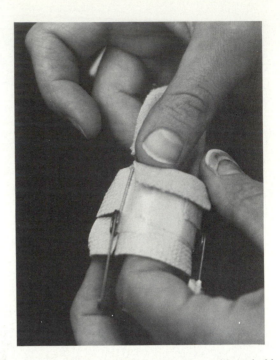

Fig. 78-22. Step 18. Covering taped areas with moleskin.

turning much easier. Cut off the wire with the end-cutting nippers after the coil is turned (Fig. 78-21).

18. Cover the taped areas with adhesive-backed moleskin, trimming it close and making sure no seams are on the inside of the splint (Fig. 78-22).

19. Apply the splint to the patient's finger, and check for proper fit, adequate circulation, and adequate distribution of pressure (Fig. 78-23).

20. Require the patient to apply and remove the splint independently. It is mandatory that the patient be able to demonstrate correct application of the splint.

Splint adjustments and modifications

As with any custom-made splint, minor adjustments and attention to detail ensure the long-term comfort of the splint on the patient. One of the most common problems is the bulbous, enlarged state of the proximal interphalangeal joint after injury. Since the finger is normally cone shaped, the enlarged proximal interphalangeal joint will receive pressure when the distal strap is tightened, since the tip of the finger is narrower than the joint (Fig. 78-24). This situation can be particularly bothersome, since the collateral ligaments of the joint frequently have been injured and direct pressure over the area elicits exquisite tenderness. This problem can be alleviated by incorporating a piece of thin plastic or cardboard material over the dorsal hood area, reinforcing it so that it becomes like an arch and does not easily compress. A small piece of splinting material molded under the distal strap so that it holds the ends of the splint apart can also alleviate this problem. It has the additional advantage of better distributing pressure at the tip. Frequently the leading edge of the Velcro strap will be constricting to the distal pulp, and this molded pad greatly increases comfort (Fig.

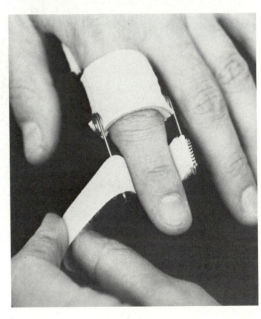

Fig. 78-23. Step 19. Applying splint to check for fit, circulation, and pressure.

78-25). An enlarged proximal interphalangeal joint may also be a problem when a spring-wire splint is fitted after a proximal phalanx fracture, since frequently the shape of the bone is deformed and one must adjust the dorsal hood piece so that it conforms to the bulbous shape of the proximal phalanx.

Although by far the most common use of a spring-wire splint is to correct a proximal interphalangeal joint flexion contracture, it can be modified to achieve other interphalangeal joint motions. It can easily be adapted to fit the interphalangeal joint of the thumb (Fig. 78-26). The direc-

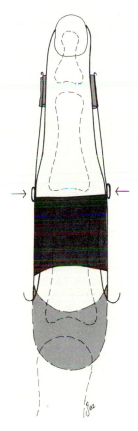

FIG. 78-24. Pressure occurs over bulbous collateral ligament area when distal strap is tightened.

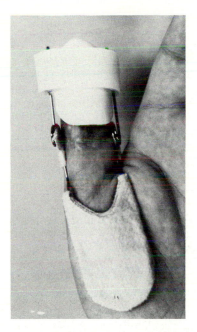

FIG. 78-25. Use of a piece of thermoplastic splinting material to maintain width of splint and better distribute pressure over distal part of pulp.

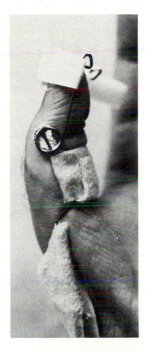

FIG. 78-26. Use of spring wire in reverse direction to achieve first ranges of flexion of interphalangeal joint of thumb.

tion of pull may be reversed for either thumb or finger interphalangeal joint flexion. It is important to note, however, that this design is effective to gain only the first ranges of flexion, since the line of pull will force the splint to slide off the finger in the latter ranges of flexion. Numerous other splint designs using spring wire are applicable to hand splinting, for which one should refer to other authors.[1,4]

CONCLUSION

The low-profile spring-wire splint first described by Capener is of significant clinical value because of its easy tolerance by the patient, which is due to its adjustability. A custom-made splint that exactly fits the length of the finger and applies force at the axis of the joint frequently offers advantages over a commercially available splint. The steps for construction are offered with the hope that this splint can become part of the armamentarium of the skilled hand therapist.

REFERENCES

1. Barr, N.: The hand: principles and techniques of simple splintmaking in rehabilitation, Boston, 1978, Butterworth Publishers.
2. Bowers, W.H., Wolf, J.W., Jr., Nehil, J.L., and Bittinger, S.: The proximal interphalangeal joint volar plate. I. Anatomical and biomechanical study, J. Hand Surg. 5:79, 1980.
3. Bunnell, S.: Active splinting of the hand, J. Bone Joint Surg. 28:732, 1946.
4. Capener, N.: Lively splints, Physiotherapy 53:371, 1967.
5. Capener, N.: Physiological rest, Br. Med. J. 2:761, 1946.
6. Kuczynski, K.: The proximal interphalangeal joint: anatomy and causes of stiffness in the fingers, J. Bone Joint Surg. 50B:656, 1968.
7. Mackin, E.J., and Maiorano, L.: Postoperative therapy following staged flexor tendon reconstruction. In Hunter, J.M., Schneider, L.H., Mackin, E.J., and Bell, J.A., editors: Rehabilitation of the hand, St. Louis, 1978, The C.V. Mosby Co., pp. 247-261.
8. McCue, F.C., Honner, R., Johnson, M.C., and others: Athletic injuries of the proximal interphalangeal joint requiring surgical treatment, J. Bone Joint Surg. 52A:937, 1970.
9. Wilson, R.E., and Carter, M.S.: Joint injuries in the hand: preservation of proximal interphalangeal joint function. In Hunter, J.M., Schneider, L.H., Mackin, E.J., and Bell, J.A., editors: Rehabilitation of the hand, St. Louis, 1978, The C.V. Mosby Co.
10. Wilson, R.E., and Carter, M.S.: Management of hand fractures. In Hunter, J.M., Schneider, L.H., Mackin, E.J., and Bell, J.A., editors Rehabilitation of the hand, St. Louis, 1978, The C.V. Mosby Co.
11. Wynn Parry, C.B.: Rehabilitation of the hand, ed. 3, Boston, 1978, Butterworth Publishers.
12. Wynn Parry, C.B., Harper, D., Fletcher, I., and others: New types of lively splints for peripheral nerve lesions affecting the hand, Hand 2:31, 1970.

79

Plaster cylinder casting for contractures of the interphalangeal joints

JUDITH A. BELL

Plaster cylinder serial casting of the interphalangeal joints of the fingers began as an idea in The Hand Rehabilitation Center established in the 1950s in Vellore, India, by Paul Brand, M.D.[1] It began in the concept of the "inevitability of gradualness" that was to be the hallmark of the center and of Dr. Brand's work. Familiar with the traditional use of force and then of "wedge casting" of clubfeet in children, Dr. Brand began to understand that the early benefits of force were often undone by later contraction of the deep tissue scarring. He felt sure that there must be a way of correcting a deformity without such force on the tissues and on the child. Under his direction, the infant was not fed before having treatment but was put to nursing while Gypsona* plaster of paris was placed in single layers directly on the foot to be corrected. While the plaster was setting, the foot was gradually moved into a corrective position until the child turned his eyes and "looked" without stopping its feeding. Correction of the foot would always stop before the point at which the child would begin to cry. The foot would be held in this position gently but firmly, and the plaster allowed to set. Successive and frequent recastings would be by the same procedure. The method was so successful that the idea was applied to the interphalangeal joints of severely clawed hands found in patients with leprosy. (Patients with leprosy often develop a neuritis of the peripheral nerves resulting in an anesthetic clawed hand with essentially normal extrinsic musculature.) The technique met with equal success and has continued as a successful treatment technique for interphalangeal joint stiffness in India up to now (Fig. 79-1).

As explained by Brand, the technique is not one of progressive "stretching" but of "growth."[†] The cells of the contracted tissue are stimulated to grow and become internally rearranged or modified by being held in the maximum possible extension. This is why the process takes time and the position must be held for a period of time—there is no chance for the remodeling to take place in an hour or two. Each day or every other day the joint can be recast, having

gained a few more degrees, taking advantage of the vital living cell modification.

Steve Kolumban,[3,4] a therapist working with Brand at the Christian Medical College and Hospital in Vellore, India, conducted two studies with leprosy patients supportive of the cylinder casting of contracted proximal interphalangeal joints of the hand in 1967. In a study of 50 samples from 24 outpatients with contractures of the interphalangeal joints, Kolumban compared splinting with regular physiotherapy technique. Regular physiotherapy given to 25 of the patients consisted of wax baths, oil massage, and exercise (passive and active-assistive). At the end of the study the group with the splinting was significantly superior. The percentage of degrees straightened from the total possible number was 45.7% with splinting and 0.9% without splinting. Out of the 25 fingers in the group without splinting, 12 joints ended with a greater contracture than that with which they began.

In a study of 26 patients with 52 samples of contracted interphalangeal joints, Kolumban compared cylinder serial casting with dynamic splinting.[2] An attempt was made in the study to match fingers from both groups into pairs of six variables: age, contracture angle, joint resiliency, length of the finger, length of splinting, and applied straightening force. A straightening force of 250 gm was applied in both

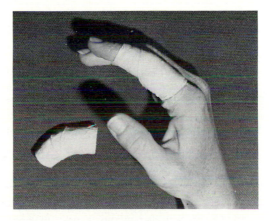

FIG. 79-1. Progressive casting of index interphalangeal joint into extension.

*Acme Cotton Products Co., Inc., Valley Stream, NY 11582.
†Brand, P.W.: The reconstruction of the hand in leprosy, Ann. R. Coll. Surg. Engl. 11:350, 1952.

875

methods of splinting. At the end of the study, the results showed a strong indication that the casting was superior to dynamic splinting. The percentage of degrees straightened from the total possible with serial cylinder casting was 47.8% and with dynamic splinting, 34.9%. Injuries from splinting (many of the patients had anesthetic hands) were none for the cylinder splinting and 7 for the dynamic splinting.

Brand brought the technique for cylinder serial casting of the joints to the United States in the treatment of leprosy patients at the United States Public Health Service Hospital in Carville, Louisiana. The adaptation of this technique of treatment for joint stiffness from causes other than leprosy was always advocated by Brand, and under his influence the technique began to be utilized for patients with a wide variety of conditions resulting in joint contractures of the hand. The technique was used at the New Orleans United States Public Health Service Hospital in 1973, and later at the Hand Rehabilitation Center, Ltd., in Philadelphia, Pennsylvania. Conditions in which the casting has been used successfully to reduce contractures include arthritis, reflex sympathetic dystrophy, Dupuytren's contracture, congenital contractures, joint dislocations, burns, boutonnière deformities, swan-neck deformities, and contractures after fractures and tendon repairs.

INDICATIONS FOR CASTING

As in the use of any type of splinting, the casting is not used for patients responding well to simple positioning, range of motion, and physiotherapy techniques. For patients with mild contractures, often a simple augmentation to therapy using night gutter splints or traction splints will be all that is necessary to achieve desired results. For moderate-to-severe contractures, in most cases I prefer cylinder casting. I have used dynamic splinting methods since 1968 and cylinder casting since 1973. Experience with the casting teaches the following:

1. The supplies needed are simple and readily available, making the method of treatment available and adaptable to a variety of circumstances—hospital wards, intensive care units, and so on.

2. Once the plaster is applied, the joint has no choice except to stay at the position casted, whereas dynamic splinting comes out of adjustment easily either by itself or by the patient. Dynamic splinting has to be continually checked to assure that traction is at the angle desired and the specific gram traction desired. The one certain thing about rubber bands used for traction is that they do get old quickly and must be changed frequently. Even after slow traction with splinting, the tissues often will not tolerate enough traction to prevent an annoying recurrence of joint stiffness that can compromise an otherwise expected progressive improvement in range.

3. Swelling is never increased by the plaster cast and is often decreased because the cast keeps the joint quiet for periods of rest. Dynamic splinting can cause an increase in swelling—if not by the amount of traction, then by decreased circulation resulting from the restriction of the finger cuff.

4. Since casting is not a stretching or a wedging, pain is not increased by cylinder casting and is often decreased.

This is particularly important in patients with reflex sympathetic dystrophy, where even a slight increase in pain is a step in the wrong direction. Traction by dynamic splinting can cause soreness, particularly with hypersensitive fingers.

5. Cylinder casting can be used over lacerations and ulcers. The technique is used in leprosy patients to protect insensitive fingers so that they can heal without further trauma.

6. Cylinder casting can be used in the treatment of old fixed deformities and in fact is indicated where the use of dynamic traction often fails.

TECHNIQUE

Supplies needed

1. Twelve- to 15-inch strip of plaster bandage, 1 inch wide
2. Scissors—suture or small bandage
3. Water—small paper cup
4. Paper towel
5. Tube of lanolin or other oil

Instructions

1. Prepare finger to be casted with lanolin.
2. Dip the plaster strip in water and drain excess water on paper towel.
3. Fold ⅛-inch edge on plaster strip for 2 inches to make a smooth edge (Fig. 79-2).
4. Begin wrapping the finger with the folded edge of the plaster strip just distal to the metacarpophalangeal joint. Overlap the plaster strip as you wrap distally to the fingertip. Two overlapping wraps of plaster is enough to make a firm cast (Fig. 79-3).
5. Support the finger in extension while wrapping if trying for interphalangeal extension; support the finger in flexion while wrapping if trying for interphalangeal flexion.
6. Use a constant motion of your fingers and thumb in a clockwise direction to maintain the position of the finger and to smooth the cast (Fig. 79-4).
7. Wrap to the distal interphalangeal crease if later distal interphalangeal movement with use of the cast is desired. Wrap past the distal interphalangeal crease if
   a. The profundus tendon is tight when casting for extension.
   b. The extensor mechanism is tight when casting for flexion.
   c. The improvement in range of movement is also desired at the distal interphalangeal joint.
8. To finish the cast at the distal tip, fold the edge of plaster strip under to make a smooth edge.
9. After wrapping is completed, continue to support the finger in the desired position of correction by continued clockwise movement of the fingers, avoiding any point pressure until the cast is firm.

OR

Apply *slight* traction to the finger by placing the metacarpophalangeal joint in flexion, supporting the palm with the thumb of one hand while holding the distal tip of the casted finger (uncasted portion) in corrected position with your index finger and thumb until the cast is firm (Fig. 79-5).

I should emphasize that the method described is not intended to wedge cast the finger or to apply force other than a slight traction to the joint. Too much force applied during casting will shortly be apparent in an angry-looking interphalangeal joint with red, shiny skin. Used correctly, casting is a very nontraumatic way of gaining additional flexion or extension range.

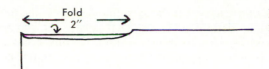

FIG. 79-2. Plaster strip 1 inch wide (cut from 2-inch wide plaster).

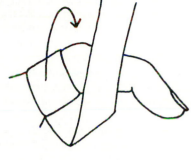

FIG. 79-3. Wrapping of plaster. Finger may be wrapped distal to proximal if believed necessary, but it is usually not necessary because plaster is for positioning of joint only and wrapping should not compress tissue.

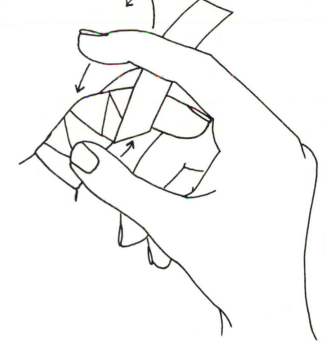

FIG. 79-4. Wrapping of finger while it is being supported in position.

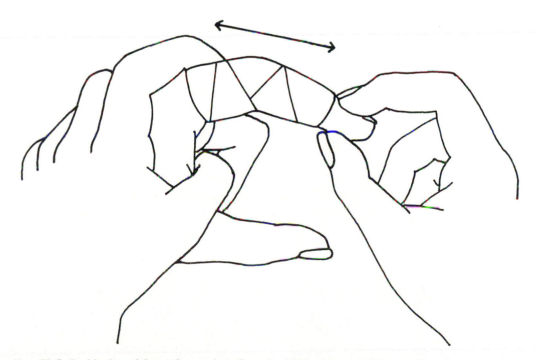

FIG. 79-5. Positioning of finger for traction. Care should be taken to avoid any point pressure on plaster.

Brand[1] recommends, when possible, that the cast be left on and removed only for exercise in therapy. The casting is most effective if it is left on continually and changed every day or every other day. It can be changed every day if possible, but it must be changed at least twice a week and the joints exercised to maintain their full mobility. After exercise, a new cast can be applied in what will probably be a few degrees more extension.

Although the cast is a total-contact plaster, one can easily remove it at the time of therapy by immersing the hand in water and unwrapping it or by squeezing the cast from side to side, which easily cracks the eggshell thickness and makes the whole splint quite pulpy and soft. At this stage it is easy to find the end of the plaster bandage and it is unwrapped. Some therapists just mark the end of the bandage or even fold the end back at the time the cast is applied so that the end will be easy to find.

The casting may be repeated as long as improvement is being maintained. Wax baths and oil rubbed into the fingers at exercise times are considered of value.

REMOVABLE CYLINDER CASTS

Occasions have arisen in which it has been necessary to make the cylinder casts removable. The most obvious cases are those in which it is most important to move the tendons frequently to prevent adhesions, as in the weeks after a tendon repair or in cases in which the patient can attend therapy only infrequently. In addition, my experience has been that casting is often not used because of a fear on the part of the surgeon or therapist that flexion of the finger in question will be lost. Flexion is not usually lost with casting, and careful measurements will assure that this is not a problem. However, by making the cylinder casts removable one can often increase flexion range of motion by flexion exercises while casting the finger into extension.

The application technique is the same as has already been described, except that the cast is removed.

Instructions

1. After the cast is firm, grasp along the length of the cast and gently loosen and remove it from the finger. IMPORTANT: The cast must be removed at this point if it is going to be removable for exercise of the joint (Fig. 79-6).
2. Check the finger and cast for point pressure. If need be, trim the edge of the cast for clearance of metacarpophalangeal or distal interphalangeal flexion.
3. Clean the excess plaster off the finger, apply another light coat of lanolin to the finger, and replace the cast.
4. If the interphalangeal joint is too swollen to allow easy removal of the cast, a slight cut can be made in the dorsal radial portion of the cast at the proximal phalanx. This cut is extended toward the interphalangeal joint until the cast can be removed (Fig. 79-7).
5. Once the cast is removed, the cut edges can be trimmed slightly and the cast replaced without losing its correction (Fig. 79-8).
6. If the finger is in a position of too much flexion to allow removal of the cast, one can make a window in the cast with scissors by first making cuts in the dorsoradial and dorsoulnar sides of the cast at the proximal phalanx. The flap is lifted,

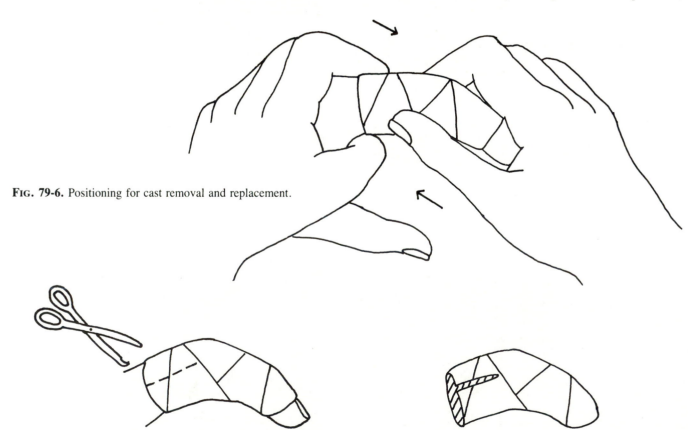

FIG. 79-6. Positioning for cast removal and replacement.

FIG. 79-7. Cast removal for swollen interphalangeal joint.

FIG. 79-8. Trimming of cast for replacement.

and the cast is removed. The flap is trimmed with scissors, and the cast can then be replaced and secured at the proximal phalanx with a small strip of adhesive tape (Fig. 79-9).

7. Once joint correction is achieved, the final cast can be worn as a retainer at night until after that period of time when joint contracture tends to recur.

8. The cast can be made to last an indefinite period of time by being coated with lacquer or fingernail polish once the plaster is dry.

ADAPTIVE CASTING

The use of the plaster casts can be coordinated with other conventional forms of therapy and splinting. The casting is particularly helpful in the treatment of fingers that require correction in two planes of movement, such as fingers with swan-neck deformities (Fig. 79-10) and contracted fingers as seen in nerve injuries and reflex sympathetic dystrophy (Fig. 79-11).

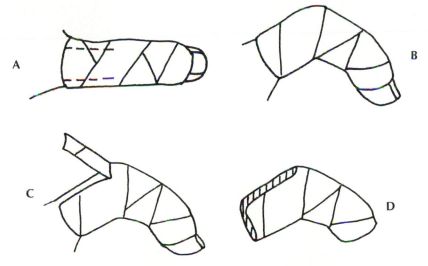

FIG. 79-9. Cast removal for severely flexed interphalangeal joint. **A,** Dorsal view. **B,** Lateral view. **C,** Flap. **D,** Cast.

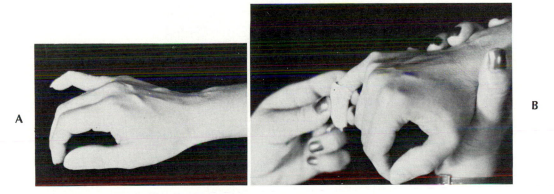

FIG. 79-10. A, Swan-neck deformity of left fifth digit with fixed hyperextension of interphalangeal joint. **B,** Technique of casting for correction in two planes. Once distal interphalangeal joint is casted into maximum possible extension, proximal interphalangeal joint is flexed and casted into maximum possible flexion with cast extending over casted distal interphalangeal joint.

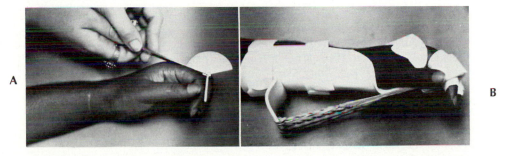

FIG. 79-11. A, Maximum extension of interphalangeal joints and maximum flexion of metacarpophalangeal joints after reflex sympathetic dystrophy. **B,** Same patient as progressively casted into extension of interphalangeal joints and as placed into flexion traction at metacarpophalangeal joints.

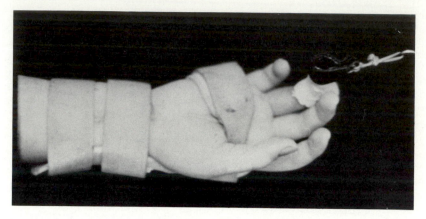

FIG. 79-12. Casting to increase extension of distal interphalangeal joint and traction to increase extension of proximal interphalangeal joint in patient with residual flexion contracture 8 weeks after second-stage flexor tendon graft.

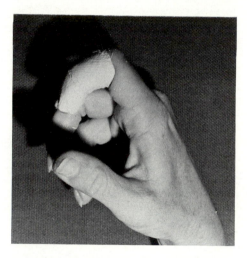

FIG. 79-13. Casting of distal interphalangeal joint to transfer power of profundus flexion to stiff proximal interphalangeal joint.

Casting of individual joints can also be used to block or transfer power of movement to other joints. After silicone rubber implants of the metacarpophalangeal joints, the patient will often begin early movement of the fingers by flexing only the interphalangeal joints. By casting the interphalangeal joints one restricts the power of flexion at the interphalangeal joints and transfers it to the metacarpophalangeal joints, until the patient is able to accomplish active flexion of the metacarpophalangeal joints. By casting a boutonnière deformity of the finger into extension at the interphalangeal joint, the lateral bands become slightly relaxed, and the power of flexion can be concentrated at the distal interphalangeal joint. Casting of the distal interphalangeal joint can be utilized to apply traction at the interphalangeal joint (Fig. 79-12) or to increase power of movement at the interphalangeal joint (Fig. 79-13).

REFERENCES

1. Brand, P.W.: The reconstruction of the hand in leprosy, Ann. R. Coll. Surg. Engl. **11:**350, 1952.
2. Kolumban, S.L.: The use of dynamic and static splints in straightening contracted proximal interphalangeal joints in leprosy patients: a comparative study, Paper read at the 47th annual conference of the American Physical Therapy Association, Washington, D.C., 1960.
3. Kolumban, S.L.: M.A. Thesis, New York University, 1967.
4. Kolumban, S.L.: The role of static and dynamic splints, physiotherapy techniques and time in straightening contractures of the interphalangeal joints, Leprosy in India, p. 323-328, Oct. 1969.

80

Static splinting and temperature assessment of the injured insensitive hand

ANNE B. BLAKENEY, HARRY T. BERGTHOLDT, and HELEN WOOD RAMSAMMY

Generally, one does not think of the loss of pain as a handicap requiring constant compensation. However, certain diseases cause loss of tactile sensation, specifically light touch, pain, and temperature, but do not significantly diminish motor functioning. Among these diseases are syringomyelia, hereditary sensory radicular neuropathy, congenital indifference to pain, diabetes, myelomeningocele, and Hansen's disease. In addition, trauma may cause peripheral nerve damage resulting in loss of sensation.

Frequently there may be an associated motor loss such as paralysis of the intrinsic hand muscles, while the extrinsic muscles continue to function. This causes an imbalance in motor performance. The "clawhand" deformity is a typical example of such an imbalance. In addition, there is generally associated damage to the autonomic nerve fibers causing loss of sweating in the insensitive areas. This results in dry, inelastic skin and increases susceptibility to injuries.

HOW INJURIES OCCUR

The total impact of such losses may at first appear minimal to the individual. His hand still functions to manipulate objects in his environment, though his grasp may have to be altered to compensate for a loss of opposition. This means that certain areas of the hand will receive repeated stresses they were not anatomically designed to tolerate. A common example typically seen with the clawhand deformity is the so-called key pinch. Repeated forceful use of an already structurally imbalanced hand may result in further deformities such as tissue trauma, subluxations, and bony changes.

The lack of pain further compounds these problems. There is now no warning system to alert the person to stop when too much force is being exerted on soft tissues or when a burn or a cut has occurred. Dr. Paul Brand has pointed out that each of us has a "built-in splint" that limits our movements when we have sustained an injury.[4] This "splint" is, of course, the pain we feel when attempting to move an injured part. We unconsciously avoid further trauma to the area because we are constantly reminded that it hurts. We therefore protect it and do not use it until it is healed.

With the loss of this vitally important warning system, it is possible to injure the hands through common daily activities and to continue using them. Burns occur while cooking, washing, or smoking a cigarette. Cuts are possible with the simplest objects: exerting extreme force on a key to open a door; holding a comb too tightly and receiving a puncture wound in the palm; pricking the finger while sewing; or blistering while sweeping or gardening. Almost any activity provides a potential hazard. In addition, calluses occur and may become a problem. It is necessary to soak dry, insensitive hands in water for at least 20 minutes daily. After this, petrolatum, or any hand cream, is applied to seal in the moisture. When calluses form, they must be trimmed. If this daily routine is not followed, these calluses can become dangerous, especially in the palmar flexion creases where they may eventually crack open. Hematomas are also common injuries, perhaps more subtle, but eventually destructive over a long period of time.

WHY SPLINT AN INJURY?

With each injury, there is no pain to warn the person that he is in danger and must stop using that injured part. There is no unconscious protection provided by the body. A small blister may develop into an open, infected ulcer as a result. Therefore it is imperative that an external splint be applied promptly to every injury to prevent the onset or spread of infection and eventual tenosynovitis, osteomyelitis, and absorption of the bone that will otherwise result. The external splint must put the injured part at rest and protect the damaged tissues from additional pressures and trauma. Infection must be prevented, if possible. If already present, the infection must not be allowed to spread to other areas of the body. The splint, through immobilization, will allow the infection to localize and promote healing. In addition to these obvious acute problems, the splint serves the purpose of preventing eventual deformity and loss of function, which result when injuries are left untreated.

SPECIAL PRECAUTIONS

Static splinting is used for injuries because immobilization is the desired goal. There are several general precautions that one must consider when applying a splint to an insensitive limb. Excessive pressure must be avoided because this can lead to additional problems. Therefore almost all removable splints will require some type of padding. When using a removable splint, always check for possible pressure points ½ to 2 hours after the initial application. If any redness is present, make appropriate adjustments to alleviate the pressure and reevaluate hourly. All edges must be smoothed and sharp points eliminated. Beware of completely encircling a part that is already edematous. Adaptations can be made in the splint to allow for the possibility of additional swelling. The splint must not fit too tightly because of the possibility of constricting the blood supply. However, caution must be taken to assure that it is not too loose because movement can then occur, causing friction that will result in another injury.

TYPES OF SPLINTS USED

Although each injury requires individual assessment and care, there are general guidelines that can be applied when splinting certain common problems. A general rule always followed with burns is maintaining the blister intact whenever possible. This is achieved by padding it with cotton and then adding a stiff protective splint such as one made with fiberglass material. The patient will wear this splint until the fluid in the blister is resorbed. If the blister is already broken and an ulcer is present, the possibility of infection is greater. It is then necessary to immobilize the total area involved. Thermoplastics or plaster may be used for this. The splint is applied over the dressing, which can be changed daily.

An open cut or puncture wound allows the introduction of bacteria and the possibility of infection. If this type of injury is on the dorsum, particularly over a joint, splint the hand in a flexed position. If on the palmer surface, position in extension and splint. Always allow sufficient space to incorporate necessary dressings. Make sure the same amount of dressing is reapplied each day to ensure continued fit of the splint.

Because of dryness, flexion crease cracks often occur and are difficult to immobilize. Once healed, these cracks may recur when the slightest force is exerted over the joint. Therefore immobilization needs to be continued beyond the point of initial healing. Lack of sweating and failure to soak and oil the hands daily causes dryness. Increased use causes callus formation. These calluses must be trimmed regularly. Failure to soak the hands and trim calluses results in loss of elasticity in the skin over an area that constantly moves. Eventually stretching is impossible and the callus breaks open, sometimes exposing the tendon sheath beneath.

Plaster casting has proved to be the most effective method of healing such injuries. It provides total contact and immobilization. The crack is first covered with a small gauze dressing. It must be held in an open position to allow healing at all levels, as opposed to superficial closure only at the surface, and to maintain extension capability. The plaster must be carefully applied, with small strips being combined over the crack itself with a circular application to provide necessary strength and to assure immobility. During application, caution is taken not to pull the plaster too tightly around the finger. During the setting time, pressing tightly in any one area is avoided to prevent localized pressure. To maintain the desired position, use an even pressure with all fingers and keep them continually moving over the plaster, thereby preventing a possible pressure point.

Once the wound has healed, an effort must be made to keep the skin moist and to keep the callus trimmed. A thermoplastic gutter splint may be used for 2 to 3 weeks to protect a recently healed crack. With chronic, recurring cracks, a skin graft or possible fusion of the joint may be necessary.

Patients with hematomas are generally not splinted for healing. However, when the therapist or patient notes their continued presence over a specific area, some method of protection is developed to prevent them. A protective cap may be made for fingers with this problem. Thermoplastics are ideal for this. The cap is molded directly on the finger, after the material has cooled sufficiently so that it will not burn the patient. This is secured with tape. Often the patient will discover that it is only one particular activity that causes the hematoma, such as his job. When this is the case, he applies the cap only when doing that activity.

If the hematoma is in an area on the hand that cannot be easily covered with a cap, such as a metacarpophalangeal joint on the dorsum or any area of the palm, an effort is made to adapt any equipment used that may cause this or to teach the patient a new way of using his hand to prevent this constant trauma. In addition, an effort is made to teach the patient to exert less force when holding any object. Patients must learn to estimate how tightly they are holding things in order to prevent excessive pressures to tissues. The absence of tactile sensation makes this extremely difficult. As a result, they may exert great force in order to have sensory feedback from deeper structures.

METHODS OF ASSESSMENT

Objective measurements must be used to evaluate the fit and effectiveness of splints on insensitive extremities. These include physical inspection, volume displacement, and temperature assessment. Regular assessments are used to determine when changes or adaptations in the splinting program are required. The use of objective methods is also necessary to help the patient understand and appreciate the purpose of a protective splint.

Physical inspection

The physical examination includes visually inspecting and palpating the skin under the area covered by the splint. The therapist must look for redness as evidence of localized high pressure or tightness. Before application of a splint, redness and edema may also indicate the presence and extent of inflammation or infection. Initially it may be necessary to immobilize more proximal joints to prevent the spread of infection. The patient also must be taught the danger signs of an improperly fitting splint and follow daily self-care evaluation techniques.

Volume displacement

The presence of edema may be objectively followed by the use of a tank that measures hand volume by water displacement.[1] This technique is employed before splint fabrication and periodically as indicated until the splinting program is discontinued. One may chart progress with a graph to note upward or downward trends in swelling. A rising curve may indicate a splint was removed before adequate healing occurred, or that the type of splint initially applied is not effectively immobilizing an injury. Appropriate corrections are then made.

Temperature assessment

Temperature assessment is another objective measurement of particular value in monitoring injuries on insensitive hands. In the absence of pain, another sign of inflammation and infection must be monitored to measure the effectiveness of splinting. Is the splint maintaining the necessary immobilization? Is it time to remove the splint? Did the patient fail to heed advice to wear the splint while working? All these questions can frequently be answered with temperature assessment. Inflamed tissue is warmer than normal tissue, and infected tissue demonstrates local heat and increased heat proximally as well.

Temperature assessment refers to the determination of skin temperature of any area in question and comparison of it to the temperature of a normal area. In normal hands a symmetric thermal pattern exists. The palm is warm with the fingers cooler distally or the hand may be of uniform temperature. Normal temperature patterns are illustrated by Travis Winsor.[9] If there is a paralysis in which the sympathetic nervous system is involved, characteristic cool patterns are noted.[6] For any hand a characteristic thermal pattern remains unchanged unless an injury or change in a pathologic condition occurs.

The hand and especially the fingers act as "radiators" to regulate body temperature, and day-to-day variations in hand temperature can be great. This presents a problem when one is using the temperature of an injured part as a guide to monitor progress. Therefore it is urgent that the temperature be compared to other normal tissue temperature. This temperature difference (ΔT) is used as an index to measure the progress of injury splinting. If large variations in the normal tissue temperature are noted, it may be necessary to utilize the "Thermal Circulation Index" developed by Burton[5] and explained by Winsor.[9] This index has proved valuable. The index difference (ΔTCI) is obtained between the temperature of the injured area and the temperature of the normal tissue (usually the contralateral site). This unit has been most helpful in the winter when fluctuations in external temperatures may be more than 20° C, causing large variations in hand temperatures.

Several methods of temperature assessment are available. The best, but unfortunately very expensive, method is infrared thermography. Infrared radiation is measured by an infrared thermography unit that displays a picture of temperature. The thermal patterns of an entire hand and lower arm are depicted, and with special "isotherm displays" the temperature of any specific area can be determined.[7] Another type of infrared detector is a radiometer, which produces a temperature readout in degrees. The cost is much more reasonable and it is easily used in a clinic. The thermistor is an excellent clinical unit, which is the least expensive of all. Using a heat-sensitive probe, it delivers an accurate spot temperature when it touches the skin for 10 to 15 seconds. Even the human hand can detect several degrees of difference between two areas. The therapist's hand is certainly capable of gross assessment by palpation

and can be valuable in assessing injury splinting.

More detailed discussions of equipment and methods are in the literature.[2,3,8] The case studies that follow demonstrate the usefulness of temperature assessment when combined with a splinting program.

CASE STUDIES

Case No. 1. A patient presented with an ainhum deformity at the distal interphalangeal joint of his ring finger. The skin eventually cracked, and the finger became infected (Fig. 80-1). The patient was unaware of the opening initially, and extensive swelling and inflammation occurred. When he was first seen with fever and chills, a problem in this finger was suspected. Temperature assessment revealed an approximate increase of 9° C in that hand when compared with the opposite extremity, indicating the presence of an acute infection. A plaster splint was made, which incorporated the metacarpophalangeal joint (Fig. 80-2). The finger was only partially enclosed with plaster, leaving an area on the dorsum open to allow for the possibility of additional swelling. The splint was applied over necessary dressings. The patient wore the splint for 2 weeks. At that time, the acute inflammation and edema had subsided and a thermoplastic gutter splint was applied to protect the finger and allow complete healing.

Case No. 2. This case demonstrates the problems that often arise from a single, small, chronic ulcer that remains untreated for a long period of time. Because these ulcers are not painful in insensitive hands, patients often apply only Band-Aids over them and continue to use their hands, allowing infection and additional trauma to occur.

This patient had such an ulcer on the tip of his shortened ring finger. Because of previous absorption, only the proximal phalanx remained in this finger. When the patient was referred for treatment, visual observation did not indicate

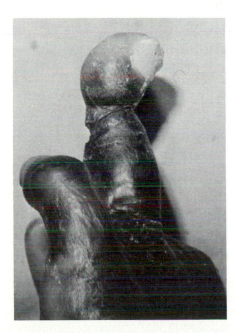

FIG. 80-1. Ainhum deformity (dactylolysis spontanea) with acute infection.

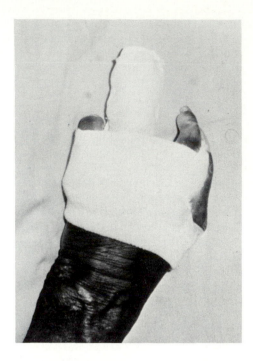

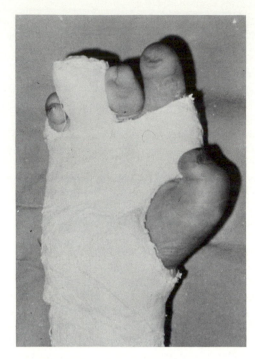

FIG. 80-2. Plaster cast used on hand in Fig. 80-1.

FIG. 80-3. Cast that extended to elbow on patient with chronic ulcer on fourth finger.

the presence of widespread infection because there was no inflammation demonstrated through redness of the skin. However, temperature assessment revealed the ring finger to be 8° C warmer than the ring finger of the opposite hand, with a ΔTCI of 15° C. Roentgenograms indicated osteomyelitis in the remaining phalanx. Temperatures were elevated from the fingertip into the forearm and elbow.

A plaster cast was applied, which provided immobilization of the hand and forearm (Fig. 80-3). After 1 week in this cast, temperatures decreased and the acute infection in the forearm, wrist, and hand appeared to have subsided. A plaster cylinder was applied to the infected finger only and changed every 2 to 3 days for a period of 3 months. The infected bone fragment eventually sloughed and the remaining tissues then healed quickly. As this case demonstrates, when osteomyelitis is already a factor, these ulcers require a much longer period of treatment than acute injuries.

Case No. 3. The last case is that of a patient with a severely deformed insensitive hand who sustained an injury on the dorsum of the hand when a pin punctured the skin, with resulting acute cellulitis and gross edema. The entire hand and forearm were splinted with a bivalved plaster cast. Appropriate antibiotic medication was instituted. Frequent temperature recordings were made to monitor the progress of the splinting. No major improvement was noted in 2 days, and so an incision was made on the palmar surface and drains were applied. Immediate improvement was noted both visually and in the temperature recordings (Fig. 80-4). Within 2 weeks the wounds were closed. Twenty-eight days after initiation of treatment, the temperatures suddenly

increased while the patient was wearing a splint on the hand only. The healing wounds had probably become irritated by his habitually hitting walls or his wheelchair with his injured hand. The resulting forces would have created intolerable pain for a hand with normal sensation. Damage to the tissues was clearly evidenced by the increase of the ΔTCI from 1 to 2 units to 13 units. A splint was applied, which again incorporated both the hand and forearm. Antibiotic medication was started again. As the condition improved, smaller, removable splints were used. Temperature assessment proved valuable in monitoring the progress of healing. This patient had many other severe deformities of his hands and feet yet had a great desire for independence and often was unwilling to follow the recommended therapy regime. Demonstrating the seriousness of his injury by temperature assessment helped his awareness and increased his cooperation.

SUMMARY

Because of certain chronic disease processes or trauma, persons with insensitive hands often suffer injuries that are not painful and do not initially diminish function. However, continued use of an injured hand will allow infection to occur, which may eventually lead to tenosynovitis, osteomyelitis, bone absorption, deformity, and, finally, loss of function. To prevent this chain of events, it is necessary to splint each injury in order to protect and immobilize the infected area and allow healing to occur.

Applying a splint to an insensitive hand must be done very carefully so that additional injuries are not caused by the splint itself. Special precautions are followed by both

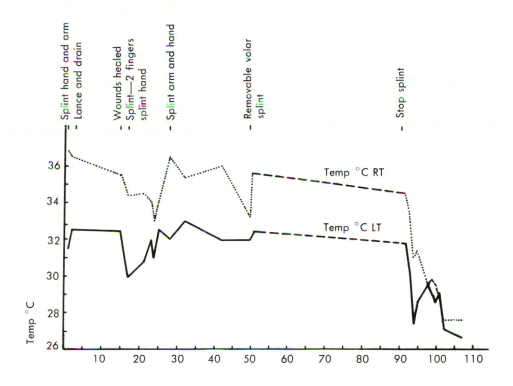

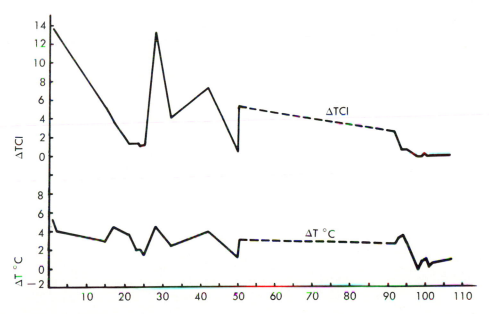

FIG. 80-4. Case No. 3. Graph of temperatures and temperature differences (ΔT, ΔTCI) for dorsum of left and right hands during course of treatment.

the therapist and the patient to prevent potential problems.

Objective measurements are used to assess the effectiveness of splints. Physical evaluation, volumetric changes, and temperature assessment provide basic information that is recorded and used in determining necessary changes in a splinting program. Of these methods, temperature assessment has proved to be the most useful. Initially, it indicates the total area requiring immobilization, and later it serves to monitor the changes in temperature as healing occurs. It is also useful in demonstrating to patients the value of splints in healing injuries and therefore helps motivate them to wear their splints for the necessary time period.

REFERENCES

1. Beach, R.: Measurement of extremity volume by water displacement, Phys. Ther. **57:**286, 1977.
2. Bergtholdt, H.T., and Brand, P.W.: Thermography: an aid in the management of insensitive feet and stumps, Arch. Phys. Med. Rehabil. **56:**205, 1975.
3. Bergtholdt, H.T., and Brand, P.W.: Temperature assessment and plantar inflammation. Lepr. Rev. **47:**211, 1976.
4. Brand, P.W.: Lecture given at the USPHS Hospital, Carville, Louisiana, February 5, 1975.
5. Burton, A.: Application of theory of heat flow, J. Nutr. **7:**497, 1934.
6. Enna, C., and Bergtholdt, H.: Temperature studies of the hand and its claw deformities due to peripheral nerve paralysis in leprosy, Hand **5**(1):14, 1973.
7. Ryan, J.: Thermography, Aust. Radiol. **13:**23, 1969.
8. Uematsu, S., editor: Medical thermography, theory and clinical applications, Los Angeles, 1976, Brentwood Publishing Corporation.
9. Winsor, T.: Peripheral vascular disease, an objective approach, Springfield, Ill., 1959, Charles C Thomas, Publisher.

XVI

THE INDUSTRIAL WORKER IN
A HAND REHABILITATION SETTING

81

The work tolerance program of the Hand Rehabilitation Center in Philadelphia

PATRICIA L. BAXTER and SHARON L. FRIED

Work therapy is active participation by the patient in prescribed therapeutic exercises and activities to achieve short- and long-term goals. It is a necessary process to promote active use, to minimize physical complications from disuse, and most importantly to increase the patient's physical abilities, which facilitate his return to work and to his former avocational activities.

Work therapy is an integral part of the hand rehabilitation program at the Hand Rehabilitation Center in Philadelphia. There are two main services provided in the hand therapy program. The primary care section provides postoperative management, splinting, sensory evaluations, and instruction in patient exercise programs. The work therapy section provides therapeutic exercises, therapeutic activities, physical capacity evaluations, functional evaluations, and public relations communication to insurance companies and rehabilitation companies (Fig. 81-1). The staff of the work therapy section consists of a registered occupational therapist, who is the full-time supervisor, a staff occupational therapist, and a certified occupational therapy assistant. A full-time industrial arts instructor instructs the patients in woodworking techniques. An art instructor from a local art college instructs patients in wood-carving techniques twice weekly.

A patient may be referred directly to work therapy by a hand surgeon for a work tolerance program. Other referring sources include primary care therapists, insurance companies, rehabilitation companies, and employers. The patient's surgeon must communicate to the therapist the amount of stress or resistance the patient's injured structures can tolerate. Wound healing, fracture stability, the type of surgical procedure, and the amount of time since the injury or surgery are considered before one starts the patient in the work tolerance program.

Each patient is assigned therapeutic activities and therapeutic exercises according to his individual condition. The patient may be referred initially to the work tolerance program based on the following general time schedule:

Condition	Time of initiation of work therapy
Tendon repairs	4 to 8 weeks after surgery
Crush injury	3 to 6 weeks after injury
Partial amputation of digits	3 weeks after injury

Condition	Time of initiation of work therapy
Replantations	6 to 8 weeks after injury
Amputation of hand	4 to 6 weeks after injury
Fractures	4 to 6 weeks after injury
Nerve compression releases	3 weeks after surgery
Burns	3 to 6 weeks after surgery
Tendon transfers	4 to 8 weeks after surgery
Reflex sympathetic dystrophy	3 to 6 weeks after injury
Soft-tissue lacerations	2 weeks after injury
Muscle/ligament injuries	4 to 6 weeks after injury
Nerve injury	6 to 8 weeks after injury
Joint fusion	8 to 12 weeks after surgery
Dupuytren's disease	4 to 6 weeks after surgery
Frostbite	3 to 4 weeks after injury

The work tolerance activities and exercises have been divided into five levels of resistance. When the surgeon refers the patient for work therapy, he frequently will order the patient to be started in a level rather than a certain activity or exercise. The patient can be referred for participation in various levels at the same time. The surgeon may order the patient to begin level 1 activities if he does not want the patient to perform activities of more than 1 pound of resistance. The purpose of level 1 activities is to promote early motion for purposeful use of the injured hand. Level 2 activities provide resistance of 1 to 3 pounds. The purpose of level 2 activities is to promote progressive prehension and coordination and initiate strengthening. Level 3 activities are between 3 and 20 pounds of resistance. The purpose of level 3 activities is to increase strength and endurance through the execution of moderately resistive activities. Level 4 activities are between 20 and 60 pounds of resistance. Level 4 activities provide moderate to heavy resistive exercise to encourage maximum strengthening and improve the patient's work tolerance. Level 5 activities are between 60 and 100 pounds of resistance. The purpose of this level of activity is to promote heavy resistive exercise, which simulates physical demands of the patient's job to prepare the patient to return to work.

EVALUATION

The patient is introduced to the work therapy staff, and an initial interview and evaluation are conducted. His diagnosis and past progress, together with a detailed job de-

889

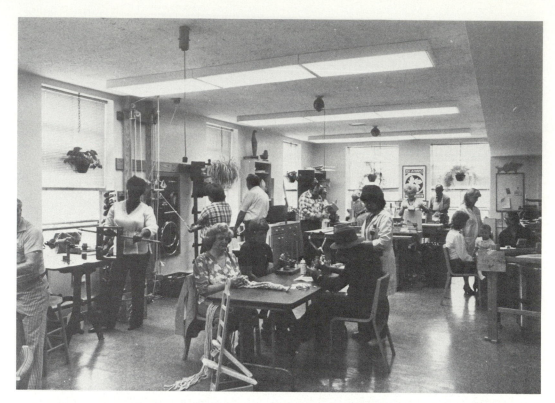

FIG. 81-1. Work therapy staff instructs patients to ensure appropriate safe performance of therapeutic activities and exercises.

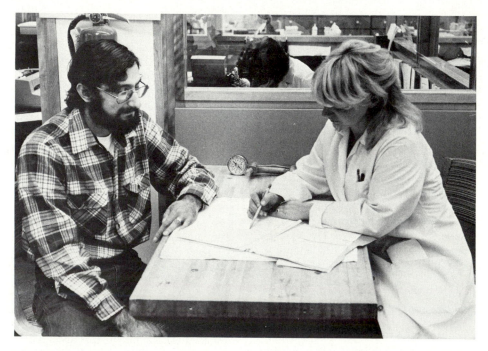

FIG. 81-2. Patient is informed of his initial hand function measurements, and a treatment plan is developed.

scription, are important for planning his program and eventual return to work. His range of motion, grip, pinch, sensibility and hand-volume measurements are included in the evaluation (Fig. 81-2). The work therapy supervisor reviews the evaluation and assigns the patient to a staff therapist (Fig. 81-3). An initial treatment program is developed from the evaluation. Therapeutic activities and therapeutic exercises are introduced to the patient. Most patients are scheduled to attend work therapy three times each week. The patient is monitored closely throughout his time in work therapy, and the amount of time of each session is increased as his work tolerance improves. The length of therapy is

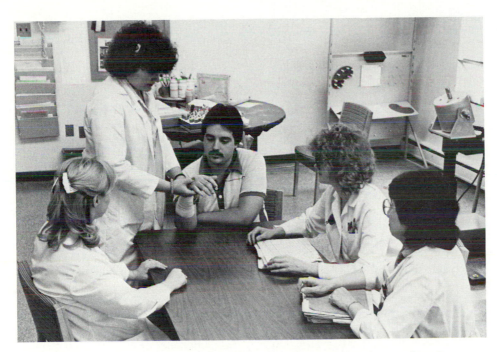

FIG. 81-3. Daily brief staff meetings are conducted to assign patients to therapist.

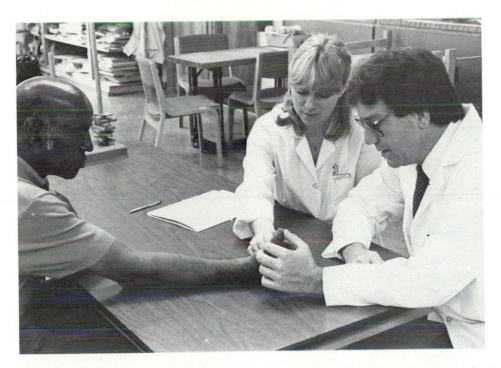

FIG. 81-4. Communication between surgeons and therapists is convenient and frequent and ensures good patient care.

determined by the patient's progress and physical endurance. He is required to perform progressive resistive exercises and activities as he improves. Performance of job-simulated tasks is incorporated into the program as soon as the patient can tolerate them. The goal of work therapy is to help the patient regain (in the most cost-effective time schedule) strength, coordination, and endurance so that he can perform his former job or a modified job.

Communication between the patient, the surgeon, and the therapist is essential to a successful program (Fig. 81-4). The patient is encouraged to ask questions regarding his program. The work therapy staff maintains ongoing communication between the patient, his primary care therapist, and his physician during the patient's rehabilitation program.

THERAPEUTIC ACTIVITIES AND THERAPEUTIC EXERCISES
Levels 1 and 2

Level 1 and level 2 activities are designed to promote active use, promote coordination, and initiate strengthening. Dr. Robert Beasley in the book *Hand Injuries* stated that the patient must be an active participant in his therapy if it is to be of lasting benefit. The patient cannot drop off his hand for therapy and collect it an hour later. This tendency by some patients must be prevented or corrected early through patient education, evaluation, and close supervision as therapeutic tasks are performed.[1] Prehension tasks, such as prehension of wooden blocks or blocks on dowels, are provided (Fig. 81-5). Games are used to encourage active motion.

Macramé is used to encourage active motion, reduce edema, and promote bilateral use of the upper extremities (Fig. 81-6). Macramé can be taught to patients with catastrophic hand injuries while they are in the acute stage of wound healing and also to patients who have sustained amputations and who are learning to use early-fitting prostheses. The difficulty of this activity can increase as the patient progresses, by having him perform the projects in elevation rather than on a flat surface and by reducing the size of the cord. Macramé is easily taught to patients. This activity is frequently an integral part of a patient's home program.

Leatherwork is used when increased resistance is allowed by the surgeon. The size of the project and the selection of lacing, stamping, or carving determine its grading (that is, level of difficulty). Generally, lacing increases elbow range of motion and digital flexion; stamping encourages bilateral digital flexion; and carving encourages three-point pinch (Fig. 81-7). Leatherwork is a good project for desensitization and for prosthetic training. Patient projects include belts, wallets, and other personal items.

Ceramics is frequently prescribed for patients to increase their active motion and strength. It is versatile and easily graded. Patients make ceramics using hand-molding techniques of coil, pinch pot, or slab. Slab projects encourage digital flexion and elbow extension and flexion. Coil projects promote digital extension. Pinch-pot projects encourage digital flexion and thumb opposition.

Throwing clay on a potter's wheel is more resistive than hand molding (Fig. 81-8). This activity requires bilateral coordination, wrist extension, and digital extension and opposition. Potter's-wheel projects can be adapted to a specific patient's needs, whether a patient needs flexion or extension. The importance of the improved self-esteem of the patients who finish a ceramic project cannot be underestimated.

Wax sculpture is less resistive than ceramics and is ac-

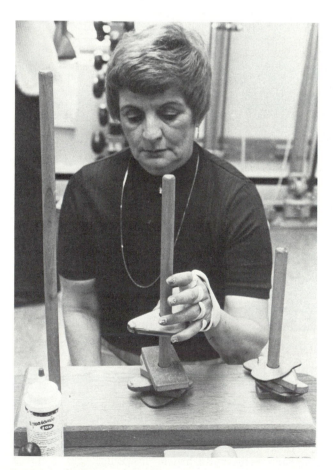

FIG. 81-5. Prehension tasks encourage patient to use his injured hand.

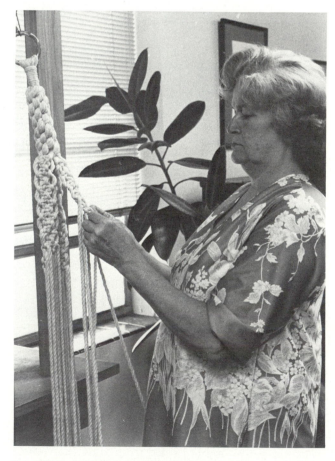

FIG. 81-6. As patient works with her arms elevated, edema is reduced.

ceptable to patients who are tactilely sensitive to clay (Fig. 81-9). The foundry wax is made pliable by submersion in warm water (98° to 100° F). The patient works the warm wax and returns it to the warm water to maintain its softness. Wax sculpture promotes gross grasp, pinch strength, and digital flexion and opposition. Patients with arthritis and reflex sympathetic dystrophies are frequently instructed in wax sculpture.

Desensitization of scar tissue and hypersensitive injured peripheral nerves is initiated during the patient's first therapy sessions if hypersensitivity is a problem to him. Hypersensitivity can cause a patient to decrease functional use of the affected hand, resulting in weakness, stiffness, and a longer period of recovery. Patients are taught to rub the sensitive area several times each hour with textures such as fur, yarn, rice, styrofoam, or BB's (Fig. 81-10). Patients are instructed to continue this process at home with textures such as rough towels, clothing, dry beans, or rice, or by tapping on hard surfaces.

Because of peripheral nerve injuries, many patients have difficulty in cold weather. Down mittens and thermal liners for gloves are provided to protect the patient's hands in 30-degree-below-zero weather or during performance of job tasks that require exposure to cold temperatures.

Coordination training may be essential if the patient has sustained a peripheral nerve injury or a severe injury that affects the biomechanical balance of the hand or wrist. Coordination training should be provided if the patient's job requirements include fine dexterity, repetitive motion, or manipulation of tools and small objects. Gross-coordination training should be initiated first. Activities such as buttoning, tying, and manipulating various mechanisms can be used to increase the patient's gross-coordination ability. Specific tasks such as writing must be practiced in a systematic way.

The initial phase of coordination training is to perform the task accurately with no regard for speed. The patient will regain coordination slowly as he performs the task accurately. Next, speed of coordination is practiced for short periods. The patient should be supervised closely to ensure that he is not using substitution motions as he performs quickly. As the patient's coordination improves, the length of time the activity is performed is increased. The Valpar Work Samples are used to evaluate and train the patient who requires coordination to perform job tasks.

Patients with difficulty in activities of daily living (ADL)

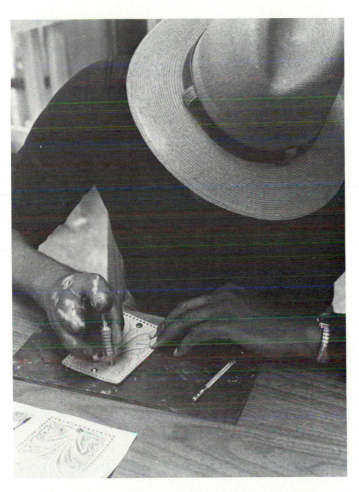

FIG. 81-7. Leather carving promotes three-point pinch.

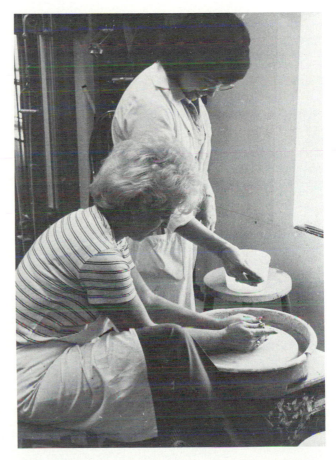

FIG. 81-8. Therapist instructs patient in therapeutic techniques on potter's wheel.

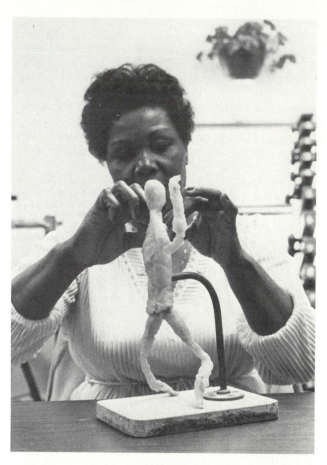

Fig. 81-9. Wax sculpture encourages finger flexion and pinch strength.

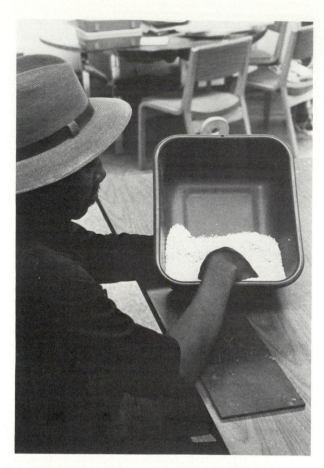

Fig. 81-10. Patient desensitizes himself by rubbing his injured hand in dry rice.

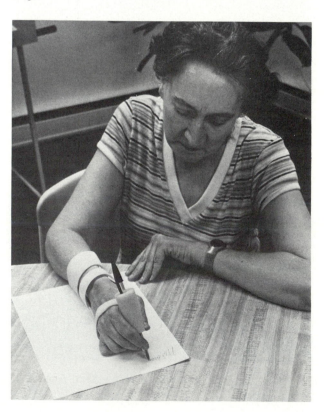

are referred by the surgeon or primary-care therapist to the certified occupational therapy assistant. An ADL checklist is completed by the patient. During the evaluation, direct questioning by the therapist may identify additional problems. All problems are discussed, suggestions are made if necessary, and adaptive equipment is provided. Instructions are given orally and in writing for the use of any equipment. Postoperative patients usually need only instructions in one-handed techniques; however, the patients with more severe injury may need adaptive equipment and suggestions in energy conservation (Fig. 81-11). Special adaptive equipment is ordered as necessary from various medical supply sources. Rocker knives and button hooks are frequently ordered for amputees. Supplies to build up tool and utensil handles include black foam tubing, foam hair rollers, and styrofoam cylinders. A small supply of inexpensive stainless flatware is kept for use in universal cuffs and for short-term adaptations.

Training in food preparation is available when necessary. A kitchen area is located adjacent to the work therapy area

Fig. 81-11. Adaptive equipment may assist patients to become independent after an injury.

for cooking training. A private treatment room is used if privacy is needed for dressing training.

An arthritic patient may be referred by his surgeon or primary care therapist to the certified occupational therapy assistant for joint protection instruction. Inabilities to perform activities of daily living are outlined and discussed. Adaptive equipment is issued as necessary. Joint protection information is discussed and reinforced by written instructions. A joint protection booklet published by Evelyn Rossky, of the Moss Rehabilitation Hospital of Philadelphia, is used.[2] The reasons for compliance and encouragement to change slowly to a joint protective life-style are explained. Arthritic patients are encouraged to call if they have questions concerning the program and the use of equipment. The patients are instructed to incorporate joint-protection techniques as they are observed performing activities such as macramé, foundry wax sculpture, and clay sculpture. It is vital to encourage the patients to make joint-protective techniques a habit.

Levels 3 to 5

Levels 3 to 5 of the work therapy program provide progressive resistive exercises and activities to facilitate the return of a patient's strength and endurance. Trombley and Scott state that muscle strength is related to the maximum tension that can be produced by a muscle during voluntary contraction.[3] The principle used to increase muscle strength is to require a maximum, or near-maximum, contraction of weak muscles. This implies use of resistance. As resistance increases, an increasing number of motor units are recruited, thereby increasing the strength of contraction.

Strengthening exercises include isometric, isotonic, and isokinetic exercises. The benefits and contraindications of the various types of strengthening exercise are considered for each patient. Isometric exercise involves performance of a static contraction of muscle by either pushing or pulling against an immovable object or by sustaining muscle tension as the patient holds a weight. This type of exercise is prescribed for patients who require strengthening early after injury, when their injured structures cannot tolerate resistance throughout the full range of joint motion. Patients who experience pain with other strengthening exercises are instructed in isometric exercises.

The patient is instructed to perform isometric exercise by lifting a weight and sustaining his muscle tension as he counts to 6. He is instructed to repeat the exercise until he fatigues. Progressive repetitions are required daily. There is one precaution: isometric exercises cause an increase in systolic blood pressure; therefore patients with high blood pressure should not perform isometrics.

Isotonic exercise involves physically lifting an object to a set position and then returning the object to its original position. Rapid improvement in muscle strength is possible if the patient can tolerate frequent increases of the weight. Progressive resistive exercises constitute the isotonic regimen used at the Hand Rehabilitation Center. The Delorme technique has been used in many rehabilitation settings. However, hand-injured patients appear to fatigue less with the modified Oxford technique of progressive resistive exercises.[4]

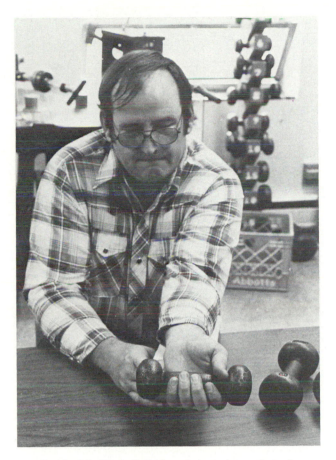

FIG. 81-12. Modified Oxford technique is used to increase strength.

With this technique, the patients are required to lift three weights 10 times each, lifting the heaviest weight first and decreasing the resistance as exercise is continued. The appropriate weights are selected on the basis of the patient's grip-strength measurements taken on the second level of the Jamar Dynamometer. The heaviest weight is identified according to the following guidelines: patient's grip strength 1 to 10 pounds—maximum weight to lift, 1 to 3 pounds; grip strength 10 to 20 pounds—maximum weight to lift, 3 to 5 pounds; grip strength 25 to 45 pounds—maximum weight to lift, 5 to 7 pounds; grip strength 45 to 60 pounds—maximum weight to lift, 7 to 10 pounds; grip strength 60 pounds or above—maximum weight to lift, 10 pounds. The patient is instructed to perform the exercise in wrist flexion, wrist extension, and radioulnar deviation (Fig. 81-12). Also the exercise can be performed in elbow flexion and extension.

There are two considerations in selecting isotonic exercise. First, the maximum weight the patient can tolerate is limited to the maximum weight he can move at the weakest angle throughout his range of motion. This may limit the patient's ability to increase the maximum weight and slow his progress considerably. Another problem with isotonic exercise is that patients may experience muscle soreness. This is attributable to the patient's performance of concentric and eccentric muscle contractions in the isotonic exercise.

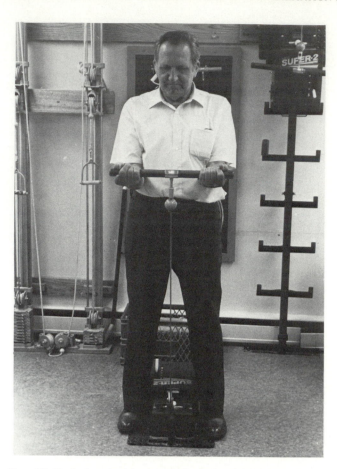

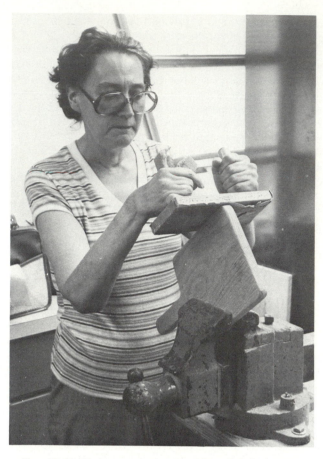

FIG. 81-13. Patient is able to exercise on a Mini-Gym placed on floor or mounted on wall.

FIG. 81-14. Patient works in elevation to control edema.

Muscle soreness is not a contraindication for performance of this type of activity; however, the patient should be educated as to the expected soreness.

Isokinetic exercise is performed on an exerciser. The force is exerted by the patient, and the speed of exercise is controlled by the exerciser. Controlled speed of performance promotes use of muscle units throughout the patient's full range of motion. Isokinetic exercise is performed on a specially designed exerciser such as a Mini-Gym or a Cybex unit. The Mini-Gym has a pulley mechanism that provides resistance equal to the force being exerted by the patient throughout the full range of the exercise being performed (Fig. 81-13). Various handles are available for this exerciser. The patient is instructed to perform exercises pulling as hard as possible throughout his full range of joint motion. If the patient has pain in one point of his range of motion, he will not exert as much force, and the resistance is decreased automatically. As the painful point is passed, the patient can continue exercising, applying maximum resistance throughout the remaining range of motion.

Isokinetic exercise is performed at a speed regulated by the Minigym. The controlled speed promotes maximum muscle contractions throughout the full range of motion. Patients who perform heavy manual labor can regain strength and endurance as they exert up to 500 pounds of force on the machine. They are instructed to perform mul-

tiple repetitions of each exercise. There is one precaution when one is considering isokinetic exercises for the patient: people with cardiovascular problems should not perform isokinetic exercises, because they increase systolic blood pressure.

Endurance training is an integral part of a therapeutic activity program. The principle of treatment to increase endurance is to grade the activity to involve moderate resistance and to require performance of a greater number of repetitions. Strengthening gain will also occur if the activity is repeated to the point of fatigue. The most frequently used activities to increase strength and endurance are activities that require sustained grip and repetitive movements.

Woodworking is an excellent therapeutic activity to increase strength and endurance. As the patient performs sustained grip of tool handles, his muscle strength improves without requiring excessive stress on injured structures, such as tendons. The activity can be initiated earlier than weight lifting. Patients with edema can work in an elevated position to encourage edema reduction (Fig. 81-14). This activity is therapeutic for several diagnoses because it can be easily graded and adapted.

Several ways of grading woodworking are possible. Grading can be achieved through the use of soft or hard wood for projects and by the type of tool selected (a hand sander requires the patient to use less force than a file, rasp, or

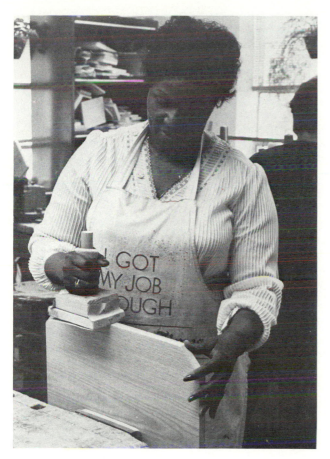

FIG. 81-15. Unilateral, bilateral, and built-up handled sanders are provided.

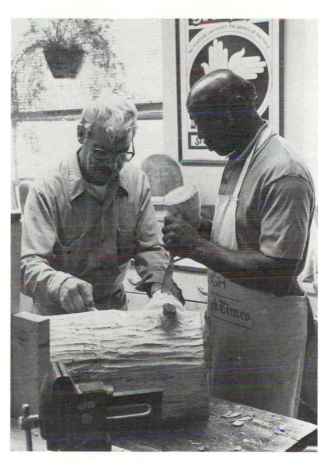

FIG. 81-16. Patient learns proper wood-carving techniques from instructor.

hand saw). Sanders are fabricated to allow adaptation to the patient's particular problem (Fig. 81-15). Handles that require digital flexion are used most commonly; they can be either unilateral or bilateral. Sanders that require digital extension, wrist supination, or active flexion during use have been designed. A common adaptation of woodworking tools is built-up handles. The adapted handle should provide total surface contact to encourage individual tendon excursion. The use of adhesive-backed foam and styrofoam cylinders enables the therapist to modify the tool handles.

Wood carving facilitates increased endurance because it is more resistive than woodworking. A patient may be given a wood-carving project when he has adequate grip strength (approximately 40 pounds) to hold the tools. Performance of wood carving demands that the patient hold a chisel in his nondominant hand and a mallet in his dominant hand. The patient carves a log by hammering, chiseling, rasping, filing, and sanding. A wood-carving instructor from a local college of art designs the projects and instructs the patient (Fig. 81-16). Refer to Chapter 82 for further details.

Another form of endurance training is performance of job-simulated tasks. The goal of the work tolerance program is to prepare the injured worker to return to his former job. The worker must regain the physical capacity to perform

the physical demands of his job. The physical demands of each job are the physical movements that are required to perform the job. For example, if the patient's job requires the lifting of 100 pounds, he is instructed to lift progressively greater weights as his capacity improves. Job simulation differs from therapeutic weight lifting in that the patient is required to carry a weighted box for repetitive sessions (Fig. 81-17). Other physical job tasks, such as handling tools and working in various postures, are duplicated as the patient uses the Valpar Work Samples. Refer to Chapter 7 for further details.

The Work Simulator provides appropriate job simulation. The Work Simulator (see Chapter 83) is a therapeutic instrument that provides resistance to the patient at specific job levels as he performs physical movements that simulate job tasks. There are 14 tool attachments that are used to simulate actual tools used for performance of physical tasks in several thousand jobs. On the Work Simulator, the patient works against progressively greater amounts of resistance for increasingly longer periods of time to improve his strength and endurance. The patient performs job simulation on the Work Simulator at an exercise level that is challenging but comfortable (Fig. 81-18). The patient's performance of each job-simulated task is plotted on a graph to indicate his improvement in work capacity and endurance.

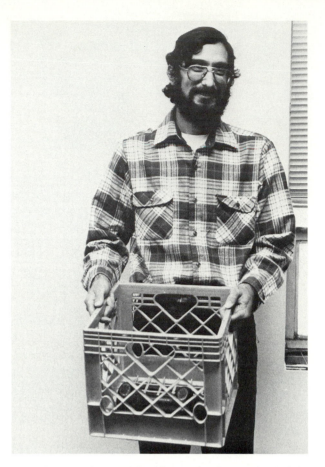

FIG. 81-17. Lifting weighted boxes simulates patient's job.

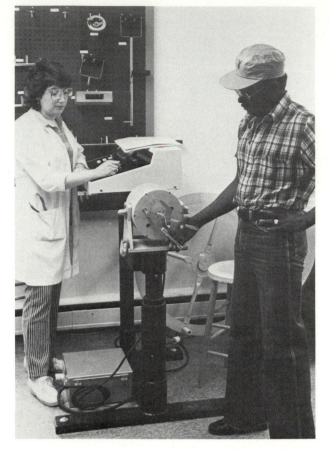

FIG. 81-18. Job-simulated tasks can be duplicated with various tool attachments of Work Simulator.

HOME PROGRAMS

Since a few hours of intensive therapy is not enough to achieve excellent hand function, each patient must be given a home program. Patients from a five-state area are seen at the Hand Rehabilitation Center in Philadelphia; some patients live beyond commuting distance and may attend therapy only once a week for evaluation and follow-up instructions. Each patient must perform activities and exercises several times each day at home to obtain optimum function. Full instructions are given to each patient, and his ability to carry out the program must be demonstrated. Verbal, written, and graphic instructions may be necessary. Home programs have been found to build confidence, morale, and compliance with the therapy program itself.

Several individualized home programs are available; they are designed based upon the patient's upper extremity dysfunction. If a patient has a hypersensitive scar, his home program may consist of only desensitization techniques. If a patient has weakness, stiffness, or edema, light prehension activities in a macramé project are suggested. Simple prehension tasks may include grasping various-sized common household objects.

Macramé performed in elevation is an excellent initial activity for early active movement and reduction of edema. It is easily transported. Macramé can be hung on a shower-curtain hook or a cabinet door at home to provide the elevation needed for work. Macramé provides goal-directed activity for improved morale just at a time when a patient may need it most. A patient is given a specific stopping point to be reached by the next therapy session. In this way, the therapist can control the amount of activity and can easily check the project for compliance and mistakes at the next therapy session.

Foundry wax and clay sculpture are used as more resistance is needed for building strength endurance. Foundry wax is softer and less resistive than clay. Patients with arthritis or reflex sympathetic dystrophy find the warmth of wax submerged in warm water more appropriate for exercise than cold clay. A small ball of either wax or clay can be put in a plastic bag for transporting.

As the patient's strength and ability to tolerate resistance improves, sustained grip activities such as woodworking are selected. Precut and stored in the work therapy department are several small projects, such as candle holders, plant stands, and cutting boards, in soft and hard woods. Frequently tools for woodworking, such as a bilateral sander or a C clamp are provided for patients for home use. The patient may make a weight well as his first home woodworking project. It is made from a 1-inch dowel 24 inches in length (soft wood, such as pine) and a 36-inch piece of

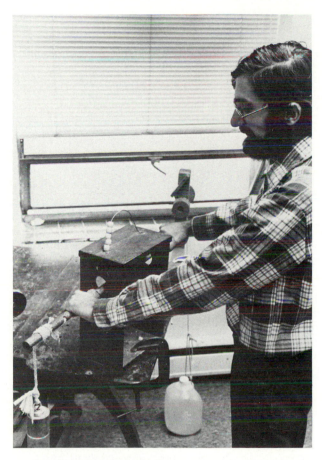

FIG. 81-19. Patient used weight well to increase finger flexion.

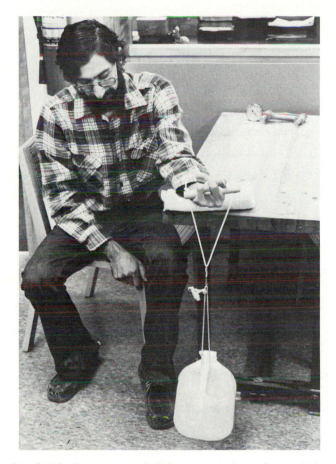

FIG. 81-20. Common household items are used to perform resistive exercises.

cord. At home, light weights may be connected to the rope and dowel, such as plastic milk containers or socks filled with coins or canned goods. Thumb, wrist, and finger exercises can be performed on the weight well (Fig. 81-19).

Isometric and isotonic exercises with weights are prescribed for home use. Since dumbbells are not usually available, patients are instructed to use a plastic gallon container attached to a wooden dowel with a rope and a shower-curtain hook (Fig. 81-20). A written home program is given to each patient to illustrate proper technique for performance of isometric or isotonic weight lifting at home. Other resistive exercises frequently suggested for home use include use of exercise putty and hand-helper exercises. In the final stages of the therapy program, job-simulated tasks such as repetitive lifting or tool handling are included in the patient's home program to prepare him to return to work.

REFERENCES

1. Beasley, R.: Hand injuries, Philadelphia, 1981, W.B. Saunders Co.
2. Rossky, E.: Protection of arthritic joints (patient pamphlet), Department of Occupational Therapy, Moss Rehabilitation Hospital, Philadelphia, Pa.
3. Trombley, C.A., Scott, A.D.: Occupational therapy for physical dysfunction, Baltimore, 1977, The Williams & Wilkins Co.
4. Zinovieff, A.N.: Heavy resistance exercises—the Oxford technique, Br. J. Phys. Med. **14:**129-132, 1951.

BIBLIOGRAPHY

Blodgett, M.: Occupational therapy and rehabilitation in the United States Public Health Service, Am. J. Occup. Ther. **2:**53, 1948.
Hunter, J.: The rehabilitation of function in injuries of the hand, Med. Clin. North Am. **49**(5):1425-1440, 1965.
Patterson, L.M.: Productivity, work study and occupational therapy, Canad. J. Occup. Ther. **30:**53-60, 1963.
Rosenberg, B., and Wellerson, T.: A structured pre-vocational program, Am. J. Occup. Ther. **14:**57-60, 1960.

82

Wood carving as therapy

ADOLPH DIODA

Wood carving is a most beneficial form of therapy for patients recovering from hand surgery. The patient is prepared for his venture into wood carving by the hand therapist. Generally, patients for whom wood carving is prescribed as a therapeutic activity have already been engaged in lighter woodworking and have learned to work with such basic tools as hammers, saws, hand drills, and screwdrivers. Carving, however, allows for more control and a more varied manipulation of tools without strain. The total carving process takes considerable time, and the progression from cutting to rasping to sanding affords the hand a wide range of strengthening exercises.

Practice in carving develops the knack for working with the devious grain in wood while strengthening the long flexors of both forearms. In using the mallet and chisel (Fig. 82-1), the patient can rapidly recover both joint function and muscle power. This is also an excellent means of strengthening the chisel-holding, or non-dominant, hand. At the beginning, the voluntary motion is tedious and requires complete concentration.

Not only does the exercise benefit the patient physically, but the feeling of accomplishment contributes to his general sense of well-being. Wood carving, in contrast to more traditional modes of therapy, excites the patient's interest. Because accomplishment is immediately visible, the patient's self-confidence is promoted. Praise and encouragement by the hand therapy personnel and interaction among patients, with their mutual assistance and advice, help sustain this feeling.

WORK AREA

The recommended height of the workbench is 28 inches. This allows the carver to work down on his piece with far less effort than that required at more conventional bench heights (Fig. 82-2). Three foot-controlled rope slings along the bench's 8-foot length are used to secure work in progress (Fig. 82-3). The slings are simple loops of ½-inch rope that issue from a pair of ¾-inch holes, 12 inches apart on the far side of the table. The ends of the rope have been secured by being knotted below the bench top. When a log is placed on the bench, the loop is easily raised, passed over the log, and dropped to the floor, where a foot placed in the loop and on the rope controls rope tension. Wedges may then be placed under the log for additional stabilization.

WOOD SELECTION AND INITIAL PREPARATION

Carving is started on freshly cut logs (Fig. 82-4), preferably of cherry or elm. Because of the moisture content, green wood is fairly easy to carve. Logs in this state are stored in plastic bags, a procedure that slows down drying and prevents the development of checks. The logs are removed from the bags daily to permit evaporation of surface moisture and are then returned. This allows the outer surface to absorb the internal moisture and subsequently permits the gradual shrinkage of the total log. Additionally, this prevents the formation of wood-discoloring mold.

Basswood, yellow poplar, and weeping willow (medium-hard woods) are ideal for sculptural projects. White oak, rock maple, beech, and cherry, although hard woods, are easily carved in the wet state but require more effort in finishing as the wood dries. Also suitable for our purposes are mahogany, white pine, and yellow poplar (tulipwood), available in board form at local lumber yards. Blocks can be made by lamination of sections of plank together to form pieces of desired size. Joined pieces should be placed in such a position that all grain runs in the same direction.

TOOLS AND SUPPLIES

Few tools and relatively simple equipment are needed for carving (Fig. 82-5). The chisels we use at the Hand Rehabilitation Center in Philadelphia include a 1-inch-deep veiner, a ½-inch-deep veiner, and a 1-inch, half-round gouge.

Cutting edges on tools used for carving soft and green woods should have a long bevel on the underside of the blade for a thin, tapering edge. Such a blade produces clean cuts and will not tear the wood. Steel used in wood carving is very brittle. For hard woods, a blunt edge is required. Thin edges tend to break when forced into a more resistant material.

Mallets are made of discarded bowling pins, two from each pin. Centering the pin in a lathe, one reshapes the neck to approximate the form of a Coca-Cola bottle. Sizes may vary from 1¼ inches to 1¾ inches at the handle's fullest diameter. This range in sizes permits the patient to choose the size that most comfortably fits his hand. A 2-inch-deep hole, ¾ inch in diameter, is drilled in the center of the remaining pin half. A dowel, 8 inches long and with a

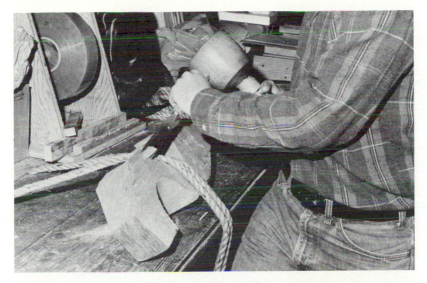

FIG. 82-1. Patient using mallet and chisel. Woodcarving is excellent activity to strengthen nondominant hand holding chisel.

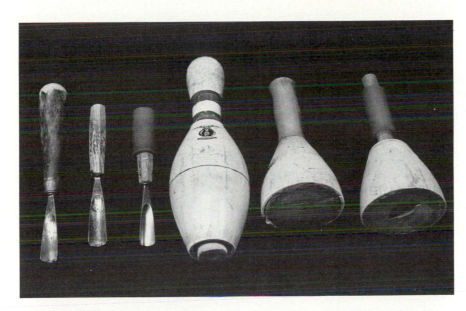

FIG. 82-2. Few tools and relatively simple equipment are needed for woodcarving.

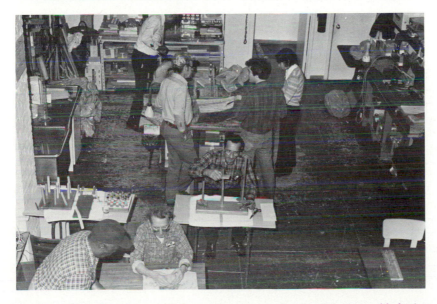

FIG. 82-3. Work bench is 28 inches high, permitting carver to work down on his piece with far less effort than that required at more conventional bench heights.

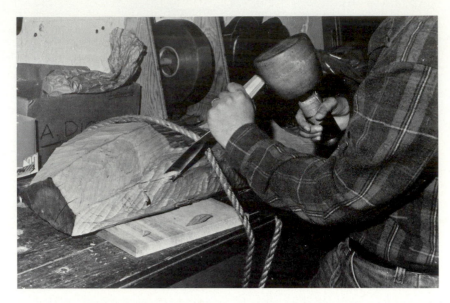

FIG. 82-4. Three foot-controlled rope slings along bench's 8 foot length are used to secure work in progress.

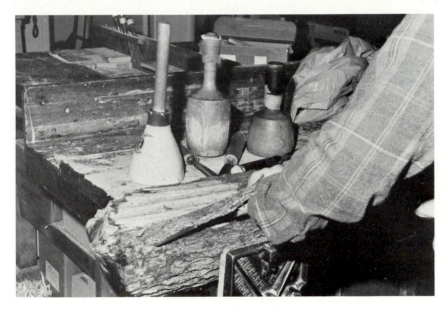

FIG. 82-5. Carving is started on freshly cut logs.

diameter to match the hole, is glued and forced into the drilled hole, thus completing the second mallet. Sections of foam rubber tubing can be slipped over these handles to cushion them. The bowling pin's plastic cover is retained. It will serve to protect the mallet head. A Surform rasp with a half-round blade attached is a most indispensable tool. Cabinetmaker's rasps are equally valuable, and an ample supply of sandpaper of various grits is very useful.

CARVING

Patients selected for wood-carving sessions are shown photographs of contemporary carvings in which elimination of details and simplicity of form are stressed, an approach that makes the activity of carving attractive. The initial piece is often a nonobjective free form where movement and wood grain are prominent. This approach encourages graduation to more complex projects, usually abstract representations that maintain the intrinsic nature of the wood.

With mallet and chisel, the patient begins his project by first stripping the bark from the selected log. The time involved depends on the physical condition of the disabled hand. The first session is usually short. Sessions that follow are lengthened by degrees as manual strength and flexibility increase. After stripping is done, the log's shape, knobs,

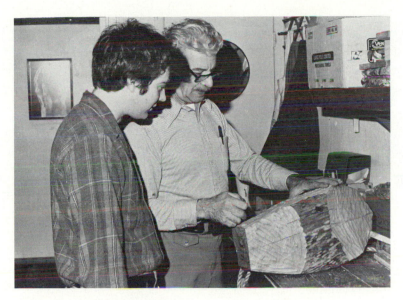

FIG. 82-6. Front and side contours are blocked.

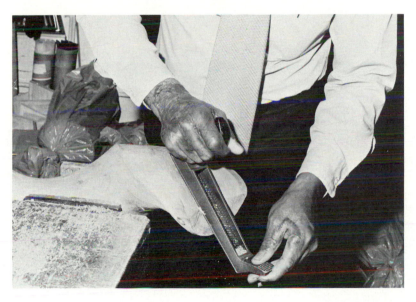

FIG. 82-7. Surface of wood is rasped and reduced to its final form.

protuberances, and so on are noted for possible inclusion in the final carved form. The bottom of the log is then cut so that the log stands in balance. Next, front and side contours are blocked (Fig. 82-6). With the silhouette defined from all visual angles, the process of determining the change of direction of surface planes follows. As work progresses, changes are made to accommodate the unexpected defect. The surface at this stage is rasped and reduced to its final form (Fig. 82-7). The final surface is accomplished in stages as one works from coarse to medium to fine sandpapers (Fig. 82-8). Drying out and cutting away have reduced moisture and bulk, but the sanded piece may require even

more time in its plastic bag to ensure absolutely thorough drying. It is imperative that the plastic bag be examined periodically for holes. The presence of these may cause a too-rapid loss of moisture from the log. When cracks, or checks, develop, insertion of long wedges of the same wood into the opening remedies the condition. These wedges are cut to the length of the opening, dipped in a solution of two parts water and one part white glue, and forced into the check. On the following day, any wedge portion projecting above the sculpture's surface can be shaved away and then sanded.

Patients are encouraged to visit Philadelphia's fine mu-

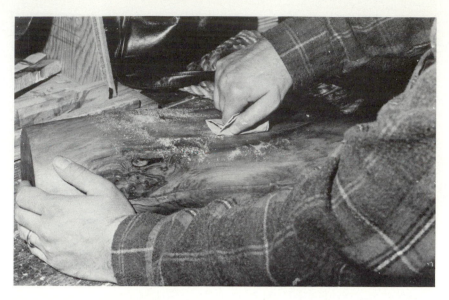

FIG. 82-8. Surface refinement is accomplished in stages working with coarse to medium to fine sandpaper.

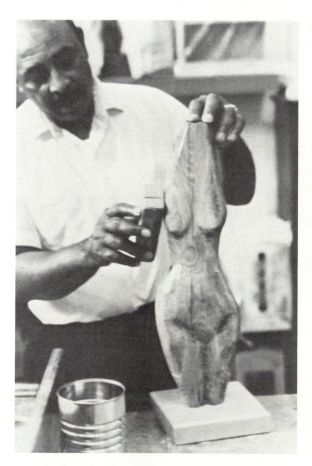

FIG. 82-9. Final sanding of sculpture by patient.

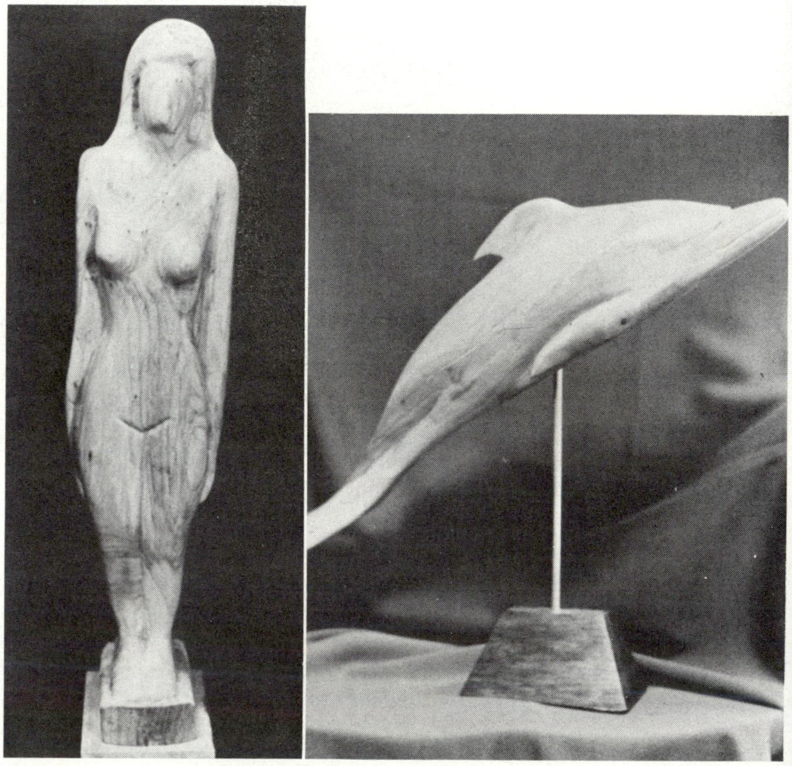

FIG. 82-10. Two pieces of sculpture completed by patients.

seums and art galleries, where exposure to great collections of contemporary, ancient, and primitive sculpture often serve to intensify budding interest. Involved in the creation of sculpture themselves, they find they are better able to relate to the vision of other artists in a totally new and unique way, often engendering a very special insight that may alter for all time the way each relates to every new experience (Figs. 82-9 and 82-10).

83

The Work Simulator

RAYMOND M. CURTIS, GAYLORD L. CLARK, and RUTH ANNE SNYDER

The Work Simulator (Fig. 83-1) was developed for the Hand Rehabilitation Center at The Union Memorial Hospital in Baltimore, Maryland, by John Engalitcheff.[1] Its purpose is to allow for the rehabilitation and testing of injured upper limbs without requiring varied types of machinery for this process. There are certain predictable and measurable patterns of use of the muscles and joints of the hand and the upper limb. These motions are used in the day-to-day activities of all people within an average population. When injury or disease alters this pattern of motion, physicians and therapists find it difficult to assess the degree of impairment and then design a program for rehabilitation to gain and document maximum functional recovery. It is not feasible or practical in any rehabilitation center to have the innumerable machines and tools used in industry and at home. To resolve this problem, a single compact instrument with a limited number of attachments was designed to provide for specific repetitive upper limb motions against measurable resistances over a measurable period of time.

Also of importance is the Work Simulator's ability to document in a numerical way the work output of the patient (Fig. 83-2). In this way periodic comparisons can be made. Such capability is not only helpful to the therapists responsible for the patients' treatment programs but also to the patients themselves, since it enables them to realize their abilities and limitations.

The hand surgeon has been continually challenged by cases in which the degree of recovery from injury or disease is guesswork on his part or the patient's. He has been unable to determine when maximum benefit from all forms of treatment has been reached and whether treatment has been effective. The tools that have been standard in making these assessments are the pinch meter, the grip-strength dynamometer, and the goniometer for measuring joint ranges of motion. Although these are excellent devices, they have many limitations and do not measure work output. Preoperative and postoperative testing methods have been essentially limited to these instruments. Now the Work Simulator can be added to this group.

The Work Simulator can provide a more accurate designation of diagnosis for persons with nonspecific symptoms who are seeking secondary gain by malingering or whose condition has a psychological cause, since this instrument uses spaced serial testings that can yield confirmatory information from erratic and inconsistent work-output figures.

In addition, physical-impairment percentage ratings for disabled hands and arms may be made with greater accuracy by use of static-power and endurance-output measurements formulated after testing with the Work Simulator.

The formula for the numerical determination of work output is based on the equation for horsepower. The work of the human hand cannot be measured in horsepower units; therefore a modification called an "engal" has been devised by Mr. Engalitcheff. The formula reads as follows:

$$\text{Power} = \frac{\text{Resistance} \times \text{Distance}}{\text{Time}}$$

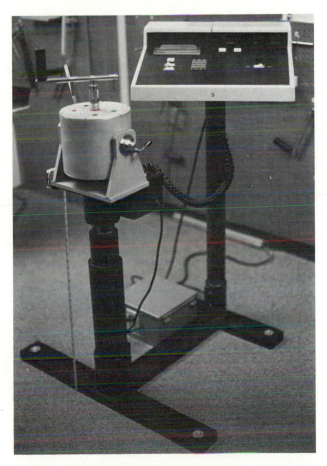

FIG. 83-1. Model of Work Simulator currently in use at Union Memorial Hospital, Baltimore, Md.

```
PAT. ID              98562
DATE                 04/10/82
TOOL NO.             161
MODE                 AUTO
EXER. LEV.           029
FORCE (in-lbs)             028
DIST.  (deg)               1299
EXER. TIME (sec)           30
WORK  (in-lb/deg)    000 037 409
POWER (engals)             001 246
STOP TIMED      13:20
```

FIG. 83-2. Sample of printed data output calculated by Work Simulator.

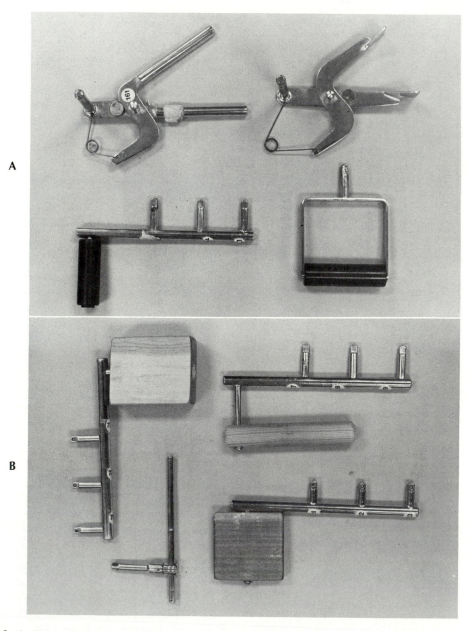

FIG. 83-3. A, Work Simulator attachment for grip, three-point pinch, pronation, supination, and wrist flexion and extension. **B,** Adapted simulator attachments for ulnar and radial deviation and elbow flexion and extension.

In terms of engals, therefore, the Work Simulator has the capability of measuring the power output of the operator. The instrument is basically an electrical braking system that can deliver varying degrees of resistance to an axial shaft. This gives the first factor in the formula. The second factor, distance traveled, is measured by degrees of arc turned on the axis of the apparatus, with 360 degrees being one complete revolution. The third factor, time, is measured by the built-in computer or by the therapist. The current model, with its computer console, automatically computes the power output and the factors that are entered into that computation.

A variety of tool attachments is available (Fig. 83-3). The basic set has 20; however, new ones may be devised and added, depending on the skill and experience of the therapist. Some tools currently in use are for the following:

Precision pinch with rotation: adjusting a key in the bit of a drill press

Lateral pinch with rotation: turning a key in a lock

Three-point prehension: squeezing a tube of toothpaste

Spheric grasp: turning a door knob

Compound wrist motion: adjusting a lathe handle

Parallel grip with supination and pronation: using a screwdriver

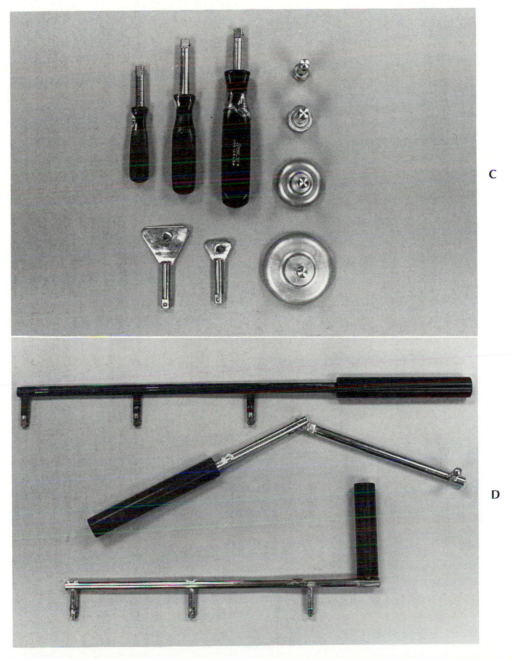

FIG. 83-3, cont'd. C, Work Simulator attachments for cylindric grip with pronation, supination, and lateral pinch. **D,** Work Simulator attachments for elbow flexion and extension with shoulder motion.

Power grip: using pliers

Perpendicular grip with pronation and supination: use of a shovel with a grip handle

Elbow flexion and extension with handgrip: turning an armature by gripping its axle

Elbow flexion and extension and shoulder motion with cylindric grasp: working control levers on heavy equipment

Two-handed shoulder and elbow motion with T handle: digging a ditch

Two-handed shoulder and elbow motion with cylindric grasp: hoeing in the garden

Composite upper extremity motion with handgrip: steering a car or turning large valves

Two-handed shoulder, elbow, and wrist motion with handgrip: drilling a hole as with an offset brace and bit

These attachments have many applications related to job tasks and upper extremity movements. Adaptations can be made on the attachments, in addition to adjustment of the height of the brake, the angle of the shaft, and the position of the patient.

In The Union Memorial Hospital Hand Rehabilitation Center we have rehabilitated house painters to use paint rollers, carpenters to use saws, longshoremen to heave bags of grain, electricians to grasp wire cutters, mechanics to use wrenches, tractor-trailer drivers to use levers for securing equipment on flat beds, bus drivers to handle the vehicle's steering wheel, and machine operators to develop skills to operate their machinery. The Work Simulator is also useful in helping the housewife, the hobbyist, and the craftsman gain strength and endurance.

There are limitations to the Work Simulator that have not yet been overcome, the most common of which is that a very strong individual could overpower the machine, making accurate recordings impossible. There are restrictions on the positioning of the equipment, such as for height or angle for working overhead or at floor level. Despite these limitations, it is believed that the Work Simulator is of great value in rehabilitation, patient evaluation, and clinical research.

Initiating the treatment of a patient on the Work Simulator requires a therapist's careful analysis of the person's physical limitations and work requirements. Goals are then established.

A typical case history is that of a 37-year-old longshoreman who in February 1980 sustained a crush injury to the right thumb, resulting in a laceration on the radial side from interphalangeal joint to under the nail and a fracture of the tuft of the distal phalanx. This was treated by proper immobilization until the fracture and the laceration healed; however, a residual stiffness was present, with discomfort during pinching. The patient's job required him to handle 150-pound bags of coffee, making it necessary for him to dig his thumbs into the bags in order to throw them onto a pallet. He was also required to climb ladders, haul on lines, drive a towmotor, and pull on levers. The major problem to be resolved was throwing the bags of coffee.

After an initial evaluation and job analysis in April 1980, it was determined that most of the Work Simulator attachments were applicable to the job-skill requirements. Modification of a level tool attachment by application of a heavy cloth bag over its handle afforded simulation of lifting bags of coffee against high resistance. After 8 weeks of appropriately supervised use of the Work Simulator, the patient declared he was ready and capable of returning to his Longshoreman job and has not required further care.

Another case involved a 45-year-old right-handed house painter who fell from his ladder, sustaining a displaced Colles' fracture of his right wrist. He was unable to work, because of severe wrist pain, and his tolerance for any type of repetitive wrist motion was greatly diminished. Because of x-ray evidence of advanced posttraumatic osteoarthritis of that joint, a successful wrist fusion was performed. After roentgenologic confirmation of a solid bony union, the patient was started on the Work Simulator. Simulation of skills required by a house painter were designed, including the use of brushes, rollers, and ladder climbing. After 12 weeks of treatment the patient returned to his regular work, 2 years after the initial injury and 6 months after the wrist fusion.

Occasionally it is necessary for the therapist or surgeon to visit job sites to observe the kinds of skills required to return a patient to a specific form of work. In instances where this type of visit is not possible, industry has provided videotapes and descriptions of the work requirements. These tapes are used for repeated viewing by therapist, patient, and surgeon.

Although not the complete answer to restoration of hand and upper limb function, the Work Simulator adds a new dimension to the hope of persons with hand injury or disease that they may restore their manual skills and return to their work with confidence.

ACKNOWLEDGMENTS

We are indebted to Douglas Browning and Jack Doub of Baltimore Therapeutic Company for their skills in developing the Work Simulator.

REFERENCE

Curtis, R.M., and Engalitcheff, J., Jr.: A Work Simulator for rehabilitating the upper extremity—preliminary report, J. Hand Surg. **6**(5):499-501, 1981.

84

Physical capacity evaluation

PATRICIA L. BAXTER and **PAMELA M. McENTEE**

Physicians and therapists treating patients with hand injuries are often faced with the question of whether these patients will return to their previous occupations. The physical capacity evaluation has been developed to provide concrete information to assist in this determination. This chapter describes the tests utilized by therapists at the Hand Rehabilitation Center in Philadelphia to assess the hand-injured worker's ability to return to his previous occupation. Interpretation of results and recommendations for return to work with or without job modifications are discussed.

Before beginning the evaluation, the patient is informed of its purpose and duration. At the Hand Rehabilitation Center, this evaluation takes approximately 3 hours to administer, and 1 hour is needed to interpret the results and prepare a written report. No two physical capacity evaluations are alike. The tests selected are based on the physical demands included in the patient's job description. Information about the patient's job can be obtained in several ways. Before the initial patient interview, the therapist may obtain the patient's job description from the *Dictionary of Occupational Titles*. The therapist should also request a complete job analysis from the rehabilitation specialist if one is assigned to the patient's case. These two sources and a thorough patient interview provide the therapist with the necessary information to select appropriate tests needed to complete the evaluation.

HAND FUNCTION EVALUATION

The physical capacity evaluation begins with a hand function assessment. Range of motion, pinch and grip strength, hand volume, activities of daily living, and sensibility testing constitute this part of the evaluation. One or all of these assessments may be used, depending on the patient's condition.

Range of motion, both active and passive, is measured with a goniometer by the standard methods of measuring and recording as described in *Joint Motion*, published by the American Academy of Orthopedic Surgeons.[1] Lateral, tip, and three-point pinch are measured on a pinch meter. Grip strength is tested on a Jamar Adjustable Dynamometer.* This dynamometer has five handle positions to allow the patient to perform a full-fisted grip on the first position and a wider grip on each of the other four positions. Research by Hook has indicated that if the patient is exerting maximum effort on each grip test on each position of the instrument, the measurements will be lowest for the first and fifth levels and highest on the second to fourth levels.[4] If all of the measurements are similar, the patient may not be exerting his maximum effort.

Hand-volume measurements are recorded before the patient performs the remaining parts of the physical capacity evaluation and after he has completed the 3-hour test. The volumeter, a specifically designed water-filled container, is used for measurement of edema.[2] The patient is instructed to submerge his hand in the volumeter, and hand volume is measured by the amount of water displaced (Fig. 84-1).

The patient's ability to use his hand for daily prehension activities is evaluated through the use of a Jebson[5] Hand Function Evaluation in conjunction with an interview. The Jebson test measures one's ability to perform daily functions such as writing, eating, and picking up small objects (Fig. 84-2).

When the sensibility function of an injured hand is questioned, tests such as two-point discrimination, light-touch perception, and the Moberg Pickup Test are essential in completing the hand function evaluation.

WORK PERFORMANCE EVALUATION

The second part of the physical capacity evaluation consists of a combination of observational and standardized tests. The therapist must refer to the patient's job analysis and the *Dictionary of Occupational Titles* to accurately simulate the physical demands of the patient's job. Physical demands are defined as those physical activities required of a worker in a job.[6] The patient must possess physical capabilities at least equal to the physical demands made by the job in order to be released for work. Table 84-1 lists and defines the various physical demands inherent in many jobs. Guidelines for the tools needed and techniques used for this part of the evaluation are also included in Table 84-1. The therapist can perform this section of the evaluation through observation of the patient performing physical tasks only (Fig. 84-3). However, we recommend that such observation be combined with standardized tests. The use of

---

*Asimow Engineering Co., 1414 So. Beverly Glen Blvd., Los Angeles, Calif. 90024.

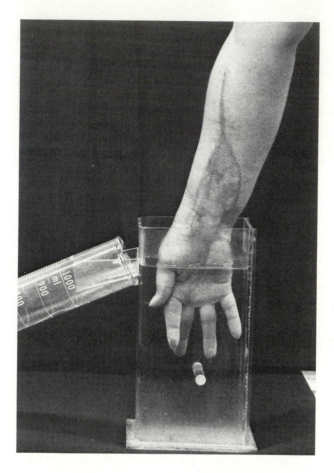

FIG. 84-1. Hand edema is measured with hand volumeter.

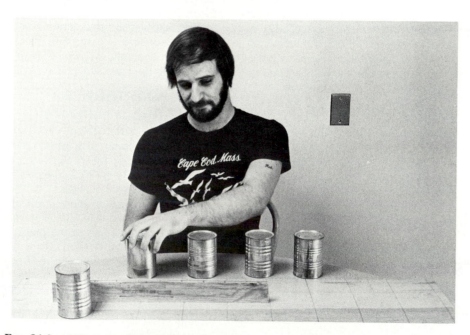

FIG. 84-2. Ability to perform prehension tasks is assessed with Jebson Hand Function Test.

TABLE 84-1. Guidelines for the work performance evaluation

Physical demands	Tools	Technique
Lifting: raising or lowering object from one level to another*	Box with weights; use maximum weight required on job; start with 10 pounds and progress to maximum weight	Observe patient performing repetitive weight lifting unilaterally and bilaterally for a period of time up to 1 hour depending on patient's job
Pushing: exerting force upon object so that object moves away from force*	Box with weights, dolly or pulley	Observe repetitive pushing and pulling on a table top, pulley, or dolly for a period of time up to 1 hour depending on patient's job
	Work Simulator	Observe patient on Work Simulator using handle nos. 801, 701, 901, and 111
Pulling: exerting force on object so that the objective moves toward the force*	Same tools as used for physical demand of pushing	Same techniques as used for physical demands of pushing
Climbing: ascending or descending using feet, legs, hands, or arms*	Stairs	Observe patient ascend and descend stairs three times
	Ladder	Observe patient ascend and descend ladder three times
Stooping: bending body downward and forward by bending spine at waist*	1- and 3-pound cans	Observe patient transferring cans from table to floor while bending body downward at waist
	Valpar Whole Body Range of Motion Work Sample	Standardized technique of Valpar Whole Body Range of Motion Work Sample
Kneeling: bending legs at knees to come to rest on knees*	1- and 3-pound cans	Observe patient transferring cans from table to floor while he is kneeling for 3 minutes
	Valpar Whole Body Range of Motion Work Sample	Standardized technique of Valpar Whole Body Range of Motion Work Sample
Crouching	1- and 3-pound cans	Observe patient transferring cans from table to floor while crouching for 3 minutes
	Valpar Whole Body Range of Motion Work Sample	Standardized technique of Valpar Whole Body Range of Motion Work Sample
Crawling		Observe patient crawl 10 feet
Sitting		Observe patient sitting during test
Standing		Observe patient standing during test
Walking		Observe patient walking during test
Reaching	Box, 1-pound cans	Observe patient reaching overhead to place cans in box; repeat with box at waist level and on the floor
	Valpar Work Samples: Whole Body Range of Motion Upper Extremity Range of Motion Simulated Assembly Work Sample	Standardized Technique of Valpar Work Samples
	Work Simulator	Observe patient on Work Simulator attachments 801, 701, 131, 901, and 141 in automatic mode
Handling: seizing, holding, grasping, turning, primarily with hand or hands*	Tools and pipe structure	Observe patient handling tools while assembling and disassembling pipe structure
	Minnesota Rate of Manipulation Test	Standardized technique of Minnesota Rate of Manipulation Test
	Valpar Work Samples: Simulated Assembly Small Tools Mechanical Upper Extremity Range of Motion Whole Body Range of Motion	Standardized techniques of Valpar Work Samples
	Work Simulator	Observe patient on Work Simulator attachments 302, 501, 502, 503, 601, 701, 111, 901, and 161 in automatic mode

*U.S. Department of Labor: Dictionary of occupational titles, ed. 3, Washington, D.C., 1968, U.S. Government Printing Office.   *Continued.*

TABLE 84-1. Guidelines for the work performance evaluation—cont'd

Physical demands	Tools	Technique
Manipulating: picking, pinching, or otherwise working with fingers primarily*	Small nuts and bolts: small tools	Observe patient manipulating small objects with and without tools
	Valpar Work Samples: Upper Extremity Range of Motion Small Tools Mechanical Whole Body Range of Motion Simulated Assembly	Standardized techniques of Valpar Work Samples
	Work Simulator	Use Work Simulator attachments 101, 102, 201, 400, and 151 in automatic mode
Feeling: perceiving such attributes of objects and materials as size, shape, temperature, and texture, by means of receptors in skin, particularly to fingertips*	Moberg Pickup Test	Observe patient's prehension pattern with vision occluded
	Valpar Work Samples: Upper Extremity Range of Motion Whole Body Range of Motion	Standardized technique of Valpar Work Samples
Talking, hearing, and seeing: Endurance: ability to work over a period of time		Observation of patient
	Valpar Work Samples: Whole Body Range of Motion Simulated Assembly Small Tools Mechanical	Standardized techniques of Valpar Work Samples
	Work Simulator	Use Work Simulator in automatic mode for 3 minutes with the tool attachments appropriate to patient's job

standardized tests provides quantitative information on the patient's ability to perform job tasks.

Valpar work samples

The Valpar Work Samples* are one set of instruments used at the Hand Rehabilitation Center to provide quantitative measurement of a patient's ability to perform job-related tasks. These standardized tests are designed to evaluate specific physical demands, such as reaching, handling, and manipulating various objects, that are inherent in many industrial jobs.

The use of standardized norms facilitates comparison of the patient's work performance to that of the uninjured worker population. During performance of a work sample, a patient is given the opportunity to report physical discomfort or fatigue he experiences, and this information is recorded on a chart designed by the Valpar Corporation (Fig. 84-4). The work samples also provide the therapist the opportunity to document worker characteristics, such as ability to complete tasks according to instructions.

The Valpar Corporation has developed 18 work samples for use by therapists and vocational evaluators. The following four work samples are utilized most frequently for phys-

ical capacity evaluations of hand-injured patients at our center.

The Valpar Upper Extremity Range of Motion Work Sample tests one's ability to reach, handle, and manipulate nuts, which must be placed onto bolts inside a 1 foot by 1 foot box (Fig. 84-5). The work sample is designed so that the patient must manipulate the nuts inside the box with his vision occluded. The patient's performance using his dominant hand is compared to his performance using his nondominant hand. The work sample is valuable for assessing patients who perform manual jobs, including machinery repair, plumbing, and construction.

The Valpar Whole Body Range of Motion Work Sample measures the patient's ability to handle various-sized objects while standing, stooping, crouching, and reaching overhead (Fig. 84-6). The work sample is appropriate for assessing patients who are required to perform the physical demands of their jobs in a variety of positions. Painters, roofers, carpenters, and welders are some of the many patients who fall in this category.

The Valpar Small Tools Work Sample is designed to measure the patient's ability to work with small tools such as pliers, screwdrivers, and wrenches of various sizes (Fig. 84-7). Patients who are electricians, automobile mechanics, appliance repairmen, and machine setters can be evaluated with this work sample.

The Valpar Simulated Assembly Work Sample evaluates manual dexterity as related to production-line work. The patient's bilateral use of his upper extremities can be ob-

---

*Valpar Work Samples, Valpar Corp., 3801 E. 34th Street, Tucson, Ariz. 85713.

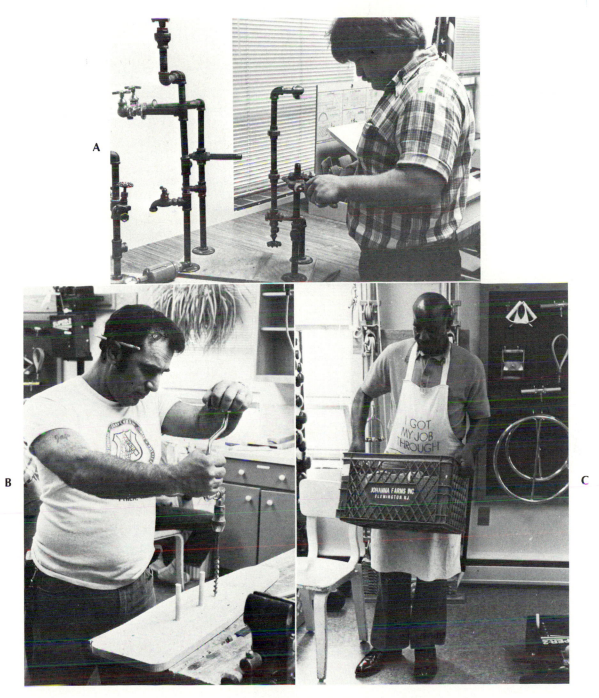

FIG. 84-3. Patient is observed as he performs physical demands of his job.

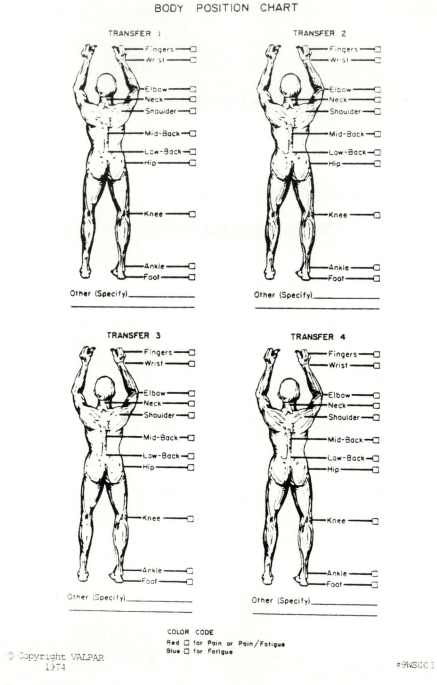

FIG. 84-4. Valpar Body Position Chart is used to record patient's subjective complaints.

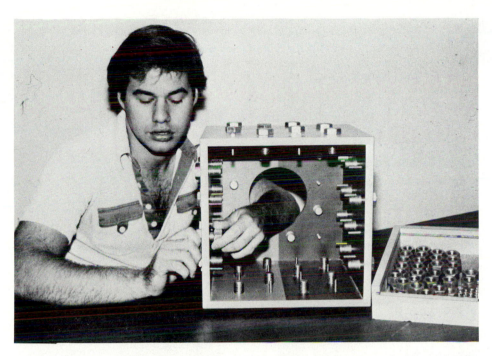

FIG. 84-5. Valpar Upper Extremity Range of Motion Work Sample assesses manipulative ability.

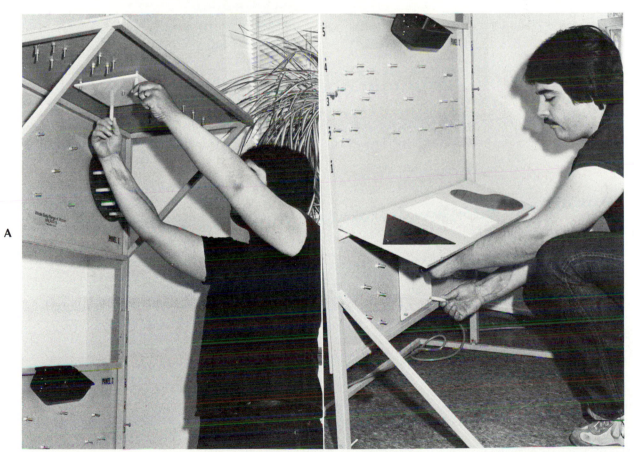

FIG. 84-6. A, Patient's endurance to work overhead is tested with this Valpar work sample. **B,** Patient stoops as he manipulates objects with his vision occluded.

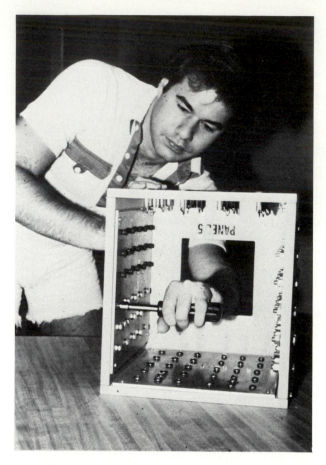

FIG. 84-7. Tool handling is assessed through this Valpar work sample.

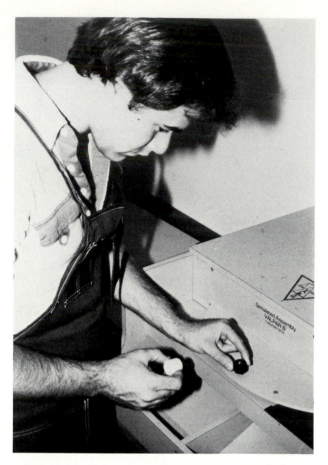

FIG. 84-8. Patient performs repetitive assembly tasks on this Valpar work sample.

served. This work sample is ideal for assessment of inspectors, line assemblers, bakery laborers, and injection molding machine tenders (Fig. 84-8).

The Work Simulator

The therapist utilizes the Work Simulator as an observational test of the patient's ability to perform the physical demands of his job. The Work Simulator (see Chapter 83) is a mechanical device designed to simulate upper extremity motions required during performance of job tasks (Fig. 84-9). The Work Simulator has 18 tool attachments. These attachments are numbered to promote universal use of the tools and to facilitate research that can be conducted in multiple clinical studies. Tool attachment numbers and the function of each one are listed in Table 84-2 and will enable the therapist to follow the guidelines for evaluating the patient's performance of the physical demands for his job, which are listed in Table 84-1. Tool attachments are selected to simulate the patient's job.

The Work Simulator has a calibrated resistance device that each tool is attached to so that the patient can work against resistance. The patient must exert force equal to the resistance set on the Work Simulator to move the tool attachment. As the patient moves the tool attachment, the Work Simulator calculates the work the patient performs by multiplying the force the patient exerts by the distance he moves the tool attachment connected to the shaft.[3] The Work Simulator also calculates the patient's endurance by dividing the work produced by the time he is able to work.

The patient is instructed to exert his maximum effort as he moves the tool attachment for a 3-minute test period. Both the dominant hand and the nondominant hand are tested in the same manner. The numerical calculations for the work and endurance of each hand are compared. The results are interpreted by comparing the patient's dominant hand to his nondominant hand. The dominant hand should exhibit greater work and endurance capacity than the nondominant hand. The Work Simulator provides objective calculations that can be used to identify the patient's capabilities and limitations in regard to upper extremity motions inherent in his job.

RECOMMENDATIONS

Based on the patient's strength, speed, coordination, and endurance, and on safety during performance of job-simulated tasks, a report with recommendations is completed regarding his return to work. The report is reviewed by the patient's physician, and final recommendations are established by the therapist and the physician.

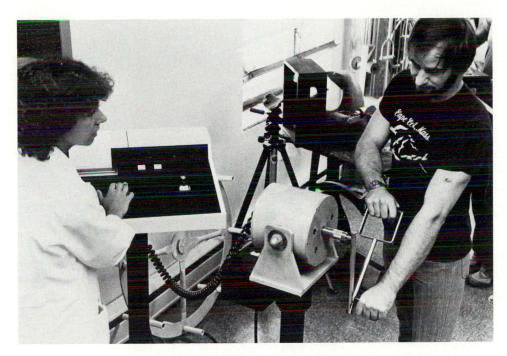

FIG. 84-9. Work Simulator assesses each patient's ability to perform his job tasks.

TABLE 84-2. Work Simulator tool attachments

Tool attachment numbers	Function of tool attachment
101	Small tip pinch
102	Medium tip pinch
201	Small lateral pinch
202	Medium lateral pinch
151	Three-point prehension
161	Power grip
111	Power grip, elbow flexion and extension
131	Combined upper extremity motion with power grip (car steering wheel)
141	Combined upper extremity motion with power grip (truck steering wheel)
302	Precision grip, wrist ulnar deviation (jar lid)
400	Lateral pinch and wrist circumduction (crank)
501	Small power grip with supination and pronation (small screwdriver)
502	Medium power grip with supination and pronation (medium screwdriver)
503	Large power grip with supination and pronation (large screwdriver)
601	Power grip with supination and pronation
701	Elbow flexion and extension with power grip
801	Elbow flexion and extension and shoulder motion with power grip
901	Two-handed shoulder and elbow motion with T handle

Recommendations vary according to each patient's performance. If the patient performs all aspects of the physical capacity evaluation without difficulty, he is released to return to his regular duties. Patients who experience pain or weakness and are unable to complete adequately all aspects of the physical capacity evaluation are placed in a work tolerance program for a specified period of time to upgrade their physical capabilities (Fig. 84-10). These patients often return to their previous occupations after an intense program of 1- to 3-months' duration. Patients with permanent impairment, such as diminished sensibility or amputation of digits, often return to their previous jobs if job modifications are permitted by their employers. One of the most common recommendations for job modification is restriction of the patient with sensory losses from working in extreme temperatures or with moving machinery. Other examples of job modifications include use of adaptive equipment and recommendations for assistance with lifting of heavy objects beyond the patient's capabilities. Some patients cannot adequately perform the majority of their former job tasks. These patients must seek jobs that do not require strenuous use of their injured hands. Recommendations for jobs for these patients, based on job history, educational level, interests, and aptitudes, may be made by the therapist. When it is appropriate, a patient is also referred to a vocational evaluator for further testing and job placement.

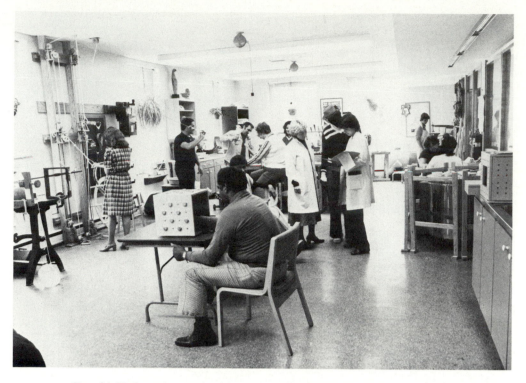

FIG. 84-10. Intensive work tolerance program reconditions industrial workers.

REFERENCES

1. American Academy of Orthopaedic Surgeons: Joint motion, method of measuring and recording, Chicago, 1965.
2. Brand, P., and Wood, H.: Hand volumeter instruction sheet, U.S. Public Health Service Hospital, Carville, La., 1978.
3. Curtis, R.M., and Engalitcheff, J., Jr.: A work simulator for rehabilitating the upper extremity—preliminary report, J. Hand Surg. **6**(5):499-501, 1981.
4. Hook, T.: The grip strength of patients tested on the Jamar Dynamometer, Presented at the American Society of Hand Therapists third annual meeting, Feb. 6 and 7, 1980, Atlanta, Ga.
5. Jebson, R.H., Taylor, N., Trieschman, R.B., Trotter, M.J., and Howard, L.A.: An objective and standardized test of hand function, Arch. Phys. Med. Rehabil. **50**:311-319, 1969.
6. U.S. Department of Labor: Dictionary of occupational titles, ed. 3, Washington, D.C., 1968, U.S. Government Printing Office.

BIBLIOGRAPHY

American Society for Surgery of the Hand: The hand—examination and diagnosis, Aurora, Colo., 1978, The Society.
Bly, B., and Michael, R.: On the job evaluations in a general hospital, Rehabil. Lit. **34**(12):364-368, Dec. 1973.
Chaffin, D.: Ergonomics guide for the assessment of human static strength, Am. Ind. Hyg. Assoc. J. **36**:505-511, 1975.
Cromwell, F.: A procedure for pre-vocational evaluation, Am. J. Occup. Ther. **13**(1):1-4, 1959.
DeVore, G., and Hamilton, G.: Volume measuring of the severely injured hand, Am. J. Occup. Ther. **22**:16-18, 1968.
Institute for the Crippled and Disabled: TOWER: testing, orientation and work evaluation in rehabilitation, New York, 1967, The Institute.
Kellor, M., Frost, J., and Silberberg, N., and others: Hand strength and dexterity, Am. J. Occup. Ther. **25**:77-83, 1971.
Kirkpatrick, J.E.: Evaluation of grip loss: a factor of permanent partial disability in California, Industr. Med. Surg. **26**:285-289, 1957.
Wegg, L.S.: The essentials of work evaluation, Am. J. Occup. Ther. **14**:65-69, 1960.

85

Industrial hand injuries: prevention and rehabilitation

SIDNEY J. BLAIR, JANE BEAR-LEHMAN, and EVA McCORMICK

The purposes of this chapter are to outline the incidence of industrial hand injuries, patterns of their occurrence, and methods of prevention, and to discuss problems experienced by returning workers.

Industrial upper extremity injuries gravely affect the lives of the patient and the members of his family and increase the costs to the community. The National Safety Council's *Accident Facts* reported that in 1979 there were approximately 2.3 million disabling work injuries.[1] Of these 13,200 were fatal and 80,000 resulted in permanent impairment. According to state labor department reports, trunk injuries occurred most frequently, followed by injuries to the thumb and finger. Arm injuries totalled 210,000, hands 160,000, and fingers 340,000. Total arm, hand, and finger injuries constituted 20% of the compensation costs of all injuries. The cost of all accidents in 1980, including motor vehicle, work, home, and public, came to 83 billion dollars. Work accidents cost 30 billion dollars, with 20% of them involving the upper extremity.

How accidents occur has been tabulated by the U.S. Department of Labor,[17] the U.S. Consumer Products Safety Commission,[13] and other organizations. Insurance carriers tabulate lists of occurrences. According to one survey, 22% of the emergency room patients with finger amputations gave up their original jobs. The Occupational Safety and Health Administration (OSHA), part of the United States Department of Labor, was created by the Occupational Safety and Health Act of 1970. The purpose of the act is to encourage employers and employees to reduce hazards in the work place. Most employers are covered under this act. OSHA often conducts work-place inspections without advance notice. OSHA has brought about a decrease in the occurrence of accidents, although they are still prevalent.

There are many tools with which a worker can injure his hands. In 1973, the United States had 290,000 power presses, 455,00 drill presses, 280,000 milling machines, and 195,000 cut-off saws, all of which present potential danger. Furthermore, safeguarding is a problem. Safety standards have been established, and organizations make safety equipment and conduct education programs, yet accidents, especially those involving power presses, still occur. For example, an investigation from February to July of 1979 conducted by the Office of Standards Development reported 50 amputations. They occurred in heavily industrial areas, mainly in the northeastern United States.[8]

Education of supervisors and redesigning of equipment are essential to the reduction of accidents. The medical community, represented by hand surgeons and others, can help to reduce injuries by contacting local safety groups and industries and by developing committees to investigate injuries. In the Chicago metropolitan area, hand surgeons have developed a cooperation with the National Safety Council's local committee and have started meeting to organize educational programs for the reduction of injuries.

RING INJURIES

Many industrial accidents involve a worker catching his ring on an object and then falling from a height. A fall from a height greater than 5 feet often produces an avulsion of all of the soft tissues of the ring finger. A ring can strip back the soft tissues of the wearer's finger, constrict circulation of bone and joint, and disrupt the skin flap. Amputation is the common result. Dr. William Frackelton of Columbia Hospital, Department of Surgery, Milwaukee, Wisconsin, developed modifications to make a ring safer for its wearer. This simple, inexpensive method slots the ring in three quadrants, thereby protecting the wearer in case of an accident. Caught on a projection, the ring spreads open, and the finger is spared (Fig. 85-1). If one were to send out this diagram to jewelers so that they could implement the design, ring avulsion injuries could be effectively reduced.

GRAIN AUGER INJURIES

There is a high prevalence of injuries among agricultural workers. In 1974, the Bureau of Labor Statistics reported that one in 10 farm workers suffered an occupational injury. Although power takeoff and grain auger injuries account for 50% of all farm machinery deaths, little is written about the grain auger. The National Safety Council report of 1979 stated that 22% of farm machinery injuries involved a grain auger and that 18% involved a corn picker. The augers are fitted with protective devices, yet 50% of the injured farm workers admitted removing or altering them for efficiency purposes. Most sustained upper extremity injuries, and about 50% suffered significant permanent disability and could not return to work. The grain auger is now being used in factories producing ground coal and plastic beads. Unfortunately, grain auger–related injuries are now prevalent among both farm and factory workers. In an effort to reduce

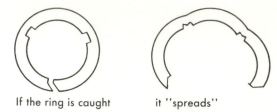

If the ring is caught   it "spreads"

FIG. 85-1. Safety ring designed by William H. Frankelton, Milwaukee, Wis.

grain auger injuries in southern Illinois, a media blitz focusing on increased awareness of the hazards of grain auger misuse was initiated in 1980. The report brought a significant reduction in injuries.

OCCUPATIONAL NERVE ENTRAPMENTS

The National Institute for Occupational Safety and Health (NIOSH) reports that more than 23,000 manual laborers from manufacturing or similar industries, including production, garment, assembly, upholstery, meat cutting, and letter sorting, are annually afflicted with carpal tunnel syndrome.[14] It is suspected that the actual incidence may significantly exceed the reported occurrences. Many injuries may be related to an overuse syndrome that results in a tenosynovitis in the hand, including the carpal canal. Entrapment of the ulnar nerve may also occur, because of repetitive elbow motion.

RAYNAUD'S PHENOMENON

Exposure to vibration may be an etiologic factor in Raynaud's phenomenon.[18] In vibration-induced Raynaud's phenomenon, commonly referred to as "vibration-induced white finger (VWF)," the symptoms are initially mild. Symptoms usually begin with the experience of frequent episodes of cold-induced numbness and blanching of the fingers. A decrease in blood supply causes fingers to become white and numb because of a spasm of the small vessels. The tip of one finger becomes white and numb when the hand is exposed to extreme cold. As the condition progresses, the symptoms occur more frequently and additional fingers become involved. The disease may occur in workers who repeatedly use air hammers, grinding tools, and chain saws, because the operation of vibrating hand tools has been shown to increase the risk of developing Raynaud's phenomenon. More than 500 studies in the medical literature have reported increased incidences of these symptoms in workers using these tools. Studies conducted among British and Scandinavian foundry chippers, grinders, and loggers who use chain saws show Raynaud's phenomenon ranging from 20% to 90%, depending on work force, length of employment, and daily severity of vibration exposure.

ERGONOMICS[10]

Ergonomics experts have joined the fight to reduce industrially related injuries. The field of ergonomics originated in Poland over a hundred years ago, and not until 1950 was it introduced into England. The term was coined from the Greek words *ergon*, meaning "work," and *nomos*, meaning "law" or "custom." Ergonomics is a branch of industrial engineering that aims to humanize jobs by fitting the work to the worker by studying man and his relationship to machines. It is an interdisciplinary approach composed of engineering, physiology, and psychology, with philosophical ideas also included in the general theory. Ergonomics revolves around a simple idea: adapt the man-made world to man, instead of the other way around. Ergonomics blends human characteristics with the living and working environment.

Ergonomics experts apply their knowledge to the design and use of hand tools, making the following recommendations:

1. The tool should be designed for operation with a straight wrist; the tool should be bent, not the wrist.
2. Workers should use power tools whenever feasible.
3. Tools should be light, and heavy tools should be suspended or otherwise counterbalanced.
4. Tools should be balanced with handles that are aligned at the center of the mass, so that no rotational moments of torque act on the hand.
5. Tools should be usable with either hand.
6. The grip span of a one-hand tool is best at about 2 inches and should not exceed 4 inches.
7. Handles of tongs and pliers should be designed so that the user will not pinch hands or fingers.
8. The handle surfaces should be so shaped as to contact the largest possible surface of the inner hand and fingers, thereby distributing forces evenly to resist creation of pressure points.

One improvement in hand tools was originated by John Bennett, of Peoria, Illinois. He studied the handle and noticed that with a closed hand there is an ellipse formed by the bottom of the hand and the knuckles of the closed fingers. From that he created a 19-degree angle for most tools, which, according to Bennett, contours the hand properly (Fig. 85-2).

Ergonomics experts have begun to investigate industries and have successfully achieved reductions in repetitive trauma disorders, including strains, tendonitis, irritation, ganglions, and carpal tunnel syndrome.[2] Methods of reduction include a task force for direction, training for education, engineering for prevention, and medical prevention and treatment. The engineering controls have led to changes being made in tools. Training consists in explanations of pertinent disorders and exploration of methods of alternative upper extremity postures and movements for work services, elevations, and orientations. Medical personnel have kept careful records to pinpoint sections of departments that have problems. By proper medical management, work restrictions, education of employee and section chiefs regarding the basic mechanics of the repetitive trauma process, and involvement of the product and biomechanical engineers to alter work positions and tool design, repetitive motion disorders have been decreased. Ergonomics engineers have also found that women have a greater risk of developing carpal tunnel syndrome and related tendon disorders than men do. Further research, however, has suggested that the

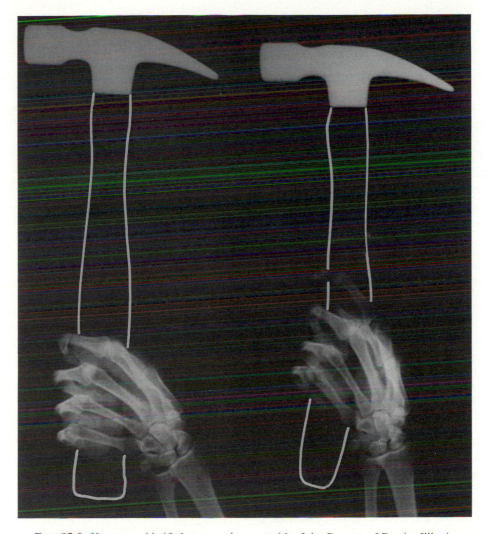

FIG. 85-2. Hammer with 19-degree angle, created by John Bennett of Peoria, Illinois.

gender variable is less important than work patterns, segmental vibrations, and hand stress.

DISABILITY AND RECOVERY

Workmen's compensation laws were enacted in the United States in 1911. They require employers to assume the cost of occupational disability. Financial losses resulting from worker disability are part of the cost of production. The basic purposes of the workmen's compensation law are as follows:

1. To encourage safety and effective delivery of benefits
2. To provide medical and rehabilitative services
3. To cover work-related injuries and protect income

Some believe that workmen's compensation influences a patient's response to treatment for a work-related injury, as well as the degree of residual disability. According to this point of view, compensated patients get more treatment and have greater residual disability than noncompensated patients. Disability is learned behavior. Since disability is what determines compensation, compensation is based upon learned behavior.

In many ways financial compensation does not help the patient or the employer. It can discourage the patient from returning to work. The appeals process can increase the duration of disability. The open claim can inhibit a return to work; thus recovering patients are often unable to return to work. How can ineffective therapy be terminated and claims closed so that recovery is maximized and the patient can return to work? In order to encourage and facilitate the return, rehabilitation centers have developed in the United States. Rehabilitation experts act as a liaison between the worker and the company. The problems of trying to locate appropriate jobs and getting a worker back to his previous employment present no easy solution.

ROLE OF THE HAND THERAPIST IN PREVENTION AND REHABILITATION
Safety and prevention task force

An American Society of Hand Therpists (ASHT) task force was formed in 1981 to study the relevance of hand therapy to the issues of safety and prevention for the injured industrial worker. The task-force consisted of volunteers from the ASHT who either work in industry or who have direct relationships with industries in their communities for the purpose of returning injured employees to work. Initial goals included identifying the present state of practice with regard to safety and prevention, establishing both evaluation and treatment goals for the incorporation of safety and prevention into a treatment regimen, increasing awareness, demonstrating how safety and prevention are part of the hand therapist's domain, and, finally, starting a resource file that includes a bibliography of references for the therapist.

Evaluation treatment

In addition to the acute care management of the hand-injured worker, the hand therapist provides evaluation and treatment directed toward return to work. The work of Baxter,[3] Matheson,[11] and Smith[16] has broadened our attention so that we are concerned not only with acute care hand therapy but also with the development of physical capacity evaluation, on-site evaluation, and the use of work therapy.[11] Implicit in such hand therapy programs during the rehabilitation phase is the concept of safe work. In regard to safe work, the following questions are raised. Does the patient employ proper body mechanics? Does he use his hand appropriately? Does he have an adequate number of rest periods? Does he know when he has done too much? These programs promote the rehearsal of work and worklike behaviors to minimize injury.

Safety and the role of hand therapy in safety are not limited to the minimizing of repeated injury. Therapists, including Rehms,[12] Johnson,[9] Douglas,[7] and Slack,[15] have been linking repeated episodes of specific injuries to a particular industries or machines; for example, tenosynovitis and carpal tunnel syndrome, have been linked to the use of crimpers in microassembly and electronics. Therapists have been establishing preventive exercise programs with the industries to diminish the incidence of these injuries. Most of these prevention programs occur in an industrial setting under the supervision of a therapist. Up to now, contacts with industry to encourage the establishment of preventive programs have been limited and on an individual basis. Interaction with ergonomics experts and exercise physiologists can be helpful when this type of program is being planned.

The objective findings from evaluative measurements are combined with clinical observations of the patients. Work therapy programs provide valuable information for predicting the ability to return to work safely and for minimizing the chances that an injury will be repeated. Review of the total clinic populations in hand therapy centers could suggest trends in occupational injury that may contribute to the achievement of prevention goals. Continued education in the principles of ergonomics, including emphasis on preparing an injured worker for a safe return to work, facilitates communication between the medical and industrial communities.

To consider the challenges that prevail in this area, we must begin by using the tools of hand therapy to gather information about our patients' work in the beginning stages of treatment. Our evaluation tools provide us with a patient's functional status, and information about the patient's job

requirements is acquired from him and confirmed by the use of the *Dictionary of Occupational Titles.*[6] Information needs to be gathered early and communicated to the medical team, the insurance carrier, and the employer in order to form a plan for return to work. Efficiency is tantamount to cost effectiveness.

The therapist at this point must decide whether his or her role as a practitioner is to facilitate the return to work through other professionals, with the therapist remaining in the acute care arena, or whether he or she feels comfortable providing the direct care through the longer rehabilitation phase.[5] The ingredients required to fulfill this second phase include the following:

1. Knowledge of industries in the local area and their specific job requirements
2. Ability to assess the patient's readiness to return to work
3. Understanding of the therapist's role in the system that now includes the industrial sector, the legal process, and all the rules and regulations that apply

With continued interest and investment in this phase of the rehabilitation of injured workers, perhaps we can further the concept of work as therapy and transfer it from hand centers to the actual work places. The use of modified work set-ups through supervision may help to minimize the confusion caused in the blanket referral of "return to work—light duty."

Although great strides have been made in reducing the number of hand injuries in the United States, there is much to be done. We need to know where the bulk of acute injuries occur. In addition, we wonder about the true number of repetitive hand injuries and the true incidence of carpal tunnel syndrome. A task force of hand therapists from the American Society of Hand Therapists and hand surgeons from the American Society for Surgery of the Hand is attempting to find ways to respond to the need for prevention of injuries. With ergonomists, labor leaders, employers, safety engineers, hand surgeons, and hand therapists working as a team, great strides can be made.

REFERENCES

1. Accident facts, Chicago, Ill., 1980, National Safety Council.
2. Armstrong, T.J., Foulke, J.A., Joseph, B.S., and Goldstein, S.A.: Investigation of cumulative trauma disorders in a poultry processing plant, Am. Ind. Hyg. Assoc. J. **43**(2):103-116, 1982.
3. Baxter, P.: A focus on work, therapy, and vocational direction. In Hunter, J.M., Schneider, L.H., Mackin, E.J., and Bell, J.A., editors: Rehabilitation of the hand, St. Louis, 1978, The C.V. Mosby Co., pp. 694-709.
4. Beatty, M.E., Zook, E.G., Russell, R.C., and Kinkead, L.R.: Grain auger injuries: the replacement of the corn picker injury? Plast. Reconstr. J. **69**(1):96-102, Jan. 1982.
5. Cantor, S.G.: Occupational therapy and occupational medicine—a merger, Am. J. Occup. Ther. **33**(10):631-634, Oct. 1979.
6. Dictionary of occupational titles, U.S. Department of Labor, Washington, D.C., 1977, U.S. Government Printing Office.
7. Jan Douglas: Personal communication, Chicago, 1982.
8. Investigation and analysis of fifty reports of injury to operators of mechanical power presses, Office of Standard Development, final report, Washington, D.C., Nov. 1975, U.S. Department of Labor (OSHA).
9. Barbara Johnson: Personal communication, United Hospitals of St. Paul, St. Paul, Minn., 1982.

10. Leamon, T.B.: The introduction of ergonomics: a problem of industrial practice, Applied Ergonomics 11(3):161-164, Sept. 1980.
11. Matheson, L.N.: Work capacity evaluation, Trabuco Canyon, Calif., 1982, Rehabilitation Institute of Southern California.
12. Rosemary Rehm: Personal communication, San Jose, Calif., 1982.
13. Report of the U.S. Consumer Products Safety Commission, Washington, D.C., 1980, U.S. Government Printing Office.
14. Sager, M.: Hazards in the workplace, The Washington Post, Feb. 22, 1982, pp. D1-D-5.
15. Slack, D.A.: Occupational therapy in industrial rheumatology, Presented at American Occupational Therapists Association, 1982.

16. Smith, S.L.: Physical capacity evaluation. In Hopkins, H.L., and Smith, H.D., editors: Willard and Spackman's occupational therapy, Philadelphia, 1978, J.B. Lippincott Co., pp. 213-218.
17. U.S. Department of Labor, Bureau of Labor Statistics, 1974, Washington, D.C.
18. Vibration white finger disease in U.S. workers using pneumatic chipping and grinding hand tools, Section I. Epidemiology; Section II. Engineering Testing (NIOSH), U.S. Department of Health and Human Services, Washington, D.C., 1981, 1982, U.S. Government Printing Office.

XVII
DEVELOPMENT OF HAND CENTERS

86

Model of a hand rehabilitation center

VERNON L. NICKEL and CAROL McGOUGH

REHABILITATION

The use of the word "rehabilitation," derived from the word *rehabilitāre,* "to restore," is most appropriate. The first documented efforts at rehabilitation were led in large measure by Sir Robert Jones in the care of crippled children in the era just before World War I and also in the care of the large number of amputees that resulted from combat in World War I. From World War I to World War II, rehabilitation as a concept, except in connection with poliomyelitis, was progressively less active. It was the care of the amputee after World War II that once again brought focus to the need for an organized team approach. For the first time the professional engineer was included as a member of the rehabilitation team. This comprehensive approach led to increased interest in prosthetics, and with supportive research money, a pronounced improvement occurred in rehabilitation of the traumatic amputee.

HAND REHABILITATION

Since the presentation of "The Model of A Hand Rehabilitation Center" at the Philadelphia Symposium on Rehabilitation of the Hand, in 1976, and the publication of the first edition of the present book, in 1978, most significant changes have occurred in the team concept of care of the complex upper limb. The word "model" that was emphasized previously is no longer valid in the same context. This necessitates an in-depth evaluation of what hand rehabilitation is and certainly warrants a reexploration of terminology in order to depict the progress that has been achieved. The use of the word "model"* is not so important as it was in 1976. By definition, this word provides limits to which we are now forced to go beyond. "Model" is no longer an appropriate word to describe our current concept of hand rehabilitation, that is, the creation of an *environment* in which needed disciplines concentrate their attention on the complex upper limb, both in a diagnostic and a therapeutic sense.

An excellent hand rehabilitation environment can be created (1) by a therapist working with a hand surgeon in his or her private office setting; (2) in a hospital environment, where an area is identified and staffed with personnel appropriate to a hand rehabilitation service (this is the most common situation); or (3) in one of the very complex and highly sophisticated diagnostic, therapeutic, and research centers that are now organized in various facilities, both in the United States and in other nations. With the growth in the number and reputation of hand rehabilitation centers, it is anticipated that every major medical center will eventually have a designated, recognizable hand center of excellence.

PAST ACCOMPLISHMENTS

It is probably true that rehabilitative efforts for patients with complex, multiorgan-system disabilities such as poliomyelitis or spinal cord injury nurtured the use of the team care concept for the complex upper limb problem. These totally devastating disabilities challenged allied health professionals to increase their understanding of the physiologic and neurologic disease processes and enhanced their ability to deal effectively with residual disabilities. These professionals now excelled not only in their personal professional disciplines, such as occupational therapy and physical therapy, but they also gained expertise in specific problem areas. Specialization, in the therapeutic mode, began to take on a much more significant meaning. In the area of poliomyelitis, the physical therapist was not only an excellent "generalist," but also gained special knowledge and experience specific to the treatment of poliomyelitis. The occupational therapist gained recognition in efforts to provide positioning and treatment programs specialized to the upper limbs of persons with spinal cord injury. These are two examples of the evolution of specialization, and the many contributions that physical and occupational therapists have made in rehabilitation. Interest and enthusiasm for specialization in the upper limb have brought us to where we are today, with the specialty area of "hand rehabilitation" and the professional title of "hand therapist."

The contribution of hand rehabilitation to our current "state of the art" standard of care for hand injuries has been enormous. Prevention is now dominant in the thinking of all the professionals dealing with such problems, and rather than most therapy being remedial and reactive, it is now actively preventive as well as actively therapeutic. This, in the aggregate, makes an enormous difference in the care and in the cost of achieving an optimal outcome. Whereas

---

*1. A representation of something, usually idealized and modified to make it conceptually easier to understand. 2. Something to be imitated. (*Stedman's Medical Dictionary,* ed. 23, 1976.)

preventable contractual deformities (as one example of many that could be cited) were usual in times past, they are now becoming progressively more unusual. An example is the much more aggressive and early intervention after reconstructive surgery in rheumatoid disease. Postoperative casts are often removed within a very few days, and dynamic splinting is applied much earlier and is more effective than heretofore believed possible.

It is now common practice for the hand surgeon to have the opportunity of participating in the care of upper limb disabilities in the environment of a hand rehabilitation center. Thus these surgeons are much more aware of the advantages of this type of environment and will be more aggressive in assuming leadership of such therapeutic entities. Similarly, occupational therapists and physical therapists who as students and therapists have had the opportunity of participating in this type of environment are much more likely to stimulate the development of hand rehabilitation centers of excellence.

THE HAND REHABILITATION TEAM

The membership of the hand rehabilitation team can vary considerably, depending on the type of problem dealt with, the availability of professional personnel, the physical plant, and numerous other factors.

Characteristically, the most common model of the hand rehabilitation team at this time consists of the hand surgeon as leader and occupational and/or physical therapists (now commonly described as hand therapists) as important members. In 1976 it was emphasized that the rehabilitation team working in the hand rehabilitation center should exercise the same discipline and demand the same high scientific standards that experienced hand surgeons customarily have learned to demand in their office and operating room personnel. This goal has been frequently met. The level of excellence that is characteristic of such centers is one to be envied by other rehabilitation efforts. There has been, however, in our opinion less than optimal use of the psychosocial disciplines, such as social service, clinical psychology, and vocational counseling. Obviously the number of persons on the team should not be excessive, but in centers that have a strong emphasis in the psychosocial disciplines these services can add immensely to the provision of total care to the patient. The increasing use of professional orthotists and rehabilitation engineers is discussed in another chapter.

The hand surgeon

The hand surgeon has been established as the unquestioned and unchallenged leader of the rehabilitation team. Without such leadership there is no hand program, and several attempts to constitute such a team without this leadership have failed. The hand surgeon has such a wide background in operative and nonoperative care that the interposition of other physicians in this team is entirely inappropriate, is clearly unnecessary, and, in fact, can be most destructive. To establish his or her reputation, the surgeon should be not only a first-class physician, but also a particularly fine technical hand surgeon. However, the surgeon needs more than this. He or she must be a team leader who is able to recognize and readily accept capabilities in others, to delegate responsibilities, and to maintain discipline.

The occupational or physical therapist

The exact roles of occupational therapists and physical therapists have not been clearly established, and there is considerable overlap. It is certainly true that both groups have made major contributions to this therapeutic effort, and the use of the word "hand therapist" implies that this person may come from either background. This has proved quite satisfactory and probably has enhanced the service as a whole. Both of these types of specialists, because of their historical and educational backgrounds, bring unique qualifications that are most desirable. The optimal situation is when the two disciplines can work, as they frequently do, in a totally collaborative manner. Graduate programs that combine occupational therapy and physical therapy are increasing in number and are adding enormously to the intellectual achievement of these specialties. At least one master's degree program in hand therapy has been established, and it will be most interesting to see the progress of this specialized graduate degree.

FUTURE CHALLENGES

It is a fact that the majority of patients treated in a hand rehabilitation center are there as a result of trauma. Much less widespread has been the care of those with very serious upper limb disability as the result of central nervous system disorders. It is our conviction that if these disabilities, which are very large in number, such as stroke, head injury, spinal cord injury, cerebral palsy, and rheumatoid disease, had had the intense intellectual attention of the hand rehabilitation team, further progress would have occurred. Some centers are now becoming interested in applying the same level of expertise that has been achieved in the area of the traumatic hand to those persons with central nervous system involvement. This, indeed, promises an improvement in the quality of care provided to persons who heretofore have not received sufficient attention.

One change that has occurred during the last few years has been the increasing interest of the hand rehabilitation specialist in the care of the quadriplegic patient. This has been stimulated in large measure by the work of Rancho Los Amigos Hospital, in Downey, California, and by the work of Moberg[2] and Lamb.[1] The widely accepted concept of using "sensibility" as a method of documenting and predicting outcomes, which has been done largely within the framework of the hand rehabilitation center concept, shows great promise for improving prognostic accuracy and encouraging the introduction of new concepts of care in cases involving severely disabled upper limbs.

Mention of acute inpatient hospitalization is also appropriate when one is thinking of future challenges. As mentioned previously, the concept of prevention, rather than remediation, has put greater responsibility on the acute care team to provide an early environment for hand rehabilitation. This change shows great potential and will improve the transition from inpatient care to outpatient care. It also will help to instill early the concept of patients taking responsibility for the management of their care—a fundamental concept in hand rehabilitation.

In summary, the evolutionary circle is being completed: early experience in the generalized inpatient rehabilitation setting has nurtured interest in outpatient hand rehabilitation. The specialized knowledge and expertise gained are now returning to our acute rehabilitation care. This brings true meaning to the word "comprehensive" in describing not only what we should offer, but also what we must offer to our patients.

We, as professionals, have grown away from the word "model" to creating an *environment,* and it may well be appropriate to consider now our use of the term "hand rehabilitation." More appropriate terminology, once again, must be explored to depict fully the intense interest and challenges that lie ahead. "Upper extremity rehabilitation" or "upper limb rehabilitation" may be more valid. *Upper extremity rehabilitation in a comprehensive environment* may well be the key words to our future.

The experience of hand rehabilitation has been universally a very positive one. Its reputation is outstanding, and its tradition of excellence in professional efforts, patient care, teaching, and research is certainly exemplary. This tradition provides an abundance of potential for the future.

REFERENCES

1. Lamb, D.W., and Landry, R.: The hand in quadriplegia, Hand **3:**31, 1971.
2. Moberg, E.: The upper link in tetraplegia: a new approach to surgical rehabilitation, Stuttgart, 1978, Georg Thieme Verlag.

87

Psychological motivation in successful hand therapy

LOIS SUSAN KEMPIN

Successful rehabilitation inevitably involves not only the body but the mind and spirit as well. The total concept of the hand center would be lost if we failed to mention the psychological effect of both the hand impairment and the atmosphere of the hand rehabilitation center on the patient. First, the team at the rehabilitation center must understand the patient and be ready to give support not only for physical needs but also for associated psychological difficulties. For whatever physical reason the patient comes to the center, be it an inherited handicap, accidental injury, disease, birth injury, or degenerative changes of old age, apprehension and anxiety are always involved. Anxiety about his state and capabilities may set back a patient's chances of recovery; therefore the rehabilitation team must allay not only his own fears but also those of his family.

Pain is a factor to some degree in almost every person coming to a hand center. Pain tolerance varies from person to person. Fear of pain is a powerful emotion, and it tends to block one's ability to reason and cooperate. The therapist must understand this and be sympathetic.

Meeting the patient's physical need is of prior importance in helping to allay the fear of falling out of the accepted pattern of life, which primarily involves continuing his current occupation. Also there is an apprehension as to the degree of rehabilitation and recovery possible.

Finally, but also of importance, there is a possible fear of reduced social acceptance. The patient should be encouraged to accept whatever handicap he may still have after rehabilitation.

Beginning with the initial contact at the hand center, the patient should be made to feel that he is an integral part of the rehabilitation team (the most important member of the team) and that his fullest cooperation is necessary for the ultimate amount of recovery. Any negative feelings and fears need to be changed to positive attitudes.

The physical decor of the hand center must be cheerful, well-lighted, clean, and comfortably well arranged, with a relaxed, pleasant atmosphere. Adequate and functional equipment produces a sense of security that provision has been made to meet the needs of recovery.

The therapist, on seeing the patient for the first time, must establish a positive rapport on an individual basis. The therapist should have a relaxed, pleasant approach in the initial greeting. Through active listening and verbal and nonverbal contact, one can learn to sense the patient's feelings, tensions, and fears. Thus it is possible to regulate the amount and degree of time and attention necessary for each patient. A brief time should be spent in educating the patient in simple anatomy and the functions of the hand that pertain to his injury. The approach of the treatment depends on the nature of each person's impairment and personality. Supportive and gentle firmness will help motivate the patient to full cooperation both at the hand center and in home therapy; it will also bolster his morale. Both a sense of empathy and caring must permeate all contact with the patient. The therapist must convince the patient that he understands him intimately and is dedicated to his welfare; this enhances the patient's expectancy of help.

Patient-to-patient contact within the hand center is a nonstructured form of group therapy. Communications and free-flowing interaction between patients are morale-boosting forms of therapy. The sharing of experiences, both positive and negative, is excellent motivation for acceptance of one's injury and also for acceptance of necessary therapy for recovery. Sharing experiences over a cup of coffee, seeing other injured hands, and watching others in rehabilitative therapy often calms tense nerves, allays deep-rooted fears, and motivates the desire to cooperate with the therapeutic treatments. The degree that the patient is involved emotionally in the process of treatment parallels his chances of successful treatment.

88

Hand therapy as an integral part of the surgical office

RICHARD L. PETZOLDT and MARY C. KASCH

It is our strong belief that hand therapy plays a significant and important part in the success of hand surgery. Typically, the surgeon may assume this responsibility himself, send the patient off to a therapist, or simply leave the patient to his own devices. However, if the surgeon attempts to play this dual role, he soon finds that he must spend an inordinate amount of time with the patient, explaining the nature of the problem and the necessity and techniques of therapy and attempting to supervise his progress. From the standpoint of the therapist working in a separate unit, there may be a lack of communication with the surgeon regarding the initial trauma or surgery involved and the treatment goals and timetables. This may then result in inadequate or inappropriate treatment for the patient. Further, if the patient does not receive proper and specific instructions for therapy, he feels uncertain about his responsibilities and participation postoperatively and fails to obtain the full potential benefit of both the surgery and the therapy.

We believed that a much better and more satisfying relationship could exist if the surgeon, the therapist, and the patient all worked together in the same setting. With this concept (Fig. 88-1), we established therapy as an integral part of our office.

PROBLEMS

Our office is small. Our staff consists of one hand surgeon, one hand therapist, and two medical assistants who do both front and back office work. In addition to the usual reception, clerical, and private consultation areas, we have three examination rooms with a total office area of 840 square feet. The problems of time and space are apparent. We solved the time problem by dovetailing our schedules during the week: the surgeon sees patients in the office full days on Tuesdays and Thursdays, and the therapist works with patients in the office on Mondays, Wednesdays, and Fridays. The space problem is solved by utilization of a common examination and therapy table in each of the examination rooms (Fig. 88-2).

Ideally, an office would have sufficient space for separate but concurrent use by the surgeon and the therapist. However, we have found that it is possible and practical to utilize common space in the manner described.

COMMUNICATION

Communication is the key to success of the concept of a three-way interchange between the surgeon, the therapist, and the patient. A direct relationship is established and continued between surgeon and patient and between therapist and patient during respective visits. Communication between the surgeon and the therapist includes regular meetings to discuss new patients to be referred for therapy and periodic follow-up reviews on all therapy patients (Fig. 88-3).

The most important form of communication is the patient's chart. This contains the history and physical examination, impressions, problems, treatment goals and plans, roentgenograms, operative reports, and other relevant material (Fig. 88-4). A problem-oriented approach is used. Specific problems are defined, as well as treatment goals and methods. Dates of initiation and termination of treatment techniques can be entered on the patient's chart. This establishes a clear progression of treatment goals and results. Progress notes are made individually by the surgeon and therapist on separate color-coded sheets, which permit a continuing means of written exchange.

To further simplify communication and to assure optimum progress and integration of efforts, standard protocols are used for all major and common operative procedures. These are developed together by the surgeon and therapist and include the specific techniques and timetables that may be employed for each problem. In this way, there is complete understanding of the treatment goals, and the therapist can still alter the methods and pace as necessary for the best progress of any one patient toward those goals.

It is very important that the patient has some understanding of the nature of his problem. He must also have sufficient motivation to actively participate in his rehabilitation program for optimal results. To help in both these respects, we use a detailed plastic model of the hand as a teaching device to point out and describe in layman's terms the significant structures and relationships and the importance of the patient's own therapy efforts (Fig. 88-5). Simple line drawings are often used for the same purpose.

In addition to the verbal and visual communication, the patient receives printed copies of his individualized home care program and some of the more standard procedures.

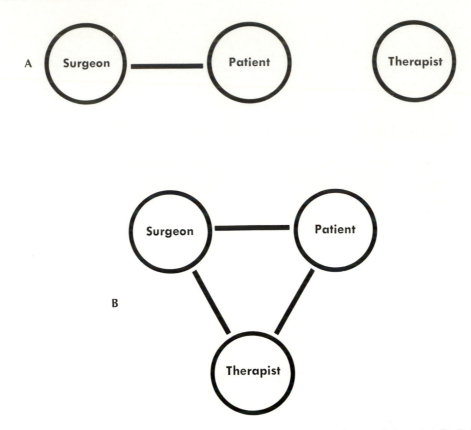

FIG. 88-1. **A,** Typical and often indefinite relationship between surgeon, patient, and therapist. **B,** Relationship that exists when therapy is made integral part of office.

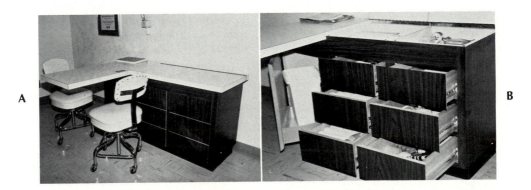

FIG. 88-2. **A,** Hand table used by both surgeon and therapist. (Design modified after others.) **B,** Each table is equipped identically with diagnostic tools, dressing supplies, therapy equipment in hinged-top compartments, and sliding drawers.

For example, before hospitalization for an elective procedure, the patient is given a printed instruction form to reinforce verbal instructions regarding his postoperative responsibilities for elevation and dressing care.

The patient also communicates with us. An injury to the hand affects the patient psychologically as well as physically. We find that by providing a supportive atmosphere in which the patient is given a structured program and responsibility for his own rehabilitation and in which he is free to verbalize his feelings, negative attitudes are minimized and more positive efforts are achieved.

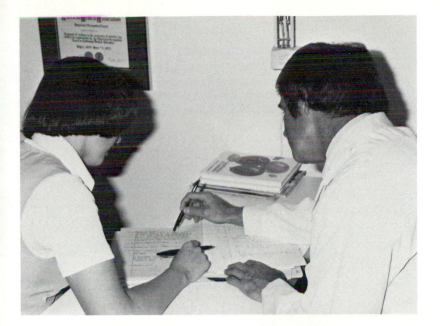

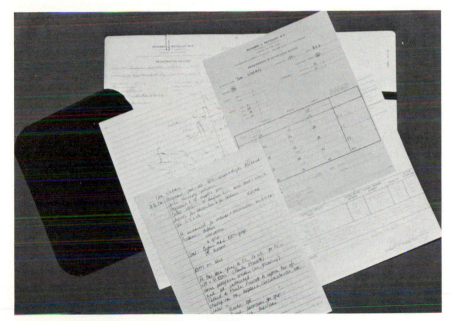

FIG. 88-3. Surgeon and therapist discuss treatment goals and timetables for each therapy patient.

FIG. 88-4. Patient's chart provides common means of communication, coordination, and documentation for surgeon and therapist.

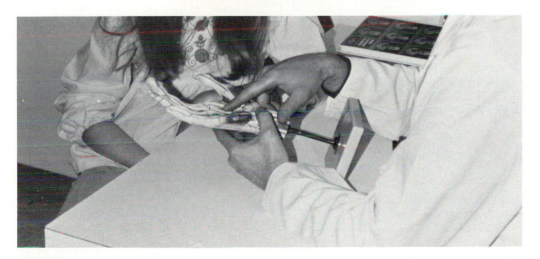

FIG. 88-5. Hand model is useful to help explain fundamental problem to patient, which increases his interest and cooperation.

REHABILITATION

Not all hand surgery patients require special therapy consideration. We reserve participation of the therapist to those cases where such therapy and rehabilitation are considered or become necessary for an improved postinjury or postoperative course.

For those patients referred for therapy, the therapist becomes involved at an early stage. For elective surgery cases she frequently does evaluations preoperatively and then works with the patient closely postoperatively for active continuation of his rehabilitation. For elective and trauma cases, she sees the patient as soon as the initial dressings are removed. She reviews the chart and the treatment goals with the surgeon and then initiates a rehabilitation program designed specifically for the patient.

The frequency of patient appointments varies according to individual requirements. Some therapy patients require only one or two visits to receive supplemental instructions, supervision for simpler problems, and splints. More complex or resistant problems of stiffness or weakness require more frequent appointments, which are then decreased as improvement is obtained. The therapist assumes the responsibility for determining the frequency of appointments based on the patient's treatment goals and progress.

Therapy sessions may provide a variety of evaluations and treatment techniques to meet each person's requirements. These may include a selective combination of heat, cryotherapy, vibration, and other facilitation techniques. In addition, the patient's program may include splinting, edema-control techniques, muscle reeducation and strengthening, reeducation of sensibility, desensitization, functional and prevocational activities, activities of daily living, and work hardening.

At appropriate intervals, the therapist remeasures ranges of joint motion, individual muscle and grip strengths, sensory status, and hand volume. Patterns of hand use are observed and recorded. Objective data are recorded and reviewed with the patient, consecutive figures are compared, and red ink is used to record gains, providing a vivid indication to the patient of his progress (Fig. 88-6). Range-of-motion flow sheets and graphs of range of motion and grip strength are used to demonstrate relative progress to help motivate the patient. In addition, the surgeon has available a ready record of the patient's progress without having to repeat all the measurements at each visit.

The fabrication, fitting, and adjustment of splints are also accomplished during therapy sessions. These may include custom-made splints of lightweight plastic material with adjustable straps and dynamic outriggers, webbing straps to improve passive motion, traction gloves, and finger trappers made of Tubigauze or Velcro. Commercial splints may be provided after careful evaluation, and adjustments are made.

The patient's home therapy program is considered the most important aspect of therapy, and the goal is to train

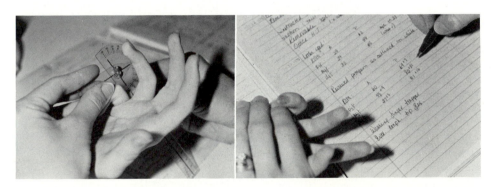

FIG. 88-6. A, Therapist periodically measures and records ranges of motion. **B,** Respective gains or losses are reviewed with patient, which provides stimulus for continued effort.

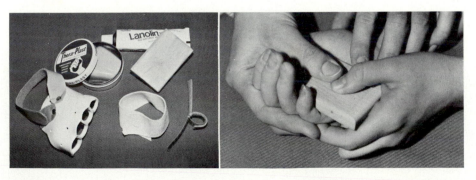

FIG. 88-7. A, Equipment for home therapy varies according to patient's needs but is always kept simple. **B,** Patient receives full instructions for use of any specific device and must demonstrate his understanding of it.

the patient sufficiently so that he may continue on his own at home on a daily basis. This is done with the oral, visual, and written techniques mentioned previously. The patient is thoroughly instructed in the use of each piece of equipment he is given as well as the proper positioning, extent of exercising, and danger signals (Fig. 88-7). His program is reviewed by the therapist frequently to assure proper techniques and progress and to make any necessary adjustments.

As part of rehabilitation, the therapist evaluates the patient's hand use in relation to his work and devises exercises and activities to simulate those needs. A patient who is unable to return to his former job may be assigned to a vocational rehabilitation counselor. We assist these counselors by recommending job limitations and by analyzing work requirements in terms of hand use.

Approximately 70% of the therapy patients are industrial compensation cases, and most of the rest are insured privately. Therapy is a financially self-sustaining function of the office. The billing is done through the office, and the therapist is salaried as an employee of the surgeon. With the availability of therapy in our own office, it is possible to offer it to those patients who need it but cannot pay and who otherwise would not have the benefit of it.

ADVANTAGES

As a result of this concept and working relationship, certain advantages for the surgeon, the therapist, and the patient have become apparent. For the surgeon, the biggest single advantage is the amount of time saved in activities that do not require his specific expertise. Basic and initial instruction for therapy is still given personally to the patient by the surgeon, but the more detailed and follow-up visits can be spaced alternately with the therapist and surgeon,

thus decreasing the total number of visits with the surgeon. The longer and more tedious evaluations and the making of splints can also be done by the therapist, decreasing the total time of any one visit with the surgeon.

There are also multiple advantages for the therapist. Since many postoperative regimens are standardized in our office, treatment goals and timetables are clearly established. However, the therapist retains the flexibility to adapt modalities and treatment to the individual patient. Time is more efficiently used for the therapist and patient because of limited paperwork and decreased patient waiting time. The patient places a greater value on the importance of therapy because of the surgeon's positive attitude toward it. As a result, his attendance is more regular, he follows through on his home program more diligently, and he cooperates more fully with the therapist.

The patient derives advantages from the continuity of care. When he goes from the surgeon to the therapist in the same office, he recognizes the team approach and the existence of a common effort in his behalf. The patient also feels that everything possible is being done to help him on his road to recovery. With the continued reinforcement from both the surgeon and the therapist, the patient progresses at an optimal rate and to an optimal level.

CONCLUSION

The goal of the hand surgeon is to obtain the best result possible for the patient. The therapist has the same goal but has not always had the opportunity to contribute the full potential of his or her abilities. By combining the two disciplines in the same office we believe we have come closer to achieving this common goal.

89

The hand rehabilitation unit in a hospital setting

GAYLORD L. CLARK and RODNEY W. SCHLEGEL

The formation of a center for the management of upper extremity and hand problems goes beyond the traditional surgical approach to disease or injury. As our collective knowledge increases and our technical capability grows, we find that it is often impossible for one person to render optimum care to the complex hand cases. It is this realization that stimulated us to create the Raymond M. Curtis Hand Center at The Union Memorial Hospital in Baltimore, Maryland. The center is designed to care for hand patients efficiently by means of the expertise of specialists interested in the field.

SURGICAL TEAM

The hand surgeon is the major catalyst in crystallizing the formation of a center. We believe that a team of surgeons is necessary, and their surgical backgrounds should be varied. The general surgeon, the orthopedic surgeon, and the plastic surgeon constitute the ideal team. Each member of this team should be highly skilled in his own right but should be able to call freely for the help of any other team member should he believe there is a need for it. The members of the surgical team should be capable of working interchangeably with each other, either in or out of the operating theater.

THERAPISTS

Closely allied with the surgical team in planning and implementing treatment for the care of the patient are the physical and occupational therapists on the hand team. Their knowledge of the function and dynamics of the hand has increased along with ours, and their skills are now highly refined. These therapists should have a flexible attitude regarding their identification with physical or occupational therapy, in order that they may freely exchange certain skills and concepts. This therapy team is fully included in the activities and conferences of the center. The therapists' working area must be furnished with adequate equipment in order that they be able to carry out their assigned tasks properly. The equipment will be different from center to center and should reflect the specific needs of a particular region as well as the ingenuity of the therapy group.

Within the hand therapy department, a distinction is maintained between physical and occupational therapists. Members of these two specialty groups, however, have overlapping treatment and teaching responsibilities, regardless of their backgrounds. An in-house educational program includes coordination of lectures, patient rounds, acquiring guest lectureships, supervision and guidance of therapy students, and staff development. This system allows for the maximum use of individual talent and encourages cooperation in areas of mutual interest.

Physical therapists

1. General responsibilities
   a. Patient education
   b. Heat and cold modalities
   c. Hydrotherapy
   d. Range-of-motion exercises (active, passive, and resistive)
   e. Massage
   f. Edema management
2. Specific responsibilities
   a. Range-of-motion measurements
   b. Muscle testing and grading
   c. Electrical stimulation for pain control
   d. Noninvasive vascular testing
   e. Biofeedback
   f. Progressive plaster casting for joint contractures
   g. Electrodiagnostic evaluation
   h. Isokinetic evaluation

Occupational therapists

1. General responsibilities
   a. Patient education
   b. Splinting (dynamic, static, and assistive)
   c. Activities of daily living
   d. Work simplification instruction
   e. Joint protection instruction
2. Specific responsibilities
   a. Light-duty workshop supervision
   b. Heavy-duty workshop supervision
   c. Grip and pinch strength measurements
   d. Sensory evaluation
   e. Sensory reeducation
   f. Desensitization for pain control
3. Further responsibilities
   a. Prevocational assessment
   b. Job-site visits
   c. Home visits

INDUSTRIAL SCIENCE SPECIALISTS

A new category of personnel has been added to our unit, the industrial science specialist, whose job is to work exclusively in the heavy-duty workshop. The responsibilities of these specialists are as follows:

1. Patient education
2. Implementation of projects and safety measures in the workshop and on the job
3. Patient direction on Work Simulator (refer to Chapter 83) for the development of strength, endurance, and work tolerance

SOCIAL WORK SERVICE

Social workers perform a very important function in the hand treatment center. It is apparent that we are learning more about the psychological aspects of hand injury than we have recognized in previous years. The reason for this appears to be that as a therapist works and talks with a patient, the patient begins to discuss his concerns with the therapist. These concerns may be in a variety of areas, including economic worry, marital or family instability, job and work insecurity, and loss of normal sexual performance. If a concern is of sufficient significance, a trained social worker must be available for consultation. This worker in turn must have the option to request the advice of a psychiatrist or even to refer the patient for psychiatric treatment if it is necessary.

Social workers
1. General responsibilities
   a. Patient education
   b. Financial status evaluation
   c. Evaluation of marital and family stability
   d. Psychiatric screening
2. Specific responsibilities
   a. Alcoholism and drug abuse counseling
   b. Detection of depression or suicidal tendencies
   c. Malingering versus hysterical conditions
   d. Self-hypnosis for pain control

VOCATIONAL REHABILITATION SPECIALISTS

Our unit also includes vocational rehabilitation specialists, whose responsibilities are as follows:
1. Patient education
2. Evaluation of work capabilities
3. Retraining programs
4. Financial support for surgery and rehabilitation

OTHER MEDICAL PERSONNEL

Various other medical personnel also play important roles, in particular the physician interested in infectious diseases. It is with this physician's knowledge of the sophisticated use of antibiotic therapy for unusual cases of infection, or potential infection, that the patient can be best cared for. A rheumatologist is also necessary to the center, to give advice concerning the care of patients having connective-tissue disease.

HAND POLICY COMMITTEE

A combined physical and occupational therapy committee has worked well for us in administering the Raymond M. Curtis Hand Center. This committee includes the director of the center as its chairman, plus three other hand surgeons and the therapist who is the director of hand rehabilitation. A hospital administrator and a nurse attend for proper li-

aison. The committee meets monthly, and special guests are invited as deemed important. We have had as guests representatives of various insurance carriers, industrial nurses, State of Maryland Crippled Children's Fund representatives, and other persons who would be interested in our work.

The responsibilities of the hand policy committee are as follows:
1. Direction of the Raymond M. Curtis Hand Center
2. Raising and administration of funds regarding donations and grants
3. Entertainment of business and insurance company representatives
4. Initiation and approval of research projects
5. Administration of Division of Hand Surgery and its quality assurance policies.

LOCATION OF CENTER

Ideally, a hand center is based in a hospital. If this is not possible, it should be situated close to a hospital. There must be appropriate space and strong administrative backing. The need for a hand center must be apparent in order to justify its existence, particularly in this day of economy-conscious regulatory boards. The need is usually dependent on the type of patient population and the density of this population. These factors will also influence the major types of cases being treated. Our tie-in with the Maryland Institute of Emergency Medical Services Systems (MIEMSS) brings to the center patients with major hand trauma, for acute management, and patients requiring later reconstructive surgery and therapy.

OVERNIGHT FACILITY

A number of low-cost overnight beds are needed for patients living at a distance and requiring daily therapy treatments. The number will vary with the center's patient load, and we consider 10 beds to be correct for our purposes.

SOURCES OF PATIENTS

Patients come from a wide area and from various sources. These sources may fluctuate from time to time but generally consists of the following: individual referrals from the local medical community, the State of Maryland Emergency Medical Services, local business and industry, national or local insurance carriers, and self-referrals.

The services of this rehabilitation center do not require staff privileges at our hospital and are open to all physicians in the local community, the state, and the nation. A physician must provide, with referral of a patient, full information about the patient's medical, surgical, or accident history. If a patient is housed in the overnight unit, a staff physician must be assigned to that patient for legal coverage while he is undergoing treatments.

EQUIPMENT

The center must have the capability of microsurgical methods. This includes the appropriate instrumentation in the operating room, with qualified nurses to care for and use the equipment. It is essential that a microsurgery laboratory be available for the surgeons to practice their art, to develop new techniques, and to carry out certain animal experimentation. For the efficient functioning of such a laboratory a qualified technician must be in charge to care for the animal population and the equipment and to prepare various surgical procedures. This laboratory should be available for the use of all surgeons interested in microsurgery, not just for the use of hand surgeons.

TRAINING PROGRAMS

Training programs are also incorporated into the center's activities. A residency or fellowship in hand surgery is an active part of it. Where there is teaching there is excellence of care. This form of training is best conducted when there is a close association with a medical school or university hospital. Teaching in the therapy areas is important for training new, developing therapists. Paramedical personnel are instructed by the center's staff when requested to do so and frequently are very important referral sources for the center. Ongoing education for all those working in the center is necessary and must be maintained. This brings into play occasional outside speakers, regularly scheduled clinical presentations, and local speakers with specialized interests as the occasion demands.

A library is available, with a current collection of journals and textbooks. It also accommodates audiovisual techniques for learning.

SUMMARY

The hand center is a relatively new phenomenon, but it is needed and offers the best skills available in the community for the treatment of hand problems. This center includes an area for the treatment of acute problems as well as offering the best services in rehabilitation that can be assembled.

It takes time and effort on the part of those interested to put together this type of center. We have had substantial private financial support and also the confidence and encouragement of private insurance companies, many of whom are involved with workmen's compensation cases. Our plan is to give a quality of care that cannot otherwise be achieved, and this goal is being realized. It is probable that small versions of what has been described can be established and probably should be. It must be understood that with today's sophisticated knowledge, no one person can offer total care by himself to all of his patients.

90

The Hand Rehabilitation Center in Philadelphia: a private comprehensive program

PAMELA M. McENTEE, WANDRA K. MILES, CATHERINE A. CAMBRIDGE, SHARON L. FRIED, and MELANIE S. BALLARD

The Hand Rehabilitation Center in Philadelphia is a privately owned corporation. It had its beginnings 15 years ago in a surgeon's small office. Its personnel consisted of a hand surgeon, a nurse receptionist, and one part-time physical therapist. Today the Hand Rehabilitation Center serves a tristate area and has evolved to the point where a three-story building became necessary to house a growing staff of 54 people (Fig. 90-1). At this time, the staff consists of four hand surgeons, four hand fellows, four hand residents, a nurse, 17 therapy personnel, a business administrator, and 23 office personnel (Fig. 90-2). The therapy staff consists of eight occupational therapists, five physical therapists, one certified occupational therapy assistant, and three aides. Although the Hand Rehabilitation Center is privately owned, it maintains a close affiliation with Thomas Jefferson University Hospital, where the majority of its hand surgery is performed.

The high incidence of industrial hand injuries and many other hand impairments as well necessitates the need for a center that specializes in the comprehensive care of the upper extremity. Approximately 70% of the patients treated at the center have sustained hand injuries through industrial accidents. There are many advantages in working within the framework of a specialized medical facility. The availability by proximity of the surgeon, therapist, and patient enhances effective communication between all concerned. This not only benefits the patient by improving care, but also the free exchange of the ideas stimulates innovative treatment approaches, research, and program development. Formal weekly conferences are held to allow for joint presentations by surgeons and therapists on educational topics and research development. Presently, research data are made available for retrieval through the use of a diagnostic filing system. Future plans for data collection include the use of a computerized collection and retrieval system.

Initial referrals of patient to the Hand Rehabilitation Center come from a variety of sources, including physicians, lawyers, insurance companies, and self-referrals. All new patients are seen by an attending surgeon for an initial evaluation and treatment recommendations. When appropriate, patients are referred to the hand therapy department through oral and written orders.

PHYSICAL PLANT

The total area of the center is 16,500 square feet. The first floor consists of a combination conference room and library and business offices. The second floor includes eight doctors' examining rooms, x-ray room (Fig. 90-3), the reception and waiting area, and additional offices. The third floor is entirely utilized by the therapy department and includes a primary care area (Fig. 90-4, A) for wound care, exercise, splinting, modalities, and prosthetics, and also a therapeutic activities workshop (Fig. 90-4, B), a work evaluation room, a sensibility evaluation room, an electromyography and nerve conduction room, an examination room, a photography lab, therapists' offices, and a kitchen. A photography table is set up in the primary care section for documentation of treatment techniques and patient progress. Videotape equipment is also available for filming of patients, and tapes are used for educational purposes. The doctors' examining room area and the therapy department are accessible through a nonpublic spiral staircase that facilitates quick consultations between therapist and surgeon (Fig. 90-5).

HAND THERAPY DEPARTMENT
Primary care

On the initial visit to the hand therapy department (Fig. 90-6) a patient is assigned to a therapist for an evaluation and treatment. The patient begins a therapy program immediately, and a written home program is routinely given. Progress notes are dictated weekly or more often if necessary.

Wound care and exercise. Many patients begin therapy before their wounds are healed. Early movement is often necessary if maximum function is to be accomplished after healing is complete. An individualized exercise program is developed for each patient by his primary care therapist, based on the goals established by the therapist and the referring surgeon. The exercise program in therapy is complemented and reinforced by a written home program.

Splinting. When indicated, splinting is an important and vital part of the patient's overall care. Patients are referred by the surgeon for splinting throughout the treatment day, and referrals are both oral and written. The design of each

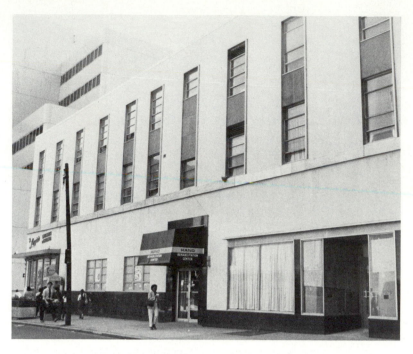

FIG. 90-1. The Hand Rehabilitation Center.

splint is based on the individual patient's needs and discussed with the surgeon before fabrication. To fabricate the splint on the day it is prescribed, each therapist is assigned a period of time during the week for splinting.

The splint area is designed so that two therapists can fabricate splints simultaneously (Fig. 90-7). Splinting tools and materials are duplicated on either side of the splinting counter. Once a splint is completed, the patient is given oral and written instructions for its use and care. The patient is requested to wear the splint for a half hour before he leaves the clinic so that necessary modifications can be made before the patient goes home. As a final check, the patient is brought to the doctors' examining area so that the referring surgeon can approve the splint.

Modalities. At the Hand Rehabilitation Center, physical therapy modalities are utilized as an adjunct to the primary care when specific indications for their use are present. Ultrasound, high-voltage galvanic stimulation, and phonophoresis, are used for specific hand problems. Biofeedback and electrical stimulation are used for muscle reeducation. Patients with pain problems are evaluated for transcutaneous nerve stimulation (TNS), and if suitability is established, patient instruction is provided. The usefulness for modalities lies in their ability to make the involved area more amenable to an active therapy program. They are not total treatments unto themselves.

Prosthetics. The majority of prosthetic patients seen at the Hand Rehabilitation Center have had partial or complete traumatic amputations of the upper extremity. A small percentage of patients have congenital losses. The prosthetic area is designed with modifications such as a tile floor and a plaster trap sink for fabrication for an early-fit prosthesis.

The majority of amputee patients seen at the Hand Rehabilitation Center are routinely fitted with an early-fit prosthesis.

Amputees are evaluated whenever possible preoperatively and routinely postoperatively for range of motion and strength. The information gained from this evaluation is discussed at a monthly prosthetic conference, during which a determination is made as to whether the patient is a candidate for a conventional or myoelectric prosthesis. The conference is attended by a surgeon, a therapist, a prosthetist, the patient, and family members.

Therapeutic activities workshop

The therapeutic activities workshop (Fig. 90-8), referred to at the Hand Rehabilitation Center as "work therapy," provides a structured program of activities to increase strength and endurance for the upper extremity–injured patient. The ultimate goal of work therapy is to return the patient to gainful employment through the use of job-simulated tasks and strengthening activities.

A patient is referred to work therapy with the approval of his surgeon. A member of the work therapy staff evaluates the patient and orients him to the department. The initial evaluation includes range of motion, pinch and grip measurements, volumeter measurements, and a detailed job description.

The workshop is staffed by a full-time occupational therapy supervisor, a staff occupational therapist, a certified occupational therapy assistant, and a woodworking instructor. All primary care therapists rotate through work therapy to ensure a comprehensive approach to their care of the hand-injured patient.

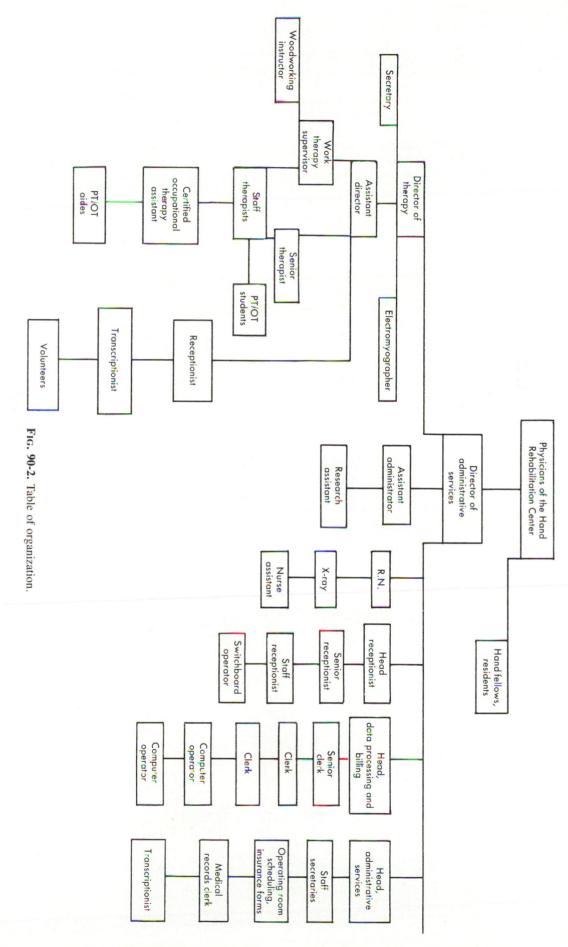

Fig. 90-2. Table of organization.

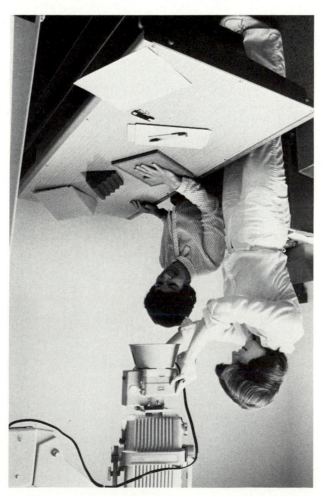

Fig. 90-3. X-ray technician with patient.

Therapeutic activities are divided into five levels. Levels 1 and 2 include light resistive activities, such as macramé and leatherwork. Levels 3 through 5 include more resistive activities such as ceramics, woodworking, and wood carving. Isokinetics and progressive resistive exercises are incorporated into the patient's work therapy program. Some special equipment utilized in work therapy include the Valpar Work Samples,* the Mini-Gym,† and the Work Simulator,‡ along with woodworking and ceramic equipment.

Specialized evaluations

Every patient seen for hand therapy receives an evaluation before initiation of his treatment. Frequently the referring surgeon requests an in-depth examination of one or more facets of the patient's disability beyond the scope of the initial evaluation. These specialized evaluations include sensory evaluation, electromyographic and nerve-conduction studies, physical capacity evaluation, and evaluation of ability to perform activities of daily living (ADL).

Sensibility evaluation. The sensibility evaluation done at the Hand Rehabilitation Center consists of a battery of tests to provide an overview of a patient's perception of tactile input. The purpose of a formal sensory evaluation is to assist the surgeon in determining diagnoses such as carpal tunnel and thoracic outlet syndromes. They are also used in assessing the progression of nerve regeneration after injury or surgical repair.

Referrals for sensory evaluations are written by the surgeon. A specific time period of 1½ hours of the therapist's weekly schedule is set aside regularly for sensory evaluations. This allows the therapist adequate time to review the medical chart, perform the evaluation, and record the results. Sensibility testing is done in a "quiet room" where the necessary instruments are readily available (Fig. 90-9). When appropriate, recommendations are made to the referring surgeon regarding initiation of a sensory reeducation program. Instructions for sensory reeducation are provided by a therapist. Sensory reeducation relies heavily on patient participation at home.

Electromyographic and nerve-conduction studies. Electrophysiologic evaluations are done on the premises at the Hand Rehabilitation Center for patients with upper ex-

*Valpar Corp., 3801 E. 34th Street, Tucson, Ariz. 85713.
†MGI Strength Systems, 1617 Valley Drive, West Chester, Pa. 19380.
‡Baltimore Therapeutic Equipment Co., 1201 Bernard Drive, Baltimore, Md. 21223.

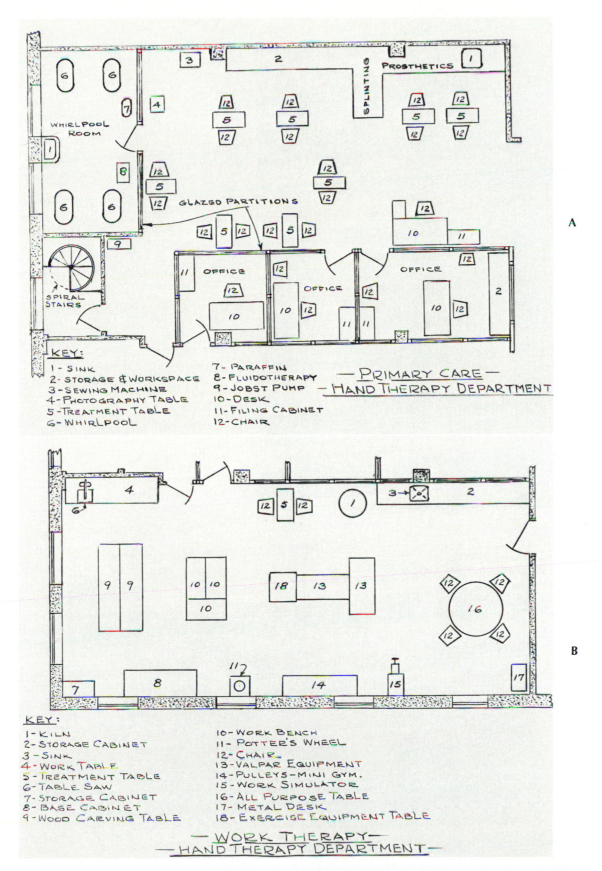

FIG. 90-4. **A,** Floor plan of primary care area. **B,** Floor plan of work therapy area.

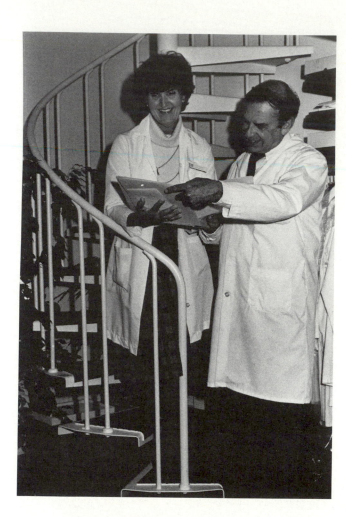

FIG. 90-5. Surgeon and therapist conferring near spiral staircase.

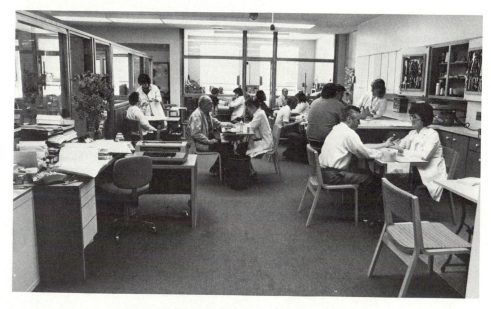

FIG. 90-6. Primary care area.

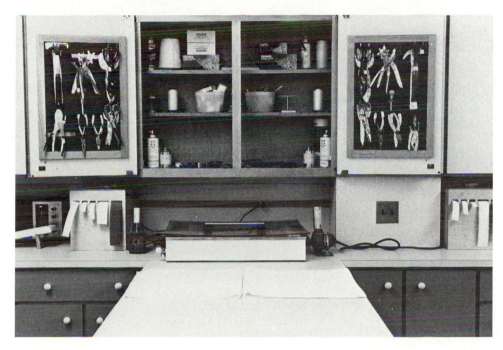

FIG. 90-7. Splinting area.

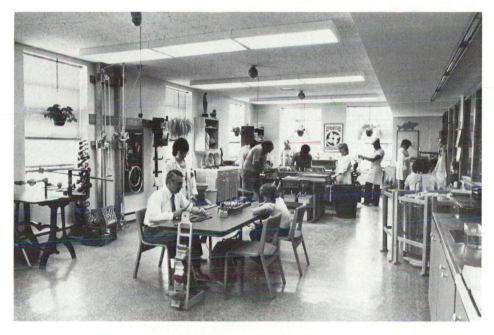

FIG. 90-8. Therapeutic activities workshop.

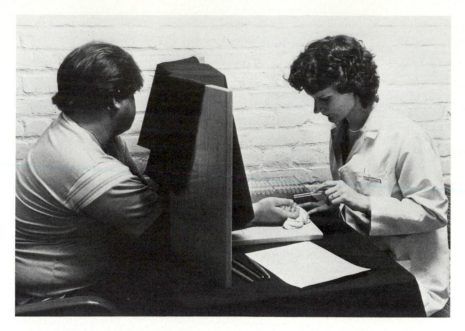

FIG. 90-9. Sensory evaluation room.

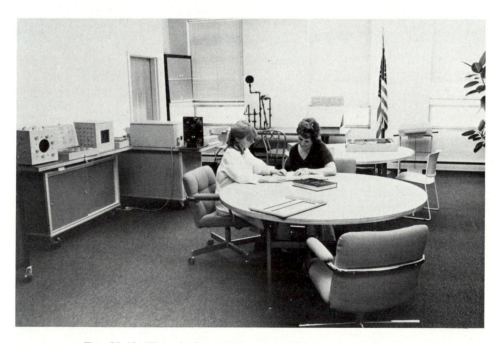

FIG. 90-10. Therapist interviewing patient in work evaluation room.

tremity injuries. For this purpose a room was specially constructed to house the equipment used to perform electrophysiologic assessments.

Electrophysiologic evaluations have two primary functions at the Hand Rehabilitation Center. They assist the physician in arriving at diagnoses such as isolated nerve injuries, brachial plexus injuries, and entrapment syndromes. They are sometimes done serially to demonstrate progression of nerve regeneration after injury or surgical repair.

Physical capacity evaluation. The physical capacity evaluation plays an integral part in the therapeutic management of hand injuries. The evaluation offers objective and subjective measurements of an individual's potential to return to a former position or a modified job, or to secure vocational counseling for job retraining. A physician, lawyer, insurance representative, or vocational counselor may refer an individual for physical capacity evaluation.

The content of each evaluation is geared to the individual. Evaluees are interviewed with regard to the physical demands and current responsibilities of their occupations (Fig. 90-10). The evaluation consists of two parts. The first part is a hand function assessment and includes hand volume, strength, ADL, and sensibility. The second part is an assessment of the patient's ability to perform simulated work requirements. Observation of the patient performing simulated work tasks and utilization of standard tests complete this part of the evaluation.

ADL evaluation. When appropriate, patients are referred to the certified occupational therapy assistant for ADL evaluation and training. An ADL checklist is used in conjunction with the patient's demonstrated abilities, to determine whether training and/or provision of equipment are needed. A kitchen area is available for training as part of this program.

SUMMARY

This chapter provides an overview of the operation of a privately run hand rehabilitation center. It is hoped that knowledge gained from this overview will provide surgeons and therapists with a working model in establishing new hand rehabilitation centers.

91

Research in a clinical setting

CHRISTINE A. MORAN

Many authors have cited the need for clinical research studies to substantiate clinical practice as both a science and an art.[4,8,15] Several reasons for the lack of clinical studies up to now have been reported.[2,13] However, as these authors have indicated, clinical research can establish standards of clinical practice through quantitative assessment of current treatment methods and techniques.

This chapter presents guidelines for the development and implementation of clinical research. Material in this chapter is directed to the therapist interested in initiating clinical research.

COMPONENTS OF RESEARCH STUDY
Question

All research studies begin with an idea, problem, or topic to pursue. However, this is not the research question in its most complete form. The object of the research study must be identified clearly and placed in a question format.[8,15,18]

Formulation of the answerable research question requires that it be specific rather than general.[11] First, carefully review pertinent journal articles that will assist you in the development of the question. Second, identify both the practical benefit and the clinical relevance of your proposed question.[15] In its final form, the research question must include the problem to be addressed, the patients to be studied, the specific variable under study, and a general outline of how the study will be executed.

After development of the research question in both correlational and experimental studies, the hypothesis statement is developed.[8] The hypothesis states what the question asks and clearly identifies the relationship between the study variables. Hypotheses in these studies are written in the null form. "Null" means without value, without significance, and implies that the difference between the different variables of the study is equal to zero.[8] Hypotheses are used to explain collected data and dependent variables using statistical analyses.

Design

The design is the framework from which the researcher conducts the study or, as Slater noted, "a way to organize the procedure and the techniques of your study that will maximize efficiency, control variables, and minimize error".[20] In a way, the design is the continuation and the expansion of the research question. The design should ex-

plain in great detail the actual steps of the study itself. Therefore it is necessary to take ample time for review of appropriate literature to assist in determining the optimal test situation, equipment, data collection, and other related components of the study design. Also involved are possible ethical and moral issues when one is deciding within the confines of the design what treatments may be withheld from certain patients of the study.

There are three major types of design methodologies: descriptive, analytical, and experimental.[14] The design methodology selected for your research study determines how the data will be collected, the grouping of subjects or patients, and statistical analysis. The descriptive research design allows observation without alteration of the setting, conditions of the observation, or direct influences through treatments or controls upon the subject.[8,14,16] This research methodology does not seek to control the subject or sample being studied but rather to give the researcher the opportunity to describe clearly and report the focus of the observations. Observations or data in descriptive research studies are gathered through surveys, checklists, or detailed case studies, and may be retrospective or prospective.

The experimental design allows for careful testing of the causal relationship existing within the study itself.[10] This design is prospective and requires that all variables of the study be identified and controlled, except for the variable being studied. Many different experimental designs can be used; which design is used depends on the subjects or patients being studied and the question being answered. Some examples of these designs are as follows: pretest/posttest control group design, Solomon four-group design, posttest-only design, and sequential medical trials. (See references 3, 5-8, 14, 16, 18, and 20 for detailed explanations of designs.)

The method of sequential medical trials, in particular, offers a controlled design plan for clinical studies.[1] Advantages of this design are as follows: appreciable reduction of the amount of study data, analysis of data as soon as collected, possible elimination of statistical computation, financial feasibility, fitting with mode of patient care, length of data collection being variable rather than fixed, and allowance for ethical considerations of patient involvement.[1,6,7] This research design is well suited for analysis of acute patient care and permits a quick decision, based on

data, to continue or stop treatment as soon as the significance is achieved.

Determination of study significance is obtained by use of graphs such as Fig. 91-1 (other graphs are available for different levels of significance). The graph is used in the following fashion after development of the question, criteria for significance, and other design components discussed earlier. Patients accepted for study are paired and randomly assigned to the old or new treatments being studied. When the criteria for significance are met or the time limit is reached, an X is placed along the vertical axis if the new treatment is significant, along the horizontal axis if the old treatment is significant, or along the diagonal axis if both treatments are equal or of no significance.[7] The starting place for X placement is adjacent to the X already located on the graph.

This plotting procedure is followed for each subsequent pair of patients until a marked X falls outside a barrier line. As noted on this graph, a significance of 0.05 is achieved for the new or old treatments if the marked X crosses the barrier into that designated space. If the X crosses into the midspace, no difference between treatments is found.

Patient criteria

As part of the design development, criteria for subject or patient selection are developed.[8,18] Criteria determination must be made before the initiation of the study for all patients or subjects who will be included. Such items as age, sex, diagnosis, surgical procedure, occupation, and symptoms, and as many other criteria as are needed to define the patients in the study completely are listed at this point in the design development.

Sampling

Many different methods can be used in the selection of subjects for the study sample, as cited by Currier.[8] Suffice it to say that the importance lies in the selection of a sampling technique that will diminish sources of error in the study. Sampling also strengthens the probable outcome of the study and controls for homogeneity of the subjects, researcher bias, and other sources of error. Types of sampling include random sampling, systematic sampling, and sampling of convenience.[8,9] Random sampling can be accomplished through the use of a numbers table, available in most statistics or research books, or simply the drawing of numbers from a hat. Systematic sampling is achieved when a complete number of a particular population is known and can be divided by the desired sample size. Thus one arrives at a quotient that can be used for the selection of the desired sample from the known population. Last, sampling of convenience is most often used when there are limited numbers of patients who can be chosen for a particular study. Though this method permits little choice in the selection of patients, it is most often used in clinical research.

Definitions

All terms identified thus far in the development of the research study require specific definition within the study's context, that is, an operational definition.[8,18] These specific definitions describe how a particular term or phrase will be

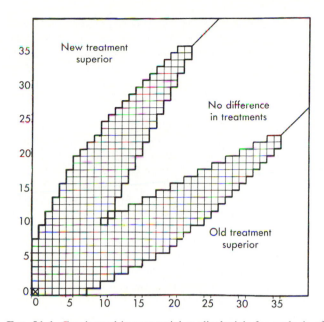

FIG. 91-1. Graph used in sequential medical trials for analysis of data. This graph is designed for data analysis at significance level of 0.05. (From Bross, I.: Biometrics **8:**189-205, 1952.)

used within the study's framework. For example, resting position of the wrist means 0 degrees to some clinicians and 5 to 10 degrees of wrist extension to other clinicians. In a study where the resting position of the wrist is important, it would be necessary for that researcher to describe in detail what is meant by resting position within the context of that particular study. Operational definitions may also be established definitions or the description of observed measurements.

Variables

There are two types of variables in research: independent and dependent.[14] Independent variables include treatments provided, stimulus, or anything that causes or influences the outcome. The dependent variable, on the other hand, is the response, or outcome, and is dependent on how the input, or independent variables, are manipulated in the study. Therefore the dependent variable is the measured outcome of a clinical study. It is imperative in all study designs that every variable involved be identified and controlled, except for the dependent variable. If it is not possible to control an independent variable—for example, home exercise compliance—then that variable should at least be identified.

Sources of error

Equally important are the sources of error that can be derived from the study itself, the researcher, and the environment. These include random error, such as elasticity of a tape measure; researcher error, such as inappropriate instrument selection; experimental error, such as delay in collecting data over a long period; systematic error, such as rounding raw numbers for convenience of the researcher.[8] These sources of error, as well as uncontrolled variables, affect both the internal and external validity of a research study. Internal validity, as noted by Lehmkuhl, is affected by changes within the study, such as sampling errors and patient attrition.[16] Gonnella divided internal validity into four groups: factors of history, maturation, testing, and instrumentation.[12] An example of the factor of history would be an uncontrolled event that occurs before or during the testing that would have a bearing on the results of the study, such as patient noncompliance with splinting. Maturation would include those processes operating within a person, such as aging or fatigue, while testing would involve the learning of a test over time by a participating patient. Instrumentation, on the other hand, includes not only the sensitivity of the instruments used but also reliability and validity.[8,12] External validity encompasses the likelihood or generalization of the study to other patients, settings, or conditions.[16] Internal validity and external validity cannot be strengthened simultaneously. Therefore a decision must be made at the time of design planning to strengthen one type of validity over the other, depending on the desired outcome of the research study.

Assumptions and limitations

Assumptions of a clinical research study are what the researcher takes for granted.[14] For example, an assumption of one study might be that the patient will not know which testing technique is considered more beneficial. Another assumption might be that equipment used in a study will remain calibrated during an entire testing session. On the other hand, limitations are the constraints of the study. An example of a limitation would be the fact that the results of a study on rheumatoid arthritic patients could not be extrapolated to patients with osteoarthritis if the study examined the effects of the use of a certain drug during splinting.

DATA COLLECTION

There are four types of data that can be collected in research studies.[11] These types, or levels, of measurement are nominal, ordinal, interval, and ratio. Frequently, interval and ratio levels of measurement are combined and called "metric."[18] Nominal data are measurements collected in an either/or expression. Examples of this measurement include names and yes or no. Ordinal data are assigned in order of

sequence, and each datum is not discrete. These data are in relative relationship to each other, such as the grades of manual muscle testing (normal, good, fair, poor, trace). Interval data include units of measurement that have been established, such as inches. Ratio data are values measured from an absolute designated zero point, such as Celsius degrees. In the planning stages of the research study, as well as in data collection, it is very important to record the data in the nominal, ordinal, interval, or ratio form rather than altering the data type. Thus the data points coincide not only with the design but also with the selected statistical analysis.

All clinicians collect data every day using various measurement techniques. In a research study, the conditions and the method of data collection are altered. For example, the design has designated and outlined the frequency of measurement, the conditions of measurement, and how the measurement itself will be performed. Data collection can only begin when every detail of measurement is determined. In addition to the details mentioned above, recording forms and measurement tools must be developed and collected before the actual day of collection. Careful preparation for data collection prevents time lost in repeated measurements, elimination of incomplete data forms, and delayed collection sessions. In addition, measurement error can be reduced by use of accepted standardized tests and tools. Keep in mind the definitions of reliability and validity.[8,14,18]

ANALYSIS

The evaluation or analysis of the collected data and the interpretation of the data are dependent on the study design and the type of data collected.[14,21] Many research and statistic books are available and offer specific information in this area.[1,8,14,17-19] In addition, Table 91-1 displays several statistics that can be used with the appropriate levels of measurement collected. Therefore helpful guidelines in data analysis and interpretation will be described here rather than detailed explanations of the appropriate statistical tests.

First, the study design, the type of data collected or level of measurement, and the statistical test must be either all qualitative or quantitative.[10] For example, if a descriptive study was undertaken using a survey to gather the data, percentages and descriptive explanations are used, not the

TABLE 91-1. Statistical tests that can be used for analysis of specific data or levels of measurement

Level of measurement	Classification of statistical test	
	Nonparametric	**Parametric**
Nominal	Mode, chi square, Cochran Q	
Ordinal	Median, rank correlation, Friedman two-way analysis, Wilcoxan matched pairs	
Interval or ratio		Mean, standard deviation, Pearson correlation, Student *t* tests, analysis of variance, regression analysis

Student *t* test. Second, statistical tests analyze data relative to frequency and tendency but do not interpret the results. Interpretation is performed by you, the researcher, based on the conditions of the study. You must decide how important each result is within the total picture of the study. A significant result may be less significant if an uncontrolled variable such as patient attrition has altered either the study design or data collection. Third, do not overload the study with statistical analyses in place of common sense and clear thinking.[18] A statistical test is a tool and not the study itself. When reviewing the data and statistical analyses, be constantly asking yourself, "Is the difference really a difference?"

CONCLUSION

This chapter has focused on the development and execution of a clinical research study. The components of a research study have been presented, and data collection and data analysis have been discussed. Through the use of results gathered from clinical research studies, one can provide patients with critically tested techniques and therapeutic treatments rather than treatments based upon clinical opinion.

REFERENCES

1. Armitage, T.: Sequential medical trials, New York, 1975, John Wiley & Sons, Inc.
2. Ballin, A.J., Breslin, W.H., Wierenga, K.A.S., and Sheppard, K.F.: Research in physical therapy: philosophy, barriers to involvement and use among California physical therapists, Phys. Ther. **60**:888, 1980.
3. Ballinger, W.F., editor: Research methods in surgery, Boston, 1964, Little, Brown & Co.
4. Basmajian, J.V.: Research or retrench: the rehabilitation profession's challenge, Phys. Ther. **55**:607, 1975.
5. Bolton, B.: Introduction to rehabilitation research, Springfield, Ill., 1974, Charles C Thomas, Publisher.
6. Bross, I.: Sequential clinical trials, J. Chronic Dis. **8**:349, 1958.
7. Bross, I.: Sequential medical plans, Biometrics **8**:189, 1952.
8. Currier, D.: Elements of research in physical therapy, Baltimore, 1979, The Williams & Wilkins Co.
9. Daniel, W.W., and Coogler, C.E.: Sampling in physical therapy research, Phys. Ther. **55**:1326, 1975.
10. Ethridge, D., and McSweeney, M.: Research in occupational therapy, Am. J. Occup. Ther. **24**:490, 1970.
11. Geitgey, D.A., and Metz, E.A.: A brief guide to designing research proposals, Nurs. Res. **18**:339, 1969.
12. Gonnella, C.: The method: what and why, Phys. Ther. **50**:382, 1970.
13. Griffin, J.E.: How can physical therapists be stimulated to engage in simple research? In which areas is clinical research most needed? Phys. Ther. **50**:259, 1970.
14. Leedy, P.: Practical research: planning and design, New York, 1974, MacMillan Publishing Co., Inc.
15. Lehmkuhl, D.: The question: what and why? Phys. Ther. **50**:61, 1970.
16. Lehmkuhl, D.: Experimental design: what and why? Phys. Ther. **50**:1716, 1970.
17. Osborne, J.F.: Statistical exercises in medical research, New York, 1979, John Wiley & Sons, Inc.
18. Payton, O.D.: Research: the validation of clinical practice, Philadelphia, 1979, F.A. Davis Co.
19. Siegel, S.: Non-parametric statistics for the behavioral sciences, New York, 1956, McGraw-Hill Book Co.
20. Slater, S.B.: The design of clinical research, Phys. Ther. **46**:265, 1966.
21. Wolery, M., and Harris, S.: Interpreting the results of single-subject research designs, Phys. Ther. **62**:445, 1982.

92

The nurse and hand surgery

CHERYL MUELLER FRIEDMAN

With the increasing complexity of hand surgery, the nurse requires knowledge of specific skills necessary in dealing with this specialty. This chapter briefly deals with hand surgery in the operating room and includes an explanation of the preparation of the hand for a surgical procedure, the care and use of specialized equipment for hand surgery, the proper technique for the handling of prosthetic implants, and the importance of communication with the patient who is awake during surgery. In addition, the nursing care during the immediate postoperative period (24 to 48 hours) is discussed.

PHYSICAL PREPARATION

Although the hand is well vascularized and is not prone to infection, if a nidus of infection does occur, the result may be permanent dysfunction of the hand. Therefore adequate surgical preparation is imperative.

The concept of antiseptic surgery had its beginnings with Louis Pasteur, Joseph Lister, and Ignaz Semmelweis. Contained in the basic works of Pasteur is the concept that viable bacteria are heat labile. From that, present-day criteria for instrument sterilization have arisen. Lister, a surgeon, experimented with a disinfectant, carbolic acid (phenol). He used this in a weak solution on gauze dressings and as a spray in the operating room. This decreased the incidence of infection in his surgical patients. Semmelweis observed that handwashing was an important factor in lowering the mortality rates in the hospital wards. This concept has led to the use of sterile gowns and gloves, handwashing, and the practice of aseptic technique in surgery.

In the operating room today, the cornerstone for any surgical procedure is the concept of aseptic technique. The nurse is the one primarily responsible for the maintenance of asepsis.

The skin is the first line of defense. Once it is penetrated, the underlying tissues are exposed and vulnerable to bacterial invasion. Although skin cannot be completely sterilized, the use of bactericidal agents can greatly reduce the number of bacteria on its surface. At our institution, Betadine, a povidone iodine–based solution is used. The patient's arm is shaved the night before; however, some may choose to shave it just before surgery. After shaving, a 10-minute scrub of the extremity with the Betadine solution is performed. The nails are cleansed and trimmed unless dy-

namic traction is to be used postoperatively. The morning of surgery the arm is scrubbed for an additional 10 minutes with the Betadine solution. If the patient is sensitive to this solution, Hibiclens or another bactericidal agent may be substituted. Then the arm is dried and wrapped in sterile towels that are taped shut. The patient arrives in the operating room with the arm prepared in this manner.

PSYCHOLOGICAL PREPARATION

Even as a nurse, one's initial introduction to the operating room can be disorienting. It is not difficult to imagine the anxiety of a nonmedically exposed patient, who is already experiencing a loss of control by being in an unfamiliar environment. This is further compounded by feelings of euphoria because of preoperative medications. Consequently, simple explanations by the nurse the night before surgery when the patient is unsedated and in a familiar environment seem to be an effective mode in the patient's psychological preparation.

Since the operating room nurse is usually the first member of the surgical team to greet the patient, the impression the nurse leaves will be a lasting one. After introducing himself or herself, checking the patient's identification, permit, and surgical site, the nurse will attempt to allay the patient's fears by clarifying any questions. Knowing what to expect will augment the patient's feelings of control and help decrease anxiety.

THE HAND TABLE

To facilitate surgery on the hand, a hand table was designed. It is composed of a smooth, flat, wooden surface whose sides are cut out to form a resting place for the surgeon's and assistant's arms while performing surgery. The patient's hand is placed in the center of the table for easy access. Two sturdy metal legs are attached to this surface to provide a wide stable base. The hand table can be firmly attached to the operating room table so that it is immovable. Fig. 92-1 shows the prepared arm on the hand table.

Draping techniques vary with linen supplies and hospital preferences. Principally, a waterproof base on the hand table should be present because of copious amounts of irrigant used throughout surgical procedures.

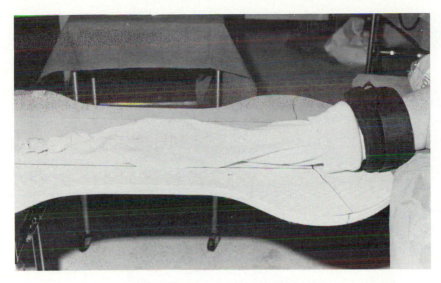

FIG. 92-1. Patient's arm draped with stockinette and resting on hand table.

TOURNIQUET APPLICATION

There are few circumstances in which a tourniquet is not used for hand surgery. The tourniquet produces a bloodless field, which is essential for the visual clarity necessary for such meticulous work. The cuff of a pneumatic tourniquet is placed around the upper arm. This is preferred over a penrose or Esmarch's tourniquet alone because it maintains an accurate, steady, measurable, and even pressure over the entire extremity. This pressure can be adjusted according to the surgeon's needs. After a Betadine preparation of the skin and the application of a sterile stockinette, the limb is exsanguinated either by elevation or wrapping a sterile rubber Esmarch's tourniquet around the extremity. The pressure in the tourniquet box is then raised to 300 mg Hg for adults, and the Esmarch's tourniquet is removed. Note that the presence of a tumor or infection would preclude the use of Esmarch's tourniquet because it may force bacteria or tumor cells into the general circulation. Elevation alone is sufficient in these cases.

Tourniquet time is precious, and so the marking out of skin incisions should be done before elevation of the tourniquet. Limits on tourniquet time vary with the discretion of the surgeon, but, in general, tourniquet times are usually less than 2 hours.

PREFERENCE CARDS

The nurse must be familiar with the surgeon's basic routine. This can be facilitated through the use of procedure cards. These are surgeon preference cards, which include special suture and instruments required for each surgical procedure. This affords better utilization of equipment and avoids unnecessary waste and expense for the patient and hospital. Therefore communication with the surgeon is vital. Teamwork will result in a shorter, less traumatic operation that will benefit everyone.

CARE OF EQUIPMENT AND INSTRUMENTS

Special care is given to any sharp instruments to ensure their quality. Delicate sharp instruments are separately bagged and gas sterilized. The sharp tips are covered with rubber protectors. This type of sterilization extends their life-span. Instruments are routinely checked for precision and repaired or replaced when necessary.

The basic instruments needed for most surgical procedures of the hand are listed on p. 955 (see also Fig. 92-2). These instruments are wrapped and steam sterilized. The sterilization is done in a high-pressure autoclave. Metal instruments are autoclaved at a temperature of 270° F at 30 pounds of pressure for 3 minutes. These autoclaves are checked daily for accuracy and ability to kill spores. At our institution, an Attest, which is a capsule containing a bacterial species, is placed in each autoclave and sterilized for 3 minutes. They are then incubated for 24 hours at which time they are checked for growth. This method enables us to test the sterilization power of each autoclave.

Power instrumentation is an adjunct to hand surgery that will shorten procedures such as arthroplasties and arthrodeses (Fig. 92-3). It is important to read the maintenance manuals that accompany each drill. Periodic maintenance checks should be carried out to ensure a safely working instrument. Electrical equipment should also have periodic checks. Fig. 92-4 depicts one type of bipolar cautery machine used at our institution. The complementary forceps and cord are shown in Fig. 92-5.

HANDLING PROSTHETIC IMPLANTS

Special consideration should be given to the care and handling of prosthetic implants during hand surgery. For example, the Hunter Silastic tendon implant is frequently used during tendon reconstructive surgery. The operating room receives this prosthesis in a sterile package from the manufacturer. To ascertain the proper-sized implant to be used, one should assemble a tendon-sizing kit before surgery. It contains one of each size of tendon, which is sterilized by the nurse in the following manner: The sizers are washed in a non–oil-based soap such as Ivory and rinsed copiously with distilled water. They are air dried and packaged in lint-free plastic bags for gas (ethylene oxide) ster-

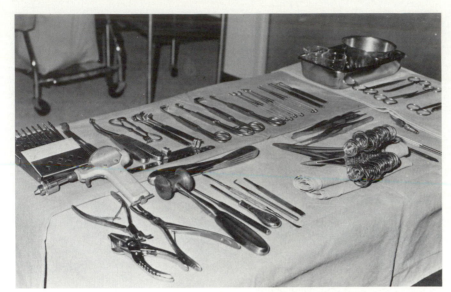

FIG. 92-2. Basic instruments for hand surgery.

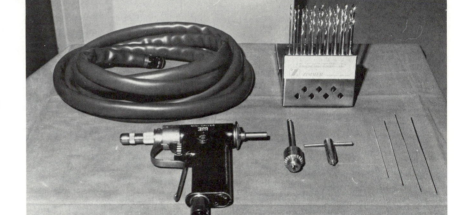

FIG. 92-3. Power drill, K-wires, and drill bits with adapter.

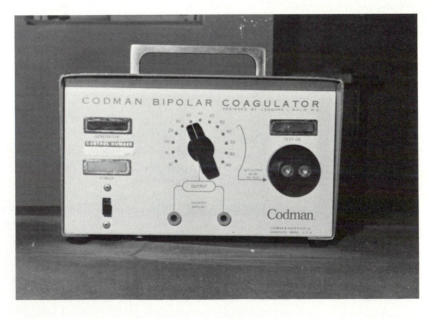

FIG. 92-4. Bipolar machine.

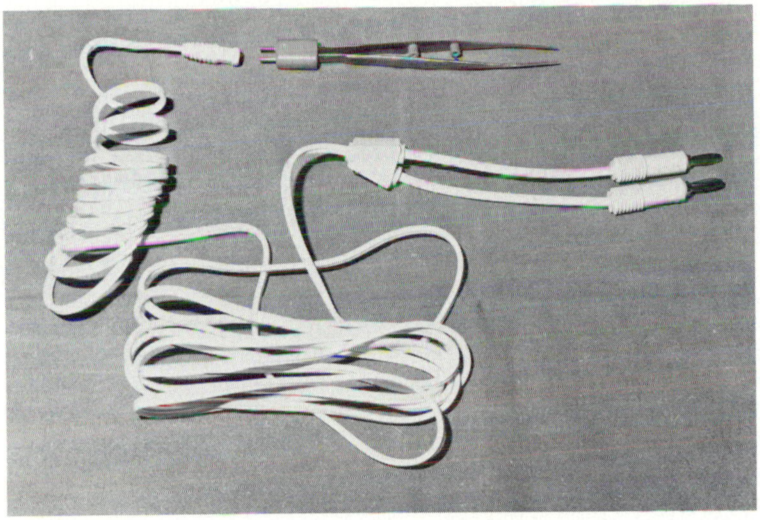

FIG. 92-5. Bipolar forceps and cord.

List of basic hand instruments

12	Halstead straight mosquito hemostats, 4¾ inch
12	Halstead curved mosquito hemostats, 4¾ inch
1	Rochester pean curved hemostat
1	Baby Mixer hemostatic forceps
1	Rochester-Oschner, 7¼ inch (Kocher)
3	Baby-Oschner (Kocher)
4	Allise clamp
1	Mayo-Hegar needle holder, 8 inch
3	Webster needle holders, 5½ inch
10	Backhaus towel clips, 5¼ inch
1	Carroll bone holding clamp
1	Diamond-edge straight Mayo scissor, 6¾ inch
1	Curved Metzenbaum scissors, 5½ inch
1	Straight plastic scissor
1	Straight Stevens scissor, 4¾ inch
1	Curved Stevens scissor, 4¾ inch
1	Curved plastic scissor, 5 inch
1	Wire suture scissor
1	Bunnell hand drill with Jacobs chuck
1	Box of drill bits—17 Zimalite twist drills
1	Berbecker pliers, 5½ inch
1	Beyer rongeur, 7 inch
1	Shearer rongeur, 5½ inch
2	Spratt bone curets, 00 and 000
1	Lucae mallet
1	No. 3 Bard-Parker knife handle
2	Beaver knife handles KD, 5 inch
2	Single tooth Adson forceps
1	Brown-Adson forceps
2	Smooth Adson forceps
1	Fine smooth forceps
2	Finger Bennett retractors
2	Carroll hand rake retractors
2	Volkman rakes, 4 inch, 4-prong blunt
2	Small reverse retractors
1	Carroll bone awl
1	Frazier suction No. 10
1	Carroll-Bunnell periosteal elevator
1	Key periosteal elevator
1	Bunnell dissecting probe, 5¾ inch
1	Freer elevator, 7½ inch, double ended
1	Metric ruler, 6 inch
2	Medium eyelid retractors
2	Small eyelid retractors
2	Meyerding smooth finger retractors—blades, ¼ inch × 11/16 inch
2	Meyerding smooth finger retractors—blades, 5/32 inch × ⅜ inch
2	Meyerding rake finger retractors—blades, 3/16 inch × ⅝ inch
2	Meyerding rake finger retractors—blades, ⅛ inch × ¼ inch
2	Singer skin hooks, 6 inch
2	Double skin hooks, 6 inch—Rollet
2	Knapp 4-prong skin hooks
2	Joseph hooks, 10 mm wide
2	Joseph hooks, 5 mm wide

ilization. They are then aerated to eliminate the remaining gas vapors from the prosthesis, for these vapors could cause damage to normal body tissues. At the time of surgery, the plastic bag is aseptically opened and the sizers are placed in a sterile basin of antibiotic solution. This "triple solution" is composed of bacitracin, 50,000 USP; neomycin, 0.5 gm; polymixin B, 500,000 units in 1 liter of lactated Ringer's solution.

Debris of any kind, whether it be powder from gloves or lint, may increase the risk of infection or cause additional adhesion formation. Using a wet sponge to remove the powder from the sterile gloves is advised before one handles any prosthesis.

When the proper-sized prosthesis has been found, the nurse opens the bag containing the silicone rubber (Silastic) tendon and places it in the basin of triple solution. The prosthesis is handled as infrequently as possible and is constantly kept moist. The implant becomes electrically charged when dry and will attract lint and dust from the surroundings. If it must be handled, atraumatic forceps should be used. This prevents weakening or tearing of the implant, so that optimal results may be obtained.

VISUAL AIDS IN HAND SURGERY

Magnification is now an accepted and necessary part of hand surgery. It ranges from 2.5 to 30 magnification. Binocular loupes with 2.5 and 4 magnification are shown in Fig. 92-6. They should be cleaned and placed in an appropriate receptacle when not in use.

A microscope can provide very high powers of magnification, which are especially useful for nerve repairs. It should be cleaned daily using the guide provided by the manufacturer. The exterior can be wiped down with alcohol to control dust collection. The foot pedal should be protected with a plastic bag from dust and moisture. Lens cleaner and cotton swabs are recommended for cleaning eyepieces and the objective lens. A periodic check should be done to ensure good working condition.

PATIENT UNDER LOCAL ANESTHESIA: THE NURSE'S ROLE

Not all patients will be asleep during their surgery. Regional blocks and local anesthetics are being used more and more often, even for involved and lengthy procedures such as tenolysis and carpal tunnel surgery. Local anesthesia has many benefits over general. The patient's airway is not compromised nor is the cardiovascular system affected with small doses as it is with systemic drugs. For the elderly, diabetic, or hypertensive patient this is the safest form of anesthesia.

Usually 1% or 2% lidocaine (Xylocaine) is injected locally, and its anesthetic effect soon ensues. Informing the patient that a temporary burning sensation may be felt relieves unnecessary anxiety. The nurse is therefore the liaison between the surgeon, who is concentrating on the procedure, and the patient behind the drapes. By keeping the patient informed of what is happening, the nurse can elicit better cooperation.

Other problems that may be encountered with an awake patient are tourniquet pain and unwanted movement. Tourniquet pain cannot be controlled through a local injection of xylocaine. Supplemental sedation with diazepam (Valium) may be necessary if pain is intolerable. However, talking with the patient may act as a distraction and thereby decrease the patient's awareness of pain and his need for more medication. Unwanted movement can be handled by making the patient as comfortable as possible before surgery and asking for his cooperation during surgery. The use of a stabilizing device, such as a lead hand, will help deter unwanted movement. Fig. 92-7 shows a lead hand that is malleable and will conform to the patient's hand. This assists in immobilizing the patient's unaffected fingers while surgery is performed.

Finally, the nurse is responsible for patient teaching. Postoperative instructions should be made simple and clear, especially if the patient has been sedated. It is advisable to write down instructions such as the time the patient should return for a checkup and a phone number where the patient can contact his surgeon if necessary.

The necessity for nurse-patient communication in the operating room can be seen with a patient undergoing local anesthesia. The nurse fulfills a role beyond that of a technician. Through the concept of a team approach, in which the patient is the center of the team, the combined efforts of the physician, nurse, therapists, and other personnel can provide the most effective mode of patient care.

IMMEDIATE POSTOPERATIVE MANAGEMENT

The nurse plays an integral role in the prevention and early detection of complications after hand surgery. In general, to avoid complications, the goal postoperatively is to promote primary wound healing followed by early motion. To promote primary wound healing, there has to be adequate circulation in the hand. A neurovascular flow sheet can be used to document innervation and circulation of the hand postoperatively. Listed below are six factors that should be considered:

1. Color: *pink* (normal), *white* (arterial insufficiency), *purple* (venous congestion)
2. Temperature: hot, normal, cold
3. Capillary refill: normal (1 to 2 seconds), sluggish, absent
4. Pulse: rate, strong or weak, absent
5. Edema: mild, moderate, severe
6. Pain: absent or present (If present, describe how severe. If pain persists even after medication given, call doctor.)

The following factors will cause decreased blood flow to the hand: edema, pain, smoking, and constricting dressings. Edema can be reduced by elevation of the hand above the level of the heart immediately postoperatively. Triamcinolone acetonide (Kenalog), 10 mg, is sometimes given locally to a patient after extensive dissection, to minimize postoperative swelling. If swelling is kept to a minimum, the patient will experience less pain. Usually a mild sedative or narcotic given postoperatively will greatly reduce the patient's discomfort.

Smoking should be strongly discouraged. Most patients are cooperative if they are told why they should not smoke. Nicotine causes blood vessels to constrict.

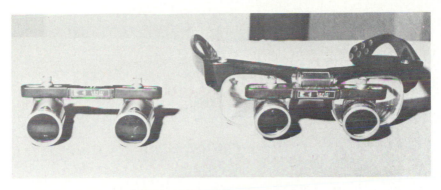

FIG. 92-6. Binocular loupes with 2.5 and 4 power.

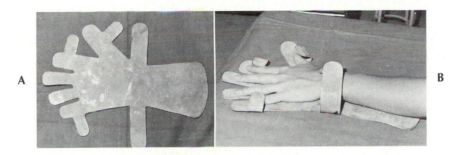

A

B

FIG. 92-7. A, Lead hand. **B,** Lead hand in use.

To ensure that a splint or cast is applied properly, ask the patient to wiggle his fingers. Check for signs of impaired circulation by using the flow sheet. Observation of the skin integrity around areas of the splint or cast edges is important. Make certain these areas are well padded. Also, any foreign body protruding through the skin such as a Kirschner wire or pin can be a locus of infection. Keep this area clean and dry. Use of an antibacterial ointment such as Betadine ointment at the pin site is strongly recommended to prevent infection.

During the immediate postoperative period patients are feeling very dependent and helpless and their anxiety is increased. The nurse can minimize patient anxiety by anticipating the patient's needs. Cut food and open containers when bringing in a meal. Place the call bell within easy reach of the patient. Remember the patient will need assistance with most activities that require two hands.

Establishing a good rapport with the patient's family is essential when one is offering psychological support. This aspect is especially important for patients undergoing tendon, nerve, or reconstructive surgery. The nurse should have the patient and family set realistic goals. During the patient's rehabilitation, range-of-motion exercises and isometrics are essential to maintain muscle strength and prevent stiffness.

Finally, patient education is crucial. Give patients written instructions before discharge. Have the patient demonstrate that he understands the instructions. Teach patients about the signs of infections—tenderness, fever, and yellowish discharge—and what to do if they occur. The most successful results occur when the patient takes an active role in his recovery. The nurse should assist the patient in achieving this goal.

BIBLIOGRAPHY

Boyes, J.H.: Bunnell's surgery of the hand, ed. 5, Philadelphia, 1970, J.B. Lippincott Co.

Flynn, J.E.: Hand surgery, Baltimore, 1966, The Williams & Wilkins Co.

93

The microsurgical nurse

ALBIE MORRIS

The goals of this chapter are to present (1) the microsurgical team concept in patient care, (2) the role of the microsurgical nurse, (3) a guideline for the psychological support of the patient preoperatively, intraoperatively, and postoperatively, and (4) a guideline for the necessary equipment and instrumentation utilized in microsurgery.

THE TEAM CONCEPT

Of all the members of the microsurgical team, the patient must be regarded as the most important member. The ultimate goal of every team member is to rehabilitate the patient to his optimal level of function. Several key personnel are necessary to achieve this goal. The surgeon, with his or her technical skills, and the surgical fellows, residents, and other assistants are vital parts of the team. The microsurgical nurse has numerous responsibilities throughout the course of care. The anesthesiologist and the nurse anesthetist play major intraoperative roles. An important team member both preoperatively and postoperatively is the therapist, who significantly contributes to the success of the surgery.

Since so many are involved in the total care of the patient, open lines of communication are essential to the hand team. The importance of maintaining a pleasant and harmonious working environment cannot be sufficiently stressed, particularly when team members are on an emergency call schedule, involving 24-hour availability.

INTRAOPERATIVE TEAM RESPONSIBILITIES

Intraoperative functions of the team are geared toward the patient's physical well-being. He should be kept free from pain and discomfort. Maintenance of a stable circulatory state, which may require the infusion of blood products, and maintenance of a normal fluid and electrolyte balance, which requires intravenous therapy, are also essential to his physical care. For extended procedures, the patient's body temperature must be maintained; this is achieved by use of a hyperthermia unit. Providing for urinary drainage, usually accomplished by an indwelling urethral catheter and drainage system, is also imperative.

The microsurgical nurse has an important role at this time. To perform this role, he or she must have a good working knowledge of all the equipment and instrumentation utilized in hand surgery. The microsurgical nurse is responsible for keeping everything in excellent working condition. By providing reference materials and procedure cards that specify surgeon preferences for various types of surgery, and sharing his or her knowledge with other nursing personnel, the microsurgical nurse teaches others so that they can function on the hand team.

The duties of the microsurgical nurse are not limited to the operating room, however. The full scope of this nurse's responsibilities enables him or her to follow the patient throughout the entire rehabilitation program.

PREOPERATIVE DUTIES OF THE MICROSURGICAL NURSE

Before surgery, the patient can benefit immensely from a visit by the nurse, who can be of great assistance in acquainting him with the unfamiliar surroundings of the hospital and in informing him of the sequence of events leading to surgery. If the patient is confused or uncertain about what his physician has explained to him, the nurse can be of value in clarifying these statements. This is one more example of the necessity for open lines of communication—in this instance, between the surgeon and the nurse.

Before the nurse visits the patient, he or she should check the patient's hospital chart for the following items:
1. The operative permit, noting the procedure for which the patient has signed
2. The history and physical report, noting any other physical problems, any allergies, and any previous surgery

Upon entering the room, the nurse should introduce herself, check the patient's identification, and offer a brief explanation of the purpose of the visit. Certain information should be imparted to the patient concerning preoperative laboratory studies, the interview by a member of the anesthesia department, and the necessity of eating or drinking nothing after midnight before the day of surgery. An explanation of the events on the day of surgery should include the following:
1. Surgical preparation of the extremity to disinfect the skin (usually with a microbicide, such as a 10% povidine-iodine solution)
2. Injection of preoperative sedation before leaving the room
3. Arrival into the operating room suite, at which time an intravenous line will be introduced

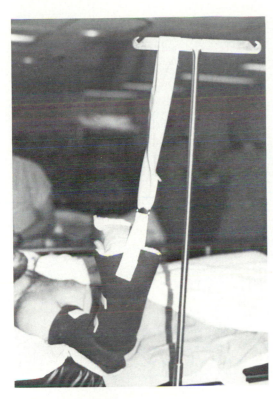

FIG. 93-1. Elevation of upper extremity with a Zimmer arm sling.

4. Final move to the operating room itself, where the major anesthetics will be administered
5. Postoperative period in the recovery room
6. Brief explanation of the immediate postoperative course, including plaster splinting, arm elevation with a sling (Fig. 93-1), and any exercises that should begin on the day of surgery

While imparting all this information to the patient, the nurse must allow equal time for him to speak, so that his questions are answered satisfactorily, and his anxieties allayed.

When the patient is scheduled for emergency surgery, very little time is allotted for preoperative support. Therefore the surgeon, the anesthesiologist, the holding-area nurse, and the microsurgical nurse must coordinate the implementation of a quick and efficient plan of care for his psychological and physical well-being.

Intraoperative duties of the microsurgical nurse

As soon as the patient arrives in the operating room, the nurse should introduce himself or herself, check the patient's identification, and check the operative permit. The nurse should tend to the patients comfort and warmth and see that he is safely positioned on the surgical table. Since excessive noise, disorganization or confusion of the surgical team, or large numbers of people present can increase the patient's anxiety, it is of utmost importance to maintain a quiet, friendly, and professional atmosphere. Unnecessary talking and unnecessary personnel in the room should be avoided for aseptic purposes and in consideration of the patient's emotional state.

This environment should be maintained throughout the surgical procedure, particularly if the patient is having a type of anesthesia other than general. For various reasons, an axillary block or local infiltration with intravenous sedation may be the anesthesia of choice. In such instances, when the patient is at least partially alert, the nurse acts as a coordinator among the anesthesiologist, the patient, and the surgeon, to provide a comfortable clinical environment.

Aside from meeting the patient's needs, the nurse is responsible for preparing the operating room with the required equipment and instruments.

BASIC HAND SURGERY EQUIPMENT
Tourniquet

During surgery a bloodless field is desirable, to provide an optimal view of the anatomic structures of the extremity. This is accomplished by use of a tourniquet. An arm cuff that is 24 inches long and secured with a Velcro strip provides continuous, even pressure over the extremity. Cotton muslin should be applied around the upper arm before the tourniquet cuff is applied for skin protection. This should be free of wrinkles. Caution must be taken not to allow any iodine prep solution to accumulate under the tourniquet cuff. The cuff is attached to the tourniquet box with rubber tubing. The tourniquet box that can be attached to a continuous supply of compressed air is preferable to those that require pressure-refill cylinders, for obvious reasons. The pressure reading on the box must be checked for accuracy at least once daily, but ideally before each surgical procedure (Fig. 93-2).

Before inflation of the tourniquet cuff, a latex rubber (Esmarch*) bandage should be wrapped securely around the elevated extremity, from the fingertips to the upper arm, to drain blood from the operative site. After inflation of the cuff, the Esmarch is removed. The time during which the tourniquet is inflated should be observed and recorded accurately. The surgeon should be notified when the tourniquet has been inflated for a period of 1 hour, and again notified every 15 minutes thereafter.

Hand table

A smooth, flat, sturdy working surface is essential in hand surgery. One hand table that provides such a surface is the Boyes-Parker† hand table. It has sliding shelves that can be opened to accommodate an irrigating pan. The tapered edges allow the surgeons sufficient proximity to the operative site while providing adequate working space and arm space. The legs are made of metal and are adjustable in height (Fig. 93-3).

Cautery

When the control of bleeding becomes necessary during surgery, an electrical cautery is utilized. A bipolar Bovie coagulator is valuable in controlling bleeding in small and

---

*Latex Esmarch Rubber Bandage, Richards, 1450 Brooks Rd., Memphis, Tenn. 38116.
†Boyes-Parker hand table, Richards, 1450 Brooks Rd., Memphis, Tenn. 38116.

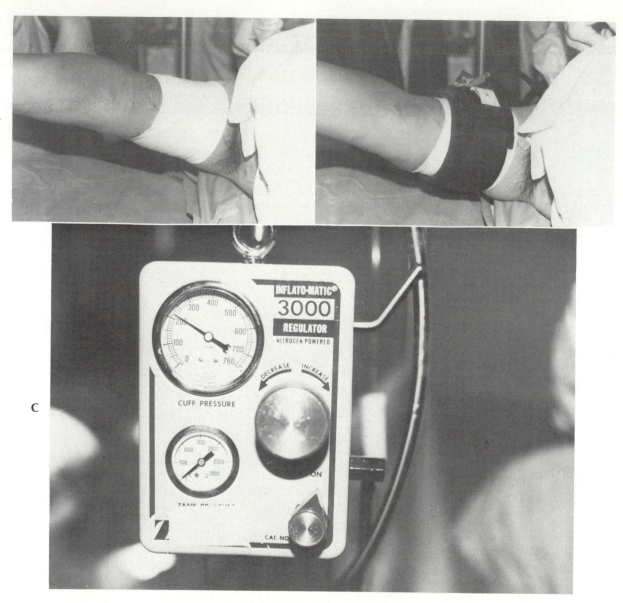

FIG. 93-2. **A,** Cotton muslin applied to upper arm before tourniquet cuff. **B,** Tourniquet cuff in place. **C,** Tourniquet box that is attached to a continuous supply of compressed air.

delicate areas without interfering with the integrity of surrounding structures (Fig. 93-4).

Suction

Because of the amount of irrigating solution used in hand surgery, suction apparatus must be supplied. If bleeding should occur, it can also be used to clear the field of blood so that the bleeding vessel can be identified and cauterized.

Organizing this equipment in the operating room involves placing everything on the side of the room that is opposite the operative site. This allows adequate space for the sterile field around the operative site—the hand table with sterile drapes, the sterile instrument tables, and the scrubbed surgeon and assistants seated at the field (Fig. 93-5).

Power instrumentation

Power drills are frequently used in hand surgery, as with arthroplasties or arthrodeses. Nitrogen tanks should be readily available as power sources.

The micro-oscillating saw* removes damaged bone and smooths rough bone edges. It is essential that blades are discarded after each use and replaced with new ones (Fig. 93-6, *A*). The Hall drill,* used with Swanson burs, reams out the remaining bone, creating a tunnel to accept an artificial implant. Used burs must be cleaned thoroughly to remove bone remnants, preferably with a wire brush. Worn burs should be replaced (Fig. 93-6, *B*). A wire-driving drill,

*Zimmer, Inc., Product Service Center, Boggs Industrial Park, Warsaw, Ind. 46580.

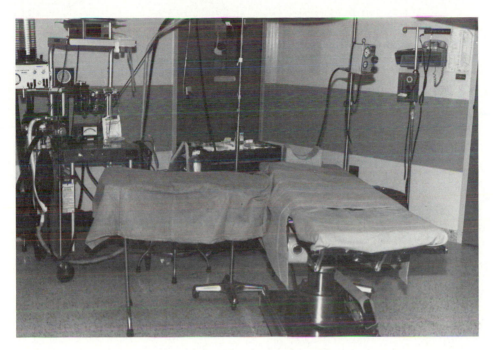

FIG. 93-3. Boyes-Parker hand table.

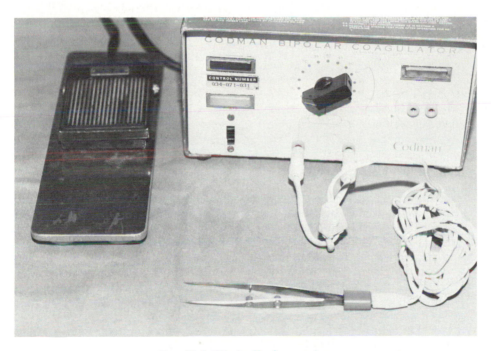

FIG. 93-4. Bipolar Bovie coagulator.

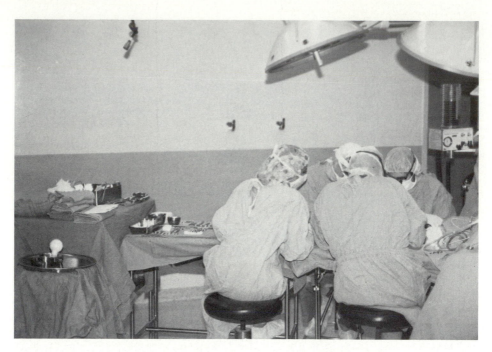

FIG. 93-5. Sterile operating field.

such as the 3M Mini-Driver,* is used to insert Kirschner wires to provide bone stabilization (Fig. 93-6, *C*).

After each use, all power equipment should be thoroughly cleansed but not immersed in water. The head of each drill should be lubricated with a lubricating oil recommended by the manufacturer before it is prepared for sterilization. This assures proper functioning when it is again utilized.

MICROSURGERY

In addition to the previously mentioned equipment and instruments, microsurgery of the hand requires high-powered magnification equipment and fine, delicate instrumentation. The surgeon and the assistants wear magnifying loupes for other procedures as well as microsurgery (Fig. 93-7). Often, however, loupes are inadequate for this type of work, and a microscope is necessary.

The hand microscope

One of the most advanced microscopes for hand surgery is the OPMI 7 P/H Microscope, a product of Zeiss.† Its advantages include a foot control and electric focus, a foot-control zoom, and a foot control *x-y* movement. The surgeon and his assistant can see the same field. There is a third head attachment for a second assistant, which can be removed to accommodate a camera attachment and camera. Other accessory equipment includes a movie camera and videorecorder. The base is electrically controlled to accommodate the accessory items (Fig. 93-8).

Before surgery begins, the microscope should be positioned on the operative side of the operating room table. The foot controls and light source should be checked so that

a proper working condition is assured. The surgeon and his assistants should adjust their respective eyepieces on the scope before scrubbing, so that minimal adjustments are required later during surgery. At the beginning of the procedure, when the microscope is not needed, the arm is rotated away from the field and the foot controls and light source are in the off position. When the microscope is needed, the nurse should rotate the arm over the operative field and switch on the controls.

In our institution (Thomas Jefferson University Hospital, in Philadelphia), the use of sterile microscope drapes is discouraged because they can easily be contaminated in a busy working environment. Ideally the use of sterile silicone-elastic cylindric covers over the eyepieces allows the surgeons and the assistants to make adjustments without fear of contamination. Sterile and nonsterile areas are better delineated on the scope with this method.

At the end of the procedure, the foot and light controls should be switched off, but the light fan is left on to cool and prolong the life of the bulb.

After the patient has left the room, the nurse is responsible for cleaning the microscope. All controls should now be off and all cords unplugged. An acceptable hospital disinfectant can be used to clean the base and arm. The lens and eyepieces require special care. They should be cleaned with a lens solution and lens paper to avoid scratching the delicate surfaces. For any imbedded debris on or around the edges of the lens and eyepieces, cotton-tip applicators and solution should be used. The microscope is then returned to its storage area, which should be near the operating room. The lens and eyepieces should be covered with a large linen or plastic bag to prevent the accumulation of dust particles on them. The base should be locked, and the electrical cords and foot control neatly hung on the base of the scope. The

---

*3M Mini-Driver, 3M Company, 225 E. Baker St., Costa Mesa, Calif. 92626.
†Carl Zeiss, Inc., 444 Fifth Avenue, New York, N.Y. 10018.

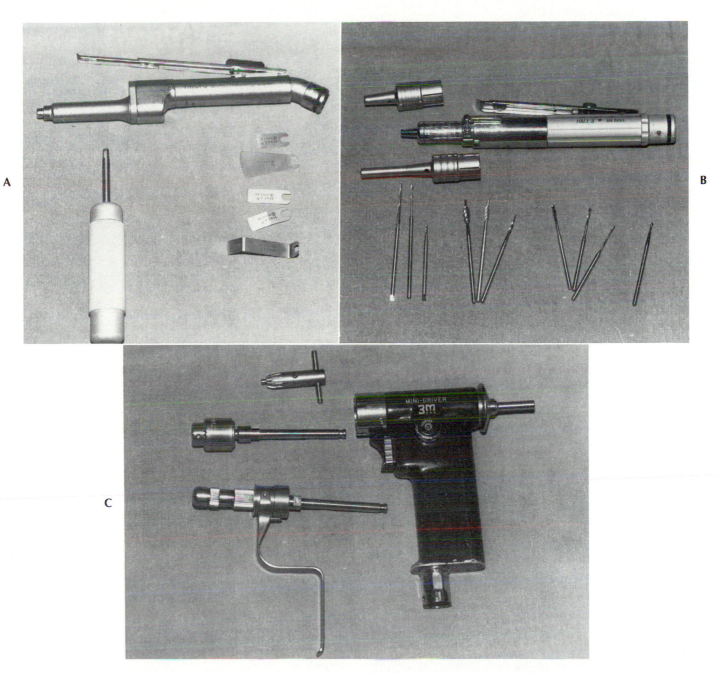

FIG. 93-6. A, Micro-oscillating saw head and blades. **B,** Hall drill with bur guards and Swanson burs. **C,** The 3M Mini-driver head and attachments.

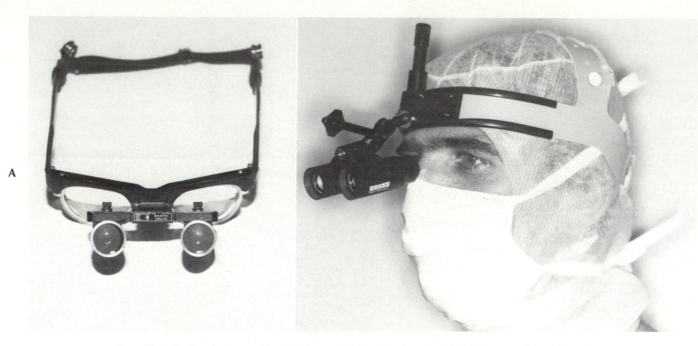

FIG. 93-7. A, Eyeglass magnification loupes. **B,** Headset loupes with high-powered magnification.

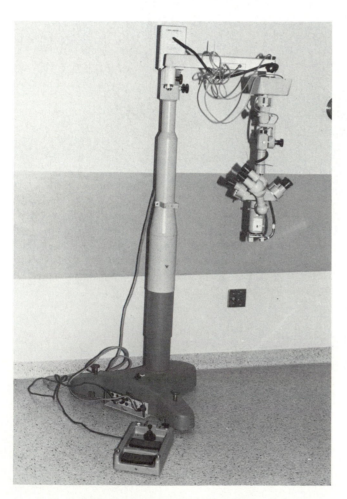

FIG. 93-8. OPMI 7 P/H microscope.

foot control should be left uncovered to prevent moisture collection, which could short circuit these controls.

Microsurgical instruments

Following is a list of basic microsurgical instruments (Fig. 93-9):

1. Fine-tip jeweler's forceps (sizes 3 and 5)
2. Microtying forceps (small and large)
3. Microdissecting and suture scissors
4. Microneedle holders, nonlocking
5. Vascular clamps—single, straight, and curved
6. Vascular clamps—double, mounted on a bar, with a mechanism for adjusting the distance between the two clamps
7. Vascular clip applier (the vascular clamps should never be opened farther than the applier allows, because doing so could strain the delicate spring mechanisms of the clamps)
8. Microsurgical bipolar cautery forceps

When not in use, these instruments should be stored in a covered metal tray with protective caps on the fine tips. One can steam sterilize them for immediate use by removing the metal cover of the tray and placing them in a high-speed autoclave for 10 minutes at 270° F and a pressure of 30 pounds per square inch.

The instruments are kept in the metal tray on the sterile field for protection until requested by the surgeon. Sterile water should also be present on the field to cleanse the instruments during surgery, to prevent the accumulation of organic debris. Saline solution should never be used on these instruments, because it causes them to rust. If a large amount of debris or blood should collect and harden, particularly in the vascular clamps, flushing with heparin solution in a tuberculin syringe will provide a thorough cleansing.

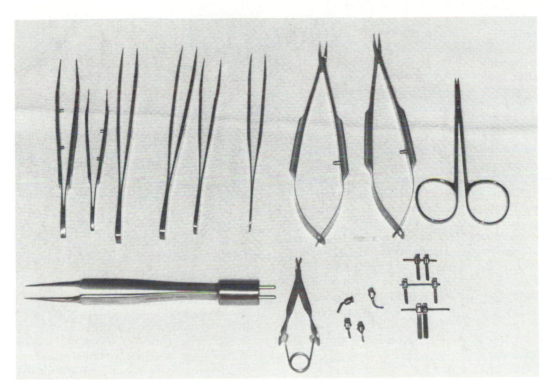

FIG. 93-9. Basic microvascular instruments.

Everyone who has contact with these instruments must be especially careful to prevent damaging their delicate tips. A backup supply of each instrument should be available in case damage does occur.

At the end of the surgical procedure, the nurse is responsible for the terminal cleaning of the microinstruments. A hemolytic cleaning solution, such as Haemo-Sol,* is effective in thoroughly cleansing and dissolving organic debris. One must give special attention to the jaws and springs of the vascular clamps, making sure the solution comes into contact with all surfaces. The instruments should be rinsed with distilled water, dried carefully, and replaced in the metal tray with protective caps on the tips. Allowing the instruments to remain damp or placing them in a moist tray could lead to rust formation.

Replantation considerations

To be prepared for replant surgery, the amputated part requires proper preservation to prolong tissue life. It should first be covered with sterile gauze, if available, and then placed in a plastic bag. A second plastic bag, filled with ice, should encase the first plastic bag. The direct contact of the amputated part with the ice must be avoided, to prevent freezing of the tissue.

In many instances, the amputated part will arrive in the operating room before the patient. A separate sterile table, containing a few of the basic hand instruments and microsurgical instruments, should be ready so that the surgeon

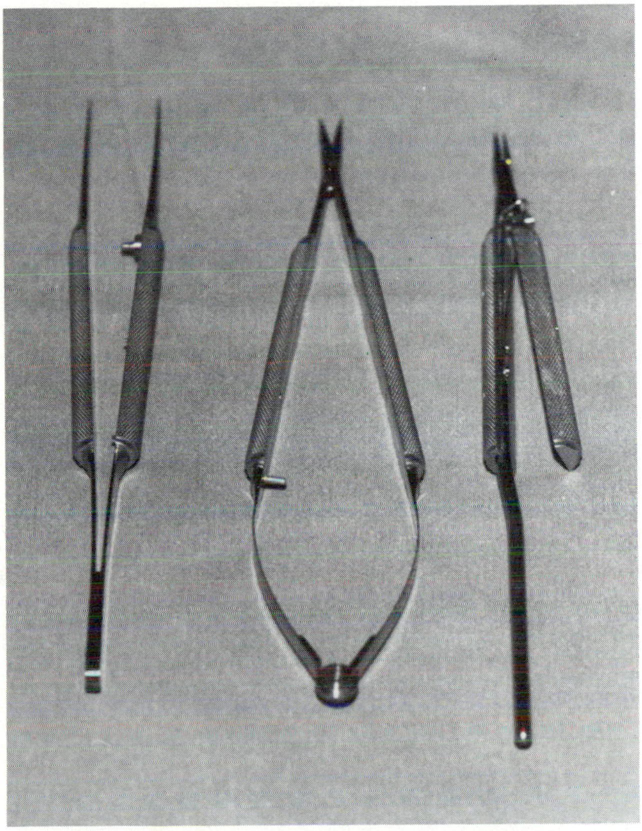

---

*Haemo-Sol, Inc., P.O. Box 6882, Baltimore, Md. 21204.

FIG. 93-10. Keeler microsurgical instrumentation.

or his assistant can begin working on this part. A predissection set, containing these instruments, is used for this procedure to avoid disruption of the major setup. An irrigating solution, usually antibiotic, should also be on this table. Microsuture of the surgeon's choice is necessary for the tagging of vessels and nerves on the amputated part to prepare it for replantation (Fig. 93-10).

Microsurgical sutures

Because of the minute size of the microsurgical needle and suture material, the utmost caution must be exercised when it is used. The exchange of the suture between surgeon and nurse is critical. The suture material should remain affixed to the cardboard square that is in the sterile package, and handed to the surgeon in this way, separate from the nonlocking needle holder. The surgeon should return the suture and the needle holder in the same fashion. The nurse places a sterile white towel in front of the surgeon on the field while the surgeon is using this suture. If the needle is disengaged accidentally from the needle holder, it is clearly visible on the white towel, whereas it would not be on the darker drapes.

The location of all needles must be ascertained throughout the surgery, to prevent an unnoticed needle from being left in the open wound. The surgeon and the nurse are responsible for a correct needle count.

Miscellaneous microsurgical supplies

Several other items have proved to be beneficial during microsurgery (Fig. 93-11). Microsurgical spears are necessary to sponge away minute oozing when work is done under the microscope. A nerve background, which is a small piece of blue or yellow rubber, can be placed under a damaged nerve that is to be repaired. Better visualization of the nerve is thus achieved by isolation of it from surrounding anatomic structures. A small Weck blade for trimming and smoothing rough nerve edges before anastomosis may also be needed. When a certain structure is to be saved on the field for use later in the surgery, such as a tendon or nerve graft, it is usually kept moist in a wet sponge. To prevent inadvertently discarding this sponge, one should wrap it in a large piece of red rubber, called a "red flag." Fogarty catheters should be available for the removal of clots in reanastomosed vessels.

Drugs and solutions

Certain drugs are needed in microsurgery. Often an intravenous antibiotic, such as cefazolin, is given before the inflation of the tourniquet. The dose may be repeated at 4- or 6-hour intervals if the procedure is extensive.

An antibiotic irrigating solution is necessary for disinfecting, particularly with a fresh traumatic injury. In our institution, a preparation of 50,000 units of bacitracin, 0.5

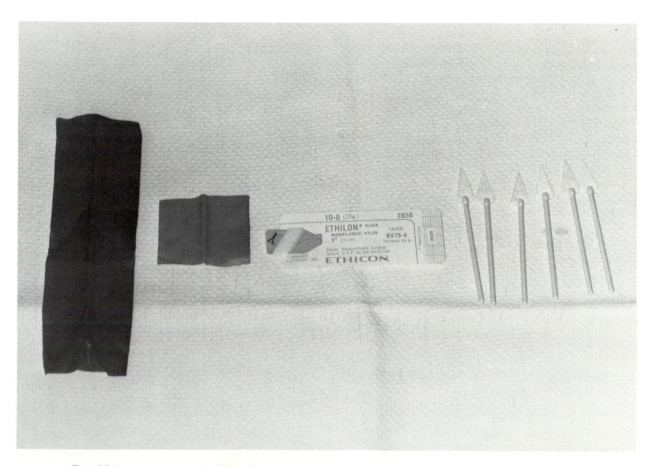

FIG. 93-11. *Left to right,* Red flag, nerve background, microsurgical suture, Weck-Cel surgical spears.

gm of neomycin, and 500,000 units of polymixin B, added to 1 liter of sterile saline or lactated Ringer's solution, is used.

A heparin irrigating solution of 5 ml of heparin, 1:1000 units, added to 500 ml of sterile saline or lactated Ringer's solution, works as an effective anticoagulant in anastomosed vessels.

Bupivacaine (Marcaine), 0.5% plain, is necessary for its antispasmodic effect on the vessels.

Dextran 40 inhibits the sludging of red blood cells, thereby preventing clot formation in the vessels. This drug should be easily accessible during microvascular surgery.

There are different methods of instilling these vascular drugs. Two methods are used in our institution. One way is to have one 20-ml syringe, with a Teflon intravenous catheter attached to its tip, for each drug used. Another way is to use the sterile 15-ml balanced salt solution ophthalmic containers. These can be emptied and the appropriate drugs introduced, which can then be instilled into vessels by attachment of ophthalmic irrigating tips to the containers. Each container or syringe must be labeled with its content to avoid confusion and error.

POSTOPERATIVE PRIORITIES

When surgery has ended, it is time for the patient to play an active role in his recovery. The microsurgical nurse who visited him preoperatively should see him again the day after his surgery. During this visit, the nurse should check the patient's physical and psychological status, reinforce any teaching presented preoperatively, and answer any questions. The patient's response to the entire experience should be observed and recorded. If any further assistance is needed or any problems have arisen, they should also be noted.

The patient's postoperative hospitalization is often brief.

He is usually discharged, with immediate follow-up at the hand rehabilitation center. Here is where the nurse's observations can be of value. The nurse should be very familiar with the hand center and visit it frequently. It is in this environment that the surgeon, the therapist, and the nurse can share information and gain a total picture of the patient. All can work together to produce a more effective rehabilitation plan.

The nurse should not limit his or her visits to postoperative follow-up, however. Preoperatively, the nurse can participate in the teaching with the therapist and the surgeon and be better prepared to impart accurate information to the patient later in the hospital. Likewise, the therapist should be encouraged, whenever possible, to observe the surgical procedure. This would be a great aid in planning postoperative therapy.

SUMMARY

The involvement of all team members throughout the course of hospitalization and rehabilitation is essential in providing the patient with an effective, organized, thorough, and comprehensive plan of care. To accomplish this, each member of the team must be proficient in his or her specific area and able to maintain open lines of communication with all other members. The microsurgical nurse has an important role. Together with other members of the team, he or she must be able to instill in the patient a sense of self-worth and the initiative to play a major role in his rehabilitation.

BIBLIOGRAPHY

American Academy of Orthopaedic Surgeons: Symposium on Microsurgery, practical use in orthopaedics, St. Louis, 1979, The C.V. Mosby Co.

O'Brien, B.M.: Microvascular reconstructive surgery, Edinburgh, 1977, Churchill Livingstone.

are legal and ethical if they are to market insurance products at affordable prices. To make a profit for their stockholders, insurance companies realize that they must return people to work if possible. In recent years loss in insurance operations has reached billions of dollars. Inflation in medical costs, hospital costs, wages, and other items that constitute insurance claims has been largely responsible for these losses, in addition to a highly competitive marketplace. If this trend is not controlled, there could be a serious loss of capacity in the world insurance marketplace. A single workers' compensation claim can exceed a million dollars in medical costs and lost wages. Settlements and court verdicts in the millions of dollars are commonplace today. Prevention of loss and control of the loss after its occurrence are tools available to insurers to minimize losses from their operations. This trend has been reinforced by legislative mandates that medical and vocational rehabilitation be covered and made available in workers' compensation and automobile no-fault cases.

SUMMARY

Insurance companies are good customers of rehabilitation centers and facilities throughout the United States and Canada. Insurance companies pay their bills and pay them promptly. It is not the building but the staff of a rehabilitation center that is important. A dedicated professional staff gets results. In choosing a center for an individual case, we believe it is advisable to send the person as close to home as possible; however, the facility must be responsive to the needs of that particular person and that particular disability. We believe, of course, that it is better to use a center where everything is under one roof and where everyone is working together as a team. But there could be strong psychological or family needs that may complicate the move to a facility. Imaging trying to move a person 100 or 200 miles after a physical disaster; it is quite a touchy matter. We want the best result in the least possible time. We want to work with the staff of the facility and to attend the staff conferences of the center. We have as much to give during a staff conference as we take away. We are all after the same thing—the rehabilitation of the patient.

There is no single hero in rehabilitation. I have never seen a case of successful rehabilitation in which one person was solely responsible for that rehabilitation. It is really a team effort. If we all work together—the insurance industry, the medical profession, the business community—there will be a new world dawning in rehabilitation. The Rehabilitation Act of 1973 set forth affirmative action for employment of the handicapped. This has been a big help in placement of the disabled. Affirmative action in regard to the handicapped is good if it is administered properly.

In the future we can expect the insurance industry to be a part of the rehabilitation team and to add to the dedicated efforts of that team.

95

The insurance rehabilitation nurse as a team member

MARIE TRUSKOWSKY

Through the years it has been the experience of insurance companies that timely and appropriate rehabilitation saves money. This savings is realized because good care results in fewer complications and reduced disability. If an insurance company has a responsibility to reimburse all or part of wages lost as a result of an inability to work, good rehabilitation further increases the savings by facilitating a safe and timely return to work. The claims person, however, does not have the time and often does not have the expertise to identify problems early, direct the injured to the best care facility, or follow up on treatment plans and arrange for a successful return to work. Because of this insufficiency, many insurance companies have hired nurses to handle these areas. These insurance rehabilitation nurses may be ''in-house''—that is, full-time employees of a particular insurance company—or insurance companies may work through a private rehabilitation company that supplies insurance rehabilitation nurses to work on a case-by-case basis.

Let us examine the goals of insurance rehabilitation nurses and some of the services they perform.

GOALS

Insurance rehabilitation nurses have the same basic goals in working with any disabled client. Briefly these goals are as follows:

1. Gathering information for the insurance company so that financial reserves may be established
2. Evaluating the injured person, recommending the most appropriate and specialized care providers, and then directing the patient to them
3. Acting as liaison for the client, family, doctor, treating team, employer, and community
4. Facilitating follow-up care
5. Assessing and coordinating return-to-work activities

Basic as these goals may seem, they are not easy to achieve and require multifaceted skills. Beyond basic medical knowledge, a registered nurse utilizes the strategies of psychology, family dynamics, social work, vocational counseling, and financial management.

Insurance rehabilitation nurses perform no direct nursing, and therefore our role is frequently questioned, sometimes misunderstood, and, to the uninitiated, enormously vague. The nontangible service we provide can perhaps be made more understandable if we consider the steps and activities we pursue while working with a client.

INITIAL EVALUATION

Client. The insurance rehabilitation nurse visits the injured person by appointment. This may take place in the hospital, but more frequently takes place in the home. We obtain information regarding the person's diagnosis and his perception of the prognosis, the treatment plan, and the injury in general. In addition, we interview the person in regard to his educational background, hobbies or interests, and work history. We discuss his financial status, medical history, and family situation. This fact-finding and developing a rapport are essential and basic in achieving our goals. Medical, financial, behavioral, and vocational aspects of an injured person's life may affect the rehabilitation process positively or negatively. The relevance of much of this information does not become evident at the treatment center, but such information can be vital to an overall positive outcome. For example, financial concern may lead to depression, which may lead to lack of follow-up with therapy.

We secure the client's written consent to speak with his employer and his physician and any others involved in his care.

Employer. The insurance rehabilitation nurse visits the employer. Our focus is to engage the employer as a member of the rehabilitation team and to do an analysis of the physical tasks and demands of the client's job. When our client has an upper extremity injury, we pay particular attention to the job functions that require upper extremity activities. We assess what is required regarding handling, pushing, pulling, turning, lifting, and fine and gross motor movements. We measure handles, tools, knobs, and so on. We discuss with the employer what areas of the job may possibly be modified or changed to accommodate the employee if he or she is unable to perform all the previous job tasks. At this time, we can ascertain skills of the job that can be transferred to other jobs.

With an industrial injury, there is frequently a fear on the part of the injured person to return to the same work site, and so we probe for other areas of the operation that may be suitable or acceptable for a return to work.

Physician. The insurance rehabilitation nurse may frequently see the treating physician at the time of a client's appointment. At this time, basic information is requested of the physician, including diagnosis, treatment plan and goals, length of disability, potential limitations, and the date

971

of projected return to work. In addition, the insurance rehabilitation nurse may request, for the insurance carrier, written reports, the physician's projection of future costs, and, if a medical plateau has been reached, a disability rating.

Some physicians may perceive that this is asking a lot; however, at this time, the insurance rehabilitation nurse shares appropriate information he or she has gathered from the job analysis. Provided with this knowledge, the physician may be better able to individualize treatment plans to facilitate a return to work or may alter his or her decision about the patient's returning to work at a modified job.

In addition, the insurance rehabilitation nurse shares pertinent information regarding the home situation and about problems and concerns that may affect treatment. The insurance rehabilitation nurse, acting as the patient's advocate, can ask the physician questions that the client has been reluctant or too timid to ask.

With the input from the physician, the insurance rehabilitation nurse can facilitate approval from the insurance company for hospitalization, treatment, equipment, prostheses, transportation, and payment of bills.

• • •

Armed with all the information the insurance rehabilitation nurse has obtained from the three sources during the initial evaluation, the nurse formulates what needs to be accomplished in follow-up activities for the client. Depending on the needs of the particular case, the insurance rehabilitation nurse visits the client and family at home to reinforce the progress of the treatment plan and remains always alert to the vocational, financial, and behavioral changes that may affect the rehabilitation process, solving problems as needed. The insurance rehabilitation nurse ensures that the client does attend appointments with the physician, the physical therapist, and the occupational therapist, so that no patients are lost to care or have their care prolonged by not following therapy plans.

We continue to keep the employer informed and to pave the way for a return to work, but in some cases a person cannot return to his previous employment. If this is known early during the recovery, the insurance rehabilitation nurse begins vocational counseling at that time. First steps include interest identification and possible job alternatives, résumé preparation, interviewing techniques, and how and where to search for a job.

Not all hand surgeons have the luxury of a fully developed occupational therapy program, with work-tolerance testing and so on. So once again the insurance rehabilitation nurse can look into job alternatives and obtain the insurance company's approval for outside testing if required.

Of course, not all patients with hand injuries were employed at the time of injury, but our goal remains the same—assisting patients to be as independent as possible in their vocational areas. And so we view housework or schoolwork in the same way that we view a paying job.

As insurance rehabilitation nurses, we feel that we are a part of the total rehabilitation team, with the patient-client as the core of that team. We have the luxury and responsibility of seeing this important person in all aspects of his life. We can provide the time and legwork that may be needed to facilitate care and follow-up.

APPENDIX

Presidential address: The American Society of Hand Therapists, January 17, 1982

EVELYN J. MACKIN

It is a great honor to have been president of the American Society of Hand Therapists. We are responsible for the very important area of rehabilitation devoted to the care and treatment of the hand and upper extremity. We all know how important our hands have been to our own lives. We all have felt for the patient who has suffered a mutilating injury of his hand; who sees his skills destroyed, his career ruined, and his family's future placed in jeopardy.[1] We are all cognizant of what role the hand has played in the progress of man and his culture. To be entrusted with the progress of the specialty of hand rehabilitation within the allied health profession provides us with many obligations and responsibilities for our actions as a profession and as a society.

With support of a seed grant from the American Society for Surgery of the Hand during the AASH presidency of Dr. Robert M. McFarlane, six therapists lit the spark that began the American Society of Hand Therapists. This group and the succeeding leaders and members not only gave direction to our society, but also maintained those directions to build on their vision and grow further. This, I can assure you, the American Society of Hand Therapists is doing.

Through the founding members' commitment to having a society whose members have a required *level of education, professional skills,* and *personal qualities,* they began a legacy of sound principles upon which we have built and grown during the past 5 years. Our society is in good hands. It has a firm foundation and a carefully designed structure.

As you look at our 1981 by-laws, you will see that the wording of our society's purposes has remained the same as in the original by-laws. The original quality of the purpose of the American Society of Hand Therapists is unchanged. As we look at these purposes, I would like to point out some of the activities that have occurred within our society during the past year to help meet them. This brief look back at the year is good for two reasons: first, it shows all of us the many areas of our society's involvement and accomplishment and, second, it shows us the capacity for future growth that exists within our society.

PURPOSE: "To become a recognized association of hand therapists, highly specialized in the field of hand rehabilitation."

"Highly specialized" was written into our first by-laws with full understanding and belief that hand therapy was and always would be practiced at the highest level by the American Society of Hand Therapists.

PURPOSE: "To become well recognized by the medical profession."

As a member of the hand rehabilitation team, hand therapists have attained a highly professional role with the surgeons, enjoying mutual respect and responsibility.

Our ability to communicate and plan with the surgeons has expedited our collegiality with the surgeons. In 1980, a member of the ASHT was appointed to the ASSH Clinical Assessment Committee by Dr. Robert Duran, Chairman, and this year, for the first time, a member of the American Society of Hand Therapists, Judy Bell, presented at the annual meeting of the American Society for Surgery of the Hand, a paper she coauthored. The proceedings of the 1980 scientific paper session at the ASHT annual meeting were published in the May 1981 issue of the *Journal of Hand Surgery.*

It was with the support of the 1980 ASSH president, Dr. Alfred Swanson, that nine members of the ASHT traveled to Rotterdam in The Netherlands in 1980 to participate as panelists and speakers at the first congress of the International Federation of Societies for Surgery of the Hand. Approximately 200 therapists and surgeons from 10 countries crowded into a meeting room at Erasmus University in Rotterdam. The meeting was a great success.

It is with Dr. Swanson's continuing support that the ASHT will again participate in the second congress of the International Federation of Societies for Surgery of the Hand in Boston in 1983.

In an effort to promote goals of mutual interest, in 1978 ASSH president, Dr. George Omer, appointed an ASSH liaison committee to the ASHT. Dr. James Hunter, always a strong supporter of the hand therapist, was the first chairman of that ASSH committee. The ASSH-ASHT Liaison Committee has continued to meet annually.

This collegiality between surgeon and therapist cannot be legislated. It is an outgrowth of the recognition of the specialized knowledge in our respective fields.

PURPOSE: "To develop standardization of terminology and evaluation techniques."

The development of hand therapy demands accurate and valid comparison of treatment techniques and research data.

The Standardization Committee is working hard on the *ASHT Standardization Manual on Recommendations for Evaluation Techniques of the Upper Extremity.* This manual will contain chapters on the following:

1. Joint range of motion
2. Edema assessment
3. Work capacity
4. Sensibility evaluation

PURPOSE: "To research treatment techniques, modalities and terminology effective in hand rehabilitation."

A major goal of our society, as stated in our by-laws, is research. Our Research Committee has been committed to the development and improvement of clinical research in hand therapy. The *ASHT Research Newsletter,* Research Bibliography, and Annotated Research Funding Bibliography are reflections of that commitment.

The goal of fostering research to document and substantiate hand therapy techniques involves many ASHT committees—Liaison, Continuing Education, Program, Publications, and Standardization—and is interwoven through the very fabric of our society.

PURPOSE: "To participate in continuing education in the field of hand rehabilitation."

The ASSH-ASHT Liaison Committee, in 1980, launched the concept of miniconferences to be conducted on a regional basis. These meetings were designed to be 1- or 2-day low-cost meetings to attract those therapists who may be unable to attend the large city symposiums. Several such meetings have been held up to now in North Carolina, Arizona, Michigan, and California and have been highly successful.

To assist in gathering local faculty willing to speak at these meetings, a resource file was compiled by the Liaison Committee and is available through the Resource Library. This file contains the names of ASHT and ASSH members interested in teaching in miniconferences.

Our Resource Library is impressive, containing many excellent books and videotapes. We are pleased to announce the availability of our most recent additions, the *Self-Assessment Examination Booklet,* developed by the Continuing Education Committee, and the *Clinical Assessment Recommendations,* developed by Elaine Fess, OTR, and Christine Moran, RPT.

PURPOSE: "To stimulate increased interest in the field of hand rehabilitation."

From coast to coast, we observe clinical settings and consultative practices at the highest level of quality and professionalism.

It is important that the public be informed and understand our profession. To assist us in this task, we have developed a position paper defining what constitutes hand therapy, and our Publications Committee is developing a brochure to describe hand therapy to laymen and physicians.

PURPOSE: "To hold meetings in order to transact official business."

The enthusiasm, commitment, and energy of the Executive Board has been exceptional. Each member has carefully undertaken his or her responsibilities consistent with the ASHT by-laws. We have met twice this year—midyear in Phoenix and here in New Orleans yesterday.

PURPOSE: "To hold meetings of a scientific, academic nature."

This fifth annual scientific paper session is another example of the ASHT goal of providing quality continuing education.

PURPOSE: "To publish and disseminate information."

The favorable comments regarding the *ASHT Research Newsletter* are most gratifying. We have continued to expand and improve upon the newsletter by adding new sections of interest to membership.

The *ASHT Membership directory* is updated each year, and the *ASHT Correspondence Newsletter* is stimulating!

PURPOSE: "To cooperate and establish communication with other affiliated organizations or agencies to maintain continued progress and growth of the profession."

The importance of communication and relationships with other members of the health team is vital to the most important member of the team—the patient.

In this area, with our peers as with the physicians, if hand therapists are to assume a greater professional role in relation to other professions, mutual respect and recognition of responsibility is essential. To this end, two ASHT members were appointed to the AOTA/AOTF* Research Advisory Board, an ASHT member was appointed to the AOTA Commission on Practice and this year an ASHT liaison representative has been appointed to the AOTA/AOTF Research Advisory Board.

At this time I would like to look at future challenges for the ASHT.

PREVENTION AND REHABILITATION OF INDUSTRIAL HAND INJURIES

The goal of hand therapy is to restore the disabled hand to maximum function. The scope of this responsibility was emphasized by Dr. Swanson[2] in his presidential address at the ASSH annual meeting in 1980, when he discussed the Kelsey Report of Yale University, Public Health Department. The American Society for Surgery of the Hand sponsored this report to obtain data on the economic impact of upper extremity disorders in America. The data from that study indicates that one third of all injuries are involved in the upper extremities; there is a 10-billion-dollar loss to our economy because of disorders to the hand and upper extremity. These include agricultural, industrial, and sports injuries and those inflicted by consumer products. There are about 16 million significant upper extremity injuries each year, and these are responsible for 90 million days of restricted activities and 16 million days of lost work.[3]

---

*American Occupational Therapy Association and American Occupational Therapy Foundation.

Last year at the annual business meeting of the ASHT in Las Vegas, Eva McCormick brought up for discussion this important and timely topic. This year, having been appointed chairman of the ASHT Task Force on Prevention and Rehabilitation of Industrial Hand Injuries, Eva has organized a task force within our society that focuses on safety and prevention of injuries. She, along with Dr. Sidney Blair, chairman of the ASSH Ad Hoc Committee for Prevention and Rehabilitation of Industrial Hand Injuries, are involved in the Chicago Committee for Safety and Prevention. Meetings are being held—a national committee has been suggested, and there already is an International committee of interested doctors—with the objective of decreasing the incidence of industrial accidents to the hand.

The challenge lies not only with the direct provision of services to rehabilitate a patient after the injury has occurred, but also in a consultative role in which a therapist and physician can determine a man's capability to do a particular job, thereby possibly preventing an injury. The man may be required to pass a physical examination by a physician, but should he not also be required to be tested for his skill and coordination to operate a particular machine? Consider the high incidence of carpal tunnel syndrome and tendonitis among certain factory workers. Therapists are now going into factories changing tools and work positions so that an employee doesn't have to assume an awkward position doing a repetitive job. This will help prevent carpal tunnel syndrome, tendonitis, and related stress injuries. The therapist is doing what he or she does every day and does best— problem solving. Problem solving and work simplification. Industry doesn't always think of these things or listen to isolated complaints and suggestions from the workers. They are very often too busy looking at the forest rather than the trees.

The challenge also lies in pushing for stronger state and federal legislation to convict those employers who would have their employees work on unsafe machinery or have an immigrant with a language problem operate a machine when he is unable to read the safety instructions. Let us think of prevention. This is an exciting new frontier in rehabilitation. Let us be a part of it!

CONTINUING EDUCATION

At the recommendation of Pat MacBain, OTC, from Canada, the Liaison Committee this year has reallocated Canadian areas on our regional map. The reallocation of these areas will make possible ASHT-sponsored miniconferences accessible to our Canadian members.

Regional coordinators have been appointed for the purpose of implementing and assisting miniconferences in the 10 designated areas. Guidelines for course construction, evaluation, course accreditation, and sponsorship by the ASHT have been completed by our Continuing Education Committee. We view the implementation of miniconferences as a necessary and positive stimulus to ASHT development and growth.

The challenge is to all of us—to be involved in miniconferences in each of the 10 regions—and let them begin with you!

RESEARCH

The American Society of Hand Therapists has been created. We have established principles of ideas and philosophy, and we have shown our value to the world of hand rehabilitation. Belief in these things, however, is not quite enough. If we are to continue to grow and be respected, we must uphold quality care through clinical research—testing, questioning, documentation, and education—to support our techniques of practice.

ISSUES CONCERNING OCCUPATIONAL THERAPY AND PHYSICAL THERAPY

Don Wortley, at the annual meeting of the American Physical Therapy Association, stated in his 1980 presidential address that "the time has come to start thinking seriously about a closer relationship between PTs and OTs. There are many areas of overlapping interests in the two professions. Instead of battling over turf, we might consider some of the mutually beneficial arrangements that could dramatically increase our numbers and therefore our impact on Washington. There could be some knotty problems with things like licensure and professional identity, but maybe it's not too far-fetched to start thinking about ideas such as equivalency testing somewhere down the road. Perhaps we could open up the two associations to one another or merge the two together—a coalescence or a union.

Both occupational therapists and physical therapists want to advance. It need not be seen as a case of giving something up. Done properly, a truly cooperative effort could be a good thing for all."[4]

Mr. Wortley said it very well. This challenge begins with each one of us.

THIRD-PARTY REIMBURSEMENT

It was from frustration with third-party payers that the Task Force to Investigate Third-Party Reimbursement was appointed this year. Many of us have felt ineffectual in dealing with third-party people who determine what our services can be, the worth of those services, and who will be compensated for those services.

This challenge is up to all of us. Our task force is preparing a "packet" (that is, letters from physicians, insurance companies, and rehabilitation counselors, expressing how much hand rehabilitation has helped them, and slides and studies that document the dollar savings of the hand-team concept). Contact this task force, chaired by Shirley Ollos Pearson, MS, OTR, to contribute to a plan to substantiate our goal of the delivery of quality care to the hand-disabled patient. We must emphasize the need and importance of hand therapy to those third-party payers.

PUBLICATIONS

Communication with the members has been a primary goal. This has been accomplished through the *ASHT Correspondence Newsletter*. The newsletter has grown with each succeeding issue.

In our constant desire to improve communication with the membership, lies the challenge—an extension or an addition to the concept of the quarterly newsletter, a journal of the American Society of Hand Therapists. A journal would serve the needs of its members and at the same time publish those editorials and articles that substantiate the scientific basis of our profession.

I remember the words of Eugene Michels, Associate Executive Director for Research and Education, APTA, who stated that "at the heart of any profession is its unique serious intellectual component. Unless that component is put into words in a meaningful way, it cannot be shared or transmitted; that is, it cannot be professed. That these words must be written is unquestioned. The only permanent substance of any profession is its trail of written words—its literature—which it leaves as a public testimony to its deeds, ideas, and achievements."[5]

I like to think that perhaps one day our challenges will lead to my favorite challenge, an international federation of societies of hand therapists.

INTERNATIONAL FEDERATION OF SOCIETIES OF HAND THERAPISTS

Tenure for an ASHT President is short but in another way a long-lasting memorable experience. In the past year I attended meetings that took me to five other countries. It has been exciting through the years to be able to share on an international basis the expanding discipline of hand therapy with Mr. Pulvertaft in England, with Dr. Tubiana's therapists in France, with Dr. Moberg's therapists in Sweden, and with Dr. Tajima's staff in Japan. The experiences reinforced what I knew to be true, that hand therapy as a profession is reaching the far corners of the world. The ASHT today has members in Canada, Japan, Sweden, The Netherlands, Israel, and Kuwait. We have pioneered a profession that is a significant and vital part of the health care system and has only begun to spread its wings.

Many letters come across the president's desk. In fact, at Christmas, as I hung up cards around our Therapy Department, I felt that the American Society of Hand Therapists was as involved as Washington, D.C.

I read a desire in letters from therapists in other countries to meet the needs of their profession and patients through the development of their own hand-therapist societies, where knowledge can be shared and research and education furthered. Nowhere did I feel this challenge more than when I visited Maria Musur-Grieve at the Rheumatology Institute in Poland.

I envision the day when there will be an international federation of societies of hand therapists. I envision a day when we will not only have an annual meeting, but also an international meeting, held perhaps every 3 years. I envision the day when the sun will never set on our profession.

Despite the growth experienced by our society during these few years, I believe that the future holds even more exciting challenges and growth. We hold our future within our own hands to be shaped by our own collective actions. The future of our society does not lie with one officer, one committee chairperson, or committee member, but with the collective ideas and opinions of our membership. It is imperative that each member become involved so that our ideas and opinions are represented in our actions and activities.

Your opinion will be heard if you make it heard when the decisions affecting our society are being made.

I wish to give special thanks to my executive board, committee chairpersons, subchairpersons, and members of these committees with whom I have had the privilege of working and who by their efforts have contributed so much to the growth and advancement of our society and our profession. I thank also those associate and affiliate members who inconspicuously have made so much possible. At this time, I want to recognize the Program Committee, chaired by Karen Prendergast. I also want to thank Ann Galbraith, Public Relations; Judy Colditz, Local Arrangements; Donna Reist, Exhibitors; Shirley Pearson, Workshops; Judy Bell, Scientific Papers; and Shellye Bittinger, Registration, who have worked extremely hard to make this fifth annual scientific papers session a success.

Finally, I would like to thank all who have helped me at my own hand center in so many ways, who are here today: Dr. Hunter and Dr. Schneider, whose support has made my participation in this great society possible; Anne Callahan, Assistant Director of Hand Therapy at the Philadelphia Hand Rehabilitation Center; and my superb staff—Pat Baxter, Loretta Maiorano, Pam McEntee, and Sue Kempin. Wandra Miles, Cathy Cambridge, Melanie Ballard, and Sharon Fried, who are not at this meeting, also deserve my thanks. My secretary, Dorothy Malin, I must mention for her unbelievable loyalty under fire and for her many contributions to our society. Finally, my son, Glenn, for just being himself.

I hope that what I have said today will serve to stimulate your dreams and goals as mine have been stimulated and that the challenge to all of us will bring even greater fulfillment to the profession of hand therapy.

Each one of us must accept the challenges that motivated the founding members. It is up to each one of us to remember the goals of our society and our profession. It will be by the efforts of each one of us by participating in society activities that new programs or the modification of on-going programs will meet these goals. Accept the challenges. Add your own, and pass it on!

"Ideals are like the stars. We can never reach them; but like mariners at sea, we should chart our course by them."

CARL SCHURZ

Pass it on!

REFERENCES

1. Pulvertaft, R.G.: Psychological aspects of hand injuries. In Hunter, J.M., Schneider, L.H., Mackin, E.J., and Bell, J.A., editors: Rehabilitation of the hand, St. Louis, 1978, The C.V. Mosby Co.
2. Kelsey, J.L., Pastides, H., Kreiger, N., and others: Upper extremity disorders: a survey of their occurrence and cost to the nation, Yale University, New Haven, Conn.
3. Swanson, A.B.: The need for medical statesmanship in our world, J. Hand Surg. **5**(4):307-317, 1980.
4. Magistro, C.M.: The 1976 presidential address, J. Am. Phys. Ther. Assoc. **56**(11):1227-1339, 1976.
5. Wortley, B.S.: The 1980 presidential address, J. Am. Phys. Ther. Assoc. **60**(11):1430-1436, 1980.

Index